SKELETAL MUSCLE
Pathology, Diagnosis and Management of Disease

Edited by

Victor R Preedy
PhD, DSc FRCPath, FlBiol
Department of Nutrition
School of Life Sciences
King's College London
Franklin-Wilkins Building
London
UK

Timothy J Peters
PhD DSc FRCP FRCP(Edin) FRCPath
Department of Clinical Biochemistry
King's College London
London
UK

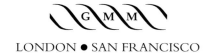

LONDON ● SAN FRANCISCO

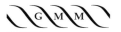

© 2002
Greenwich Medical Media
4th Floor, 137 Euston Road,
London
NW1 2AA,

870 Market Street, Ste 720
San Francisco
CA 94109, USA

ISBN 1841100293

First Published 2002

www.greenwich-medical.co.uk

Distributed worldwide by Plymbridge Distributors Ltd and in the USA by Jamco Distribution.

Printed by MPG Books Ltd, Bodmin, Cornwall

CONTENTS

CHAPTER 17

CHAPTER 18

CHAPTER 19

CHAPTER 20

CHAPTER 21

CHAPTER 22

CHAPTER 23

CHAPTER 24

CHAPTER 25

CHAPTER 35

CHAPTER 36

CHAPTER 37

CHAPTER 38

CHAPTER 39

CHAPTER 40

CHAPTER 41

CHAPTER 42

CHAPTER 43

CHAPTER 44

CHAPTER 45

CHAPTER 46

CHAPTER 47

CHAPTER 48

CHAPTER 49

CHAPTER 50

CHAPTER 51

CHAPTER 52

CHAPTER 53

CHAPTER 54

CHAPTER 55

CHAPTER 56

CHAPTER 57

CHAPTER 58

CONTRIBUTORS

Ronald Aaron
Professor of Physics
Northeastern University
Boston, USA

Louise Ada, PhD
Senior Lecturer at the School of
Physiotherapy
University of Sydney
Sydney, Australia

Anthony A. Amato, MD
Associate Professor of Neurology
Harvard Medical School
Chief of the Neuromuscular Division
Director of the Clinical Laboratory
Department of Neurology
Brigham and Women's Hospital
Boston, Massachusetts
USA

Francesa Andreetta, PhD
Department of Neuromuscular Disease
National Neurological Institute
"C.Basta"
Milan, Italy

Carlo Antozzi, MD
Department of Neuromuscular Disease
National Neurological Institute
"Carlo Besta"
Milan, Italy

Josep M. Argilés, PhD
Assistant Professor
Department de Bioquímica i Biologia
Molecular
Facultat de Biologia
Universitat de Barcelona
Barcelona, Spain

Doron Aronson, MD
Director, Cardiac Step-Down Unit
Division of Cardiology
Rambam Medical Center
Haifa, Israel

Fulvio Baggi, PhD
National Neurological Institute
"Carlo Besta"
Milan, Italy

Antonio Barbieri, MD
Fellow in Clinical Pain Research &
Neurosurgery
Pain Medicine Centre
Scientific Institute & Hospital San
Raffaele DSNP
Milan, Italy

Antoni Barrientos, PhD
Department of Biological Sciences
Columbia University
New York, USA

Sheezard Basaria, MD
Division of Endocrinology and
Metabolism
John Hopkins University School
Medicine
Bayview Medical Center
Baltimore, USA

Pia Bernasconi, PhD
National Neurological Institute
"Carlo Besta"
Milan, Italy

Ori Better, MD
Professor of Medicine
Faculty of Medicine
Crush Syndrome Center
Technion-Israel Institute of Technology
Haifa, Israel

Thomas M. Best, MD, PhD
Assistant Professor of Family Medicine
and Orthopedic Surgery
Affiliate Assistant Professor of
Kinesiology and Biomedical
Engineering
UW Medical School
Madison, USA

David A. Bluemke, MD, PhD
Department of Radiology
John Hopkins University
School of Medicine
Baltimore, USA

Leo Booij, MD, PhD, FRCA
Professor and Chairman
Department on Anestehsiology
University Medical Center Nijmegen
Academisch Ziekenhuis Nijmegen
Anesthesiologie
Nijmegen, The Netherlands

Mark B. Bromberg, MD, PhD
Professor of Neurology
Department of Neurology
University of Utah
Utah, USA

Claudio Bruno, MD
H. Houston Merritt Clinical Research
Center for Muscular Dystrophy and
Related Diseases
Department of Neurology
Columbia University
New York, USA

Colleen Canning, PhD
Lecturer at the School of
Physiotherapy

University of Sydney
Sydney, Australia

Ricardo F. Capozza, PhD
Centre for P-Ca Metabolism Studies
(CEMFoC)
University of Rosario
Buenos Aires, Argentina

Francesc Cardellach, MD
Professor of Medicine
Muscle Research Unit
Hospital Clinic
University of Barcelona
Barcelona, Spain

Paul V. Carroll, MD, MRCPI
Department of Endocrinology
St, Bartholomew's Hospital
London, UK

Jordi Casademont, MD, PhD
Department of Medicine
Hospital Clínic de Barcelona
Universitat de Barcelona
Barcelona, Spain

Ted Ciaraldi, PhD
Project Endocrinologist
University of California
VA San Diego Healthcare System
San Diego, USA

Priscilla M. Clarkson, PhD
Department of Exercise Science
University of Massachusetts
Amherst, USA

Torben Clausen, MD, Dmed
Sci
Professor
Institute of Physiology
University of Aarhus
Aarhus, Denmark

Andrew J. S. Coats, DM,
FRACP, FRCP, FACC,
FESC, MBA
Viscount Royston Professor of Clinical
Cardiology
Imperial College School of Medicine

Royal Brompton Hospital
London, UK

Gustavo R. Cointry, PhD
Centre for P-Ca Metabolism Studies
(CEMFoC)
University of Rosario
Buenos Aires, Argentina

Dane B. Cook, PhD
Assistant Professor
Center for War Related Illness and
CFS Cooperative
Research Center
VA Medical Center
East Orange, USA

Staen C. Dennis, PhD
Department of Human Biology
University of Cape Town Medical
School
Cape Town, South Africa

Elton Wayne Derman,
MBCHB, PhD
Department of Human
Sports Science Institute of South Africa
Cape Town, South Africa

Brandon K. Doan, MS
Human Performance Laboratory
Ball State University
Muncie, USA

Adrian Dobs, MD, MHS
Division of Endocrinology and
Metabolism
John Hopkins University School of
Medicine
Baltimore, USA

Inge Dørup, MD, DMedSci
Department of Cardiology
Aarhus University Hospital
Aarhus, Denmark

Mohammed Ferdjallah, PhD
Assistant Professor
Electrical & Computer Engineering
Pennsylvania State University in Erie
Erie, USA

Joaquim Fernández-Solá, MD
Muscle Research Unit
Department of Internal Medicine
Hospital Clínic,
University of Barcelona
Barcelona, Spain

José Luis Ferretti, MD, Phd
Centre for P-Ca Metabolism Studies
(CEMFoC)
University of Rosario
Metabolic Research Institute/
Foundation (IDIM/FIM)
Department of Osteology
Faculty of Medicine
Del Salvador University
Buenos Aires, Argentina

Christopher R. Forrest, MD,
MSc, FRCS(C)
Director
Centre for Craniofacial Care and
Research
The Hospital for Sick Children
Associate Professor
Division for Plastic Surgery
Department of Surgery
University of Toronto
Ontario, Canada

Hans H. Goebel, MD
Professor of Neuropathology
Department of Neuropathology
Johannes Gutenberg University
Mainz, Germany

Bret H. Goodpaster, PhD
Department of Medicine
Endocrinology and Metabolism
University of Pittsburgh
Montefiore Hospital
Pittsburgh, USA

Pierre A. Grandjean, MS
Sr Staff Scientist
Heart Failure Management
Bakken Research Centre
Maastricht, The Netherlands

Robert C. Griggs, MD
Chair, Department of Neurology

Professor of Neurology, Medicine,
Pathology, Laboratory Medicine
University of Rochester School of
Medicine and Dentistry
Rochester, New York
USA

Richard D. Griffiths, BSc, MD,
FRCP
Reader in Medicine (Intensive Care)
Intensive Care Research Group
Department of Medicine
University of Liverpool
Liverpool, UK

Manfred Gross, MD, PhD
Professor of Medicine
University of Munich
Munich, Germany

Derek Harrington, MD
Consultant Cardiologist
Sevenoaks Hospital
Sevenoaks, UK

Steven B. Heymsfield, MD
Professor of Medicine
Deputy Director
Obesity Research Center
St. Luke's-Roosevelt Hospital
Columbia University
College of Physicians and Surgeons
New York, USA

Ulrich Hoheisel, Dr rer nat
Postdoc
University Hospital
Kiel University
Kiel, Germany

Johnny Huard, PhD
Assistant Professor
Department of Orthopaedic Surgery
And Molecular Genetics and
Biochemistry
Children's Hospital and University of
Pittsburgh
Pittsburgh, USA

Ben F. Hurley, PhD
Department of Kinesiology
College of Health & Human
Performance
University of Maryland
Baltimore, USA

Hiromasa Ishii, MD
Sports Medicine Research Center
Keio University School of Medicine
Tokyo, Japan

Frederick M. Ivey, PhD
Division of Gerontology
Department of Medicine
University of Maryland School of
Medicine
Geriatric Research, Education and
Clinical Center
Baltimore V A Medical Center
Baltimore, USA

Yves Jammes, MD, D es Sci
Professor of Physiology
Laboratiore de Physiopathologie
Respiratiore EA 2201
Institût Jean Roche, Faculté de
Médecin
Marseille, France

Josep-Maria Grau Junyent, MD
Muscle Research Unit
Department of Internal Medicine
Hospital Clínic
University of Barcelona
Barcelona, Spain

Shinzo Kato, MD
Division of Gastroenterology
Department of Internal Medicine
Keio University
School of Medicine
Tokyo, Japan

Shaifali Kaushik, MD
Department of Radiology
John Hopkins University
School of Medicine

William J. Kraemer, PhD
Professor/Director of Research
Human Performance Laboratory
Department of Kinesiology
The Neag School of Education
The University of Connecticut
Storrs, USA

Kyriacos Kyriacou, PhD
Attending Electron Microscopist
Department of EM and Molecular
Pathology
The Cyprus Institute of Neurology &
Genetics
Nicosia, Cyprus

Theodoros Kyriakides, MD
Senior Consultant Neurologist
Head of Neuropathology Lab
The Cyprus Institute of Neurology &
Genetics
Nicosia, Cyprus

Robert Lee, MS
Weight Control Unit
St Luke's Roosevelt Hospital Center
New York, USA

Francisco J. López-Soriano,
PhD
Assistant Professor
Department de Bioquimica I Biologia
Molecular
Facultat de Biologia
Universitat de Barcelona
Barcelona, Spain

Renato Mantegazza, MD
Myopathology and Immunology Unit
Department of Neuromuscular Disease
Natl. Neurological Inst. "C. Besta"
Milan
Italy

David Mantle BSc PhD FRSC
FRCPath
Department of Surgery
Medical School
University of Newcastle upon Tyne
UK

Paolo Marchettini, MD
Director Pain Medicine Center
Scientific Institute & Hosptial San
Raffaele
Milan, Italy

Michael D. Menger, Prof. Dr.
med
Professor for Experimental Surgery and
Chairman
Institute for Clinical & Experimental
Surgery
University of Saarland
Homburg/Saar, Germany

Siegfried Mense, Prof. Dr. med
University Professor
Department of Antomy and Cell
Biology III
Heidelberg University
Heidelberg, Germany

Lyle L. Moldawer, PhD
Department of Surgery
University of Florida College of
Medicine
Gainesville, Florida, USA

Kanneboyina Nagaraju, MVSc,
PhD
Assistant Professor of Medicine
Division of Rheumatology
Department of Medicine
John Hopkins School of Medicine
Baltimore, USA

Setsuko Nakanishi, D. Sci
Senior Researcher
Pharmaceutical Frontier Research
Laboratories
Jaoan Tobacco Inc.
Kanagawa, Japan

Robert Newton PhD
Associate Professor
Biomechanics Laboratory
Ball State University
Muncie, USA

Shohei Ohnishi, MD
Associate Professor

Sports Medicine Research Center
Keio University
Yokohama, Japan

Cho Y. Pang, PhD
Senior Scientist
Research Institute
The Hospital for Sick Children
Departments of Surgery and
Physiology
University of Toronto
Ontario, Canada

Alistair Paice, MBBS, PhD
Honorary Post-Doctoral Researcher
Department of Clinical Biochemistry
Kings College School of Medicine and
Dentistry
London, UK

Adam M. Persky, MS
Doctoral Student
Department of Pharmaceutics
College of Pharmacy
University of Florida
Gainesville, USA

Timothy J. Peters, PhD, DSc,
FRCP, FRSA, FRCPath Edin
Head of Department
Department of Clinical Biochemistry
Guy's Kings and St Thomas School of
Medicine, London, UK

John E. Rectenwald, MD
Department of Surgery
University of Florida College of
Medicine
Gainesville, Florida, USA

Rajkumar Rajendram, MBBS
(dist), BSc (hons), AKC
Research Associate
Department of Nutrition
King's College
London, UK

Mantegazza Renato, MD
Department of Neuromuscular Disease
"Carlo Besta" National Neurological
Institute

Milan, Italy

Jack E. Riggs, MD
Professor of Neurology, Medicine, and
Community Medicine
Department of Neurology
West Virginia University School of
Medicine
West Virginia, USA

Amyn M. Rojiani, MD, PhD
Associate Professor and Director of
Neuropathology
Department of Interdisciplinary
Oncology
University of South Florida
Tampa, Florida, USA

Michael R. Rose, BSc, MD,
FRCP
Consultant and Honorary Senior
Lecturer in Neurology
King's Neurosciences Centre
Kings College Hospital and Greenwich
District Hospital
London, UK

Irit Rubinstein, DSc
Senior Investigator
Faculty of Medicine
Department of Physiology and
Biophysics and Crush Syndrome
Center
Technion-Israel Institute of Technology
Haifa, Israel

Pierre Rustin, PhD
Unité de Recherches sur les Handicaps
Génétiques de l'Enfant
Hôpital des Enfants-Malades
Paris, France

Yoshihiro Sato, MD
Department of Rehabilitation Medicine
Institute of Brain Science
Hirosaki University School of Medicine
Hirosaki, Japan

Sydney S. Schochet, Jr, MD
Professor of Pathology, Neurology, and
Neurosurgery

West Virginia University School of Medicine
West Virginia, USA

Roy J. Shephard, MD, PhD, DPE

Faculty of Physcial Education and Health
Department of Public Health Sciences
University of Toronto
Toronto Rehabilitation Centre,
Toronto, Canada

C. Shiffman, PhD

Professor of Physics
Northeastern University
Boston, USA

Stephan Sorichter, MD, Dr. med

Department of Internal Medicine
Division of Pneumology
University Hospital Freiburg
Freiburg, Germany

John D. Urschel, MD, FRCSEd

Associate Professor
Department of Surgery
McMaster University
Hamilton, Ontario, Canada

Fernando Vale, MD

Assisstant Professor
Department of Neurosurgery
University of South Florida
Tampa, Florida, USA

Jeff S. Volek, PhD, RD

Assistant Professor
Human Performance Laboratory
Department of Kinesiology
Neag School of Education
The University of Connecticut
Storrs, USA

John Vissing, MD, PhD

Director, Neuromuscular Clinic
Department of Neurology
National University Hospital
Copenhagen, Denmark

Brigitte Vollmar, Prof. Dr. med

Professor for Experimental Surgery
Heisenberg Fellow of the Deutsche
Forschungsgemeinschaft
Institute for Clinical & Experimental
Surgery
University of Saarland
Homburg/Saar, Germany

Yoshihiro Wakayama, MD, PhD

Division of Neurology
Department of Medicine
Showa University, Fujigaoka Hospital
Yokohama, Japan

Zilian Wang, PhD

Assistant Professor of Medicine
Luke's-Roosevelt Hospital
Columbia University
College of Physicians and Surgeons
New York, USA

Jacqueline J. Wertsch, MD

Physical Medicine & Rehabilitation
Department
The Medical College of Wisconsin
Milwaukee, USA

Robbin B. Wickham, MS, PT

Human Performance Laboratory
Ball State University
Muncie, USA

Greg Wilson, PhD, BPE (Hons)

North Coast Institute of TAFE
Kingscliff, Australia

Simon S. Wing, MD, FRCP (C)

Associate Professor
Department of Medicine
McGill University
Quebec, Canada

Hajime Yamazaki, MD

Sports Medicine Research Center
Keio University
Yokohama, Japan

José R. Zanchetta, MD

Metabolic Research
Institute/Fundation (IDIM/FIM)
Department of Osteology
Faculty of Medicine
Del Salvador University
Buenos Aries, Argentina

FOREWORD

Over thirty years ago I chose to explore the clinical physiology and metabolism of skeletal muscle and its diseases because I saw it as a wide open field. It seemed to me that it was paradoxical that some forty percent of the body's mass did not (and still does not) have its own clinical speciality. "Myology" as it is known in some research communities has yet little practical clinical service identity apart from the valuable work done in the very few multi–disciplinary Muscle Clinics. While diseases of muscle appear in texts of Neurology, Rheumatology, Paediatrics and Clinical Genetics, the viewpoint tends to be that from the particular clinical speciality. Reading this book re-inforces my belief that a more integrated view of the function, structure and biology of skeletal muscle is long overdue. Not only have developments in the basic sciences been very rapid and influential-genetics, imaging and spectroscopic modalities and other measurement techniques, but there is much popular interest in muscular performance in health and disease. So, unsurprisingly, skeletal muscle, the largest organ in the body and central to nutrition and fluid and electrolyte metabolism, does respond in many various, intriguing and complex ways to diseases (inherited or acquired) which, affect other body organs or systems.

In an age of "Evidence Based Healthcare" in which the randomised control trial is paramount, this intriguing field is one where, for reasons of rarity of individual cases but where the diversity is commoner than hitherto suspected, there is still need for opportunistic observation and therapeutic intervention. That the clinical research approach is thus alive and well is amply demonstrated in the fifty-eight chapters of this wide-ranging book. Its title promises much: the most important of which is the energy of exploration of the pathophysiological basis of the disorders which prevent us making the most of the human engine for life-breath, movement and physical recreation that is skeletal muscle.

I applaud the Editors and the authors of the individual Chapters and commend their concisely crafted contributions as pointers on a continuing intellectual journey. Distilled from a much larger literature in these and related biomedical science fields, such markers are of importance for enlightenment and inspiration of you and me, the readers, who may or may not be able to follow, but who are nevertheless interested in the amazing variety of gene expression and diverse responses of skeletal muscle and who still hope for effective treatment of its diseases.

Emeritus Professor RHT Edwards
Emeritus Professor of Research and Development in Health and Social Care,
University of Wales. Previously Professor of Medicine and (Founding) Director of the University of Liverpool Muscle Research and Magnetic Resonance Research Centres.

1

Metabolic myopathies: an overview

Joaquim Fernández-Solà and Josep-Maria Grau Junyent

Introduction

Metabolic myopathies constitute a diverse and hetero-geneous group of diseases with the common feature of impairment of skeletal muscle bioenergetics (Griggs et al 1995a). These myopathies may frequently lead to muscle dysfunction with progressive functional impairment of muscle strength and trophism (Wortmann 1991, Kaminski and Ruff 1994). In some cases, structural muscle damage coexists.

At present, most of the abnormalities of muscle metabolism may be specifically defined by bio-chemical or molecular lesions. Therefore, recognition of metabolic myopathies is important since some are treatable. In other cases, genetic counselling may be undertaken.

Reduced exercise tolerance is the main complaint of metabolic myopathies, frequently accompanied by intermittent muscle pain or myoglobinuria (Elliot et al 1989, Kent-Braun et al 1993). Sometimes muscle weakness is also present, although not as relevant as in muscle dystrophies or inflammatory myopathies. A metabolic myopathy may be suggested in the presence of intermittent, exercise-related muscle symptoms (Griggs et al 1995a).

Causes and mechanisms

Table 1.1 summarizes the major causes of metabolic myopathies. Only causes not otherwise referred to in this book will be described. Endocrine myopathies may also be considered as a part of the metabolic disturbance of muscle, since the final pathway involving muscle bioenergetics is common to that of other metabolic myopathies (Kaminski and Ruff 1994). The skeletal muscle system not only provides locomotion, but it is also the largest protein store in humans and plays an important role in the control of carbohydrate metabolism. Muscle diseases associated with endocrine disturbances are the paradigm of interaction between force-generating mechanisms and muscle metabolic functions. Additionally, endocrine myopathies may derange the normal intracellular and extracellular electrolyte concentrations, resulting in impaired muscle action potential and excitation-contraction coupling, and leading to muscle weakness. Thus, a clear inter-relationship between endocrine and metabolic myopathies exists. For similar reasons, we also include the toxic myopathies (George and Pourmand 1997), the syndromes of rhabdomyolysis/myoglobinuria (Knochel 1993) and that of exertional cramps (Layzer 1994) in this group of diseases.

Table 1.1— Main causes of metabolic myopathies

Endocrine myopathies
  Hyper and hypofunction of thyroid gland
  Hyper and hypofunction of adrenal cortex
  Hyper and hypofunction of parathyroid glands
  Hyper and hypofunction of pituitary gland
  Insulin resistance and myopathy
Toxic myopathies
Rhabdomyolysis/myoglobinuria syndrome
Exertional cramps syndrome
Glycogen metabolic defects (see Chapter 21)
  Lactate dehydrogenase
  Myophosphorylase
  Phosphoglycerate kinase
  Phosphoglycerate mutase
  Phosphorylase b kinase
Lipid metabolic defects (see Chapter 19)
  Carnitine palmitoyl transferase deficiency
Purine nucleotide cycle defects (see Chapter 30)
  Myoadenilate deaminase deficiency
Mitochondrial myopathies (see Chapter 20)

Muscle contraction depends on the chemical energy supplied by adenosine triphosphatase (ATP). Four major pathways supply ATP to muscle:

1. glycogen metabolism

2. lipid metabolism

3. phosphocreatine stores

4. the purine nucleotide cycle.

Thus, specific enzymatic deficits, and hormonal or toxic interferences in these pathways are the major causes of metabolic myopathies (Griggs et al 1995a).

An abnormality in glycogen metabolism may be suspected when the patient has adverse symptoms during high-intensity muscular activity. An alteration in oxidative phosphorylation may exist when the patient has difficulty performing intermittent sub-maximal aerobic exercise; in these conditions, blood flow to muscle is not impaired and oxidative phosphorylation is the major pathway for carbohydrate metabolism. A defect in muscle lipid metabolism may be evident during prolonged aerobic exercise, although it may also be present under resting conditions. When muscle symptoms appear only in limited, very high intensity exercise, the phosphocreatine and purine nucleotide-cycle pathways may also be implicated.

Clinical symptoms

Dynamic symptoms are the most prominent features in metabolic myopathies. Fatigue, exertional myalgia and muscle stiffness are frequent complaints (Elliot et al 1989, Kent-Braun et al 1993). Static symptoms (proximal fixed muscle weakness) are less prominent. In metabolic myopathies, dynamic and static symptoms may coexist to some degree, although the juxtaposition of both types of symptoms is particularly apparent in mitochondrial myopathies (Di Mauro et al 1985). Specific antecedents of toxic habits (alcoholism), use of illicit drugs (heroin, cocaine), trauma or infection, coexistence of pharmacologic treatment or other systemic diseases (renal failure) may be important.

Physical examination may also disclose specific signs such as goitre, exophthalmos, Cushing's phenotype, osteotendinous reflex abnormalities (thyroid myopathies) or skin hyperpigmentation (Addison's disease) (Kaminski and Ruff 1994). In mitochondrial myopathies, ptosis and motor ocular deficits are particularly frequent.

Diagnosis

Diagnosis of metabolic myopathies requires a systematic evaluation of the patient in a multidisciplinary approach. Only the sum of an accurate clinical assessment, exercise testing evaluation and specific complementary studies may lead to correct diagnosis (Wortmann 1991, Griggs et al 1995a). This consists of an evaluation of specific signs and symptoms of myopathy, measurement of muscle enzymes and proteins, muscle electrophysiological studies and exercise tests evaluating muscle fuel dynamics and its utilization during exercise, usually with the forearm. In some cases, a muscle biopsy is required, with conventional histology and histochemistry being essential. In selected cases, immunohistochemical, electron microscopy, biochemical or molecular muscle analysis are also required. Other complementary studies such as nuclear magnetic resonance spectroscopy may be useful in order to monitor phosphocreatine, inorganic phosphate, intracellular pH, ATP and lactate levels and, if possible, the influence of exercise on these parameters (Duboc et al 1987). Since metabolic myopathies may develop slowly, and symptoms may not be apparent in the early stages, a repeated evaluation of some tests over time may be necessary.

Endocrine myopathies

Endocrine function is essential to maintain the mechanisms of force-generation and skeletal muscle metabolism. Endocrine disorders may derange extra- and intracellular electrolyte concentration, change membrane excitability, disrupt muscle cellular repair mechanisms and influence excitation–contraction coupling (Kaminski and Ruff 1994). Thyroid dysfunction is the paradigm of endocrine myopathy, although adrenal, pituitary, parathyroid and adrenal dysfunction may also induce skeletal myopathy.

Hypothyroid myopathy

The classical picture—proximal muscle weakness, progressive muscle enlargement, slowed muscle movements in congenital hypothyroidism (Debré–Sémélaigne syndrome) or painful cramps and muscle enlargement in the adult variant (Hoffman syndrome) —is the prototype of hypothyroid myopathy (Klein et al 1991). Usually, patients with hypothyroidism may present with primary manifestations of skeletal myopathy, developing proximal weakness, fatigue, slowed muscle movements, decreased osteotendinous reflexes, stiffness, myalgia, local myoedema and, occasionally, cramps, muscle enlargement, myokymia and acute rhabdomyolysis. Severe weakness and muscle respiratory involvement occurs in few cases. Muscle disease may also occur without apparent myxoedema (Kaminski and Ruff 1994). Serum creatine kinase (CK) levels usually rise (10-fold) and reverse with thyroid hormone replacement. Electromyography (EMG) may be normal or with variable non-specific manifestations, including fibrillations, fasciculations and myotony.

Muscle structure changes in hypothyroidism include atrophy of fibres, glycogen deposition (Fig. 1.1), focal necrosis, ring fibres, interstitial fibrosis and oxidative disruption (Ono et al 1987, Monforte et al 1990). Ultrastructural studies show mitochondrial swelling and inclusions, myofibrillar disarray, glycogen and lipid accumulation, dilatation of the sarcoplasmic reticulum (SR) and autophagic vacuoles. Mitochondrial changes and abnormalities of the SR and of T tubules seem to contribute to myoedema, cramping and slow muscle contraction.

Pathophysiology

The main changes involve carbohydrate metabolism, decreasing mitochondrial oxidation capacity, muscle oxidative enzyme activity and glucose uptake, with impaired glycogenolysis and an insulin-resistant state (Argov et al 1988). Protein metabolism is also affected by reducing both protein synthesis and degradation mediated by altered DNA transcription. Altered

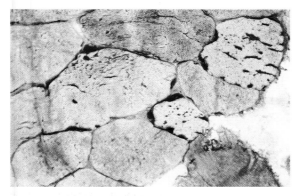

Figure 1.1—Muscle biopsy of a patient with hypothyroid myopathy. Subsarcolemmal glycogen accumulation is evident in periodic acid–Schiff reaction (PAS) staining.

myosin ATPase activity and impaired Ca^{2+}-uptake by the SR contributes to the sluggish contractions. Hypothyroidism also reduces the muscle uptake of triglycerides. This situation causes impaired energy metabolism, thus restricting the force generation mechanisms. A decrease in cardiac output and beta-adrenergic activity may also contribute to impaired exercise tolerance.

Treatment

Treatment consists in progressive replacement of the thyroid hormone. However, the disease is not always reversible in pathologic terms. In our experience, persistent histological changes in the muscle are seen even after euthyroid status is reached (Monforte et al 1990). Serum CK monitoring is a reliable marker of relapse in skeletal myopathy.

Hyperthyroid myopathy

Muscle weakness and atrophy were major complaints in Graves-Basedow's (1835) original descriptions of hyperthyroidism. However, the clinical spectrum of myopathy in hyperthyroidism is more diverse (Swanson et al 1981). The severity of muscle symptoms does not always correlate with the degree of thyroid dysfunction. Proximal weakness is present in 60–80% of patients, whereas distal weakness is less prominent and develops later. Fatigue, decreased exercise tolerance and myalgia are common, but usually less intense, as in hypothyroidism. In severe forms, the bulbar, oesophageal and respiratory muscles may be involved.

Pathophysiology

The main changes associated with thyrotoxicosis are:

1. Altered contractile response with relaxation, shortening of tendon reflexes, probably because of modification in the expression of myosin heavy chains, a shift in the Ca^{2+} sensitivity and increased Ca^{2+} uptake by the SR

2. Decreased efficiency of muscle contraction because of a derangement in glucose uptake and increased capillary density

3. Alterations in membrane excitability because of depolarization-induced Na^+-channel inactivation and altered T-tubule structure

4. Changes in intracytosolyc electrolyte concentration, with an initial increase in passive K^+ efflux, global K^+ depletion from the muscle and a compensatory upregulation of the Na^+-K^+ pumps (Schwartz and Oppenheimer 1987).

Specific forms

Specific forms of hyperthyroid myopathy include:

- **Acute thyroid myopathy** with a sudden onset of generalized weakness involving bulbar muscles (Joasoo et al 1970).
- **Association of myasthenia gravis** reflecting a common autoimmune disorder. Thyrotoxicosis usually precedes myasthenia and worsens its clinical course (Kiessling et al 1981).
- **Thyrotoxic periodic paralysis (TPP)**, is similar to that of familiar hypokalaemia periodic paralysis, with recurrent episodes of transitory focal or generalized muscle weakness (Kelley et al 1989). Serum potassium may be normal or low during the crisis. This entity was originally described in Asian countries, although it has also been reported in Western countries (Fernández-Solà et al 1992). The cause of paralysis in TPP appears to be Na^+-channel inactivation, which produces sarcolemmal depolarization.
- **Ophthalmoplegia** associated with exophthalmos. Elevation and abduction are the most severely compromised eye movements. Subsarcolemmal collection of mucopolysaccharides, together with plasma cell, mast cell or macrophage infiltrates in the extraocular muscles, may be present (Hallin and Feldon 1988).

Diagnosis

Serum muscle enzymes and myoglobin are usually normal. EMG may show short-duration motor unit potential and increased incidence of polyphasic potentials. Although non-specific, atrophy of both types of fibres, isolated necrosis of fibres with interstitial macrophage and lymphocyte infiltrates, increased number of internal nuclei, interstitial oedema and fatty infiltration are the most frequent muscle structure changes. Ultrastructural studies may show mitochondrial abnormalities, myofibrillar disarray and sub-sarcolemmal glycogen deposition (Celsing et al 1986).

Myopathy in glucocorticoid excess

Exogenous or endogenous glucocorticoid excess is a usual cause of skeletal myopathy. In the original Cushing description (1932) of endogenous glucocorticoid excess, severe proximal weakness, wasting and myalgia were present. Patients refer to difficulty in climbing stairs or combing their hair. A similar clinical picture was described by endogenous ectopic production of ACTH (Urbanic and George 1981) and in exogenous glucocorticoid administration (Picado et al 1990). These patients appear with the classical phenotype of Cushing's syndrome. Proximal weakness is of progressive onset, and usually predominates in the legs, women being more prone to present with muscle symptoms. Sphincter, oesophageal and bulbar musculature are usually preserved. There is a wide variability in the muscle effects of glucocorticoids because other factors such as nutrition and physical activity may modify the clinical course. Prolonged duration of the disease and the use of fluorinated corticoids are usually related to the more severe forms.

A specific form of acute quadriplegic myopathy in critically ill patients has been described (Miró et al 1994), usually affecting patients receiving large doses of glucocorticoids over a few days in coexistence with several of the following factors: immobilization, organ transplantation, sepsis, mechanical ventilation and neuromuscular blockade with curare-like agents (Miró et al 1999). All these factors seem to increase the potential toxic effect of glucocorticoids on skeletal muscle.

Pathophysiology

Glucocorticoid myopathy impairs protein synthesis by decreasing the total RNA content, increasing protein degradation, modifying carbohydrate metabolism by increasing muscle glycogen content and producing mitochondrial changes by interfering with the muscle oxidative capacity (Kaminski and Ruff 1994). Weakness may be induced via a reduction in Ca^{2+} release from the SR, by changing the myofibrillar

structure and altering ATP-ase activity (Laszewski and Ruff 1985). However, glucocorticoid-induced potentiation of excitation–contraction coupling may decrease the intensity of muscle symptoms and preserve the capacity for muscle force-generation.

Diagnosis

Diagnosis requires an appropriate clinical and histological approach and exclusion of other causes of myopathy (Kaminski and Ruff 1994). Serum muscle enzymes and proteins are usually normal. EMG findings are variable; non-specific low-amplitude and short-duration motor unit and occasional fibrillation potentials are observed. Selective Type II fibre atrophy is the main histological finding. Increased muscle glycogen and lipid content and mitochondrial aggregation and vacuolization are other frequent findings. In acute quadriplegic myopathy lack of reactivity in ATP-ase reaction is the pathological hallmark (Fig. 1.2). At an ultrastructural level, a selective loss of thick filaments and disarray of myofibrils is seen.

Treatment

Treatment of endogenous glucocorticoid excess, with normalization of ACTH or glucocorticoid levels, usually reverses the muscle-related symptoms. Exogenous steroid-induced myopathy requires a decrease in corticosteroid dosage to the lowest level possible. Subsequent protein replacement and exercise are necessary to prevent muscle atrophy in patients receiving steroids.

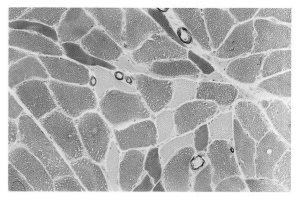

Figure 1.2—Patient receiving high-dose steroids and non-depolarizing blocking agents who developed an acute quadriplegic myopathy. Note the absence of reactivity in some muscle fibres in a pH 9.4 ATP-ase reaction.

Myopathy in hypofunction of the adrenal cortex

Muscle weakness is a classical symptom of adrenal insufficiency (Addison's syndrome). Severe generalized weakness, fatigue and muscle cramping are reported by a quarter to half of the patients with adrenal insufficiency (Mor et al 1987). Specific forms of hyperkalaemic periodic paralysis, respiratory myopathy and myasthenia gravis have been described in association with adrenal failure (Vilchez et al 1980).

Pathophysiology

Adrenal insufficiency leads to impairment in carbohydrate metabolism with depletion of muscle glycogen stores, fluid and electrolyte imbalance and altered vascular reactivity because of insensitivity to adrenergic stimulation. This results in hypovolaemia, hyponatraemia and hyperkalaemia (Kaminski and Ruff 1994). The coexistence of malnutrition also contributes to muscle damage.

Diagnosis

Serum muscle enzymes and proteins are usually normal. A decrease in muscle glycogen is the only histological evidence in these patients (Karpati and Carpenter 1984).

Treatment

Treatment of addisonian myopathy requires glucocorticoid and mineralocorticoid replacement, with prompt response. Hyperkalaemic periodic paralysis related to adrenal insufficiency also requires a decrease in serum K^+ concentrations by glucose administration.

Myopathy in pituitary dysfunction

Hypopituitarism

Global hypopituitarism (Simmonds–Sheehan's syndrome) causes marked weakness and fatigability without clear muscle atrophy, a fact presumably attributable to the deficit in thyroid and adrenocortical hormones and their synergistic effects (Isaksson et al 1985). Additionally, somatomedins (insulin-like growth factors; IGFs) appear to play a role in muscle trophism in hypopituitarism.

Acromegaly

Some patients with acromegaly develop proximal muscle weakness, wasting and hypotonia. Fatigue and exercise intolerance is present in half of the cases. Serum enzymes remain normal or slightly elevated (Khaleeli et al 1984). The EMG is normal in half of the cases and a myopathic pattern may appear in the remaining patients. In histological studies, hypertrophy of either Type I or II fibre, internal nuclei, glycogen or lipofuscin deposition, occasional necrosis, and the presence of autophagic vacuoles and tubular aggregates have been reported (Karpati and Carpenter 1984). This myopathy usually resolves when human growth hormone (hGH) levels return to normal.

Myopathy in parathyroid disorders

Hyperparathyroidism

In primary or secondary hyperparathyroidism a variable picture of proximal muscle weakness, wasting and fatigability may appear. Muscle stiffness, hypotonia, osteotendinous hyperreflexia and muscle atrophy may also be present (Laszewski and Ruff 1985). Parathyroid hormone (PTH) excess may increase muscle cytoplasmic Ca^{2+} levels, activate cytosolic proteases and reduce the Ca^{2+} sensitivity of the contractile system. CK levels are usually normal. The main EMG findings are the decreased size of motor unit potentials and an increased frequency of polyphasic potentials without spontaneous activity. Histological muscle changes are non-specific. The severity of this myopathy does not correlate with serum calcium or phosphate levels. Parathyroidectomy usually alleviates muscle symptoms (Kaminski and Ruff 1994).

Patients with secondary hyperparathyroidism resulting from chronic renal failure develop a myopathy similar to that of primary hyperparathyroidism.

Hypoparathyroidism

Hypoparathyroidism may affect muscle, inducing a hypocalcaemic and hypomagnesaemic-related tetany (Flink 1981). In these situations, the axons are hyperexcitable, thus resulting in distal numbness, paresthesia, carpopedal spasms and diffuse muscle cramping. Chvostek and Trousseau's signs are usually evident. Hyperventilation and metabolic alkalosis aggravate tetany. Occasional signs of chronic myopathy with mild weakness, CK activity elevation and slight muscle fibre atrophy have been reported in hypo- and pseudohypoparathyroidism (Yamaguchi et al 1987). Calcium, magnesium and vitamin D replacement quickly improves the muscle symptoms.

Osteomalacia

Osteomalacia usually develops with slight muscle symptoms, with proximal muscle weakness, wasting and myalgia being the most prominent (Ritz et al 1980). These symptoms resemble those of primary hyperparathyroidism, and they are independent of the aetiology of osteomalacia. Vitamin D deficiency deranges muscle protein synthesis, Ca^{2+} uptake and myofibrillar ATP-ase activity, thus resulting in impaired excitation–contraction coupling. Muscle symptoms resolve with vitamin D, but not with calcium or phosphate as the only replacement therapy.

Insulin resistance and endocrine myopathies

Insulin is a potent anabolic agent. Since aging, acromegaly, glucocorticoid excess, hypophosphataemia-associated PTH excess and hypothyroidism are conditions related to insulin resistance, a question arises as to whether insulin resistance may induce or contribute to muscle damage (DeFronzo 1979). However, it is difficult to separate the muscular effects of insulin resistance from those of the other primary endocrine diseases. A potential increase in muscle insulin sensitivity may potentially help to correct these endocrine myopathies.

Rhabdomyolysis/ myoglobinuria syndrome

Rhabdomyolysis (RML) may be defined as significant increase in muscle enzymes and proteins in the plasma, arising from muscle leakage because of structural or functional muscle membrane damage (Gabow et al 1982, Knochel 1993). This term does not necessarily imply muscle necrosis, although it is frequently present. CK is quantitatively the most important enzyme in the muscle cytosol and, therefore, the easiest to measure when rhabdomyolysis appears (Ventura-Clapier et al 1998). Usually, a 10-fold increase of normal CK activity (n.v: 150–200 IU/l) is necessary to ascertain acute rhabdomyolysis, although some authors have proposed a 100-fold increase (Fernández-Solà and Grau 1990). Other enzymes, such as lactate dehydrogenase, aldolase and glutamic-oxalacetic or glutamic-pyruvic transaminases or proteins (myoglobin) may also be helpful to monitor muscle damage and leakage to the plasma (Panteghini 1995).

Myoglobinuria (MGB) is defined by the abnormal presence of myoglobin in the urine, proceeding from muscle leakage to the plasma (Slater and Mullins 1998).

Both situations reflect a similar clinical condition. This syndrome may appear in physiological conditions such as in unusually demanding exercise. A variety of pathologic conditions including trauma, infections, metabolic and electrolyte disturbances, drug treatment, toxic ingestion and ischaemia may also be causative (Lofberg et al 1998; Table 1.2). In our experience (Fernández-Solà et al 1988) alcohol misuse is the most frequent finding related to RML, followed by inflammatory myopathies and RML related to excessive exercise or trauma.

Clinical features

Acute proximal muscle weakness, pain, tenderness, swelling and cramping of affected muscles and ecchymosis in contiguous skin areas are the most frequent features (Gabow et al 1982, Fernández-Solà et al 1988). Usually, a dark brown-pigmented urine appears, reflecting the presence of myoglobin. This syndrome may develop subclinically, only evidenced by biochemical serum or urine analysis. When the cause of

Table 1.2 — Main causes of rhabdomyolysis/ myoglobinuria syndrome

---

1. Infection
    Viral: Influenzae, Enteroviruses, human
        immunodeficiency virus (HIV)
    Bacterial: Gram-negative sepsis, *Salmonella* spp,
        Legionella spp, Mycoplasma, *Clostridium* spp.
2. Drugs
    Alcohol, cocaine, heroin, amphetamines
    Neuroleptics, barbiturates
    Succinylcholine, halothane
3. Electrolyte disturbance
    Hypokalaemia
    Hypophosphataemia
4. Trauma, compression, thermic or mechanical injury
    (crush syndrome)
5. Vigorous exercise, agitation or convulsions
6. Surgery or muscle puncture
7. Ischaemia
8. Metabolic and energetic myopathies
    Enzyme deficiencies of glycolysis/glycogenolysis
    Diabetic ketoacidosis
    Carnitine or carnitine palmytoyl transferase
    deficiencies
    Mitochondrial myopathies

RML ceases, the symptoms progressively disappear, with complete recovery. Clinical relapse is possible if re-exposure to the aetiological agent occurs. Sometimes, an additional ischaemic compromise may develop (compartmental syndrome), in addition to the original muscle damage. An acute severe form of RML/MGB syndrome has been described (Griggs et al 1995b), with an abrupt increase in serum CK activity, to as high as 100 000 IU/l, intense muscle weakness and swelling and development of acute renal failure. This may be a life-threatening situation and major life-support measures are required. Recurrent MGB may be present in some cases of mitochondrial myopathies, carnitine palmitoyl transferase and acid maltase deficiencies (Lofberg et al 1998).

Laboratory findings

The easiest way to confirm the presence of MGB is a urine dipstick test, which is negative in the presence of non-myoglobin urine pigmentation (porphyria or haemoglobinuria). Haematuria should be ruled out by microscopic examination of urine sediment. Myoglobin radioimmunoassay allows quantitative measurement of serum or urine myoglobin concentration, with normal myoglobin levels being those with less than 80 μg/ml in plasma and 12 μg/ml in urine. Visible MGB implies a minimum serum concentration of 1 mg/ml and corresponds to a previous destruction of 200 g muscle tissue. Serum CK activity is always elevated in the presence of MGB. Usually, serum CK activity ranges from 1000 to 5000 IU/l in RML and persists over 3–5 days. A concomitant rise in K^+ and uric acid parallels the CK activity peak in severe cases. CK activities do not predict acute renal failure (Kim et al 1992, Slater and Mullins 1998).

Histology

Histological findings in RML are focal or extensive necrosis, inflammation and regeneration signs and internal nuclei depending on the time of biopsy (Fernández-Solà and Grau 1990). In advanced states, muscle may appear nearly normal.

Pathophysiology

The precise mechanism of muscle injury leading to RML is still unclear. Selective depletion of ATP is presumed to predispose muscle breakdown (Knochel 1993). A particular susceptibility to damage following eccentric contraction may also contribute.

Treatment

Acute severe RML requires intensive care support with serum and electrolyte repletion and bicarbonate administration in order to avoid myoglobin deposition. Compartmental syndrome requires fasciotomy. Dialysis may correct fluid and electrolyte abnormalities (Slater and Mullins 1998). Training reduces susceptibility to RML.

Toxic myopathies

Exposure to a large variety of drug or toxic agents has been related to muscle disturbances (Table 1.3). The clinical presentation of toxic myopathy is diverse (George and Pourmand 1997). Myalgias and acute muscle weakness are usual. Mechanisms producing muscle toxicity include direct toxic effect (e.g. alco-

Table 1.3 — Main aetiological causes of toxic myopathies

Drugs
Common
   Glucocorticoids
   Cholesterol lowering agents
   Colchicine
   Cyclosporine
   Zidovudine
   Haloperidol
   Halothane
   Diuretics (inducing hypokalaemia)
   Vincristine
   Depolarizing muscle agents
Uncommon
   Rifampin
   Penicillamine
   Amiodarone
   Epsilon-aminocaproic acid
   Ipecac
   Cimetidine
   Antithyroid drugs

Toxic agents
   Alcohol
   Heroin
   Cocaine
   Barbiturates
   Amphetamines

Associations that potentiate muscle toxicity
   Immobilization and steroids
   Statins and fibrates
   Colchicine and renal failure
   Steroids and depolarizing muscle relaxants
   Age and multipharmacological treatment

hol, colchicine, zidovudine), local toxicity (injection of meperidine into muscle), production of a systemic, endocrine, metabolic or immunologic disorder (e.g. diuretic-induced hypokalaemia), depression of consciousness with resulting pressure and ischaemic necrosis of muscles (e.g. heroin) or through inducing RML/MGB syndrome (Fernández-Solà et al 1988). In most cases a careful medical record with attention to a possible temporary relationship between toxic exposure and development of muscle symptoms may be helpful (Griggs et al 1995b). Sometimes, reintroduction or re-exposure precipitates new or recurrent episodes of myopathy. It is important to assert possible precipitating conditions such as immobilization or the presence of renal failure. A mild transitory rise in serum CK activity is frequent. Muscle biopsy should be reserved for difficult or severe cases. Histological findings in muscle are usually non-specific, with a variable degree of muscle necrosis, oxidative disturbances and fibre atrophy. Some specific muscle changes may suggest the origin of the myopathy, for example, an inflammatory myopathy in penicillamine administration or vacuolar myopathy in hypokalaemic-induced agents or AZT fibres (Fig. 1.3). Cessation of exposure to the toxin, drugs or precipitating factors and rest usually reverse the muscle changes, although recovery may be slow.

Muscle cramps and contracture

Cramps

Ordinary muscle cramps are defined as a painful explosive onset of visible, palpable contraction of a

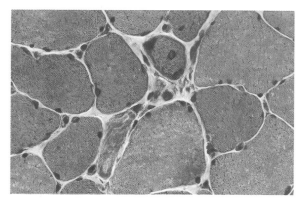

Figure 1.3—Patient with human immunodeficiency virus (HIV) infection under long-term zidovudine treatment. Some fibres appear with a ragged-red appearance (AZT fibres).

part or all muscles, with independent waxing and waning in different parts of the muscle that usually terminates spontaneously or by passive stretching (Layzer 1994). Cramps may occur spontaneously at rest, although they are often triggered by a brief contraction after a trivial movement, but also after forceful contraction, when the muscle shortens. During cramps, EMG shows high-amplitude, high-frequency typical discharges. Most of the cramping conditions are related to hyperactivity of the central or peripheral nervous system rather than primary muscle disease. In the latter case, cramps probably originate in the intramuscular portion of motor nerve terminals in relation to rapid changes of extracellular fluid. When cramps are related to muscle energy store exhaustion, McArdle disease may be suspected. A considerable number of cases remain undiagnosed. Fasciculations and cramps, although sometimes coexistent, seem to have different physiopathological mechanisms. Membrane-stabilizing agents are the only drugs which are useful in preventing cramps. Quinine is recommended to control nocturnal cramps, and clonazepam, phenytoin and carbamazepine are useful for frequent daytime cramps.

Contracture

Muscle contracture is a state of active muscle contraction unaccompanied by electrical activity. This phenomenon is a frequent cause of muscle spasms during exercise. It occurs in a few rare cases, including primary disorders of muscle relaxation such as myotonia, paramyotonia or the Lamber–Brody syndrome, endocrine myopathies (hypothyroidism) and metabolic myopathies (glycolytic and glycogenolytic deficiencies) (Layzer 1994). Slow relaxation and myotonic phenomenon may coexist with muscle contracture. A relationship has been suggested between contracture and high-energy phosphate metabolism, with focal ATP depletion presumably being responsible for muscle contracture induction.

References

Argov Z, Renshaw PF, Boden B, Winokur A, Bank WJ. (1988) Effects of hypothyroid hormones on skeletal muscle bioenergetics: In vivo phosphorus-31 magnetic resonance spectroscopy study of humans and rats. *J Clin Invest* 81: 1695–1701.

Celsing F, Bolmstrand E, Melichna J, et al. (1986) Effect of hyperthyroidism on fibre-type composition, fibre area, glycogen content and enzyme activity in human skeletal muscle. *Clin Physiol* 6: 171–181.

DeFronzo RA. (1979) Glucose intolerance and aging: evidence for tissue insensitivity to insulin. *Diabetes* 28: 1095–1101.

Di Mauro S, Bonilla E, Zeviani M, Nakagawa M, DeVivo DC. (1985) Mitochondrial myopathies. *Ann Neurol* 17: 521–528.

Duboc D, Jehenson P, Dinh ST, Marsac C, Syrola A, Fardeau M. (1987) Phosphorus NMR spectroscopy study of muscular enzyme deficiencies involving glycogenolysis and glycolysis. *Neurology* 33: 663–671.

Elliot DL, Buist NMR, Goldberg L, Kennaway NG, Powell BR, Kuehl KS. (1989) Metabolic myopathies: Evaluation by graded exercise testing. *Medicine (Balt)* 68: 163–172.

Fernández-Solà J, Grau JM, Pedro-Botet JC, et al. (1988) Rabdomiólisis no traumática: análisis clínico de 53 casos. *Med Clin (Bar)* 90: 199–202.

Fernández-Solà J, Grau JM. (1990) Significado clínico de los valores séricos de creatincinasa y sus isoenzimas. *Med Clin (Bar)* 94: 708–710.

Fernández-Solà J, Pedrol E, Galofré J, Casademont J, Grau JM, Urbano-Márquez A. (1992) Parálisis periódica tireotóxica. *An Med Intern (Mad)* 9: 294–296.

Flink EB. (1981) Magnesium deficiency: Etiology and clinical spectrum. *Acta Med Scand (Suppl)* 647: 125–137.

Gabow PA, Haehny ND, Kelleher SP. (1982) The spectrum of rhabdomyolysis. *Medicine (Balt)* 61: 141–152.

George KK, Pourmand R. (1997) Toxic myopathies. *Neurol Clin* 15(3): 711–730.

Griggs RC, Mendell JR, Miller RG. (1995a) Metabolic myopathies. In: Griggs RC, Mendell JR, Miller RG, eds. *Evaluation and treatment of myopathies*. Philadelphia: FA Davis Company, pp. 247–293.

Griggs RC, Mendell JR, Miller RG. (1995b) Myopathies of systemic disease: agents directly toxic to the muscle. In: Griggs RC, Mendell JR, Miller RG, eds. *Evaluation and treatment of myopathies*. Philadelphia: FA Davis Company, pp. 371–377.

Hallin E, Feldon SE. (1988) Grave's ophthalmopathy: correlation of clinical signs with measures derived from computed tomography. *Br J Ophthalmol* 72: 678–782.

Isaksson OGP, Eden S, Jansson JO. (1985) Mode of action of pituitary growth hormone on target cells. *Annu Rev Physiol* 47: 483–499.

Joasoo A, Murray IPC, Stteinbeck AW. (1970) Involvement of bulbar muscles in thyrotoxic myopathy. *Aust An Med* 19: 338–340.

Kaminski HJ, Ruff RL. (1994) Endocrine myopathies. In: Engel AG, Amstrong CF, eds. *Myology*. 2nd Ed, Vol 2. New York: Mc Graw-Hill, pp. 1726–1753.

Karpati G, Carpenter S. (1984) Acromegalic myopathy. In: Karpati G, Carpenter S, eds. *Pathology of skeletal muscle*. New York: Churchill Livingstone, p. 416.

Kelley DE, Gharib H, Kennedy FP, Duda RJ, McManis PG. (1989) Thyrotoxic periodic paralysis. Report of 10 cases and electromyographic findings. *Arch Intern Med* 149: 2597–2600.

Kent-Braun JA, Miller RG, Weiner MW. (1993) Phases of metabolism during progressive exercise to fatigue in human skeletal muscle. *Am J Physiol* 75: 573–580.

Khaleeli AA, Levy RD, Edwards RHT, et al. (1984) The neuromuscular features of acromegaly: A clinical and pathological study. *J Neurol Neurosurg Psychiatry* 47: 1009–1015.

Kiessling WR, Pfluehaupt KW, Ricker K, Haubitz I, Mertens HG. (1981) Thyroid function and circulating antithyroid antibodies in myasthenia gravis. *Neurology* 31: 771–774.

Kim SH, Kim CHS, Lee JS. (1992) Acute renal failure secondary to rhabdomyolysis. *Acta Radiol* 33: 573–575.

Klein I, Parker M, Shebert R, Ayyar DR, Levey GS. (1991) Hypothyroidism presenting as muscle stiffness and pseudohypertrophy: Hoffman's syndrome. *Am J Med* 70: 891–892.

Knochel JP. (1993) Mechanisms of rhabdomyolysis. *Curr Op Rheumatol* 5: 725–731.

Laszewski B, Ruff RL. (1985) The effects of glucocorticoid treatment on excitation-contraction coupling. *Am J Physiol* 248: E 363–369.

Layzer RB. (1994) Muscle pain, cramps and fatigue. In: Engel AG, Amstrong CF, eds. *Myology*. 2nd Ed, Vol 2. New York: Mc Graw-Hill, pp. 1754–1768.

Lofberg M, Jankala H, Pateau A, Harkonen M, Somer H. (1998) Metabolic causes of recurrent rhabdomyolysis. *Acta Neurol Scand* 98: 268–275.

Miró O, Grau JM, Nadal P, Picado C, Plaza V, Urbano-Márquez A. (1994) Miopatía aguda en relación con la administración de glucocorticoides y bloqueadores neuromusculares. *Med Clin (Bar)* 103: 458–461.

Miró O, Salmerón JM, Masanés F, Graus F, Mas A, Grau JM. (1999) Acute quadriplegic myopathy with myosin-deficient muscle fibres after liver transplantation. Defining the clinical picture and delimiting the risk factors. *Transplantation* 67: 1144–1150.

Monforte R, Fernández-Solà J, Casademont J, Vernet M, Grau JM, Urbano-Márquez A. (1990) Miopatia hipotiroidea; estudio prospectivo clínico e histológico de 19 pacientes. *Med Clin (Bar)* 95: 126–129.

Mor F, Green P, Wysenbeek AJ. (1987) Myopathy in Addison's disease. *Ann Rheum Dis* 46: 81–83.

Ono S, Inouye K, Mannen T. (1987) Myopathology of hypothyroid myopathy. Some new observations. *J Neurol Sci* 77: 237–248.

Panteghini M. (1995) Enzyme and muscle diseases. *Curr Opin Rheumatol* 7: 469–474.

Picado C, Fiz JA, Montserrat JM, et al. (1990) Respiratory and skeletal muscle function in steroid-dependent bronchial asthma. *Am Rev Respir Dis* 141: 14–20.

Ritz E, Boland R, Kreusser W. (1980) Effects of vitamin D and parathormone on muscle: Potential role of uremic myopathy. *Am J Clin Nutr* 33: 1522–1529.

Schwartz HL, Oppenheimer JH. (1978) Physiologic and biochemical actions of thyroid hormone. *Pharmacol Ther* 3: 349–376.

Slater, MS, Mullins RJ. (1998) Rhabdomyolysis and myoglobinuric renal failure in trauma and surgical patients: a review. *J Am Coll Surg* 186: 693–715.

Swanson JW, Kelly JJ, McConahey WM. (1981) Neurologic aspects of thyroid dysfunction. *Mayo Clin Proc* 56: 504–512.

Turken SA, Cafferty M, Silverberg SJ, et al. (1989) Neuromuscular involvement in mild, asymptomatic, primary hyperparathyroidism. *Am J Med* 87: 553–557.

Urbanic RC, George JM. (1981) Cushing's disease: 18 years experience. *Medicine (Balt)* 60: 14–24.

Ventura-Clapier R, Kuznetsov V, Veksler E, Bohem E, Anflous K. (1998) Functional coupling of creatine kinases in muscles: Species and tissue specificity. *Mol Cell Bioch* 184: 231–247.

Vilchez JJ, Cabello A, Bendito J, Vilarroya T. (1980) Hyperkalemic paralysis, neuropathy and persistent motor neuron discharges in Addison's disease. *J Neurol Neurosurg Psychiatry* 43: 818–822.

Wortmann RL. (1991) Metabolic myopathies. *Curr Opin Rheumatol* 3: 925–933.

Yamaguchi H, Okamoto K, Shooji M, Morimatsu M, Hirai S. (1987) Muscle histology of hypocalcemic myopathy in hypoparathyroidism. *J Neurol Neurosurg Psychiatry* 50: 817–818.

2

Review of skeletal muscle injuries

Doron Aronson

Introduction

Muscle injury can occur through diverse mechanisms (Table 2.1). However, at the cellular level, muscle damage usually results from a relatively few damaging processes. Furthermore, regardless of the aetiology of muscle injury, the inflammatory and regenerative responses bear significant similarities, indicating that muscle tissue can only undergo a limited number of responses to injury. This chapter will examine the cellular mechanisms that culminate in muscle damage, and the similarities between muscle cells response to different insults.

Exertion-induced injury to skeletal muscle

Several types of muscle injury fall into the broad category of exertion-induced muscle injury. Exercise, especially when it involves concentric muscle actions (Stauber et al 1990), associated with overloading (i.e. conditions where the force requirement of the muscle exceeds the habitual or functional requirements) or over-activity (i.e. the firing rate of motor neurons is increased beyond its physiological levels or duty cycles) can result in injury to skeletal muscle. While overloading occurs commonly during growth and work-induced hypertrophy, over-activity is seen most often in disease states characterized by spasticity or tetany (Stauber and Smith 1998), or after exhaustive long-term exercise (Ostrowski et al 1998a, 1998b), or with chronic electrical stimulation (Maier et al 1986). From these examples, when myofibre response has been studied, the muscle response seems to show a reproducible pattern seen also in traumatic injuries such as crush or over strain (Stauber and Smith 1998).

An activity that involves loading of muscle by external forces and subsequent lengthening of the

Table 2.1 — Etiology of skeletal muscle injury

Exercise-induced
Ischaemia/reperfusion injury
Mechanical injury (e.g. crush injury, stretch injury)
Muscular dystrophy
Biochemical disorders (e.g. carnitine deficiency)
Infectious disorders (e.g. streptococcus A, human
  immunodeficiency virus)
Drug-induced (e.g. statins)
Toxins (e.g. snake toxin, notexin)
Injury to grafted muscle

muscle as its activity develops tension (e.g. eccentric exercise) is also effective in inducing this type of damage. Naturally occurring examples are contractions in the biceps brachii as a heavy load is being slowly lowered, and the activity in the gluteus maximus that checks the forward swing of the leg during running (Cannon et al 1990). In terms of the sliding filament mechanism of muscle contraction, the myosin cross-bridges make repeated connections with the actin filaments throughout the duration of the active state in the muscle fibre. However, actin filaments instead of being propelled toward the centre of the myosin are pulled in opposite direction by the external forces on the muscle.

The sequence of events that characterize muscle injury which occurs when human muscle is subjected to eccentric exercise is:

1. Loss of strength and change in the force–frequency relationship of the muscle

2. Pain and muscle tenderness, which is not usually evident during the period of exercise but appears within the following 6–12 h, and reaches a peak 24–48 h after the exercise

3. Release of soluble muscle proteins such as into the circulation peaking at 5–6 days

4. Destruction of muscle fibres, accompanied by infiltration of inflammatory cells to the tissue, between 6 and 10 days after exercise

5. Activation of satellite cells, with the formation of myotubes and restoration of normal structure and function within 2 to 3 weeks (Armstrong et al 1983).

The inflammatory and regenerative steps in the exercise-induced injury sequence seem to follow the same general order described for other types of muscle injury (Carlson and Faulkner 1983, Armstrong et al 1991a). However, little is known about the causative factor or the cellular mechanisms involved in exertion-induced injury to skeletal muscle. Two major hypotheses have been proposed to explain the initial damage to muscle cells in this setting (Armstrong 1986, Armstrong et al 1991b).

The metabolic hypothesis assumes that metabolic overload results in Ca^{2+} overload of cells. Several observations support this hypothesis, including the resemblance of exercise-induced muscle damage to ischaemic muscle damage, and the susceptibility of patients with muscle disorders secondary to known metabolic defects to exercise-induced muscle damage. The mechanisms by which increased intracellular Ca^{2+}

results in muscle damage have been reviewed extensively elsewhere (Armstrong 1990, Smith et al 1990, Armstrong et al 1991b), and they are beyond the scope of this chapter.

The mechanical hypothesis assumes that mechanical strain on muscle fibres results in rupture of structural component (Newham et al 1987, Ebbeling and Clarkson 1990). For example, several studies have shown that muscle fibre injury results from high tensile stresses occurring during concentric contractions (McCully and Faulkner 1985, 1986). The mechanical hypothesis also leads to an elevation in intracellular Ca^{2+} through disruption of the normal permeability barrier to extracellular Ca^{2+} (Armstrong et al 1991b).

Exertion-induced skeletal muscle injury induces an acute inflammatory response (McCully et al 1985). The presumed adaptive value of this response may be related to removal of necrotic or cellular debris, which subsequently promotes repair of damaged myofibrils and extracellular matrix (Cannon and Pierre 1998). The production of cytokines from infiltrating neutrophils, monocyte/macrophages, and activated fibroblasts, plays an important role in cell proliferation, migration, and regeneration. For example, increased neutrophil concentrations in exercise-damaged muscle correlate with elevated interleukin-1 levels (Fielding et al 1993). The ability of macrophages to regulate proliferation and differentiation of satellite cells underscores their importance demonstrating that, besides their scavenger role, macrophages contribute to myoblast proliferation during muscle regeneration (Cantini et al 1994). However, even in the absence of macrophages, the response of muscle to strain injury is unaltered (Lowe et al 1995), raising the possibility that muscle cells can regulate an inflammatory response. Indeed, Ostrowski et al (1998a) have shown that inflammatory cytokines are produced locally in skeletal muscle fibres in response to prolonged intense exercise.

Cellular responses to injury

There is no evidence that the muscle is permanently impaired as a result of exertion-induced injury, and physical conditioning results in an adaptation such that all indicators of damage are reduced following repeated bouts of exercise (Schwane and Armstrong 1983, Ebbeling and Clarkson 1989). These observations suggest that the exercise-induced muscle injury is an adaptive response. Because exercise is an important stimulus for structural remodelling and functional hypertrophy of skeletal muscle (Vandenburgh and Kaufman 1979), exercise-induced injury may be a

normal precursor of muscle adaptation to increased use (Armstrong 1990). Therefore, the initiating molecular and cellular mechanisms of muscle adaptation to increased load and exercise-induced injury may bear significant similarity (Aronson et al 1998a, Boppart et al 1999). Recent studies have identified some of the intracellular signaling pathways that may mediate the biological effects observed upon increased muscle activity (Aronson et al 1997a, 1998b) and eccentric exercise (Boppart et al 1999).

The stress activated protein kinases and eccentric exercise

Exposure of cells to environmental stressors such as UV irradiation or osmotic shock evokes a series of phosphorylation events leading to the modification of transcription factors and altered gene expression (Cano and Mahadevan 1995, Raingeaud et al 1995, Kyriakis et al 1996). In mammalian cells, there are at least three related but distinct mitogen-activated protein (MAP) kinase cascades that are activated by diverse environmental stresses (Fig. 2.1). The extracellular-regulated kinase (ERK) pathway is activated by growth factors (Seger and Krebs 1995), and by cellular stresses such as hyperosmolarity (Matsuda et al 1995, Seger and Krebs 1995), and reperfusion injury (Knight and Buxton 1996; Fig. 2.1A). A second pathway uses the c-Jun NH_2-terminal kinases (JNKs) for transmitting stress signals (Kyriakis and Avruch 1996). JNKs can be stimulated by a variety of cellular stresses such as UV radiation (Dérijard et al 1994), osmotic and heat shock (Cano et al 1995), as well as by proinflammatory cytokines including tumour necrosis factor-α and interleukin-1 (Kyriakis et al 1994, Kyriakis and Avruch 1996; Fig. 2.1B). The third member of the MAP kinase family, the p38 kinase, is also regulated by stress signals such as UV light, heat shock (Rouse et al 1994), proinflammatory cytokines (Raingeaud et al 1995), and endotoxin from gram-negative bacteria (Han et al 1996). An important physiological substrate of p38 kinase is the MAP kinase-activated protein kinase-2, an enzyme that plays a role in the regulation of heat shock proteins as part of the cellular response to stress (Rouse et al 1994).

The earliest cellular response described thus far in association with exercise (Aronson et al 1997b, 1998b, Widegren et al 1998) and other forms of contractile activity (Aronson et al 1997a) is a rapid activation of the ERK and JNK pathways, detected immediately post exercise (Fig. 2.2). The activation of ERK and JNK with contractile activity is associated with the

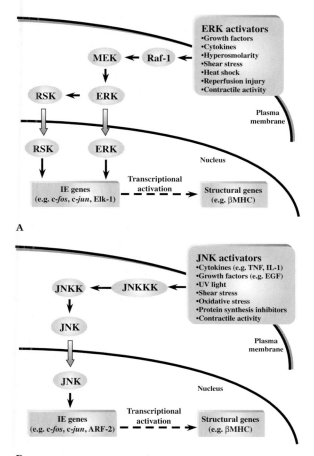

A

B

Figure 2.1—**Schematic representation of the mitogen-activated protein (MAP) kinase cascades. A** The extracellular-regulated kinase (ERK) pathway involves the sequential phosphorylation and activation of the serine kinase Raf1, the ERK kinase kinases (MEK), and two ERK isoforms (ERK1/ERK2). The ERKs can phosphorylate and activate cytosolic substrates such as the p90 ribosomal S6 kinase (RSK). A fraction of the activated ERK and RSK population translocates into the nucleus and activates several nuclear transcription factor genes, including c-*myc*, c-*fos*, and *Elk-1*. The ERK pathway is activated by growth factors, cytokines, and by cellular stresses such as hyperosmolarity, and reperfusion injury (see text). **B** The c-Jun NH$_2$-terminal kinase (JNK) pathway involves the sequential phosphorylation and activation of JNK kinase kinase (JNKKK), JNK kinase (JNKK), and JNK. Like ERKs, JNKs can translocate to the nucleus and activate a variety of transcription factors. JNKs can be stimulated by a variety of cellular stresses such as UV radiation, osmotic and heat shock, as well as by pro-inflammatory cytokines including tumour necrosis factor-α (TNF) and interleukin-1 (IL-1).

rapid induction of early response genes such as c-*jun* and c-*fos* (Aronson et al 1997a, 1998b), which constitute one of the cellular responses to injury (see below). The same signalling pathway is stimulated during

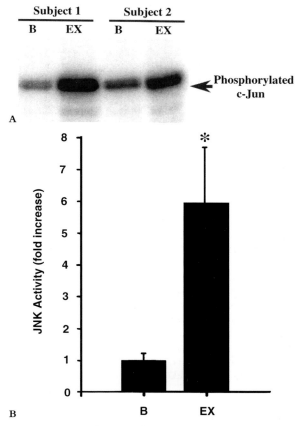

Figure 2.2—**Stimulation of the stress activated protein kinases with an acute bout of exercise on JNK activity.** Muscle extracts were immunoprecipitated with anti-JNK, and the immunoprecipitates were subjected to an in vitro kinase assay using GST-c-Jun-(1-135) as substrate. **A** Representative immunoblots of two subjects showing increased JNK activity (as reflected by increased c-Jun phosphorylation) after a 30 min bout of exercise. **B** Overall (n = 8), exercise resulted in a 5.9 ± 1.8 (mean ± SEM) fold increase in JNK activity ($p < 0.05$) B, baseline; EX, post-exercise. Modified from Aronson et al 1998b.

eccentric exercise-induced muscle injury in humans, although the magnitude of the stimulation is substantially higher (Boppart et al 1999; Fig. 2.3).

The mechanism by which contractile activity induces activation of these signalling cascades is currently unknown. The possibility that the activation of the MAP kinase pathways during exercise is primarily mediated by hormones or cytokines released systemically is unlikely since activation of these signalling pathways is confined to the exercising limb (Aronson et al 1997b, 1998b). Thus, muscle cells are intrinsically able to sense mechanical signals and respond by activation of specific signalling cues in the absence of neural

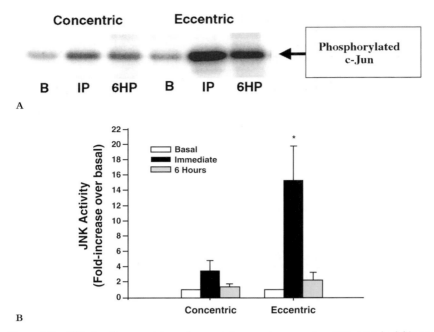

Figure 2.3 — **Effects of concentric and eccentric exercise on c-Jun NH$_2$-terminal kinase (JNK) activity. A** Reaction products from JNK activity assay from two representative subjects who underwent either concentric or eccentric exercise in the basal state (B), immediately postexercise (IP), and 6 h postexercise (6HP). **B** JNK activity (mean ± SEM) for concentric (n = 5) and eccentric (n = 5) groups. ⋆$p < 0.05$ vs concentric IP group. Note the magnitude of JNK stimulation with eccentric exercise (which was associated with evidence of muscle damage in this study) compared with concentric exercise. Adapted from Boppart et al. 1999.

or hormonal factors. This ability is also suggested by the observation that cultured skeletal muscle cells can undergo hypertrophy without participation of humoral or neural factors (Vandenburgh et al 1979). Local stimulation of the stress–activated protein kinases in the setting of muscle overuse can occur through several mechanisms.

Several studies have suggested that stretch can activate intracellular signalling pathways by releasing growth factors in an autocrine/paracrine fashion, which in turn activate their specific receptors and, subsequently, secondary messenger systems (Morrow et al 1990, Vandenburgh et al 1979, 1991). Growth factors and cytokines known to activate the stress pathways are produced by skeletal muscle cells, and their production correlates with increased muscle activity (Devol et al 1990, Morrow et al 1990). Clarke et al (1993) have shown that leakage of growth factors such as basic fibroblast growth factor (bFGF) through mechanically-induced plasma membrane disruptions can occur with contractile activity.

The extracellular matrix carries the external mechanical force to the cell surface, and its association with cytoskeletal integrins is known to regulate diverse phenomena such as muscle morphogenesis and organization of the contractile apparatus (Sastry et al 1996, Carson and Wei 2000). Integrins function in signal transducing and matrix–integrin interaction can trigger activation of stress pathways (Miyamoto et al 1995, MacKenna et al 1998). For example, JNK is activated in epithelial cells in response to disengaging the integrins and disrupting the cytoskeleton (detachment of cells); restoring attachment can prevent JNK activation (Frisch et al 1996).

Crush injury

This topic is reviewed in detail in Chapter 5. In this section, only the similarities between the molecular events observed with exercise-induced injury and with trauma will be discussed. Muscle injury induced by cutting or crushing results in a rapid and striking activation of all three stress-activated protein kinase (Aronson et al 1998a; Fig. 2.4). The marked activation of the stress cascades following muscle tissue injury

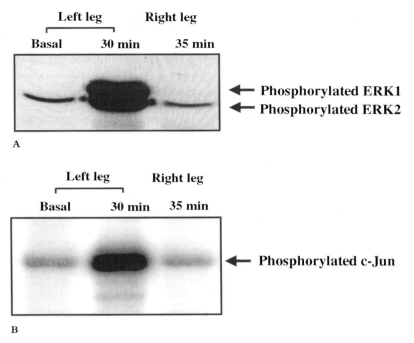

Figure 2.4—**Effects of cutting on stress-activated protein kinases in human skeletal muscle.** After cutting injury to muscle from the left leg, a striking increase in ERK isoforms activity (**A**) and JNK activity (**B**) occurs within 30 min. This response is restricted to the injured muscle and does not occur in the contralateral leg. Modified from Aronson et al 1998a.

may initiate adaptive responses that render cells more resistant to the stress of the wound environment. In NIH 3T3 and PC12 cells, Guyton et al (1996) have shown that the potential for cell survival following oxidant injury correlated with the capacity for ERK activation. MAP kinases may trigger a beneficial stress response by activating genes coding for proteins that confer protection against environmental insults. For example, work by Schreiber et al (1995) indicates that the induction of both c-*fos* and c-*jun* is part of the natural defence mechanism that increases the ability of mammalian cells to withstand UV irradiation. Several studies have demonstrated that tissue injury also causes a rapid induction of early response genes (Hengerer et al 1990, Pawar et al 1995), which are among the major nuclear targets of MAP kinases (Seger and Krebs 1995). Hengerer et al (1990) have shown that transection of the sciatic nerve rapidly increases c-*fos* and c-*jun* mRNA, with peak levels 2 h following injury. Similarly, Pawar et al (1995) have demonstrated a rapid induction of c-*fos* and *EGR-1* after scrape wounding of renal epithelial cells. Hence, activation of MAP kinases following tissue injury may represent a prototype stress response that results in an increased ability of cells to survive by activating genes coding for

proteins that confer protection against stress, or facilitate the repair of stress-damaged cells (Aronson et al 1998a). In addition, MAP kinases (especially the p38 kinase) can also regulate heat shock proteins (Rouse et al 1994), which have been shown to be involved in the response to tissue injury (Currie and White 1981) and human wound healing (Oberringer et al 1995). Heat-shock conditioning with upregulation of heat-shock proteins confers significant biochemical and ultrastructural protection against ischaemic injury in rat skeletal muscle (Garramone et al 1994).

Reperfusion injury in skeletal muscle

Prolonged periods of ischaemia produce skeletal muscle dysfunction and ultimately necrosis through loss of cellular energy and elaboration of toxic tissue metabolites. Although restoration of blood flow is essential for salvage of ischaemic muscle tissue, reperfusion elicits a complex series of events involving the production of reactive oxygen species, neutrophil accumulation, microvascular barrier disruption, and oedema formation. A significant part of total muscle injury after ischaemia is attributable to the effects of reperfusion.

Formation of reactive oxygen metabolites

Reperfusion elicits highly reactive metabolites of molecular oxygen, which may exacerbate ischaemic tissue injury. Reoxygenation of endothelial cells is associated with a burst of oxygen free-radical production both from endothelial cells and from the muscle itself (McCutchan et al 1990), peaking within minutes of reperfusion and lasting for hours thereafter. The biochemical sources of toxic species such as superoxide, hydrogen peroxide and hydroxyl anion appear to be xanthine oxidase, mitochondrial electron transport chain and recruited neutrophils (Korthuis et al 1985, Smith et al 1989, Allen et al 1995, Gute et al 1998). These highly reactive molecules may result in lipid peroxidation, membrane dysfunction, and membrane permeability. Oxygen free-radicals can promote other pathophysiological processes that play a central role in the development of reperfusion injury such as intracellular calcium overload (Allen et al 1995, Gute et al 1998) and altered arachidonic acid metabolism (Anderson et al 1990). However, the pathways by which these occurrences result in reperfusion injury are interrelated extensively (Allen et al 1995, Rubin et al 1996). The reader is referred to Chapter 35 for a more detailed discussion in free radical-mediated muscle injury.

Role of neutrophils in the pathogenesis of reperfusion injury

Leukocytes accumulate in ischaemic and reperfused skeletal muscle under the influence of chemoattractants, and they play a central role in tissue damage that occurs in the reperfused muscle (Smith et al 1991, Gute et al 1998; Fig. 2.5). Post-reperfusion necrosis can be ameliorated by depletion of circulating leukocytes (Belkin et al 1989, Crinnion et al 1994), or by monoclonal antibodies (Iwahori et al 1998, Lozano et al 1999) and ligand blockers directed against cell adhesion molecules.

Multiple cytokines act synergistically to draw leukocytes into loci of hypoxic vascular injury including IL-1, TNF, and IL-8 (see Ch. 33). Leukocyte recruitment entails a complex series of events that involves a number of adhesive molecules. Circulating neutrophils that localize to a reperfused area first adhere to the activated endothelial surface in a decelerating,

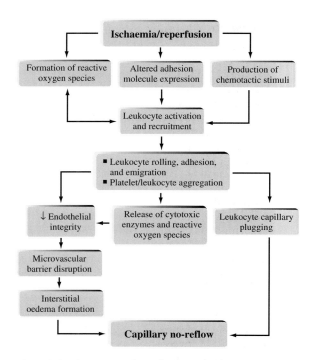

Figure 2.5—**Sequence of mechanisms leading to capillary no-reflow in reperfused skeletal muscle.**

rolling type of adhesive process mediated by endothelial P-selectin (Geng et al 1990, Mayadas et al 1993), which is rapidly expressed on endothelial cell surface during reperfusion (Weyrich et al 1993). This interaction brings neutrophils into close proximity to the endothelial surface, to promote firmer adhesive interactions mediated by molecules such as L-selectin (Lozano et al 1999), platelet activating factor (Silver et al 1996), intracellular adhesion molecule-1 (ICAM-1) on the endothelial cell, and the neutrophil β_2 integrins (CD11/CD18) (Petrasek et al 1996, Zamboni et al 1997). Neutralization of the functional epitopes of CD11/CD18 attenuates neutrophil sequestration (Carden et al 1990), microvascular barrier disruption (Jerome et al 1994a) and capillary no-reflow (Jerome et al 1993, 1994b) in skeletal muscle (Smith et al 1991).

Upon recruitment into ischaemic/reperfused tissue, neutrophils release numerous cytotoxic lysosomal enzymes, including elastase and the metalloproteases collagenase and gelatinase. In addition, under the influence of cytokines and chemotactic factors neutrophils undergo a respiratory burst, which elicits a sudden release of toxic oxygen metabolites such as the superoxide anion, hydroxyl radical, and hydrogen peroxide.

Post-ischaemic capillary no-reflow

The microcirculation is a primary target for the development of post-ischaemic reperfusion injury with manifestations of different pathophysiological events occurring within the individual segments of the microcirculation (Menger et al 1997). The lack of nutritive capillary perfusion despite reperfusion of the ischaemic tissue (termed no-reflow) is probably the most deleterious capillary dysfunction involved in reperfusion injury. This is supported by experimental studies in skeletal muscle, demonstrating that the development of capillary no-reflow is associated with prolongation of tissue hypoxia during reperfusion resulting in aggravation of ischaemic tissue injury.

Several functional and mechanical mechanisms have been suggested to promote the development of post-ischaemic no-reflow including oedema, intravascular haemoconcentration and thrombosis, swelling of endothelial cells, and plugging of capilaries with leukocytes (Allen et al 1995, Oredsson et al 1995, Menger et al 1997; Fig. 2.5). Activated leukocytes play a major role in post-ischaemic no-reflow; a strong correlation exists between the number of leukocytes present in ischaemic tissues and the percentage of capillaries exhibiting no-reflow (Gute et al 1998). Neutrophil/endothelial cell adhesive interactions are necessary for capillary no-reflow in skeletal muscle (Jerome et al 1993, 1994a). Although complete mechanical obstruction of capillary lumen is unlikely in skeletal muscle (Jerome et al 1993, Gute et al 1998), oxidants produced by activated neutrophils can induce endothelial cell damage and swelling and disrupt the microvascular barrier with subsequent increase in capillary permeability (Gute et al 1998).

References

Allen DM, Chen LE, Seaber AV, Urbaniak JR. (1995) Pathophysiology and related studies of the no reflow phenomenon in skeletal muscle. *Clin Orthop* 314: 122–133.

Anderson RJ, Cambria RA, Dikdan G, Lysz TW, Hobson RW. (1990) Role of eicosanoids and white blood cells in the beneficial effects of limited reperfusion after ischemia-reperfusion injury in skeletal muscle. *Am J Surg* 160: 151–155.

Armstrong RB. (1986) Muscle damage and endurance events. *Sports Med* 3: 370–381.

Armstrong RB. (1990) Initial events in exercise-induced muscular injury. *Med Sci Sports Exerc* 22: 429–435.

Armstrong RB, Ogilvie RW, Schwane JA. (1983) Eccentric exercise-induced injury to rat skeletal muscle. *J Appl Physiol* 54: 80–93.

Armstrong RB, Warren GL, Warren JA. (1991) Mechanisms of exercise-induced muscle fibre injury. *Sports Med* 12: 184–207.

Aronson D, Boppart MD, Dufresne SD, Fielding RA, Goodyear LJ. (1998b) Exercise stimulates c-Jun NH2 kinase activity and c-Jun transcriptional activity in human skeletal muscle. *Biochem Biophys Res Commun* 251: 106–110.

Aronson D, Dufresne SD, Goodyear LJ. (1997a) Contractile activity stimulates the c-Jun NH2-terminal kinase pathway in rat skeletal muscle. *J Biol Chem* 272: 25636–25640.

Aronson D, Violan MA, Dufresne SD, Zangen D, Fielding RA, Goodyear LJ. (1997b) Exercise stimulates the mitogen-activated protein kinase pathway in human skeletal muscle. *J Clin Invest* 99: 1251–1257.

Aronson D, Wojtaszewski JF, Thorell A, Nygren J, Zangen D, Richter EA, Ljungqvist O, Fielding RA, Goodyear LJ. (1998a) Extracellular-regulated protein kinase cascades are activated in response to injury in human skeletal muscle. *Am J Physiol* 275: C555–C561.

Belkin M, LaMorte WL, Wright JG, Hobson RW. (1989) The role of leukocytes in the pathophysiology of skeletal muscle ischemic injury. *J Vasc Surg* 10: 14–18.

Boppart MD, Aronson D, Gibson L, Roubenoff R, Abad LW, Bean J, Goodyear LJ, Fielding RA. (1999) Eccentric exercise markedly increases c-Jun NH(2)-terminal kinase activity in human skeletal muscle. *J Appl Physiol* 87: 1668–1673.

Cannon JG, Orencole SF, Fielding RA, Meydani M, Meydani SN, Fiatarone MA, Blumberg JB, Evans WJ. (1990) Acute phase response in exercise: interaction of age and vitamin E on neutrophils and muscle enzyme release. *Am J Physiol* 259: R1214–R1219.

Cannon JG, St.Pierre BA. (1998) Cytokines in exertion-induced skeletal muscle injury. *Mol Cell Biochem* 179: 159–167.

Cano E, Mahadevan LC. (1995) Parallel signal processing among mammalian MAPKs. *Trends Biochem Sci* 20: 117–122.

Cantini M, Massimino ML, Bruson A, Catani C, Dalla LL, Carraro U. (1994) Macrophages regulate proliferation and differentiation of satellite cells. *Biochem Biophys Res Commun* 202: 1688–1696.

Carden DL, Smith JK, Korthuis RJ. (1990) Neutrophil-mediated microvascular dysfunction in postischemic canine skeletal muscle. Role of granulocyte adherence. *Circ Res* 66: 1436–1444.

Carlson BM, Faulkner JA. (1983) The regeneration of skeletal muscle fibers following injury: a review. *Med Sci Sports Exerc* 15: 187–198.

Carson JA, Wei L. (2000) Integrin signaling's potential for mediating gene expression in hypertrophying skeletal muscle. *J Appl Physiol* 88: 337–343.

Clarke MS, Khakee R, McNeil PL. (1993) Loss of cytoplasmic basic fibroblast growth factor from physiologically wounded myofibers of normal and dystrophic muscle. *J Cell Sci* 106(1): 121–133.

Crinnion JN, Homer-Vanniasinkam S, Hatton R, Parkin SM, Gough MJ. (1994) Role of neutrophil depletion and elastase inhibition in modifying skeletal muscle reperfusion injury. *Cardiovasc Surg* 2: 749–753.

Currie RW, White FP. (1981) Trauma-induced proteins in rat tissues: a physiological role for a "heat shock" protein? *Science* 214: 72–73.

Devol DL, Rotwein P, Sadow JL, Novakofski J, Bechtel PJ. (1990) Activation of insulin-like growth factor gene expression during work-induced skeletal muscle growth. *Am J Physiol* 259: E89–E95.

Dérijard B, Hibi M, I-H Wu, Barrett T, Su B, Deng T, Karin M, Davies RJ. (1994) JNK1: a protein kinase stimulated by UV light and Ha-Ras that binds and phosphorylates the c-JUN activation domain. *Cell* 76: 1025–1037.

Ebbeling CB, Clarkson PM. (1989) Exercise-induced muscle damage and adaptation. *Sports Med* 7: 207–234.

Ebbeling CB, Clarkson PM. (1990) Muscle adaptation prior to recovery following eccentric exercise. *Eur J Appl Physiol* 60: 26–31.

Fielding RA, Manfredi TJ, Ding W, Fiatarone MA, Evans WJ, Cannon JG. (1993) Acute phase response in exercise. III. Neutrophil and IL-1 beta accumulation in skeletal muscle. *Am J Physiol* 265: R166–R172.

Frisch SM, Vuori K, Kelaita D, Sicks S. (1996) A role for Jun-N-terminal kinase in anoikis; suppression by bcl-2 and crmA. *J Cell Biol* 135: 1377–1382.

Garramone RR, Jr., Winters RM, Das DK, Deckers PJ. (1994) Reduction of skeletal muscle injury through stress conditioning using the heat-shock response. *Plast Reconstr Surg* 93: 1242–1247.

Geng JG, Bevilacqua MP, Moore KL, McIntyre TM, Prescott SM, Kim JM, Bliss GA, Zimmerman GA, McEver RP. (1990) Rapid neutrophil adhesion to activated endothelium mediated by GMP-140. *Nature* 343: 757–760.

Gute DC, Ishida T, Yarimizu K, Korthuis RJ. (1998) Inflammatory responses to ischemia and reperfusion in skeletal muscle. *Mol Cell Biochem* 179: 169–187.

Guyton KZ, Liu Y, Gorospe M, Xu Q, Holbrook NJ. (1996) Activation of mitogen-activated protein kinase by H_2O_2. Role in cell survival following oxidant injury. *J Biol Chem* 271: 4138–4142.

Han J, Lee JD, Jiang Y, Li Z, Feng L, Ulevitch RJ. (1996) Characterization of the structure and function of a novel MAP kinase kinase (MKK6). *J Biol Chem* 271: 2886–2891.

Hengerer B, Lindholm D, Heumann R, Ruther U, Wagner EF, Thoenen H. (1990) Lesion-induced increase in nerve growth factor mRNA is mediated by c-fos. *Proc Natl Acad Sci USA* 87: 3899–903.

Iwahori Y, Ishiguro N, Shimizu T, Kondo S, Yabe Y, Oshima T, Iwata H, Sendo F. (1998) Selective neutrophil depletion with monoclonal antibodies attenuates ischemia/reperfusion injury in skeletal muscle. *J Reconstr Microsurg* 14: 109–116.

Jerome SN, Dore M, Paulson JC, Smith CW, Korthuis RJ. (1994a) P-selectin and ICAM-1-dependent adherence reactions: role in the genesis of postischemic no-reflow. *Am J Physiol* 266: H1316–H1321.

Jerome SN, Akimitsu T, Korthuis RJ. (1994b) Leukocyte adhesion, edema, and development of postischemic capillary no-reflow. *Am J Physiol* 267: H1329–H1336.

Jerome SN, Smith CW, Korthuis RJ. (1993) CD18-dependent adherence reactions play an important role in the development of the no-reflow phenomenon. *Am J Physiol* 264: H479–H483.

Knight RJ, Buxton DB. (1996) Stimulation of c-Jun kinase and mitogen-activated protein kinase by ischemia and reperfusion in the perfused rat heart. *Biochem Biophys Res Commun* 218: 83–88.

Korthuis RJ, Granger DN, Townsley MI, Taylor AE. (1985) The role of oxygen-derived free radicals in ischemia-induced increases in canine skeletal muscle vascular permeability. *Circ Res* 57: 599–609.

Kyriakis JM, Avruch J. (1996) Sounding the alarm: protein kinase cascades activated by stress and inflammation. *J Biol Chem* 271: 24313–24316.

Kyriakis JM, Banerjee P, Nikolakaki E, Dai T, Rubie EA, Ahmad MF, Avruch J, Woodgett JW. (1994) The stress-activated protein kinase subfamily of c-Jun kinases. *Nature* 369: 156–160.

Lowe DA, Warren GL, Ingalls CP, Boorstein DB, Armstrong RB. (1995) Muscle function and protein metabolism after initiation of eccentric contraction-induced injury. *J Appl Physiol* 79: 1260–1270.

Lozano DD, Kahl EA, Wong HP, Stephenson LL, Zamboni WA. (1999) L-selectin and leukocyte function in skeletal muscle reperfusion injury. *Arch Surg* 134: 1079–1081.

MacKenna DA, Dolfi F, Vuori K, Ruoslahti E. (1998) Extracellular signal-regulated kinase and c-Jun NH_2-terminal kinase activation by mechanical stretch is integrin-dependent and matrix-specific in rat cardiac fibroblasts. *J Clin Invest* 101: 301–310.

Maier A, Gambke B, Pette D. (1986) Degeneration-regeneration as a mechanism contributing to the fast to slow conversion of chronically stimulated fast-twitch rabbit muscle. *Cell Tissue Res* 244: 635–643.

Matsuda S, Kawasaki H, Moriguchi T, Gotoh Y, Nishida E.

(1995) Activation of protein kinase cascades by osmotic shock. *J Biol Chem* 270: 12781–12786.

Mayadas TN, Johnson RC, Rayburn H, Hynes RO, Wagner DD. (1993) Leukocyte rolling and extravasation are severely compromised in P selectin-deficient mice. *Cell* 74: 541–554.

McCully KK, Faulkner JA. (1985) Injury to skeletal muscle fibers of mice following lengthening contractions. *J Appl Physiol* 59: 119–126.

McCully KK, Faulkner JA. (1986) Characteristics of lengthening contractions associated with injury to skeletal muscle fibers. *J Appl Physiol* 61: 293–299.

McCutchan HJ, Schwappach JR, Enquist EG, Walden DL, Terada LS, Reiss OK, Leff JA, Repine JE. (1990) Xanthine oxidase-derived H_2O_2 contributes to reperfusion injury of ischemic skeletal muscle. *Am J Physiol* 258: H1415–H1419.

Menger MD, Rucker M, Vollmar B. (1997) Capillary dysfunction in striated muscle ischemia/reperfusion: on the mechanisms of capillary "no-reflow". *Shock* 8: 2–7.

Miyamoto S, Teramoto H, Coso OA, Gutkind JS, Burbelo PD, Akiyama SK, Yamada KM. (1995) Integrin function: molecular hierarchies of cytoskeletal and signaling molecules. *J Cell Biol* 131: 791–805.

Morrow NG, Kraus WE, Moore JW, Williams RS, Swain JL. (1990) Increased expression of fibroblast growth factors in a rabbit skeletal muscle model of exercise conditioning. *J Clin Invest* 85: 1816–1820.

Newham DJ, Jones DA, Clarkson PM. (1987) Repeated high-force eccentric exercise: effects on muscle pain and damage. *J Appl Physiol* 63: 1381–1386.

Oberringer M, Baum HP, Jung V, Welter C, Frank J, Kuhlmann M, Mutschler W, Hanselmann RG. (1995) Differential expression of heat shock protein 70 in well healing and chronic human wound tissue. *Biochem Biophys Res Commun* 214: 1009–14.

Oredsson S, Qvarfordt P, Plate G. (1995) Polymorphonuclear leucocytes increase reperfusion injury in skeletal muscle. *Int Angiol* 14: 80–88.

Ostrowski K, Rohde T, Zacho M, Asp S, Pedersen BK. (1998a) Evidence that interleukin-6 is produced in human skeletal muscle during prolonged running. *J Physiol (Lond)* 508(3): 949–953.

Ostrowski K, Hermann C, Bangash A, Schjerling P, Nielsen JN, Pedersen BK. (1998b) A trauma-like elevation of plasma cytokines in humans in response to treadmill running. *J Physiol (Lond)* 513(3): 889–894.

Pawar S, Kartha S, Toback FG. (1995) Differential gene expression in migrating renal epithelial cells after wounding. *J Cell Physiol* 165: 556–565.

Petrasek PF, Lindsay TF, Romaschin AD, Walker PM.

(1996) Plasma activation of neutrophil CD18 after skeletal muscle ischemia: a potential mechanism for late systemic injury. *Am J Physiol* 270: H1515–H1520.

Raingeaud J, Gupta S, Rogers JS, Dickens M, Han J, Ulevitch RJ, Davis RJ. (1995) Pro-inflammatory cytokines and environmental stress cause p38 mitogen-activated protein kinase activation by dual phosphorylation on tyrosine and threonine. *J Biol Chem* 270: 7420–7426.

Rouse J, Cohen P, Trigon S, Morange M, Alonso-Llamazares A, Zamanillo D, Hunt T, Nebreda AR. (1994) A novel kinase cascade triggered by stress and heat shock that stimulates MAPKAP kinase-2 and phosphorylation of the small heat shock proteins. *Cell* 78: 1027–1037.

Rubin BB, Romaschin A, Walker PM, Gute DC, Korthuis RJ. (1996) Mechanisms of postischemic injury in skeletal muscle: intervention strategies. *J Appl Physiol* 80: 369–387.

Sastry SK, Lakonishok M, Thomas DA, Muschler J, Horwitz AF. (1996) Integrin alpha subunit ratios, cytoplasmic domains, and growth factor synergy regulate muscle proliferation and differentiation. *J Cell Biol* 133: 169–184.

Schreiber M, Baumann B, Cotten M, Angel P, Wagner EW. (1995) Fos is essential component of the mammalian UV response. *EMBO J* 14: 5338–5349.

Schwane JA, Armstrong RB. (1983) Effect of training on skeletal muscle injury from downhill running in rats. *J Appl Physiol* 55: 969–975.

Seger R, Krebs EG. (1995) The MAPK signaling cascade. *FASEB J* 9: 726–735.

Silver D, Dhar A, Slocum M, Adams JG, Jr., Shukla S. (1996) Role of platelet-activating factor in skeletal muscle ischemia-reperfusion injury. *Adv Exp Med Biol* 416: 217–221.

Smith A, Hayes G, Romaschin A, Walker P. (1990) The role of extracellular calcium in ischemia/reperfusion injury in skeletal muscle. *J Surg Res* 49: 153–156.

Smith JK, Carden DL, Korthuis RJ. (1989) Role of xanthine oxidase in postischemic microvascular injury in skeletal muscle. *Am J Physiol* 257: H1782–H1789.

Smith JK, Carden DL, Korthuis RJ. (1991) Activated neutrophils increase microvascular permeability in skeletal muscle: role of xanthine oxidase. *J Appl Physiol* 70: 2003–2009.

Stauber WT, Clarkson PM, Fritz VK, Evans WJ. (1990) Extracellular matrix disruption and pain after eccentric muscle action. *J Appl Physiol* 69: 868–874.

Stauber WT, Smith CA. (1998) Cellular responses in exertion-induced skeletal muscle injury. *Mol Cell Biochem* 179: 189–196.

Vandenburgh HH. (1992) Mechanical forces and their second messengers in stimulating cell growth in vitro. *Am J Physiol* 262: R350–R355.

Vandenburgh HH, Hatfaludy S, Karlisch P, Shansky J. (1991) Mechanically induced alterations in cultured skeletal muscle growth. *J Biomech* 24(Suppl 1): 91–99.

Vandenburgh, HH, Kaufman S. (1979) In vitro model of stretchinduced hypertrophy of skeletal muscle. *Science* 203: 265–268.

Weyrich AS, Ma XY, Lefer DJ, Albertine KH, Lefer AM. (1993) In vivo neutralization of P-selectin protects feline heart and endothelium in myocardial ischemia and reperfusion injury [see comments]. *J Clin Invest* 91: 2620–2629.

Widegren U, Jiang XJ, Krook A, Chibalin AV, Bjornholm M, Tally M, Roth RA, Henriksson J, Wallberg-Henriksson H, Zierath JR. (1998) Divergent effects of exercise on metabolic and mitogenic signaling pathways in human skeletal muscle. *FASEB J* 12: 1379–1389.

Zamboni WA, Stephenson LL, Roth AC, Suchy H, Russell RC. (1997) Ischemia-reperfusion injury in skeletal muscle: CD 18-dependent neutrophil-endothelial adhesion and arteriolar vasoconstriction. *Plast Reconstr Surg* 99: 2002–2007.

3

Inflammatory myopathies

Anthony A. Amato

Introduction

Dermatomyositis (DM), polymyositis (PM), and inclusion body myositis (IBM) are the three major categories of idiopathic inflammatory myopathy. The incidence of these inflammatory myopathies is approximately one in 100 000 (Medsger et al 1970, Dalakas 1991). Importantly, DM, PM, and IBM are clinically, histologically, and pathogenically distinct (Amato and Barohn 1997; Table 3.1). IBM, myositis related to infection (including myopathy related to human immunodeficiency virus) and connective tissue disorders, and the treatment of inflammatory myopathy are discussed in separate chapters. This chapter will focus only on DM, PM, and related disorders.

Dermatomyositis

Clinical features

Unlike PM and IBM, DM can present at any age, including childhood. Childhood DM usually presents between the ages of 5 and 14 years (Medsger et al 1970), but it can even develop during infancy (Bruguier et al 1984). Although the pathogenesis of childhood and adult DM are presumably similar, there are important differences in some of the clinical features and associated manifestations. There is a female predominance in both childhood and adult-onset DM. Weakness usually develops over several weeks, however, the onset can be more abrupt or insidious (Bohan and Peters 1975a, Tymms and Webb 1985, Hochberg et al 1986, Amato et al 1996). The earliest and most severely affected muscle groups are the neck flexors, shoulder and pelvic girdle muscles. Distal extremity muscles are also affected, although involvement is never as severe as evident in proximal muscles (Amato et al 1996). Children are more likely to present with fatigue, low grade fevers, and a rash. Muscle weakness and myalgias tend to have a more insidious onset (Pachman 1995). Approximately 30% of DM patients complain of dysphagia caused by inflammation of oropharyngeal and oesophageal muscles (Tymms and Webb 1985, Hochberg et al 1986, Pachman 1995). Rarely, difficulties with chewing can arise secondary to masseter muscle involvement. Inflammation of the pharyngeal and the tongue muscles can result in dysarthria or speech delay in children (Pachman 1995). Sensation is normal and muscle stretch reflexes are preserved until a severe degree of weakness has developed.

Table 3.1 — Idiopathic inflammatory myopathies: clinical and laboratory features

Disorder	Sex	Age of onset	Rash	Pattern of weakness	Serum CK	Muscle biopsy	Cellular infiltrate	Response to IS therapy	Common associated conditions
DM	F > M	Childhood and adult	Yes	Proximal > Distal	Increased (up to 50x normal)	Perimysial and perivascular inflammation; MAC, Ig, C deposition on vessels	CD4+ T cells; B cells	Yes	Myocarditis, interstitial lung disease, malignancy, vasculitis, other connective tissue diseases
PM	F > M	Adult	No	Proximal > Distal	Increased (up to 50x normal)	Endomysial inflammation	CD8+ T cells; macrophages	Yes	Myocarditis, interstitial lung disease, other connective tissue diseases
IBM	M > F	Elderly (>50 yrs)	No	Proximal = Distal; Predilection for: finger/ wrist flexors, knee extensors	Normal or mildly increased (< 10x normal)	Endomysial inflammation; rimmed vacuoles; amyloid deposits; EM: 15–18 nm tubulofilaments	CD8+ T cells; macrophages	None or minimal	Neuropathy autoimmune disorders (uncommon)

DM, dermatomyositis
F, female
IS, immunosuppressive
C, complement
PM, polymyositis
M, male
Ig, immunoglobulin
CK, creatine kinase
IBM, inclusion body myositis
EM, electron microscopy
MAC, membrane attack complex

From Amato AA, Barohn RJ. (1997) Idiopathic inflammatory myopathies. *Neurol Clin* 15: 615–648, with permission)

The characteristic rash of DM can accompany or precede the onset of muscle (Dalakas 1991, Engel et al 1994, Griggs et al 1995, Amato and Barohn 1997). The classic skin manifestations include a heliotrope rash (purplish discolouration of the eyelids often associated with periorbital oedema) and Gottren's sign (papular, erythematous, scaly lesions over the knuckles). In addition, a flat, erythematous, sun-sensitive rash may appear on the face, neck and anterior chest (V-sign), on the shoulders and upper back (shawl sign), and on the elbows, knees and malleoli. The nail-beds often have dilated capillary loops occasionally with thrombi or haemorrhage. Rarely, patients have the characteristic rash but never develop weakness, so-called *amyopathic dermatomyositis* (Euwer and Sontheimer 1993).

Subcutaneous calcifications develop in 30–70% of children, however, this is an uncommon complication in adults (Henriksson and Sandstedt 1982, Cohen et al 1986, Engel et al 1994, Griggs et al 1995, Pachman 1995). These lesions present as painful, hard nodules typically over pressure points (buttocks, knees, elbows). In severe cases, ulceration of the overlying skin with extrusion of calcific debri occurs. Subcutaneous calcifications can be prevented with early, aggressive treatment of the inflammatory myopathy. Once calcinosis has developed, eradication of these lesions becomes very difficult. Colchicine, probenecid, warfarin, and phosphate buffers have been tried but with only limited success (Engel et al 1994, Oddis 1994, Griggs et al 1995). Surgical removal of the calcifications can be attempted, but the lesions may reoccur or worsen.

Associated manifestations

Electrocardiographic abnormalities including conduction defects and arrhythmias occur frequently in childhood and adult DM, although patients are typically asymptomatic from a cardiac standpoint (Denbow et al 1919, Gottdiener et al 1978, Haupt and Hutchins 1982, Strongwater et al 1983, Askari 1984, Tymms and Webb 1985, Hochberg et al 1986). However, congestive heart failure, pericarditis, myocarditis can develop (Gottdiener et al 1978, Hochberg et al 1986). Echocardiography and radionucleotide scintigraphy may demonstrate ventricular and septal wall motion abnormalities and reduced ejection fractions (Gottdiener et al 1978).

Aspiration pneumonia can occur in patients with significant oropharyngeal and oesophageal weakness (Dickey and Myers 1984). Importantly, interstitial lung disease (ILD) develops in approximately 10% of DM patients (Frazier and Miller 1974, Park and Nyhan 1975, Schwartz et al 1976, Hochberg et al 1986, Pachman 1995). Dyspnoea and non-productive cough can begin abruptly or insidiously, and they often precede the development of the characteristic rash and muscle weakness. Chest radiographs reveal a diffuse reticulonodular pattern with a predilection for involvement at the lung bases. In more fulminant, abrupt-onset cases, a diffuse alveolar pattern or "ground-glass" appearance may be apparent (Dickey and Myers 1984, Griggs et al 1995). Pulmonary function tests demonstrate restrictive defects and a decreased diffusion capacity. In at least half the patients with ILD and inflammatory myopathies, antibodies directed against t-histidyl transfer RNA synthetase, so-called Jo-1 antibodies, can be found on serologic testing (Hochberg et al 1984, Targoff 1984, Love et al 1991).

Inflammation of the skeletal and smooth muscles of the gastrointestinal tract can lead to dysphagia and delayed gastric emptying. Vasculitis of the gastrointestinal tract with mucosal ulceration, perforation, and life-threatening haemorrhage is much more common in childhood DM compared with adult DM (Engel et al 1994, Griggs et al 1995, Pachman 1995). Necrotizing vasculitis may affect other tissues including the eyes (retina and conjunctiva), kidneys, and lungs. Rarely, massive muscle necrosis can develop secondary to ischaemia leading to myoglobinuria and acute renal tubular necrosis.

Arthralgias with or without arthritis are common. Arthritis involves both the large and small joints and it is typically symmetric. Pain often eases when the limbs are flexed, which leads to the development of flexion contractures across the major joints. A common early finding in childhood DM is toe-walking as a result of flexion contractures at the ankles (Engel et al 1994).

There is an increased incidence of malignancies in adult DM, ranging from 6–45% (Bohan and Peters 1975a; Bohan et al 1977, Tymms and Webb 1985, Hochberg et al 1986, Sigurgeirsson et al 1992, Callen 1994). However, a similar increased risk of cancer is not evident in childhood DM. The risk of malignancy is greater in patients over the age of 40 years and occurs in males and females with equal frequency. The majority of malignancies are identified within two years (before or after) of the clinical presentation of DM. There may be an increased risk of malignancy in patients with cutaneous vasculitis (Feldman et al 1983, Basset-Seguin et al 1990). However, the severity of the inflammatory myopathy does not appear to correlate with the presence or absence of a neoplasm. Treatment of the underlying malignancy may improve muscle strength in some patients.

A comprehensive history and annual physical

examinations, with breast and pelvic exams for women and testicular and prostate exams for men, should be performed to search for an underlying malignancy. A complete blood count (CBC), routine blood chemistries, urinalysis, and stool specimens for occult blood are obtained. Chest X-rays, mammograms and pelvic ultrasounds (to look for ovarian cancer) are the only radiographic studies that I routinely order. Other work-up (e.g., upper and lower gastrointestinal tract X-rays, CT scans) should be sign and symptom directed.

Laboratory features

Necrosis of muscle fibres results in elevations of serum creatine kinase (CK), aldolase, myoglobin, lactate dehydrogenase, aspartate aminotransferase (AST), and alanine aminotransferase (ALT). Serum CK is the most sensitive and specific marker for muscle destruction and is elevated (up to 50 times normal) in more than 90% of DM patients (Bohan and Peters 1975b, Tymms and Webb 1985, Hochberg et al 1986, Amato et al 1996). However, serum CK levels do not correlate with the severity of weakness and they can be normal even in markedly weak individuals, particularly in childhood DM. Erythrocyte sedimentation rate (ESR) is usually normal or only mildly elevated and this is not a reliable indicator of disease severity.

Antinuclear antibodies (ANA) can be detected in 24–60% of DM patients (Hochberg et al 1986, Love et al 1991, Targoff 1984). The presence of these antibodies should lead to consideration of an overlap syndrome. Some have suggested that "myositis-specific antibodies" (MSAs) are useful in predicting response to therapy and prognosis (Targoff 1984, Love et al 1991, Joffe et al 1993, Miller 1993, Plotz et al 1995). However, MSAs are demonstrated in only a minority of patients with inflammatory myopathy and they have not been studied prospectively in regards to their predictive value. Further, the pathogenic relationship of these antibodies to inflammatory myopathies is unknown; they may just represent an epiphenomena. The most common MSAs are Jo-1 antibodies which are associated with ILD (Hochberg et al 1984, Targoff 1984, Love et al 1991). Jo-1 antibodies are more common in PM than adult DM and there are only a few reports of these antibodies in childhood DM (Pachman 1995). Some have suggested that Jo-1 antibodies are associated with only a moderate response to treatment and a poor long-term prognosis (Joffe et al 1993, Plotz et al 1995), although a prospective study of treatment outcomes of myositis-ILD patients with anti-Jo-1 antibodies compared with similar patients without these antibodies has not been performed. Antibodies directed against Mi-2, a 240 kD nuclear protein of unknown function, are seen almost exclusively in DM and they can be found in 15–20% of patients (Targoff 1984, Love et al 1991, Joffe et al 1993, Plotz et al 1995). Most patients with anti-Mi-2 antibodies have an acute onset, a florid rash, a good response to therapy, and a favourable prognosis.

The characteristic features on electromyography (EMG) include:

1. increased insertional and spontaneous activity with fibrillation potentials, positive sharp waves, and occasionally complex repetitive discharges

2. short duration, small amplitude, polyphasic motor unit potentials (MUPs)

3. early recruitment of MUPs (Bromberg and Albers 1986).

Decreased recruitment (a diminished number of MUPS that are fast firing) can be seen in advanced disease secondary to the loss of muscle fibres of entire motor units. The amount of insertional and spontaneous EMG activity is reflective of ongoing disease activity, however, such activity may be decreased in later stages of the disease as destroyed muscle tissue is replaced by fat and connective tissue. In addition, long duration, high amplitude polyphasic MUPs may also be seen later in the course reflecting chronicity of the disease due to muscle fibre splitting and regeneration. EMG can be helpful in determining which muscle to biopsy in patients with only mild weakness. In addition, EMG may be useful in previously responsive myositis patients who become weaker by differentiating relapse from weakness secondary to Type II muscle fibre atrophy from disuse or chronic steroid administration. Isolated type 2 muscle fibre atrophy is not associated with EMG findings.

Magnetic resonance imaging (MRI) can provide information on the pattern of muscle (Kaufman et al 1987, Fraser et al 1991, Hernandez et al 1993, Pitt et al 1993). Signal abnormalities secondary to inflammation and oedema or replacement by fibrotic tissue are evident in affected muscles. Some have advocated MRI as a guide to which muscle to biopsy (Pitt et al 1993). However, I have found that MRI adds little to a good clinical examination and EMG in defining the pattern of muscle involvement and determining which muscle to biopsy.

Histopathology

The frequency and severity of histological abnormalities can vary within the muscle biopsy specimens

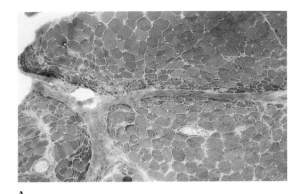

A

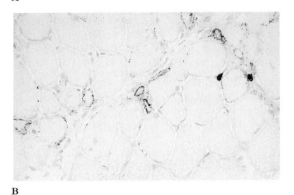

B

Figure 3.1 — Dermatomyositis. **A** Muscle biopsy demonstrates the characteristic perifascicular atrophy. Note the lack of inflammation. Modified Gomori Trichrome. **B** The earliest histological abnormality in dermatomyositis is the deposition of C5b-9 (membrane attack complex) on small blood vessels. This is not seen in polymyositis or inclusion body myositis. Membrane attack complex (MAC) can also deposit on necrotic muscle fibres. Immunoperoxidase with antibodies directed against MAC.

because the pathological process is multifocal. The characteristic histological feature in DM is perifascicular atrophy, which is evident on muscle biopsies in up to 90% of children but in less than 50% of adults (Fig. 3.1A; Dalakas 1991, Engel et al 1994, Griggs et al 1995). Within the perifascicular region, small degenerating fibres as well as atrophic and non-atrophic fibres with microvacuolation and disrupted oxidative enzyme staining are apparent. In addition, microinfarcts of muscle fascicles and scattered necrotic fibres may be seen. However, an important histological feature distinguishing DM from PM and IBM is the lack of invasion of non-necrotic fibres. Inflammatory cells are not always evident and, when present, the infiltrate is predominantly perivascular and located in the perimysium rather than the endomysium. This inflammatory infiltrate is composed primarily of macrophages, B cells, and CD4[+] (T-helper) cells (Arahata and Engel 1984, Engel and Arahata 1984).

Preceding inflammation and other structural abnormalities is the deposition of C5b-9 complement membrane attack complex (MAC) on small blood vessels (Fig. 3.1B), a feature specific for DM (Kissel et al 1986, Emslie-Smith and Engel 1990, Kissel et al 1991). In addition, other complement components (C3 and C9), IgM, and less often IgG are also deposited within the walls of intramuscular blood vessels (Whitaker and Engel 1972). As a result, these vessels necrose, and there is an overall reduction in the capillary density (Emslie-Smith and Engel 1990). Hyperplasia, microvacuolation, and cytoplasmic inclusions within the endothelium of small arterioles and capillaries are apparent on electron microscopy (EM) (Banker 1975, DeVisser et al 1989).

Pathogenesis

DM is a humorally-mediated microangiopathy resulting in ischaemia of muscle tissue. The trigger of this autoimmune attack is unknown.

Prognosis

The majority of patients with DM improve with immunosuppressive therapy. Five year mortality rates of adult DM have ranged from 7 to 30% (Hochberg et al 1983, 1986, Zhanuzakov et al 1986, Zitnan et al 1991). The survival rate in children is very high with early, aggressive treatment. Poor prognostic features are the presence of malignancy, increased age, ILD, cardiac disease, and late or previous inadequate treatment (Tymms and Webb 1985, Hochberg et al 1986, Murayabashi et al 1991, Joffe et al 1993, Chwalinska-Sadowska and Madykowa 1994).

Polymyositis

Clinical features

In contrast to DM which frequently occurs in childhood, PM generally presents in patients over the age of 20 years (Medsger et al 1970, Bohan and Peters 1975a, Hochberg et al 1986, Tymms and Webb 1985, Amato et al 1996). Although there are rare cases of myositis beginning in infancy (Kinoshita et al 1980, 1986, Thompson 1982, Roddy et al 1986, Shevell et al 1990, Nagai et al 1992), most of these cases are probably congenital muscular dystrophies (CMDs) with secondary inflammation (Morse et al 1995,

Pegoraro et al 1996). There have been several reports of patients with the classical type of CMD with prominent inflammation in which merosin (α_2 laminin) deficiency was demonstrated on muscle biopsies (Morse et al 1995, Pegoraro et al 1996, Mendell et al 1997). Mutations within the merosin gene have demonstrated in some of these cases. The majority of infants with inflammation on their biopsy probably have a form of CMD rather than a primary myositis.

Similar to DM, there is a female predominance in PM. The diagnosis of PM is often delayed compared with DM (Amato et al 1996). Patients present with neck flexor and symmetric proximal arm and leg weakness developing over several weeks or months (Bohan and Peters 1975a, Amato et al 1996). Distal muscles also are affected, but they are not as weak as the more proximal muscles. Myalgias and tenderness are common. Approximately one third of patients develop dysphagia as a result of oropharyngeal and oesophageal involvement (Tymms 1985, Hochberg et al 1986, Dalakas 1991, Engel et al 1994, Griggs et al 1995). In some patients, mild facial weakness can be demonstrated on examination. Sensory examination and muscle stretch reflexes are usually normal.

Associated manifestations

The cardiac and pulmonary complications of PM are similar to those described with DM. Inflammation of cardiac muscle results in congestive heart failure or conduction abnormalities in up to one third of patients (Gottdiener et al 1978, Denbow et al 1979, Henderson et al 1980, Kehoe et al 1981, Strongwater et al 1983, Askari 1984, Tymms and Webb 1985, Hochberg et al 1986). ILD complicates more than 10% of PM cases, half of which are associated with Jo-1 antibodies (Frazier and Miller 1974, Schwartz et al 1976, Dickey and Myers 1984, Tymms and Webb 1985, Hochberg et al 1986, Love et al 1991, Targoff 1984). ILD can present prior to the onset of muscle weakness. Polyarthritis occurs in up to 45% of PM patients (Tymms and Webb 1985). The risk of malignancy with PM is lower than that seen in DM, nevertheless, it may be slightly higher than expected in the general population (Bohan et al 1977, Tymms and Webb 1985, Sigurgeirsson et al 1992, Callen 1994).

An interesting variant of PM is granulomatous or giant cell PM (Namba et al 1974, Pazcuzzi et al 1986). Most of the reported patients also had myasthenia gravis and/or thymoma. The thymoma can be benign or malignant. The myositis can develop before or after the clinical presentation of myasthenia gravis or the diagnosis of the thymoma. Besides proximal weakness, patients with concurrent myasthenia gravis also had diplopia, ptosis, and bulbar dysfunction. Importantly, a granulomatous myocarditis can also occur in this disorder.

Laboratory features

Serum CK level is elevated 5 to 50-fold in the majority of PM cases (Bohan and Peters 1975b, Tymms and Webb 1985, Hochberg et al 1986, Amato et al 1996). However, serum CK levels can be normal in patients who are weak, and they can be elevated in those who have normal manual muscle strength and functional testing. Serum CK can be useful in monitoring response to therapy but only in conjunction with the physical exam. Similar to DM, ESR is normal in the majority of patients and does not correlate with disease activity or severity (Bohan and Peters 1975b).

PM patients have positive ANAs in 16–40% of cases (Bohan and Peters 1975b, Tymms and Webb 1985, Hochberg et al 1986, Love et al 1991). The MSAs are more common in PM than DM, specifically Jo-1 and SRP antibodies (Hochberg et al 1983, Love et al 1991, Miller 1993, Targoff 1984, Plotz et al 1995). Jo-1 antibodies are detected in as many as 20% of PM patients. Approximately 4% of PM patients have antibodies directed against signal recognition protein (SRP). Anti-SRP antibodies have been associated an acute onset of severe weakness, myalgias, myocarditis, resistant to immunosuppressive therapy, and a very poor prognosis with a 5 year survival of 25% (Targoff 1984, Love et al 1991, Miller 1993, Joffe et al 1993).

Muscle imaging studies can reveal signal changes suggestive of areas of inflammation in affected muscles (Kaufman et al 1987, Fraser et al 1991, Pitt et al 1993). EMG usually demonstrates increased insertional and spontaneous activity, small polyphasic MUPs, and early recruitment in severely affected muscles (Bromberg and Albers 1986). However, these electrophysiological findings are non-specific and they do not distinguish PM from other myopathies. The paraspinals being the most proximal muscle group are the earliest involved on EMG and should always be studied in patients suspected of having PM.

Histopathology

Muscle biopsies reveal fibre size variability, scattered necrotic and regenerating fibres, and endomysial inflammatory cells which invade non-necrotic muscle fibres (Fig. 3.2). The invaded and some of the non-invaded muscle fibres express major histocompatibility

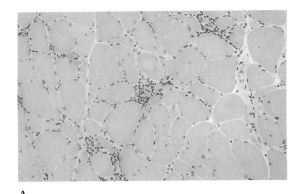

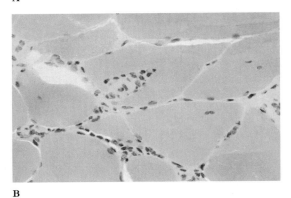

Figure 3.2— Polymyositis. **A** Muscle biopsy reveals variability in fibre size with endomyseal inflammation. **B** The endomyseal mononuclear inflammatory cells invade non-necrotic fibres. H&E.

complex class I antigen on the sarcolemma of muscle fibres—a finding not present in normal muscle (Emslie-Smith et al 1989). The inflammatory infiltrate is composed primarily of activated CD8$^+$ (cytotoxic), $\alpha\beta$ T cells and macrophages (Arahata and Engel 1984, Engel et al 1984, 1994), although there is a report of PM with CD4$^-$ CD8$^-$ $\gamma\delta$ T cells (Hohlfeld et al 1991). An oligoclonal pattern of gene rearrangement and a restricted motif in the CD3R region of the T cell receptor (TCR) is apparent in the endomysial T cells (Mantegazza et al 1993). In contrast to DM, there is no evidence of a humorally-mediated vasculopathy. In patients with granulomatous or giant cell PM, muscle biopsies reveal granulomas and multinucleated giant cells in skeletal and often cardiac muscle.

Pathogenesis

The above evidence suggests that PM is a result of a HLA-restricted, antigen-specific, cell-mediated immune response directed against muscle fibres. However, the antigen against which this autoimmune attack is generated and the trigger of this response is not known. Some posit a viral infection, but viral antigens and genomes have not been demonstrated in muscle fibres (Dalakas 1991, Leff et al 1992, Ytterberg 1994). Perhaps, a virus could indirectly trigger an autoimmune response by secondary cross-reactivity with specific muscle antigens, altering the expression of self-antigens on muscle fibres, or by the loss of physiological self-tolerance (Engel et al 1994). In this regard, PM can develop as a complication of human immunodeficiency virus (HIV) and human T-lymphocyte virus-1 (HTLV-1) infection. The myositis associated with HIV and HTLV-1 infections appears to be the result of indirect triggering of the immune response against muscle fibres.

Prognosis

Most patients with PM improve with immunosuppressive agents, however, life-long treatment is usually required (Chwalinska-Sadowska and Madykowa 1994, Tymms and Webb 1985, Hochberg et al 1983, 1984, Murayabashi et al 1991, Joffe et al 1993, Dalakas 1994, Amato et al 1996). The response in PM does not appear to be as favourable as that seen in DM (Joffe et al 1993, Amato et al 1996). Poor prognostic features include older age, ILD, cardiac disease, the presence of Jo-1 or SRP antibodies, granulomatous or giant cell myositis, and a delay in treatment or previous inadequate treatment.

Overlap syndromes

The overlap syndromes are a group of disorders in which inflammation occurs in association with another well-defined connective tissue disorder (CTD) such as scleroderma, mixed connective tissue disease, Sjögrens syndrome, systemic lupus erythematosus, and rheumatoid arthritis (Amato and Barohn 1997). Clinical and histological features of either DM and PM can develop. Some suggest the myosites associated with overlap syndromes are more responsive to immunosuppressive treatment than DM and PM (Hochberg et al 1986, Joffe et al 1993).

Eosinophilic polymyositis

Clinical features

Eosinophilic PM usually occurs as a part of the hypereosinophilic syndrome (HES) (Layzer et al 1977,

Moore et al 1985, Banker 1994). The diagnostic criteria of an HES are:

1. persistent eosinophilia of 1500 eosinophils/mm³ for at least 6 months

2. no evidence of parasitic or other recognized causes of eosinophilia

3. signs and symptoms of organ system involvement related to infiltration if eosinophils.

Eosinophilic PM is characterized by an insidious onset of muscle pain and proximal weakness. The myopathy is often accompanied by other systemic manifestations of HES including encephalopathy, peripheral neuropathy, myocarditis/pericarditis, pulmonary fibrosis, pleuritis, asthma, renal and gastrointestinal involvement, and skin changes.

Laboratory features

Hypereosinophilia, hypergammaglobulinaemia, anaemia, elevated serum CK, and rheumatoid factor are evident (Layzer et al 1977, Moore et al 1985, Banker 1994). ESR is elevated in less than 50% and ANAs are usually not present. EKG may demonstrate cardiac arrhythmias or conduction block. Chest X-ray can reveal pulmonary infiltrates. Increased insertional and spontaneous activity (e.g., fibrillation potentials, PSWs) and early recruitment of small polyphasic MUPs are seen on EMG.

Histopathology

Muscle biopsies reveal perivascular and endomysial inflammation composed predominantly of eosinophils (Layzer et al 1977, Moore et al 1985, Banker 1994). Nodular granulomas, necrotic, invaded, and regenerating muscles fibres may also be seen.

Pathogenesis

The aetiology of eosinophilic PM and HES is unknown. Tissue destruction may be related to infiltration by eosinophils and the release of toxins contained within the eosinophilic granules.

Prognosis

Early reports suggested a poor prognosis for long-term survival with fewer than 20% of patients surviving 3 years. However, these series may have been biased by the inclusion of autopsied cases. Response to corticosteroids has been inconsistent, but they have been effective in some patients in reducing the eosinophilia

and end-organ damage. Second-line cytotoxic agents should be tried if patients fail to improve with steroids.

Focal myositis

Clinical features

Focal myositis is a rare disorder which can develop in infancy to late adult life (Heffner et al 1977, 1981, Moskowitz et al 1991, Colding-Jorgenson et al 1993, Caldwell et al 1995, Moreno-Lugris et al 1996). It presents as a solitary, painful, and rapidly expanding skeletal muscle mass that often mimics a malignant soft tissue tumour. The leg is the most common site of involvement, but the upper extremities, abdomen, head and neck can also be affected. The disorder needs to be distinguished from sarcoidosis, Bechet's syndrome, and vasculitis, which can begin focally in skeletal muscle, as well as soft tissue tumours (e.g., sarcoma).

Laboratory features

Serum CK and ESR are usually normal. MRI and CT imaging demonstrates oedema within the affected muscle groups (Moskowitz et al 1991, Caldwell et al 1995, Moreno-Lugris et al 1996).

Histopathology

Mononuclear inflammatory cells composed of CD4⁺ and CD8⁺ T lymphocytes and macrophages are present in the endomysium (Caldwell et al 1995). Non-specific myopathic features include fibre size variability, necrosis, split fibres, increased central nuclei, and endomysial fibrosis. MHC class I antigens may not be expressed on muscle fibres, in contrast to typical PM.

Pathogenesis

The aetiology is unknown. Immunological studies suggest that the disorder is distinct from PM and not the result of a cell-mediated attack directed against a muscle specific antigen (Caldwell et al 1995).

Prognosis

Focal myositis usually resolves spontaneously or with treatment. There are rare cases of focal myositis generalizing to more typical polymyositis (Heffner and Barron 1981).

References

Amato AA, Barohn RJ. (1997) Idiopathic inflammatory myopathies. *Neurol Clinics* 15: 615–648.

Amato AA, Gronseth GS, Jackson CE, et al. (1996) Inclusion body myositis: Clinical and pathological boundaries. *Ann Neurol* 40: 581–586.

Arahata K, Engel AG. (1984) Monoclonal antibody analysis of mononuclear cells in myopathies. I. Quantitative of subsets according to diagnosis and sites of accumulation and demonstration and counts of muscle fibers invaded by T cells. *Ann Neurol* 16: 193–208.

Askari AD. (1984) Inflammatory disorders of muscle: Cardiac abnormalities. *Clin Rheum Dis* 12: 131–149.

Banker BQ. (1975) Dermatomyositis of childhood. Ultrastructural alterations of muscle and intramuscular blood vessels. *J Neuropathol Exp Neurol* 34: 46–75.

Banker BQ. (1994) Other inflammatory myopathies. In: Engel AG, Franzini-Armstrong C (eds). *Myology* (2nd ed). New York: McGraw Hill, pp. 1461–1886.

Basset-Seguin N, Roujeau J-C, Gherardi R, et al. (1990) Prognostic factors and predictive signs of malignancy in adult dermatomyositis: A study of 32 cases. *Arch Dermatol* 126: 633–637.

Bohan A, Peters JB. (1975a) Polymyositis and dermatomyositis. Part 1: *N Engl J Med* 292: 344–347.

Bohan A, Peters JB. (1975b) Polymyositis and dermatomyositis. Part 2: *N Engl J Med* 292: 403–407

Bohan A, Peter JB, Bowman RL, et al. (1977) A computer-assisted analysis of 153 patients with polymyositis and dermatomyositis. *Medicine* 56: 255–286.

Bromberg MB, Albers JW. (1986) Electromyography in idiopathic myositis. *Mt Sinai J Med* 55: 459–464.

Bruguier A, Texier P, Clement MC, Dulac O, Ponsot G, Arthuis M. (1984) Dermatomyosites infantiles: A propos de vingt-huit observations. *Arch Fr Pediatr* 41: 9–14.

Caldwell CJ, Swash M, Van der Walt JD, Geddes JF. (1995) Focal myositis: a clinicopathological study. *Neuromusc Disord* 5: 317–321.

Callen JP. (1994) Relationship of cancer to inflammatory muscle diseases: Dermatomyositis, polymyositis, and inclusion body myositis. *Rheum Dis Clin N Am* 20: 943–953.

Chwalinska-Sadowska H, Madykowa H. (1994) Polymyositis-dermatomyositis: 25 year follow-up of 50 patients-disease course, treatment, prognostic factors. *Mater Med Pol* 22: 213.

Cohen MG, Nash P, Webb J. (1986) Calcification is rare in adult-onset dermatomyositis. *Clin Rheumatol* 5: 512–516.

Colding-Jorgenson E, Laursen H, Lauritzen M. (1993) Focal myositis of the thigh. *Acta Neurol Scand* 88: 289–292.

Dalakas MC. (1991) Polymyositis, dermatomyositis, and inclusion body myositis. *N Engl J Med* 325: 1487–1498.

Dalakas MC. (1994) How to diagnose and treat the inflammatory myopathies. *Semin Neurol* 14: 137–145.

DeVisser M, Emslie-Smith AM, Engel AG. (1989) Early ultrastructural alterations in dermatomyositis: Capillary abnormalities precede other structural changes in muscle. *J Neurol Sci* 94: 181–192.

Denbow CE, Lie JT, Tancredi RG, et al. (1979) Cardiac involvement in polymyositis. *Arthritis Rheum* 22: 1088–1092.

Dickey BF, Myers AR. (1984) Pulmonary disease in polymyositis/dermatomyositis. *Semin Arthritis Rheum* 14: 60–76.

Emslie-Smith AM, Arahata K, Engel AG. (1989) Major histocompatibility complex 1 antigen expression, immunolocalization of interferon subtypes, and T cell-mediated cytotoxicity in myopathies. *Hum Pathol* 20: 224–231.

Emslie-Smith AM, Engel AG. (1990) Microvascular changes in early and advanced dermatomyositis: A quantitative study. *Ann Neurol* 27: 343–356.

Engel AG, Arahata K. (1984) Monoclonal antibody analysis of mononuclear cells in myopathies. II: Phenotypes of autoinvasive cells in polymyositis and inclusion body myositis. *Ann Neurol* 16: 209–215.

Engel AG, Hohlfeld B, Banker BQ. (1994) The polymyositis and dermatomyositis syndromes. In: Engel AG, Franzini-Armstrong C (eds). *Myology* (2nd ed). New York: McGraw Hill, pp. 1335–1383.

Euwer RL, Sontheimer RD. (1993) Amyopathic dermatomyositis: A review. *J Invest Dermatol* 100: 124S–127S.

Feldman D, Hochberg MC, Zizic TM, Stevens MB. (1983) Cutaneous vasculitis in adult polymyositis/dermatomyositis. *J Rheumatol* 10: 85–89.

Fraser DD, Frank JA, Dalakas M, Miller FW, Hicks JE, Plotz PH. (1991) Magnetic resonance imaging in idiopathic inflammatory myopathies. *J Rheumatol* 18: 1693–1700.

Frazier RA, Miller RD. (1974) Interstitial pneumonitis in association with polymyositis and dermatomyositis. *Chest* 65: 403–407.

Gottdiener JS, Sherber HS, Hawley RJ, Engel WK. (1978) Cardiac manifestations in polymyositis. *Am J Cardiol* 41: 1141–1149.

Griggs RC, Mendell JR, Miller RG. (1995) Inflammatory myopathies. In: *Evaluation and Treatment of Myopathies*. Philadelphia: FA Davis Co, pp. 154–210.

Haupt HM, Hutchins GM. (1982) The heart and conduction system in polymyositis-dermatomyositis. *Am J Cardiol* 50: 998–1006.

Heffner RR, Armbrustmacher VW, Earle KM. (1977) Focal myositis. *Cancer* 40: 301–306.

Heffner RR, Barron SA. (1981) Polymyositis beginning as a focal process. *Arch Neurol* 38: 439–442.

Henderson A, Cumming WJK, Williams DO, et al. (1980) Cardiac complications of polymyositis. *J Neurol Sci* 47: 425–428.

Henriksson KG, Sandstedt P. (1982) Polymyositis – treatment and prognosis. A study of 107 patients. *Acta Neurol Scand* 65: 280–300.

Hernandez RJ, Sullivan DB, Chenevert TL, Keim DR. (1993) MR imaging in children with dermatomyositis: Findings and correlations with clinical and laboratory findings. *Am J Roentgenol* 161: 359–366.

Hochberg MC, Lopez-Acuna D, Gittleshon AM. (1983) Mortality from polymyositis and dermatomyositis in the United States, 1968–1978. *Arthritis Rheum* 26: 1465–1471.

Hochberg MC, Feldman D, Stevens MB, Arnett FC, Reichlen M. (1984) Antibody to Jo-1 in polymyositis/dermatomyositis: Association with interstitial pulmonary disease. *J Rheumatol* 11: 663–665.

Hochberg MC, Feldman D, Stevens MB. (1986) Adult-onset polymyositis/dermatomyositis: Analysis of clinical and laboratory features and survival in 76 cases with a review of the literature. *Semin Arthritis Rheum* 15: 168–178.

Hohlfeld R, Engel AG, Ii K, Harper MC. (1991) Polymyositis mediated by T lymphocytes that express the gamma-delta receptor. *N Engl J Med* 324: 877–881.

Joffe MM, Love LA, Leff RL. (1993) Drug therapy of idiopathic inflammatory myopathies: Predictors of response to prednisone, azathioprine, and methotrexate and a comparison of their efficacy. *Am J Med* 94: 379–387.

Kaufman LD, Gruber BL, Gerstman DP, Kael AT. (1987) Preliminary observations on the role of magnetic resonance imaging for polymyositis and dermatomyositis. *Ann Rheum Dis* 46: 569–572.

Kehoe RF, Bauernfeind R, Tommaso C, Wyndham C, Rosen K. (1981) Cardiac conduction defects in polymyositis: Electrophysiologic studies in four patients. *Ann Intern Med* 94: 41–43.

Kinoshita M, Iwasaki Y, Wada F. (1980) A case of congenital polymyositis: a possible pathogenesis of "Fukuyama type congenital muscular dystrophy". *Clin Neurol* 20: 911–916.

Kinoshita M, Nishina M, Koya N. (1986) Ten years follow-up study of steroid therapy for congenital encephalomyopathy. *Brain Dev* 8: 281–284.

Kissel JT, Mendell JR, Rammohan KW. (1986) Microvascular deposition of complement membrane attack complex in dermatomyositis. *N Engl J Med* 314: 331–334.

Kissel JT, Halterman RK, Rammohan KW, Mendell JR. (1991) The relationship of complement-mediated micro-vasculopathy to the histologic features and clinical duration of disease in dermatomyositis. *Arch Neurol* 48: 26–30.

Layzer RB, Shearn MA, Satya-Murti S. (1977) Eosinophilic polymyositis. *Ann Neurol* 1: 65–71.

Leff RL, Love LA, Miller FW, Freenberg SJ, Klein EA, Dalakas MC, Plotz PH. (1992) Viruses in idiopathic inflammatory myopathies: Absence of candidate viral genomes in muscle. *Lancet* 339: 1192–1195.

Love LA, Leff RL, Fraser DD, Targoff IN, Dalakas MC, Plotz PH, Miller FW. (1991) A new approach to the classification of idiopathic inflammatory myopathy: Myositis-specific autoantibodies define useful homogeneous patient groups. *Medicine* 70: 360–374.

Mantegazza R, Andreetta F, Bernasconi P, Baggi F, Oksenberg JR, Simoncini O, Mora M, Cornelia F, Steinman L. (1993) Analysis of T cell receptor of muscle-infiltrating T lymphocytes in polymyositis: Restricted Vα/β rearrangements may indicate antigen-driven selection. *J Clin Invest* 91: 2880–2886.

Medsger TA Jr, Dawson WN, Masi AT. (1970) The epidemiology of polymyositis. *Am J Med* 48: 715–723.

Mendell JT, Feng B, Sahenk Z, Marcluf GA, Amato AA, Mendell JR. (1997) Novel laminin 2 mutations in congenital muscular dystrophy [abstract]. Neurology 48 (Suppl 2): A195.

Metzger AL, Bohan A, Goldberg LS, Bluestone R, Pearson CM. (1974) Polymyositis and dermatomyositis: combined methotrexate and corticosteroid therapy. *Ann Intern Med* 81: 182–189.

Miller FW. (1993) Myositis-specific antibodies. Touchstones for understanding the inflammatory myopathies. *JAMA* 270: 1846–1849.

Moore PM, Harley JB, Fauci AS. (1985) Neurologic dysfunction in the idiopathic hypereosinophilia syndrome. *Ann Intern Med* 102: 109–114.

Moreno-Lugris C, Gonzalez-Gay M, Sanchez-Andrade A, Blanco R, Basanta D, Ibanenz D, Pulpiero JR. (1996) Magnetic resonance imaging: a useful technique in the diagnosis and follow-up of focal myositis [Letter]. *Ann Rheumatol Dis* 55: 856.

Morse RP, Kagan-Hallet K, Amato AA. (1995) Congenital inflammatory myopathy: A real entity [abstract]? *J Child Neurol* 10: 162.

Moskowitz E, Fisher C, Westbury G, Parsons C. (1991) Focal myositis: a benign inflammatory pseudotumor: CT appearances. *Br J Radiol* 64: 489–493.

Murayabashi K, Saito E, Okada S. (1991) Prognosis and life in polymyositis/dermatomyositis. *Ryumachi* 31: 391.

Nagai T, Hasgawa T, Saito M, Hayashi S, Nonaka I. (1992) Infantile polymyositis: a case report. *Brain Development* 14: 167–169.

Namba T, Brunner NG, Grob D. (1974) Idiopathic giant cell polymyositis. *Arch Neurol* 31: 27–31.

Oddis CV. (1994) Therapy of inflammatory myopathy. *Rheum Dis Clin North Am* 20: 899–918.

Pachman LM. (1995) Juvenile dermatomyositis. Pathophysiology and disease expression. *Ped Rheumatol* 42: 1071–1098.

Park JH, Vital TL, Ryder NM, Hernandez-Schulman M, Partain CL, Price RR, Olsen NJ. (1994) Magnetic resonance imaging and P-31 magnetic resonance spectroscopy provide unique quantitative data useful in the longitudinal management of patients with dermatomyositis. *Arthritis Rheum* 37: 736–747.

Park S, Nyhan WL. (1975) Fatal pulmonary involvement in dermatomyositis. *Am J Dis Child* 129: 727–728.

Pazcuzzi RM, Roos KL, Phillips LH. (1986) Granulomatous inflammatory myopathy associated with myasthenia gravis. *Arch Neurol* 43: 621–623.

Pegoraro E, Mancias P, Swerdlow SH, Raikow RB, Garcia C, Marks H, Crawford T, Carver V, Di Ciamo B, Hoffman EP. (1996) Congenital muscular dystrophy with primary laminin 2 (merosin) deficiency presenting as inflammatory myopathy. *Ann Neurol* 40: 782–791.

Pitt AM, Fleckenstein JL, Greenlee RG Jr, Burns DK, Bryan WW, Haller RH. (1993) MRI-guided biopsy in inflammatory myopathy: Initial results. *Magn Reson Imaging* 11: 1093–1099.

Plotz PH, Rider LG, Targoff IN, Raben N, O'Hanlon TP, Miller FW. (1995) Myositis: immunologic contributions to understanding cause, pathogenesis, and therapy. *Ann Intern Med* 122: 715–724.

Roddy SM, Ashwal S, Peckham N, Mortensen PB. (1986) Infantile myositis: a case diagnosed in the neonatal period. *Ped Neurol* 2: 241–244.

Schwartz MI, Matthay RA, Sahn SA, Stanford RE, Marmorstein BL, Scheinhorn DJ. (1976) Interstitial lung disease in polymyositis and dermatomyositis: Analysis of six cases and review of the literature. *Medicine* 55: 89–104.

Shevell M, Rosenblatt B, Silver K, Carpenter S, Karpati G. (1990) Congenital inflammatory myopathy. *Neurology* 40: 1111–1114.

Sigurgeirsson B, Lindelöf B, Ellander E. (1992) Risk of cancer in patient with dermatomyositis or polymyositis. *N Engl J Med* 326: 363–367.

Strongwater SL, Annesley T, Schnitzer TJ. (1983) Myocardial involvement in polymyositis. *J Rheumatol* 10: 459–463.

Targoff IN. (1984) Immune manifestations of inflammatory disease. *Rheum Dis Clin North Am* 20: 857–880.

Thompson CE. (1982) Infantile myositis. *Dev Med Child Neurol* 24: 307–313.

Tymms KE, Webb J. (1985) Dermatomyositis and other connective tissue diseases: A review of 105 cases. *J Rheumatol* 12: 1140–1148.

Whitaker JN, Engel WK. (1972) Vascular deposits of immunoglobulin and complement in idiopathic inflammatory myopathy. *N Engl J Med* 286: 332–338.

Ytterberg SR. (1994) The relationship of infectious agents to inflammatory myositis. *Rheum Clin North Am* 20: 995–1015.

Zhanuzakov MA, Vinogradova OM, Soleva AP. (1986) Effect of corticosteroids on survival of patients with idiopathic dermatomyositis. *Ter Arkh* 58: 102–105.

Zitnan D, Rovensky J, Lukac J. (1991) Systemic connective tissue diseases-prognostic conclusions on a 30 year study. *Vnitr Lek* 37: 853.

4

Muscle crush syndrome: pathogenesis and management of casualties

Ori S. Better and Irit Rubinstein

Abreviations

ACS	acute compartment syndrome
ARF	acute renal failure
ATP	adenosine triphosphate
bNOS	brain (neuronal) nitric oxide synthase
ECF	extracellular fluid
eNOS	endothelial nitric oxide synthase
ET	endothelin
GFR	glomerular filtration rate
iNOS	inducible nitric oxide synthase
i.u.	intravenous
LPS	lipopolysaccharide
MCS	muscle crush syndrome
mRNA	messenger ribonucleic acid
NO	nitric oxide
NOS	nitric oxide sythase
PLA$_2$	phospholipase A$_2$
PTS	proximal tubule segment
RBF	renal blood flow
ROI	reactive oxygen intermediates
TNF	tumour necrosis factor
VSMC	vascular smooth muscle cell

Introduction

Extensive skeletal muscle injury, whether caused by mechanical crush or by extreme physical exertion or by ischaemia, is incompatible with life, unless treated immediately and vigorously. The early cause of morbidity in the crush syndrome is leakiness of the sarcolemmal membrane to cardiotoxic or nephrotoxic cations and metabolites (K$^+$, phosphate, myoglobin and urate) from the sarcoplasma and simultaneous rapid massive uptake by the muscles of Na$^+$ and Ca^{2+} and extra cellular fluid, leading to profound hypovolaemic and hypocalcaemic shock. Based on animal experiments it is postulated that muscle crush in humans activates the inducible nitric oxide synthase (iNOS) resulting in exaggerated nitric oxide (NO) generation. Such trauma–induced sustained NO generation in muscles would cause vasodilatation with aggravation of the hypovolaemic shock. Excessive NO generation could also suppress muscular cellular respiration and thus accentuate and propagate rhabdomyolysis. Casualties who survive the early (hours) cardiotoxicity of steep hyperkalaemia and arterial hypotension are susceptible to myoglubinuric acute renal failure owing mainly to the combination of vasomotor nephropathy, nephrotoxicity and tubular obstruction by myoglobin plugs and urate. Management includes immediate (prehospital) intravenous vigorous volume replacement followed (in hospital) by mannitol-alkaline diuresis. The alkali regimen ameliorates the acidosis associated with shock and hyperkalaemia, and it protects against the nephrotoxicity of myoglobin and urate by alkalinization of the urine. Mannitol, through its impermeant hyperoncotic properties, decompresses and mobilizes muscle oedema and promotes renal tubular flow, thus flushing myoglobin plugs and enhancing urinary elimination of nephrotoxic metabolites. With this regimen, and when necessary also with the use of dialysis, a substantial salvage of lives, limbs, and kidney function has been achieved in the last 20 years.

Background

Mass disasters such as the "blitz" of London in the autumn of 1940 (Bywaters et al 1941, Bywaters 1990), or following the major earthquake in Armenia on December 7, 1988 (Collins 1989) inflict a heavy loss of lives and leave in their wake hundreds of casualties suffering myoglobinuric acute renal failure (ARF) resulting from renal involvement in muscle crush syndrome (MCS). Although MCS and myoglobinuric ARF were described early this century and a prophylactic regimen for the prevention of the type of ARF was suggested in 1944 (Bywaters 1990) and implemented in 1982 (Better et al 1990), their general acceptance by the world medical community has been slow (Bywaters 1990, Better et al 1997). Consequently, during the course of the recent rescue of casualties of the January 17, 1995 earthquake in Kobe Japan (Oda et al 1997) there were 372 casualties suffering from myoglobinuric ARF secondary to MCS. Apparently, these survivors did not benefit from adequate early volume replacement because the rescuers, by their own account, were not familiar with MCS and its current management (see discussion in Oda et al 1997, p. 476). These casualties in Kobe were, therefore, susceptible to the excessive dangers of hypovolaemic shock, hyperkalaemia, and myoglobinuric ARF (Oda et al 1997). These lethal complications are potentially preventable. It is, therefore, timely to review recent advances in the understanding of the profound circulatory collapse of the MCS, the attendant derangement of electrolyte and acid–base metabolism and the causation and prevention of the associated pigment nephropathy. For more detailed background information, the readers are referred to four previous reviews (Knochel 1981, Better et al 1990, 1992, Vanholder et al 2001).

Skeletal muscles and their susceptibility to rhabdomyolysis

The muscles are the largest organ of the body (~40–50% of total body weight) and maximal muscular blood perfusion may exceed 20 L/min. Unlike the brain and the vital internal organs, the skeletal muscles lack extensive bony protection, and they are highly exposed to mechanical trauma. In addition to their sheer bulk, the muscles contain the largest single pool of body water (~30 l in an adult), of body potassium (~70%) and the largest concentration of membranal Na^+K^+ ATPase pumps. It is, therefore, not surprising that widespread skeletal muscle injury may unleash the most extreme disturbances seen in clinical medicine in plasma electrolyte concentrations and in the size of body fluid compartments. These extreme metabolic perturbations particularly hyperkalaemia may be lethal within 1–2 h of injury, and yet they are potentially reversible with vigorous early medical intervention (Bywaters 1990, Better et al 1990, 1992).

The sarcolemma (the membrane of muscle cells) under normal conditions is almost entirely impermeable to extra-cellular fluid (ECF) and its cations and thus protects the relatively hyperoncotic cytosol from being flooded by the ECF and its solutes down their steep electrochemical gradients (Better et al 1990). Any minor physiological sarcolemmal leak is compensated by the Na^+K^+ ATP sarcolemmal cationic pumps, which maintain cytosolic electronegativity and sequester K^+ intracellularly and extrude Na^+. Sarcolemmal damage—by mechanical injury, stretch (Heppenstall et al 1986, Better et al 1990), excessive physical exertion, hyperthermia or metabolic lesions—interferes with sarcolemmal integrity and impermeability and causes a two way overwhelming leak: Ca^{2+} and Na^+ followed by water penetrate the cytosol and possibly the interstitium causing depletion of the ECF and hypovolaemic hypocalcaemic shock. Potassium, phosphate, purines (precursors of urate), myoglobin and other proteins leak into the ECF (Better et al 1997). With the exception of K^+, these metabolites or their derivatives are highly nephrotoxic, particularly on the background of renal vasoconstriction and aciduria, and increased urinary concentration, all of which are invariably seen in casualties with hypovolaemic shock.

Entry of Ca^{2+} into the cytosol of damaged myocytes and ultimately into the mitochondria causes mitochondrial damage that interferes with their function and with their ability to generate ATP, which is vital

to all normal cellular functions. In this respect muscle mitochondrial dysfunction secondary to stretch definitely occurs earlier than mitochondrial impairment secondary to ischaemia (3–4 h) (Heppenstall et al 1986).

Nitric oxide involvement

In the early 1990s a new regulator of skeletal muscle function and blood supply was described. This regulator is the NO system. It has been demonstrated that NO, the small gaseous molecule, regulates contractility of skeletal muscle (Kobzik et al 1994, 1995) as well as blood vessel tone and blood flow (Moncada et al 1991, 1993). Human skeletal muscle, under normal conditions, contains the two constitutive types of nitric oxide synthase (NOS), the enzyme that regulates NO metabolism: the brain (neuronal) NOS (bNOS) and the endothelial NOS (eNOS) (Frandsen et al 1996), but it lacks the inducible form (iNOS). bNOS immunoreactivity was found in the sarcolemma and cytoplasm of all human skeletal muscle fibres. It was detected in all fibre types, adjacent the cellular locations of the mitochondria. eNOS immunoreactivity was observed in the endothelium of blood vessels—larger vessels as well as microvessels of the muscles. It should be noted that in rats eNOS was detected in the cytoplasm in mitochondria rich fibres and within the mitochondrium.

A major known function of NO is regulation of blood vessel tone and, therefore, of blood flow (Moncada et al 1991, 1993). Studies from humans and animals (Vallance et al 1989, Rubinstein et al 1998) have shown that NO is involved in skeletal muscle perfusion through its vasodilatory action. The stimulus for NO release from vascular endothelial cells in skeletal muscle may be shear stress of increased blood flow (Pohl et al 1991). Another function of NO is to regulate the contractile force of skeletal muscles (Kobzik et al 1994, 1995). Myocyte function is sensitive to redox modulation under basal conditions. Reactive oxygen intermediates (ROI) and NO are two classes of molecules that modulate muscle function under physiological conditions (Reid 1996). The ROI promote excitation – contraction coupling and appear to be obligatory to optimal contractile function (Reid et al 1993, Reid 1996). NO opposes the action of ROI. The dynamic balance between production and inactivation of ROI and NO maintains redox homeostasis within the cell. NOS activity has a decisive influence on the effectiveness of excitation – contraction coupling. Inhibitors of NOS increase twitch and submaximal tetanic force production in skeletal muscles, whereas NO donors decrease force production (Kobzik et al 1994).

Following endotoxin administration, mouse skeletal muscle shows ability to induce the synthesis of iNOS mRNA and protein and it has iNOS activity (Thompson et al 1996). Rubinstein et al (1998) also found an excessive induction of iNOS, and increased immunoreactivity, following muscle crush injury in the rat model. Mechanically crushed muscle contains macrophages (Rubinstein et al 1998). iNOS is induced by macrophages, as well as by certain cytokines like TNF and interleukins, and by lipopolysaccharides (LPS) acting through the release of cytokines. Cytokines regulate iNOS, some promoting and others inhibiting the induction of the enzyme (Moncada et al 1995). iNOS is responsible for the excess generation of NO, which may exert an autocytotoxic effect, as well as a cytotoxic effect on other cells in the vicinity (Moncada et al 1993, 1995). The induction of iNOS in the macrophages results in the sustained production of NO. There the NO combines with iron–sulphur centres in key enzymes of both the mitochondrial respiratory cycle and the DNA synthesis pathway. In normal situations, NO is capable of rapidly and reversibly inhibiting the mitochondrial respiratory chain; but when NO is generated by iNOS, it may change the pattern of inhibition to a prolonged one (Brown et al 1994, Cleeter et al 1994). Such enzymatic inhibition may cause cellular hypoxia, in spite of intact circulation. The end result of mitochondrial failure is myocytic anoxia and acidosis, which may be lethal. The impact of excess NO production on muscle perfusion might have a further influence on muscle function and possibly on systemic haemodymanics. Extreme vasodilatation, caused by sustained vascular NO production, may lead to haemodynamic-hypovolaemic shock, which is the hallmark of the crush syndrome in man. Increased NO formation (by induction of iNOS) may also cause oxidant peroxinitrite devastating damage to the muscular tissue (Anggard 1994), either directly or via its metabolite, and thus aggravate and possibly propagate rhabdomyolysis. iNOS is similarly responsible for the sustained increased levels of NO in septic shock characteristically often complicated by ARF. In view of the clear evidence that mechanical trauma to muscles induces NO production, it can be speculated that NO is involved in the pathogenesis of MCS.

Acute compartment syndrome

Acute compartment syndrome (ACS) is a devastating local complication of posttraumatic or postexertional

Table 4.1 — Causes of haemodynamic shock in muscle crush syndrome[a]

- Internal volume losses resulting from sequestration of fluid and solute in traumatized muscles ("third spacing") may reach 10–18 l/day.
- External volume losses resulting from dehydration (excessive sensible and insensible losses, during exertion or prostration in hot, arid environments, hyperthermia, vomiting, and diarrhoea).
- Cardiovascular depression caused by the combination of hyperkalaemia and hypocalcaemia and the action of cytokines and endotoxin.
- Vasodilatation of crushed muscles because of excessive increase in the activity of inducible nitric oxide synthase and nitric oxide production (Rubinstein et al 1998).

---

[a]Better et al 1990

rhabdomyolysis. Its clinical manifestation is a rapid painful turgid swelling of the affected limb. In extreme cases ACS may be accompanied by local neurologic motor and/or sensory deficits and by myoglobinuric ARF (Blick et al 1986, Schwartz et al 1989). The aetiologic hallmark of ACS is a steep increase in the intra-compartmental interstitial pressure from the normal of 0.0 ± 2.0 mmHg to pressures that may exceed the mean arterial pressure.

The cause of the intra-comparmental "hypertension" in the ACS is interstitial oedema and hyperoncotic swelling of muscle cells within muscle compartments covered by tight sheaths of fibrous fascia with relative low compliance. In subacute compartment syndrome further increase in intra-compartmental pressure may conceivably be a result of hyperperfusion and pressure secondary to stimulation, local production of NO and vasodilatation (Rubinstein et al 1998). Increase in intra-compartmental pressure will block the venous drainage out of the compartment. This imbalance between blood inflow and outflow to the affected compartment would lead to its swelling and ultimately turgidity and tamponade. Thus, within hours to days ACS will superimpose ischaemic myopathy damage to muscles on traumatic rhabdomyolysis.

It is obvious that management of ACS is immediate decompression. The prevailing textbook view is that early fasciotomy is mandatory in ACS (Mubarak and Hargens 1981).

Before 1982 results with fasciotomy by our orthopaedic surgeons for ACS in combat casualties from the

South Lebanon arena were dismal, with prohibitory loss of limbs and even lives (Better et al 1990). Therefore since 1982 we became conservative with the indications for fasciotomy and perform it only rarely. Moreover non-surgical decompression of the ACS has been achieved with intravenous (i.v.) hypertonic mannitol in the ACS in man (Daniels et al 1998), in dogs (Better et al 1991) and in rabbits (Oredsson et al 1994). Our suggestion at present for casualties with ACS who are candidates for fasciotomy is that they first be given a trial of i.v. mannitol (20%; Table 4.2). If i.v. mannitol results in symptomatic relief and reduction of the circumference of the affected swollen limb, then fasciotomy can be postponed or pre-empted altogether.

It is interesting to note that fasciotomy was associated with increased mortality and morbidity in victims of the extensive earthquake in Iran in 1990, which claimed 43 390 injured (Nadjafi et al 1997). These authors, therefore, question, based on their vast personal experience, the advisability of fasciotomy in the management of ACS. Furthermore fasciotomy doubled the rate of septicaemia and increased the requirement of blood transfusions in casualties of the August 17th 1999 Maramara disaster (Vanholder et al 2001, Sever 2000).

Another promising potential for non-surgical approach to the management of ACS, at least in the dog, was the use of hyperbaric oxygen treatment (Strauss et al 1983). Our preliminary experimental results suggest that hyperbaric oxygen treatment in rat model of crush injury has a protective effect on the crushed muscle, and it may, in the future, serve as a therapeutic adjunct in severe cases of the crush syndrome and ACS in humans.

Plasma electrolyte disorder in muscle crush syndrome

Within 2 h of extrication of live buried casualties, they may manifest hyperkalaemia, hypocalcaemia, hyperphosphataemia, hyperuricaemia and metabolic acidosis ("extra renal uraemic pattern"). The hypocalcaemia aggravates the cardio-toxicity of hyperkalaemia, and it has a suppressive effect on the entire cardiovascular tree. Hyperphosphataemia intensifies the hypocalcaemia and further undermines kidney function (Zager 1996; see Table 4.1).

Table 4.2—Suggested volume replenishment during extrication of young adults from under collapsed buildings[a] or resuscitation from prolonged coma

- When a limb is extricated, start imediately with intravenous (i.v.) saline at a rate of 1 l/h. The entire extrication stage may last 4–8 h. Once the patient is freed, monitor arterial blood pressure, central venous pressure, and urinary output.
- Following extrication, continue i.v. infusion with 500 ml saline alternating with 5% glucose, 1 l/h.
- Once the patient is admitted to hospital, add sodium bicarbonate ampules of 50 meq/l to each second or third bottle of glucose, so that the pH of the urine is maintained above 6.5 (usual requirement for bicarbonate: 200–300 meq/l for the first day).
- Once there is evidence of urine flow, add a 20% solution of mannitol at a rate of 1–2 g/kg body weight over 4 h.
- Keep urine flow at least 8 l/day. This will generally require an infusion of 12 l/day. The positive balance of 4 l/day will be due to oedema mainly in the limbs, which is an acceptable risk in young adults. Elderly traumatized patients may require lower and slower volume replacements.
- The amount of mannitol required to maintain a urinary flow of 8 l/day should not exceed 200 g/day. Plasma osmolar gap should remain below 55 mOsm/kg corresponding to 1000 mg/dl (10 g/l) of mannitol in the blood (Better 1997).
- If bicarbonate administration has produced metabolic alkalosis (arterial blood pH above 7.45), use acetazolamide as a bolus i.v. of 500 mg.
- The above regimen should be continued until urinary myoglobin has disappeared, usually by the third day.
- If the patient is anuric, a bolus of 20 g mannitol combined with 120 mg furosemide may be tried to initiate urinary output. If all of the above measures do not result in urinary flow, dopamine infusion will not reverse the situation. Yet some authorities suggest administration of a "renal dose" of dopamine, 1–2 μg/kg body weight/min.
- Mannitol should *not* be given to casualties with established anuria.[a]
- As anihyperkalaemic defence, the following may be considered: inhalation of beta 2 agonists—for example salbuterol (albuterol), i.v. 10% glucose and insulin and/or i.v. calcium 1gr and as 10% solution.

[a]Better et al 1990

Circulatory failure of muscle crush syndrome

Casualties suffering from MCS usually are in a profound state of haemodynamic shock. The main reason for this circulatory collapse is massive uptake of ECF by the crushed muscle. Practically the entire 14 l of the ECF can be sequestered in the crushed muscles within hours of injury. The depleted circulation is further depressed by the combination of hyperkalaemia and hypocalcaemia, which are negatively inotropic and chronotropic. The hyperkalaemia of MCS may reach extreme levels of well above 10 meq/l (!) in casualties who suffered from the combined effects of exertional and traumatic rhabdomyolysis (Schaller et al 1990). Even excessive muscle damage resulting from marathon-type exertion in *normal* trained athletes may cause hyperkalaemia approaching 9.0 meq/l (McKechie et al 1967). Furthermore, the volume depletion and arterial hypotension of MCS would probably be aggravated by profuse vasodilatation in the crushed muscles. Such crush-induced vasodilatation has been demonstrated in our laboratory in experimental animals, and it was a result of increased iNOS generation and NO production in the muscle (Rubinstein et al 1998).

The circulatory collapse in untreated MCS triggers, via the baroreceptors, the release of powerful systemic vasoconstrictors such as noradrenaline (norepinephrine), angiotensin II, endothelin (ET) and thromboxan, which tend to cause renal cortical vasoconstriction and hypoperfusion hypofiltration and ischaemia. Such renal vasoconstriction is intensified by myoglobin which chelates renal vasodilatory NO (Zager 1996). It is interesting to note that extreme renal cortical ischaemia, following extensive muscle injury, may occur even in animals whose muscles lack myoglobin such as the rabbit (Trueta et al 1947). Therefore, the nephrotoxicity of myoglobinuria is not a prerequisite for renal failure caused by trauma to muscles.

There are two main components to myoglobinuric ARF: vasomotor (renal vasoconstriction and renal ischaemia) and nephrotoxic—obstructive due to tubular cast formation of muscle metabolites (myoglobin, urate and phosphate) leaked from disintegrating muscle into the circulation and the kidneys. Aciduria and hyperstenuria potentiate the nephrotoxicity of both myoglobin and urate in myoglobinuric ARF (Bywaters et al 1944).

Morphologic alterations in the kidneys

Myoglobinuric ARF in humans and experimental animals is characterized by striking morphologic changes which include:

1. formation of haem casts in the distal nephron

2. proximal tubular necrosis and detachment of epithelial cells from the basement membrane (Zager 1996).

Tubular casts obstruct the luminal flow and thus impair kidney function (Baker and Dodds 1925, Jaenike 1967). Tubular obstruction apparently occurs in the first few hours after the induction of pigment nephropathy, whereas the established phase of ARF is associated with collapsed tubules (Ruiz-Guninazu et al 1967, Jaenike 1969). Therefore, the relative importance of the nephrotoxic vs the obstructive elements in the pathogenesis of ARF is still being debated.

Zager and Gamelin (1989) suggested that haemprotein cytotoxicity plays a critical role in tubular epithelial damage during myoglobinuria. In this condition, formation of casts causes luminal obstruction and stasis. Such stasis further enhances cast formation, and it allows increased cast contact with tubular epithelium. Urinary concentration and acidity in MCS aggravates not only the nephrotoxicity of myoglobin and of urate but also the myoglobin–Tamm Horsfall polymers in the distal tubules (Zager 1996).

Mechanisms of the renal impairment following acute myopathy

Two factors are considered to play a pivotal role in the initiation of this insult: renal ATP depletion and oxidant stress (Zager 1996, Zager and Gamelin 1989).

Ischaemic damage and ATP depletion

As with other forms of ARF, available evidence suggests that myoglobinuric renal injury is largely secondary to the ischaemic as well as toxic renal insults induced by haem proteins. A reduction in renal perfusion has been consistently reported in experimental models of myohaemoglobinuric ARF (Vetterlein et al 1995). This effect is attributed to haem protein-induced renal vasoconstriction and hypoperfusion.

Trifillis et al (1981) have demonstrated that ATP content in the renal cortex of rats with glycerol-induced myoglobinuric ARF is decreased. Renal ATP depletion is caused not only by ischaemia, but in large part also by leakage of ATP precursors (adenosine, inosine and hypoxanthine within hours of glycerol injection) as a result of the increased permeability of the injured tubular cells. This drain of precursors will render the generation of ATP "costlier" and slower (Simon 1995). Therefore, the provision of ATP or its precursors, or inhibitors of the enzymes that convert nucleotides to nucleosides and bases, accelerates recovery of this type of ARF (Fischereder et al 1994). Depletion of cellular ATP, which usually accompanies ischaemia, impairs energetic metabolism and the function of sarcolemmal ionic pumps (Zager 1996). The end result is an increase in cytosolic Ca^{2+} due to the following mechanisms:

1. failure of Ca^{2+}-ATPase driven Ca^{2+} efflux due to ATP depletion

2. interference with intracellular Ca^{2+} sequestration

3. increased Na^+/Ca^{2+} exchange following intensive Na^+ influx, which further depletes precariously low cytosolic ATP content.

Interestingly, when myoglobin was infused into rats in the presence of iron chelator, ATP levels (Zager 1991) remained intact. Similar results were obtained when free iron–low molecular weight proteins (~17 kD) were infused into experimental animals, indicating that iron plays a critical role in haem-protein ATP depletion.

Oxidant tissue stress

Haem proteins appear to be toxic to the proximal tubular cells (Zager 1996). This notion stems from the observations that pretreatment of rats prior to renal artery occlusion with non-toxic doses of myoglobin or haemoglobin, potentiates the induction of ischaemic ARF (Yuile et al 1945, Badenoch and Darmady 1948, Lowe 1996). The mechanisms underlying this phenomenon are incompletely understood. However, since non-iron containing proteins were also able to intensify the cytotoxicity of ischaemia, Zager et al (1987) concluded that endocytic protein uptake, and not necessarily cell iron loading per se, is largely responsible for nephrotoxicity of haem proteins. These authors have further supported their theory by experimental data involving in vitro incubations of proximal tubule segments (PTS), derived from either normal or haem-infused mice/rats, with exogenous

phospholipase A_2 (PLA_2), a critical determinant of ischaemia-induced cellular damage. While normal PTS were not affected by this enzyme, haem-loaded PTS were severely damaged. This indicates that haem proteins directly sensitize these cells to lethal injury.

Reactive oxygen and non-oxygen based radicals were implicated in the pathogenesis of a variety of renal diseases including myoglobinuric ARF (Zager 1996). The first step in this pathway is proximal tubular cell transport and accumulation of poryphrin rings. Within the proximal epithelial cells the rings undergo degradation resulting in iron release, which is eliminated within several weeks (Bunn and Jandl 1969a). The extension and site of iron release are critically dependent on the concentration of haem protein in the lumen of proximal tubules (Bunn and Jandl 1969a, Bunn et al 1969b). For example, when the filtered load of either myoglobin or haemoglobin exceeds the absorptive capacity of proximal tubules they congest the tubules, and subsequently iron is released in the lumen (Bunn and Jandl 1969a, Zager 1992). Regardless of the controversy about the nephrotoxicity of iron, the fact that iron is an intermediate accelerator in the generation of free radicals, and it could itself become a free radical, contributes to the pathogenesis of ARF. This notion—"iron-induced oxidant stress"—is supported by numerous studies where administration of iron chelators, such as deferoxamine, or scavengers of reactive oxygen metabolites, such as glutathione, can protect against haemoglobinuric ARF (Paller et al 1984, Shah and Walker 1988, Abul-Ezz et al 1991, Zager 1996,). Moreover, the production of hydrogen peroxide (H_2O_2) in rat kidney increased following myohaemoglobinuric procedure (Paller 1988, Guidet and Shah 1989). Considering that hydrogen peroxide constitutes an important source for radical formation, and it may itself promote the release of iron from intracellular sites, these findings indicate that hydroxyl radical formation (most likely in the mitochondria) plays a critical role in haem-induced nephrotoxicity.

Renal vasoconstriction

The renal perfusion is regulated by the interaction of vasoactive endothelial metabolites. Chief among these are vasoconstrictors such as endothelin and vasodilators such as prostacyclin and NO (Moncada et al 1991, Kohan 1997).

Endothelin

ET plays an important role in the pathophysiology of

the ischaemic and myoglobinuric varieties of ARF (Brooks 1997, Kohan 1997). Intrarenal administration of ET leads to steep reduction in renal blood flow (RBF) and glomerular filtration rate (GFR) resembling the early ischaemic pattern of experimental ARF. Furthermore the levels of ET-1 and its renal binding sites are increased in the rat ischaemic ARF model (Firth and Ratcliffe 1992). Similarly, Karam et al (1995) reported that plasma ET-1 levels, as well as urinary ET excretion, were increased 24 h after intramuscular glycerol injection in rats (myoglobinuric model). The increased immunoreactivity of both ET-1 and ET–mRNA following these renal insults is considered to be secondary to renal hypoxia and exaggerated production of oxygen radicals. Most ET receptor antagonists were able to ameliorate the renal hypoperfusion/hypofiltration and excretory function in the rat myohaemoglobinuric ARF and ischaemic ARF models. Pretreatment with Bosentan, a novel potent non-peptide ET_A/ET_B receptor antagonist, restored almost completely RBF in the myoglobinuric rats (Karam et al 1995). Taken together, these findings indicate that activation of systemic and renal ET system contributes to renal vasoconstriction in myoglobinuric and other types of rat ARF.

Nitric oxide

Originally described as the endothelial-derived relaxing factor, NO is a diffusable gaseous molecule produced in endothelial cells of renal and non-renal vasculature, as well as in tubular epithelial and mesangial cells, from its precursor, L-arginine (Baylis et al 1990, King and Brenner 1991, Luscher et al 1991, Moncada et al 1991, Bachrnan et al 1994). NO exerts a tonic vasodilatory action on renal microcirculation, primarily in the afferent arteriole and to mediate the renal vasorelaxant action of acetylcholine and bradykinin. In addition to its vascular effects, NO also affects renal function by modulating tubuloglomerular feedback, renin release and tubular salt reabsorption (Luscher et al 1991, Moncada et al 1991, Bachman 1994). In addition, NO is capable of inhibiting the migration and proliferation of vascular smooth muscle cells (VSMC) and the aggregation of platelets (Luscher 1991, Moncada et al 1991, Bachmann and Mundel 1994). Given the importance of NO in the defence of RBF, the role of the NO system in myoglobinuric ARF should be examined. Indeed, renal NO production is impaired in response to many renal insults including ischaemia and exposure to haem proteins (Simon 1995, Peters and Noble 1996). Renal

ischaemia can impair vasodilator generation, and it can stimulate production of vasoconstrictors. Furthermore, the ischaemic kidney is almost exclusively dependent on NO synthesis for maintenance of RBF, GFR and medullary oxygenation (Agmon et al 1994). This protective role of NO in the face of renal vasoconstriction can be augmented by providing L-arginine—the metabolic NO donor (Wakabayashi and Kikawada 1996). Haem proteins derived from disintegrating muscles are powerful NO scavengers. In the kidney they thus deplete NO stores, and consequently undermine renal ability to counteract ET-induced vasoconstriction. Moreover, there is growing evidence that NO and its metabolic product peroxinitrite (ONOO) are involved in the pathophysiology of both toxic-induced and hypoxia–reperfusion-induced injury (Noiri et al 1996). Liebertal (1997) showed that suppression of tubular NO production aggravates ischaemic nephrotoxicity. The locally produced NO in the tubular cells is most likely generated via iNOS activity. It should be emphasized that both free myoglobin and haemoglobin are toxic, and they may induce iNOS (Liebertal 1997). Schwartz et al (1997) demonstrated that NO, generated by iNOS after lipopolysaccharide administration, inhibited eNOS, a renal vasodilator. Selective inhibition of iNOS prevented the decrease in GFR following lipopolysaccharide administration, suggesting that excess iNOS is detrimental to kidney function, probably via excessive production of NO. Furthermore, NOS is strongly induced by several cytokines including tumour necrosis factor (TNF) (Kone 1997). Plasma levels of TNF are increased in rats during glycerol-induced ARF, suggesting a role for TNF, probably through iNOS, in the pathogenesis of this experimental form of ARF (Kone 1997). Infusion of neutralizing anti-TNF-α antiserum immediately prior to glycerol injection significantly protected kidney function (Shulman et al 1993). Similarly anti-TNF-α improves myocardial recovery after ischaemia and reperfusion (Gurevich et al 1997). In summary, similar to other forms of ARF, rhabdomyolysis–induced ARF is associated with reduced endothelium-derived NO production, which causes renal vasoconstriction. Furthermore increased NO generation in the tubular cells by iNOS exacerbates the deleterious effects of ischaemia and endotoxin. This may explain the controversial reports about the role of NO donors and NOS inhibitors in prevention of ARF. Therefore, any future modulation of NO activity in ARF must be directed toward preservation of eNOS activity, while suppressing iNOS action, to protect the kidney against ischaemia.

Management of casualties with impending myoglobinuric acute renal failure (post-traumatic and post-exertional)

Casualties with massive muscle crushing classically seen following earthquakes suffer from profound hypo-volaemic shock (Table 4.1). Therefore, the mainstay of management of these casualties is early, massive, volume replacement started preferably in the field. This is followed in the hospital stage by forced solute (mannitol)–alkaline diuresis (Table 4.2), which alkalanises the urine and protects the kidney against the nephrotoxicity of myoglobin and urate. The iatrogenic mild metabolic alkalosis and the increase in blood bicarbonate by itself may ameliorate, during this regimen, hyperkalaemia—an early potentially lethal complication of MCS. Furthermore the hyperosmotic effect of mannitol may decompress oedematous muscles and protect them against further rhabdomyolysis. Such presumed "muscle sparing" effect of mannitol would decrease the muscular leak of myoglobin, purines and phosphate and lower the burden of these nephrotoxic metabolytes on the kidney. Mannitol diuresis increases intratubular pressure and flow, and it flushes toxic tubular pigment plugs. Therefore, by increased urinary elimination as well as by suppressing leak from muscles, mannitol reduces plasma pool of nephrotoxic muscle metabolytes. If the regimen suggested in Table 4.2 is started less than 6 h following extrication of trapped casualties myoglobinuric ARF can be completely prevented, even in those buried for up to 32 h. This salvage should be contrasted with the 100% mortality associated with myoglobinuric ARF in casualties buried for 3–4 h in London in 1940 (Bywaters and Beal 1941). The therapeutic potential of mannitol in the prevention of myoglobinuric ARF as well as its limitation and contra-indications have recently been reviewed (Better 1997). Interestingly, the majority of survivors with established myoglobinuric ARF have spontaneous, ultimately full, recovery of renal function even following prolonged dialysis treatment.

References

Abul-Ezz SR, Walker PD, Shah SV. (1991) Role of glutathione in an animal model of myoglubinuric acute renal failure. *Proc Natl Acad Sci USA* 88: 9833–9837.

Agmon Y, Peleg H, Greenfeld Z, Rosen S, Brezis M. (1994) Nitric oxide and prostanoid protect the renal outer medulla from radiocontrast toxicity in the rat. *J Clin Invest* 94: 1069–1075.

Anggard, E. (1994) Nitric oxide: mediator, murderer and medicine. *Lancet* 343: 1199–1206.

Bachmann S, Mundel P. (1994) Nitric oxide in the kidney: Synthesis, localization and function. *Am J Kidney Dis* 24: 112–129.

Badenoch AW, Darmady EM. (1948) The effect of stroma free hemoglobin on the ischemic kidney of the rabbit. *Br J Exp Pathol* 29: 215–223.

Baker SL, Dodds EC. (1925) Obstruction of the renal tubules during the excretion of haemoglobin. *Br J Exp Pathol* 6: 247–260.

Baylis C, Harton P, Engels K. (1990) Endothelial derived relaxing factor controls renal hemodynamics in the normal rat kidney. *J Am Soc Nephrol* 1: 875–881.

Better OS, Rubinstein I, Winaver JM, Knochel JP. (1997) Mannitol therapy revisited (1940–1997). *Kidney Intl* 51: 886–894.

Better OS, Rubinstein I, Winaver J. (1992) Recent insights into the pathogenesis and early management of the crush syndrome. *Sem Nephrol* 12: 217–222.

Better OS, Zinman C, Reis DN, Har-Shai Y, Rubinstein I, Abussi Z. (1991) Hypertonic mannitol ameliorates inter-compartmental tamponade in model compartment syndrome in the dog. *Nephron* 58: 344–346.

Better OS, Abassi Z, Rubinstein I, Marom S, Winaver Y, Silberman M. (1990) The mechanism of muscle injury in the crush syndrome: Ischemic versus pressure-stretch myopathy. *Miner Electrolyte Metab* 16: 181–184.

Better OS. (1997) History of the crush syndrome: from the earthquake of Messina, 1909 to Armenia, 1988. *Am J Nephrol* 17: 392–394.

Better OS, Stein JH. (1990) Early management of shock and prophylaxis of acute renal failure in traumatic rhabdomyolysis. *N Engl J Med* 322: 825–829.

Blick SS, Brumback RJ, Poka A, Burgess AR, Ebraheim NA. (1986) Compartment syndrome in open tibial fractures. *J Bone Joint Surg* 68A: 1348–1353.

Brooks DP. (1997) Endothelin: "the prime suspect" in kidney disease. *News Physiol Sci* 12: 83–89.

Brown GC, Cooper CE. (1994) Nanomolar concentrations of nitric oxide reversibly inhibit synaptosomal respiration by competing with oxygen at cytochrome oxidase. *FEBS Lett* 345: 50–54.

Bunn HF, Jandl JH. (1969a) The renal handling of hemoglobin. II Catabolism. *J Exp Med* 129: 925–934.

Bunn HF, Eshman WT, Bull RW. (1969b) The renal handling of hemoglobin. I. Glomerular filtration. *J Exp Med* 129: 909–924.

Bywaters EGL, Stead JK. (1944) The production of renal failure following injection of solution containing myohaemoglobin. *Q J Exp Physiol* 33: 53–70.

Bywaters EGL, Beal D. (1941) Crush syndrome with impairment of renal function. *Brit Med J* 1: 427–432.

Bywaters EGL. (1990) 50 years on: The crush syndrome. *Brit Med J* 301: 1412–1415.

Cleeter MWJ, Cooper CE, Drley-Usmar VM, Moncada S, Schapira AHV. (1994) Reversible inhibition of cytochrome C oxidase, the terminal enzyme of the mitochondrial respiratory chain, by nitric oxide. Implications for neurodegenerative disease. *FEBS Lett* 345–50–54.

Collins AJ. (1989) Kidney dialysis treatment for victims of the Armenian earthquake. *N Engl J Med* 320: 1291–1292.

Daniels M, Reichman J, Brezis M. (1998) Mannitol treatment for acute compartment syndrome. *Nephron* 79: 492–493.

Firth JD, Ratcliffe PJ. (1992) Organ distribution of the three rat endothelin messenger RNAs and the effects of ischemia on renal gene expression. *J Clin Invest* 90: 1023–1031.

Fischereder M, Trick W, Nath KA. (1994) Therapeutic strategies in the prevention of acute renal failure. *Semin Nephrol* 14: 41–52.

Frandsen U, Lopez-Figueroa M, Hellsten Y. (1996) Localization of nitric oxide synthase in human skeletal muscle. *Biochem Biophys Res Commun* 227: 88–93.

Guidet B, Shah SV. (1989) Enhanced in vivo H_2O_2 generation by rat kidney in glycerol–induced acute renal failure. *Am J Physiol* 257: F440–F445.

Gurevitch J, Frolkis I, Yuhas Y, Lifschitz-Mercer B, Berger E, Paz Y, Matsa M, Kramer A, Mohr R. (1997) Anti tumor necrosis factor alpha improves myocardial recovery after ischemia and reperfusion. *J Am Coll Cardiol* 30: 1554–1561.

Heppenstall B, Scott R, Sapega A, Park YS, Chance B. (1986) A comparative study of the tolerance of skeletal muscle to ischemia. *JBJS* 68A(6): 820–828.

Jaenike JR. (1967) The renal lesion associated with hemoglobinuria: a study of the pathogenesis of the excretory defect in the rat. *J Clin Invest* 46: 378–387.

Jaenike JR. (1969) Micropuncture study of methemoglobin-induced acute renal failure in the rat. *J Lab Clin Med* 73: 459–468.

Karam H, Bruneval P, Clozel J-P, Loffler B-M, Bariety J, Clozel M. (1995) Role of endothelin in acute renal failure due to rhabdomyolysis in rats. *J Pharmacol Exp Therap* 274: 481–486.

King AJ, Brenner BM. (1991) Endothelium-derived relaxing factor and renal vasculature. *Am J Physiol* 260: R653–R662.

Knochel JP. (1981) Rhabdomyolysis and myoglobinuria. *Sem Nephrol* 1: 75–86.

Kobzik L, Reid MB, Bredt DS, Stamler JS. (1994) Nitric oxide in skeletal muscle. *Nature* 372: 546–548.

Kobzik L, Stringer B, Balligand J-L, Reid MB, Stamler JS. (1995) Endothelial type nitric oxide synthase in skeletal muscle fibers: mitochondrial relationships. *Biochem Biophys Res Commun* 211: 375–381.

Kohan DE. (1997) Endothelin in the normal and diseased kidney. *Am J Kidney Dis* 29: 2–26.

Kone BC. (1997) Nitric oxide in renal health and disease. *Am J Kidney Dis* 30: 311–333.

Lieberthal W. (1997) Biology of acute renal failure: therapeutic implications. *Kidney Intl* 52: 1102–1115.

Lowe MB. (1966) Effects of nephrotoxins and ischemia in experimental hemoglobinuria. *J Pathol Bact* 92: 319–323.

Luscher TF, Bock HA, Yang Z, Diederich D. (1991) Endothelium–derived relaxing and contracting factors. Perspectives in nephrology. *Kidney Intl* 39: 575–590.

McKechnie JK, Leary WP, Joubert SM. (1967) Some electrocardiographic and biochemical changes recorded in marathon runners. *S African Med J* 41: 722–725.

Moncada SR, Palmer RM, Higgs EA. (1991) Nitric oxide: Physiology, pathophysiology, and pharmacology. *Pharmacol Rev* 43: 109–142.

Moncada S, Higgs A. (1991) Endogenous nitric oxide: Physiology, pathology and clinical relevance. *Eur J Clin Invest* 21: 361–374.

Moncada S, Higgs A. (1993) The L-arginine-nitric oxide pathway. *N Engl J Med* 329: 2002–2012.

Moncada S, Higgs A. (1995) Molecular mechanisms and therapeutic strategies related to nitric oxide. *FASEB J* 9: 1319–1330.

Mubarak SJ, Hargens AR. (1981) Compartment syndromes and volkmann's contracture. Saunders Monographs in Clinical Orthopaedics, Vol. III.

Nadjafi I, Atef MR, Broumand B, Rastegar A. (1997) Suggested guidelines for treatment of acute renal failure in earthquake victims. *Renal Failure* 19(5): 655–664.

Noiri E, Peresleni T, Miller F, Goligorsky M.S. (1996) In vivo targeting of inducible NO synthase with oligodeoxynucleotides protects rat kidney against ischemia. *J Clin Invest* 97: 2377–2383.

Oda J, Tanaka H, Yoshioka T, Iwai A, Yanmamura H, Ishikawa K, Matsuoka T, Kuwagata, Y, et al. (1997) Analysis of 372 patients with crush syndrome caused by the Hanshin-Awaji earthquake. *J Trauma* 42: 470–476.

Oredsson S, Plate G, Qvarfordt P. (1994) The effect of mannitol on reperfusion injury and postischemic compartment pressure in skeletal muscle. *Eur J Vasc Surg* 8: 326–331.

Paller MS, Hoidal JR, Ferris TF. (1984) Oxygen free radicals in ischemic acute renal failure in the rat. *J Clin Invest* 74: 1156–1164.

Paller MS. (1988) Hemoglobin- and myoglobin-induced acute renal failure in rats: Role of iron in nephrotoxicity. *Am J Physiol* 255: F539–F544.

Peters H, Noble NA. (1996) Dietary L-arginine in renal disease. *Sem Nephrol* 16: 567–575.

Pohl U, Herlan K, Huang A, Bassenge E. (1991) Platelet inhibition by an L-arginine-derived substance released by IL-1β treated vascular smooth muscle cells. *Am J Physiol* 261: H2016–2023.

Reid MB, Khawli FA, Moody MR. (1993) Reactive oxygen in skeletal muscle. III. Contractility of unfatigued muscle. *J Appl Physiol* 75: 1081–1087.

Reid MB. (1996) Reactive oxygen and nitric oxide in skeletal muscle. *News Physiol Sci* 11: 114–119.

Rubinstein I, Abassi Z, Coleman R, Milman F, Winaver J, Better OS. (1998) Involvement of Nitric Oxide System in Experimental muscle crush injury. *J Clin Invest* 101: 1325–1333.

Ruiz-Guninazu A, Coelho JB, Paz RA. (1967) Methemoglobin-induced acute renal failure in the rat. *Nephron* 4: 257–275.

Schaller MD, Fischer AP, Perret CH. Hyperkalemia. (1990) A prognostic factor during hypothermia. *JAMA* 264: 1842–1845.

Schwartz D, Mendonca M, Schwartz I, Xia Y, Satriano J, Wilson CB, Blantz R. (1997) Inhibition of constitutive nitric oxide synthase (NOS) by nitric oxide generated by inducible NOS after liposaccaride administration provokes renal dysfunction. *J Clin Invest* 100: 439–448.

Schwartz Jr JT, Brumback RJ, Lakatos R, Poka A, Bathon GH, Burgess AR. (1989) Acute compartment syndrome of the thigh. *J Bone Joint Surg* 71A: 392–400.

Sever MS (2000) Personal Communication

Shah SV, Walker PD. (1988) Evidence suggesting a role for hydroxyl radical in glycerol-induced acute renal failure. *Am J Physiol* 255: F438–F443.

Shulman LM, Yuhas Y, Frolkis I, Gavendo S, Knecht A, Eliahou HE. (1993) Glycerol induced ARF in rats mediated by tumor necrosis factor-alpha. *Kidney Intl* 43: 1397–1401.

Simon E. (1995) New aspects of acute renal failure. *Am J Med Sci* 310: 217–221.

Strauss MB, Hargens AR, Gershuni DH, Greenberg DA, Crenshaw AG. (1983) Reduction of skeletal muscle necrosis using intermittent hyperbaric oxygen in a model compartment syndrome. *J Bone Joint Surg* 65(A): 656–662.

Thompson M, Becker L, Bryant D, Williams G, Levin D, Margraf L, Goroir BP. (1996) Expression of the inducible nitric oxide synthase gene in diaphragm and skeletal muscle. *J Appl Physiol* 81: 2415–2420.

Trifillis AL, Kahng MW, Trump BF. (1981) Metabolic studies of glycerol-induced acute renal failure in the rat. *Exp Molec Pathol* 35: 1–13.

Trueta J, Barclay AE, Franklin KJ, Daniel PM, Prichard MML. (1947) *Studies of the renal circulation.* Blackwell Scientific Publication, Oxford.

Vallance P, Collier J, Moncada S. (1989) Effects of endothelium-derived nitric oxide on peripheral arteriolar tone in man. *Lancet* 997–1000.

Vanholder R, Sever MS, Desmet M, Erek E, Lameire N. (2001) Intervention of the renal disaster relief task force in 1999 Marmara earthquake. *Kidney Internat* 59: 783–791.

Vetterlein R, Hoffmann F, Pedina J, Neckel M, Schmidt G. (1995) Disturbances in renal microcirculation induced by myoglobin and hemorrhagic hypotension in anesthetized rat. *Am J Physiol* 268: F839–F846.

Wakabayashi Y, Kikawada R. (1996) Effect of L-arginine on myoglobin-induced acute renal failure in the rabbit. *Am J Physiol* 270: F784–F789.

Yuile CL, Gold MA, Hinds EG. (1945) Hemoglobin precipitation in renal tubules. *J Exp Med* 82: 36–374.

Zager RA. (1991) Myoglobin depletes renal adenine nucleotide pools in the presence and absence of shock. *Kidney Intl* 39: 111–119.

Zager RA. (1992) Combined mannitol and deferoxamine therapy for myohemoglobinuric renal injury and oxidant stress. Mechanistic and therapeutic implications. *J Clin Invest* 90: 711–719.

Zager RA. (1996) Rhabdomyolysis and myohemoglobinuric acute renal failure. *Kidney Intl* 49: 314–326.

Zager RA, Gamelin LM. (1989) Pathogenetic mechanisms in experimental hemoglobinuric acute renal failure. *Am J Physiol* 256: F446–F455.

Zager RA, Teubner EJ, Adler S. (1987) Low molecular weight proteinuria exacerbates experimental ischemic renal injury. *Lab Invest* 56: 180–188.

Zager RA, Burkhart K, Conrad DS, Gmur DJ. (1995) Iron, heme oxygenase, and glutathione: Effects on myohemoglubinuric proximal tubular injury. *Kidney Intl* 48: 1624–1634.

Zager RA, Burkhart K, Conrad DS, Gmur DJ, Iwata M. (1996) Phospholipase A2 induced cytoprotection of proximal tubules: Potential determinants and specificity for ATP depletion mediated injury. *J Am Soc Nephrol* 71: 64–72.

5

Muscle injury in athletics

Thomas M. Best

Introduction

The tendon–muscle fibre–tendon linkage, that connects bone to bone and is responsible for movement and limb control, is a unique component of skeletal muscle. Exercise commonly results in injury to this linkage, particularly if the exercise is intense, of long duration, or involves eccentric activity. Muscle also contains an extracellular matrix, nerves, and blood vessels, all of which can be injured during exercise; this should be kept in mind during the evaluation and treatment of injury.

Injury to skeletal muscle can occur through a variety of mechanisms: direct blunt trauma, laceration, ischaemia, and stretch-induced or muscle-overload injury. This chapter will focus on the primary injuries to muscle that occur with athletic activity: muscle strains and contusions. Muscles crossing one joint such as the soleus muscle often lie close to bone and are more responsible for postural maintenance; these muscles are most susceptible to contusion injury. Muscles crossing two joints such as the rectus femoris are more susceptible to stretch-induced damage (strain). For each injury we will discuss the mechanism, diagnosis, and factors affecting the occurrence and magnitude of injury (Table 5.1). Treatment and prevention recommendations will be reviewed, and complications such as compartment syndrome, myositis ossificans and rhabdomyolysis will also be considered.

Strain injuries

Muscle strains have been estimated to represent between 30% and 67% of athletic injuries (Herring 1990, Kibler 1990). Muscle strains are usually associated with stretch of non-activated or, more commonly, an actively contracting muscle. The latter has been termed an eccentric contraction, or perhaps more correctly a pliometric contraction (Hunter and Faulkner 1997). This is in contrast to a concentric (or miometric) contraction where the muscle shortens during activation, or an isometric contraction in which muscle length remains constant.

A continuum of muscle strain injuries exists. The most benign form is delayed onset muscle soreness (DOMS), where no acute symptoms are present. The typically more severe acute muscle strains can be partial, in which some muscle function is still present, or complete tears, which may require surgical management.

Delayed onset muscle soreness

DOMS is characterized by generalized muscle soreness and weakness 1–2 days following exercise, and rarely in long-term morbidity.

Mechanism

There is general consensus that the initial insult is mechanical damage to the contractile apparatus (Warren et al 1993). Local sarcomere overstretching can result in disruption of the sarcolemma, sarcoplasmic reticulum and myofilaments. Sarcolemmal disruption allows efflux of intracellular proteins, such as creatine phusphukinase (CPK) and Lactate Dehydrogenase (LDH), and influx of extracellular calcium. Muscle fibres contain intrinsic autodegradative and proteolytic pathways that are activated by the initial injury, and which can result in further fibre damage (Armstrong 1990). Intracellular calcium overload is thought to be an important intermediary in this process (Fig. 5.1).

DOMS injury usually occurs to a very small proportion of fibres (Friden et al 1983). A loss of labelling for the structural protein desmin, a component of Z-discs, occurs rapidly (Lieber et al 1994). Z-band streaming, A-band disruption and myofibril mis-

Table 5.1— Characteristics of major forms of muscle injury observed in athletics

Injury type	DOMS[a]	Partial strain	Complete strain (tear)	Contusion
Mechanism	Rep. stretch	Single stretch	Single stretch	Blunt trauma
Pain	After 24–72 h	Immediate	Immediate	Immediate
Site	Muscle belly	MTJ[a]	MTJ or muscle belly	Muscle belly
Bleeding	None	May escape	May escape	Confined to injury site
Surgery	No	No	Possible	Possible
Complications	Rhabdomyolysis	Sear function	Sear function	Rhabdomyolysis, compartment syndrome, myositis ossificans

[a]DOMS, delayed-onset muscle soreness; MTJ, musculotendinous junction.

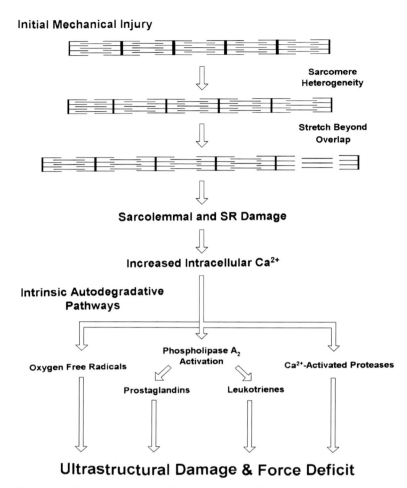

Figure 5.1 — Proposed mechanism of delayed-onset muscle soreness (DOMS) injury. The initial mechanical injury is thought to result in an increased intracellular calcium, which may activate several autodegradative pathways within the muscle fibre. (SR, sarcoplasmic reticulum)

alignment can be seen within 10 min of eccentric exercise (Armstrong et al 1983). An inflammatory response follows, and neutrophils invade the injury site, releasing cytokines that attract additional inflammatory cells. Neutrophils may also promote further damage through the release of oxygen free radicals and lysosomal proteases. Macrophages subsequently invade damaged fibres and phagocytose debris.

Diagnosis

The soreness is generally described as a dull aching pain that may be localized to the musculotendinous junction or experienced throughout the muscle.

Muscle soreness is typically maximum at 24–72 h and is usually gone by 5 to 7 days.

Other sequelae include stiffness, swelling and a reduction in range of motion (ROM) and force production. The reduction in maximal muscle force and power production may be caused by a decrease voluntary effort secondary to pain, as well as a decline in the intrinsic force-generating capacity due to fibre damage. In some animal studies, the decrease in force production follows a biphasic pattern, with an initial decrease immediately following the injury, a partial recovery 24 h later and a subsequent secondary reduction in contractile force at 48 h (McCully and Faulkner 1986).

Factors influencing occurrence and magnitude of injury

DOMS can occur following any unaccustomed physical activity. The intensity of activity is important in determining the magnitude of the damage, and several studies, primarily with animal models, have focused on isolating mechanical factors best correlated with the extent of injury. Force production deficit following protocols of repeated eccentric contractions has been correlated with both the elevated peak forces (McCully and Faulkner 1986, Warren et al 1993) and the strain imposed (Lieber and Friden 1993) during the stretch. Newham and coauthors (1988) observed a greater decline in maximal voluntary contraction force after contractions initiated from a longer initial fibre length. However, these studies are complicated by the fact that a force deficit may also result from fatigue. The fibre damage and decline in force production with eccentric exercise occur within the first 15 min of the exercise protocol (McCully and Faulkner 1986, Lieber et al 1996). One interpretation of these results is that fatigue may serve to protect muscle fibres against this form of damage, perhaps by limiting the peak forces produced.

Ageing appears to have two important effects on eccentric contraction-induced injury. Muscles from old rats are injured more than muscles from young rats, and they recover more slowly from injuries of similar magnitude (Brooks and Faulkner 1990). In fact, muscles from older animals may have deficits for months afterwards.

Training, stretching and proper warm-up are often recommended as strategies to help prevent DOMS. Prior training with eccentric exercise had been shown to protect against similar subsequent injury in humans (Friden et al 1983), rats (Schwane and Armstrong 1983), and mice (Sacco and Jones 1992). It appears that the training adaptation has a finite duration (Sacco and Jones 1992). One theory regarding the protective effect of training has been the "fragile fibre" hypothesis: fibres that are most susceptible to injury are damaged during an initial bout of eccentric contractions and then replaced with newer, more robust fibres (Armstrong et al 1983). However, in rats one 30-minute protocol of downhill running, which in itself did not result in an increase in plasma CPK, was sufficient to decrease the damage seen following subsequent downhill running (Schwane and Armstrong 1983). This would suggest that injury during training may not be necessary to produce protective effects during exercise, although it must be remembered that muscle enzyme release does not necessarily correlate with extent of injury (Newham et al 1987).

Data on stretching and warm-up and prevention of DOMS are less clear. Rodenberg and coauthors (1994) found that a combined regimen of stretching and warm-up prior to exercise, as well as massage afterwards, resulted in decreased CPK efflux and force deficit following eccentric exercise. At present it would appear that recommendations for stretching and warm-up to protect against DOMS are based primarily on individual experience.

Treatment

The initial treatment of DOMS is aimed primarily at controlling pain, swelling and stiffness. Eccentric contractions should be avoided early in the recovery period to prevent further damage. Total immobilization should also be avoided as this may increase stiffness; active and passive ROM exercises should be carried out as tolerated. Intermittent compression of the affected muscle group has been found to temporarily decrease the swelling and stiffness, but it did not attenuate strength loss (Chelboun et al 1995).

The use of non-steroidal anti-inflammatory drugs (NSAIDs) for delayed onset muscle soreness is somewhat controversial. Naproxen sodium has been shown to attenuate the muscle soreness and strength decrease following eccentric exercise in human volunteers (Dudley et al 1997, Lecomte et al 1998), although it is difficult to ascertain how much of the improved function may have been because of less soreness. On the other hand, NSAID treatment has also been shown to result in a deficit in force generation 1 month after eccentric-contraction induced injury in rabbits (Mishra et al 1995). Many clinicians advise the cautious use of non-steroidal agents and do not recommend them as a routine treatment modality for DOMS.

Further rehabilitation is guided by the individual athlete's response; both flexibility and strength deficits should be objectively measured. Concentric and isometric strengthening protocols, with progressive resistance exercises, can be resumed as tolerated. Isokinetic exercise can be particularly beneficial as the athlete can work through a full range of motion. When full range of motion and adequate strength are achieved, closed kinetic chain and sports specific activities are initiated. No specific criteria for safe return to competition have been examined, although resolution of tissue injury, full ROM, adequate strength and ability to perform sport-specific activities are typically recommended (Herring 1990).

Partial or complete muscle strain

In contrast to DOMS, acute muscle strains typically present immediately with focal pain and weakness, and they may result in significant morbidity. Various grading systems have been proposed (Kujala et al 1997) although their usefulness with regard to treatment and prognosis is not universally accepted.

Mechanism

Acute strains occur more frequently during high-velocity exercise (Best et al 1994). As with DOMS, acute strains are most commonly seen following eccentric contractions, and muscles that perform eccentric contractions to control and regulate movement are, therefore, common sites of injury. Much of the hamstring and quadriceps action during sprinting involves eccentric contractions to control deceleration of the lower extremities. Muscles that are most susceptible to acute strain cross two joints, such as the quadriceps, hamstrings and adductors. For unknown reasons, certain muscles within a particular group are more vulnerable (Speer et al 1993). These include the adductor longus in the adductor group, biceps femoris of the hamstrings, rectus femoris of the quadriceps, and medial head of the gastrocnemius in the triceps surae. Muscles that limit motion at a joint in certain limb positions are also susceptible to strains. For example, the hamstring limits knee extension when the hip is flexed, and the gastrocnemius limits dorsiflexion of the foot when the knee is extended.

Most acute strain injuries occur at or very near the musculotendinous junction (MTJ; Fig. 5.2), and it should be remembered that the MTJ can be suprisingly extensive (e.g., over half the length of the biceps femoris and semimembranosus). A significant amount of bleeding may occur; however, this often takes days to be clinically detectable. The bleeding may escape through the fascia to the subcutaneous space, in which case it often tracks distal to the injury site.

Diagnosis

The athlete usually reports a sudden and intense pain, often accompanied by a "popping" sensation and subsequent tightness in the involved muscle. Weakness and decreased range of motion are other immediate symptoms; total loss of force generation can occur with a complete rupture or tendon avulsion. Local tenderness is often observed. A palpable defect in the muscle belly may be appreciated with severe injuries, and failure of the muscle distal to the defect to contract suggests a complete tear. With complete muscle tears, there will often be an asymmetry compared with the contralateral muscle.

Other injuries may mimic acute muscle strains. For example, the differential diagnosis of hamstring strains includes apophysitis, painful unfused apophysis, acute and old bony avulsions, piriformis syndrome, gluteus medius insertion tendinitis, posterior trochanteric or ischiogluteal bursitis, tight iliotibial tract, pain radiating from the lower back, sacroilitis, ectopic muscle calcification, and pelvic stress fractures (Kujala et al 1997).

Plain X-rays are generally not necessary in the initial evaluation, unless a bony avulsion is suspected as in children with open epiphyseal plates. Plain films may be helpful in demonstrating a complete hamstring avulsion from the ischial tuberosity.

Magnetic resonance imaging (MRI) is superior to computed tomography (CT) for imaging of muscle injuries, except for late ectopic calcium deposition in injured muscle (Speer et al 1993). MRI best depicts the extent of the injury, which is often greater than first appreciated on clinical examination. The optimal time for MRI detection of injury is felt to be between 1 and 3 days post-injury, corresponding to the appearance of maximum oedema. MRI has shown some promise in predicting prognosis following acute hamstring strains (Pomeranz and Heidt 1993). In general, the routine use of MRI is not advocated, although it may be helpful in detecting muscle belly rupture or complete muscle–tendon avulsion, which may prompt surgical repair. MRI may also be helpful in chronic injuries, where scar tissue and nerve entrapment have been reported (Sallay et al 1996).

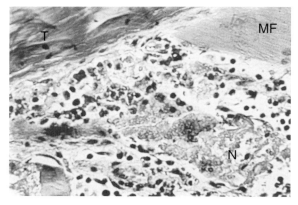

Figure 5.2 — Partial muscle strain injury located near the myotendinous junction, at 24 hours. T – muscle tendon, MF – muscle fibres, N – area of fibre necrosis. Note the presence of inflammatory infiltrate. Magnification = 100×.

Factors influencing occurrence and magnitude of injury

Muscle strains are most common in sprinters or speed athletes, and they are frequently observed in sports that require rapid velocity changes (such as football, basketball, rugby, soccer and sprinting). Common sites in addition to those mentioned earlier include: the biceps and triceps in weight lifters and baseball pitchers, the adductors in horseback riders, soccer players and bowlers, and the calf muscle in boxers, tennis players and runners (Chamout and Skinner 1986; Fig. 5.3). Affected muscles typically have a high percentage of Type II muscle fibres (Garrett 1990).

Animal models of injury following single eccentric contractions have made it possible to more precisely define the mechanical factors responsible for injury,

since single contractions do not result in fatigue. Brooks and coauthors (1995) found the most important single predictor of force production deficit to be the displacement, or magnitude, of the imposed stretch. The combination of displacement and average force produced (the work done, or energy absorbed) explained 82% of the variation in force deficit. For single eccentric contractions initiated from a range of initial fibre lengths, the best prediction of the extent of subsequent injury is the work or energy absorbed, combined with the initial fibre length (Hunter and Faulkner 1997). Others have shown that the strain experienced locally within a fibre predicts the site of injury (Best et al 1994).

Baseline muscle strength and flexibility are thought to be important factors in determining susceptibility to injury, particularly with respect to strength imbalances

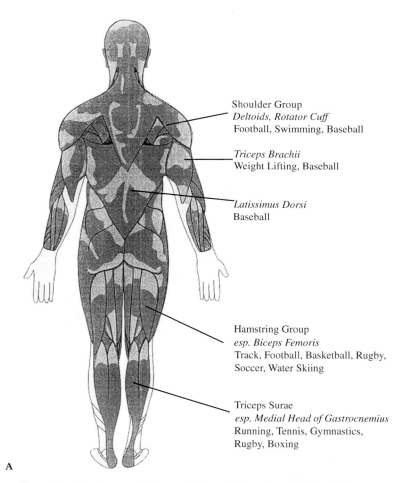

Shoulder Group
Deltoids, Rotator Cuff
Football, Swimming, Baseball

Triceps Brachii
Weight Lifting, Baseball

Latissimus Dorsi
Baseball

Hamstring Group
esp. Biceps Femoris
Track, Football, Basketball, Rugby, Soccer, Water Skiing

Triceps Surae
esp. Medial Head of Gastrocnemius
Running, Tennis, Gymnastics, Rugby, Boxing

A

Figure 5.3 — Muscles susceptible to strain injury during various athletic activities.

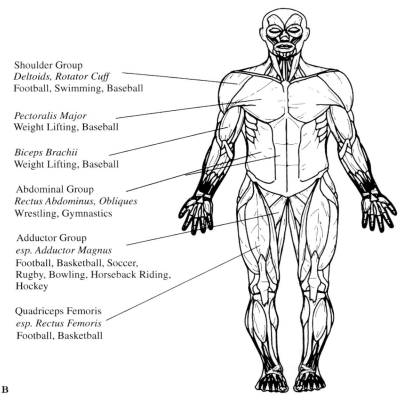

Shoulder Group
Deltoids, Rotator Cuff
Football, Swimming, Baseball

Pectoralis Major
Weight Lifting, Baseball

Biceps Brachii
Weight Lifting, Baseball

Abdominal Group
Rectus Abdominus, Obliques
Wrestling, Gymnastics

Adductor Group
esp. Adductor Magnus
Football, Basketball, Soccer,
Rugby, Bowling, Horseback Riding,
Hockey

Quadriceps Femoris
esp. Rectus Femoris
Football, Basketball

B

Figure 5.3 (continued)

between agonist and antagonist groups (Cross and Worrell 1999). A history of previous strain injury to the involved muscle is thought to be a significant risk factor for subsequent injury (Garret 1996). Ekstrand and Gillquist (1983) found that minor hamstring injuries were often followed by a more severe injury within 2 months. In addition to a loss of active force-generating ability, muscles lose tensile strength following injury (Obremsky et al 1994), and tensile strength recovers more slowly than force-generating capacity. The loss of tensile strength may predispose to further strain injury early in recovery (Garrett 1990).

Clinical observation suggests that muscle strain injuries often occur late in practice sessions or competition, leading to the hypothesis that fatigue may predispose to acute strain injuries (in contrast to DOMS, where fatigue may actually have a protective effect). Studies of rabbit muscles injured by applied stretches have noted that muscles were injured at the same length regardless of fatigue, but that it took less energy or work absorption to bring fatigued muscles to this length (Mair et al 1996).

Training, stretching, and warm-up are often recommended for the prevention of acute muscle strains, as with DOMS. There would seem to be at least some support in the literature for each of these recommendations (Safran et al 1989, Taylor et al 1990), although direct clinical studies are scarce and they often do not attempt to isolate individual risk factors. The introduction of a stretching program in a Division III football program resulted in a 48.8% decrease in the number of lower extremity strain injuries compared with the previous year (Cross and Worrell 1999).

Treatment

The vast majority of acute strain injuries can be managed non-operatively. Indications for consideration of surgical intervention include complete rupture of the muscle belly or musculotendinous junction, and avulsion of the muscle–tendon complex from bone. Examples of the latter include avulsion of the hamstring from the ischial tuberosity, adductor from the femur, and pectoralis major from the humerus (Wolfe et al 1992). Apophyseal avulsions may also occur in the paediatric population, although these rarely require surgical repair. Successful late repair of chronic complete tendon rupture has been reported (Cross et al 1998). Surgery may also be considered in cases of large intramuscular haematoma or strains involving over half of the muscle belly (Kujala et al 1997).

If conservative treatment is selected, a balance between rest and early ROM is important. Rest is important in order to protect against reinjury, and early immobilization has been shown to accelerate formation of the granulation tissue matrix (Jarvinen and Lehto 1993). However, immobilization can also lead to atrophy, stiffness, and weakness (Herring 1990), as well as deleterious effects on surrounding cartilage, ligament, bone and joint capsules. Early tensile loading of muscle and tendon may facilitate proper collagen-fibre growth, limit adhesions, and help to maintain proprioception (Herring 1990). Therefore, a reasonable recommendation is to begin early mobilization after a sufficient period (3–5 days for rat muscle) of immobilization (Jarvinen and Lehto 1993).

Icing is recommended in the first 48 h to decrease muscle spasm, pain and swelling. A compression dressing may also be used to minimize swelling. Most clinicians reserve heat application for subacute or chronic injuries. Ultrasound is widely recommended in some circles, but there are no studies to date which clearly provide a scientific rationale for its use (Kujala et al 1997). A study with contusion injuries (Rantanen et al 1999) found a promotion of satellite cell proliferation, but no significant effects on the overall morphology of muscle regeneration.

Medications including analgesics, muscle relaxants, steroids, topical anaesthetics, and NSAIDs have been used in the treatment of muscle strains. As with DOMS, the use of NSAIDs in muscle strains is debatable, and a similar recommendation to limit their use to the acute healing phase is now advocated (Kujala et al 1997). Piroxicam treatment in animal studies early in recovery (Obremsky et al 1994), but delayed muscle regeneration at the injury site (Almekinders and Gilbert 1986, Obremsky et al 1994).

Progress through the stages of rehabilitation is primarily gauged on an individual basis by the athlete's pain, although objective measures of flexibility and strength should also be monitored. As recovery proceeds, and active and passive ROM exercises are well-tolerated, strengthening can be initiated with isometric exercises. When comfortable, isotonic and isokinetic exercises with progressive resistance are instituted for both the injured and antagonist muscles.

Full ROM and adequate strength permit transition to closed kinetic chain and sport-specific activities. While specific rehabilitation of the injured muscle is being accomplished, aerobic exercise should be prescribed to maintain cardiovascular fitness.

Before return to competition, there is general agreement that joint ROM should be full compared with the uninjured side, and the athlete should be able to perform sport-specific activities without difficulty; it has been suggested that strength should be 90% of the uninjured side. Sport-specific retraining has been thought to play an important role in avoiding reinjury (Herring 1990). However, there are no studies of objective criteria for safe return to competition.

Contusion injuries

Contusions are a result of direct trauma to the involved muscle group, with subsequent bleeding leading to pain and swelling. In contrast to the bleeding seen with muscle strain, which can extravasate the area, bleeding after contusions is usually confined to within the muscle belly. Contusions are most frequently seen in contact sports, particularly football, hockey and soccer. The quadriceps and gastrocnemius groups are most often involved.

Initial treatment should emphasize aggressive control of swelling and bleeding with ice, compression, elevation, and flexion at the proximal joint (Ryan et al 1991). The resultant pain can often be significant, and narcotics may be necessary for short-term use. As with strain injuries, NSAID use is somewhat controversial as this may increase bleeding. If the girth of the injured region has not stabilized at 48 h, other injuries such as compartment syndrome or muscle rupture should be considered.

The second phase of rehabilitation, which begins after swelling has stabilized, focuses on restoration of motion. Initially, passive ROM exercises are utilized, with active ROM exercises often started within 24 h. Excessive passive stretching of a previously immobilized limb has produced myositis ossificans in animal models, but in general early ROM has resulted in reduced scar formation (Jarvinen and Lehto 1993). Isometric exercises are begun when they can be performed without pain, and weight-bearing as tolerated may be allowed. Eventually progressive resistance exercises are initiated; for quadriceps contusions, this is often done when subjects regain 90° of knee flexion.

No clinically proven objective guidelines for safe return to competition exist. Some authors (Aronen and Chronister 1992) have recommended that return to play after quadriceps contusion is possible when athletes have regained 120° or more of active knee flexion, and they show no evidence of atrophy, weakness, or asynchronous muscle function. It does appear that reinjury of an injured muscle is the major risk factor for the development of myositis ossificans (King 1998).

Traumatic myositis ossificans should be suspected when there is persistent oedema, warmth and tenderness of a contused muscle group. It occurs when severe compression of soft tissue against bone results in disruption of muscle fibres, capillaries, connective tissue and periosteum, with subsequent heterotopic bone formation (Fig. 5.4). In addition to reinjury, early massage and excessively vigorous mobilization and rehabilitation have been claimed to be risk factors (Kujala et al 1997). Clinical findings may include a tender bony mass, marked muscle atrophy, and notable restricted joint motion. Usually the lesion becomes radiographically evident 2–4 weeks following a severe contusion, and it resembles mature lamellar bone by 4–6 months. The differential diagnosis includes osteosarcoma, post-traumatic periostitis and osteomyelitis. As soon as this entity is suspected, a treatment regimen of rest, pain-free passive stretching, and NSAIDs should be prescribed. NSAID therapy (e.g., indomethacin for 6 weeks) is sometimes helpful in reducing inflammation and further bone formation. Surgery should be avoided within the first 4 months because it may exacerbate heterotopic bone formation and prolong disability. Surgical intervention should be considered only when the heterotopic bone is mature, which may take up to 1 year. Recovery of normal function is possible even in the presence of myositis ossificans.

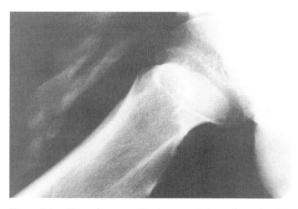

Figure 5.4— X-ray demonstrating heterotopic bone formation in a college athlete.

Compartment syndrome

Compartment syndrome occurs when interstitial pressure within a closed fascial space exceeds capillary perfusion pressure. The resulting ischaemia can cause paralysis, muscle necrosis, contractures, and permanent nerve and muscle damage. Acute compartment syndrome is seen most often in the lower extremity, but it has been observed in the anterior and posterior compartments of the thigh (Kujala et al 1997) and the flexor and pronator forearm muscles (Berlemann et al 1998). It usually occurs after trauma and contusion injury, but it can be seen after unaccustomed intense exercise without trauma.

Diagnosis should always be considered when pain is out of proportion to the injury. Compartment syndrome make take from 12 to 24 h to develop following trauma. It usually presents as a tense, swollen, tender muscle. Severe pain with passive motion should prompt one to consider the diagnosis. The presence of all five "Ps" (pain out of proportion, pain on passive motion, pulselessness, paresthesia, and pallor) is a late finding and it carries a poor prognosis. The diagnosis is confirmed by measuring compartment pressures, although some disagreement exists as to the threshold for surgical intervention. The range of values used is 30–45 mmHg, or within 10–30 mmHg of diastolic pressure. Acute compartment syndrome is a medical emergency, and consultation with an orthopaedic or vascular surgeon should be obtained so that fasciotomy can be performed if the diagnosis is confirmed.

Chronic exertional compartment syndrome (CECS) has also been described. The typical presentation is an athlete with an aching and cramping lower leg or forearm pain that comes on only during activity. Occasionally, a mild ache in the affected area may persist for a short time after activity. The gold standard for diagnosis of CECS is compartment pressure testing. Treatment recommendations are rest and cross-training; if unsuccessful, surgical fasciotomy may be necessary for relief of symptoms.

Rhabdomyolysis

Rhabdomyolysis, or muscle breakdown, may occur after contusions, strain injuries or exertional heat stroke. If severe enough, myoglobinuria results, presenting clinically as dark brown or rust-coloured urine accompanied by muscle aches, swelling, and weakness (which can be severe). Dehydration and hypokalaemia place the athlete at higher risk for myoglobinuria. The most significant potential complication is acute tubular necrosis caused by obstruction of the nephrons by myoglobin. Urine dipstick testing is positive for blood even in the absence of gross haematuria. Up to 5-fold elevations in plasma creatine kinase (CK) levels can be noted, although serum CK levels do not seem to correlate with the degree of renal failure (Campion et al 1972). Plasma creatine may rise because of both muscle breakdown and renal failure, and it is out of proportion to plasma Blood Urea Nitrogen (BUN).

Maintenance of urine output is the mainstay of treatment. For mild to moderate cases oral rehydration may be sufficient, while severe cases require aggressive intravenous hydration and occasionally diuretics such as mannitol or furosemide. Establishment of an alkaline urine by adding bicarbonate to the intravenous fluid may be helpful. Electrolyte imbalances are frequent and they should be corrected. Daily weight monitoring can be followed to assess rehydration, and the decrease in weight from baseline should be less than 3% before the next training session is allowed (Rucker and Tanner 1992). Serum CK levels should be monitored and further exercise avoided while they remain elevated. Endurance training is thought to help prevent rhabdomyolysis, and it has been shown to decrease the incidence of myoglobinuria after intense exercise in military recruits (Hurley 1989).

References

Almekinders LC, Gilbert JA. (1986) Healing of experimental muscle strains and the effects of nonsteroidal anti-inflammatory medication. *Am J Sports Med* 14: 303–308.

Armstrong RB, Ogilvie RW, Schwane JA. (1983) Eccentric exercise-induced injury to rat skeletal muscle. *J Appl Physiol* 54: 80–93.

Armstrong RB. (1990) Initial events in exercise-induced muscular injury. *Med Sci Sports Exerc* 22: 429–435.

Aronen JG, Chronister RD. (1992) Quadriceps contusions: Hastening the return to play. *Physician Sportsmedicine* 20: 130–136.

Berlemann U, al Momani Z, Hertel R. (1998) Exercise-induced compartment syndrome in the flexor-pronator muscle group. A case report and pressure measurements in volunteers. *Am J Sports Med* 26: 439–441.

Best TM, Hasselman CT, Garrett WE. (1994) Clinical aspects and basic science of muscle strain injuries. *BAM* 4: 77–90.

Best TM. (1997) Soft tissue injuries and muscle tears. *Clin Sports Med* 16: 419–434.

Brooks SV, Faulkner JA. (1990) Contraction-induced injury: recovery of skeletal muscles in young and old mice. *Am J Physiol* 258: C436–442.

Brooks SV, Zerba E, Faulkner JA. (1995) Injury to muscle fibres after single stretched of passive and maximally stimulated muscles in mice. *J Physiol* 488: 459–469.

Campion DS, Arais JM, Carter NW. (1972) Rhabdomyolysis and myoglobinuria. Association with hypokalemia of renal tubular acidosis. *JAMA* 220: 967–969.

Chammout MO, Skinner HB. (1986) The clinical anatomy of commonly injured muscle bellies. *J Trauma* 26: 549–552.

Chelboun GS, Howell JN, Baker HL, et al. (1995) Intermittent pneumatic compression effect on eccentric exercise-induced swelling, stiffness, and strength loss. *Arch Phys Med Rehab* 76: 744–749.

Cross KM, Worrell TW. (1999) Effects of a static stretching program on the incidence of lower extremity musculotendinous strains. *J Athletic Training* 34: 11–14.

Cross MJ, Vandersluis R, Wood D, Banff M. (1998) Surgical repair of chronic complete hamstring tendon rupture in the adult patient. *Am J Sports Med* 26: 785–788.

Dudley GA, Czerkawski J, Meinrod A, Gillis F, Baldwin A, Scarpone M. (1997) Efficacy of naproxen sodium for exercise-induced dysfunction muscle injury and soreness. *Clin J Sports Med* 7: 3–10.

Ekstrand J, Gillquist J. (1983) Soccer injuries and their mechanisms: a prospective study. *Med Sci Sports Exercise* 15: 267–270.

Friden J, Seger J, Sjostrom M, Ekblom B. (1983) Adaptive response in human skeletal muscle subjected to prolonged eccentric training. *Intl J Sports Med* 4: 177–183.

Friden J, Sjostrom M, Ekblom B. (1983) Myofibrillar damage following intense eccentric exercise in man. *Intl J Sports Med* 4: 170–176.

Garrett WE, Jr. (1990) Muscle strain injuries: clinical and basic aspects. *Med Sci Sports Exercise* 22: 436–443.

Garrett WE, Jr. (1996) Muscle strain injuries. *Am J Sports Med* 24: S2–8.

Herring SA. (1990) Rehabilitation of muscle injuries. *Med Sci Sports Exercise* 22: 453–456.

Hunter KD, Faulkner JA. (1997) Pliometric contraction-induced injury in mouse skeletal muscle: effect of initial length. *J App Physiol* 82: 278–283.

Hurley JK. (1989) Severe rhabdomyolsis in well conditioned athletes. *Military Med* 154: 244–245.

Jarvinen MJ, Lehto MU. (1993) The effects of early mobilisation and immobilisation on the healing process following muscle injury. *Sports Med* 15: 78–89.

Kibler WB. (1990) Clinical aspects of muscle injury. *Med Sci Sports Exercise* 22: 450–452.

King JB. (1998) Post-traumatic ectopic calcification in the muscles of athletes: a review. *Br J Sports Med* 32: 287–290.

Kujala UM, Orava S, Jarvinen M. (1997) Hamstring injuries. Current trends in treatment and prevention. *Sports Med* 32: 287–290.

Lecomte JM, Lacroix VJ, Montgomery DL. (1998) A randomized controlled trial of the effects of naproxen on delayed onset muscle soreness and muscle strength. *Clin J Sports Med* 8: 82–87.

Lieber RL, Friden J. (1993) Muscle damage is not a function of muscle force but active muscle strain. *J Appl Physiol* 74: 520–526.

Lieber RL, Schmitz MC, Mishra DK, Firdne J. (1994) Contractile and cellular remodeling in rabbit skeletal muscle after cyclic eccentric contractions. *J Appl Physiol* 77: 1926–1934.

Lieber RL, Thornell LE, Friden J. (1996) Muscle cytoskeletal disruption occurs within the first 15 min of cyclic eccentric contraction. *J Appl Physiol* 80: 278–284.

Mair SD, Seaber AV, Glisson RR, Garrett WE, Jr. (1996) The role of fatigue in susceptibility to acute muscle strain injury. *Am J Sports Med* 24: 137–143.

McCully KK, Faulkner JA. (1986) Characteristics of lengthening contractions associated with injury to skeletal muscle fibres. *J Appl Physiol* 61: 293–299.

Mishra DK, Firden J, Schmitz MD, Lieber RL. (1995) Anti-inflammatory medication after muscle injury. A treatment resulting in short-term improvement but subsequent loss of muscle function. *J Bone Joint Sur* – American Volume 77: 1510–1519.

Newham DJ, Jones DA, Clarkson PM. (1987) Repeated high-force eccentric exercise: effects on muscle pain and damage. *J Appl Physiol* 63: 1381–1386.

Newham DJ, Jones DA, Ghosh G, Aurora P. (1998) Muscle fatigue and pain after eccentric contractions at long and short length. *Clin Sci* 74: 553–557.

Obremsky WT, Seaber AV, Ribbeck BM, Garrett WE, Jr. (1994) Biomechanical and histologic assessment of a controlled muscle strain injury treated with piroxicam. *Am J Sports Med* 22: 558–561.

Pomeranz SJ, Heidt RS, Jr. (1993) MR imaging in the prognostication of hamstring injury. Work in progress. *Radiol* 189: 897–900.

Rantanen J, Thorsson O, Wollmer P, Hurme T, Kalimo H. (1999) Effects of therapeutic ultrasound on the regeneration of skeletal myofibres after experimental muscle injury. *Am J Sports Med* 27: 54–59.

Rodenberg JB, Steenbeek D, Schiereck P, Bar PR. (1994) Warm-up, stretching and massage diminish harmful effects of eccentric exercise. *Intl J Sports Med* 15: 414–419.

Rucker KS, Tanner R. (1992) Reconditioning after exertional rhabdomyolsis: Avoiding setbacks. *Physician Sportsmedicine* 20: 95–102.

Ryan JB, Wheeler JH, Hopkinson WJ, Arciero RA, Kolakowski KR. (1991) Quadriceps contusions. West Point update. *Am J Sports Med* 19: 299–304.

Sacco P, Jones DA. (1992) The protective effect of damaging eccentric exercise against repeated bouts of exercise in the mouse tibialis anterior muscle. *Exp Physiol* 77: 757–760.

Safran MR, Seaber AV, Garret WE, Jr. (1989) Warm-up and muscular injury prevention. An update. *Sports Med* 8: 239–249.

Sallay PI, Friedman RL, Coogan PG, Garrett WE. (1996) Hamstring muscle injuries among water skiers. Functional outcome and prevention. *Am J Sports Med* 24: 130–136.

Schwane JA, Armstrong RB. (1983) Effect of training on skeletal muscle injury from downhill running in rats. *J Appl Physiol* 55: 969–975.

Speer KP, Lohnes J, Garrett WE, Jr. (1993) Radiographic imaging of muscle strain injury. *Am J Sports Med* 21: 89–95.

Taylor DC, Dalton JD, Jr, Seaber AV, Garrett WE, Jr. (1990) Viscoelastic properties of muscle-tendon units. The biomechanical effects of stretching. *Am J Sports Med* 18: 300–309.

Warren GL, Hayes DA, Lowe DA, Armstrong RB. (1993) Mechanical factors in the initiation of eccentric contraction-induced injury in rat soleus muscle. *J Physiol (Lond)* 464: 457–475.

Wolfe SW, Wickiewicz TL, Cavanaugh JT. (1992) Ruptures of the pectoralis major muscle. An anatomic and clinical analysis. *Am J Sports Med* 20: 587–593.

6

Cancer cachexia

Josep M. Argilés and Francisco J. López-Soriano

Introduction

Cancer cachexia is a complex syndrome that occurs in more than two thirds of patients who die with advanced cancer, and it is responsible for nearly a third of cancer deaths. In addition, the degree of cachexia is inversely correlated with the survival time of the patient, and it always implies a poor prognosis (De Wys 1985). Cachexia is characterized by weight loss, anorexia, weakness, anaemia and asthenia. Asthenia is probably the most prevalent symptom of patients with advanced cancer and it reflects very well one of the most interesting factors involved in cancer cachexia, that of muscle wastage (Argilés et al 1992). Indeed lean body mass depletion is one of the main trends of cachexia, and it involves not only skeletal muscle but it also affects cardiac protein, resulting in important alterations in heart performance (Houten and Reilley 1980).

The complications associated with the appearance of cachexia affect both the physiological and bio-chemical balance of the patient, and they have effects on the efficiency of the anticancer treatment. At the metabolic level, cachexia is associated with loss of skeletal muscle protein together with a depletion of body lipid stores. The cachectic patient, in addition to having practically no adipose tissue, is basically subject to an important muscle wastage manifested as an excessive nitrogen loss. Different explanations can be found to account for cancer-induced cachexia. Tumour growth is associated with a malnutrition status resulting from the induction of anorexia. In addition, the competition for nutrients between the tumour and the host leads to an "accelerated" starvation state (Argilés and Azcón-Bieto 1988), which promotes severe metabolic disturbances in the host (Table 6.1). The metabolic changes are partially mediated by alterations in circulating hormone concentrations or in their effectiveness. On the other hand, a large number of observations point towards cytokines as the molecules responsible for the above referred metabolic derangements. This chapter deals with the changes in muscle metabolism that are found in the host during tumour burden, together with the possible mediators of cachexia. The role of different tumour-secreted compounds and humoral factors is discussed; among these, tumour necrosis factor-α (TNF) seems to have a key role in cachexia.

Table 6.1 — Metabolic changes induced by the presence of the tumour

Carbohydrate metabolism
Glucose intolerance
Increased hepatic gluconeogenesis
Increased Cori cycle activity
Increased glucose turnover
Decreased skeletal muscle glucose uptake
Lipid metabolism
Decreased total host lipid
Hyperlipidaemia
Increased lipolysis
Decreased white adipose tissue LPL
Protein metabolism
Increased whole body protein turnover
Increased hepatic protein synthesis
Increased skeletal muscle protein breakdown
Decreased skeletal muscle amino acid uptake
Increased BCAA turnover
Changes in circulating amino acid pattern
Main hormonal changes
Insulin resistance
Normal or decreased insulin secretion
Increased counter-regulatory hormones (cortisol, catecholamines)

Muscle wasting during cancer

Asthenia is directly related to the muscle wastage observed in cachectic states. The skeletal muscle, which accounts for almost half of the whole body protein mass, is severely affected in cancer cachexia (Lawson et al 1982), and evidence has been provided for muscle protein wastage as being associated with enhanced turnover rates (Tessitore et al 1987, Melville et al 1990). Since cachexia tends to develop at a rather advanced stage of the neoplastic growth, preventing muscle wastage in cancer patients is of great clinical interest. Whether the negative protein balance results from altered rates of synthesis or breakdown, or from changes on both sides of muscle protein turnover is still debated (Emery et al 1982, Tessitore et al 1987, Pain et al 1984). Rennie et al (1983) have suggested that, during cancer cachexia, the muscle mass is decreased as a result of a lower rate of protein synthesis, while changes in protein degradation are secondary. Conversely, studies involving the release of 3-methylhistidine (a marker of myofibrillar protein degradation) from peripheral muscle in cancer patients suggest that protein degradation is clearly increased (Lundholm et al 1982). We have demonstrated, using several experimental models, that protein synthesis is hardly altered in skeletal muscle during tumour growth and that there is a great increase in protein degradation both in vivo (Costelli et al 1993) and in vitro (García-Martínez et al 1995). The result of the enhanced proteolysis is a large release of amino acids from skeletal muscle, particularly of alanine and glutamine. The release of amino acids is also potentiated by an inhibition of amino acid transport into skeletal muscle (García-Martínez et al 1995). Alanine is mainly channelled to the liver for both gluconeogenesis and protein synthesis. Interestingly, liver fractional rates of protein synthesis are increased in tumour-bearing animals, accounting for the production of the so-called acute phase proteins, while there is a decrease in albumin synthesis (Kern and Norton 1988). Glutamine is basically taken up by the tumour to sustain both the energy and nitrogen demands of the growing mass (Medina et al 1992).

Branched-chain amino acids (BCAA) are essential nutrients for both humans and animals, making up to 40% of the minimal daily requirements of indispensable amino acids in humans (Adibi 1976). In studying the mechanism that leads to protein waste, particular interest has been given to the metabolism of these amino acids (Nair et al 1992). The carbon skeletons arising from transamination of BCAA provide a major source of metabolic fuel for skeletal muscle (Fig. 6.1). In wasting disorders plasma concentrations of BCAA are often increased and their turnover rates altered (Argilés and López-Soriano 1990b). It has been demonstrated that in vivo leucine oxidation to CO_2 is enhanced in tumour-bearing animals (Goodlad et al 1981, Argilés and López-Soriano 1990b, Costelli et al 1995b), related to an increased turnover of this amino acid. The trigger for the increased leucine oxidation remains unknown. Williams and Matthaei (1981)

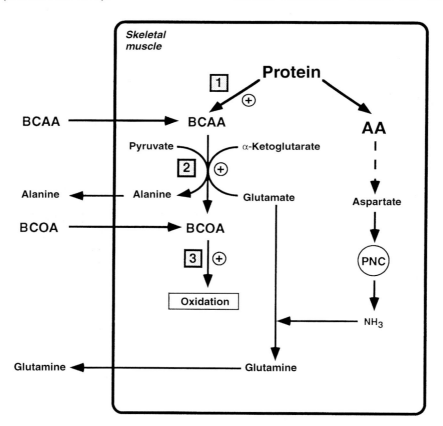

Figure 6.1—**Oxidation of branched-chain amino acids in skeletal muscle**. Both branched-chain amino acids (BCAA) from internal muscle proteolysis (1) or from circulation can be transaminated (2) and later oxidized (3) in skeletal muscle, resulting in both alanine and glutamine release. Branched-chain 2-oxo acids (BCOA) coming basically from liver can also be oxidized. During cancer cachexia, there is an activation of these processes: (1) ATP-dependent proteolysis, (2) BCAA transaminase, and (3) BCOA dehydrogenase. (AA, amino acids; PNC, purine nucleotide cycle.)

suggested that the plasma concentration of ketone bodies could modulate the extrahepatic oxidation of BCAA, and that a decrease in their levels during cancer could result in increased oxidation. However, this hypothesis is in contrast with the observation of increased plasma ketone bodies in tumour-bearing mice (Rofe et al 1986). Alternatively, uncontrolled BCAA oxidation may be due to hypoinsulinaemia (Buse et al 1976) or peripheral insulin resistance (Lundholm 1985).

Despite the controversy about the underlying molecular mechanisms of cancer cachexia, the growing tumour has a considerable demand for essential amino acids. Attempts have been made to inhibit the development of cancer by altering the diet composition of ingested amino acids, inducing a state of amino acid imbalance (Brennan 1981). In particular, it has been shown that tumour growth is delayed in rats maintained on a valine-depleted diet; however, this had a negative impact on the nutritional state of the host (Nishihira et al 1993). A tumour can increase considerably the daily need for leucine in humans, the increase having a better correlation with the clinical deterioration of the patient than the modification of carbohydrate and energy metabolism (Lazo 1985). As a result of the demand for leucine, there is an amino acid flux from muscle to the tumour associated with muscle wastage in the host. In general, however, the leucine taken up by the tumour only represents a minor part of the amino acid demand in the tumour-bearing animal (Argilés and López-Soriano 1990b). It can, therefore, be proposed that the major contribution to BCAA oxidation in cancer-bearing states is made by skeletal muscle. Indeed, BCAA are the only amino acids that are extensively degraded in skeletal muscle, and they have been shown to stimulate protein synthesis and inhibit degradation in skeletal muscle in vitro (Buse and Reid 1975, Mitch and Clark 1984) and in vivo (Smith et al 1992). It could be proposed that during cancer cachexia the response of muscle protein turnover to BCAA is altered. Interestingly, the activation of muscle proteolysis in skeletal muscle always parallels that of BCAA oxidation. We have also described that β_2-agonists (clenbuterol in particular) are able to suppress the activation of the ubiquitin-dependent proteolytic system during tumour growth (Costelli et al 1995a). In a similar manner, β_2-agonists are also able to suppress the increase in BCAA oxidation in skeletal muscle during cancer cachexia (Smith et al 1992). Concerning possible mechanisms involved in the activation of BCAA oxidation, hormonal changes could be involved. Insulin resistance is often present during cancer-

bearing states, but recently it has been demonstrated that it does not influence either protein or BCAA metabolism in cancer patients (Pisters et al 1992). The changes in muscle protein turnover are presumably induced by the combined actions of cytokines (Costelli et al 1993) alone or in combination with the so-called stress hormones such as glucagon (Hartl et al 1990), glucocorticoids (Liu et al 1994) and catecholamines.

As a result of these major changes in amino acid metabolism, plasma amino acid profiles are altered in experimental animals (Rivera et al 1987, Argilés and López-Soriano 1990a) and humans (Meguid et al 1992) during cancer-bearing states. It is observed that the concentrations of gluconeogenic amino acids are decreased, particularly in very cachectic tumours, such as those of the lung and gastrointestinal tract. Interestingly, the plasma concentration of BCAA is either normal or increased, even in the presence of severe malnutrition. This finding confirms the profound differences between cancer-induced cachexia and non-cancer malnutrition, in which both gluconeogenic and BCAA are reduced in relation to normal feeding. Another interesting finding concerning plasma amino acids in cancer relates to tryptophan. Meguid et al (1992) have found great increases in free tryptophan concentrations during tumour growth, and they have suggested this amino acid as a marker for neoplastic disease.

The role of the ubiquitin-dependent proteolytic system in muscle wasting

Muscle wasting is generally thought to be caused by an increase in protein breakdown. Indeed, protein degradation is activated in numerous pathological conditions, and it may represent an important factor in loss of body weight since skeletal muscle represents over 40% of total body mass in humans (Forbes 1987). Bearing this in mind, a growing interest has developed concerning the proteolytic systems that are activated in skeletal muscle and that are responsible for muscle wasting in pathological states. The apparent selectivity of the ATP-ubiquitin-dependent pathway makes it an attractive mechanism, which could account for the specificity of protein degradation within skeletal muscle (Fig. 6.2). Thus recent studies have focused on the role of ubiquitin in muscle in a number of patho-

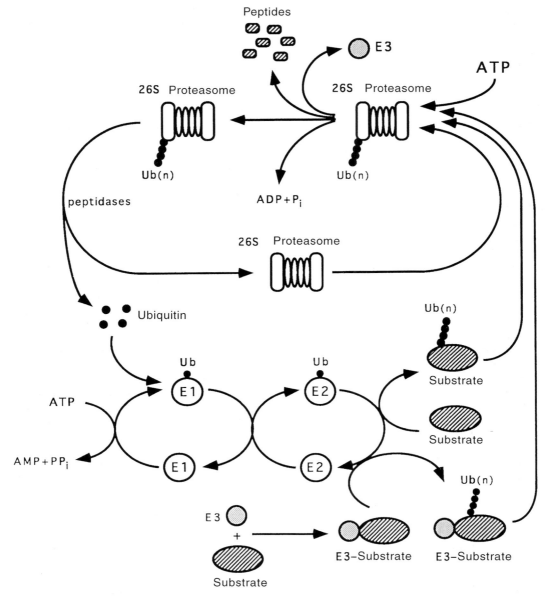

Figure 6.2 — **The ubiquitin-mediated proteolysis**. The ubiquitin-activating enzyme (E1), together with ATP, generates a high energy link (thioester bond) with ubiquitin (Ub), which is then transferred to the ubiquitin-conjugating enzyme (E2). This permits substrate recognition by the multicatalytic protease complex (26S proteasome) and, consequently, its proteolytic degradation in an ATP-dependent process. In some cases, the substrate recognition by the E2 enzyme is mediated by the formation of an ubiquitin–E3–substrate complex. Following ATP-dependent proteasome action, ubiquitin is released from the substrate by means of a peptidase or isopeptidase activity either soluble or linked to the proteasome. The specificity of the degradation pathway is mediated by both E2 and E3 enzymes. (E3, protein ligase.)

Table 6.2 — Pathological states associated with activation of the ubiquitin-dependent proteolytic system in skeletal muscle

- Muscular atrophy
- Tumour growth
- Protein deficiency
- Infection
- Exercise-induced muscle damage
- Burn injury
- Acidosis

logical states (Argilés and López-Soriano 1996, Argilés et al 1998; Table 6.2).

As previously stated, muscle wasting during cancer cachexia is generally accepted to be caused by an increase in protein breakdown with little or no change in protein synthesis (Tessitore et al 1987). Llovera et al (1994) reported that both the presence of ubiquitin conjugates and the expression of different ubiquitin genes is highly elevated in the skeletal muscle of cachectic tumour-bearing rats. In addition, incubations of skeletal muscles from tumour-bearing rats (Llovera et al 1995) revealed little or no involvement of either lysosomal cathepsin and cytosolic Ca^{2+}-dependent calpains in the increased muscle proteolysis encountered in the skeletal muscle of AH-130 Yoshida-bearing rats (Fig. 6.3). Activation of the ubiquitin system in skeletal muscle during cancer cachexia seems to be unrelated to the high circulating levels of glucocorticoids found in these animals (Costelli et al 1993), and it can be reversed by clenbuterol treatment (Costelli et al 1995a). Later work on the involvement of the ubiquitin-dependent pathway in muscle wasting during cancer cachexia has con-

firmed the initial observations (Temparis et al 1994, Baracos et al 1995). Preliminary observations made in skeletal human muscle from cachetic pancreatic patients also point towards the ubiquitin system being responsible for the activation of proteolysis in skeletal muscle.

Wing and Banville (1994) presented the first evidence of hormonal control of ubiquitin conjugation. They cloned the E214k gene responsible for the synthesis of the ubiquitin conjugating enzyme and reported increases in one of the mRNA transcripts with fasting and subsequent decrease with insulin treatment. Therefore, the mechanisms involving insulin and glucocorticoids in modulation of ubiquitin-dependent proteolysis may be completely independent, although insulin can suppress the stimulation of muscle proteolysis by glucocorticoids both in vivo and in vitro (Tomas et al 1984).

At least during fasting, the glucocorticoids seem to be involved in the activation of the proteolytic ubiquitin-dependent pathway in muscle, since adrenalectomy prevents the rise in ubiquitin conjugates after fasting (Wing and Goldberg 1993). The mechanism is unclear since the characteristic sequences found in many glucocorticoid-responsive genes are not found in the ubiquitin genes (Wiborg et al 1985). In addition, studies carried out using the glucocorticoid antagonist RU486 do not support the involvement of glucocorticoids in activating the ubiquitin system during cancer cachexia (Llovera et al 1996b).

Our research group has reported that TNF administration to rats results in an increase in skeletal muscle proteolysis both in vivo (Llovera et al 1993b) and in vitro (García-Martínez et al 1993b) and that it is associated with both an increase in the presence of ubiquitin conjugates (García-Martínez et al 1993a) and ubiquitin mRNA (García-Martínez et al 1994a). Administration of polyclonal anti-TNF antibodies to cachectic tumour-bearing rats (with high circulating TNF levels) results in a normalization of muscle weight with no signs of muscle cachexia (Costelli et al 1993) and reverses the increased muscle ubiquitin gene expression (Llovera et al 1996a). These results support the involvement of the cytokine in mediating the activation of the muscle ubiquitin system during cancer cachexia. The action of this cytokine seems to be independent of that of interleukin-1 (IL-1) since treatment of animals with IL-1 receptor antagonist is unable to reverse the increased proteolysis found after TNF treatment (Costelli et al 1995c). The action of TNF could either be indirect (through another unknown mediator) or direct. Skeletal muscle has TNF receptors (Hofmann et al 1994), and we have

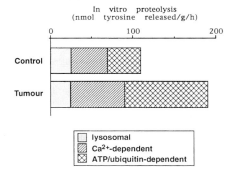

In vitro proteolysis
(nmol tyrosine released/g/h)

☐ lysosomal
▨ Ca^{2+}-dependent
▧ ATP/ubiquitin-dependent

Figure 6.3 — **Activation of ubiquitin-dependent proteolysis in tumour-bearing rats**. Increased skeletal muscle protein degradation is associated with an activation of the ATP and ubiquitin-dependent proteolytic system (adapted from Llovera et al 1995).

observed a direct effect on ubiquitin mRNA in incubations of skeletal muscles in vitro in the presence of the cytokine (Llovera et al 1997).

Mediators of muscle wasting associated with cancer cachexia

Although the search for the "cachectic" factor(s) started a long time ago, and although many efforts have been devoted to its discovery, we are still a long way from knowing the whole truth. A lot of progress has been made, however, and the suggested mediators can be divided into two categories: of tumour origin (produced and released by the neoplasm) and humoral factors (mainly cytokines).

Tumour necrosis factor-α

In 1893 Coley introduced the idea that tumour regression in human cancer patients could be accomplished by challenging them with bacterial toxins. Much later, Old (1985) identified a protein in the serum of endotoxin-treated rabbits that was responsible for the haemorrhagic necrosis of tumours. It was then named tumour necrosis factor (TNF) and later on TNF-α after the discovery of lymphotoxin or TNF-β. Kawakami and Cerami (1981) identified a molecule responsible for the wasting syndrome seen in many chronic diseases, such as cancer or chronic infection. This molecule was named cachectin, since it was responsible for the induction of cachexia, and it later proved to be identical to TNF (Beutler et al 1985).

TNF is synthesized mainly by macrophages, in response to invasive stimuli, as a 26 kDa membrane-bound precursor that is cleaved proteolytically to a mature 17 kDa form with the prosequence polypeptide remaining associated with the membrane (Jue et al 1990). The peptide is bioactive as a 51 kDa trimer, which can be recognized by two different receptors, TNFR1 or p55 (55 kDa) and TNFR2 or p75 (75 kDa). TNF is a pleiotropic factor that exerts a variety of effects such as growth promotion, growth inhibition, angiogenesis, cytotoxicity, inflammation and immunomodulation (Aggarwal and Natarajan 1996).

Episodic TNF administration has proved unsuccessful at inducing cachexia in experimental animals (Mahony and Tisdale 1988, Socher et al 1988a).

Indeed, repetitive TNF administrations initially induce a cachectic effect, but tolerance to the cytokine soon develops and food intake and body weight return to normal. Others have shown that escalating doses of TNF are necessary to maintain the cachectic effects (Tracey et al 1988). However, a very elegant approach involving the implantation of chinese hamster ovary (CHO) cells, which were transfected with the human TNF gene, in nude mice seems to indicate that TNF may have a clear and important role in the induction of cachexia (Oliff et al 1987).

Raised concentrations of TNF have been detected in the serum of patients with parasitic infections (Scuderi et al 1986) and with septicaemia (Waage et al 1986), which are pathological states where a high degree of cachexia is achieved. The increase in plasma TNF in septicaemia is likely to be caused by increased concentrations of endotoxin, which can elicit a transitory rise in plasma TNF when administered to healthy control subjects (Tracey et al 1987, Michie et al 1988). In contrast, evidence for increased TNF in the plasma of cancer patients is controversial. Balkwill et al (1987) found that 50% of serum samples from cancer patients had a positive response for TNF with an enzyme-linked immunosorbent assay, and more recently the presence of this cytokine has been observed in the serum of children with acute lymphoblastic leukaemia (Saarinen et al 1990). Other studies (Waage et al 1986, Socher et al 1988b), however, have reported no increase, even in patients with small-cell lung cancer (Selby et al 1988). Similarly, in tumour-bearing mice, no TNF could be detected in plasma with bioassays (Moldawer et al 1988). In contrast, other studies have found considerable amounts of TNF in the blood of tumour-bearing rats (Stovroff et al 1988, Costelli et al 1993). These divergent findings may be caused by different sensitivities or specificities of the assay methods, stability of TNF on storage, short half-life of TNF in vivo or localized paracrine production of TNF.

A large body of evidence suggests that TNF participates in the protein wasting associated with cachectic situations. Chronic treatment of rats with TNF resulted in a depletion of body protein compared with pair-fed control animals (Fong et al 1989). Indeed, chronic treatment with either recombinant TNF or IL-1-β resulted in a body protein redistribution and a significant decrease in muscle protein content, associated with coordinate decreases in muscle mRNA levels for myofibrillar proteins (Fong et al 1989). Studies involving administration of TNF in vivo have shown an increase in nitrogen efflux from skeletal muscle of non-weight losing humans with disseminated cancer (Warren et al 1987). Flores et al (1989) showed that chronic recombinant TNF administration significantly enhanced muscle protein breakdown in rats. Goodman (1991), measuring both tyrosine and 3-methylhistidine release by incubated rat muscles of animals acutely treated with the cytokine, concluded that TNF was involved in activating muscle proteolysis. The mechanisms underlying such actions still remain obscure. Our research group (Llovera et al 1993a,b) has demonstrated that TNF treatment enhances protein degradation measured in vivo in rat skeletal muscle. In addition, we have described that, at least during tumour growth, muscle wasting is associated with the activation of non-lysosomal ubiquitin-dependent proteases (Llovera et al 1994, 1995), and that this activation seems to be mediated via TNF (García-Martínez et al 1993a, b, 1994a). We have also reported that in vivo administration of TNF to rats results in an increased skeletal muscle proteolysis associated with an increase in both gene expression and higher levels of free and conjugated ubiquitin (García-Martínez et al 1993a, b). In addition, the in vivo action of TNF during cancer cachexia does not seem to be mediated by IL-1 (Costelli et al 1995c) or glucocorticoids (Llovera et al 1996b). Concerning a possible direct action of TNF on muscle proteolysis, the presence of both p55 and p75 receptors has been described (Tartaglia and Goeddel 1992), and we have recently demonstrated that the action of the cytokine on the induction of ubiquitin-dependent proteolysis can be direct (Llovera et al 1997). In conclusion, TNF, alone or in combination with other cytokines, seems to mediate most of the changes concerning nitrogen metabolism associated with cachectic states.

Other cytokines

Strassman et al (1993), using a murine colon adenocarcinoma, have shown that treatment with an anti-mouse IL-6 antibody was successful in reversing the key parameters of cachexia in tumour-bearing mice. These results seem to indicate that, at least in certain types of tumours, IL-6 could have a more direct involvement than TNF in the cachectic state of the animals. Conversely, other studies have revealed that IL-6 is not involved in cachexia in a very similar mouse tumour model (Soda et al 1995). In addition, in vitro studies using incubated rat skeletal muscle have shown that IL-6 had no direct effect on muscle proteolysis (García-Martínez et al 1994b).

Another interesting candidate is interferon-γ (IFN-γ). Matthys et al (1991b), using a monoclonal antibody against IFN-γ, were able to reverse the wasting syndrome associated with the growth of the Lewis lung carcinoma in mice, thus indicating that endogenous production of IFN-γ occurs and subsists in the tumour-bearing mice, and it is instrumental in bringing about some of the generalized metabolic changes characteristic of cancer cachexia. The same group has also demonstrated that severe cachexia also develops rapidly in nude mice inoculated with CHO cells constitutively producing IFN-γ, as a result of the transfection of the corresponding gene (Matthys et al 1991a).

Other cytokines, such as the leukaemia inhibitory factor (LIF; Mori et al 1991), transforming growth factor-β (TGF-β; Zugmaier et al 1991) or IL-1 (Moldawer et al 1987) have also been proposed to be mediators of cachexia. Concerning this last cytokine, although its anorectic effect is well-known (Mrosovsky et al 1989), administration of IL-1 receptor antagonist to tumour-bearing rats did not result in any improvement in the degree of cachexia (Costelli et al 1995c), thus suggesting that its role in cancer cachexia may be secondary to the actions of other mediators.

From all this information, it may be concluded that, although TNF has a very important role in the induction of cachexia, the metabolic derangement leading to this pathological state can also be influenced by other cytokines, or changes in the hormonal milieu, brought about by immune cells as a consequence of invasive stimuli.

Other factors

It is by no means intended here to give the idea that cytokines are the only molecules involved in cachexia. Many other compounds have been reported to have an important role in the cachectic state. Perhaps the first evidence of such compounds came from studies with Krebs-2 carcinoma cells in mice; inactive extracts of these cells could induce cachexia once injected in normal non-tumour-bearing mice (Costa and Holland 1966). Similarly, toxohormone L was isolated from the ascites fluid of patients with hepatoma and sarcoma-bearing mice (Masuno et al 1981), and it induces lipid mobilization and immunosuppression (Kitada et al 1980). Extracts of thymic lymphoma, conditioned medium from thymic lymphoma cell lines, and serum from lymphoma-bearing mice, cause lipid mobilization in experimental animals (Kitada et al 1980, 1982).

It is worth mentioning the studies of Todorov et al (1996) using a murine colon adenocarcinoma. They were able to purify and characterize a 24 kDa proteoglycan (also present in urine of human cachectic patients), which perhaps accounts for the loss of adipose tissue and skeletal muscle mass found in the tumour-bearing mice.

Conclusions

Bearing in mind all the information presented here, it can indeed be concluded that no definite mediator of cancer cachexia has been yet identified. However, among all the possible mediators considered here, TNF is one of the most relevant candidates. Indeed, TNF can mimic most of the abnormalities found during cancer cachexia: weight loss, anorexia, increased thermogenesis, adipose tissue dissolution, insulin resistance and muscle wastage, including activation of protein breakdown and increased BCAA metabolism. However, TNF alone cannot explain all the cachectic metabolic alterations present in different types of human cancers and experimental tumours. Another important drawback is the fact that TNF circulating concentrations are not always elevated in cancer-bearing states and, although it may be argued that in those cases local tissue production of the cytokine may be high, cachexia does not seem to be a local tumour effect. Consequently, both tumour-produced and humoral factors must collaborate in the full induction of the cachectic state. In conclusion, and because metabolic alterations often appear early after the onset of tumour growth, the scope of appropriate treatment, although not aimed at achieving immediate eradication of the tumour mass, could influence the course of the patient's clinical state or, at least, prevent the steady erosion of dignity that the patient may feel in association with the syndrome. This would no doubt contribute to improving the patient's quality of life and, possibly, prolong survival.

References

Adibi SA. (1976) Metabolism of branched-chain amino acids in altered nutrition. *Metabolism* 25: 1287–1302.

Aggarwal BB, Natarajan K. (1996) Tumor necrosis factors: developments during last decade. *Eur Cytokin Netw* 7: 93–124.

Argilés JM, Azcón-Bieto J. (1988) The metabolic environment of cancer. *Mol Cell Biochem* 81: 3–17.

Argilés JM, López-Soriano FJ. (1990a) The effects of tumour necrosis factor-α (cachectin) and tumour growth on hepatic amino acid utilization in the rat. *Biochem J* 266: 123–126.

Argilés JM, López-Soriano FJ. (1990b) The oxidation of leucine in tumour-bearing rats. *Biochem J* 268: 241–244.

Argilés JM, López-Soriano FJ. (1996) The ubiquitin-dependent proteolytic pathway in skeletal muscle: its role in pathological states. *Trends Pharmacol Sci* 17: 223–226.

Argilés JM, García-Martínez C, Llovera M, López-Soriano FJ. (1992) The role of cytokines in muscle wasting: its relation with cancer cachexia. *Med Res Rev* 12: 637–652.

Argilés JM, López-Soriano FJ, Pallarés-Trujillo J. (1998) *Ubiquitin and Disease*. p. 174. R.G. Landes Co., Austin.

Balkwill F, Burke F, Talbot D, et al. (1987) Evidence for tumour necrosis factor/cachectin production in cancer. *Lancet* 2: 1229–1232.

Baracos VE, DeVivo C, Hoyle DHR, Goldberg AL. (1995) Activation of the ATP-ubiquitin-proteasome pathway in skeletal muscle of cachectic rats bearing a hepatoma. *Am J Physiol* 268: E996–E1006.

Beutler B, Greenwald D, Hulmes JD, et al. (1985) Identity of tumor necrosis factor and the macrophage-secreted factor cachectin. *Nature* 316: 552–554.

Brennan MF. (1981) Total parenteral nutrition in the cancer patient. *N Engl J Med* 305: 375–382.

Buse MG, Reid SS. (1975) Leucine: a possible regulator of protein turnover in muscle. *J Clin Invest* 56: 1250–1261.

Buse MG, Herlong HF, Weigand DA. (1976) The effects of diabetes, insulin and redox potential on leucine metabolism by isolated rat diaphragm. *Endocrinology* 98: 1166–1175.

Coley WB. (1893) The treatment of malignant tumours by repeated inoculations of erysipelas; with a report of ten original cases. *Am J Med Sci* 105: 487–511.

Costa G, Holland JF. (1966) Effects of Krebs-2 carcinoma on the lipid metabolism of male Swiss mice. *Cancer Res* 22: 1081–1083.

Costelli P, Carbó N, Tessitore L, et al. (1993) Tumor necrosis factor-α mediates changes in tissue protein turnover in a rat cancer cachexia model. *J Clin Invest* 92: 2783–2789.

Costelli P, García-Martínez C, Llovera M, et al. (1995a) Muscle protein waste in tumor-bearing rats is effectively antagonized by a β₂-adrenergic agonist (clenbuterol). *J Clin Invest* 95: 2367–2372.

Costelli P, Llovera M, García-Martínez C, Carbó N, López-Soriano FJ, Argilés JM. (1995b) Enhanced leucine oxidation in rats bearing an ascites hepatoma (Yoshida AH-130) and its reversal by clenbuterol. *Cancer Lett* 91: 73–78.

Costelli P, Llovera M, Carbó N, García-Martínez C, López-Soriano FJ, Argilés JM. (1995c) Interleukin-1 receptor antagonist (IL-1ra) is unable to reverse cachexia in rats bearing an ascites hepatoma (Yoshida AH-130). *Cancer Lett* 95: 33–38.

De Wys WD. (1985) Management of cancer cachexia. *Semin Oncol* 12: 452–460.

Emery PW, Neville AM, Edwards RHT, Rennie MJ. (1982) Increased myofibrillar degradation and decreased protein synthesis in tumor-bearing mice. *Eur J Clin Invest* 12: 10.

Flores EA, Bistrian BR, Pomposelli JJ, Dinarello CA, Blackburn GL, Istfan NW. (1989) Infusion of tumor necrosis factor/cachectin promotes muscle catabolism in the rat. A synergistic effect with interleukin-1. *J Clin Invest* 83: 1614–1622.

Fong Y, Moldawer LL, Morano M, et al. (1989) Cachectin/TNF or IL-1α induces cachexia with redistribution of body proteins. *Am J Physiol* 256: R659–R665.

Forbes GB. (1987) In: *Human Body Composition: Growth, Aging, Nutrition and Activity*, p. 171. Springer-Verlag, New York.

García-Martínez C, Agell N, Llovera M, López-Soriano FJ, Argilés JM. (1993a) Tumour necrosis factor-α increases the ubiquitinization of rat skeletal muscle proteins. *FEBS Lett* 323: 211–214.

García-Martínez C, López-Soriano FJ, Argilés JM. (1993b) Acute treatment with tumour necrosis factor-α induces changes in protein metabolism in rat skeletal muscle. *Mol Cell Biochem* 125: 11–18.

García-Martínez C, Llovera M, Agell N, López-Soriano FJ, Argilés JM. (1994a) Ubiquitin gene expression in skeletal muscle is increased by tumour necrosis factor-α. *Biochem Biophys Res Commun* 201: 682–686.

García-Martínez C, López-Soriano FJ, Argilés JM. (1994b) Interleukin-6 does not activate protein breakdown in rat skeletal muscle. *Cancer Lett* 76: 1–4.

García-Martínez C, López-Soriano FJ, Argilés JM. (1995) Amino acid uptake in skeletal muscle of rats bearing the Yoshida AH-130 ascites hepatoma. *Mol Cell Biochem* 148: 17–23.

Goodlad GAJ, Tee MK, Clark CM. (1981) Leucine oxidation and protein degradation in the extensor digitorum longus and soleus of the tumor-bearing host. *Biochem Med* 26: 143–147.

Goodman MN. (1991) Tumor necrosis factor induces skeletal muscle protein breakdown in rats. *Am J Physiol* 260: E727–E730.

Hartl WH, Miyoshi H, Jahoor F, Klein S, Elahi D, Wolfe RR. (1990) Bradykinin attenuates glucagon-induced leucine oxidation in humans. *Am J Physiol* 259: E239–E245.

Hofmann C, Lorenz K, Braithwaite SS, et al. (1994) Altered gene expression for tumour necrosis factor-α and its receptors during drug and dietary modulation of insulin resistance. *Endocrinology* 134: 264–270.

Houten L, Reilley AA. (1980) An investigation of the cause of death from cancer. *J Surg Oncol* 13: 111–116.

Jue DM, Sherry B, Luedke C, Manogue KR, Cerami A. (1990) Processing of newly synthesized cachectin/tumor necrosis factor in endotoxin-stimulated macrophages. *Biochemistry* 29: 8371–8377.

Kawakami M, Cerami A. (1981) Studies of endotoxin-induced decrease in lipoprotein lipase activity. *J Exp Med* 154: 631–637.

Kern KA, Norton JA. (1988) Cancer cachexia. *J Parent Enteral Nutr* 12: 286–298.

Kitada S, Hays EF, Mead JF. (1980) A lipid mobilizing factor in serum of tumor-bearing mice. *Lipids* 15: 168–174.

Kitada S, Hays EF, Mead JF. (1982) Lipolysis induction in adipocytes by a protein from tumour cells. *J Cell Biochem* 20, 409–416.

Lawson DH, Richmond A, Nixon DW, Rudman D. (1982) Metabolic approaches to cancer cachexia. *Annu Rev Nutr* 2: 277–301.

Lazo PA. (1985) Tumour-host metabolic interaction and cachexia. *FEBS Lett* 187: 189–192.

Liu CC, Teh JY, Ou BR, Forsberg NE. (1994) Actions of a beta-adrenergic agonist on muscle protein metabolism in intact, adrenalectomized, and dexamethasone-supplemented adrenalectomized rats. *J Nutr Biochem* 5: 43–49.

Llovera M, López-Soriano FJ, Argilés JM. (1993a) Chronic tumour necrosis factor-α treatment modifies protein turnover in rat tissues. *Biochem Mol Biol Intl* 30: 29–36.

Llovera M, López-Soriano FJ, Argilés JM. (1993b) Effects of tumor necrosis factor-α on muscle-protein turnover in female Wistar rats. *J Natl Cancer Inst* 85: 1334–1339.

Llovera M, García-Martínez C, Agell N, Marzábal M, López-Soriano FJ, Argilés JM. (1994) Ubiquitin gene expression is increased in skeletal muscle of tumour-bearing rats. *FEBS Lett* 338: 311–318.

Llovera M, García-Martínez C, Agell N, López-Soriano FJ, Argilés JM. (1995) Muscle wasting associated with cancer cachexia is linked to an important activation of the ATP-dependent ubiquitin-mediated proteolysis. *Intl J Cancer* 61: 138–141.

Llovera M, Carbó N, García-Martínez C, et al. (1996a) Anti-TNF treatment reverts increased muscle ubiquitin gene expression in tumour-bearing rats. *Biochem Biophys Res Commun* 221: 653–655.

Llovera M, Garcia-Martínez C, Costelli P, et al. (1996b) Muscle hypercatabolism during cancer cachexia is not reversed by the glucocorticoid receptor antagonist RU 38486. *Cancer Lett* 99: 7–14.

Llovera M, García-Martínez C, Agell N, López-Soriano FJ, Argilés JM. (1997) TNF can directly induce the expression of ubiquitin-dependent proteolytic system in rat soleus muscles. *Biochem Biophys Res Commun* 230: 238–241.

Lundholm KG. (1985) Energy and substrate metabolism in the cancer-bearing host. In: *Nutrition in Cancer and Trauma Sepsis* (Bozzetti F, Dionigi R, eds.), pp. 78–95. Karger, Basel.

Lundholm K, Bennegard K, Eden E, Svaninger G, Emery PW, Rennie MJ. (1982) Efflux of 3-methylhistidine from the leg in cancer patients who experience weight loss. *Cancer Res* 42: 4807–4811.

Mahony SM, Tisdale MJ. (1988) Induction of weight loss and metabolic alterations by human recombinant tumour necrosis factor. *Br J Cancer* 58: 345–349.

Masuno H, Yamaskai N, Okuda H (1981) Purification and characterization of a lipolytic factor (toxohormone L) from cell free fluid of ascites sarcoma 180. *Cancer Res* 41: 284–288.

Matthys P, Dukmans R, Proost P, Van Damme J, Heremans H, Sobis H, Billiau A. (1991a) Severe cachexia in mice inoculated with interferon-γ-producing tumor cells. *Intl J Cancer* 49: 77–82.

Matthys P, Heremans H, Opdenakker G, Billiau A (1991b) Anti-interferon-γ antibody treatment, growth of Lewis lung tumours in mice and tumour-associated cachexia. *Eur J Cancer* 27: 182–187.

Medina MA, Sánchez-Jiménez F, Márquez J, Rodriguez-Quesada A, Núñez de Castro I. (1992) Relevance of glutamine metabolism to tumor cell growth. *Mol Cell Biochem* 113: 1–15.

Meguid MM, Muscaritoli M, Beverly JL, Yang ZJ, Cangiano C, Rossifanelli F. (1992) The early anorexia paradigm: changes in plasma free tryptophan and feeding indexes. *J Parent Enteral Nutr* 16: S56–S59.

Melville S, McNurlan MA, Graham Calder A, Garlick PJ. (1990) Increased protein turnover despite normal energy metabolism and responses to feeding in patients with lung cancer. *Cancer Res* 50: 1125–1131.

Michie HR, Manogue KR, Spriggs DR, et al. (1988) Detection of circulating tumor necrosis factor after endotoxin administration. *N Engl J Med* 318: 1481–1486.

Mitch WE, Clark AS. (1984) Specificity of the effects of leucine and its metabolites on protein degradation in skeletal muscle. *Biochem J* 222: 579–586.

Moldawer LL, Georgieff M, Lundholm K. (1987) Interleukin-1, tumour necrosis factor-α/cachectin and the pathogenesis of cancer cachexia. *Clin Physiol* 7: 263–274.

Moldawer LL, Drott C, Lundholm K. (1988) Monocytic production and plasma bioactivities of interleukin-1 and tumour necrosis factor in human cancer. *Eur J Clin Invest* 18: 486–492.

Mori M, Yamaguchi K, Honda S, et al. (1991) Cancer cachexia syndrome developed in nude mice bearing melanoma cells producing leukemia-inhibitor factor. *Cancer Res* 51: 6656–6659.

Mrosovsky N, Molony LA, Conn CA, Kluger MJ. (1989) Anorexic effects of interleukin 1 in the rat. *Am J Physiol* 257: R1315–R1321.

Nair KS, Schwartz RG, Welle S. (1992) Leucine as a regulator of whole body and skeletal muscle protein metabolism in humans. *Am J Physiol* 263: E928–E934.

Nishihira T, Takagi T, Mori S. (1993) Leucine and manifestation of antitumor activity by valine-depleted amino acid imbalance. *Nutrition* 9: 146–152.

Old LJ. (1985) Tumor necrosis factor (TNF). *Science* 230: 630–632.

Oliff A, Defeo-Jones D, Boyer M, et al. (1987) Tumors secreting human TNF/cachectin induce cachexia in mice. *Cell* 50: 555–563.

Pain VM, Randall DP, Garlick PJ. (1984) Protein synthesis in liver and skeletal muscle of mice bearing an ascites tumor. *Cancer Res* 44: 1054–1057.

Pisters PWT, Cersosimo E, Rogatko A, Brennan MF. (1992) Insulin action on glucose and branched-chain amino acid metabolism in cancer cachexia: differential effects of insulin. *Surgery* 3: 301–310.

Rennie MJ, Edwards RHT, Emery PW, Halliday D, Lundholm K, Millward DJ. (1983) Depressed protein synthesis is the dominant characteristic of wasting and cachexia. *Clin Physiol* 3: 387–398.

Rivera S, López-Soriano FJ, Azcón-Bieto J, Argilés JM. (1987) Blood amino acid compartmentation in mice bearing Lewis lung carcinoma. *Cancer Res* 47: 5644–5646.

Rofe AM, Bais R, Conyers RAJ. (1986) Ketone body metabolism in tumor-bearing rats. *Biochem J* 233: 485–491.

Saarinen UM, Kosfelo EK, Teppo AM, Simes MA. (1990). Tumor necrosis factor in children with malignancies. *Cancer Res* 50: 592–595.

Scuderi P, Lam KS, Ryan KJ, et al. (1986) Raised serum levels of tumour necrosis factor in parasitic infections. *Lancet* 2: 1364–1365.

Selby PJ, Hobbs S, Niner C, Jackson E, Smith IE, McElwain TJ. (1988) Endogenous tumour necrosis factor in cancer patients. *Lancet* 1: 483.

Smith K, Barua JM, Watt PW, Scrimgeour CM, Rennie MJ. (1992) Flooding with L-[1-^{13}C]leucine stimulates human muscle protein incorporation of continuously infused [1-^{13}C]valine. *Am J Physiol* 262: E372–E376.

Socher SH, Friedman A, Martinez D. (1988a) Recombinant human tumor necrosis factor induces acute reductions in food intake and body weight in mice. *J Exp Med* 167: 1957–1962.

Socher SH, Martinez D, Craig JB, Kuhn JG, Oliff A. (1988b) Tumour necrosis factor nondetectable in patients with cancer cachexia. *J Natl Cancer Inst* 80: 595–598.

Soda K, Kawakami M, Kashii A, Miyata M. (1995) Manifestations of cancer cachexia induced by colon 26 adenocarcinoma are not fully ascribable to interleukin-6. *Intl J Cancer* 62: 332–336.

Stovroff MC, Fraker DL, Norton JA. (1988) Cachectin activity in the serum of cachectic, tumor-bearing rats. *Arch Surg* 124: 94–99.

Strassmann G, Fong M, Freter CE, Windsor S, D'Alessandro F, Nordan RP. (1993) Suramin interferes with interleukin-6 receptor binding in vitro and inhibits colon-26-mediated experimental cancer cachexia in vivo. *J Clin Invest* 92: 2152–2159.

Tartaglia LA, Goeddel DV. (1992) Two TNF receptors. *Immunol Today* 13: 151–153.

Temparis S, Asensi M, Taillandier D, et al. (1994) Increased ATP-ubiquitin-dependent proteolysis in skeletal muscles of tumor-bearing rats. *Cancer Res* 54: 5568–5573.

Tessitore L, Bonelli G, Baccino FM. (1987) Early development of protein metabolic perturbations in the liver and skeletal muscle of tumour-bearing rats. *Biochem J* 241: 153–159.

Todorov P, Cariuk P, McDevitt T, Coles B, Fearon K, Tisdale M. (1996) Characterization of a cancer cachectic factor. *Nature* 22: 739–742.

Tomas FM, Murray AJ, Jones LM. (1984) Interactive effects of insulin and corticosterone on myofibrillar protein turnover in rats as determined by N-methylhistidine excretion. *Biochem J* 220: 469–479.

Tracey KJ, Fong Y, Hesse DG, et al. (1987) Anticachectin/ TNF monoclonal antibodies prevent septic shock during lethal bacteraemia. *Nature* 330: 662–664.

Tracey KL, Wei H, Manogue KR, et al. (1988) Cachectin/ tumor necrosis factor induces cachexia, anemia and inflammation. *J Exp Med* 167: 1211–1227.

Waage A, Espevik T, Lamvik J (1986) Detection of tumor necrosis factor–like cytotoxicity in serum from patients with septicaemia but not from untreated cancer patients. *Scan J Immunol* 24: 739–743.

Warren RS, Starnes HF, Jr, Gabrilove JL, Oettgen HF, Brennan MF. (1987) The acute metabolic effects of tumor necrosis factor administration in humans. *Arch Surg* 122: 1396–1400.

Wiborg O, Pederson MS, Wind A, Berglund LE, Marcker KA, Vuust J. (1985) The human ubiquitin multigene family: some genes contain multiple directly repeated ubiquitin coding sequences. *EMBO J* 4: 755–759.

Williams JF, Matthaei KI. (1981) Cancer induced body wasting. A review of cancer cachexia and a hypothesis concerning the molecular basis of the condition. *ASEAN J Clin Sci* 2: 158–173.

Wing SS, Banville D (1994) 14-kDa ubiquitin-conjugating enzyme: structure of the rat gene and regulation upon fasting and by insulin. *Am J Physiol* 267: E39–E48.

Wing SS, Goldberg AL. (1993) Glucocorticoids activate the ATP-ubiquitin-dependent proteolytic system in skeletal muscle during fasting. *Am J Physiol* 264: E668–E676.

Zugmaier G, Paik S, Wilding G, et al. (1991) Transforming growth factor β1 induces cachexia and systemic fibrosis without an antitumor effect in nude mice. *Cancer Res* 51: 3590–3594.

7

Effect of hypoxia on skeletal muscle

Yves Jammes

Introduction

The oxygen supply to muscles is mostly a diffusion-limited system. So, the delivery of oxygen to muscle fibres depends on the driving pressure of this gas (PO_2), which dramatically falls from atmosphere to mitochondria. The major steps of PO_2 fall during the oxygen transport by convection in the lungs and the cardiovascular system are represented in Fig. 7.1A. Then, intracellular PO_2 continues to decrease, reaching 2 to 4 mmHg close to the mitochondria (Fig. 7.1B) (Gayeski and Honig 1986). The boundary between cellular normoxia and hypoxia is thus very narrow. Hypoxia results from different mechanisms. The first one is characterized by the sole reduction of arterial PO_2 (hypoxaemia), a circumstance encountered at high altitude and most often in patients with respiratory insufficiency. The second major cause of hypoxia is a reduced blood oxygen content (ischaemia) resulting from lowered cardiac output or decreased peripheral muscle blood flow in patients suffering from cardiovascular diseases, and also during shock. Hypoxia may also result from a decrease in blood oxygen carrier only (anaemia) and/or from an impaired function of haemoglobin (CO poisoning and abnormal haemoglobins).

This study first reviews the consequences of hypoxia on muscle blood flow and metabolism, then the maximal mechanical performances at work as well as the associated changes in myoelectrical activity. Finally, the consequences of muscle hypoxia on its sensorimotor control will be examined

Effects of hypoxia on muscle blood flow

It is clear that skeletal muscle blood flow is not homogeneous within the muscle fibre types in a given muscle, the capillary density in the region of slow-oxidative fibres being higher than that of fast-glycolytic ones (Wittenberg and Wittenberg 1989). In animals, acute hypoxaemia results in a marked decline in muscle blood flow and thus in systemic oxygen transport to muscles (Marshall 1995). As for healthy humans, echodoppler measurements reveal that muscle blood flow in the *medial gastrocnemius* artery decreased during a 10-min period of breathing a low oxygen gas mixture ($FiO_2 = 0.09$; unpublished observations). After the subjects inhaled the ambient air again, this effect persisted during the first 2 min; it was followed by a marked transient increase in muscle

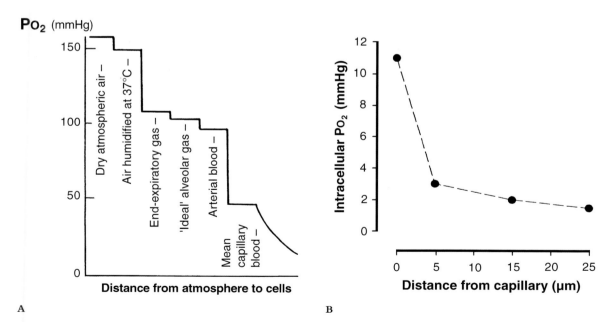

A   **B**

Figure 7.1 — The fall in the partial pressure of oxygen (PO_2) between atmosphere and cells (A) and between the cell membrane and mitochondria (B) (From data reported by Gayeski and Honig 1986). Please note that the X-scale on A is virtual because the length varies from cm to μm.

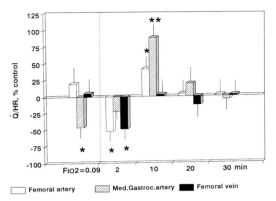

Figure 7.2 — During acute normobaric hypoxia muscle blood flow, measured by echodoppler and normalized to heart rate changes (Q/HR), begins to decrease. This response persists for the first 2 min of re-oxygenation. It is then followed by a marked increase in muscle perfusion (Barthelemy et al 2001). Asterisks denote significant hypoxia-induced changes.

perfusion (Fig. 7.2). These effects are a result of the variations in cross-sectional area of muscle artery. Animal studies have indicated that the peripheral vasodilatation that follows acute muscle hypoxaemia is caused by the local release of potassium, adenosine and nitric oxide (NO) by the endothelial cells as well as by the muscle fibres (Marshall 1995). Hypoxia-induced vasospasm is attributed to a catecholamine release, which may result from a direct stimulating effect of hypoxia on the sympathetic system or a pressor reflex due to the activation of group IV muscle afferents. The consequences of hypoxia on muscle afferent pathways will be examined later.

Metabolic consequences of hypoxia

Numerous human studies during acute (Stenberg et al 1966, Zattara-Hartmann and Jammes 1996a) or chronic (West et al 1983, Cerretelli and Hoppeler 1996) exposure to hypoxia as well as studies in animal muscles contracting under acute hypoxic conditions (Gutierrez et al 1989, Stainsby et al 1990) have shown that reduced oxygen supply to working muscles significantly lowers the maximal oxygen uptake. This is not true in resting hypoxic muscles, in which acute hypoxaemia has no effect on oxygen uptake (VO_2). In the same way, acute hypoxaemia increases the glucose transport through the membrane of perfused rat limb muscles (Cartee et al 1991). Therefore, reduced VO_2 under hypoxaemic conditions cannot be attributed to reduced energy supply to muscles. There are also

marked effects of hypoxaemia on the early muscle energetics, assessed by a slowed time constant for VO_2 change (Engelen et al 1996). This effect was attributed to a greater breakdown of phosphocreatine (PCr) by contracting muscles in dog (Hogan et al 1992). ^{31}P-magnetic resonance studies during sustained handgrip in humans (Bendahan et al 1998) show that, for a given increase in myoelectrical activity, PCr consumption was greater and intramuscular pH (pH_i) lower in acute hypoxaemia compared with normoxia (Fig. 7.3). The slowed time constant for VO_2 changes at the beginning of exercise under hypoxaemic conditions may also have a non-metabolic origin. Indeed, we have shown a slower rate of increase in minute ventilation and heart rate at the beginning of hypoxic cycling exercise in humans (Zattara-Hartmann and Jammes 1996b), attributed to a hypoxia-induced depression of the neurogenic components of the cardiorespiratory response to exercise.

It is commonly observed that general hypoxaemia does not markedly increase muscle lactate concentration in animal and human skeletal muscles at rest (Sahlin and Katz 1989, Zattara-Hartmann and Jammes 1996a). By contrast, at a given exercise intensity, acute hypoxia in humans (Stenberg et al 1966, Zattara-Hartmann and Jammes 1996a) and animals (Stainsby et al 1990, Gutierrez et al 1993) markedly increases the blood lactate concentration (Fig. 7.4). This is associated with a lowered anaerobic threshold during progressive cycle exercise in hypoxia, an effect which is proportional to the PaO_2 fall (Zattara-Hartmann and Jammes 1996a). The facilitating effect of acute hypoxaemia on lactic acid release is attenuated by alkalaemia (Gutierrez et al 1993), and this may explain why, after acclimatization to high altitude (chronic hypoxaemia associated with alkalaemia), blood lactate concentration at a given workload tends to return to values measured at sea level (Cerretelli and Hoppeler 1996). Other explanations for a reduced production of lactate by contracting muscle fibres in chronic hypoxaemic subjects could be:

1. an increased mobilization and use of free fatty acids, resulting in reduced anaerobic paths, sparing of muscle glycogen (Jones et al 1972, Young et al 1982)

2. changes in the proportion of muscle fibres (muscle plasticity).

Some studies suggest that chronic exposure to hypoxia modifies the muscular metabolic paths towards an increased level of oxidative enzymes in high-altitude adaptive animals (Hochachka 1994). However, human studies in sea-level natives after an

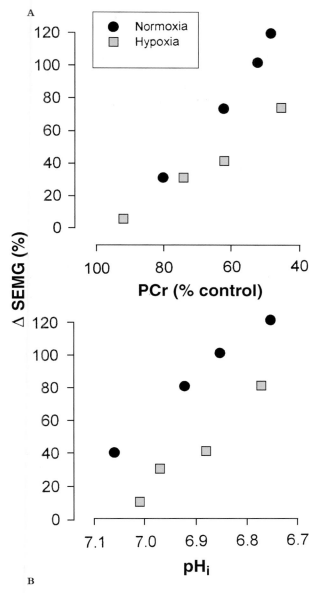

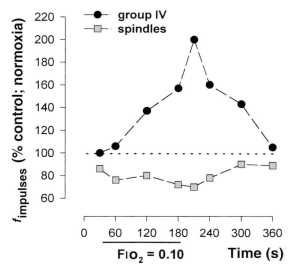

Figure 7.4—In resting cat muscle, acute hypoxia exerts opposing influences on the sensory pathways (from data published by Lagier-Tessonnier et al 1993). The baseline activity of group IV muscle afferents (called metaboreceptors) markedly increases, whereas the afferent discharge of proprioceptors, elicited by high-frequency tendon vibrations, is significantly depressed.

Figure 7.3—Acute normobaric hypoxia modifies the relationships between the quantitative surface electromyography (SEMG) changes and the corresponding phosphocreatine (PCr) consumption (A) or the fall in pH_i (B) during sustained handgrip (from data reported by Bendahan et al 1998). For a given myoelectrical activity, hypoxia accentuates the PCr decrease and muscle acidosis. For the same energetic level, hypoxia depresses the SEMG changes.

18-day residence at 4300 m (Young et al 1984) or during the simulated Everest II operation (Green et al 1989), as well as in high-altitude (3600 m) natives (Desplanches et al 1996), did not confirm animal observations. They even suggested that high-altitude natives had a reduced capillarity and muscle tissue oxidative capacity compared with sea-level natives (Desplanches et al 1996). Moreover, one study by Desplanches et al (1993) clearly indicates that training at the same relative workload in normoxia and hypoxia ($FIO_2 = 0.10$) has similar effects on muscle tissue. Consequently, biochemical and histoenzymatic studies in normal subjects cannot serve to explain the consensus that chronic exposure to hypoxia reduces the post-exercise muscle acidosis. In patients with chronic respiratory insufficiency, biochemical studies have shown reduced ATP and PCr levels in skeletal muscles at rest and a lowered recovery of PCr resynthesis after exercise (Payen et al 1993). This suggests an impairment of cellular metabolism related to hypoxaemia. In addition, the same study has demonstrated that reoxygenation of hypoxaemic patients significantly improved the indices of muscular oxidative metabolism (P_i/PCr ratio and pH_i) at the end of exercise.

In addition to the aforementioned changes in muscle metabolism, acute hypoxia is also suspected to enhance oxygen free radical generation during strenuous exercise (Sjödin et al 1990, Sen 1995). Indeed, intense muscular activity causes a metabolic stress, similar to that occurring during ischaemia, an effect amplified when oxygen supply to muscle is already lowered under hypoxaemic condition. Increased delivery of oxygen free radicals in exercising muscles is responsible for membrane lipid peroxydation and also for the activation of cyclooxygenase and lipo-oxygenase enzymes, resulting in the local synthesis of prostaglandins and thromboxan. During the Everest III Comex '97 experiment we measured a significant increase in blood content of indices used to character-ize an increased synthesis of oxygen free radicals (thiobarbituric acid reactive compounds, TBARCs; Joanny et al 2001). This effect was already significant at 6000 m, and it was markedly accentuated when subjects exercised at high altitude. In addition, increased blood content of TBARCs persisted, and was even accentuated, 24 hours after the subjects had returned to sea level, a response which was similar to that found in myocytes and brain cells during tran-sients from ischaemia to reperfusion.

Effects of hypoxia on muscle force generation and endurance time to fatigue

In humans, data in the literature are often contradic-tory. During chronic exposure to hypobaric hypox-aemia (real or simulated high altitude), Bowie and Cumming (1971), Fulco et al (1994), Garner et al (1990), Orizio et al (1994) and Young et al (1980) reported no change in maximal voluntary contraction (MVC) nor in endurance time to sustained fatiguing efforts. By contrast, during acute exposure to hypox-aemia (inhalation of a 10% oxygen gas mixture) Kaijer (1970) reported a significant decrement (−55%) in dynamic forearm work time; Eiken and Tesch (1984) observed a decreased quadriceps peak torque and Badier et al (1994) noted a 26% MVC decrease in the *adductor pollicis*. These discrepancies between acute and chronic exposure to hypoxia in healthy subjects are confirmed by Fulco et al (1994) who have shown in the same individuals that acute (1 day), but not chronic (13 days), altitude exposure (4300 m) leads to a rapid decline in *adductor pollicis* MVC. The conse-quences of pathological chronic hypoxaemia on force generation by skeletal muscles are much more pronounced than those exerted by acute hypoxia in healthy subjects (Zattara-Hartmann et al 1995). Compared with normal individuals of the same age and weight, patients suffering from severe respiratory insufficiency (PaO_2 = 57 mmHg) developed reduced

MVC by the *adductor pollicis* (−30%) and *vastus lateralis* (−35%). Oxygen breathing in these chronic hypox-aemic patients restored normal PaO_2 value. Then, within 10 min, MVC generated by the two muscles was markedly enhanced, but this improvement was only found when PaO_2 was equal to or higher than 80 mmHg.

Effects of hypoxia on neuromuscular transmission of myopotentials

Hypoxia-induced alterations in evoked compound muscle potentials (M wave) during and after fatiguing contractions are still debated. Garner et al (1990) reported no change in M wave during a 20 Hz stimu-lation of ankle dorsiflexor at simulated Everest alti-tude, whereas we found, under the same experimental conditions, a significant decline in M wave amplitude with prolonged conduction time from the altitude of 7000 m, the effects being even accentuated during 10-min epochs of transient reoxygenation (Caquelard et al 2000). There are very few studies on the conse-quences of acute hypoxia on the M wave characteris-tics. Mortimer et al (1970) found a significant decline in M wave in contracting ischaemic or hypoxaemic muscle. During progressive dynamic leg exercise executed above the anaerobic threshold, we reported a positive correlation between declined M wave amplitude and decreased blood pH, which reflects the anaerobic metabolic paths (Jammes et al 1997). However, the changes in M wave measured at high exercise levels were only significant in untrained individuals whereas they were absent or insignificant in trained cyclists. This clearly indicates that large interindividual differences in M wave response to muscular metabolic changes may be expected.

Effects of hypoxia on sensorimotor control

Failure of muscle force during rhythmic or sustained contractions at high force level is associated with a shift of electromyography (EMG) power spectrum towards lower frequencies (i.e. a decline in median frequency (MF) of the power spectrum). Numerous observations strongly suggest that the declined MF value during fatiguing muscle contractions results from depressed firing rate of motor neurons by a peripheral reflex originating in response to fatigue-induced metabolic changes in muscles (central fatigue) (Enoka and Stuart 1992), a phenomenon called *muscle wisdom*. This leads to the preferential recruitment of low-frequency motor units (i.e. slow-oxidative, fatigue-resistant muscle fibres) which delates muscle failure. The enhancement of afferent pathways carried by the group III-IV muscle endings, also called metaboreceptors, is the major candidate for the inhibitory influences exerted on alpha motor neurons. Acute hypoxaemia exerts an overall depressor influence on EMG variations during isometric contractions sustained at the same muscle strength by the *adductor pollicis*, the diaphragm (Badier et al 1994) and the forearm flexor (Bendahan et al 1998), but it does not accentuate the rate of MF decrease. During chronic exposure to hypoxia, there is also a significant reduction in integrated EMG activities, but no significant accentuation of MF decrease during isometric contractions in the elbow (Orizio et al 1994) and forearm flexors (unpublished observations in Everest III Comex'97). In cat hindlimb muscles at rest, acute hypoxaemia elicits a long-lasting activation of group III and mostly of group IV muscle endings (Hill et al 1992, Lagier-Tessonnier et al 1993), and it also attenuates the response of muscle mechanoreceptors to muscle contraction (Lagier-Tessonnier et al 1993; Fig. 7.4). The combination of increased inhibitory influences carried by group III-IV muscle afferents and reduced facilitatory proprioceptive pathways may depress the discharge of alpha motor neurons when muscles get tired. It is tempting to speculate that acute hypoxaemia, which increases anaerobic muscle metabolism, may potentiate the fatigue-induced activation of group IV muscle afferents. However, our recent observations in rabbit hindlimb muscles show that acute hypoxaemia does not enhance the response of group IV muscle afferents to fatigue but, on the contrary, markedly depresses it (Fig. 7.5). This corroborates the aforementioned observations in humans that acute as well as chronic hypoxaemia does not accentuate the filtering effects on the motor drive to contracting muscles. Therefore, animal and human data strongly suggest that *muscle wisdom* could be depressed under hypoxic conditions.

Re-oxygenation of chronic hypoxaemic patients markedly improved muscle performances and attenuated EMG variations in the *adductor pollicis* during fatiguing contractions (Zattara-Hartmann et al 1995). Based on these observations, the existence of an excitation–contraction uncoupling in chronic hypoxaemic patients (i.e. an increased ratio of integrated EMG activity to muscle force) is suspected. So, the benefits of re-oxygenation may be to improve the excitation–contraction coupling, with the immediate consequences of reduced myoelectrical-to-force ratio.

Marked discrepancies are found between the consequences of acute and chronic hypoxia on skeletal muscles. Acute hypoxia increases the anaerobic metabolic path, reduces MVC and endurance time to fatigue, and it lowers the motor unit recruitment at the same muscle strength. Chronic hypoxia in high-altitude natives or subjects acclimatized to high altitude has little metabolic influence, and the changes in MVC and endurance time values are weak or absent. By contrast, chronic hypoxaemia in severely ill patients markedly reduces MVC, shortens the endurance time to fatigue and affects the muscle metabolism. Only in these patients, re-oxygenation improves the mechanical muscle performances and reduces the metabolic disturbances. This brief review of the effects of hypoxia on muscles shows that numerous studies are still needed to understand better the handicap associated with reduced oxygen supply to muscle fibres.

Low-frequency fatigue

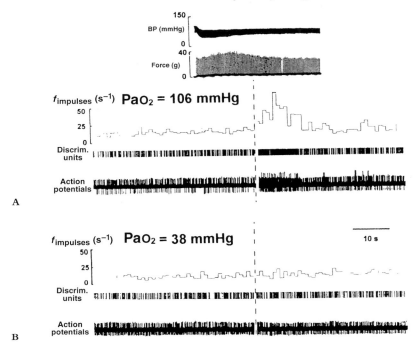

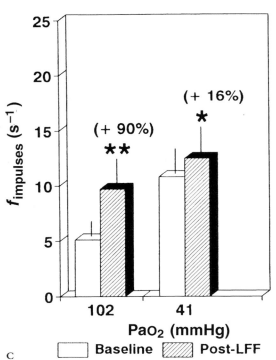

Figure 7.5—In contracting rabbit muscle, electrically-induced fatigue (LEF) induces a marked, prolonged activation of group IV muscle afferents in normoxic condition (A). This response is severely depressed in acute hypoxemic condition (B). Panel C: asterisks indicate the significance of post-fatigue changes in nerve discharge; this figure also shows that acute hypoxaemia increases the baseline activity of thin fibre afferents.

References

Badier M, Guillot Ch, Lagier-Tessonnier F, Jammes Y. (1994) EMG changes in respiratory and skeletal muscles during isometric contraction under normoxic, hypoxemic or ischemic condition. *Muscle Nerve* 17: 500–508.

Barthelemy P, Bregeon F, Zaltara-Hartmann MC, Humbert-Gena C, Jammes Y. (2001) The changes in leg blood flow during and after mild on severe acute hypoxaemia in healthy humans. *Clin Physiol* 21: 308–315.

Bendahan D, Badier M, Jammes Y, et al. (1998) Metabolic and myoelectrical effects of acute hypoxaemia during isometric contraction of forearm muscles in humans: a combined ^{31}P-magnetic resonance spectroscopy – surface electromyogram (MRS-SEMG) study. *Clin Sci* 94: 279–286.

Bowie W, Cumming GR. (1971) Sustained handgrip-reproducibility: effects of hypoxia. *Med Sci Sports* 3: 24–31.

Caquelard F, Burnet H, Tagliernin F, Cauchy E, Richalet JP, Jammes Y. (2000) Effects of prolonged hyobaric hypoxia on human skeletal muscle function and electro-myographic events. *Clin Sci* 98: 329–337.

Cartee GD, Douen AG, Ramlal T, Klip A, Holloszy JO. (1991) Stimulation of glucose transport in skeletal muscle by hypoxia. *J Appl Physiol* 70: 1593–1600.

Cerretelli P, Hoppeler H. (1996) Morphologic and metabolic responses to chronic hypoxia: the muscle system. In: Fregly MJ, Blatteis CM (eds.) *Handbook of Physiology, section 4 Environmental Physiology, vol II*. New-York: Oxford University Press, pp. 1155–1181.

Desplanches D, Hoppeler H, Linossier MT, et al. (1993) Effects of training in normoxia and normobaric hypoxia on human muscle ultrastructure. *Eur J Appl Physiol* 25: 263–267.

Desplanches D, Hoppeler H, Tüscher L, et al. (1996) Muscle tissue adaptations of high-altitude natives to training in chronic hypoxia or acute normoxia. *J Appl Physiol* 81: 1946–1951.

Eiken O, Tesch PA. (1984) Effects of hyperoxia and hypoxia on dynamic and sustained performance of the human quadriceps muscle. *Acta Physiol Scand* 122: 629–633.

Engelen M, Porszasz J, Riley M, Wasserman K, Maehara K, Barstow TJ. (1996) Effects of hypoxic hypoxia on oxygen uptake and heart rate kinetics during heavy exercise. *J Appl Physiol* 81: 2500–2508.

Enoka RM, Stuart DG. (1992) Neurobiology of muscle fatigue. *J Appl Physiol* 72: 1631–1648.

Fulco CS, Cymerman A, Muza SR, Rock PB, Pandolf KB, Lewis SF. (1994) Adductor pollicis muscle fatigue during acute and chronic altitude exposure and return to sea level. *J Appl Physiol* 77: 179–183.

Garner SH, Sutton JR, Burse RL, McComas AJ, Cymerman A, Houston CS. (1990) Operation Everest II: neuromuscular performance under conditions of extreme simulated altitude. *J Appl Physiol* 68: 1167–1172.

Gayeski TE, Honig CR. (1986) Oxygen gradient from sarcolemma to cell interior in red muscle at maximal oxygen uptake. *Am J Physiol* 251: H789–H799.

Green HJ, Sutton JR, Cymerman A, Young PM, Houston CS. (1989) Operation Everest II: adaptations in human skeletal muscle. *J Appl Physiol* 66: 2454–2461.

Gutierrez G, Pohil RG, Narayana P. (1989) Skeletal muscle oxygen consumption and energy metabolism during hypoxemia. *J Appl Physiol* 66: 2117–2123.

Gutierrez G, Hurtado FJ, Gutierrez AM, Fernandez E. (1993) Net uptake of lactate by rabbit hindlimb during hypoxia. *Am Rev Respir Dis* 148: 1204–1209.

Hill JM, Pickar JG, Parrish MD, Kaufman MP. (1992) Effects of hypoxia on the discharge of group III and IV muscle afferents in cats. *J Appl Physiol* 73: 2524–2529.

Hochachka PW. (1994) *Muscles as molecular and metabolic machines*. Boca Raton: CRC Press.

Hogan MC, Nioka S, Brechue WF, Chance B. (1992) A ^{31}P-NMR study of tissue respiration in working dog muscle during reduced oxygen delivery conditions. *J Appl Physiol* 73: 1662–1670.

Jammes Y, Zattara-Hartmann MC, Caquelard F, Arnaud A, Tomei Ch. (1997) Electromyographic changes in vastus lateralis during dynamic exercise. *Muscle Nerve* 20: 247–249.

Joanny P, Steinberg J, Rabaoh P, Richalet JP, Gortan C, Gardetten B, Jammes Y. (2001) Operation Everest III (Comex '97): the effect of simulated severe hypobaric hypoxia on lipid peroxidation and antioxidant defence systems in human blood at rest and after maximal exercise. *Resuscitation* 49: 307–314.

Jones NL, Robertson DG, Kane JW, Heart RA. (1972) Effect of hypoxia on free fatty acid metabolism during exercise. *J Appl Physiol* 33: 733–738.

Kaijer L. (1970) Limiting factors for aerobic muscle performance. *Acta Physiol Scand Suppl* 346: 1–98.

Lagier-Tessonnier F, Balzamo E, Jammes Y. (1993) Comparative effects of ischaemia and acute hypoxemia on muscle afferents from *tibialis anterior* in cats. *Muscle Nerve* 16: 135–141.

Marshall JM. (1995) Skeletal muscle vasculature and systemic hypoxia. *NIPS* 10: 274–280.

Mortimer JT, Magnusson R, Petersen I. (1970) Conduction velocity in ischemic muscle: effect on EMG frequency spectrum. *Am J Physiol* 219: 1324–1329.

Orizio C, Esposito F, Veicsteinas A. (1994) Effect of acclimatization to high altitude (5,050 m) on motor unit activation pattern and muscle performance. *J Appl Physiol* 77: 2840–2844.

Payen JF, Wuyam B, Levy P, et al. (1993) Muscular metabolism during oxygen supplementation in patients with chronic hypoxemia. *Am Rev Respir Dis* 147: 592–598.

Sahlin K, Katz A. (1989) Hypoxaemia increases the accumulation of inosine monophosphate (IMP) in human skeletal muscle during submaximal exercise. *Acta Physiol Scand* 136: 199–203.

Sen Ch K. (1995) Oxidants and antioxidants in exercise. *J Appl Physiol* 79: 675–686.

Sjödin B, Westing YH, Apple FS. (1990) Biochemical mechanisms for oxygen free radical formation during exercise. *Sports Med* 10: 236–254.

Stainsby WN, Brechue WF, O'Drobinak DM, Barclay JK. (1990) Effects of ischemic and hypoxic hypoxia on VO_2 and lactic acid output during tetanic contractions. *J Appl Physiol* 68: 574–579.

Stenberg J, Ekblom B, Messin R. (1966) Hemodynamic response to work at simulated altitude 4,000 m. *J Appl Physiol* 21: 1589–1594.

West JB, Boyer SJ, Graber DJ, et al. (1983) Maximal exercise at extreme altitudes on Mount everest. *J Appl Physiol* 55: 688–698.

Wittenberg BA, Wittenberg JB. (1989) Transport of oxygen in muscle. *Ann Rev Physiol* 51: 857–878.

Young AJ, Evans WJ, Cymerman A, Pandolf KB, Knapik JJ, Maher JT. (1982) Sparing effect of chronic high-altitude exposure on muscle glycogen utilization. *J Appl Physiol* 52: 857–862.

Young AJ, Evans WJ, Fisher EL, Sharp RL, Costill DL, Mahar JT. (1984) Skeletal muscle metabolism of sea-level natives following short-term high-altitude residence. *Eur J Appl Physiol* 52: 463–466.

Young A, Wright J, Knapick J, Cymerman A. (1980) Skeletal muscle strength during exposure to hypobaric hypoxia. *Med Sci Sports Exercise* 12: 330–335.

Zattara-Hartmann MC, Badier M, Guillot Ch, Tomei Ch, Jammes Y. (1995) Maximal force and endurance to fatigue of respiratory and skeletal muscles in chronic hypoxaemic patients: the effects of oxygen breathing. *Muscle Nerve* 18: 495–502.

Zattara-Hartmann MC, Jammes Y. (1996a) Cardiorespiratory response to progressive leg exercise under acute normobaric hypoxia. *Arch Physiol Bioch* 104: 272–281.

Zattara-Hartmann MC, Jammes Y. (1996b) Acute hypoxaemia depresses the cardiorespiratory response during phase I constant load exercise and unloaded cycling. *Arch Physiol Bioch* 104: 212–219.

8

Biochemical aspects of aging of skeletal muscle injuries

Antoni Barrientos, Jordi Casademont, Pierre Rustin and Francesc Cardellach

Introduction

The primary purpose of skeletal muscle is to convert chemical energy into work. Because muscle-working capacity appears to be compromised with aging, major attention has been given to the energy-generating pathways of the muscle cell as the source of age-related biochemical changes that would explain such decay. Indeed, the observation that human beings tend to be less energetic with age would be perfectly accounted for by a decreased ability of the cells to generate ATP. Since the 1960s, this has been the simple rationale for a continuous search for biochemical lesions in elderly people that might underlie a putative shortage in ATP production.

The aim of this chapter is to give a general description of some of the changes in skeletal muscle metabolism (in energy-utilization pathways, and especially in energy-generation pathways) that have been reported to be associated with age. We have tried to look at these changes from the perspective of their physiological effects, a necessity in this controversial field for any biochemical finding to be taken into consideration. Major attention has been paid to changes in the mitochondrial oxidative phosphorylation (OXPHOS) system, and the effect of environmental factors on its modulation has also been considered. For an excellent earlier review on bioenergetics in aging the reader is referred to Hansford (1983), whose conclusions remain valid today.

Age-related physiological and structural changes in skeletal muscle as the starting point for a biochemistry of aging

A glance at the literature on aging-associated changes in metabolic parameters of skeletal muscle depicts a scenario saturated with conflicting findings. To avoid accumulation of data without a clear interpretation, the biochemist should try to provide a mechanism at the biochemical level only after convincing identification of age-related physiological and structural changes.

The identification of possible factors contributing, primarily or secondarily, to age-related changes in

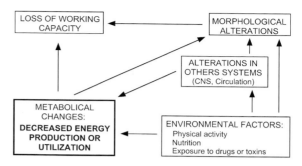

Figure 8.1— Possible factors contributing to age-related changes in skeletal muscle. This simple scheme represents the complexity of the cause–effect relationship among them.

skeletal muscle is complex (Fig. 8.1). Aging would result in a gradual loss of muscle function, associated with muscle atrophy. The loss of muscle mass has been postulated to result from a decrease in fibre number or size, or both (Lexell et al 1988, Holloszy et al 1991). Type II fibres may be the most affected (Lexell et al 1988, Kinderdall and Garrett 1998). Major factors underlying a loss of muscle fibres are denervation (Flanigan et al 1998, Kinderdall and Garrett 1998) and changes in the microcirculation, in part caused by a reduced vasodilatory capacity and a decreased capillarization (Degens 1998). All these changes would account for the observed decline in maximal oxygen uptake (reviewed in Paterson and Cunningham 1999), which would affect the aerobic pathways of muscle metabolism. If all these changes occur, a shift in the metabolism of the tissue should also be expected.

However, the extent of muscle mass loss varies from one individual to another, and from muscle to muscle (Tomonaga 1977, Rogers and Evans 1993, Lynch 1999). There is now good evidence to suggest that these losses could be the result of conditions frequently found in old age, like nerve entrapments, ischaemia, latent chronic diseases, malnutrition and, fundamentally, muscle disuse. This is illustrated by studies of the apparent age-related decline of physiological performance, and of structural and metabolic parameters; however, these can be minimized, or even reversed, with training (Rogers and Evans 1993, Kirkendall and Garrett 1998, Reimers et al 1998). If physiologists can not consider a decline in the muscle's force-producing capacity as an inevitable consequence of aging, changes in biochemical parameters defining muscle metabolism should never be interpreted as a primary cause of aging, but as a consequence of this process.

Effects of age on ATP utilization during contraction–associated processes

Metabolism is closely coupled to muscle performance, the ultimate chemical driving reaction being the breakdown of ATP, which is used in several biochemical reactions associated with muscle contraction (Fig. 8.2).

The significance of age-related alterations in contractility at the biochemical level is controversial. The maximal velocity of muscle shortening is directly proportional to the actin activated ATPase activity of myosin. Early studies in rats showed some decrease in actomyosin ATPase activity (Syrovy and Gutmann 1970), but in general no significant changes have been reported (Larsson et al 1978, Florini and Ewton 1989), which correlates with an also unchanged intrinsic velocity of shortening of the whole muscle (Faulkner

et al 1990). The Ca^{2+} pump work in the sarcoplasmic reticulum is mediated by a $Ca^{2+}Mg^{2+}ATPase$, the activity of which remains unchanged with age (Narayanan et al 1996).

In general, contractility seems not to be biochemically impaired during aging, although electrophysiological experiments provide different results depending on the muscle studied (Doherty and Brown 1997, Hunter et al 1999).

Effects of age on the enzymatic pathways leading to ATP generation

Chemical energy reaches the muscle in the form of glucose and fatty acids, and it may be stored as glycogen. These substances are metabolized to produce ATP, the primary energy supplier. The supply of ATP is secured in at least three ways operating on different time scales:

- phosphorylation by phosphocreatine, which is a short-term store of high energy
- anaerobic glycolysis as a medium-term supply
- aerobic respiration as a long-term supply.

Next sections will comment on age-related changes in these pathways.

Lohmann reaction

In the Lohman reaction, ATP is regenerated directly by transphosphorylation from phosphocreatine to ADP (Fig. 8.2). Creatine phosphokinase activity has been reported to decline progressively with age, apparently mainly due to muscle disuse (Steinhagen-Thiessen and Reznick 1987, McCully et al 1993). Reports showing no significant changes in its activity also appear in the literature (Ermini 1976). In addition, studies on changes in resting phosphocreatine and ATP concentrations, and on the capacity to restore phosphocreatine after exercise, show contradictory results (Ermini 1976, Taylor et al 1984, Cady et al 1989, Klitgaard et al 1989). Phosphocreatine resynthesis is regulated by an isozyme of creatine phosphokinase bound to the outer mitochondrial membrane, and the initial rate of recovery is proportional to the rate of mitochondrial oxygen consump-

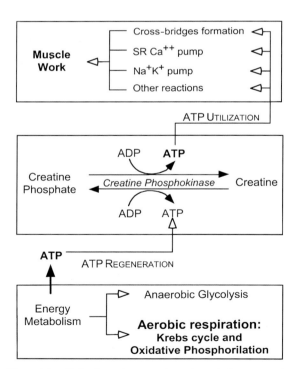

Figure 8.2—Skeletal muscle energetics and metabolism. In working muscle, the reserve of creatine phosphate is drawn on, and is recharged by energy metabolism after the muscle return to rest. SR, sarcoplasmic reticulum. *Is the ATP provision or utilization compromised with aging, leading a limitation in the working capacity?*

tion (Mahler et al 1985, Kemp et al 1993, Thompson et al 1994). It seems likely that the lag in the reestablishment of creatine phosphatase levels to the resting values reported for some aged muscles, reflects more an impairment in ATP generation than a decrease in creatine kinase activity. Nevertheless, easy associations are not possible in this field: we are also far from a clear demonstration of an universal decrease in mitochondrial respiratory capacity with age (see below).

Anaerobic glycolysis

Creatine phosphatase is quickly exhaustible, and further processes to replenish the ATP supply are needed. In the anaerobic glycolysis pathway, glycogen is metabolized via glucose-6-phosphate to lactic acid, yielding only two ATP molecules per unit of glucose. This pathway is much less productive than the aerobic degradation of glucose, but it may represent a significant source of ATP, particularly in white muscle fibres.

An age-related change in the relative type composition of muscle fibres, as has been postulated, would reflect a switch in the metabolic characteristics of the tissue. There are few reports dealing with age-related alterations in glycolytic enzymes. No changes or non-consistent changes have been found in phosphofructokinase, phosphorylase, aldolase or hexokinase activities (Larsson et al 1978, Schlenska and Kleine 1980, Aniansson et al 1986, Borges and Essen-Gustavsson 1989). Some studies have reported a significant decrease in lactate dehydrogenase activity (Coggan et al 1992). This is a very interesting enzyme since it is functionally placed between the anaerobic (end of glycolysis) and aerobic energy metabolism (NAD+ dependence). Nevertheless these changes were attributed to muscle disuse. Studies in rats have shown that age-related changes can be manifested differently in the various fibre and muscle types (Holloszy et al 1991). In general, it seems that glycolytic enzyme activities are not adversely affected by aging. As a consequence, the hypothesis of a general shift in skeletal muscles from a basically aerobic to a more glycolytic metabolism should be observed with caution.

Aerobic degradation of glucose: Krebs cycle and oxidative phosphorylation system

The aerobic degradation of glucose via the citric acid cycle and oxidative phosphorylation, yielding 38 ATP molecules per molecule of glucose, constitutes the main source of ATP for skeletal muscle. For this reason, much of the studies devoted to age-related changes in ATP generation have focused on the characterization of potential mitochondrial OXPHOS impairment. OXPHOS results from the concurrent activities of the four electron transfer chain complexes (complexes I–IV) and of the ATPase (complex V; Fig. 8.3).

The biochemical demonstration of skeletal muscle OXPHOS impairment obviously represents the corner stone of any theory endowing mitochondria the key role in a putative age-dependent decrease of muscle ATP production, and it should constitute a preliminary requirement before establishing any search for underlying alterations in possibly related genes.

Unfortunately, despite 40 years of intensive effort to clarify the situation, no general agreement about the existence of age-related OXPHOS alterations has been reached in the scientific community so far. Similar approaches still produce apparently irreconcilable sets of data on human skeletal muscle. As a result, there are still tenets that a gross impairment of the mitochondrial OXPHOS takes place with age in human skeletal muscle (Cardellach et al 1989, Trounce et al 1989, Boffoli et al 1994, Lezza et al 1994, Lefai et al 1995), whereas others conclude that OXPHOS is substantially not changed in the elderly (Zucchini et al 1995, Barrientos et al 1996, Brierley et al 1996). Most of these studies rely on statistical analyses of putative age-dependent decreases of mitochondrial OXPHOS enzyme activities, trying to correlate

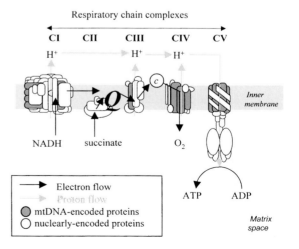

Figure 8.3— The mitochondrial respiratory chain. Q, ubiquinone (CoQ$_{10}$); c, cytochrome c.

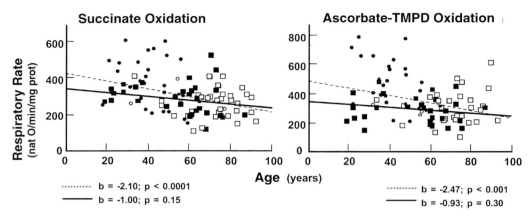

Figure 8.4—Relationship between respiratory rates of substrate oxidation in human skeletal muscle mitochondria (modified from Barrientos et al 1996). The continuous line represents the relationship between age and oxygen consumption rates once controlled for confounding variables physical activity and tobacco consumption. Dotted line figures a simple linear regression analysis. Although we made an effort to consider the influence of confounding variables, the distribution of values obtained suggests the necessity to consider parameters other than respiratory rates and statistical analyses other than regression lines. Solid dots: smokers with normal physical activity. Empty dots: smokers with limited physical activity. Solid squares: non-smokers with normal physical activity. Empty squares: non-smokers with limited physical activity.

activities with age by using linear regression analyses. Loss of cytochrome *c* oxidase (COX) activity, the terminal oxidase of the respiratory chain, is now the most frequently reported age-dependent change. How similar analyses of relatively large cohorts of control individuals can lead to opposite conclusions is a quite intriguing question. In an attempt to solve this puzzle, we and others have evidenced factors that interfere with the determination of enzyme activity levels, or respiratory rates, in human skeletal muscle (Barrientos et al 1996, Brierley et al 1996; Fig. 8.4). But even before considering such factors, one should question the statistical significance of the analysis of enzyme activity values. Strikingly large ranges of absolute activities of OXPHOS enzymes are actually measured in human skeletal muscle, even for a given age class (Boffoli et al 1994, Lefai et al 1995, Barrientos et al 1996). Noticeably, zero value often falls within two standard deviations of the mean value! This has led us to analyse the type of statistical distribution of OXPHOS activities in control individuals. Such analysis regularly shows non-Gaussian distribution of OXPHOS enzyme activities for a given age class. From this simple observation, it follows that attempts: i) to use means and standard deviations in quantifying OXPHOS enzyme activities and ii) to establish a correlation between age and OXPHOS enzyme activity through the calculation of the linear

regression coefficient and the associated *p* values, are essentially meaningless.

The use of additional parameters to characterize the activity of the OXPHOS pathway, therefore, appears imperative. It is a general observation that, echoing the virtually constant cytochrome composition of the respiratory chain spectra, relative activities of the respiratory chain complexes are consistently conserved in functional mitochondria (Rustin et al 1991, Chretien et al 1998). A tight balance between respiratory chain activities is indeed required to allow concurrent oxidation of various substrates to proceed and to avoid significant leakage of free radicals from the respiratory chain. Therefore, respiratory chain activity ratios, which present a Gaussian distribution in the control population (see *inset* of Fig. 8.5), constitute confident parameters to diagnose subtle changes in the activity of any of the respiratory chain complexes. Based on this observation, we have analysed, in the largest cohort of individuals investigated so far, the correlation of skeletal muscle OXPHOS enzyme activities with age. The absence of any statistically significant, and specific, variation with age in the enzymatic activity of any of the respiratory chain complex has been unambiguously established by using this approach (Chretien et al 1998; Fig. 8.5). After reviewing 270 papers related to bioenergetics of aging in 1983, a similar verdict was returned by RG Hansford who stated

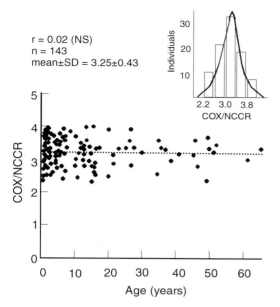

r = 0.02 (NS)
n = 143
mean±SD = 3.25±0.43

Figure 8.5— Absence of age-related changes of cytochrome *c* oxidase (COX) to NADH-cytochrome *c* reductase (NCCR) activity ratio in human skeletal muscle mitochondria. *Inset*: The normal distribution of COX/NCCR activity ratios in the control population.

in his conclusion that "Credence can no longer be given to the results of experiments showing grossly impaired oxidative phosphorylation in suspensions of mitochondria from senescent animals... mitochondria are substantially undamaged both biochemically and morphologically...".

The conclusion that the capacity of OXPHOS complexes is not grossly impaired with age does not preclude that changes might occur in vivo in the use of this capacity to produce ATP. A reduced availability of substrate to the mitochondrial dehydrogenases, a downregulation of the activity of specific mitochondrial enzymes (pyruvate crossroad, Krebs cycle, fatty acid oxidation, etc), or even a physiological regulation of respiratory chain complex activities, all might concur in vivo leading to a slowing down of ATP production. One should also keep in mind that behavioural characteristics of aged individuals (i.e. decreased physical activity) might largely affect the cell energy demand (Zamora et al 1995; see below), a factor known to directly affect the overall mitochondrial activity. Therefore, a putative decrease in energy production in vivo may well be the result, rather than the consequence, of age.

Once settled that no gross loss of OXPHOS enzyme activities are observed with age, it has to be mentioned that some investigators have shown—by

using the polymerase chain reaction (PCR)—an age-related appearance of a low percentage of mutant mitochondrial DNA (mtDNA) species (Cortopassi and Arnheim 1990, Wallace et al 1995, Cortopassi and Wong 1999). It should be noted that, in patients with respiratory chain defects originating from mtDNA mutations, tissues with less than 20% of mutant mtDNA generally do not show any OXPHOS defect, while in some cell types up to 90% of mutant mtDNA may be necessary to produce any biochemical defect! (Bourgeron et al 1993). The biochemical and physiological consequences in the skeletal muscle syncytium of a very limited amount of mutant mtDNA species may, therefore, reasonably be considered as negligible. It is, however, worth noting that this might actually not hold true for specific cells, such as neurons, that could be more sensitive to mtDNA mutations and even go into apoptosis or necrosis in case of mitochondrial OXPHOS impairment.

Modulation of some biochemical parameters by environmental factors

The majority of metabolic, structural and physiological alterations of skeletal muscles affected by disuse, malnutrition, diseases, drugs and injuries are similar, if not identical, to changes that are observed in old age (reviewed in Carmeli and Reznick 1994). Since these factors interfere directly or indirectly with mitochondrial function they can be confused with the age factor, which could explain the considerable controversy concerning age-related changes in skeletal muscle's mitochondrial metabolism.

There are a number of factors to be considered.

Exercise

Physical training and exercise have, in particular, been proven to largely control the level of OXPHOS activity in skeletal muscle mitochondria (Zamora et al 1995). The importance of taking into account the individual's physical activity habits in studies of age-related changes in OXPHOS function is illustrated by an already cited work in which we analysed a large number of individuals from 15 to 95 years (Barrientos et al 1996). We found an inverse correlation between age and substrate oxidation rates that, however, disappeared when physical activity was taken into consideration as a confounding variable (Fig. 8.4).

Moreover, no significant differences in any respiratory parameter were found between young and elderly athletes (Brierley et al 1997), indicating that, probably, active muscles do not suffer any significant age-related OXPHOS alteration. Although strenuous exercice is characterized by an increased oxygen consumption and disturbance of intracellular prooxidant–antioxidant homeostasis (Ji et al 1998), this delicate balance seems to be maintained in elderly people who undergo mild exercise.

Drugs

A large number of drugs have a deleterious effect on mitochondria through different mechanisms: inhibition of DNA synthesis, inhibition of β-oxidation, uncoupling of oxidative phosphorylation and electron transport, inhibition of respiratory chain substrate oxidation or changing the membrane properties. Some of them, especially antiviral agents of the nucleoside analogues group (e.g. zidovudine; Dalakas et al 1990) are toxic to skeletal muscle in a dose dependent manner. Mitochondrial function alterations have also been described with anaesthetics (Miró et al 1999), neuroleptic medications (Barrientos et al 1998), non-steroidal anti-inflamatory drugs (Moreno-Sánchez et al 1999), and many other agents (reviewed in Cardellach et al 1998). Although people take these drugs in a different manner, it is obvious that many elderly use some of them. In consequence, all studies on mitochondrial function in aging should take into account this potential confounding variable.

Toxins

Some common toxins also can affect OXPHOS function. Tobacco smoke causes a general substrate oxidation inhibition in rats (Pryor et al 1992). Studies performed in human skeletal muscle mitochondria have shown decreased complex I and IV activities (Larsson and Orlander 1984, Smith et al 1993), and increased endogenous production of oxygen free radicals (Kalra et al 1991) in smokers. Studies in human lymphocytes have shown that in smokers complex IV activity is decreased, and succinate oxidation increases probably as a compensatory mechanism (Miró et al 1999). Similar effect on oxidation seems to occur in human skeletal muscle (Barrientos et al 1996; Fig. 8.4). Chronic alcoholism also has a deleterious effect on muscles. It is commonly associated with chronic myopathy of skeletal muscle and cardiomyopathy (Rubin 1979, Urbano-Márquez et al 1989;

Ch. 23), but the involvement of the mitochondria in the pathogenesis of the lesions is not clearly established (Cardellach et al 1992, Haida et al 1998).

Nutrition

The importance of nutrition in delaying the aging process is well recognized. Caloric restriction has been suggested to reduce oxidative stress and effectively increases the life span of animals by causing a metabolic shift towards increased protein turnover and decreased macromolecular damage (Lee et al 1999). Specific dietary habits will contribute to maintaining an appropriate cellular antioxidant defence system, and a correct supply of substrates necessary for mitochondrial function. In keeping with this, some specific myopathies with mitochondrial abnormalities are a consequence of specific dietary element deficiencies, like selenium (Osaki et al 1998) and copper (Mao et al 1998).

Other factors

The consideration of all these aforementioned factors, in addition to those putative mitochondrial-associated diseases in elderly, like Parkinson's disease (Cardellach et al 1993), is crucial for the understanding of the role of mitochondria in the pathogenesis of aging and also to diagnose confidently patients with an OXPHOS deficiency (Barrientos et al 1996, Chretien et al 1998).

Conclusions

With age, people tend to become less energetic. During the last 30 years biochemists have focused on the description of metabolic alterations to explain age-associated changes in skeletal muscle physiology and structure. These changes are expressed in a different manner and to a different degree in different fibres, muscles and individuals, questioning their categorization as primary effectors of aging. On the other hand, conflicting findings are abundant in the literature on the influence of age on the skeletal muscle system. This is especially true for studies seeking changes based on biochemical parameters related to muscle energetics and enzymology. A number of factors may account for the conflicting results: measurement of biochemical parameters that are not appropriate, differences in experimental designs, including the selection of muscle type examined, or in statistical analyses. In addition, a multitude of extraneous factors, such as the health status of the subjects and animals used, their life style, or the influence of changes in systems other than muscle, modulate skeletal muscle metabolism, and the biochemist is not always able to control their influence. Their importance is illustrated by the fact that, for example, most biochemical changes (and their physiological and structural consequences) can totally or in part be compensated for by physical activity; this questions again the primary effect of aging compared with exercise deficiency, or in a more general way, if biochemical changes are cause or effect of senescence. No firm evidence of general alterations in biochemical pathways implicated in ATP breakdown in muscle contraction-associated processes, or in enzymatic pathways sustaining the generation of ATP (Lohmann reaction, anaerobic and aerobic glucose degradation) has been yet convincingly reported. It is a fact that mitochondria, the main actors in respiratory processes, remain basically unchanged at biochemical level during aging, questioning the validity of some aspects of theories of aging based on OXPHOS dysfunction.

References

Aniansson A, Hedberg M, Henning GB, Grimby G. (1986) Muscle morphology, enzymatic activity, and muscle strength in elderly men: a follow-up study. *Muscle Nerve* 9: 585–591.

Barrientos A, Casademont J, Rotig A, et al. (1996) Absence of relationship between the level of electron transport chain activities and aging in human skeletal muscle. *Biochem Biophys Res Commun* 229: 536–539.

Barrientos A, Marin C, Miró O, et al. (1998) Biochemical and molecular effects of chronic haloperidol administration on brain and muscle mitochondria of rats. *J Neurosci Res* 53: 475–481.

Boffoli D, Scacco SC, Vergari R, Solarino G, Santacroce G, Papa S. (1994) Decline with age of the respiratory chain activity in human skeletal muscle. *Biochim Biophys Acta* 1226: 73–82.

Borges O, Essen-Gustavsson B. (1989) Enzyme activities in type I and II muscle fibres of human skeletal muscle in relation to age and torque development. *Acta Physiol Scand* 136: 29–36.

Bourgeron T, Chretien D, Rötig A, Munnich A, Rustin P. 1993. Fate and expression of the deleted mitochondrial DNA differ between heteroplasmic skin fibroblast and Epstein-Barr virus-transformed lymphocyte cultures. *J Biol Chem* 268: 19369–19376.

Brierley EJ, Johnson MA, James OF, Turnbull DM. (1996) Effects of physical activity and age on mitochondrial function. *Q J Med* 89: 251–258.

Brierley EJ, Johnson MA, Bowman A, et al. (1997) Mitochondrial function in muscle from elderly athletes [published erratum appears in *Ann Neurol* (1997) 41(5): 698]. *Ann Neurol* 41: 114–116.

Cady EB, Jones DA, Lynn J, Newham DJ. (1989) Changes in force and intracellular metabolites during fatigue of human skeletal muscle. *J Physiol* 418: 311–325.

Cardellach F, Galofré J, Cussó R, Urbano-Márquez A. (1989) Decline in skeletal muscle mitochondrial respiration chain function with aging. *Lancet* 2: 44–45.

Cardellach F, Galofré J, Grau JM, et al. (1992) Oxidative metabolism in muscle mitochondria from patients with chronic alcoholism. *Ann Neurol* 31: 515–518.

Cardellach F, Martí MJ, Fernandez-Solà J, et al. (1993) Mitochondrial respiratory chain activity in skeletal muscle from patients with Parkinson's disease. *Neurology* 43: 2258–2262.

Cardellach F, Casademont J, Urbano-Márquez A. (1998) [Secondary mitochondrial diseases]. *Rev Neurol* 26: S81–86.

Carmeli E, Reznick AZ. (1994) The physiology and biochemistry of skeletal muscle atrophy as a function of age. *Proc Soc Exp Biol Med* 206: 103–113.

Chretien D, Gallego J, Barrientos A, et al. (1998) Biochemical parameters for the diagnosis of mitochondrial respiratory chain deficiency in humans, and their lack of age-related changes. *Biochem J* 329: 249–254.

Coggan AR, Spina RJ, King DS, et al. (1992) Histochemical and enzymatic comparison of the gastrocnemius muscle of young and elderly men and women. *J Gerontol* 47: B71–76.

Cortopassi GA, Arnheim N. (1990) Detection of a specific mitochondrial DNA deletion in tissues of older humans. *Nucleic Acids Res* 18: 6927–6933.

Cortopassi GA, Wong A. (1999) Mitochondria in organismal aging and degeneration. *Biochim Biophys Acta* 1410: 183–193.

Dalakas MC, Illa I, Pezeshkpour GH, Laukaitis JP, Cohen B, Griffin JL. (1990) Mitochondrial myopathy caused by long-term zidovudine therapy. *N Engl J Med* 322: 1098–1105.

Degens H. (1998) Age-related changes in the microcirculation of skeletal muscle. *Adv Exp Med Biol* 454: 343–348.

Doherty TJ, Brown WF. (1997) Age-related changes in the twitch contractile properties of human thenar motor units. *J Appl Physiol* 82: 93–101.

Ermini M. (1976) Aging changes in mammalian skeletal muscle: biochemical studies. *Gerontology* 22: 301–316.

Faulkner JA, Brooks SV, Zerba E. (1990) Skeletal muscle weakness and fatigue in old age: underlying mechanisms. *Annu Rev Gerontol Geriatr* 10: 147–166.

Flanigan KM, Lauria G, Griffin JW, Kuncl RW. (1998) Age-related biology and diseases of muscle and nerve. *Neurol Clin* 16: 659–669.

Florini JR, Ewton DZ. (1989) Skeletal muscle fibre types and myosin ATPase activity do not change with age or growth hormone administration. *J Gerontol* 44: B110–117.

Haida M, Yazaki K, Kurita D, Shinohara Y. (1998) Mitochondrial dysfunction of human muscle in chronic alcoholism detected by using ^{31}P-magnetic resonance spectroscopy and near-infrared light absorption. *Alcohol Clin Exp Res* 22: 108S–110S.

Hansford RG. (1983) Bioenergetics in aging. *Biochim Biophys Acta* 726: 41–80.

Holloszy JO, Chen M, Cartee GD, Young JC. (1991) Skeletal muscle atrophy in old rats: differential changes in the three fibre types. *Mech Aging Dev* 60: 199–213.

Hunter SK, Thompson MW, Ruell PA, et al. (1999) Human skeletal sarcoplasmic reticulum Ca^{2+} uptake and muscle function with aging and strength training. *J Appl Physiol* 86: 1858–1865.

Ji LL, Leeuwenburgh C, Leichtweis S, et al. (1998) Oxidative stress and aging. Role of exercise and its influences on antioxidant systems. *Ann N Y Acad Sci* 854: 102–117.

Kalra J, Chaudhary AK, Prasad K. (1991) Increased production of oxygen free radicals in cigarette smokers. *Intl J Exp Pathol* 72: 1–7.

Kemp GJ, Taylor DJ, Radda GK. (1993) Control of phosphocreatine resynthesis during recovery from exercise in human skeletal muscle. *NMR Biomed* 6: 66–72.

Kirkendall DT, Garrett WE, Jr. (1998) The effects of aging and training on skeletal muscle. *Am J Sports Med* 26: 598–602.

Klitgaard H, Brunet A, Maton B, Lamaziere C, Lesty C, Monad H. (1989) Morphological and biochemical changes in old rat muscles: effect of increased use. *J Appl Phyiol* 67: 1409–1417.

Larsson L, Sjodin B, Karlsson J. (1978) Histochemical and biochemical changes in human skeletal muscle with age in sedentary males, age 22–65 years. *Acta Physiol Scand* 103: 31–39.

Larsson L. (1978) Morphological and functional characteristics of the aging skeletal muscle in man. A cross-sectional study. *Acta Physiol Scand Suppl* 457: 1–36.

Larsson L, Orlander J. (1984) Skeletal muscle morphology, metabolism and function in smokers and non-smokers. A study on smoking-discordant monozygous twins. *Acta Physiol Scand* 120: 343–352.

Lee CK, Klopp RG, Weindruch R, Prolla TA. (1999) Gene expression profile of aging and its retardation by caloric restriction. *Science* 285: 1390–1393.

Lefai E, Terrier-Cayre A, Vincent A, Boespflug-Tanguy O, Tanguy A, Alziari S. (1995) Enzymatic activities of mitochondrial respiratory complexes from children muscular biopsies. Age-related evolutions. *Biochim Biophys Acta* 1228: 43–50.

Lexell J, Taylor CC, Sjostrom M. (1988) What is the cause of the aging atrophy? Total number, size and proportion of different fibre types studied in whole vastus lateralis muscle from 15- to 83-year-old men. *J Neurol Sci* 84: 275–294.

Lezza AM, Boffoli D, Scacco S, Cantatore P, Gadaleta MN. (1994) Correlation between mitochondrial DNA 4977-bp deletion and respiratory chain enzyme activities in aging human skeletal muscles. *Biochem Biophys Res Commun* 205: 772–779.

Lynch NA, Metter EJ, Lindle RS, et al (1999) Muscle quality. I. Age-associated differences between arm and leg muscle groups. *J Appl Physiol* 86: 188–194.

Mahler M. (1985) First-order kinetics of muscle oxygen consumption, and an equivalent proportionality between QO2 and phosphorylcreatine level. Implications for the control of respiration. *J Gen Physiol* 86: 135–165.

Mao S, Medeiros DM, Wildman RE. (1998) Cardiac hypertrophy in copper-deficient rats is owing to increased mitochondria. *Biol Trace Elem Res* 64: 175–184.

McCully KK, Fielding RA, Evans WJ, Leigh JS, Jr., Posner JD. (1993) Relationships between in vivo and in vitro measurements of metabolism in young and old human calf muscles. *J Appl Physiol* 75: 813–819.

Miró O, Barrientos A, Alonso JR, et al. (1999) Effects of general anaesthetic procedures on mitochondrial function of human skeletal muscle. *Eur J Clin Pharmacol* 55: 35–41.

Miró O, Alonso JR, Jarreta D, Casademont J, Urbano-Márquez A, Cardellach F. (1999) Smoking disturbs mitochondrial respiratory chain function and enhances lipid peroxidation on human circulating lymphocytes. *Carcinogenesis* 20: 1331–1336.

Moreno-Sanchez R, Bravo C, Vasquez C, Ayala G, Silveira LH, Martinez-Lavin M. (1999) Inhibition and uncoupling of oxidative phosphorylation by nonsteroidal anti-inflammatory drugs: study in mitochondria, submitochondrial particles, cells, and whole heart. *Biochem Pharmacol* 57: 743–752.

Narayanan N, Jones DL, Xu A, Yu JC. (1996) Effects of aging on sarcoplasmic reticulum function and contraction duration in skeletal muscles of the rat. *Am J Physiol* 271: C1032–C1040.

Osaki Y, Nishino I, Murakami N, et al. (1998) Mitochondrial abnormalities in selenium-deficient myopathy. *Muscle Nerve* 21: 637–639.

Paterson DH, Cunningham DA. (1999) The gas transporting systems: limits and modifications with age and training. *Can J Appl Physiol* 24: 28–40.

Pryor WA, Arbour NC, Upham B, Church DF. (1992) The inhibitory effect of extracts of cigarette tar on electron transport of mitochondria and submitochondrial particles. *Free Radic Biol Med* 12: 365–372.

Reimers CD, Harder T, Saxe H. (1998) Age-related muscle atrophy does not affect all muscles and can partly be compensated by physical activity: an ultrasound study [published erratum appears in *J Neurol Sci* (1999) 162(2): 211]. *J Neurol Sci* 159: 60–66.

Rogers MA, Evans WJ. (1993) Changes in skeletal muscle with aging: effects of exercise training. *Exerc Sport Sci Rev* 21: 65–102.

Rubin E. (1979) Alcoholic myopathy in heart and skeletal muscle. *N Engl J Med* 301: 28–33.

Rustin P, Chretien D, Bourgeron T, et al. (1991) Assessment of the mitochondrial respiratory chain. *Lancet* 338: 60.

Schlenska GK, Kleine TO. (1980) Disorganization of glycolytic and gluconeogenic pathways in skeletal muscle of aged persons studied by histometric and enzymatic methods. *Mech Aging Dev* 13: 143–154.

Smith PR, Cooper JM, Govan GG, Harding AE, Schapira AH. (1993) Smoking and mitochondrial function: a model for environmental toxins. *Q J Med* 86: 657–660.

Steinhagen-Thiessen E, Reznick AZ. (1987) Effect of short- and long-term endurance training on creatine phosphokinase activity in skeletal and cardiac muscles of CW-1 and C57BL mice. *Gerontology* 33: 14–18.

Syrovy I, Gutmann E. (1970) Changes in speed of contraction and ATPase activity in striated muscle during old age. *Exp Gerontol* 5: 31–35.

Taylor DJ, Crowe M, Bore PJ, Styles P, Arnold DL, Radda GK. (1984) Examination of the energetics of aging skeletal muscle using nuclear magnetic resonance. *Gerontology* 30: 2–7.

Thompson LV. (1994) Effects of age and training on skeletal muscle physiology and performance. *Phys Ther* 74: 71–81.

Tomonaga M. (1977) Histochemical and ultrastructural changes in senile human skeletal muscle. *J Am Geriatr Soc* 25: 125–131.

Trounce I, Byrne E, Marzuki S. (1989) Decline in skeletal muscle mitochondrial respiratory chain function: possible factor in aging. *Lancet* 1: 637–639.

Urbano-Márquez A, Estruch R, Navarro-López F, Grau JM, Mont L, Rubin E. (1989) The effects of alcoholism on skeletal and cardiac muscle. *N Engl J Med* 320: 409–415.

Wallace DC, Shoffner JM, Trounce I, et al. (1995) Mitochondrial DNA mutations in human degenerative diseases and aging. *Biochim Biophys Acta* 1271: 141–151.

Zamora AJ, Tessier F, Marconnet P, Margaritis I, Marini JF. (1995) Mitochondria changes in human muscle after prolonged exercise, endurance training and selenium supplementation. *Eur J Appl Physiol* 71: 505–511.

Zucchini C, Pugnaloni A, Pallotti F, et al. (1995) Human skeletal muscle mitochondria in aging: lack of detectable morphological and enzymic defects. *Biochem Mol Biol Intl* 37: 607–616.

9

Steroid misuse in athletes: effects on skeletal muscle

Priscilla M. Clarkson and Adam M. Persky

Introduction

For decades athletes have used synthetic derivatives of testosterone to increase muscle mass and exercise performance. Because these drugs still maintain some androgenic (masculinizing) effects of testosterone, they are referred to as anabolic–androgenic steroids (AAS) (Wagner 1991). The types of athletes who use AAS have traditionally been men who participate in activities requiring force and bulk, such as football, weight lifting and some track sports. However, to gain a competitive edge more and more athletes are using steroids with legal implications (Gimson 2000).

This chapter will review data on the prevalence of AAS use and the mechanism of steroid action. We will also provide an overview of the effectiveness of AAS on increasing muscle mass and strength. Lastly, we will briefly discuss the effects of steroids on health as well as athletes' perceptions of their physiological benefits.

Types of anabolic–androgen steroids

Athletes' choice of AAS can depend on the anabolic–androgenic balance of the drug and the route of administration desired. Testosterone and testosterone analogues have low oral bioavailability and, therefore, are formulated for intramuscular administration. Oral bioavailability of the steroid molecule is accomplished after alkylation at the 17-α position on the steroid ring, thus reducing first-pass metabolism.

The anabolic–androgenic balance is inherent in the molecular structure and no one drug has been synthesized to be fully anabolic or androgenic. For example, fluoxymesterone (Halotestin) is an oral steroid with strong androgenic properties. However methandrostenolone (Dianabol) is an oral steroid with strong anabolic properties. Other commonly used steroids are injectable nandrolone decanoate (Deca-Durabolin), stanozolol (Winstrol) as an injectable and oral formulation, the oral steroid oxandrolone (Anavar), injectable and oral methenolone (Primbolan), and several testosterone esters (e.g., testosterone-enanthate, -cypionate, -propionate). Injectable testosterone is esterified at the 17-β position. Despite the various molecular arrangements to accommodate the desired effects, or desired route of administration, the mechanism by which AAS work is universal.

In 1991, Catlin and Hatton reported that there were over 40 synthetic AAS marketed worldwide. Based on results of positive drug tests for AAS, the most commonly found oral AAS were methandrostenolone, oxandrolone, stanozolol, oxymetholone (Anadrol, considered one of the most anabolic oral steroid), and methyltestosterone. The most common injectable AAS were esters of nandrolone (Anadur, Deca-Durabolin, Durabolin, Dynabolin, Laurabolin), testosterone, and methenolone. Catlin and Hatton (1991) also noted the presence of veterinarian AAS such as Boldenone (Equipoise—used for horses and cattle), mibolerone, and injectable stanozolol as well as AAS not FDA approved such as trenbolone (Finaject, Parabolan), furazabol (Miotolan), and formebolone (Esiclene) in urine samples from athletes.

Prevalence of use

We know little about the prevalence of current steroid use in elite or collegiate athletes. Because these drugs are banned by many national governing bodies, including the International Olympic Committee and the National Collegiate Athletic Association, athletes are unlikely to want to report using them for fear of being discovered and disqualified. The number of positive drug tests are not an accurate reflection of use; athletes know how long they have to stop taking the steroids in order not to test positive, and they know how to use masking agents. Prevalence of use by those in the general public is also difficult to assess because these drugs are illegal if not prescribed by a physician. Thus, the data provided below are probably an underestimation of actual use.

Competitive athletes

Surveys done in the 1970s indicated that 61% of track and field athletes who participated in the 1972 Olympic Games had used AAS in the past 6 months (Silvester 1972). Thirty-one per cent of elite track and field athletes and 75% of the throwers in Sweden admitted to prior steroid use (Ljunqvist 1975). Few data exist on current use of AAS by elite athletes. However, in a newspaper survey of 147 Olympians from 1932–1984 Winter Games, 75% of 45 medalists responded that more athletes in 1992 used enhancing drugs compared with when they competed (Pearson 1994).

Other competitive athletes taking AAS are the bodybuilders (Lindström et al 1990, Perry et al 1990, Auge and Auge 1999). In 1990, Lindstrom report that 75% of those competing in a body building competition were considered to be taking AAS. Curry and

Wagman (1999) sent questionnaires to 26 US Powerlifting Team members who had competed since 1988: 15 questionnaires were returned, and of these, 10 admitted to using AAS and 5 admitted to beating the International Olympic Committee's doping control procedures.

In a review of studies of US Collegiate athletes, Yesalis and Bahrke (1995) noted a range of steroid use of about 1–10%, with the highest incidence in the football players. A survey of college athletes during 1988–1989 showed that 5% of Division 1 athletes reported steroid use (Anderson et al 1991). Because of the problem with underestimation, Yesalis et al (1993) took a different approach and asked over 1600 collegiate athletes at Division 1 institutions to estimate their competitor's AAS use. The results showed that these athletes estimated a 14.7% use for males and a 5.9% use for females, with male football players at 29.3%.

Stilger and Yesalis (1999) reported that of 873 high school football players, 6.3% had taken steroids, and the average age at time of first use was 14 years. Fifteen per cent began taking steroids before the age of 10 years. About half of the users reported that they could obtain the steroids when they wanted, and they listed their sources as other athletes, physicians and coaches.

Although there are a fair number of females using AAS (Strauss et al 1985, Cordova 1996, Gruber and Pope 2000), the incidence of use for females is usually less than one third that for the males. From the summary tables presented in the review by Yesalis and Bahrke (1995), an average AAS use of 3.7% for college male athletes and 0.4% for college female athletes was calculated. Most females are taking steroids to improve athletic performance in those sports that required strength (Cordova 1996).

General public and recreational athletes

Yesalis et al (1993) reported data on AAS use obtained from the 1991 National Household Survey on Drug Abuse. They estimated that over 1 million Americans were using or had used AAS. While there may be some therapeutic use for these drugs, and some users may be taking the drugs to enhance performance, another reason for taking these drugs is to increase muscle mass for appearance. The ideal man towards the end of the 20th century demonstrated some muscle development, but over the years the ideal has become very muscular. This is seen in today's popular images of men, and it is clearly depicted in the profound muscularity of GI Joe doll today compared with when the doll was introduced in 1964 (Lee 1996, Nurse 1998). In fact, the pressure for males to achieve this muscular body type is now associated with the disorder "muscle dysmorphia". Individuals with this disorder become pathologically preoccupied with their degree of muscularity (Pope et al 1993, 1997, Wroblewski 1997).

In a survey of a private fitness club, of 184 individuals surveyed, 27 indicated steroid use (Kersey 1993). When asked why they were resistance training, 20.4% said they wanted to get more fit/stronger and 19% said they wanted to look better. Another survey of 1310 men attending a fitness club indicated that 9.1% had taken AAS and the reasons given were to increase muscle mass, increase strength and train harder (Korkia 1996). Of 1010 male college students surveyed in 1988, 17 reported using steroids and of these, 6 were not varsity athletes (Pope et al 1988).

The change in societal views of the ideal male along with the desire to increase athletic prowess has probably pressured younger males to try steroids. In 1988, Buckley et al reported that 6.6% of 12th grade (modal age 17 yrs) males (n = 3403) had used AAS. In a later report from the same survey (Wang et al 1994), 47% of the high school boys desired to gain weight, 24% were not sure about the dangers of using steroids, and 74% believed that other males in their class used steroids. A survey of 1028 male high school students in 1990 indicated that 6.5% used steroids (Terney and McLain 1990), and similar results were found in a 1993 study showing that 6.5% of high school boys taking a compulsory health-science class (mean age = 14.9 yrs) boys had used steroids (DuRant et al 1993). In 1994, 2.4% of 1013 male high school studies reported steroid use (Corbin et al 1994). A study of middle school students found that 5.3% of 128 boys indicated that they had used steroids (Nutter 1997). From the summary tables presented in the review by Yesalis and Bahrke (1995), an average AAS use of 6.8% for middle and high school males and 1.8% for females was calculated. Kindlundh et al (1999) noted from their survey of 2742 high school students that use of doping agents involved more than the desire to enhance muscle mass and sport performance, and it was related to use of alcohol, tobacco and psychotropic drugs.

Mechanism of action

Although AAS have target effects on various tissues—including reproductive tissue (Feinberg et al 1997), bone (Katznelson et al 1996), adipose (Hislop et al 1999), brain (Rubinow and Schmidt 1996), prostate (Jin et al 1996), liver (Boada et al 1999) and kidney

(Martorana et al 1999)—it is the effects on skeletal muscle that is of primary interest to athletes. The main effect that athletes desire is increased muscle mass. It was long believed that AAS acted directly on skeletal muscle through the androgen receptor as part of the steroid hormone receptor superfamily. This superfamily includes receptors for glucocorticoids, estradiol, retinoids, thryoid hormone, progesterone and mineralocorticoids (Brinkman et al 1999). Recent evidence suggests androgens and AAS can act indirectly on skeletal muscle to control muscle mass (Sheffield-Moore 2000).

In general, steroid hormones partition into target cells via diffusion because of the lipophilic nature of the molecule. Steroid molecules can then interact with intracellular receptors to control the synthesis of mRNA and proteins. The androgen receptor is encoded on the X chromosome, and it is mediated by testosterone and its metabolite 5α-dihydrotestosterone. In the case of skeletal muscle, testosterone is a more important mediator because skeletal muscle's ability to produce the 5α metabolite is minimal (Wilson and Gloyna 1970).

The main effect of testosterone and AAS on the body is positive nitrogen balance. The increase in nitrogen balance can be the result of increases in protein synthesis or decreases in protein catabolism. Sheffield-Moore et al (1999) examined the effects of 5 day administration of 15 mg oral oxandrolone on protein synthesis in males. They found a 44% increase in the fractional synthetic rate (FSR) but no change in protein breakdown rates. This group also found testosterone enanthate increased net protein synthesis (Ferrando et al 1998). These finding agree with other studies that found testosterone administration increases protein synthesis (Griggs et al 1989, Urban et al 1995, Brodsky et al 1996). The changes in protein synthesis may be attributable to direct interaction with the androgen receptor, but changes in catabolism may result from indirect actions.

Although some pharmacological aspects of AAS are mediated directly through steroid receptors, AAS can act indirectly on skeletal muscle. Indirect actions of AAS can include induction or modulation of secondary transcription factors that indirectly regulate genes in the target tissue or modulate gene expression by controlling autocrine or paracrine mediators via membrane receptors (Verhoeven and Swinnen 1999). AAS could also mediate effects by changing secretion of other hormones such as insulin-like growth factor (IGF-1). Gayan-Ramirez et al (2000) found that 7.5 mg/kg of nandrolone deconate increases IGF-1 mRNA by 77% in rodent diaphragm. Other investigators have found increases in IGF-1 mRNA (Urban et al 1995) and circulating IGF-1 (Arnold et al 1996) with AAS administration.

AAS have shown to have antiglucocorticoid actions (Hickson et al 1990). Glucocorticoids have demonstrated catabolic effects on skeletal muscle and, therefore, antagonists of glucocorticoids would reduce muscle catabolism and result in positive nitrogen balance. In vitro work with testosterone, fluoxymesterone, methandorstenolone, norethandrolone, and 17α-methyl testosterone demonstrated the ability to abolish dexamethasone binding to glucocorticoid receptors (Mayer and Rosen 1975). However, the in vivo data have been equivocal, with some AAS demonstrating no inhibition of glucocorticoid binding (Capaccio et al 1987, Danhaive and Rousseau 1988) or decreased glucocorticoid binding (Mayer and Rosen 1975, Danhaive and Rousseau 1988, Sharpe et al 1986). Despite the lack of agreement about the action of AAS on glucucorticoid binding, clinical administration of testosterone enanthate to burn patients has been shown to reduce protein catabolism but not to affect protein synthesis (Sheffield-Moore 2000). Bates et al (1987) found that stanazolol increased RNA and inhibited the reduction of RNA by corticosterone. Finally, an alternative route by which androgens may inhibit glucocorticoid actions is at the gene level by binding to glucocorticoid response elements on DNA (Hickson et al 1990).

AAS can increase muscle mass by regulating both protein synthesis and catabolism. Synthesis can be increased as a direct result of androgen-receptor interaction or by stimulation of IGF-1 synthesis. The reduction in protein catabolism can be regulated indirectly by AAS, acting as a glucocorticoid antagonist. The full understanding of how AAS may regulate gene transcription, beyond the site of the interaction with its receptor, has yet to be elucidated.

Effects of steroid use on muscle mass and strength

In the 1970s, several investigators examined whether AAS use would alter body composition. Casner et al (1971) reported a significantly larger increase in body weight between subjects taking 2 mg stanozolol for 21 days compared with those taking the placebo, with some subjects in the AAS group gaining up to 11 lbs (5 kg). Ward (1973) reported similar results with subjects taking 10 mg Dianabol daily for 4 weeks. In contrast, others (Fahey and Brown 1973, Crist et al 1983) reported no increase in lean body weight in subjects injected approximately every week or every 2 weeks with nandrolone decanoate, and Hervey et al (1976, 1981) questioned whether the weight gain with AAS was caused by an accretion of lean muscle mass. The conflicting study results probably result from differences in the type of drug administered, length of the treatment and lack of controls (Yesalis and Bahrke 1995).

Griggs et al (1989) examined the effect of a pharmacological dose of testosterone enanthante (3 mg/kg/wk) for 12 weeks on muscle protein synthesis determined from whole-body leucine flux/oxidation and from biopsy samples. They found a 27% increase in muscle protein synthesis, which they suggested was responsible for the increase in muscle mass. In a well-controlled study, Bhasin et al (1996) injected men with supraphysiological doses of testosterone (600 mg) or placebo for 10 weeks. Subjects were placed into one of 4 groups: resistance training/drug, resistance training/placebo, no exercise/drug, no exercise/placebo. Muscle size was assessed with magnetic resonance imaging (MRI), and body composition was assessed using hydrostatic weighing. They found that the subjects who both exercised and were injected with testosterone gained the most body weight, which was reflected in fat-free mass (a gain of 6.1 kg in 10 weeks). Also, the increase in cross-sectional area of the triceps and quadriceps muscle was greatest for the exercise/drug group.

Increased skeletal muscle fibre size with AAS use has also been reported (Alén et al 1984, Kadi et al 1999). Biopsies were taken from the trapezius muscle of two groups of high-level powerlifters: those who reported use of AAS in high doses for several years and those who never used AAS (Kadi et al 1999). The fibre type composition was similar in both groups, but the mean fibre area was larger in the steroid users. There was also a greater number of fibres expressing developmental protein isoforms in the steroid users, indicating the presence and formation of new fibres (Kadi et al 1999). However, the results could also be explained by differences in genetic makeup, or other confounding differences, between the groups.

Several studies examined whether there was a performance-enhancing effect of steroids, and the results have been inconsistent (see these review papers: Blue and Lombardo 1999, Braunstein 1997, Clarkson and Thompson 1997, Haupt and Rovere 1984, Lamb 1984, Sturmi and Diorio 1998, Yesalis and Bahrke 1995, Yesalis et al 1989). Yesalis and Bahrke (1995)

cite problems with previous studies including use of doses perhaps too low to be effective, different drugs used, lack of control of diet, no placebo and inappropriate outcome measures. Elashoff et al (1991) reviewed studies of steroid effect on strength and concluded that the nine studies of trained athletes supported the claim of improved strength. In a position stand by the American College of Sports Medicine, the overall conclusion drawn was that AAS especially with strength training facilitate increases in strength (American College of Sports Medicine 1984). Bhasin et al (1996), in the study described above, found that supraphysiological doses of injected testosterone alone significantly increase strength and muscle mass, although these effects were enhanced when combined with resistance training. For example, the increase in squatting strength was 3 kg for the placebo/no exercise groups, 13 kg for the testosterone/no exercise group, 25 kg for the placebo/exercise group, and 38 kg for the testosterone/exercise group.

The results of Bhasin et al (1996) confirm what athletes who used these drugs have reported. However, the amount of increase in strength and muscle mass may underestimate what is actually occurring in the field. Athletes are likely taking even higher doses and often "stack" various types of AAS as well as other anabolic drugs (Burkett and Falduto 1984). Athletes use AAS in cycles of 6–12 weeks and can use an average of five different steroids, mixing oral and injectable forms, as well as including growth hormone, human chorionic gonadotropin, anti-oestrogens, and clenbuterol. Because AAS are banned by several sport governing bodies, athletes will cycle off them prior to competition (Sturmi and Diorio 1998).

Adverse effects associated with steroid use

Adverse effects that have been attributed to steroid use are testicular atrophy, sterility, virilization, and gynaecomastia (Cowan 1994). Also, in adolescents there is the possibility for premature closing of the epiphyseal plates and hence a reduced growth potential. Several studies reported a lower level of high-density lipoprotein (HDL) cholesterol in men who were taking steroids (Zuliani et al 1988, Frohlich et al 1989, Baldo-Enzi et al 1990). Hepatic haematoma and intra-abdominal haemorrhage has been found in a case report of an AAS user (Schumacher et al 1999). Also observed are infections related to non-sterile injection techniques (Rich et al 1999). DuRant et al (1993) reported that 25% of adolescents who used steroids were sharing needles.

Several cases of myocardial infarction associated with AAS use have been recorded. Goldstein et al (1998) reported a case of a 26 year-old man with no risk factors for coronary heart disease who had an acute myocardial infarction after taking both clen-buterol and AAS. Power athletes taking large doses of AAS were found to have altered myocardium, as indicated by increased QT dispersion despite short QT intervals from electrocardiographic repolarization indexes (Stolt et al 1999). Steroid use has been associated with hypertension, ischaemic heart disease, hypertrophic cardiomyopathy and sudden death (Sullivan et al 1999). Sullivan (1999) reported a case of a young male bodybuilder who took large doses of AAS and presented to the emergency room with rapid atrial fibrillation. This condition did not reoccur after discontinuation of the drugs.

Depression, psychosis and behavioural problems occur with steroid use (Bahrke et al 1996). Pope and Katz (1988) noted major psychiatric symptoms in a group of male bodybuilders who were taking steroids, and Gruber and Pope (2000) demonstrated psychiatric disorders in women athletes using AAS. Multiple drug use or "stacking" was particularly associated with severe hostility and aggression (Choi et al 1990). Pope et al (2000) used a randomized, placebo-controlled study to examine the effect of up to 600 mg testosterone/week for 6 weeks on psychiatric outcome measures. The testosterone treatment significantly increased manic scores and aggressive responses. However the responses demonstrated a large inter-subject variability such that most of the men taking the drug showed little psychological changes, while a few developed prominent effects.

AAS use has been linked to premature death (Parssinien et al 2000). Thiblin et al (2000) investigated deaths of 34 males who were known to use AAS. Of these, 9 were homicide victims, 11 committed suicide, 12 were accidental, and 2 were undetermined. The results indicated an increased risk of violent death from impulsive, aggressive or depressive behaviour associated with steroid use. In two of the accidental deaths, the deaths were a result of lethal polypharmacia. Those individuals who use steroids often use other potentially dangerous drugs; Arvary and Pope (2000) suggested that AAS use may serve as a "gateway" to other drugs such as opioids, leading to substantial morbidity and mortality. A recent article stated that AAS users were taking nalbuphine (an opioid agonist/antagonist analgesic), and those with nalbuphine dependence reported widespread nalbuphine use in the weight training centres that they frequented (Wines et al 1999).

Athletes' perception of anabolic–androgenic steroid effects

Sturmi and Diorio (1998) stated in their review paper that the physical side-effects of AAS use "have been historically overstated". They go on to say that most of the adverse events are minor and reversible following cessation of use. Yet, they do acknowledge that use of multiple substances is dangerous. Certainly, from the section above, it is clear that serious side-effects do occur, and they occur most seriously in those athletes who are "stacking". However, like for any drug, there is a large inter-subject variability in the response to AAS.

AAS users believe that these drugs enhance physical strength, athletic ability, confidence, assertiveness, feelings of sexuality and feelings of optimism (Schwerin and Corcoran 1996). A relationship has been established between narcissistic personality traits and AAS use (Porcerelli and Sandler 1995). Olich and Ewing (1999) examined the perceptions of 10 young resistance-training men who were using or had used AAS. Nine of these described steroid use in a very favourable manner; they perceived increases in muscle mass, strength, peer recognition, social status, sexual performance and vocational performance. Schwerin et al (1996) stated that the AAS users in their study presented an appearance of healthfulness, strength, sex appeal and physical attractiveness. They noted that AAS are the only addictive substances that over the short to middle-term will "enhance a user's physical appearance and whose purpose is to allow the user to work hard and longer".

Anshel and Russell (1997) surveyed 291 competitive track and field athletes, who were registered with the New South Wales Track and Field Association, concerning their knowledge of the health consequences of AAS use and their attitudes about using steroids. The results of that study showed that increased knowledge of the deleterious side-effects of steroid use was not significantly related to negative attitudes about use of these drugs. Athletes' beliefs concerning the positive and favourable effects of steroid use outweighs their concern over any long-term consequences.

Summary

The initial synthesis of testosterone analogues back in the 1930s led to their use by athletes desiring to enhance muscle mass and strength. Russian weightlifters were first described to be using AAS in the 1950s, and worldwide use by competitive athletes began in the 1960s (Braunstein 1997). Despite bans of AAS by several sport governing bodies, such as the International Olympic Committee and the National College Athletic Association, athletes continue to use them, from high school to the professional level. Research has corroborated the anecdotal reports from athletes that AAS can increase muscle mass and strength, especially when accompanied by resistance training.

There are many adverse effects associated with AAS, but not every athlete who uses steroids experiences negative effects. Serious adverse events are generally associated with multiple drug use. Mostly, athletes report enhanced physical strength, athletic ability, confidence, assertiveness, feelings of sexuality and feelings of optimism from AAS use, and they are persuaded that these benefits outweigh the risks. Societal pressure to achieve extreme muscularity and athletic prowess in males is a strong driving force behind AAS use. Of great concern is the use of AAS by adolescents and the suggestion that AAS use is the gateway to using even more dangerous drugs.

References

Alén M, Häkkinen K, Komi PV. (1984) Changes in neuromuscular performance and muscle fiber characteristics of elite power athletes self-administering androgenic and AAS. *Acta Physiol Scand* 122: 535–544.

American College of Sports Medicine. (1984) Position stand on the use of anabolic-androgenic steroids in sports. *Med Sci Sports Exerc* 19: 534–539.

Anderson W, Albrecht M, McKeag D, et al. (1991) A national survey of alcohol and drug use by college athletes. *Phys Sportsmed* 19: 91–104.

Anshel MH, Russell KG. (1997) Examining athletes' attitudes toward using AAS and their knowledge of the possible effects. *J Drug Educ* 27(2): 121–145.

Arnold AM, Peralta JM, Thonney ML. (1996) Ontogeny of growth hormone, insulin-like growth factor-I, estradiol and cortisol in the growing lamb: effect of testosterone. *J Endocrinol* 150(3): 391–399.

Arvary D, Pope HG, Jr. (2000) Anabolic-androgenic steroids as a gateway to opioid dependence. *N Engl J Med* 342(20): 1532.

Auge WK, Auge SM. (1999) Sports and substance abuse – naturalistic observation of athletic drug-use patterns and behavior in professional-caliber bodybuilders. *Subs Use Misuse* 34: 217–249.

Bahrke MA, Yesalis III CE, Wright JE. (1996) Psychological and behavioural effects of endogenous testosterone and anabolic-androgenic steroids: An update. *Sport Med* 22(6): 367–390.

Baldo-Enzi G, Giada F, Zuliani G, et al. (1990) Lipid and apoprotein modifications in body builders during and after self-administration of AAS. *Metabolism* 39: 203–207.

Bates PC, Chew LF, Millward DJ. (1987) Effects of the anabolic steroid stanozolol on growth and protein metabolism in the rat. *J Endocrinol* 114(3): 373–381.

Bergman R, Leach RE. (1995) The use and abuse of AAS in olympic-caliber athletes. *Clin Orthop* 198: 169–172.

Bhasin S, Storer TW, Berman N, et al. (1996) The effects of supraphysiologic doses of testosterone on muscle size and strength in normal men. *N Engl J Med* 335(1): pp 1–7.

Blue JG, Lombardo JA. (1999) Steroids and steroid-like compounds. *Clin Sports Med* 18(3): 667–689.

Boada LD, Zumbado M, Torres S, et al. (1999) Evaluation of acute and chronic hepatotoxic effects exerted by anabolic-androgenic steroid stanozolol in adult male rats. *Arch Toxicol* 73(8–9): 465–472.

Braunstein GD. (1997) The influence of anabolic steroids on muscular strength. *Molecular and Cellular Pharmacology* (Series: Principles of Medical Biology) JAI Press Inc, USA 8B: 465–474

Brinkmann AO, Blok LJ, de Ruiter PE, et al. (1999) Mechanisms of androgen receptor activation and function. *J Steroid Biochem Mol Biol* 69(1–6): 307–313.

Brodsky IG, Balagopal P, Nair KS. (1996) Effects of testosterone replacement on muscle mass and muscle protein synthesis in hypogonadal men—a clinical research center study. *J Clin Endocrinol Metab* 81(10): 3469–3475.

Bronson FH, Nguyen KQ, De La Rosa J. (1996) Effect of anabolic steroids on behavior and physiological characteristics of female mice. *Physiol Behav* 59(1): 49–55

Buckley WE, Yesalis CE III, Friedl KE, Anderson WA, Streit AL, Wright JE. (1988) Estimated prevalence of AAS use among male high school seniors. *JAMA* 260: 3441–3445.

Burkett LN, Falduto MT. (1984) Steroid use by athletes in a metropolitan area. *Phys Sportsmed* 12: 69–74.

Capaccio JA, Kurowski TT, Czerwinski SM, Chatterton RT, Jr., Hickson RC. (1987) Testosterone fails to prevent skeletal muscle atrophy from glucocorticoids. *J Appl Physiol* 63(1): 328–334.

Casner Jr SW, Early RG, Carlson RR. (1971) AAS effects on body composition in normal young men. *J Sports Med* 11: 98–103.

Catlin DH, Hatton CK. (1991) Use and abuse of anabolic and other drugs for athletic enhancement. *Adv Intern Med* 36: 399–424.

Choi PYL, Parrott AC, Cowan D. (1990) High-dose AAS in strength athletes: Effects upon hostility and aggression. *Human Psychopharmacol* 5: 349–356.

Clarkson PM, Thompson HT. (1997) Drugs and sport: Research findings and limitation. *Sports Med* 24(6): 366–384.

Corbin CB, Feyrer-Melk SA, Phelps C, Lewis L. (1994) AAS: a study of high school athletes. *Ped Exer Sci* 6: 149–158.

Cordova ML. (1996) Steroid use and the female athlete. *J Strength Cond Res* April: 17–18.

Cowan DA. (1994) Drug abuse. In: Harries M, Williams C, Standish WD, Micheli LJ, editors. *Oxford Textbook of Sports Medicine*. New York: Oxford University Press, pp. 314–329.

Crist DM, Stackpole PJ, Peake GT. (1983) Effects of androgenic-AAS on neuromuscular power and body composition. *J Appl Physiol* 54: 366–370.

Curry LA, Wagman DF (1999) Qualitative description of the prevalence and use of anabolic androgenic steroids by United States powerlifters. *Percept Mot Skills* 88: 224–233.

Danhaive PA, Rousseau GG. (1988) Evidence for sex-dependent anabolic response to androgenic steroids mediated by muscle glucocorticoid receptors in the rat. *J Steroid Biochem* 29(6): 575–581.

Dobs AS. (1999) Is there a role for androgenic AAS in medical practice? *JAMA* 281(14): 1326–1327.

DuRant RH, Rickert VI, Ashworth CS, Newman C, Slavens G. (1993) Use of multiple drugs among adolescents who use AAS. *N Engl J Med* 328(13): 922–926.

Elashoff JD, Jacknow AD, Shain SG, Braunstein GD. (1991) Effects of anabolic-androgenic steroids on muscular strength. *Ann Int Med* 115: 387–393.

Evans NA. (1997) Gym and tonic: a profile of 100 male steroid users. *Br J Sports Med* 31: 54–58.

Fahey TD, Brown CH. (1973) The effects of an AAS on the strength, body composition and endurance of college males when accompanied by a weight training program. *Med Sci Sports Exerc* 5: 272–276.

Feinberg MJ, Lumia AR, McGinnis MY. (1997) The effect of anabolic-androgenic steroids on sexual behavior and reproductive tissues in male rats. *Physiol Behav* 62(1): 23–30.

Ferrando AA, Tipton KD, Doyle D, Phillips SM, Cortiella J, Wolfe RR. (1998.) Testosterone injection stimulates net protein synthesis but not tissue amino acid transport. *Am J Physiol* 275(5 Pt 1): E864–E871.

Frohlich J, Kullmer T, Urhausen A, Bergmass R, Kindermann W. (1989) Lipid profile of body builders with and without self-administration of AAS. *Eur J Appl Physiol* 59: 98–103.

Gayan-Ramirez G, Rollier H, Vanderhoydonc F, Verhoeven G, Gosselink R, Decramer M. (2000) Nandrolone decanoate does not enhance training effects but increases IGF-I mRNA in rat diaphragm. *J Appl Physiol* 88(1): 26–34.

Gimson A. (2000) International:E German who doped swimmers fined. *The Daily Telegraph (London)* January 13, 18.

Goldstein DR, Dobbs T, Krull B, Plumb VJ. (1998) Clenbuterol and AAS: A previously unreported cause of myocardial infarction with normal coronary arteriograms. *South Med J* 91(8): 780–784.

Griggs RC, Kingston W, Jozefowicz RF, Herr BE, Forbes G, Halliday D. (1989) Effect of testosterone on muscle mass and muscle protein synthesis. *J Appl Physiol* 66(1): 498–503.

Gruber AJ, Pope HG, Jr. (2000) Psychiatric and medical effects of anabolic-androgenic steroid use in women. *Psychother Psychosom* 69(1): 19–26.

Haupt HA, Rovere GD. (1984) AAS: a review of the literature. *Am J Sports Med* 12: 469–484.

Haussinger D, Roth E, Lang F, Gerok W. (1993) Cellular hydration state: an important determinant of protein catabolism in health and disease. *Lancet* 341(8856): 1330–1332.

Hervey GR, Hutchinson I, Knibbs AV, Burkinshaw L, Jones PRM, Norgan NG, Levell MJ. (1976) "Anabolic" effects of methandienone in men undergoing athletic training. *Lancet* 2: 699–702.

Hervey GR, Knibbs AV, Burkinshaw L, et al. (1981) Effects of methandienone on the performance and body composition of men undergoing athletic training. *Clin Sci* 60: 457–461.

Hickson RC, Czerwinski SM, Falduto MT, Young AP. (1990) Glucocorticoid antagonism by exercise and androgenic-anabolic steroids. *Med Sci Sports Exerc* 22(3): 331–430.

Hislop MS, Ratanjee BD, Soule SG, Marais AD. (1999) Effects of anabolic-androgenic steroid use or gonadal testosterone suppression on serum leptin concentration in men. *Eur J Endocrinol* 141(1): 40–46.

Jin B, Turner L, Walters WA, Handelsman DJ. (1996) The effects of chronic high dose androgen or estrogen treatment on the human prostate [corrected] [published erratum appears in *J Clin Endocrinol Metab* (1997) 82(2): 413]. *J Clin Endocrinol Metab* 81(12): 4290–4295.

Kadi F, Eriksson A, Holmner S, Thornell LE. (1999) Effects

of AAS on the muscle cells of strength-trained athletes. *Med Sci Sports Exerc* 31(11): 1528–1534.

Katznelson L, Finkelstein JS, Schoenfeld DA, Rosenthal DI, Anderson EJ, Klibanski A. (1996) Increase in bone density and lean body mass during testosterone administration in men with acquired hypogonadism. *J Clin Endocrinol Metab* 81(12): 4358–4365.

Kersey RD. (1993) Anabolic-androgenic steroid use by private health club/gym athletes. *J Strength Cond Res* 7(2): 118–126.

Kindlundh AMS, Isacson DGL, Berglund L, Nyberg F. (1999) Factors associated with adolescent use of doping agents:anabolic-androgenic steroids. *Addiction* 94(4): 543–553.

Korkia P. (1996) Use of AAS has been reported by 9% of men attend gymnasiums. *Br Med J* 313: 1009.

Lamb DR. (1984) AAS in athletics: how well do they work and how dangerous are they? *Am J Sports Med* 12: 31–38.

Lee S. (1996) Once "too violent" GI Joe now seen as a regular guy. *Chicago Tribune* September 20: 1.

Lindström M, Nilsson AL, Katzman PL, Janzon L, Dymling JF. (1990) Use of anabolic-androgenic steroids among body builders—frequency and attitudes. *J Intern Med* 227(6): 407–411.

Ljungquist A. (1975) The use of anabolic steroids in top Swedish atheletes. *Br J Sports Med* 9(2): 82.

Martorana G, Concetti S, Manferrari F, Creti S. (1999) Anabolic steroid abuse and renal cell carcinoma. *J Urol* 162(6): 2089.

Mayer M, Rosen F. (1975) Interaction of anabolic steroids with glucocorticoid receptor sites in rat muscle cytosol. *Am J Physiol* 229(5): 1381–1386.

Nurse D. (1998) G.I. Joe: Classic action figure finding new roles. *The Atlanta Journal and Constitution* August 21: 09JJ.

Nutter J. (1997) Middle school students' attitudes and use of AAS. *J Strength Cond Res* 11(1): 35–39.

Olich TW, Ewing ME. (1999) Life of steroids: Bodybuilders describe their perceptions of the anabolic-androgenic steroid use period. *Sport Psychol* 13(3): 299–312.

Parssinien M, Kujula U, Vartiainen E, Sarna S, Seppala T. (2000) Increased premature mortality of competitive powerlifters suspected to have used anabolic agents. *Intl J Sports Med* 21(3): 225–227.

Pearson M. (1994) Olympians of winters past. *USA Today* February 7.

Perry PJ, Andersen KH, Yates WR. (1990) Illicit AAS use in athletes. *Am J Sports Med* 18(4): 422–428.

Pope HG, Jr, Gruber AJ, Choi P, Phillips KA. (1997) Muscle dysmorphia. An underrecognized form of body dysmorphic disorder. *Psychosomatics* 38(6): 548–557.

Pope HG, Jr, Katz DL. (1988) Affective and psychotic symptoms associated with AAS use. *Am J Psychiatry* 145(4): 487–490.

Pope H, Jr, Katz D, Champoux R. (1988) Anabolic-androgenic steroid use among 1010 college men. *Phys Sportsmed* 16(7): 75–81.

Pope HG, Jr, Katz DL, Hudson JI. (1993) Anorexia nervosa and "reverse anorexia" among 108 body builders. *Compr Psychiatry* 34(6): 406–409.

Pope HG, Jr, Kouri EM, Hudson JI. (2000) Effects of supraphysiological doses of testosterone on mood and aggression in normal men – a randomized controlled trial. *Arch Gen Psychiatry* 57(2): 133–140.

Porcerelli JH, Sandler BA. (1995) Narcissism and empathy in steroid users. *Am J Psychiatry* 152(11): 1672–1674.

Rich JN, Dickinson BP, Flanigan TP, Valone SE. (1999) Abscess related to anabolic-androgenic steroid injection. *Med Sci Sports Exerc* 31(2): 207–209.

Rubinow DR, Schmidt PJ. (1996) Androgens, brain, and behavior. *Am J Psychiatry* 153(8): 974–984.

Schumacher J, Müller G, Klotz E-F. (1999) Large hepatic hematoma and intraabdominal hemorrhage associated with abuse of AAS. *N Engl J Med* 340(14): 1123–1124.

Schwerin MJ, Corcoran KJ. (1996) Beliefs about steroids: user vs. non-user comparisons. *Drug Alcohol Depend* 40: 221–225.

Schwerin MJ, Corcoran KJ, Fisher L, et al. (1996) Social physique anxiety, body esteem, and social anxiety in bodybuilders and self-reported AAS users. *Addict Behav* 21(1): 1–8.

Sharpe PM, Buttery PJ, Haynes NB. (1986) The effect of manipulating growth in sheep by diet or anabolic agents on plasma cortisol and muscle glucocorticoid receptors. *Br J Nutr* Jul 56(1): 289–304.

Sheffield-Moore M, Urban RJ, Wolf SE, et al. (1999) Short-term oxandrolone administration stimulates net muscle protein synthesis in young men. *J Clin Endocrinol Metab* 84(8): 2705–2711.

Sheffield-Moore M. (2000) Androgens and the control of skeletal muscle protein synthesis. *Ann Med* 32: 181–186.

Stilger VG, Yesalis CE. (1999) Anabolic-androgenic steroid use among high school football players. *J Community Health* 24: 131–145.

Stolt A, Karila T, Viitasalo M, Mantysaari M, Kujala UM, Karjalainen J. (1999) QT interval and QT dispersion in endurance athletes and in power athletes using large doses of AAS. *Am J Cardiol* 84(3): 364–366.

Strauss RH, Liggett MT, Lanese RR. (1985) AAS use and perceived effects in ten weight-trained women athletes. *JAMA* 253(19): 2871–2873.

Sturmi JE, Diorio DJ. (1998) Anabolic agents. Sports Pharmacology. *Clin Sports Med* 17(2): 261–282.

Sullivan ML, Martinez CM, Gallagher EJ. (1999) Atrial fibrillation and AAS. *J Emerg Med* 17(5): 851–857.

Sylvester LJ. (1973) Anabolic steroids and the Munich Olympics. *Scholastic Coach* 43: 90–92.

Terney R, McLain LG. (1990) The use of AAS in high school students. *Am J Dis Child* 144: 99–103.

Thiblin I, Lindquist O, Rajs J. (2000) Cause and manner of death among users of anabolic androgenic steroids. *J Forensic Sci* 45(1): 16–23.

Urban RJ, Bodenburg YH, Gilkison C, et al. (1995) Testosterone administration to elderly men increases skeletal muscle strength and protein synthesis. *Am J Physiol* 269(5 Pt 1): E820–826.

Verhoeven G, Swinnen JV. (1999) Indirect mechanisms and cascades of androgen action. *Mol Cell Endocrinol* 151(1–2): 205–212.

Wagner JC. (1991) Enhancement of athletic performance with drugs. *Sports Med* 12: 250–265.

Wang MQ, Fitzhugh EC, Yesalis CE, Buckley WE. (1994) Desire for weight gain and potential risks of adolescent males using AAS. *Percept Mot Skills* 78: 267–274.

Ward P. (1973) The effect of an AAS on strength and lean body mass. *Med Sci Sports Exerc* 5: 277–282.

Wilson JD, Gloyna RE. (1970) The intranuclear metabolism of testosterone in the accessory organs of reproduction. *Recent Prog Horm Res* 26: 309–336.

Wines JD, Jr, Gruber AJ, Pope HG, Jr, Lukas SE. (1999) Nalbuphine hydrochloride dependence in AAS users. *Am J Addict* 8(2): 161–164.

Wroblewski AM. (1997) Androgenic—AAS and body dysmorphia in young men. *J Psychosom Res* 42(3): 225–234.

Yesalis CE, Wright JE, Lombardo JA. (1989) Anabolic-androgenic steroids: a synthesis of existing data and recommendations for future research. *Clin Sports Med* 1: 109–134.

Yesalis CE, Kennedy NJ, Kopstein AN, Bahrke M. (1993) Anabolic-androgenic steroid use in the United States. *JAMA* 270: 1217–1221.

Yesalis CE, Bahrke MS. (1995) Anabolic—androgenic steroids. *Sports Med* 19: 326–340.

Zuliani U, Bernardini B, Catapano A, Camoana M, Cerioli G, Spattini M. (1988) Effects of AAS, testosterone and HGH on blood lipids and echocardiographic parameters in body builders. *Intl J Sports Med* 10: 62–88.

10

Skeletal muscle changes in heart disease

Andrew J.S. Coats and Derek Harrington

Introduction

Cardiac involvement in primary myopathic disorders is not uncommon. In contrast, primary myopathy is rare in heart diseases, although secondary alterations in a variety of aspects of skeletal muscle structure and function are increasingly recognized in chronic heart diseases, most notably in chronic heart failure, a subject upon which this chapter will concentrate. In the majority of cardiac illnesses, even those in which there is primary cardiac muscle disease, there are no clinically significant muscle changes. As a result cardiologists have in the past paid little or no attention to skeletal muscle. Chronic heart failure (CHF) is, however, an exception. Recently this disease has become viewed as a clinical syndrome encompassing the central haemodynamic changes and a number of peripheral alterations. The most prominent of these peripheral changes are changes in the skeletal musculature, recognized now to be a major cause of symptomatic limitation in this condition.

In this chapter we will review what is known of the muscular changes occurring in CHF and consider the possibility that in CHF these muscle changes are not simply the inevitable consequence of the central haemodynamic dysfunction, but rather that they represent a specific response by the body to the neurohormonal and metabolic abnormalities seen as a consequence of CHF, and furthermore, that they may contribute to the pathophysiology of the underlying condition.

Skeletal muscle abnormalities

Skeletal muscle atrophy

Although muscular atrophy is well recognized in cardiac cachexia, muscle bulk is also reduced in CHF patients without obvious wasting or documented weight loss. Mancini et al (1992), using a creatinine/height index and mid-arm muscle circumference, found severe muscle atrophy in 68% of patients. They were, however, unable to show significant abnormalities of protein synthesis (using serum albumin, pre-albumin or transferrin) or of body fat stores (using triceps skin fold thickness, or percentage ideal body weight). Using differing techniques including magnetic resonance imaging (MRI; Minotti et al 1993) and computer tomography (CT; Harrington et al 1997) of the thigh muscles and dual energy X-ray

absorptiometry (DEXA) of the leg other investigators have confirmed these findings.

Skeletal muscle strength

With the observed reduction in muscle bulk, abnormalities of muscle performance might be expected (Table 10.1). Early small studies reported variable results: some noting significant weakness (Lipkin et al 1988, Buller et al 1991) and others observing preservation of maximal strength (Minotti et al 1991, 1993). In a subsequent larger study we observed significant weakness that occurred as a result of both muscle atrophy and a reduction in muscle quantity (Harrington et al 1997). No significant weakness has been demonstrated in adductor pollicis, foot dorsiflexors or the wrist flexors (Wilson et al 1985, Lipkin et al 1988, Minotti et al 1992), suggesting that in the majority of patients the abnormalities in small non-weight bearing muscle may be less marked.

Skeletal muscle fatigue

Using various protocols, all groups have reported an increase in skeletal muscle fatigue in CHF (Buller et al 1991, Minotti et al 1993, Harrington et al 1997). Wilson et al (1992) have confirmed this using surface electromyograms. In normal individuals electromyography suggests recruitment of new fibres to assist fatiguing fibres at the maximal and preceding stage of exercise. In CHF patients, similar changes are observed, although at significantly lower workloads suggesting an earlier onset of muscular fatigue. This reduced endurance does not appear to be a result of impaired neuromuscular transmission. A superimposed tetanic stimulus, given either during a maximal foot dorsiflexion or after a maximal contraction has decayed to 60%, results in similar increases in force generation in both normal and CHF patients (Minotti et al 1992). Similarly the changes are not explained by reduced muscle blood flow. During ischaemic conditions (obtained by inflating a thigh cuff to a suprasystolic pressure) differences between patients and controls persist (Minotti et al 1991).

Histology

With the observed abnormalities of skeletal muscle function various groups have attempted to define a characteristic underlying histological pattern. Most reports have been of leg muscle histology (generally quadriceps) obtained using a needle biopsy technique

Table 10.1—Skeletal muscle function in chronic heart failure

Authors	Muscle group	Number of patients	Strength	Correlation with peak V_{O_2}	Strength per unit muscle	Fatigue resistance	Correlation with peak V_{O_2}
Magnusson et al (1994)	Quadriceps	8	⇓ (ISK/ISM)		⇔	⇓	
Minotti et al (1993)	Quadriceps	21	⇔ (ISK/ISM)	No	⇔	⇓	
Lipkin et al (1988)	Quadriceps	9	⇓ (ISM)	Yes			
Buller et al (1991)	Quadriceps	15	⇓ (ISM)	Yes	⇔	⇓	Yes
Buller et al (1991)	Adductor pollicis	15	⇔ (ISM)			⇔	
Minotti et al (1991)	Quadriceps	16	⇔ (ISK/ISM)	No		⇓	Yes
Wilson et al (1985)	Wrist flexors	9	⇔				
Minotti et al (1992)	Foot dorsiflexors	9	⇔			⇓	
Harrington et al (1997)	Quadriceps	100	⇓ (ISM)	Yes	⇓	⇓	No

ISK, isokinetic; ISM, isometric; V_{O_2}, oxygen consumption.

(results are summarized in Table 10.2); a few reports describe other muscle groups including the diaphragm. An increase in the percentage of type II fibres present has generally been observed (Lipkin et al 1988, Yancy et al 1989, Sullivan et al 1990, Drexler et al 1992), with similar changes reported in animal models (Sabbah et al 1993). When type II fibres have been sub-typed, the alteration in distribution appears to result from an increase in type IIB fibres with no alteration in type IIA frequency. Type I fibres are mostly reported to be reduced or have a strong trend towards reduction.

While Lipkin et al (1988) report atrophy of both Type I and II fibres, other investigators have described a reduction only in type II fibre size. The sub-type affected varies: some report that only type IIB fibres are reduced in size (Sullivan et al 1990), while others describe a reduction in the size of both sub-types (Mancini et al 1989, Belardinelli et al 1995). Despite these alterations in muscle composition and fibre size,

Table 10.2—Skeletal muscle histology and metabolism in chronic heart failure

Authors	Number of patients	Fibre type				Glycolytic pathway	Krebs cycle	Lipid oxidation	Capillary density	
		I	IIa	IIb	IIc				/fibre	/mm²
Lipkin et al (1988)	9	⇓	⇑ᵃ							⇔
Yancy et al (1989)	6	⇓	⇑ᵃ			⇔	⇓		⇓	⇓
Mancini et al (1989)	22	⇔	⇓	⇑	⇑	⇔	⇔	⇓	⇔	⇑
Sullivan et al (1990)	11	⇓	⇔	⇑	⇔	⇔	⇓	⇔	⇓	⇔
Drexler et al (1992)	57	⇓	⇑ᵃ			⇔		⇓		⇓
Belardinelli et al (1995)	27	⇓	⇑ᵃ							

[a]Studies in which Type II fibres were not sub-typed, data is given for all type II fibres.

Mancini et al (1989) noted in their study that the percentage of the total muscle area occupied by each fibre type was normal.

The vascularity of skeletal muscle has been assessed although reports are inconsistent. Initially normal capillary numbers were reported (Lipkin et al 1988). Subsequent investigators have reported a reduction in capillaries per fibre but a normal number per unit area (Sullivan et al 1990), a reduction in capillaries per unit volume of muscle (Drexler et al 1992), no change in capillary number per fibre but an increase in capillaries per unit area (Mancini et al 1989) and a reduction in all measures of capillary density (Yancy et al 1989). Despite these inconsistencies the net effect of the majority of these changes, when taken in concert with reduced muscle bulk, is a reduction in skeletal muscle vascular conductance.

Muscle mitochondria are abnormal in CHF patients. Drexler et al (1992) calculated the volume density of mitochondria (mitochondrial volume fraction per unit volume of muscle tissue) and the surface density of mitochondrial cristae (surface fraction of mitochondrial cristae per unit volume of muscle). They observed that both of these indices were reduced in CHF patients compared with normal controls.

Histological studies thus suggest a reduced aerobic capacity. The marked differences in histology reported may be partially explained by the small number of patients studies and by the variation in the severity of heart failure.

Skeletal muscle metabolism in chronic heart failure

Muscle metabolism has been studied at rest and during exercise by analysing biopsies, measuring metabolites in femoral venous blood, and using magnetic resonance spectroscopy.

Biopsy studies

Enzyme and metabolite levels have been measured in muscle homogenates and by staining biopsies for enzymes of the metabolic pathways. Muscle composition assessments have suggested normal protein and myoglobin content, with normal or reduced high-energy phosphate levels (Sullivan et al 1990, Broquist et al 1994). Reduced glycogen levels associated with normal levels of glycolytic intermediates and lactate but with increased pyruvate levels suggest an increased level of glycolysis (Mancini et al 1989, Sullivan et al 1990). Most studies have reported a decrease in the oxidative enzymes of Krebs cycle (Yancy et al 1989, Sullivan et al 1990, Drexler et al 1992) although Mancini et al (1989) report normal citrate synthetase activity. The ability to oxidize fat also appears impaired since β-Hydroxyacyl CoA Dehydrogenase levels are reduced (Mancini et al 1989, Sullivan et al 1990). The activity of the glycolytic pathway, however, has been consistently reported as normal (Mancini et al 1989, Yancy et al 1989, Sullivan et al 1990).

Magnetic resonance spectroscopy

Using ^{31}P magnetic resonance spectroscopy, skeletal muscle metabolism has been monitored non-invasively both at rest during exercise in patients with CHF. Analysis of the spectra allows the evaluation of the relative concentrations of inorganic phosphate (P_i), phosphocreatine (PCr) and adenosine triphosphate (ATP) in intact tissues in vivo. Additionally the technique can be used to assess intracellular pH and the rate of PCr utilization. Mitochondrial respiration is closely related to adenosine diphosphate (ADP) level, which in turn is directly related to the P_i/PCr ratio. This ratio correlates linearly with the velocity of mitochondrial oxidation. Thus, the relationship between P_i/PCr and power output (or workload) is also linear (at least at low workloads) and it is an index of metabolic efficiency.

Initial studies in CHF patients analysed the forearm muscles during protocols of gradually increasing workload (Wilson et al 1985, Massie et al 1987b). Although resting spectra were normal, with low level exercise PCr decreased and P_i increased. The changes (reflected in the P_i/PCr ratio) were much greater in CHF patients despite equivalent workloads, resulting in a significantly higher slope in the relationship between the P_i/PCr ratio and power output. In normal individuals there was no change in pH until the peak workload, while in CHF patients there was a progressive decrease in pH at all workloads, although pH at peak exercise was similar. Subsequently, similar observations have been reported in the legs (Mancini et al 1988, Arnolda et al 1990, Mancini et al 1992).

Reduced blood flow could account for these observations, and patients with peripheral vascular disease have abnormalities of phosphocreatine metabolism similar to those seen in CHF (Hands et al 1986). However, at low level exercise forearm blood flow is normal (assessed using occlusion plethysmography) despite the presence of metabolic abnormalities (Wiener et al 1986, Massie et al 1987b). Massie et al (1987b) also noted no difference in blood flow at a specific workload, post-ischaemic blood flow or rate of increase of flow when comparing patients who have normal and abnormal PCr metabolism. The observation that during ischaemic exercise differences persist, with an earlier and greater fall in pH in CHF patients, also suggests an abnormality independent of flow (Massie et al 1988). Other factors that may play a role are metabolic deficiencies such as a depletion in mitochondrial oxidative enzymes and the effects of insulin resistance.

Lactate production during exercise

An early onset of lactic acid release associated with CHF has been recognized for many years (Meakins and Lang 1927, Huckabee and Judson 1958, Donald et al 1961), and it has been a consistent finding amongst more recent investigations (Wilson et al 1984, Weber and Janicki 1985, Sullivan et al 1988). It has, therefore, been suggested that the nutritive blood flow to skeletal muscle (as assessed by lactate production) is reduced (Wilson et al 1984). This could occur as a result of decreased oxygen delivery (potentially as a result of a reduced cardiac output response to exercise, or deficient local vasodilatation) or as a result of an impaired ability of exercising muscle to utilize oxygen. Wilson et al (1984) considered 23 patients, grading them according to their peak oxygen consumption. They measured leg blood flow using femoral venous catheters and observed that with increasing exercise tolerance there was a progressively earlier increase in femoral venous lactate associated with a lower cardiac output response to exercise, a lower leg blood flow and a higher leg vascular resistance. Their results suggested that the reduced nutritive flow could be explained both by a pump failure and by impaired vasodilatation in the exercising muscle group. However further work has suggested that the early onset of lactate production is not solely a result of reduced muscle perfusion. Wilson et al (1993) identified a subgroup of previously studied patients who had normal leg blood flow responses during exercise. Compared with other CHF patients, this group had a better cardiac output response to exercise, and their leg arterio-venous oxygen differences were normal. Despite this they had a persistently abnormal lactate response to exercise suggesting that, in some patients at least, the early lactate release is a result of intrinsic muscle abnormalities and not simply a consequence of impaired muscle perfusion. Further

evidence for these intrinsic metabolic abnormalities comes from experiments in which leg blood flow has been acutely improved. Hydralazine and dobutamine increase cardiac output and leg blood flow both at rest and during exercise in CHF (Wilson et al 1983, 1984, Maskin et al 1983). Infusion of either of these drugs is not associated with any change in lactate production, while leg oxygen extraction is decreased, suggesting that the increased oxygen supplied as a consequence of increased flow is not utilized by the muscle.

In summary, metabolic studies suggest that in CHF patients exercising muscle exhibits increased glycolytic metabolism, and it appears to be metabolically less efficient in relation to external work performed. These observations cannot be explained on the basis of abnormal blood flow alone, although chronic flow impairment could play a role in the genesis of the changes.

Respiratory muscle abnormalities

Given the documented abnormalities of skeletal muscle in CHF, and the often severe dyspnoea that patients suffer, abnormalities of the respiratory musculature have been sought. Reduced maximal inspiratory and expiratory mouth pressures (MIP, MEP) have been observed in CHF patients (Hammond et al 1990, McParland et al 1992, Ambrosino et al 1994, Chua et al 1995, Evans et al 1995) compared with controls. Although some only describe a trend towards MIP and MEP weakness (Mancini et al 1992, 1994) or the presence of weakness only in more symptomatic patients (Nishimura et al 1994). Table 10.3 summarizes these results.

Using the twitch interpolation technique of Bellemare and Bigland-Richie (1984), a technique which measures diaphragmatic strength interdependent of volition, diaphragm strength has been assessed. Mancini et al (1992) reported normal transdiaphragmatic peak pressure differences, and no abnormality of maximal rate of contraction or relaxation. However the time–tension index for the diaphragm (an index of diaphragmatic work defined as the fraction of a breathing cycle spent in inspiration multiplied by the mean transdiaphragmatic pressure, divided by the maximal voluntary transdiaphragmatic pressure) was significantly greater in patients at rest and throughout exercise, as was the transdiaphragmatic pressure. Although they concluded that this increased work of breathing could contribute to the sensation of breath-

Table 10.3 — Respiratory muscle function in chronic heart failure

Authors	Number of patients	MIP	MEP	Correlation with exercise capacity
Hammond et al (1990)	16	⇓	⇓	
McParland et al (1992)	9	⇓	⇓	Yes (MIP and Mahler dyspnoea index)
Evans et al (1995)	20	⇓	⇓	No
Ambrosino et al (1994)	45	⇓	⇓	
Chua et al (1995)	20	⇓	⇔ (Trend to ð)	Yes (MIP and peak $\dot{V}O_2$)
Mancini et al (1992)	10	⇔ (Trend to ð)	⇔ (Trend to ð)	
Mancini et al (1994)	15	⇔ (Trend to ð)	⇔ (Trend to ð)	
Nishimura et al (1994)	23	⇓ (In NYHA III/IV)	⇔	Yes (MIP and peak $\dot{V}O_2$)

MIP, maximum inspiratory pressure; MEP, maximum expiratory pressure; $\dot{V}O_2$, oxygen consumption; NYHA, New York Heart Association class.

lessness, and hence exercise limitation, more recent work by this group does not support this concept (Mancini et al 1996). The diaphragm and respiratory muscles fatigue. Following exercise, Davies et al (1990) observed a fall in MIP and MEP in patients alone, while others describe similar falls in mouth pressures in both patients and controls (Mancini et al 1992). Maximal voluntary ventilation and maximal sustainable ventilation (ventilation using a 3 min incremental work rate programme, while maintaining isocapnia), both indices of diaphragm endurance, are significantly reduced in CHF (Mancini et al 1994).

Abnormalities of skeletal muscle structure, function and metabolism have been documented in CHF. The abnormalities are present in patients with heart failure resulting from ischaemic heart disease and dilated cardiomyopathy. It is, therefore, unlikely that, as previously suggested, they are simply a reflection of a generalized myopathy.

The aetiology of muscle changes in chronic heart failure

Inactivity results in alterations in skeletal muscle superficially similar to those observed in CHF. It is possible to envisage a cycle in which muscle change leads to inactivity, which in turn leads to greater change in skeletal muscle. Regular exercise training is, at least in part, able to reverse the muscle abnormalities in CHF (Adamoupolos et al 1993). Inactivity does not, however, explain all the observed changes. Abnormalities have been documented in the hand flexors, a muscle group in which normal use may be expected (Buller et al 1991). Moreover abnormalities of the respiratory musculature have been documented, even though these muscles are more likely to experience increased rather than decreased usage.

Some authors have suggested malnutrition as a potential cause, and they have documented a reduced calorific intake or a negative net energy balance in some patients. However dietary supplementation has not been demonstrated to produce any improvement in the muscle abnormalities or exercise capacity (Broquist et al 1994). Muscle blood flow is abnormal (Zelis and Flaim 1982), and a reduced blood flow may play an important role. However, as discussed, many of the observed metabolic and functional abnormalities appear to be independent of blood flow, and these can persist in a situation in which blood flow is temporarily halted.

A final possible explanation is that CHF constitutes a catabolic state and that the observed muscle changes are a result of this. There is sympathetic activation and, in addition to documented insulin resistance (Swan et al 1997), catabolic factors such as Tumour Necrosis Factor are known to be elevated in severe CHF (McMurray et al 1991, Anker et al 1997). CHF clearly can become a catabolic state with the development of the severe muscle wasting seen in cardiac cachexia.

Significance of the changes in chronic heart failure

CHF is characterized by exercise intolerance usually associated with breathlessness or fatigue. It was believed that this exercise intolerance was simply a reflection of the central haemodynamic disturbance. However, many investigators have demonstrated a poor correlation between central haemodynamic disturbance and exercise capacity (Franciosa et al 1981, Higginbotham et al 1983, Szlachcic et al 1985). These findings, in addition to the observation that an acute increase in cardiac output did not immediately increase exercise capacity (Maskin et al 1983, Wilson et al 1993, 1984), have led to a search for an alternative source of exercise limitation in CHF. The possibility that the muscular changes outlined are not simply a consequence of the disturbed haemodynamics of CHF, but that they may contribute to the generation of symptoms in this disabling condition, has been considered (Drexler 1992, Minotti et al 1993, Coats et al 1994, Wilson 1995). There is some evidence to support such a concept. Indices of skeletal muscle structure and function in some instances correlate well with exercise intolerance as measured by peak oxygen consumption, and exercise training can improve exercise capacity in the absence of improvement in the haemodynamic disturbance (Belardinelli et al 1995). The muscular changes occurring with training correlate well with the degree of improvement in exercise capacity. In addition, adding arm exercise to near-peak leg exercise results in an increase in peak oxygen consumption in CHF patients but not in controls. The mechanisms whereby skeletal muscle changes cause exercise fatigue in heart failure are easy to understand, but the recent finding that ergo- or metabo-reflex responses from the metabolically abnormal muscle in heart failure can cause exaggerated reflex responses (including sympathoexcitation and a heightened ventilatory response to muscular exercise) may indicate alternative mechanisms whereby the skeletal muscle may be important in the syndrome of CHF (Piepoli et al 1996).

The question of the potential value of "treating" the muscle abnormalities thus arises. Although training programmes are successful, to date, pharmacological intervention aimed at reversing the muscle changes has not improved exercise capacity (Harrington et al 1997b). Interestingly, however, dietary creatine supplementation does attenuate the abnormal metabolic response to exercise and improves forearm muscle endurance (Andrews et al 1998).

Conclusions

CHF is associated with widespread changes in the skeletal musculature that result in impaired muscular function and in a reduced muscular oxidative capacity. It is possible that these abnormalities contribute to the pathophysiology of CHF. Such a hypothesis, if true, is important since it would provide a novel area for therapeutic intervention.

References

Adamopoulos S, Coats AJS, Brunotte F, et al. (1993) Physical training improves skeletal muscle metabolic abnormalities in patients with chronic heart failure. *J Am Coll Cardiol* 23: 1101–1106.

Ambrosino N, Opasich C, Crotti P, Cobelli F, Tavazzi L, Rampulla C. (1994) Breathing pattern, ventilatory drive and respiratory muscle strength in patients with chronic heart failure. *Eur Respir J* 7: 17–22.

Andrews R, Greenhaff P, Curtis S, Perry A, Cowlet AJ. (1998) The effect of dietary creatinine supplementation on skeletal muscle metabolism in congestive heart failure. *Eur Heart J* 19: 617–622.

Anker SD, Swan JW, Chua TP, et al. (1997) Hormonal changes and catabolic/anabolic imbalance in chronic heart failure: The importance for cardiac cachexia. *Circulation* 96: 526–534.

Arnolda L, Conway M, Dolecki M, et al. (1990) Skeletal muscle metabolism in heart failure: a 31P nuclear magnetic resonance spectroscopy study of leg muscle. *Clin Sci* 9: 583–589.

Belardinelli R, Georgiou D, Scocco V, Barstow TJ, Puracaro A. (1995) Low intensity exercise training in patients with chronic heart failure. *J Am Coll Cardiol* 26: 975–982.

Bellemare F, Bigland-Richie B. (1984) Assessment of human diaphragm strength and activation using phrenic nerve stimulation. *Respir Physiol* 58: 263–277.

Broquist M, Arnquist H, Dahlstrom U, Larsson J, Nylander E, Permert J. (1994) Nutritional assessment and muscle energy metabolism in severe chronic heart failure – effects of long term dietary supplementation. *Eur Heart J* 15: 1641–1650.

Buller NP, Jones D, Poole-Wilson PA. (1991) Direct measurements of skeletal muscle fatigue in patients with chronic heart failure. *Br Heart J* 65: 20–24.

Chua TP, Anker SD, Harrington D, Coats AJS. (1995) Inspiratory muscle strength is a determinant of maximum oxygen consumption in chronic heart failure. *Br Heart J* 74: 381–385.

Coats AJS, Adamopoulos S, Radaelli A, et al. (1992) Controlled trial of physical training in chronic heart failure: exercise performance, hemodynamics, ventilation, and autonomic function. *Circulation* 85: 2119–2131.

Coats AJS, Clark AL, Piepoli M, Volterrani, Poole-Wilson. (1994) Symptoms and quality of life in heart failure: The muscle hypothesis. *Brit Heart J* 2(suppl): S36–S39.

Davies SW, Jordan SSL, Pride NB, Lipkin DP. (1990) Respiratory muscle failure in chronic heart failure. *Circulation* 82(Suppl III): III–24.

Donald KW, Gloster J, Harris EA, Reeves J, Harris P. (1961) The production of lactic acid during exercise in normal subjects and patients with rheumatic heart disease. *Am Heart J* 62: 494–510.

Drexler H, Riede U, Mnzel T, Knig H, Funke E, Just H. (1992) Alterations of skeletal muscle in chronic heart failure. *Circulation* 85: 1751–1759.

Drexler H. (1992) Skeletal muscle failure in heart failure. *Circulation* 85: 1621–1623.

Evans SA, Watson L, Hawkins M, Cowley AJ, Johnston IDA, Kinnear WJM. (1995) Respiratory muscle strength in chronic heart failure. *Thorax* 50: 625–628.

Franciosa JA, Park M, Levine TB. (1981) Lack of correlation between exercise capacity and indexes of resting left ventricular performance in heart failure. *Am J Cardiol* 47: 33–39.

Hammond MD, Bauer KA, Sharp JT, Rocha RD. (1990) Respiratory muscle strength in congestive heart failure. *Chest* 98: 1091–1094.

Hands LJ, Bore PJ, Galloway G, Morris PJ, Radda GK. (1986) Muscle metabolism in patients with peripheral vascular disease, investigated by 31-P nuclear magnetic resonance spectroscopy. *Clin Sci* 71: 283–290.

Harrington D, Anker SD, Chua TP, et al. (1997) Skeletal muscle function and its relation to exercise tolerance in chronic heart failure. *J Am Coll Cardiol* 30: 1758–1764.

Harrington D, Chua TP, Poole-Wilson PA, Coats AJS. (1997b) Respiratory muscle strength is increased in chronic heart failure by salbutamol a β2 adreno receptor agonist. *J Am Coll Cardiol* 29 (Suppl A): 424A.

Higginbotham MB, Morris KG, Conn EH, Coleman RE, Cobb FR. (1983) Determinants of exercise performance among patients with congestive heart failure. *Am J Cardiol* 1: 52–60.

Holloszy JO, Coyle EF. (1984) Adaptations of skeletal muscle to endurance exercise and their metabolic consequences. *J Appl Physiol* 56: 831–838.

Huckabee WK, Judson WE. (1958) The role of anaerobic metabolism in the performance of mild muscular work. I. Relationship to oxygen consumption and cardiac output and the effect of congestive heart failure. *J Clin Inv* 37: 1577–1592.

Lipkin D, Jones D, Round J, Poole-Wilson P. (1988) Abnormalities of skeletal muscle in patients with chronic heart failure. *Intl J Cardiol* 18: 187–195.

Magnusson G, Isberg B, Karlberg K, Sylven C. (1994) Skeletal muscle strength and endurance in chronic congestive heart failure secondary to idiopathic dilated cardiomyopathy. *Am J Cardiol* 73: 307–309.

Mancini DM, Coyle E, Coggan A, et al. (1989) Contribution of intrinsic skeletal muscle changes to 31P NMR skeletal muscle abnormalities in patients with chronic heart failure. *Circulation* 0: 1338–1346.

Mancini DM, Ferraro N, Nazzaro D, Chance B, Wilson JR. (1991) Respiratory muscle deoxygenation during exercise in patients with heart failure demonstrated with near-infrared spectroscopy. *J Am Coll Cardiol* 8: 492–498.

Mancini DM, Ferraro N, Tuchler M, Chance B, Wilson JR. (1988) Detection of abnormal calf muscle metabolism in patients with heart failure using phosphorus-31 nuclear magnetic resonance. *Am J Cardiol* 62: 234–1240.

Mancini DM, Henson D, LaManca J, Levine S. (1994) Evidence of reduced respiratory muscle endurance in patients with heart failure. *J Am Coll Cardiol* 4: 972–981.

Mancini DM, Henson D, LaManca J, Levine S. (1992) Respiratory muscle function and dyspnoea in patients with chronic congestive heart failure. *Circulation* 86: 909–918.

Mancini DM, LaManca J, Donchez L, Henson D, Levine S. (1996) The sensation of dyspnoea is not determined by the work of breathing in patients with heart failure. *J Am Coll Cardiol* 8: 391–395.

Mancini DM, Walter G, Reichnek N, et al. (1992) Contribution of skeletal muscle atrophy to exercise intolerance and altered muscle metabolism in heart failure. *Circulation* 85: 1364–1373.

Maskin CS, Forman R, Sonnenblick EH, Frishman WH, LeJemtel TH. (1983) Failure of dobutamine to increase exercise capacity despite haemodynamic improvement in severe chronic heart failure. *Am J Cardiol* 51: 177–182.

Massie BM, Conway M, Rajagopalan BM, et al. (1988) Skeletal muscle metabolism during exercise under ischaemic conditions in congestive heart failure. Evidence for abnormalities unrelated to blood flow. *Circulation* 78: 320–326.

Massie BM, Conway M, Yonge R, et al. (1987b) Skeletal muscle metabolism in patients with congestive heart failure: relation to clinical severity and blood flow. *Circulation* 76: 9–19.

Massie BM, Conway M, Yonge R, et al. (1987) 31P nuclear magnetic resonance evidence of abnormal skeletal muscle metabolism in patients with congestive heart failure. *Am J Cardiol* 60: 309–315.

McMurray J, Abdullah I, Dargie HJ, Shapiro D. (1991) Increased concentrations of tumour necrosis factor in 'cachectic' patients with severe chronic heart failure. *Br Heart J* 66: 356–358.

McParland C, Krishnan B, Wang Y, Gallagher CG. (1992) Inspiratory muscle weakness and dyspnoea in chronic heart failure *Am Rev Respir Dis* 146: 467–472.

Meakins J, Lang CNH. (1927) Oxygen consumption, oxygen debt and lactic acid in circulatory failure. *J Clin Inv* 273–293.

Minotti JR, Christoph I, Oka R, Weiner MW, Wells L, Massie BM. (1991) Impaired skeletal muscle function in patients with congestive heart failure. Relationship to systemic exercise performance. *J Clin Invest* 88: 2077–2082.

Minotti JR, Pillay P, Chang L, Wells L, Massie BM. (1992) Neurophysiological assessment of skeletal muscle fatigue in patients with congestive heart failure. *Circulation* 86: 903–908.

Minotti JR, Pillay P, Oka R, Wells L, Christoph I, Massie BM. (1993) Skeletal muscle size: relationship to muscle function in heart failure. *J Appl Physiol* 75: 373–381.

Nishimura Y, Maeda H, Tanaka K, Nakamura H, Hashimoto Y, Yokoyama M. (1994) Respiratory muscle strength and hemodynamics in chronic heart failure. *Chest* 105: 355–359.

Piepoli M, Clark AL, Volterrani M, Adamopoulos S, Sleight P, Coats AJ. (1996) Contribution of muscle afferents to the hemodynamic, autonomic, and ventilatory responses to exercise in patients with chronic heart failure: effects of physical training. *Circulation* 93: 940–952.

Sabbah HN, Hansen-Smith F, Sharov VG, et al. (1993) Decreased proportion of type I myofibres in skeletal muscle of dogs with chronic heart failure. *Circulation* 87: 1729–1737.

Sullivan MJ, Green HJ, Cobb FR. (1990) Skeletal muscle biochemistry and histology in ambulatory patients with long-term heart failure. *Circulation* 81: 518–527.

Sullivan MJ, Higginbotham MB, Cobb FR. (1988) Exercise training in patients with severe left ventricular

dysfunction: hemodynamic and metabolic effects. *Circulation* 78: 506–516.

Swan JW, Anker SD, Walton C, et al. (1997) Insulin resistance in chronic heart failure: Relationship to severity and etiology of heart failure. *J Am Coll Cardiol* 30: 527–532.

Szlachcic J, Massie BM, Kramer BL, Topic N, Tubau J. (1985) Correlates and prognostic implication of exercise capacity in chronic congestive heart failure. *Am J Cardiol* 55: 1037–1363.

Weber KT, Janicki JS. (1985) Lactate production during maximal and submaximal exercise inpatients with chronic heart failure. *J Am Coll Cardiol* 6: 717–724.

Wiener DH, Fink LI, Maris J, Jones RA, Chance B, Wilson JR. (1986) Abnormal skeletal muscle bioenergetics during exercise in patients with heart failure: role of reduced muscle blood flow. *Circulation* 73: 1127–1136.

Wilson JR, Fink L, Maris J, et al. (1985) Evaluation of energy metabolism in skeletal muscle of patients with heart failure with gated phosphorous-31 nuclear magnetic resonance. *Circulation* 71: 57–62.

Wilson JR, Mancini DM, Dunkman WB. (1993) Exertional fatigue due to skeletal muscle dysfunction in patients with heart failure. *Circulation* 87: 470–475.

Wilson JR, Mancini DM, Simson M. (1992) Detection of skeletal muscle fatigue in patients with heart failure using electromyography. *Am J Cardiol* 70: 488–493.

Wilson JR, Martin JL, Ferraro N. (1984) Impaired skeletal muscle nutritive flow during exercise in patients with congestive heart failure: role of cardiac pump dysfunction as determined by the effect of dobutamine. *Am J Cardiol* 53: 1308–1315.

Wilson JR, Martin JL, Schwartz D, Ferraro N. (1984) Exercise intolerance in patients with chronic heart failure: role of impaired nutritive flow to skeletal muscle. *Circulation* 69: 1079–1087.

Wilson JR. (1995) Exercise Intolerance in heart failure Importance of skeletal muscle. *Circulation* 91: 559–561.

Yancy CW, Jr, Parsons D, Lane L, Carry M, Firth BG, Blomqvist CG. (1989) Capillary density, fiber type and enzyme composition of skeletal muscle in congestive heart failure. *J Am Coll Cardiol* 13(suppl): 38A.

Zelis R, Flaim SF. (1982) Alterations in vasomotor tone in congestive heart failure. *Prog Cardiovase Dis* 24: 437–459.

11

Skeletal muscle dysfunction in renal failure

Simon S. Wing

Clinical and laboratory manifestations of muscle dysfunction in renal failure

Muscular complaints are frequent among patients suffering from renal failure. In a study of patients on dialysis (Fahal et al 1997), all patients complained of fatigue and weakness and many complained of muscle pains or cramps (Table 11.1). Most, however, were able to manage with movements fundamental to daily living such as getting out of bed or climbing stairs. Objectively, though, approximately half of these patients manifested muscle wasting in upper and/or lower extremities, and this wasting was often associated with some weakness on examination.

Laboratory findings in these patients confirmed the presence of muscle dysfunction (Fahal et al 1997). Although electrical stimulation studies indicated normal excitation–contraction coupling, most patients did show some impaired generation of force. This was particularly apparent in older and malnourished patients, identified as those with low serum albumin levels. Muscle biopsies in this study and others revealed abnormal findings in a majority of subjects (Floyd et al 1974, Ahonen 1980, Guarnieri et al 1983, Fahal et al 1997). A variety of abnormalities have been observed. Most commonly, there is increased

Table 11.1 — Neuromuscular characteristics in a study of 49 dialysis patients (modified from Fahal et al 1997, used with permission of the publisher)

Proportion of patients with history of:	
Fatigue	100%
Weakness	100%
Muscle pain or cramps	53%
Muscle stiffness	4%
Bone pain	6%
Proportion of patients who are able to:	
Sit up in bed unaided	100%
Climb stairs	100%
Raise arms above head	100%
Rise from chair	96%
Squat	84%
Proportion of patients with evidence on examination of:	
Upper limb wasting	47%
Lower limb wasting	43%
Upper limb weakness	20%
Lower limb weakness	33%

variation in fibre diameter. This is usually associated with atrophy of Type II fibres and either normal or hypertrophic Type I fibres. Occasionally more dramatic abnormalities such as necrotic, moth-eaten or whorled fibres have been described (Floyd et al 1974, Ahonen 1980). Biochemical parameters measured in muscle biopsies are consistent with atrophy of fibres. Protein content and RNA content is diminished (Guarnieri et al 1983), as occurs in many other muscle atrophic conditions.

Molecular basis of muscle weakness

Several mechanisms may explain the muscle weakness found in patients with chronic renal failure (Table 11.2). The most evident one is impaired force generation from decreased muscle bulk in these patients. The decreased muscle bulk is a direct consequence of the atrophy of muscle fibres. Since myofibres consist primarily of contractile proteins, this atrophy must represent increased loss of muscle protein. Like proteins in all compartments of the body, muscle proteins are constantly being turned over. Since the body normally turns over about 4 gm protein per kg body weight per day, a small excess in protein loss can result in significant depletion of body protein over a period of several weeks.

Muscle protein loss arises from a fall in the rate of protein synthesis and/or an increase in the rate of protein degradation (Fulks et al 1975). In vivo rates of protein synthesis can be estimated from rates of labelled amino acid uptake into tissues. Rates of muscle protein synthesis in patients with renal failure were found not to be suppressed, but actually increased compared with controls indicating increased overall protein turnover (Garibotto et al 1996). However, as measured by several approaches, rates of muscle protein degradation are elevated. In vivo measurements of the rate of appearance of phenylalanine across the forearm muscle bed showed elevated rates

Table 11.2 — Abnormalities in muscle that may cause weakness

Loss of contractile proteins from activation of protein degradation
Activation of amino acid oxidation
Carnitine deficiency
Lower activities of enzymes involved in generating ATP
Abnormal levels of intracellular electrolytes

of muscle protein degradation (Garibotto et al 1996). Furthermore, a net release of alanine from muscle has been observed in uraemic patients (Garibotto et al 1994) as well as in rats in whom renal failure has been induced (Garber 1978). Finally, increased 3-methyl histidine production (a post-translationally modified histidine found uniquely on myofibrillar proteins and which is not metabolized, but excreted in the urine) has been observed in uraemic acidotic patients (Williams et al 1991). Use of animal models has permitted more detailed characterization of protein turnover in muscles. Rates of protein synthesis and protein degradation have been measured in isolated muscles from uraemic rats (Clark and Mitch 1983). Similar to the in vivo data in patients, muscle protein catabolism arises from accelerated protein degradation as rates of protein synthesis were unchanged.

Activation of protein breakdown is, therefore, the principal cause of the muscle protein loss. This is similar to many other catabolic conditions such as fasting, sepsis and cancer (Wing and Goldberg 1993, Temparis et al 1994, Baracos et al 1995, Voisin et al 1996). The biochemical mechanisms by which muscle breaks down protein have only recently become better understood. Muscle like all eukaryotic cells contains multiple pathways of protein catabolism. Lysosomes are organelles that contain numerous hydrolytic enzymes (Bohley and Seglen 1992). Lysosomal proteolysis is primarily non-specific in that the principle mode of uptake of proteins into lysosomes is by autophagy, which involves sequestration of random portions of cytoplasm. This pathway does not appear to be involved in the muscle catabolism. Inhibition of the pathway in the isolated muscles from uraemic rats does not block the activation of protein breakdown seen, compared with normal rats (Mitch et al 1994). Calcium-dependent proteases (Sorimachi et al 1997) are apparently involved in more selective proteolysis in cells, but they too do not appear to be involved in the catabolic process, as their inhibition also does not abrogate the activation of protein breakdown (Mitch et al 1994). Interestingly, the activation of protein breakdown in muscles is blocked when they are depleted of ATP suggesting that some energy-dependent process is involved in the activation of catabolism. To date, the only eukaryotic non-lysosomal ATP-dependent proteolytic process known is the ubiquitin-dependent system (Hershko and Ciechanover 1998). In this proteolytic pathway, ubiquitin, an 8 kDa peptide found in all eukaryotic cells, becomes covalently linked to target proteins marking them for recognition and degradation by the 1.5×10^6 Da proteolytic complex, the 26S proteasome.

Interestingly, the activation of protein breakdown seen in uraemic rats can be blocked by incubating the muscles in the presence of an inhibitor of the proteasome (Fig. 11.1), arguing strongly for a role for this pathway in the degradative process (Bailey et al 1996). In further support of the activation of the ubiquitin-dependent system, there is increased transcription of ubiquitin genes as well as increased mRNA expression of some subunits of the proteasome in the atrophying muscles (Mitch et al 1994). Thus, activation of protein breakdown in the uraemic state is most likely caused by activation of the ubiquitin proteasome dependent pathway, and the accelerated proteolysis causes muscle protein loss and fibre atrophy. This is probably a major cause of the muscle weakness.

Other disturbances of amino acid metabolism may also contribute to the negative nitrogen balance. There are abnormalities in distribution of amino acids, both in the circulation and within the muscle fibres. Patients have low plasma concentrations of essential amino acids and high concentrations of non-essential amino acids (Swendseid and Kopple 1973). Similar disturbances in the intramuscular levels of these amino acids have also been observed (Bergstrom et al 1978, 1990). After a meal, absolute uptake of essential amino

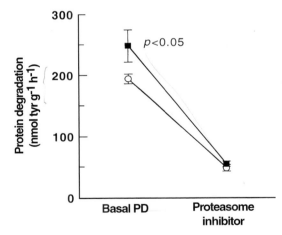

Figure 11.1—The chronic renal failure induced increase in muscle protein degradation in rats is prevented by an inhibitor of the proteasome. Both epitrochlearis muscles were isolated from rats subjected to near total nephrectomy (filled squares) or sham operated (open circles) and incubated in vitro. The basal rate of protein degradation (PD) was measured in one epitrochlearis muscle and compared with values measured in the contralateral muscle incubated with the proteasome inhibitor, MG132. The difference in protein degradation between chronic renal failure and sham operated control muscles in the absence of inhibitor was statistically significant by t test ($p < 0.05$); there was no difference when the inhibitor was present. (From Bailey et al 1996, used with permission of the publisher.)

acids is normal, but there is increased uptake of non-essential amino acids (Garibotto et al 1995). In uraemia, the acidotic state produces activation of muscle branched-chain keto acid dehydrogenase activity (Hara et al 1987). Branched-chain amino acids are the most important essential amino acids with respect to protein metabolism, and they make up 50% of dietary amino acids. Absolute values of uptake of these amino acids in chronic renal failure patients are similar to controls (Garibotto et al 1995), but intracellular oxidation is increased in these patients leading to decreased muscle levels of these amino acids. Indeed, intramuscular valine levels correlate inversely with severity of metabolic acidosis in humans (Reich et al 1992). Furthermore, these amino acids, in particular leucine, play an important role in suppressing muscle proteolysis (Tischler et al 1982), and so their intracellular deficiency can aggravate muscle protein loss.

Mitochondria are the energy generators of the cell and an adequate supply of ATP is critical for normal muscle function. Muscle ATP levels as well as creatine phosphate levels, measured by nuclear magnetic resonance (NMR), are lower in renal failure patients on dialysis than in normal controls (Thompson et al 1994, Pastoris et al 1997). Carnitine levels are low in muscles of patients on dialysis (Boemer et al 1978, Wanner and Horl 1988). Since carnitine is required as a cofactor in the transport of free fatty acids into the mitochondrion for oxidation to generate ATP, its deficiency is an attractive mechanism for explaining the low ATP levels and the abnormal force generation. However, there is no accumulation of cytoplasmic lipid, which is a typical finding of isolated carnitine deficiency. Measurements of various enzymatic activities in muscle have also demonstrated decreased cytochrome oxidase activity, which can result in decreased oxidative phosphorylation, thereby also contributing to decreased levels of ATP (Pastoris et al 1997).

Various abnormalities of intracellular electrolytes such as higher sodium and chloride and decreased potassium contents (Cotton et al 1979) have been described. The significance of these findings, particularly as they relate to the impairment of muscle function, remains unclear.

Pathophysiology of muscle dysfunction in renal insufficiency

How renal insufficiency results in these many abnormalities of muscle composition and function is an

Table 11.3 — Potential mechanisms by which renal failure causes muscle dysfunction

Metabolic acidosis
Insufficient caloric intake
Insufficient protein intake
Insulin resistance
IGF-1[a] resistance/lower IGF-1 bioactivity
High levels of glucocorticoid hormones
Inflammatory cytokines
Hyperparathyroidism

[a]IGF-1, insulin-like growth factor 1

intriguing question. Renal failure results in multiple derangements of normal homeostasis. Therefore, multiple factors are likely involved, possibly acting in concert to mediate the muscle dysfunction (Table 11.3). One critical factor in the defective homeostasis is metabolic acidosis, a major feature of the uraemic state. Studies in animals have shown that, at degrees of acidaemia typical of uraemic patients, there is intracellular acidosis (Bailey et al 1996). Consequently, many intracellular functions may be altered by the change in pH. The metabolic acidosis results in activation of protein degradation, and this can be reversed by treatment with alkali (Fig. 11.2) (Reich et al 1993). Indeed in a study of nine patients, there was an

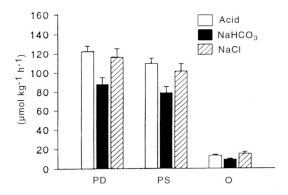

Figure 11.2 — Correction of acidosis in patients with chronic renal failure decreases protein degradation and amino acid oxidation. Rates of whole body protein degradation (PD), protein synthesis (PS) and amino acid oxidation (O) were measured by leucine kinetics prior to treatment (Acid) and subsequent to 4 weeks of treatment with sodium bicarbonate (NaHCO$_3$) or sodium chloride (NaCl). Statistical significance – PD: Acid vs NaHCO$_3$, $p<0.01$; NaHCO$_3$ vs NaCl, $p<0.01$, Acid vs NaCl, NS; PS: Acid vs NaHCO$_3$, $p<0.01$; NaHCO$_3$ vs NaCl, $p<0.01$, Acid vs NaCl, NS; O: Acid vs NaHCO$_3$, $p<0.05$, NaHCO$_3$ vs NaCl, $p<0.01$; Acid vs NaCl, NS. (NS, non-significant. From Reich et al 1993, used with permission of the publisher.)

inverse relationship between plasma bicarbonate and protein balance (Garibotto et al 1996). Negative nitrogen balance and the increased excretion of methylhistidine can also improve with the correction of metabolic acidosis (Papadoyannakis et al 1984). Metabolic acidosis alone can also lead to activation of branched-chain amino acid dehydrogenase and yield increased amino acid oxidation, thereby also leading to amino acid loss. These observations have been made both in human subjects (Reaich et al 1992, 1993) and in animal models (Hara et al 1987).

Patients are often somewhat anorexic and so can suffer from malnutrition. In one survey of 35 patients, approximately 25% of patients reported caloric intakes of less than 70% of recommended allowances (Kopple 1978). The inadequate caloric intake can itself lead to activation of muscle protein loss. The dialysis procedure itself also results in loss of nutrients. It has been estimated that 5–8 g of free amino acids, 3–4 g of bound amino acids and 20–50 g of glucose may be lost during a 4 h haemodialysis session (Kopple 1978).

Patients, particularly those awaiting dialysis, are generally treated with a low protein diet. Normal subjects usually respond to a low protein diet by initially suppressing amino acid oxidation to ensure an adequate supply of essential amino acids for protein synthesis. Subsequently, rates of protein degradation are also suppressed, maintaining nitrogen balance (Motil et al 1981, Tom et al 1995). Whether patients suffering from renal failure have defects in these adaptive mechanisms remains controversial. Non-acidotic patients in renal failure (Goodship et al 1990), or those stably managed with dialysis and supplemented with amino acids or keto acids (Tom et al 1995), appear to respond normally to restrictions in protein intake with decreases in whole body protein turnover and amino acid oxidation. Although those studies demonstrated that urinary nitrogen losses (reflective of total body protein) fell with protein restriction, a study in which urinary 3-methylhistidine was also followed as a marker of muscle protein loss showed that this index of protein degradation remained elevated (Williams et al 1991). This suggests that although overall body protein catabolism may be suppressed, muscle protein degradation may remain elevated.

Abnormal hormonal physiology may also play a role in the pathogenesis of muscle wasting. Glucose turnover studies have demonstrated the presence of insulin resistance, seen mainly as decreased rates of insulin-stimulated glucose uptake and non-oxidative glucose metabolism, the latter reflecting glycogen synthesis (Foss et al 1996). Correction of metabolic acidosis can improve insulin action (Reaich et al 1995). Similar defects have been identified in rats with chronic renal failure (May et al 1985). Insulin plays an important role in regulating body protein turnover, by suppressing protein degradation (Gelfand and Barrett 1987). However, studies to date suggest that insulin resistance appears specific to glucose metabolism, and it does not affect protein metabolism.

Insulin-like growth factor I (IGF-1) is an anabolic hormone, and it is the key mediator of post-natal growth. It stimulates muscle protein synthesis and inhibits protein degradation (Kettelhut et al 1988). In rat models of chronic renal failure, decreased IGF-1 levels have been observed (Ding et al 1996). Measurements of serum IGF-1 levels in patients with kidney failure though, have not revealed any deficiency (Blum et al 1991, Filho Divino et al 1998). However, increased levels of some IGF-binding proteins have been observed (Filho Divino et al 1998) and, therefore, it is quite possible that levels of free IGF-1, the bioactive form, are low and may contribute to a catabolic state. Finally, administration of IGF-1 to rats with uraemia results in impaired suppression of plasma amino acids (Ding et al 1996) suggesting resistance to the action of IGF-1 in this condition.

In rats, uraemia induces increased production of adrenal glucocorticoid hormones (May et al 1987). These hormones are well known to suppress protein synthesis and under certain conditions activate protein breakdown in skeletal muscle (reviewed in Kettelhut et al 1988). Furthermore, inhibition of glucocorticoid production in these animal models can blunt or prevent the activation of muscle protein degradation (May et al 1986). However, increased glucocorticoids alone are unable to activate proteolysis, indicating that they are necessary but not sufficient. It is unclear in humans, though, whether there is chronic excess glucocorticoid production in the uraemic state.

Inflammatory cytokines such as interleukin-1 (IL-1) and tumour necrosis factor-α (TNF-α) are recognized to stimulate protein catabolism (Goodman 1991, Zamir et al 1991, Llovera et al 1993). Whether levels of such cytokines are increased in patients with renal failure, particularly those treated with haemodialysis where the dialysis membrane may activate complement, is controversial (Herbelin et al 1990, Pereira et al 1994). Some of these conflicting results may reflect times of sampling as levels may be transiently increased, such as during haemodialysis treatments. However, endogenous inhibitors of cytokine action also appear increased in these patients (Pereira et al 1994), and therefore the net effect of these abnormalities remains unclear.

Patients with renal failure generally have high circulating parathyroid hormone levels in response to hypocalcaemia from hyperphosphataemia and 1,25-dihydroxy-vitamin D deficiency. This hyperparathyroidism may contribute to the muscle dysfunction. Administration of parathyroid hormone to rats mimicked some of the muscle abnormalities seen in uraemia, such as decreased concentrations of creatine phosphate and ATP (Baczynski et al 1985). Exposure of isolated rat muscles to parathyroid hormone resulted in net amino acid release arising from decreased rates of protein synthesis and increased rates of protein degradation (Garber 1983).

Treatment

Maintenance of adequate nutrition is essential. Sufficient calories are essential and protein intake needs to be optimized. Patients, particularly those not requiring dialysis, are often on protein-restricted diets to decrease progression and minimize symptoms of uraemia. If normal homeostatic responses to suppress protein turnover are not effective, a catabolic state may ensue. Several studies indicate that protein balance can be maintained on protein-restricted diets by supplementation with essential amino acids or a keto acid mixture (Abras and Walser 1982, Masud et al 1994, Van der Niepen et al 1998). Careful assessments need to be made on a regular basis to verify adequate caloric and protein intakes.

Patients should also be adequately dialysed. Optimization of dialysis was observed to improve electromyographic parameters of muscle function (Sobh et al 1998). Haemodialysis can also ameliorate the insulin resistance seen in uraemic patients, and it blunts the amino acid abnormalities (Foss et al 1996). Such optimization of dialysis will also partly treat the metabolic acidosis that clearly causes many of the metabolic abnormalities seen in renal failure. In short-term studies, bicarbonate therapy can suppress the activated branched-chain amino acid oxidation and protein degradation in muscle (Papadoyannakis et al 1984, Reaich et al 1993, Bailey et al 1996). Its use may be helpful in patients awaiting dialysis or those who are inadequately dialysed. Attention must be paid to possible adverse effects, such as hypertension from the sodium content.

Pharmacological therapy for muscle wasting remains investigative at this time. Growth hormone administration to six chronically wasted patients on haemodialysis resulted in increased rates of muscle protein synthesis and net protein balance (Garibotto et al

1997). A double-blind medium-term study involving 40 subjects (Jensen et al 1996) confirmed that growth hormone can produce an increase in lean body mass and improve sense of well being. However, there were no detectable changes in laboratory measurements of muscle contraction force in treated patients. Of concern, though, treatment resulted in increased left ventricular mass. Growth hormone is also recognized to have lipolytic effects, and it can worsen insulin resistance. Whether therapy results in long-term, clinically apparent improvements of function without significant side-effects remains to be determined. Therapy with IGF-1 has been considered but not studied in detail in uraemia (Kopple et al 1995). However, when used in the catabolic state of human immunodeficiency virus (HIV) infection, the improvements in protein balance have generally been transient (Lieberman et al 1994, Lee et al 1996). Anabolic steroids have proven beneficial in stimulating significant improvements in muscle size and function in patients suffering from other catabolic disorders (Bhasin et al 1996, Rabkin et al 1997, Ferreira et al 1998). However, because of the lack of pure anabolic steroids without androgenic effects, such therapy would appear limited to men at this time. However, 'designer' steroids with anabolic but without androgenic activities may be developed and such agents could be useful in women. Megestrol acetate has often been used in other anorectic conditions and found to stimulate appetite and weight gain (Oster et al 1994, Von Roenn et al 1994). However, most of the weight gain is in the form of adipose tissue (Oster et al 1994). Combination therapy with anabolic steroids may be useful, though, and studies are underway in other wasting conditions to evaluate this combination.

Carnitine supplements have been studied, although small studies yielded conflicting results: some showed decreases in muscle symptoms in treated patients (Sakurauchi et al 1998) and small increases in diameter of Type I and Type IIa muscle fibres (Giovenali et al 1994), while others found no changes in oxidative capacity in these muscles and no functional im-

Table 11.4 — Treatment approaches to muscle dysfunction

Adequate nutrition
Adequate dialysis
Sodium bicarbonate for acidosis
Anabolic agents (experimental) – Growth hormone, IGF-1[a], androgens
Supplements – carnitine, amino acids, ketoacids

[a]IGF-1, insulin-like growth factor 1

provements (Thompson et al 1997). A multicentre randomized, placebo-controlled trial did show, in carnitine-treated patients, fewer muscle cramps, increased oxygen consumption during progressive exercise and increases in mid-arm circumference as a measure of muscle mass (Ahmad et al 1990).

Anaemia is a prominent feature of uraemia, and it has previously been suggested as a potential cause of muscle dysfunction by limiting oxygen delivery to muscles. However, improvement of the anaemia by erythropoietin therapy has not resulted in clear improvement in muscle function (Painter and Moore 1994, Thompson et al 1996).

Summary

The metabolic derangements associated with uraemia, in particular metabolic acidosis, play a key role in activation of protein breakdown and oxidation of branched-chain amino acids in skeletal muscle. These disturbances of nitrogen metabolism lead to net protein loss in skeletal muscle and atrophy of muscle fibres. The resulting loss of bulk may contribute significantly to the observed decrease in muscle force generation and to the muscular weakness experienced by many patients. Adequate dialysis and sufficient caloric and protein intake are important factors in minimizing muscle protein wasting. Other therapeutic modalities, such as amino acid supplementation and anabolic agents, are currently being evaluated, and these may be useful adjuncts in improving strength, functional capacity and overall well being in these patients.

References

Abras E, Walser M. (1982) Nitrogen utilization in uremic patients fed by continuous nasogastric infusion. *Kidney Int* 22: 392–397.

Ahmad S, Robertson T, Golper TA, et al. (1990) Multicenter trial of L-carnitine in maintenance hemodialysis patients. II. Clinical and biochemical effects. *Kidney Int* 38: 912–918.

Ahonen RE. (1980) Light microscopic study of striated muscle in uremia. *Acta Neuropathol* 49: 51–55.

Baczynski R, Massry SG, Magott M, El-Belbessi S, Kohan R, Brautbar N. (1985) Effect of parathyroid hormone on energy metabolism of skeletal muscle. *Kidney Int* 28: 722–727.

Bailey JL, England BK, Long RC, Mitch WE. (1996) Influence of acid loading, extracellular pH and uraemia on intracellular pH in muscle. *Miner Electrolyte Metab* 22: 66–68.

Bailey JL, Wang X, England BK, Price SR, Ding X, Mitch WE. (1996) The acidosis of chronic renal failure activates muscle proteolysis in rats by augmenting transcription of genes encoding proteins of the ATP-dependent ubiquitin-proteasome pathway. *J Clin Invest* 97: 1447–1453.

Baracos VE, DeVivo C, Hoyle DH, Goldberg AL. (1995) Activation of the ATP-ubiquitin-proteasome pathway in skeletal muscle of cachectic rats bearing a hepatoma. *Am J Physiol* 268: E996–E1006.

Bergstrom J, Alvestrand A, Furst P. (1990) Plasma and muscle free amino acids in maintenance hemodialysis patients without protein malnutrition. *Kidney Int* 38: 108–114.

Bergstrom J, Furst P, Noree L-O, Vinnars E, Widstrom A. (1978) Intracellular free amino acids in muscle tissue of patients with chronic uremia: effect of peritoneal dialysis and infusion of essential amino acids. *Clin Sci Mol Med* 54: 51–60.

Bhasin S, Storer TW, Berman N. (1996) The effects of supraphysiologic doses of testosterone on muscle size and strength in normal men. *N Engl J Med* 335: 1–7.

Blum WR, Ranke MB, Kietzmann K, Tonshoff B, Mehls O. (1991) Growth hormone resistance and inhibition of somatomedin activity by excess of insulin-like growth factor binding protein in uremia. *Ped Nephrol* 5: 539–544.

Boemer T, Bergrem H, Eiklid K. (1978) Carnitine deficiency induced during intermittent hemodialysis for renal failure. *Lancet* i: 126–128.

Bohley P, Seglen PO. (1992) Proteases and proteolysis in the lysosome. *Experientia* 48: 151–157.

Clark AS, Mitch WE. (1983) Muscle protein turnover and glucose uptake in acutely uremic rats. *J Clin Invest* 72: 836–845.

Cotton JR, Woodard T, Carter NW, Knochel JP. (1979) Resting skeletal muscle membrane potential as an index of uremic toxicity. *J Clin Invest* 63: 501–506.

Ding H, Gao X, Hirschberg R, Vadgama JV, Kopple JD. (1996) Impaired actions of insulin-like growth factor 1 on protein synthesis and degradation in skeletal muscle of rats with chronic renal failure. *J Clin Invest* 97: 1064–1075.

Fahal IH, Bell GM, Bone JM, Edwards RH. (1997) Physiological abnormalities of skeletal muscle in dialysis. *Nephrol Dialysis Transplantation* 12: 119–127.

Ferreira IM, Verreschi IT, Nery LE, et al. (1998) The Influence of 6 months of oral anabolic steroids on body mass and respiratory muscles in undernourished COPD patients. *Chest* 114: 19–28.

Filho Divino JC, Hazel SJ, Furst P, Bergstrom J, Hall K. (1998) Glutamate concentration in plasma, erythrocyte and muscle in relation to plasma levels of insulin-like growth factor (IGF)-I, IGF binding protein-1 and insulin in patients on haemodialysis. *J Endocrinol* 156: 519–527.

Floyd M, Ayyar DR, Barwick DD, Hudgson P, Weightman D. (1974) Myopathy in cronic renal failure. *Quarterly J Med* XLI: 509–524.

Foss MC, Gouveia LM, Moyses Neto M, Paccola GM, Piccinato CE. (1996) Effect of hemodialysis on peripheral glucose metabolism of patients with chronic renal failure. *Nephron* 73: 48–53.

Fulks R, Li JB, Goldberg AL. (1975) Effects of insulin, glucose, and amino acids on protein turnover in rat diaphragm. *J Biol Chem* 250: 290–298.

Garber A. (1978) Skeletal muscle protein and amino acid metabolism in experimental chronic uremia in the rat. Accelerated alanine and glutamine formation and release. *J Clin Invest* 62: 623.

Garber AJ. (1983) Effects of parathyroid hormone on skeletal muscle protein and amino acid metabolism in the rat. *J Clin Invest* 71: 1806–1821.

Garibotto G, Barreca A, Russo R, Sofia A, Araghi P, Cesarone A. (1997) Effects of recombinant human growth hormone on muscle protein turnover in malnourished haemodialysis. *J Clin Invest* 99: 97–105.

Garibotto G, Deferrari G, Robaudo C, Saffioti S, Sofia A, Russo R. (1995) Disposal of exogenous amino acids by muscle in patients with chronic renal failure. *Am J Clin Nutr* 62: 136–142.

Garibotto G, Russo R, Sofia A, et al. (1994) Skeletal muscle protein synthesis and degradation in patients with chronic renal failure. *Kidney Int* 45: 1432–1439.

Garibotto G, Russo R, Sofia A, Sala MR, Sabatino C, Moscatelli P. (1996) Muscle protein turnover in chronic renal failure patients with metabolic acidosis or normal acid base balance. *Miner Electrolyte Metab* 22: 58–61.

Gelfand RA, Barrett EJ. (1987) Effect of physiologic hyperinsulinemia on skeletal muscle protein synthesis and breakdown in man. *J Clin Invest* 80: 1–6.

Giovenali P, Fenocchio D, Montanari G, et al. (1994) Selective trophic effect of L-carnitine in type I and IIa skeletal muscle fibres. *Kidney Int* 46: 1616–1619.

Goodman MN. (1991) Tumor necrosis factor induces skeletal muscle protein breakdown in rats. *Am J Physiol* 260: E727–E730.

Goodship T, Mitch W, Hoerr R, Wagner D, Steinman T, Young V. (1990) Adaptation to low-protein diets in renal failure: leucine turnover and nitrogen balance. *J Am Soc Nephrol* 1: 66–75.

Guarnieri G, Toigo G, Situlin R, et al. (1983) Muscle biopsy studies in chronically uremic patients: Evidence for malnutrition. *Kidney Int* 24: S187–S193.

Hara Y, May RC, Kelly RA, Mitch WE. (1987) Acidosis,

not azotemia, stimulates branched-chain, amino acid catabolism in uremic rats. *Kidney Int* 32: 808–814.

Herbelin A, Nguyen AT, Zingraff J, Urena P, Descamps-Latscha B. (1990) Influence of uremia and hemodialysis on circulating interleukin-1 and tumor necrosis factor α. *Kidney Int* 37: 116–125.

Hershko A, Ciechanover A. (1998) The ubiquitin system. *Annu Rev Biochem* 67: 425–479.

Jensen PB, Hansen TB, Oxhoj H, Froberg K, Ekelund B, Nielsen FT. (1996) What are the clinical benefits of correcting the catabolic state in haemodialysis patients? *Br J Clin Practice Supplement* 85: 47–51.

Kettelhut IC, Wing SS, Goldberg AL. (1988) Endocrine regulation of protein breakdown in skeletal muscle. *Diabetes/Metabolism Rev* 4: 751–772.

Kopple JD. (1978) Abnormal amino acid and protein metabolism in uremia. *Kidney Int* 14: 340–348.

Kopple JD, Ding H, Gao XL. (1995) Altered physiology and action of insulin-like growth factor 1 in skeletal muscle in chronic renal failure. *Am J Kid Dis* 26: 248–255.

Lee PD, Pivarnik JM, Bukar JG, et al. (1996) A randomized, placebo-controlled trial of combined insulin-like growth factor I and low dose growth hormone therapy for wasting associated with human immunodeficiency virus infection. *J Clin Endocrinol Metab* 81: 2968–2975.

Lieberman SA, Butterfield E, Harrison D, Hoffman AR. (1994) Anabolic effects of fecombinant insulin-like growth factor-I in cachectic patients with the acquired immunodeficiency syndrome. *J Clin Endocrinol Metab* 78: 404–410.

Llovera M, Lopez-Soriano FJ, Argiles JM. (1993) Effects of tumor necrosis factor-alpha on muscle protein turnover in female Wistar rats. *J Natl Cancer Inst* 85: 1334–1339.

Masud T, Young VR, Chapman T, Maroni BJ. (1994) Adaptive responses to very low protein diets: The first comparison of ketoacids to essential amino acids. *Kidney Int* 45: 1182–1192.

May RC, Clark AS, Goheer MA, Mitch WE. (1985) Specific defects in insulin-mediated muscle metabolism in acute uremia. *Kidney Int* 28: 490–497.

May RC, Kelly RA, Mitch WE. (1987) Mechanisms for defects in muscle protein metabolism in rat with chronic uremia. Influence of metabolic acidosis. *J Clin Invest* 79: 1099–1103.

May RC, Kelly RA, Mitch WE. (1986) Metabolic acidosis stimulates protein degradation in rat muscle by a glucocorticoid-dependent mechanism. *J Clin Invest* 77: 614–621.

Mitch WE, Medina R, Grieber S, et al. (1994) Metabolic acidosis stimulates muscle protein degradation by activating the adenosine triphosphate-dependent pathway involving ubiquitin and proteasomes. *J Clin Invest* 93: 2127–2133.

Motil KJ, Matthews DE, Bier DM, Burke JF, Munro HN, Young VR. (1981) Whole-body leucine and lysine metabolism: response to dietary protein intake in young men. *Am J Physiol* 240: E712–E721.

Oster MH, Enders SR, Samuels SJ, et al. (1994) Megestrol acetate in patients with AIDS and cachexia. *Ann Inter Med* 121: 400–408.

Painter P, Moore GE. (1994) The impact of recombinant human erythropoietin on exercise capacity in hemodialysis patients. *Advances Renal Replacement Therapy* 1: 55–65.

Papadoyannakis NJ, Stefanidis CJ, McGeown M. (1984) The effect of the correction of metabolic acidosis on nitrogen and potassium balance of patients with chronic renal failure. *Am J Clin Nutr* 40: 623–627.

Pastoris O, Aquilani R, Foppa P, Bovio G, Segagni S, Baiardi P. (1997) Altered muscle energy metabolism in post-absorptive patients with chronic renal failure. *Scand J Urol Nephrol* 31: 281–287.

Pereira BJG, Shapiro L, King AJ, Falagas ME, Strom JA, Dinarello CA. (1994) Plasm levels of IL-1β, TNFα and their specific inhibitors in undialyzed chronic renal failure, CAPD and hemodialysis patients. *Kidney Int* 45: 890–896.

Rabkin JG, Rabkin R, Wagner GJ. (1997) Testosterone treatment of clinical hypogonadism in patients with HIV/AIDS. *Intl J STD AIDS* 8: 537–545.

Reaich D, Channon SM, Scrimgeour CM, Daley SE, Wilkinson R, Goodship THJ. (1993) Correction of acidosis in humans with CRF decreases protein degradation and amino acid oxidation. *Am J Physiol* 265: E230–E235.

Reaich D, Channon SM, Scrimgeour SM, Goodship THJ. (1992) Ammonium chloride-induced acidosis increases protein breakdown and amino acid oxidation in humans. *Am J Physiol* 263: E735–E739.

Reaich D, Graham KA, Channon SM, et al. (1995) Insulin-mediated changes in PD and glucose uptake after correction of acidosis in humans with CRF. *Am J Physiol* 268: E121–E126.

Sakurauchi Y, Matsumoto Y, Shinzato T, Takai I, Nakamura Y, Sato M. (1998) Effects of L-carnitine supplementation on muscular symptoms in hemodialyzed patients. *Am J Kid Dis* 32: 258–264.

Sobh MA, Sheashaa H, Tantawy A, Ghoneim MA. (1998) study of effect of optimization of dialysis and protein intake on neuromuscular function in patients under maintenance hemodialysis treatment. *Am J Nephrol* 18: 399–403.

Sorimachi H, Ishiura S, Suzuki K. (1997) Structure and

physiological function of calpains. *Biochem J* 328: 721–732.

Swendseid ME, Kopple JD. (1973) Nitrogen balance, plasma amino acid levels and amino acid requirements. *Trans NY Acad Sci* 35: 471.

Temparis S, Asensi M, Taillandier D, et al. (1994) Increased ATP-ubiquitin-dependent proteolysis in skeletal muscles of tumor-bearing rats. *Cancer Res* 54: 5568–5573.

Thompson CH, Irish AB, Kemp GJ, Taylor DJ, Radda GK. (1997) The effect of propionyl L-carnitine on skeletal muscle. *Clin Nephrol* 47: 372–378.

Thompson CH, Kemp GJ, Barnes PR, Rajagopalan B, Styles P, Taylor DJ. (1994) Uraemic muscle metabolism at rest and during exercise. *Nephrol Dialysis Transplantation* 9: 1600–1605.

Thompson RT, Muirhead N, Marsh GD, Gravelle D, Potwarka JJ, Driedger AA. (1996) Effect of anaemia correction on skeletal muscle metabolism. *Nephron* 73: 436–441.

Tischler ME, Desautels M, Goldberg AL. (1982) Does leucine, leucyl-tRNA, or some metabolite of leucine regulate protein synthesis and degradation in skeletal and cardiac muscle? *J Biol Chem* 257: 1613–1621.

Tom K, Young VR, Chapman T, Masud T, Akpele L, Maroni BJ. (1995) Long-term adaptive responses to dietary protein restriction in chronic renal failure. *Am J Physiol* 268: E668–E677.

Van der Niepen P, Allein S, Verbeelen D. (1998) Muscle metabolism in uremia and the effect of amino acid supplementation. *Nephron* 79: 387–398.

Voisin L, Breuille D, Combaret L, et al. (1996) Muscle wasting in a rat model of long-lasting sepsis results from the activation of lysosomal, Ca^{2+}-activated, and ubiquitin-proteasome proteolytic pathways. *J Clin Invest* 97: 1–8.

Von Roenn JH, Armstrong D, Kotler DP, et al. (1994) Megestrol acetate in patients with AIDS-related cachexia. *Ann Inter Med* 121: 393–399.

Wanner C, Horl WH. (1988) Carnitine abnormalities in patients with renal insufficiency. *Nephron* 50: 89–102.

Williams B, Hattersley J, Layward E, Walls J. (1991) Metabolic acidosis and skeletal muscle adaptation to low protein diets in chronic uremia. *Kidney Int* 40: 779–786.

Wing SS, Goldberg AL. (1993) Glucocorticoids activate the ATP-ubiquitin-dependent proteolytic system in skeletal muscle during fasting. *Am J Physiol* 264: E668–E676.

Zamir O, Hasselgren PO, von Allmen D, Fischer JE. (1991) The effect of interleukin-1 alpha and the glucocorticoid receptor blocker RU38486 on total and myofibrillar protein breakdown in skeletal muscle. *J Surg Res* 50: 579–583.

12

The effect of non–insulin dependent diabetes on skeletal muscle

Ted Ciaraldi

Morphological/ structural changes

Fibre type composition can be an important determinant of the substrate utilization of human skeletal muscle. Red, slow twitch oxidative (Type I) muscle is the most insulin sensitive (Essen et al 1975, James et al 1985). White, fast twitch muscle fibres are classed as oxidative (Type IIA) and glycolytic (IIB). While studied in only a few muscle types, fibre type composition is fairly uniform in non-diabetic individuals, with Type I representing the major class at 44–58% and Type IIB the least abundant (Table 12.1). Fibre type composition is altered in muscle from Type 2 diabetic individuals. The major difference is an increase in Type IIB fibres (Table 12.1), which could contribute to a lower capacity to utilize glucose in response to insulin. This behaviour is observed in both the rectus abdominus (Hickey et al 1995) and vastus lateralis (Marin et al 1994, Nyholm et al 1997) but not the gastrocnemous muscles (Hickey et al 1995). The impact of fibre type on metabolism is also seen in a correlation between the percentage of Type IIB fibres and insulin resistance that holds for diabetic and non-diabetic individuals (Hickey et al 1995). First degree relatives of Type 2 diabetic subjects, who are insulin resistant, also display an elevated content of Type IIB fibres (Nyholm et al 1997), suggesting fibre type may be an intrinsic or genetic property of diabetic muscle. Like many matters concerning Type 2 diabetes, variations in muscle fibre type composition are not found by all investigators (Kelley and Simoneau 1994), testimony to the considerable heterogeneity of the disease.

Another factor that can influence muscle metabolism is the capillary density. There are reports of the presence of lower than normal capillary densities in a number of insulin resistant states, including Type 2 diabetes (Marin et al 1994) and insulin-resistant, non-diabetic Pima Indians (Lillioja et al 1987). Capillary density was found to be inversely related to muscle insulin action (Marin et al 1994). Low capillary density would appear to be an acquired defect, for the first degree relative of Type 2 diabetic subjects mentioned above displayed normal skeletal muscle capillary density (Nyholm et al 1997).

Vascular reactivity

Beyond capillary density, a major determinant of substrate utilization in skeletal muscle is blood flow (ter Maaten et al 1998, Baron et al 1994). Insulin has been shown to increase blood flow by dilating the skeletal muscle vasculature (Anderson et al 1991, Baron and Brechtel 1993, Vollenweider et al 1995). Such a response would increase the tissue delivery of both glucose and insulin. A vasodilatory response to insulin that occurs at physiological hormone levels and with a time frame similar to insulin's effects on glucose disposal has been reported (Laasko et al 1990a, 1990b, Baron 1996, ter Maaten et al 1998); however, this behaviour has not been observed by all investigators (Utriainen et al 1995, 1997, Dela et al 1995). Besides

Table 12.1— Effect of diabetes and obesity on muscle fibre type composition

Muscle	Subjects	Fibre type proportion (%) Type			Reference
		I	IIa	IIb	
vastus lateralis	ND[a]	51	34	9	(Marin et al 1994)
	T2[b]	42	29	28★	(Marin et al 1994)
	ND	44	34	21	(Ohtani et al 1996)
	1° relatives of T2	41	29	29★	(Ohtani et al 1996)
	obese ND	58	30	12	(Niskanen et al 1996)
	obese ND (insulin resistant)	39	30	30	(Kriketos et al 1996)
rectus abdominus	lean ND	50	38	12	(Hickey et al 1995)
	obese ND	40	45	15	(Hickey et al 1995)
	obese T2	32	49	19★	(Hickey et al 1995)

[a]ND, non-diabetic
[b]T2, Type 2 diabetic
★significantly different from non-diabetic group in same study

this vasodilatory effect, insulin can also influence blood flow by opposing the vasopressive response to noradrenaline (norepinephrine) (Baron et al 1994, Vollenweider et al 1995, Tack et al 1996). Both of these means by which insulin regulates skeletal muscle blood flow are impaired in insulin-resistant states, including Type 2 diabetes (Laasko et al 1990b, Baron et al 1994, Vollenweider et al 1995, Tack et al 1996). Insulin-mediated vasodilatation is reduced in obese diabetic subjects to a greater extent than in weight-matched obese individuals (Laasko et al 1990a, 1990b), indicating a further impact of the diabetic state. There is a strong correlation between markers of insulin resistance and the impairment of vasodilatation (Baron 1994, ter Maaten et al 1998).

Alterations in glucose metabolism

Glucose disposal in muscle

In the fasting (basal) state, the majority of glucose disposal occurs in non-insulin-sensitive tissues, the most important being brain, accounting for ~50% of total disposal (Baron et al 1985, Eastman et al 1990). Skeletal muscle is responsible for 15–20% of the glu-

cose utilization, as lipid is the preferred fuel under these conditions (Saloranta and Groop 1996). Glucose uptake and utilization in the brain and other non-insulin-sensitive tissues is not altered in diabetes (Baron et al 1985, Eastman et al 1990, Kumagai 1999). Although glucose utilization in the heart is insulin responsive, this response is also not altered in diabetes (Utriainen et al 1998). Given the modest contribution of skeletal muscle to basal glucose utilization, the reduction in fasting glucose disposal that occurs in diabetic muscle (Alzaid et al 1994, Taniguchi et al 1994, Nielson et al 1998) has little impact on whole body glucose disposal. Following a meal skeletal muscle becomes more important, and it is responsible for disposal of 50–60% of the glucose load (DeFronzo 1992) and essentially all of the impairment in whole body glucose utilization (Baron et al 1988, Sugden et al 1993, Nielson et al 1998).

Specific pathways of glucose utilization

The multiple pathways by which glucose is metabolized in muscle are outline in Figure 12.1. The major fates are storage in glycogen, non-oxidative disposal, and glycolysis to pyruvate and generation of lactate, or complete oxidation. A small portion of glucose is utilized through the hexosamine pathway, to generate

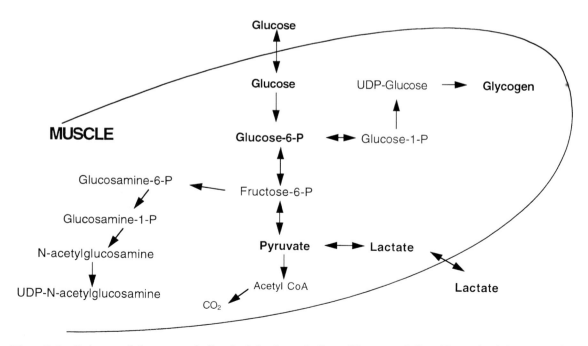

Figure 12.1 — **Pathways of glucose metabolism in skeletal muscle**. Reversible steps are indicated by two headed arrows. Multiple arrows between fructose-6-P and pyruvate are omitted for space reasons. (UDP, uridine diphosphate; CoA, coenzyme A; P, phosphate.)

UDP-*N*-acetyl-glucosamine. In the fasting state there is essentially no glycogen production, with ~60% of glucose proceeding to lacatate, ~40% oxidized through the tricarboxylic acid (TCA) cycle, and 2–3% directed through the hexosamine pathway (Andres et al 1956, DeFronzo 1988). After a glucose load, insulin stimulates both oxidative and non-oxidative metabolism with glycogen synthesis accounting for 90% of non-oxidative utilization (Shulman et al 1990, Sugden et al 1993).

Besides decreases in total glucose utilization, this balance between oxidative and non-oxidative disposal is perturbed in diabetic muscle. The evidence is overwhelming that glucose entry into the cell is impaired in Type 2 diabetes (Bonadonna et al 1993, Rothman et al 1995), which would reduce flux through all pathways. When glucose entry is adjusted to match normal rates, such as by the mass action effect of increasing glucose levels, glycogen synthesis remains impaired (Thonburn et al 1990). It is a common finding that non-oxidative disposal and glycogen synthesis are defective in diabetes, in both the absence and presence of insulin (Butler et al 1990, Rothman et al 1995). Flux through the hexosamine synthetic pathway might be augmented, both because of the mass action effect of hyperglycaemia and because the rate limiting enzyme for entry of glucose into the hexosamine pathway (glutamine:fructose-6-phosphate amidotransferase) is elevated in diabetic muscle (Daniels et al 1996, Yki-Jarvinen et al 1996). This later change may be important because increased flux through the hexosamine biosynthetic pathway has been associated with the development of insulin resistance (reviewed in McClain and Crook 1996). What is less certain is the impact of diabetes on glucose oxidation. There is evidence that oxidative glucose disposal in diabetic muscle is reduced to the same extent as non-oxidative disposal (Kelley et al 1993). Others have found little or no change in glucose oxidation in diabetes (Butler et al 1990). There is also a report that the activities of glycolytic enzymes are elevated in diabetic muscle (Simoneau and Kelley 1997), which would divert glucose from complete oxidation. Confounding the understanding of diabetes-induced changes in glucose oxidation is the influence of elevated lipid levels and increased lipid oxidation on glucose oxidation (see below).

Regulation of specific steps in glucose metabolism

Key proteins involved in glucose metabolism are outlined in Figure 12.2. The next section will attempt to detail the impact of Type 2 diabetes on specific processes in glucose metabolism and the proteins or enzymes mediating those processes.

Glucose transport/glucose transporters

The initial, and generally rate-limiting, step in muscle glucose utilization is glucose entry into the muscle cell (Ziel et al 1988). Whether glucose uptake under fasting conditions, in the absence of insulin stimulation, is altered in diabetes is difficult to ascertain in vivo, as net uptake reflects the mass action effect of elevated glucose levels. Glucose effectiveness (S_G) determined from the frequently sampled intravenous glucose tolerance test can account for this difference (Taniguchi et al 1994) and provide a comparative measure of basal glucose uptake. S_G was found to be impaired in diabetic subjects (Taniguchi et al 1994). Basal glucose uptake measured in isolated muscle strips, where glucose and insulin levels can be tightly controlled, was reported to be essentially normal (Dohm et al 1988), or only slightly lower (Andréasson et al 1991), in diabetic compared with normal muscle. On the other hand, basal glucose uptake in muscle cells cultured from Type 2 diabetic subjects was ~50% of the activity measured in non-diabetic muscle cells (Ciaraldi et al 1995).

Whole body studies using stable isotopes (Rothman et al 1995) and the triple isotope forearm balance technique (Bonadonna et al 1993, Saccomani et al 1996) have established that insulin-stimulated glucose uptake is impaired in diabetic skeletal muscle. The insulin-induced increment in uptake in diabetic muscle is 0–50% of that in normal muscle (Bonadonna et al 1993, Rothman et al 1995). Both the final capacity and the affinity of the transport system for glucose are reduced (Baron et al 1991). Diabetes-related defects in insulin-stimulated glucose transport are also observed in isolated muscle strips (Dohm et al 1988, Andréasson et al 1991) and cultured muscle cells (Ciaraldi et al 1995). Therefore, insulin resistance for glucose transport is a defining characteristic intrinsic to Type 2 diabetic muscle, and it is not solely the result of the in vivo metabolic environment.

Glucose transport is a function of the number, activity and intracellular localization of glucose transport proteins. In skeletal muscle, three members of the family of facilitated glucose transporters, GLUT1, GLUT3 and GLUT4, mediate entry into the tissue (Mueckler 1994). Numerous investigators have shown that the total content of GLUT4 protein is normal in skeletal muscle of Type 2 diabetic subjects (Handberg et al 1990, Eriksson et al 1992, Garvey et al 1992).

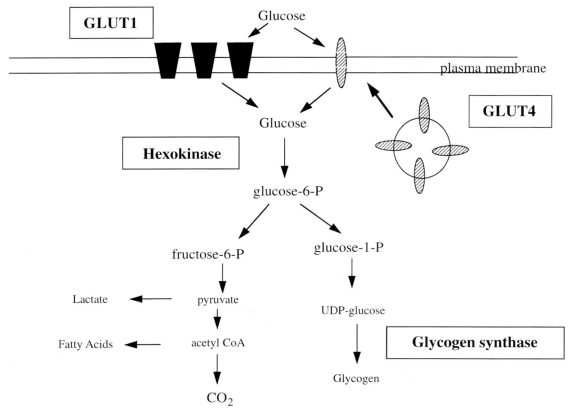

Figure 12.2 — **Sites of regulation of glucose metabolism in skeletal muscle**. Key proteins are indicated by bold text in boxes. (GLUT1, GLUT4, glucose transporters; P, phosphate; CoA, coenzyme A; UDP, uridine diphosphate.)

This is in contrast to the situation in adipose tissue, where GLUT4 content is reduced in diabetics (Garvey et al 1991, Sinha et al 1991). While GLUT1 routinely resides on the cell surface, in the basal state GLUT4 is sequestered in specific intracellular vesicles (Rea and James 1997). Upon insulin stimulation, GLUT4 proteins move to the cell surface (translocation) where they are inserted in the plasma membrane and can then transport additional glucose into the cell (reviewed in St-Denis and Cushman 1998). Subfractionation of muscle into plasma membrane and intracellular components has provided evidence that the magnitude of insulin-induced GLUT4 translocation in skeletal muscle is reduced, or totally absent, in diabetic subjects (Lund et al 1993, Zierath et al 1996, Garvey et al 1998). Thus, while diabetic muscle retains a normal compliment of GLUT4 proteins, a smaller portion moves to the cell surface in response to insulin.

Glucose phosphorylation/hexokinase

In skeletal muscle phosphorylation of glucose after transport into the cell is performed by hexokinase (HK) (Cardenas et al 1998). Muscle contains two isozymes of hexokinase: HKI and HKII (Cardenas et al 1998). In human these are present in near equal amounts (Vestergaard et al 1995). Insulin effects on hexokinase involve a rapid redistribution of HKII from the cytosol to association with the mitochondria (Vogt et al 1998) and a later (4–6 h) increase in HKII expression and activity (Mandarino et al 1995). Both events would result in augmented hexokinase activity.

There are several reports that total HKII expression and activity are reduced in diabetic muscle (Vestergaard et al 1995, Kruszynska et al 1998, Vogt et al 1998), as is the response to chronic insulin. As hexokinase activity is usually highest in Type I fibres (Essen et al 1975), the lower expression might partially reflect the greater proportion of Type II fibres seen in diabetes (Marin et al 1994, Hickey et al 1995, Nyholm et al 1997). Whatever the mechanism, the end result would be that both glucose transport and phosphorylation would be impaired in diabetic muscle. However, it should be noted that there are also reports of normal hexokinase expression and insulin responsiveness in diabetic muscle (Kelley et al 1996).

Glycogen synthase/related kinases and phosphatases

The majority of insulin-stimulated glucose disposal in skeletal muscle occurs via non-oxidative pathways (Sugden et al 1993), primarily storage into glycogen (Shulman et al 1995). This non-oxidative disposal is impaired in diabetic muscle (Shulman et al 1990, Butler et al 1990). More specifically, glucose incorporation into muscle glycogen (in vivo glycogen synthesis) is reduced in Type 2 diabetes subjects (Butler et al 1990, Shulman et al 1990, Rothman et al 1995). Therefore, it is clear that glycogen synthesis represents a major defect in diabetes.

The final, rate-determining step in glycogen synthesis is mediated by glycogen synthase (GS). Regulation of the enzyme occurs at the levels of allosteric control, covalent modification and expression (Lawrence and Roach 1997). The sequence of the GS gene has been found to be normal in several insulin-resistant populations (Bjorbaek et al 1994, Majer et al 1996, Hansen et al 1997). Regulation of GS expression does not appear to be a major mechanism in diabetes as both elevations (Lofman et al 1995) and reductions (Majer et al 1996) have been observed in diabetic muscle, while mRNA levels are either normal (Lofman et al 1995) or decreased (Vestergaard et al 1991). Rather than expression, it is the activity of GS that is the point of control. Insulin acutely activates GS via a dephosphorylation mechanism to increase the affinity for allosteric regulators and substrate (Lawrence and Roach 1997). Insulin stimulation/activation of GS is routinely lower in diabetic muscle (Bak et al 1992, Barriocanal et al 1995). This impaired insulin responsiveness of GS is also observed in cultured fibroblasts (Wells et al 1993) and muscle cells (Henry et al 1996) from diabetic subjects, as well as in non-insulin resistant first-degree relatives of diabetic subjects (Vaag et al 1992), indicating that insulin resistance for GS is a genetic property of Type 2 diabetes.

Insulin can activate GS through two primary mechanisms: activation of protein phosphatase 1 (PP1), which dephosphorylates and activates GS (Barriocanal

et al 1995), and inhibition of glycogen synthase kinase 3 (GSK3), which phosphorylates and deactivates GS (Eldar-Finkelman et al 1996). PP1 activity is both reduced in diabetic muscle (Chen et al 1994) and displays a delayed reponse to insulin (Barriocanal et al 1995), yet expression at the mRNA level is normal (Chen et al 1994). PP1 regulation of GS is dependent upon a glycogen targeting subunit, $PP1G_M$, that brings PP1 and glycogen synthase in proximity in glycogen particles. Polymorphisms in the sequence of $PP1G_M$ are more prevalent in a diabetic Japanese population (Maegawa et al 1999), and correlate with whole body glucose oxidation (Hansen et al 1995), as if utilization were shunted away from storage into glycogen. In addition, GSK3 activity and expression are elevated in diabetic skeletal muscle (Nikoulina et al 2000), which would lead to a reduced activation state of glycogen synthase. Thus, it appears that the balance between dephosphorylation/activation and phosphorylation/deactivation of GS is shifted in diabetic muscle toward deactivation, reducing glucose storage into glycogen.

Insulin signalling pathways

The presence of normal levels of key effector proteins, such as GLUT4 and GS, in diabetic muscle, suggests that the insulin resistance of these responses may involve insulin signalling pathways. Key events in insulin signalling (Fig. 12.3) involve binding to the insulin receptor on the cell surface, with activation of the tyrosine kinase activity intrinsic to the receptor, and initiating phosphorylation/dephosphorylation cascades (reviewed in Taha and Klip 1999, Virkamaki et al 1999). A crucial event is phosphorylation of adapter molecules such as insulin receptor substrates (IRSs), permitting association of IRSs with other molecules, including the regulatory subunit of phosphatidylinositol 3-kinase (PI3-K). One target of PI3-K is protein kinase B (PKB), which is activated by PI3-K (Downward 1998). Activated PKB has been shown to be involved in insulin stimulation of glucose transport and glycogen synthase (Shepherd et al 1997).

Insulin receptor protein levels are normal in diabetic muscle (Caro et al 1987, Obermaier-Kusser et al 1989). The insulin receptor (IR) exists in two isoforms, the products of alternative splicing (Sesti et al 1992), in which exon 11 is either present (IR-B) or absent (IR-A). Insulin receptor isoform expression is tissue specific, with IR-A the most abundant in normal muscle. In diabetic muscle the expression of IR-B is greatly increased (Mosthaf et al 1991, Kellerer et al 1993, Norgren et al 1993, 1994), though not all investigators observe this behaviour (Anderson et al 1993,

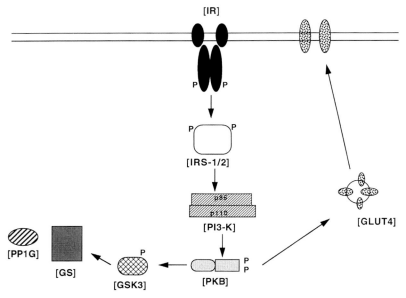

Figure 12.3 — **Selected steps in insulin signalling leading to metabolic responses.** Names of key proteins are indicated in brackets. (P, site of phosphorylation, not all sites are indicated; IR, insulin receptor; IRS, insulin receptor substrate; PI3-K, phosphatidylinositol 3-kinase; PkB, protein kinase B; GS, glycogen synthase; GSK3, glycogen synthase kinase 3; PP1G, protein phosphatase 1 glycogen targeting subunit; GLUT4, glucose transporter.)

Hansen et al 1993). Studies suggest that IR-B may be less efficient in signalling (Kosaki and Webster 1993), which could contribute to impaired insulin action. Both autophosphorylation and the tyrosine kinase activity of the insulin receptor in diabetic muscle are impaired (Maegawa et al 1991, Handberg et al 1993, Kellerer et al 1995).

At the next stage in signalling, numerous variants have been found in the genes for IRS-1 and IRS-2 (Almind et al 1993), but none appear to be associated with the presence of diabetes in the general population (Whitehead et al 1998, Bektas et al 1999, Lei et al 1999), though a link may exist in Japanese diabetics (Ura et al 1996). IRS-1 levels are normal in diabetic muscle (Bjornholm et al 1997), but tyrosine phosphorylation in response to insulin is impaired (Bjornholm et al 1997). Levels of the primary regulatory subunit of PI3-K, p85, are reduced in diabetic muscle (Krook et al 1998). Most importantly, a reduction in insulin stimulation of PI3-K activity is a common finding in diabetic muscle (Krook et al 1998, Kim et al 1999). In some reports the insulin effect is totally lost (Bjornholm et al 1997). In spite of this defect, stimulation of PKB activity is normal at physiological insulin levels (Krook et al 1998, Kim et al 1999), inferring that other targets downstream of PI3-K may contribute to insulin resistance.

Alterations in lipid metabolism

There are two concerns about the regulation of lipid metabolism in diabetic muscle. The first is the role of the balance between glucose and lipid oxidation, where, through substrate competition and accumulation of intracellular intermediates, high levels of lipid oxidation reduce glucose oxidation—the Randle cycle. Lipid oxidation is inversely related to glucose oxidation (Felber et al 1987). Lipid oxidation is elevated in Type 2 diabetics, while glucose oxidation is lower than normal (Vaag et al 1995, 1996). Elevating free fatty acid (FFA) levels reduces both oxidative and non-oxidative glucose disposal (Kelley et al 1993). Conversely, lowering FFA levels in diabetics improves muscle glucose utilization, glucose oxidation and glycolysis, but it has no effect on glycogen synthesis (Piatti et al 1996). Thus substrate availability in muscle can play a large role in determining both absolute fluxes and the balance between glucose and lipid metabolism.

The second concern is the intrinsic capacity of diabetic muscle to utilize lipid, independent of substrate levels. In the most complete study of this question, Kelley and Simoneau (1994) found that lipid extraction and oxidation by muscle in the postabsorptive state were reduced in Type 2 diabetic, while glucose oxidation was increased. Muscle FFA uptake is suppressed in the postprandial state; this response is impaired in diabetics (Kelley and Simoneau 1994). The evidence suggests that both glucose and lipid metabolism, as well as the mechanisms controlling the balance between the two, are perturbed in skeletal muscle in Type 2 diabetes.

References

Almind K, Bjorbaek C, Vestergaard H, Hansen T, Echwald S, Pedersen O. (1993) Aminoacid polymorphisms of insulin receptor substrate-1 in non-insulin-dependent diabetes mellitus. *Lancet* 342: 828–832.

Alzaid AA, Dinneen SF, Turk DJ, Caumo A, Cobelli C, Rizza RA. (1994) Assessment of insulin action and glucose effectiveness in diabetic and nondiabetic humans. *J Clin Invest* 94: 2341–2348.

Anderson CM, Henry RR, Knudson PE, Olefsky JM, Webster NJG. (1993) Relative expression of insulin receptor isoforms does not differ in lean, obese, and non-insulin-dependent diabetes mellitus subjects. *J Clin Endocrinol Metab* 76: 1380–1382.

Anderson EA, Hoffman RP, Balon TW, Sinkey CA, Mark AL. (1991) Hyperinsulinemia produces both sympathetic nerve activation and vasodilation in normal humans. *J Clin Invest* 87: 2246–2252.

Andréasson K, Galuska D, Thörne A, Sonnenfeld T, Wallberg-Henriksson H. (1991) Decreased insulin-stimulated 3-O-methylglucose transport in *in vitro* incubated muscle strips from type 11 diabetic subjects. *Acta Physiol Scand* 142: 255–260.

Andres R, Cader G, Zierler KL. (1956) The quantitatively minor role of carbohydrate in oxidative metabolism by skeletal muscle in intact man in the basal state. Measurements of oxygen and glucose uptake and carbon dioxide and lactate production in the forearm. *J Clin Invest* 35: 671–682.

Bak JF, Moller N, Schmitz O, Saaek A, Pedersen O. (1992) In vivo insulin action and muscle glycogen synthase activity in Type 2 (non-insulin dependent) diabetes mellitus: effect of diet treatment. *Diabetologia* 35: 777–784.

Baron AD. (1994) Hemodynamic actions of insulin. *Am J Physiol* 267: E187–E202.

Baron AD. (1996) Insulin and the vasculature-old actors, new roles. *J Investigative Med* 44: 406–412.

Baron AD, Brechtel G. (1993) Insulin differentially regulates systemic and skeletal muscle vascular resistance. *Am J Physiol* 265: E61–E67.

Baron AD, Brechtel G, Johnson A, Fineberg N, Henry DP, Steinberg HO. (1994) Interactions between insulin and norepinephrine on blood pressure and insulin sensitivity: studies in lean and obese men. *J Clin Invest* 93: 2453–2462.

Baron AD, Brechtel G, Wallace P, Edelman SV. (1988) Rates and tissue sites of non-insulin- and insulin-mediated glucose uptake in humans. *Am J Physiol* 255: E769–E774.

Baron AD, Kolterman OG, Bell J, Mandarino LJ, Olefsky JM. (1985) Rates of noninsulin-mediated glucose uptake are elevated in Type II diabetic subjects. *J Clin Invest* 76: 1782–1788.

Baron AD, Lasko M, Brechtel G, Edelman SV. (1991) Reduced capacity and affinity of skeletal muscle for insulin-mediated glucose uptake in noninsulin-dependent diabetic subjects. *J Clin Invest* 87: 1186–1194.

Baron AD, Steinberg H, Brechtel G, Johnson A. (1994) Skeletal muscle blood flow independently modulates insulin-mediated glucose uptake. *Am J Physiol* 266: E248–E253.

Barriocanal LA, Borthwick AC, Stewart M, et al. (1995) The effect of acute (60 minute) insulin stimulation upon human skeletal muscle glycogen synthase and protein phosphatase-1 in non-insulin-dependent diabetic patients and control subjects. *Diabetes Med* 12: 1110–1112.

Bektas A, Warram JH, White MF, Krolewski AS, Doria A. (1999) Exclusion of insulin receptor substrate 2 (IRS-2) as a major locus for early-onset autosomal dominant type 2 diabetes. *Diabetes* 48: 640–642.

Bjorbaek C, Echwald SM, Hubricht P, et al. (1994) Genetic varients in promoters and coding regions of the muscle glycogen synthase and the insulin responsive GLUT4 genes in NIDDM. *Diabetes* 43: 976–983.

Bjornholm M, Kawano Y, Lehtihet M, Zierath JR. (1997) Insulin receptor substrate-1 phosphorylation and phosphatidylinositol 3-kinase activity in skeletal muscle from NIDDM subjects after in vivo insulin stimulation. *Diabetes* 46: 524–527.

Bonadonna RC, Del Prato S, Saccomani MP, et al. (1993) Transmembrane glucose transport in skeletal muscle of patients with non-insulin-dependent diabetes. *J Clin Invest* 92: 486–494.

Butler PC, Kryshak EJ, Marsh M, Rizza RA. (1990) Effect of insulin on oxidation of intracellularly and extracellularly derived glucose in patients with NIDDM. *Diabetes* 39: 1373–1380.

Cardenas ML, Cornish-Brown A, Ureta T. (1998) Evolution and regulatory role of the hexokinases. *Biochem Biophys Acta* 1401: 242–264.

Caro JF, Sinha MK, Raju SM, et al. (1987) Insulin receptor kinase in human skeletal muscle from obese subjects with and without noninsulin dependent diabetes. *J Clin Invest* 79: 1330–1337.

Chen YH, Hansen L, Chen MX, et al. (1994) Sequence of the human glycogen-associated regulatory subunit of Type I protein phosphatase and analysis of its coding region and mRNA level in muscle from patients with NIDDM. *Diabetes* 43: 1234–1241.

Ciaraldi TP, Abrams L, Nikoulina S, Mudaliar S, Henry RR. (1995) Glucose transport in cultured human skeletal muscle cells. Regulation by insulin and glucose in non-diabetic and non-insulin-dependent diabetes mellitus subjects. *J Clin Invest* 96: 2820–2827.

Daniels MC, Ciaraldi TP, Nikoulina S, Henry RR, MeClain DA. (1996) Glutamine:fructose-6-phosphate amidotransferase activity in cultured human skeletal muscle cells. *J Clin Invest* 97: 1235–1241.

DeFronzo RA. (1988) Lilly Lecture. The triumvirate: β-cell, muscle, liver. A collusion responsible for NIDDM. *Diabetes* 37: 667–687.

DeFronzo RA. (1992) Pathogenesis of type 2 (non-insulin-dependent) diabetes mellitus: a balanced overview. *Diabetologia* 35: 389–397.

Dela F, Larsen JJ, Mikines KJ, Galbo H. (1995) Normal effect of insulin to stimulate leg blood flow in NIDDM. *Diabetes* 44: 221–226.

Dohm GL, Tapscott EB, Pories WJ, et al. (1988) An in vitro human muscle preparation suitable for metabolic studies. *J Clin Invest* 82: 486–494.

Downward J. (1998) Mechanisms and consequences of activation of protein kinase B/Akt. *Curr Op Cell Biol* 42: 262–267.

Eastman RC, Carson RE, Gordon MR, et al. (1990) Brain glucose metabolism in non-insulin dependent diabetes mellitus: a study in Pima Indians using positron emission tomography during hyperinsulinemia with euglycemic clamp. *J Clin Endocrinol Metab* 71: 1602–1610.

Eldar-Finkelman H, Argast GM, Foord O, Fischer EH, Krebs EG. (1996) Expression and characterization of glycogen synthase kinase-3 mutants and their effect on glycogen synthase activity in intact cells. *Proc Natl Acad Sci USA* 93: 10228–10233.

Eriksson J, Franssila-Kallunki A, Ekstrand A. (1989) Early metabolic defects in persons at increased risk for non-insulin-dependent diabetes mellitus. *N Engl J Med* 321: 337–357.

Eriksson J, Koranyi L, Bourey R, et al. (1992) Insulin resistance in Type 2 (non-insulin-dependent) diabetic patients and their relatives is not associated with a defect in the expression of the insulin-responsive glucose transporter (GLUT4) gene in human skeletal muscle. *Diabetologia* 35: 143–147.

Essen B, Jansson E, Henriksson J, Taylor AW, Saltin B. (1975) Metabolic characteristics of fiber types in human skeletal muscle. *Acta Physiol Scand* 95: 153–165.

Felber J-P, Ferrannini E, Golay A, et al. (1987) Role of lipid oxidation in pathogenesis of insulin resistance of obesity and Type II diabetes. *Diabetes* 36: 1341–1350.

Garvey WT, Maianu L, Hancock JA, Golichowski AM, Baron A. (1992) Gene expression of GLUT4 in skeletal muscle from insulin-resistant patients with obesity, IGT, GDM, and NIDDM. *Diabetes* 41: 465–475.

Garvey WT, Maianu L, Huecksteadt TP, Birnbaum MJ, Molina JM, Ciaraldi TP. (1991) Pretranslational suppression of GLUT4 glucose transporters causes insulin resistance in type II diabetes. *J Clin Invest* 87: 1072–1081.

Garvey WT, Maianu L, Zhu J-H, Brechtel-Hook G, Wallace P, Baron AD. (1998) Evidence for defects in the trafficking and translocation of GLUT4 glucose transporters in skeletal muscle as a cause of human insulin resistance. *J Clin Invest* 101: 2377–2386.

Handberg A, Vaag A, Damsbo P, Beck-Nielson H, Vinten J. (1990) Expression of Insulin-regulatable glucose transporters in skeletal muscle from Type 2 (non-insulin-dependent) diabetic patients. *Diabetologia* 33: 625–627.

Handberg A, Vaag A, Vinten J, Beck-Nielsen H. (1993) Decreased tyrosine kinase activity in partially purified insulin receptors from muscle of young non-obese first degree relatives of patients with Type 2 (non-insulin-dependent) diabetes mellitus. *Diabetologia* 36: 668–674.

Hansen L, Arden KC, Rasmussen SB, et al. (1997) Chromosomal mapping and mutational analysis of the coding region of the glycogen synthase kinase-3alpha and β isoforms in patients with NIDDM. *Diabetologia* 40: 940–946.

Hansen L, Hansen T, Vestergard H, et al. (1995) A widespread amino acid polymorphism at codon 905 of the glycogen-associated regulatory subunit of protein phosphatase-1 is associated with insulin resistance and hypersecretion of insulin. *Hum Mol Gen* 4: 1313–1320.

Hansen T, Bjorbaek C, Vestergaard H, Gronskov K, Bak JF, Pedersen O. (1993) Expression of insulin receptor spliced variants and their functional correlates in muscle from patients with non-insulin-dependent diabetes mellitus. *J Clin Endocrinol Metab* 77: 1500–1505.

Henry RR, Ciaraldi TP, Abrams-Carter L, Mudaliar S, Park KS, Nikoulina SE. (1996) Glycogen synthase activity is reduced in cultured skeletal muscle cells of non-insulin-dependent diabetes mellitus subjects. *J Clin Invest* 98: 1231–1236.

Hickey MS, Carey JO, Azevedo JL, et al. (1995) Skeletal muscle fibre composition is related to adiposity and in vitro glucose transport rate in humans. *Am J Physiol* 268: E453–E457.

Hickey MS, Weidner MD, Gavigan KE, Zheng D, Tyndall GL, Houmard JA. (1995) The insulin action-fibre type relationship in humans is muscle group specific. *Am J Physiol* 269: E150–E154.

James DE, Jenkins AB, Kraegen EW. (1985) Heterogeneity of insulin action in individual muscles in vivo: euglycemic clamp studies in rats. *Am J Physiol* 249: E567–E574.

Kellerer M, Coghlan M, Capp E, et al. (1995) Mechanism of insulin receptor kinase inhibition in non-insulin-dependent diabetes mellitus patients. *J Clin Invest* 96: 6–11.

Kellerer M, Sesti G, Seffer E, et al. (1993) Altered pattern of insulin receptor isotypes in skeletal muscle membranes of Type 2 (non-insulin-dependent) diabetic subjects. *Diabetologia* 36: 628–632.

Kelley DE, Mintun MA, Watkins SC, et al. (1996) The effect of non-insulin-dependent diabetes mellitus and obesity on glucose transport and phosphorylation in skeletal muscle. *J Clin Invest* 97: 2705–2713.

Kelley DE, Mokan M, Simoneau J-A, Mandarino LJ. (1993) Interaction between glucose and free fatty acid metabolism in human skeletal muscle. *J Clin Invest* 92: 91–98.

Kelley DE, Simoneau J-A. (1994) Impaired free fatty acid utilization by skeletal muscle in non-insulin-dependent diabetes mellitus. *J Clin Invest* 94: 2349–2356.

Kim Y-B, Nikoulina SE, Ciaraldi TP, Henry RR, Kahn BB. (1999) Normal insulin-dependent activation of Akt/protein kinase B, with diminished activation of phosphoinositide 3-kinase, in muscle in type 2 diabetes. *J Clin Invest* 104: 733–741.

Kosaki A, Webster NJG. (1993) Effect of dexamethasone on the alternative splicing of the insulin receptor mRNA and insulin action in HepG2 hepatoma cells. *J Biol Chem* 268: 21990–21996.

Kriketos AD, Pan DA, Lillioja S, et al. (1996) Interrelationships between muscle morphology, insulin action, and adiposity. *Am J Physiol* 270: R1332–R1339.

Krook A, Roth RA, Jiang XJ, Zierath JR, Wallberg-Henriksson H. (1998) Insulin-stimulated Akt kinase activity is reduced in skeletal muscle from NIDDM subjects. *Diabetes* 47: 1281–1286.

Kruszynska YT, Mulford MI, Baloga J, Yu JG, Olefsky JM. (1998) Regulation of skeletal muscle hexokinase II by insulin in nondiabetic and NIDDM subjects. *Diabetes* 47: 1107–1113.

Kumagai AK. (1999) Glucose transport in brain and retina: implications in the management and complications of diabetes. *Diabetes Metab Res Rev* 15: 261–273.

Laasko M, Edelman SV, Brechtel G, Baron AD. (1990a) Decreased effect of insulin to stimulate muscle blood flow in obese man: a novel mechanism for insulin resistance. *J Clin Invest* 85: 1844–1852.

Laasko M, Edelman SV, Brechtel G, Baron AD. (1990b) Impaired insulin-mediated skeletal muscle blood flow in patients with NIDDM. *Diabetes* 41: 1076–1083.

Lawrence JC, Roach PJ. (1997) New insights into the role and mechanism of glycogen synthase activation by insulin. *Diabetes* 46: 541–547.

Lei H-H, Coresh J, Shuldiner AR, Boerwinkle E, Brancati FL. (1999) Variants of the insulin receptor substrate-1 and fatty acid binding protein 2 genes and the risk of type 2 diabetes, obesity, and hyperinsulinemia in African Americans. *Diabetes* 48: 1868–1872.

Lillioja S, Young A, Cutler CL, et al. (1987) Skeletal muscle capillary density and fiber type are possible determinants of in vivo insulin resistance in man. *J Clin Invest* 80: 415–424.

Lofman M, Yki-Jarvinen H, Parkkonen M, et al. (1995) Increased concentrations of glycogen synthase protein in skeletal muscle of patients with NIDDM. *Am J Physiol* 32: E27–E32.

Lund S, Vestergaard H, Andersen PH, Schmitz O, Gotzsche LBH, Pedersen O. (1993) GLUT-4 content in plasma membrane of muscle from patients with non-insulin-dependent diabetes mellitus. *Am J Physiol* 265: E889–E897.

Maegawa H, Shi K, Hidaka H, et al. (1999) The 3′-untranslated region polymorphism of the gene for skeletal muscle-specific glycogen-targeting subunit of protein phosphatase 1 in the type 2 diabetic Japanese population. *Diabetes* 48: 1469–1472.

Maegawa H, Shigeta Y, Egawa K, Kobayashi M. (1991) Impaired autophosphorylation of insulin receptors from abdominal skeletal muscles in nonobese subjects with NIDDM. *Diabetes* 40: 815–819.

Majer M, Mott DM, Mochizuki H, et al. (1996) Association of the glycogen synthase locus on 19q13 with NIDDM in Pima indians. *Diabetologia* 39: 314–321.

Mandarino LJ, Printz RL, Cusi KA, et al. (1995) Regulation of hexokinase II and glycogen synthase mRNA, protein, and activity in human muscle. *Am J Physiol* 269: E701–E708.

Marin P, Andersson B, Krotkiewski M, Bjorntorp P. (1994) Muscle fiber composition and capillary density in women and men with NIDDM. *Diabetes Care* 17: 382–386.

McClain DA, Crook ED. (1996) Hexosamines and insulin resistance. *Diabetes* 45: 1003–1009.

Mosthaf L, Vogt B, Häring H, Ullrich A. (1991) Altered expression of insulin receptor types A and B in the skeletal muscle of non-insulin-dependent diabetes mellitus patients. *Proc Natl Acad Sci USA* 88: 4728–4730.

Mueckler M. 1994. Facilitative glucose transporters. *Eur J Biochem* 219: 713–725.

Nielsen MF, Basu R, Wise S, Caumo A, Cobelli C, Rizza RA. (1998) Normal glucose-induced suppression of glucose production but impaired stimulation of glucose disposal in type 2 diabetes. *Diabetes* 47: 1735–1747.

Nikoulina SE, Ciaraldi TP, Mudaliar S, Mohideen P, Carter L, Henry RR. (2000) Role of glycogen synthase kinase 3 in skeletal muscle insulin resistance of Type 2 diabetes. *Diabetes* 49: 263–271.

Niskanen L, Uusitupa M, Sarlund H, Siitonen O, Paljarvi L, Laasko M. (1996) The effects of weight loss on insulin sensitivity, skeletal muscle composition and capillary density in obese non-diabetic subjects. *Intl J Obesity Rel Metabolic Disorders* 20: 154–160.

Norgren S, Zierath J, Galuska D, Wallberg-Henriksson H, Luthman H. (1993) Differences in the ratio of RNA encoding two isoforms of the insulin receptor between control and NIDDM patients. *Diabetes* 42: 675–681.

Norgren S, Zierath J, Wedell A, Wallberg-Henriksson H, Luthman H. (1994) Regulation of human insulin receptor RNA splicing in vivo. *Proc Natl Acad Sci USA* 91: 1465–1469.

Nyholm B, Qu Z, Kaal A, et al. (1997) Evidence of an increased number of type IIb muscle fibers in insulin-resistant first-degree relatives of patients with NIDDM. *Diabetes* 46: 1822–1828.

Obermaier-Kusser B, White MF, Pongrantz DE, et al. (1989) A defective intramolecular autoactivation cascade may cause the reduced kinase activity of skeletal muscle insulin receptor from patients with non-insulin-dependent diabetes mellitus. *J Biol Chem* 264: 9497–9504.

Piatti PM, Monti LD, Davis SN, et al. (1996) Effects of an acute decrease in non-esterified fatty acid levels on muscle glucose utilization and forearm indirect calorimetry in lean NIDDM patients. *Diabetologia* 39: 103–113.

Rea S, James DE. (1997) Moving GLUT4. The biogenesis and trafficking of GLUT4 storage vesicles. *Diabetes* 46: 1667–1677.

Rothman DL, Magnusson I, Cline G, et al. (1995) Decreased muscle glucose transport/phosphorylation is an early defect in the pathogenesis of non-insulin-dependent diabetes mellitus. *Proc Natl Acad Sci USA* 92: 983–987.

Saccomani MP, Bonadonna RC, Bier DM, DeFronzo RA, Cobelli C. (1996) A model to measure insulin effects on glucose transport and phosphorylation in muscle: a three tracer study. *Am J Physiol* 270: E170–E185.

Saloranta C, Groop L. (1996) Interactions between glucose and FFA metabolism in man. *Diabetes Metab Rev* 12: 15–36.

Schalin-Jantti C, Harkonen M, Groop LC. (1992) Impaired activation of glycogen synthase in people at increased risk for developing NIDDM. *Diabetes* 41: 598–604.

Sesti G, Marini M, Montemurro A, et al. (1992) Evidence that two naturally occurring human insulin receptor α-subunit variants are immunologically distinct. *Diabetes* 41: 6–11.

Shepherd PR, Nave BT, Rincon J, et al. (1997)

Involvement of phosphoinositide 3-kinase in insulin stimulation of MAP-kinase and phosphorylation of protein kinase-B in human skeletal muscle: implications for glucose metabolism. *Diabetologia* 40: 1172–1177.

Shulman GI, Rothman DL, Jue T, Stein P, DeFronzo RA, Shulman RG. (1990) Quantitation of muscle glycogen synthesis in normal subjects and subjects with non-insulin-dependent diabetes by 13C nuclear magnetic resonance spectroscopy. *N Engl J Med* 322: 223–228.

Shulman RG. (1996) Nuclear magnetic resonance studies of glucose metabolism in non-insulin-dependent diabetes mellitus. *Mol Med* 2: 533 – 540.

Shulman RG, Bloch G, Rothman DL. (1995) In vivo regulation of muscle glycogen synthase and the control of glycogen synthesis. *Proc Natl Acad Sci USA* 92: 8525–8542.

Simoneau JA, Kelley DE. (1997) Altered glycolytic and oxidative capacities of skeletal muscle contribute to insulin resistance in NIDDM. *J Appl Physiol* 83: 166–171.

Sinha MK, Raineri-Maldonado C, Buchanan C, et al. (1991) Adipose tissue glucose transporter in NIDDM: decreased levels of muscle/fat isoform. *Diabetes* 40: 472–477.

St-Denis JF, Cushman SW. (1998) Role of SNARE's in the GLUT4 translocation response to insulin in adipose cells and muscle. *Basic Clin Physiol Pharmacol* 9: 153–165.

Sugden MC, Howard RM, Munday MR, Holness MJ. (1993) Mechanisms involved in the coordinate regulation of strategic enzymes of glucose metabolism. *Adv Enz Reg* 33: 71–95.

Tack CJ, Smits P, Wollemsen JJ, Lenders JW, Thein T, Lutterman JA. (1996) Effects of insulin on vascular tone and sympathetic nervous system in NIDDM. *Diabetes* 45: 15–22.

Taha C, Klip A. (1999) The insulin signaling pathway. *J Membrane Biol* 169: 1–12.

Taniguchi A, Nakai Y, Doi K, et al. (1994) Glucose effectiveness in two subtypes within impaired glucose tolerance. *Diabetes* 43: 1211–1217.

Taniguchi A, Nakai Y, Fukushima M, et al. (1994) Insulin sensitivity, insulin secretion, and glucose effectiveness in subjects with impaired glucose tolerance: a minimal model analysis. *Metabolism* 43: 714–718.

Taniguchi A, Nakai Y, Fukushima M, et al. (1992) Pathogenic factors responsible for glucose intolerance in patients with NIDDM. *Diabetes* 41: 1540–1546.

ter Maaten JC, Voorburg A, de Vries PM, ter Wee PM, Donker AJ, Gans RO. (1998) Relationship between insulin's haemodynamic effects and insulin-mediated glucose uptake. *Eur J Clin Invest* 28: 279–284.

Thornburn AW, Gumbiner B, Bulacan F, Wallace P, Henry RR. (1990) Intracellular glucose oxidation and glycogen synthase activity are reduced in non-insulin dependent

(Type II) diabetes independent of impaired glucose uptake. *J Clin Invest* 85: 522–529.

Ura S, Araki E, Kishikawa H, et al. (1996) Molecular scanning of the insulin receptor substrate-1 (IRS-1) gene in Japanese patients with NIDDM: identification of five novel polymorphisms. *Diabetologia* 39: 600–608.

Utriainen T, Nuutila P, Takala T, et al. (1997) Intact insulin stimulation of skeletal muscle blood flow, its heterogeneity and redistribution, but not of glucose uptake in non-insulin-dependent diabetes mellitus. *J Clin Invest* 100: 777–785.

Utriainen T, Malmstrom R, Makimattila S, Yki-Jarvinen H. (1995) Methodological aspects, dose–response characteristics and causes of interindividual variation in insulin stimulation of limb blood flow in normal subjects. *Diabetologia* 38: 555–564.

Utriainen T, Takala T, Luotolahti M, et al. (1998) Insulin resistance characterizes glucose uptake in skeletal muscle but not in the heart in NIDDM. *Diabetologia* 41: 555–559.

Vaag A, Alford F, Beck-Nielsen H. (1996) Intracellular glucose and fat metabolism in identical twins discordant for non-insulin-dependent diabetes mellitus (NIDDM): acquired versus genetic metabolic defects? *Diabetic Med* 13: 806–815.

Vaag A, Alford F, Henriksen FL, Christopher M, Beck-Nielsen H. (1995) Multiple defects of both hepatic and peripheral intracellular glucose processing contribute to the hyperglycemia of NIDDM. *Diabetologia* 38: 326– 336.

Vaag A, Henriksen JE, Beck-Nielsen H. (1992) Decreased insulin activation of glycogen synthase in skeletal muscles in young nonobese caucasian first-degree relatives of patients with non-insulin-dependent diabetes mellitus. *J Clin Invest* 89: 783–788.

Vestergaard H, Bjorbaek C, Andersen PH, Bak JF, Pedersen O. (1991) Impaired expression of glycogen synthase mRNA in skeletal muscle of NIDDM patients. *Diabetes* 40: 1740–1745.

Vestergaard H, Bjorbaek C, Hansen T, Larsen FS, Granner DK, Pedersen O. (1995) Impaired activity and gene expression of hexokinase II in muscle from non-insulin-dependent diabetes mellitus patients. *J Clin Invest* 96: 2639–2645.

Virkamaki A, Ueki K, Kahn CR. (1999) Protein-protein interaction in insulin signaling and the molecular mechanisms of insulin resistance. *J Clin Invest* 103: 931–943.

Vogt C, Yki-Jarvinen IP, Pipek R, et al. (1998) Effects of insulin on subcellular localization of hexokinase II in human skeletal muscle in vivo. *J Clin Endocrinol Metab* 83: 230–234.

Vollenweider L, Tappy L, Owlya R, Jequier E, Nicod P, Scherrer U. (1995) Insulin-induced sympathetic activation and vasodilation in skeletal muscle. Effects of insulin resistance in lean subjects. *Diabetes* 44: 641–645.

Wells AM, Sutcliffe IC, Johnson AB, Taylor R. (1993) Abnormal activation of glycogen synthesis in fibroblasts from NIDDM subjects. *Diabetes* 42: 583–589.

Whitehead JP, Humphreys P, Krook A, et al. (1998) Molecular scanning of the insulin receptor substrate 1 gene in subjects with severe insulin resistance. *Diabetes* 47: 837–883.

Yki-Jarvinen H, Daniels MC, Virkamaki A, Makimattila S, DeFronzo RA, McClain D. (1996) Increased glutamine: fructose-6-phosphate amidotransferase activity in skeletal muscle of patients with NIDDM. *Diabetes* 45: 302–307.

Ziel FH, Venkatesan N, Davidson MB. (1988) Glucose-transport is rate limiting for skeletal muscle glucose metabolism in normal and STZ-induced diabetic rats. *Diabetes* 37: 885–890.

Zierath JR, He L, Guma A, Wahlstrom EO, Klip A, Wallberg-Henriksson H. (1996) Insulin action on glucose transport and plasma membrane GLUT4 content in skeletal muscle from patients with NIDDM. *Diabetologia* 39: 1180–1189.

13

The effect of magnesium and potassium deficiencies on skeletal muscle

Inge Dørup and Torben Clausen

Introduction

Although often overlooked, magnesium (Mg^{2+}) and potassium (K^+) deficiencies occur frequently in both underdeveloped and developed communities.

In the Third World, nutritional inadequacy of Mg^{2+} and K^+ together with infectious diarrhoea and anorexia contribute to these deficiency states, which are common among malnourished children (Caddell and Goddard 1967, Waterlow 1992, Singla et al 1998).

In the wealthier part of the World, Mg^{2+}- and K^+-deficiencies are not likely to develop as a result of nutritional inadequacy alone but rather in conditions with pathological faecal or renal losses, as seen in patients with chronic diarrhoea, in alcoholics, or in patients treated with diuretics. In spite of increasing focus during the last decade on electrolyte deficiencies, both deficiencies are often overlooked. This is because the commonly used measurements on plasma samples do not give adequate information about the total body content, and measurements of tissue contents are not yet widely available.

Diagnosis of magnesium and potassium deficiency

Extracellular Mg^{2+} and K^+ accounts for less than 2% of the total body content, and neither plasma Mg^{2+} nor plasma K^+ are generally good indicators of the total body content. The plasma levels are usually kept stable within a narrow range by shifts between extra- and intracellular compartments, and by renal control; conditions with definite tissue deficiencies may often be accompanied by normal plasma values. Measurement of the renal excretion of Mg^{2+} following an intravenous test load has been recommended, but this is time-consuming, tedious and requires normal renal handling of Mg^{2+}. It is, therefore, inappropriate in diabetic patients, and in patients ingesting agents influencing the renal excretion of Mg^{2+}, such as alcohol, diuretics or β_2-agonists.

About 75% of the total body pool of K^+ and 25–30% of the total pool of Mg^{2+} is located in skeletal muscle, suggesting that measurements of muscle concentrations could be a useful marker for Mg^{2+}–K^+-status. Indeed, as described below, several studies have demonstrated reduced muscle concentrations of Mg^{2+} and K^+ in patients with deficiencies due to alcoholism or diuretic treatment, as well as the subsequent repletion after Mg^{2+} supplementation (Lim and Jacob 1972a, 1972b, Dyckner et al 1988, Widman et al 1988, Dørup et al 1988a, 1993a, Ravn and Dørup 1997).

Bergström (1962) was the first to describe a method for determining electrolytes in small samples of human muscle. Biopsies weighing 20–50 mg were obtained from the vastus lateralis muscle using a special biopsy needle, dried, extracted for fat, and ashed with nitric acid. We have developed a less time-consuming and simpler method, based on extraction of the electrolytes by homogenization of the wet biopsy in trichloroacetic acid (0.3 M), followed by centrifugation, dilution and direct measurement of Mg^{2+} by atomic absorption and of K^+ and Na^+ by flame photometry (Dørup et al 1988b). A light compressing bandage around the thigh prevents the development of haematoma and minimizes eventual discomfort in relation to the biopsy procedure. The procedure is easily carried out on outpatients, who can continue with their physical activity, work, bicycling etc. immediately after the biopsy procedure.

Main causes of magnesium and potassium deficiency in skeletal muscle

Alcohol abuse

Alcohol ingestion increases the renal Mg^{2+} excretion acutely by 167–260% (McCollister et al 1960, Kalbfleish et al 1963), and a steady alcohol intake leading to a continuous urinary loss of Mg^{2+} may, together with an inadequate nutritional intake, lead to overt Mg^{2+} depletion. In chronic alcoholics skeletal muscle Mg^{2+} is reduced by 16–32% (Jones et al 1969, Lim and Jacob 1972a, Anderson et al 1980), and hypomagnesaemia is frequent (Ellisaf et al 1998), although normal plasma Mg^{2+} does not exclude Mg^{2+} deficiency. Alcoholism may also be accompanied by K^+ deficiency (Jones et al 1969, Lim and Jacob 1972a, Aaggaard et al 1999).

Diuretic treatment and β_2-agonists

Diuretic treatment is a cornerstone in the treatment of congestive heart disease and arterial hypertension, both of which are very common disorders in the industrialized world. In the Copenhagen City Heart Study (1989), comprising around 20 000 men and women above 20 years of age, 9% were treated continuously with diuretics. Both thiazides and loop diuretics produce a significant increase in the renal excretion of Mg^{2+} and K^+ (Dørup 1994). Several studies have documented an average loss of Mg^{2+} and K^+ from skeletal muscles of 14–23% in patients on long-term diuretic therapy for arterial hypertension or congestive heart failure, and the values were below the control range in 41–55% of all patients (Lim and Jacob 1972b, Dyckner and Wester 1987, Dørup et al 1993a). However, in 22% of the patients in our study, muscle Mg^{2+} and K^+ were reduced by more than 25% (Fig. 13.1). In spite of this, only 7% of the patients showed subnormal plasma Mg^{2+} or K^+ (Dørup et al 1993a).

In patients with chronic obstructive lung disease (COLD), who received diuretic treatment, even more pronounced reductions of skeletal muscle Mg^{2+} and K^+ were seen, amounting to an average of 28% and 27%, respectively (Ravn and Dørup 1997). However, COLD patients not treated with diuretics also showed significant reductions in muscle Mg^{2+} and to a lesser degree in muscle K^+ (Ravn and Dørup 1997). This could be caused by treatment with β_2-agonists, which favour the renal loss of Mg^{2+} (Bos et al 1988), or by inadequate intake of Mg^{2+} (Britton et al 1994).

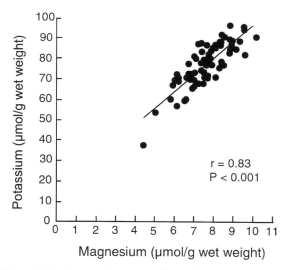

Figure 13.1—Relation between Mg^{2+} and K^+ contents in biopsies of vastus lateralis muscle from 76 patients receiving diuretics. Each point represents mean of measurements performed on 2-4 specimens obtained from each patient. Reproduced, with permission, from Dørup 1994.

Effects of magnesium and potassium deficiencies

Interrelation between magnesium and potassium

The concentrations of Mg^{2+} and K^+ often show close correlation in muscle biopsies; this has been demonstrated in patients treated with diuretics (Fig. 13.1), in COLD patients and in normal subjects (Dyckner and Wester 1978, Johansson 1979, Dørup et al 1993b, Ravn and Dørup 1997). Furthermore, in patients with concurrent Mg^{2+} and K^+ deficiency, such as patients in long-term diuretic treatment, Mg^{2+} supplementation leads to normalization of both muscle Mg^{2+} and K^+ (Dyckner and Wester 1979, Dyckner et al 1988, Dørup et al 1993b).

Primary Mg^{2+} deficiency favours the renal loss of K^+ leading to a general deficiency in Mg^{2+} and K^+ in animals and in human subjects (Shils 1969, Ryan et al 1973). Rats maintained on Mg^{2+}-deficient fodder develop a concomitant net loss of both Mg^{2+} and K^+ (Dørup and Clausen 1993b), and in soleus and extensor digitorum longus muscles from such animals, the concentration of Mg^{2+} and K^+ are closely correlated (Fig. 13.2A). This correlation would appear to reflect a close association between the renal excretion of Mg^{2+} and K^+. However, when isolated rat muscles are incubated in Mg^{2+}-free buffer, a net loss of both Mg^{2+} and K^+ takes place, leading to a similar correlation between Mg^{2+} and K^+ contents. Even more pronounced and equally correlated losses of Mg^{2+} and K^+ are elicited by including the Mg^{2+} and calcium (Ca^{2+}) chelators EDTA and EGTA as well as the Mg^{2+}/Ca^{2+}-ionophore A23187 in the buffer (Fig. 13.2B).

Since Mg^{2+} depletion in vitro was found to produce an acute increase in the rate of K^+ efflux, it is likely, therefore, that the effect of general Mg^{2+} deficiency on muscle K^+ content reflects an effect of Mg^{2+} on K^+ homeostasis in muscle. This view is strongly supported by the observation that the correlation between Mg^{2+} and K^+ contents in skeletal muscle is very similar in muscles from patients treated with diuretics, in muscles from rats receiving Mg^{2+}-deficient fodder or in isolated muscles exposed to Mg^{2+} depletion in vitro (Table 13.1). Moreover, a more comparative review on Mg^{2+} and K^+ deficiency showed that in human skeletal muscle the molar Mg^{2+}/K^+ ratio only varied from 0.082 to 0.109 in 11 different studies (Hosseini and Elin 1991).

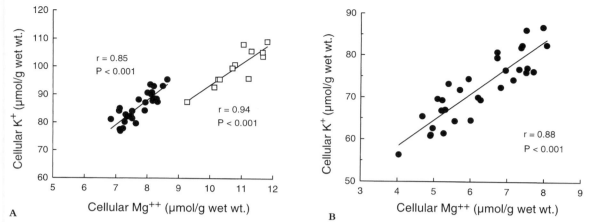

Figure 13.2—Correlations between cellular Mg^{2+} and K$^+$ contents in vivo (A) and in vitro (B). In vivo Mg^{2+}-depletion was achieved by maintaining rats on Mg^{2+}-deficient fodder for 21 days. Each point represents Mg^{2+} and K$^+$ contents in soleus (filled circles, n = 27) or extensor digitorum longus (EDL; open squares, n = 12) from one animal. In vitro Mg^{2+}-depletion (B) was achieved by incubating isolated solcus muscles for 145–300 min in standard Krebs Ringer buffer or in Ca^{2+}-Mg^{2+}-free Krebs-Ringer Buffer with the Mg^{2+} and Ca^{2+} ionophore A23287 or the Mg^{2+} and Ca^{2+}-binding agents EDTA and EGTA. Each point represents Mg^{2+} and K$^+$ contents in one soleus muscle (n = 41). Adapted, with permission, from Dørup and Clausen, 1993b.

Table 13.1 — Comparison of correlations between cellular concentrations of magnesium (Mg^{2+}) and potassium (K$^+$) in human muscle biopsies and in rat muscles Mg^{2+} depleted in vivo or in vitro (Reproduced from Dørup and Clausen 1993b, with permission).

Parameters[a]	Human muscle biopsies[b]	In vivo Mg^{2+}-depleted[c]		In vitro Mg^{2+}-depleted Soleus[d]
		Soleus	EDL	
r	0.83	0.85	0.94	0.95
a	8.16	8.80	7.70	7.98
b (μmol/g wet wt)	15.5	17.5	16.2	22.2
n	76	27	12	41

[a] r, correlation coefficient; a, slope; b, intercept with y-axis. These values are from the regression lines correlating muscle Mg^{2+} and K$^+$ levels for given muscles.
[b] Data from Figure 13.1.
[c] Data from Figure 13.2A.
[d] Data from Figure 13.2B.

It has repeatedly been shown that Mg^{2+} favours inward rectification of several K$^+$ channels—the inward rectifier K$^+$ channel (Matsuda 1991); the ATP-sensitive K$^+$ channel (Horie et al 1987a) and the muscarinic receptor-mediated K$^+$ channel (Horie et al 1987a). Hence, in Mg^{2+}-deficient muscle, loss of inward rectification leads to higher net efflux of K$^+$ from the muscle cells.

Effect on sodium–potassium-homeostasis and sodium–potassium-pumps

Primary K$^+$ deficiency, as well as that elicited by Mg^{2+} deficiency, is associated with an almost equivalent gain of Na$^+$ in skeletal muscle (Nørgaard et al 1981, Dørup and Clausen 1993b). In both Mg^{2+} and K$^+$ deficiency, the concentration of Na$^+$-K$^+$-pumps in skeletal muscle is downregulated in proportion to the loss of K+. K+ deficiency induced by mineralocorticoids was also found to be associated with downregulation of the concentration of Na+–K+-pumps in skeletal muscle (Fig. 13.3; Dørup and Clausen 1997). In diuretic treated patients, Mg2+, K+ deficiency of skeletal muscle was associated with a decrease in the concentration of Na+–K+-pumps, which correlated with the muscle K+ concentration (Dørup et al 1988a). Furthermore, the concentration of Na+–K+-pumps was restored after correcting the electrolyte contents of the muscles (Dørup and Clausen 1993b).

As pointed out in the review by McDonough and Thompson (1996), K+ deficiency in general seems to elicit reduced synthesis and degradation of the α_2-isoform of Na+–K+-ATPase in skeletal muscle.

Effect on muscle function

It is well-known that K+ deficiency is associated with fatigue that can be quite pronounced. Measurement of contractile performance have shown that in K+-deficient dogs tetanic and twitch force of the anterior calf muscles were reduced by 90 and 71 respectively (Hazeyama & Sparks 1979). In rats, K+ deficiency was shown to lead to a marked reduction in physical endurance (Bollaert et al 1993). Little is known, however, about the mechanisms underlying the contractile failure.

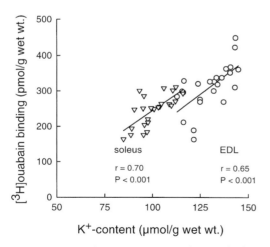

Figure 13.3 — Relationship between muscle K+ and Na+,K+-pump concentration ([3H]ouabain binding sites) in 24 rats infused with vehicle or aldosterone (0.02–0.5 mg/kg body weight per day) for 7 days. Each point represents values obtained from one animal (n=24). Reproduced, with permission, from Dørup and Clausen, 1997.

The downregulation of Na+–K+-pumps in skeletal muscle is associated with reduced capacity for performing active Na+–K+-transport (Clausen et al 1987), interfering with the ability to restore Na+–K+-gradients during and after exercise. This, in turn, is likely to cause impairment of excitability and contractile performance (Clausen et al 1998). Indeed, during continuous electrical stimulation, soleus muscles obtained from K+-deficient rats showed a more than two-fold faster rate of force decline (118%) than muscles from control animals (Fig. 13.4). In these muscles, the concentration of Na+–K+-pumps was reduced by 54%. When a similar reduction (63%) in the Na+–K+-pump capacity was induced by pretreatment with ouabain (10^{-6} M) for 2 h in vitro, the rate of force decline was increased to almost the same extent (Fig. 13.4).

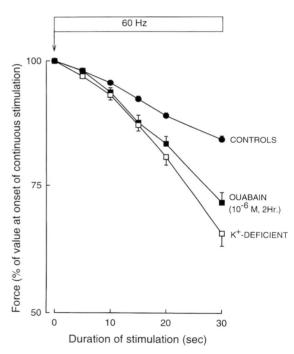

Figure 13.4 — Effect of ouabain and K+-deficiency on the relative changes in contractile endurance of rat soleus muscle during 30 sec of continuous stimulation at 60 Hz. Control muscles obtained from 4-week-old rats were preincubated without ouabain for 1 h before time zero. The effects of reducing the Na+,K+-pump capacity was examined using either: a) muscles preincubated for 2 h with ouabain (10^{-6} M), leading to blockade of 63% the Na+,K+-pumps, or b) muscles prepared from K+-deficient rats, where the concentration of Na+,K+-pumps was reduced by 54%. Symbols indicate mean and SEM of observations on between 8 and 20 muscles. Reproduced, with permission, from Nielsen & Clausen, 1996.

Such experiments performed using varying periods of pretreatment with different concentrations of ouabain showed that the rate of force decline is correlated to the Na^+–K^+-pump capacity over a wide range. This indicates that muscle endurance and physical performance depends on the concentration of Na^+–K^+-pumps in skeletal muscle.

In patients with chronic heart failure a poor correlation between haemodynamics and the degree of symptoms has been demonstrated (Lipkin et al 1986), and it has been proposed that abnormal skeletal muscle composition can account for many symptoms of this condition (Coats et al 1994). The reduced concentration of Na^+–K^+-pumps in skeletal muscle may contribute to the fatigue often experienced by patients with Mg^{2+}–K^+-deficiency induced by diuretics or prolonged intake of alcohol.

Effect on plasma potassium level and cardiac glycoside distribution

Another implication of downregulation of Na^+–K^+-pump concentration in skeletal muscle is impaired capacity to clear K^+ from the plasma and the extracellular water space. Skeletal muscles contain the largest single pool of Na^+–K^+-pumps in the body and, therefore, they play a decisive role in counterbalancing increases in extracellular K^+ elicited by exercise or by the ingestion or infusion of K^+. Thus, in hypothyroid rats, where the concentration of Na^+–K^+-pumps in skeletal muscle is considerably reduced, intravenous infusion of potassium chloride induced more than a two-fold greater increase in plasma K^+ than in euthyroid controls (Kubota and Ingbar 1990).

The reduction in the pool of Na^+–K^+-pumps in skeletal muscle induced by K^+ deficiency leads to a corresponding decrease in the peripheral binding of digitalis glycosides. Therefore, a larger fraction of a given dose of digitalis will be available for distribution in the extracellular space, resulting in a higher plasma concentration. In K^+-deficient rats, where the concentration of Na^+–K^+-pumps in skeletal muscle was reduced by 63%, the injection of ^3H-ouabain produced a 77% greater increase in plasma ^3H-activity than in control animals (Clausen et al 1982) given the same dose of ^3H-ouabain. This relationship explains the well-known clinical experience that in K^+-deficient patients, the sensitivity to digitalis is increased (Surawicz 1985).

Effects on growth and protein synthesis

If an animal receives a diet with insufficient contents of either Mg^{2+} or K^+, but which is otherwise adequate, the response is a marked and rapid inhibition of growth (Dørup et al 1991a, Flyvbjerg et al 1991). This is seen within a few days, and following repletion with the element lacking, growth rate is promptly increased. The ability to fully catch up in weight may, however, be compromised in young animals, and repeated episodes of deficiency may lead to lasting stunting of weight as well as of height (Fig. 13.5) (Dørup et al 1991a, Flyvbjerg et al 1991). In Third World children, repeated episodes of diarrhoea leading to significant losses of Mg^{2+} and K^+ may contribute to the long-term stunting of growth often seen in these children (Dørup 1994).

Dietary Mg^{2+} and K^+ deficiencies are both followed by compromised muscle protein synthesis demonstrated by reduced amino acid incorporation into muscle protein (Dørup and Clausen 1989, Dørup et al 1991a). In isolated muscles, K^+ depleted in vitro, the reduction of ^3H-leucine incorporation into muscle protein correlated with the K^+ concentration of the muscles. In animals, K^+ depleted or Mg^{2+} depleted in vivo by feeding them low-K or low-Mg^{2+} diets, however, the inhibition of protein synthesis occurred almost instantaneously, and became significant before a decrease in tissue K^+ and Mg^{2+} levels could be

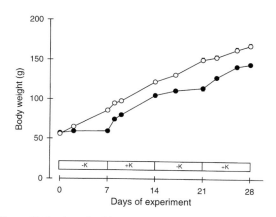

Figure 13.5 — 4-week-old rats were maintained on fodder with normal K^+ content (○) or in periods of 1 week on K^+-deficient fodder (●). Periods on K^+-deficient fodder are reflected in growth retardation, whereas the restoration of normal K^+ contents of the fodder leads to rapidly increasing growth rates. The effect of K^+-deficient fodder is pronounced in the young rats, and repeated periods of K^+ deficiency may lead to permanent stunting. Adapted, with permission, from Dørup 1994.

detected (Dørup and Clausen 1989). Therefore, the inhibition of protein synthesis seems to be a response to a general deficiency rather than to any local deficiency. This response may be mediated by reduced circulating and locally produced insulin-like growth factor-1 (IGF-1) (Dørup et al 1991b, Flyvbjerg et al 1991, Hsu et al 1997). In keeping with this, human malnutrition is characterized by poor growth and reduced serum IGF-1 levels, and it may be accompanied by specific deficiencies of Mg^{2+} and K^+ (Caddel and Goddard 1967, Waterlow 1992, Singla et al 1998). In the past, only little attention has been paid to mineral repletion of severely malnourished children, but it has been acknowledged in the more recent recommendations (Briend and Golden 1993).

Conclusion

Mg^{2+} and K^+ deficiencies are widely encountered in clinical medicine, developing mainly as a result of malnutrition, diarrhoea, alcohol abuse or diuretic treatment. Deficiencies and repletion are easily detected by measurements on skeletal muscle biopsies. Mg^{2+} and K^+ levels are closely correlated in skeletal muscle, and deficiencies lead to downregulation of the concentration of Na^+–K^+-pumps, to interference with muscle endurance and physical performance as well as to increased sensitivity to digitalis. In young individuals Mg^{2+} and K^+ deficiencies lead to inhibition of growth and protein synthesis. Repletion of these deficiencies is simple, and it can be achieved by an oral Mg^{2+}-supplement, provided this is maintained for at least 6 months (Dørup et al 1993).

Acknowledgements

The present study was supported by grants from the Danish Medical Research Council (J. No 12-1336), The Danish Biomembrane Center and Aarhus University Research Foundation.

References

Aagaard NK, Dørup I, Andersen H, Borre M, Clausen T, Vilstrup H, Jakobsen J. (1999) Reduced skeletal muscle concentrations of magnesium, potassium and sodium, potassium pumps in alcoholic liver disease. *J Hepatol* 30(Suppl. 1): 149 (abstract).

Anderson R, Cohen M, Haller R, Elms J, Carter NW, Knochel JP. (1980) Skeletal muscle phosphorus and magnesium deficiency in alcoholic myopathy. *Miner Electrolyte Metab* 4: 106–112.

Bergström J. (1962) Muscle electrolytes in man. *Scan J Clin Lab Invest* 14(Suppl 68): 1–110.

Bollaert PE, Robin-Lherbier B, Mallie JP, Guilland JC, Straczek J, Larcan A. (1993) Effect of chronic potassium depletion on muscle bioenergetics in rats. *J Lab Clin Med* 121: 668–674.

Bos WJW, Postma DS, Doormaal JJ. (1988) Magnesiuric and calciuric effects of terbutaline in man. *Clin Sci* 74: 595–597.

Briend A, Golden MHN. (1993) Treatment of severe child malnutrition in refugee camps. *Eur J Clin Nutr* 47: 750–754.

Britton J, Pavord I, Richards K, Wisniewski A, Knox A, Lewis S, et al. (1994) Dietary magnesium, lung function, wheezing, and airway hyperreactivity in a random adult population sample. *Lancet* 344: 357–362.

Caddell JL, Goddard DR. (1967) Studies in protein–calorie malnutrition. 1. Chemical evidence for magnesium deficiency. *N Engl J Med* 276: 533–535.

Clausen T, Hansen O, Kjeldsen K, Norgaard A. (1982) Effect of age, potassium depletion and denervation on specific displaceable 3H-ouabain binding in rat skeletal muscle in vivo. *J Physiol (London)* 333: 367–381.

Clausen T, Everts ME, Kjeldsen K. (1987) Quantification of the maximum capacity for active sodium-potassium transport in rat skeletal muscle. *J Physiol* 388: 163–181.

Clausen T, Nielsen OB, Harrison AP, Flatman JA, Overgaard K. (1998) The Na^+, K^+ pump and muscle excitability. *Acta Physiol Scand* 162: 183–190.

Coats AJS, Clark AL, Piepoli M, Volterrani M, Poole-Wilson PA. (1994) Symptoms and quality of life in heart failure: the muscle hypothesis. *Br Heart J* 72(Suppl): S36–39.

Dørup I, Skajaa K, Clausen T, Kjeldsen K. (1988a) Reduced concentrations of potassium, magnesium, and sodium-potassium pumps in human skeletal muscle during treatment with diuretics. *Br Med J* 296: 455–458.

Dørup I, Skajaa K, Clausen T. (1988b) A simple and rapid method for the determination of the concentrations of magnesium, sodium, potassium and sodium, potassium pumps in human skeletal muscle. *Clin Sci* 74: 241–248.

Dørup I, Clausen T. (1989) Effects of potassium deficiency on growth and protein synthesis in skeletal muscle and the heart. *Br J Nutr* 62: 269–284.

Dørup I, Clausen T. (1991a) Effects of Mg^{2+}- and Zn deficiency on growth and protein synthesis in skeletal muscle and the heart. *Br J Nutr* 66: 493–504.

Dørup I, Flyvbjerg A, Everts ME, Clausen T. (1991b) Role of insulin-like growth factor-1 and growth hormone in growth inhibition induced by Mg^{2+}- and Zn-deficiency. *Br J Nutr* 66: 505–521.

Dørup I, Skajaa K, Thybo NK. (1993a) Oral magnesium supplementation restores the concentrations of magnesium, potassium and sodium, potassium pumps in skeletal muscle of patients in diuretic treatment. *J Int Med* 233: 117–123.

Dørup I, Clausen T. (1993b) Correlation between magnesium and potassium contents in muscle – role of Na^+-K^+ pump. *Am J Physiol (Cell Physiol)* 264: C457–C463.

Dorup I. (1994) Magnesium and potassium deficiency – its diagnosis, occurrence and treatment in diuretic therapy and its consequences for growth, protein synthesis and growth factors. Doctoral Thesis. *Acta Physiol Scand* 150: 1–55 (Suppl. 618).

Dørup I, Clausen T. (1997) Effects of adrenal steroids on the concentration of Na^+,K^+-pumps in rat skeletal muscle. *J Endocrinol* 152: 49–57.

Dyckner T, Wester PO. (1978) The relation between extra- and intracellular electrolytes in patients with hypokalemia and/or diuretic treatment. *Acta Med Scand* 204: 269–282.

Dyckner T, Wester PO. (1979) Ventricular extrasystoles and intracellular electrolytes before and after potassium and magnesium infusions in patients on diuretic treatment. *Am Heart J* 97: 12–17.

Dyckner T, Wester PO. (1987) Plasma and skeletal muscle electrolytes in patients on longterm diuretic therapy for arterial hypertension and/or congestive heart failure. *Acta Med Scand* 222: 231–236.

Dyckner T, Wester PO, Widman L. (1988) Effects of peroral magnesium on plasma and skeletal muscle electrolytes in patients on long-term diuretic treatment. *Int J Cardiol* 19: 81–87.

Elisaf M, Bairaktari E, Kalaitzidis R, Siamopoulos KC. (1998) Hypomagnesemia in alcoholic patients. *Alcoholism: Clin Exp Res* 22: 134.

Flyvbjerg A, Dørup I, Everts ME, Ørskov H. (1991) Evidence that potassium deficiency induces growth retardation through reduced somatomedin C production. *Metabolism* 40: 769–775.

Hazeyama Y, Sparks HV. (1979) Exercise hyperemia in potassium-depleted dogs. *Am J Physiol* 236: H480–H486.

Horie M, Irisawa H, Noma A. (1987a) Voltage-dependent Mg^{2+} block of adenosine triphosphate-sensitive K^+ channels in guinea-pig ventricular cells. *J Physiol* (London) 387: 251–272.

Horie M, Irisawa H. (1987b) Rectification of muscarinic K^+ current by Mg^{++} ion in guinea pig atrial cells. *Am J Physiol* 253 (Heart Circ Physiol 22): H210–H214.

Hosseini JM, Elin RJ. (1991) Letter. *Scand J Clin Lab Invest* 51: 497–498.

Hsu FW, Tsao T, Rabkin R. (1997) The IGF-1 axis in kidney and skeletal muscle of potassium deficient rats. *Kidney Int* 52: 363–370.

Johansson G. (1979) Magnesium metabolism. *Scand J Urol Nephr Suppl* 51: 1–73.

Jones JE, Shane SR, Jacobs VM, Flink EB. (1969) Magnesium balance studies in chronic alcoholism. *Ann NY Acad Sci* 162: 934–946.

Kalbfleish L, Lindeman RD, Ginn HE, Smith W. (1963) Effects of ethanol administration on urinary excretion of magnesium and other electrolytes in alcoholic and normal subjects. *J Clin Invest* 42: 1471–1475.

Kubota K, Ingbar SH. (1990) Influences of thyroid status and sympathoadrenal system on extrarenal potassium disposal. *Am J Physiol* 258: E428–E435.

Lim P, Jacob E. (1972a) Magnesium status of alcoholic patients. *Metabolism* 21: 1045–1051.

Lim P, Jacob E. (1972b) Magnesium deficiency in patients on long-term diuretic therapy for heart failure. *Br Med J* 3: 620–622.

Lipkin DP, Canepa-Anson R, Stephens MR, Poole-Wilson PA. (1986) Factors determining symptoms in heart failure: Comparison of fast and slow exercise tests. *Br Heart J* 55: 439–445.

Matsuda H. (1991) Magnesium gating of the inwardly rectifying K^+ channel. *Annu Rev Physiol* 53: 289–298.

McCollister RJ, Flink EB, Doe RP. (1960) Magnesium balance studies in chronic alcoholism. *J Lab Clin Med* 55: 98–104.

McDonough AA, Thompson CB. (1996) Role of skeletal muscle sodium pumps in the adaptation to potassium deprivation. *Acta Physiol Scand* 156: 295–304.

Nørgaard A, Kjeldsen K, Clausen T. (1981) Potassium depletion decreases the number of ^{3}H-ouabain binding sites and the active Na^+-K^+ transport in skeletal muscle. *Nature* 293: 739–741.

Ravn HB, Dørup I. (1997) Glucocorticoid treatment upregulates the skeletal muscle concentration of Na^+,K^+-pumps in patients with chronic obstructive lung disease. *J Intern Med* 241: 23–29.

Ryan MP, Whang R, Yamalis W. (1973) Effect of magnesium deficiency on cardiac and skeletal muscle potassium during dietary potassium restriction. *Proc Soc Exp Biol Med* 143: 1045–1047.

Shils ME. (1969) Experimental human magnesium depletion. *Medicine* 48: 61–85.

Singla PN, Chand P, Kumar A, Kachhawaha JS. (1998) Serum magnesium levels in protein-energy malnutrition. *J Trop Ped* 44: 117–119.

Surawicz B. (1985) Factors affecting tolerance to digitalis. *J Am Coll Cardiol* 5: 69A–81A.

The Copenhagen City Heart Group. Østerbroundersogelsen. (1989) Appleyard M (Ed). *Scand J Soc Med* Suppl 41: 1–160.

Waterlow JC. (1992) *Protein-energy malnutrition*. London: Edward Arnold.

Widman L, Dyckner T, Wester PO. (1988) Effects of triamterene on serum and skeletal muscle electrolytes in diuretic treated patients. *Eur J Clin Pharmacol* 33: 577–579.

14

Mitochondrial myopathies

John Vissing

Mitochondrial evolution, metabolism and genetics

Mitochondria are, with a few exceptions, present in all animal cells, usually in numbers of hundreds or thousands per cell. These organelles are unique because they contain a separate genome that is a relic of the mitochondrion's evolutionary past. Many studies have affirmed the eubacterial origin of this genome (Gray et al 1999). Mitochondrial DNA (mtDNA) was discovered in 1963 by Nass and Nass, and the genome was fully sequenced in 1981 (Anderson et al). Soon after sequencing the human mtDNA, the evolutionary antecedents of human mitochondria were traced to a single ancestor in a subgroup of the α-proteobacteria (Yang et al 1985).

Mitochondria generate most of the energy needed for cell survival via the process of oxidative phosphorylation (OXPHOS). In this process, electrons are passed along a series of carrier molecules, called the electron transport chain, which consists of four respiratory enzyme complexes (complexes I–IV). The electrons are generated from reduced nicotinamide adenine dinucleotide (NADH), which is formed during oxidation of fuels, and they are transferred to molecular oxygen. The electron transport chain is embedded in the inner mitochondrial membrane, and is arranged so that the passage of electrons through these complexes releases energy that is stored as a proton gradient across the membrane (Saraste 1999). In turn, this energy is used by the fifth mitochondrial complex, ATP synthase, to produce ATP from ADP and phosphate.

The mitochondrial genome only codes for about 15% of the 83 polypeptides that make up the respiratory chain (Table 14.1). In addition, the small genome codes for the 22 transfer RNAs (tRNA) and 2 ribosomal RNAs (rRNA) needed for mitochondrial translation. All other polypeptides needed for mito-chondrial metabolism are encoded by nuclear genes. Besides the 70 subunits of complexes I–V, this includes two small electron carriers (coenzyme Q10 and cytochrome c), the DNA and RNA polymerases, the mtDNA regulatory factors, the enzymes of Kreb's cycle and the ribosomal proteins. In accordance with the endosymbiotic origin of human mtDNA, the genome is circular. The genome is double-stranded and consists of 16 569 base-pairs (bp). The two strands are designated the heavy (H) and light (L) strands because the H strand contains the bulk of the encoding genes (12 of the 13 polypeptide-encoding genes, 14 of the 22 tRNA and both rRNA genes; Fig. 14.1). The mtDNA is very compact. In contrast to nuclear genes, mtDNA does not contain introns and all coding sequences lack significant untranslated flanking regions. Two stretches of mtDNA, approximately 1000 bp on the H-strand and 30 bp on the L-strand that contain the origin of H and L strand replication and promoters for the transcription of the two strands, are the only non-coding regions of the mtDNA.

Each mitochondrion contains 1–10 copies of the mitochondrial genome. In skeletal muscle, which is rich in mitochondria, this means that each cell usually contains several thousand copies of the genome, a condition called polyplasmy. Normally, all mtDNA in the organism will be identical (homoplasmy). However, mtDNA has a high mutation rate, which can lead to a condition where wild-type and mutated mtDNA coexist in the cell, a condition known as heteroplasmy. The mitochondria are randomly distributed to the daughter cells (replicative segregation), which can give rise to variable mutation loads in the different tissues of the body (mosaicism). A deleterious effect of a mutation depends on the energy requirements of the tissue in question, the degree of heteroplasmy and the nature of the mutation. Each tissue has a threshold for phenotypic expression of a mutation, which for skeletal muscle usually is in the range of 60 to 90% mutant mtDNA before symptoms emerge.

Table 14.1 — Number and genetic origin of polypeptide subunits in the respiratory chain

Enzyme complex		Number of subunits	
		Total	Encoded by mtDNA
I	(NADH–ubiquinone oxidoreductase)	41	7 (ND1–6 and ND4L)
II	(Succinate–ubiquinone oxidoreductase)	4	0
III	(Ubiquinol–cytochrome c oxidoreductase	11	1 (cytochrome b)
IV	(Cytochrome c oxidase)	13	3 (COI–III)
V	(ATP synthase)	14	2 (ATPase 6 and 8)

At these levels of mutant mtDNA, the defective or lacking products resulting from mutant mtDNA can no longer be complemented by coexisting wild-type mtDNA.

Mitochondrial genetics is complex, which complicates genetic counselling. Mitochondrial disease may be sporadic or transmitted by autosomal recessive, autosomal dominant, X-linked recessive or maternal inheritance. In the following, different clinical syndromes that include skeletal muscle symptoms, will be described according to a classification of mitochondrial disorders by the genetic defect.

Mitochondrial myopathies

Mitochondrial disease most frequently results in multisystem disorders. The most affected organs are typically those that have a high oxygen need (i.e. skeletal muscle, heart, nervous tissue). In this context skeletal muscle is unique because in the healthy state mitochondrial OXPHOS can increase more than 50-fold from rest to exercise, a range of oxygen requirement that is unmatched by any tissue in the body. For this reason, exercise intolerance is a clinical hallmark of nearly all mitochondrial diseases. The pronounced symptoms from skeletal muscle have led to the term mitochondrial myopathies, although most of these myopathies also have symptoms from other organs.

Most of the mitochondrial myopathies that we know today are caused by mutations in mtDNA that directly encodes subunits of complexes I–V or the RNA machinery needed to transcribe these subunits. A smaller, but increasingly recognized, number are caused by mutations in nuclear DNA (nDNA) that either encode subunits of the respiratory chain directly or encode proteins that indirectly affect OXPHOS. Other more recently recognized disorders associated with mitochondrial dysfunction are caused by nuclear mutations that encode non-OXPHOS mitochondrial proteins. Most of these disorders (i.e. Friedreich's ataxia, hereditary spastic paraplegia, Wilson's disease, sideroblastic anaemia, Mohr–Tranebjaerg syndrome) do not cause mitochondrial myopathy, and these will not be covered in this chapter, but have been reviewed recently (Leonard and Schapira 2000a, Schapira 2000).

Mitochondrial myopathy caused by mutations of mtDNA

Identical mtDNA mutations can cause very different phenotypes, and different mutations can produce identical phenotypes. A good example of the variable relationship between genotype and phenotype in mitochondrial disease is Leigh syndrome. Leigh syndrome can be phenocopied by defects in non-OXPHOS enzymes and nDNA (Loeffen et al 1998, Tiranti et al 1998, Triepels et al 1999) and by mtDNA encoded defects of complexes I, II, IV and V (Santorelli et al 1993, Bourgeron et al 1995). On the other hand, a mtDNA mutation causing Leigh syndrome may also present as neurogenic weakness, ataxia and retinitis pigmentosa (NARP; Santorelli et al 1993).

Luft et al (1962) were the first to link human disease to dysfunction of mitochondria. But it was not until 1988 when the landmark discoveries of mtDNA mutations leading to disease were made (Holt et al 1988, Wallace et al 1988), that the scene was set for a "gold rush" search for mutations in the small mitochondrial genome. This search, which is far from over, has resulted in the discovery of more than 100 different mutations in the mitochondrial genome (Servidei 2000).

Point mutations of mtDNA

Point mutations of mtDNA have a strict maternal inheritance (Giles et al 1980). Although paternal leakage of small amounts of mtDNA may occur from sperm to the ovum (Gyllensten et al 1991), it appears that an active elimination process of sperm mtDNA occurs as the cells divide (Manfredi et al 1997a). Pathogenic point mutations in mtDNA are characterized by being heteroplastic, by changing highly conserved nucleotides in mtDNA, and by higher levels of mutant versus wild type mtDNA in ragged red or cytochrome oxidase-negative (COX-negative) fibres compared with histological normal looking fibres. The mutations may afffect tRNA genes, and thus translation of all mitochondrial proteins encoded by mtDNA, or genes encoding specific respiratory chain subunits giving rise to specific defects of the enzyme complexes. The clinical spectrum that point mutations of mtDNA cause is remarkable. Even the number of phenotypes that a single specific mutation may cause in different individuals is bewildering. In the following, some common clinical syndromes are described.

Mitochondrial encephalomyopathy, lactic acidosis and stroke-like episodes (MELAS)
This clinical picture is usually associated with the most common mtDNA point mutation at nucleotide position 3243 (A3243G) in the tRNA gene for leucine, but other mtDNA point mutations may give a similar

phenotype (Chinnery et al 1997a, Servidei 2000). As implied by the acronym, the hallmark of this syndrome is stroke-like episodes usually occurring in childhood or early adulthood. The episodes present as hemianopia or hemiparesis, and they do not represent strokes on a thromboembolic or arteriosclerotic vascular basis, but rather local abnormalities of mitochondrial metabolism in brain or brain vessels (Hasegawa et al 1991). Other common symptoms in this syndrome are exercise intolerance, diabetes mellitus, lactic acidosis, headaches, seizures and hearing impairment. More rarely patients have retinitis pigmentosa or sensory neuropathy, or they are demented. There is a considerable overlap of symptoms with an other common clinical syndrome, MERRF (Chinnery et al 1997a).

Myoclonic epilepsy with ragged red fibres (MERRF)

This clinical picture is usually associated with the common mtDNA point mutation at nucleotide position 8344 (A8344G) in the tRNA gene for lysine. The condition is associated with progressive cerebellar ataxia, myoclonic epilepsy, exercise intolerance, muscle weakness and hearing impairment.

Neurogenic weakness, ataxia and retinitis pigmentosa (NARP)

This clinical picture is usually associated with a common mtDNA point mutation at nucleotide position 8993 (T8993G) in the ATPase subunit 6 gene. Onset is usually in adulthood with weakness, ataxia and retinitis pigmentosa as the acronym indicates. If the degree of heteroplasmy is high (>95%), however, patients typically develop symptoms in early childhood with a Leigh syndrome phenotype (maternally inherited Leigh syndrome; MILS). Leigh syndrome is characterized by hypotonia, seizures, pyramidal signs, delayed psychomotor development and focal symmetric lesions in the thalamus, brainstem and posterior column of the spinal cord. Although weakness in NARP usually is attributed to a neurogenic cause, it is evident that generalized myopathy, including progressive external ophthalmoplegia (PEO), also occurs in patients with the T8993G mtDNA mutation (Uziel et al 1997).

Leber hereditary optic neuropathy (LHON)

Three mtDNA point mutations, all in genes encoding complex I subunits, usually cause this syndrome; the G11778A mutation in the ND4 gene (subunit 4 of complex I), the T14484C mutation in the ND6 gene (subunit 6 of complex I), and the G3460A mutation in the ND1 gene (subunit 1 of complex I). The syndrome is characterized by bilateral, sudden loss of central vision due to optic neuropathy. Onset is usually in the second or third decade, and men are affected more frequently (higher penetrance) than women. The syndrome apparently is very organ-specific with exclusive visual symptoms. However, muscle OXPHOS is also impaired as indicated by muscle histology and phosphorous magnetic resonance spectroscopy of working skeletal muscle (Lodi et al 1997), and some may also have cardiac conduction defects or dystonia.

Although most mitochondrial diseases are associated with multisystem manifestations, skeletal muscle is almost invariably involved, and in many cases symptoms are exclusive to skeletal muscle. Both mtDNA mutations in tRNA and respiratory chain subunit genes may cause pure muscle symptoms. Particular attention has been drawn to mutations in the mtDNA-encoded cytochrome b gene, which have been claimed to be associated with a homogenous phenotype of pure muscle symptoms with exercise intolerance, weakness or myoglobinuria (Andreu et al 1999a). However, a severe multisystem involvement in a patient with a novel cytochrome b gene mutation has recently been reported (Wibrand et al 2001), indicating that the spectrum of clinical presentation in cytochrome b gene mutations is broad, as in most other mtDNA mutations. Other mutations associated with pure exercise intolerance or myoglobinuria have been described in the tRNA gene for phenylalanine (Chinnery et al 1997b) and in the respiratory chain subunit genes ND4 (Andreu et al 1999b), COXIII (Keightley et al 1996) and COXI (Karadimas et al 2000).

Large-scale mtDNA rearrangements

Rearrangements of mtDNA are usually sporadic in nature. Exceptions are the maternally-inherited duplication/deletions of mtDNA giving rise to diabetes (Rötig et al 1992, Dunbar et al 1993) and rarely deafness (Ballinger et al 1992) and myopathy (Manfredi et al 1997b). Large-scale single deletions of mtDNA are usually flanked by duplications of variable length. It appears, however, that the duplications play no direct role in pathogenesis (Manfredi et al 1997b). Almost all large-scale deletions are localized between the end of the D-loop region and Origin L (Fig. 14.1). The deletions always affect more than one gene, including tRNA genes, and thus typically result in a translationally incompetent mtDNA, where the remaining intact genes can only be translated if wild-type mtDNA is contained in the same mitochondrion. Experiments in cell cultures indicate that if the mitochondrial content of mutant mtDNA exceeds 60% then translational capability is lost (Hayashi et al 1991).

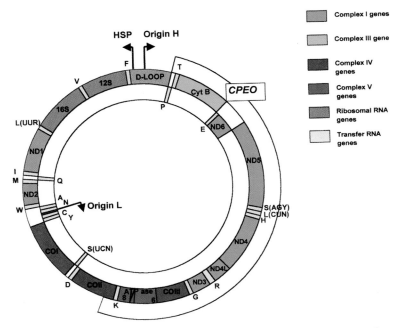

Figure 14.1—The human mitochondrial genome. Encoding-genes on the H and L strands are coloured according to the enzyme complex they contribute to. Transfer RNA (tRNA) genes are light blue and each have a letter according to the amino acid they transfer. The semi-circle designated CPEO, is the region of mtDNA where deletions occur.

Large-scale single deletions give rise to three main clinical pictures:

1. Chronic progressive external ophthalmoplegia (CPEO) is the most common presentation, and indeed one of the most common mitochondrial disorders. This condition is characterized by exercise intolerance and, as the name implies, external ophthalmoplegia with pronounced ptosis that often requires surgical treatment. Additionally, the condition may be associated with mild cognitive impairment and proximal limb weakness. Life-expectancy is only mildly affected.

2. Kearns–Sayre syndrome (KSS) is a multiorgan disorder that is much less common that CPEO. The condition is defined by an onset before age 20, pigmentary retinopathy and PEO. Typically, the patients also develop dementia, ataxia, cardiac conduction disturbances and have elevated cerebrospinal fluid (CSF) protein levels. The condition is very progressive with death usually occurring before the age of 30.

3. Pearson's syndrome (PS) is a very rare condition of infancy. In contrast to KSS and CPEO, skeletal muscle involvement is less prominent in PS. The primary symptoms of PS are sideroblastic anaemia and exocrine pancreas dysfunction. Usually, the bone marrow dysfunction leading to pancytopenia is lethal, but interestingly, the few children that survive go on to develop a picture of KSS (Rötig et al 1990).

Rearranged mtDNA is normally present in oocytes of healthy individuals (Chen et al 1995). The reason why similar deletions can result in these three clinically different syndromes is probably related to a skewed segregation of rearranged mtDNA molecules in the different germ layers of the early embryo. In CPEO patients, deleted mtDNA preferentially or exclusively segregates to the myogenic lineage, whereas in PS and KSS more germ layers are involved, with particular involvement of the haemopoietic lineage in PS. For the same reason, deleted mtDNA usually can not be detected in blood of CPEO patients, but always in skeletal muscle.

Nuclear encoded mitochondrial myopathies

Considering that most mitochondrial proteins are encoded by nDNA, it should be expected that most mitochondrial disorders were caused by defects in nDNA and not mtDNA. The fact is, however, that mtDNA mutations today account for a much higher number of known cases of mitochondrial disease than nDNA mutations do. Reason for this may be as follows.

- The mtDNA is small, easily sequenced and all genes code for proteins related to mitochondrial metabolism. In contrast, nuclear mitochondrial genes, although far outnumbering mtDNA genes, only make up a tiny fraction of all nuclear genes, which makes mitochondrial nDNA mutations hard to locate.
- The mtDNA has a higher propensity to mutate than nDNA because of poor mtDNA repair system (protective proteins like histones are lacking), and production of mutagenic oxygen radicals near the inner mitochondrial membrane may promote mutations.

Still, an increasing number of nuclear defects are associated with mitochondrial defects, and probably we have only seen the top of the iceberg when it come to nDNA mutations causing mitochondrial disease.

Although nDNA mutations cause many of the same clinical features as those caused by mtDNA mutations, nDNA mutations often are associated with more multiorgan manifestations. In many cases, clinical myopathy may be secondary to the severe central nervous system (CNS) disorders. The first reported nDNA mutation, was in a gene encoding a flavoprotein of complex II, which caused a phenotype of Leigh syndrome (Bourgeron et al 1995). Subsequent reports of other nDNA mutations also giving rise to a Leigh syndrome phenotype have followed. These mutations are associated with defects in the COX assembly genes SCO2 (Papadopoulou et al 1999) and SURF-1 (Tiranti et al 1998, Zhu et al 1998), and defects in complex I (Loeffen et al 1998, Van den Heuvel et al 1998, Schuelke et al 1999, Triepels et al 1999).

A number of nuclear mutations give rise to defects in intergenomic signalling and cause mtDNA depletion and multiple mtDNA deletions. The genetic defect has only been defined in one of these conditions, mitochondrial neurogastrointestinal encephalomyopathy (MNGIE). This autosomal recessive condition is associated with multiple deletions and depletion of mtDNA (Hirano et al 1994, Papadimitriou et al 1998, Nishino et al 1999), and a homogenous clinical picture of gastrointestinal manifestations (borborygmi, pain, diarrhoea), peripheral neuropathy, cachexia, and myopathy with ophthalmoplegia and ptosis (Nishino et al 2000). The condition is caused by mutations in the gene on chromosome 22 that codes for thymidine phosphorylase (Nishino et al 1999). The accumulation of thymidine, induced by the metabolic block, is thought to impair mtDNA replication or repair by altering the deoxynucleoside and nucleotide pools (Nishino et al 1999, 2000). Other autosomal dominant and recessive mitochondrial myopathies associated with multiple mtDNA deletions are characterized by PEO and limb weakness. Typically, recessive forms have onset in childhood and are associated with multisystem dysfunction, whereas dominant forms have adult onset and usually pure myopathic features. The dominant myopathic forms have been linked to chromosome 3p14.1–21.2, 4q34–35 and 10q23.3–24.3 (Suomalainen et al 1995, Kaukonen et al 1996, 1999). Primary mitochondrial depletion is a condition of infancy with a presumed autosomal recessive inheritance, associated with multisystem failure and usually death before the age of one year.

Other mitochondrial myopathic conditions caused by still undefined autosomal recessive defects are; primary Q10 deficiency associated with encephalomyopathy, exercise intolerance and recurrent myoglobinuria (Ogasahara et al 1989, Sobreira et al 1997), the Larsson–Linderholm syndrome, where patients have isolated severe exercise intolerance and myoglobinuria (Haller et al 1989, 1991, Haller and Vissing 1999) and defects in iron–sulphur proteins (Hall et al 1993, Drugge et al 1995).

In recent years it has become evident that neurological diseases as different as Wilson's disease, Huntington's chorea, Friedreich's ataxia and the chromosome 16-linked hereditary spastic paraparesis are nuclear genome encoded mitochondrial disorders. Although abnormal skeletal muscle morphology, biochemistry and OXPHOS are clearly present in Huntington's chorea, Friedreich's ataxia and the chromosome 16-linked hereditary spastic paraparesis (Koroshetz et al 1997, Arenas et al 1998, Lodi et al 1999), the myopathic features of these conditions are secondary to the primary neurological deficits caused by CNS symptoms.

Diagnostic evaluation of suspected mitochondrial myopathies

Muscle biopsy

The number of clinical syndromes associated with mitochondrial disorders is bewildering, and, therefore, patients with mitochondrial disease may present themselves to many disciplines of medicine. Patients with exercise intolerance, which is present in more than 95% of mitochondrial diseases caused by mtDNA mutations, should have a needle muscle biopsy examined and a stress test performed before more specific and expensive genetic and biochemical examinations are carried out. A muscle biopsy is important, not only for the histological investigations, but also for subsequent genetic and biochemical analyses. Ragged red fibres (RRFs) are the histological hallmark of mitochondrial myopathies. RRFs can be visualized in the Gomori trichrome and succinate dehydrogenase stain (Fig. 14.2), and they represent accumulation of abnormal mitochondria. RRFs often stain negative for COX, except when caused by mtDNA mutations in complex I, III or V genes. The accumulation of RRFs increases with age, and typically they are less pronounced in muscle biopsies from children with mitochondrial myopathy. A small number of RRFs (<1%) can be observed with aging, and in other disorders unrelated to mitochondrial disorders such as human immunodeficiency virus (HIV) patients treated with antiretroviral reverse-transcriptase inhibitors, muscular dystrophies, ischaemia and polymyositis (Rowland et al 1991). A level of more than 2% RRF muscle is a major indicator of primary mitochondrial disease. The level of RRFs (and COX-negative fibres) in muscle, however, varies greatly between mutation types. Patients with large-scale mitochondrial deletions often have a high number of both, whereas patients with point mutations and mild exercise intolerance generally have fewer RRFs and COX-negative fibres (Collins et al 1995). Patients with the common A3243G mtDNA mutation often have no RRFs. Electron microscopic evidence of mitochondrial myopathy (i.e. mitochondria with altered cristae structure or size and crystal inclusions) can not be considered as convincing evidence for mitochondrial disease, unless there is light-microscopic evidence as well.

Exercise stress tests

Cycle ergometry: The main purpose of a cycle ergometry test is to determine the maximal oxygen uptake (VO_{2max}) and lactate response to an incremental cycle test to exhaustion. It is important to have a sense of the patient's work capacity before the test, so that the increments in workload will result in a total exercise duration of approximately 15 min. Patients with mitochondrial myopathy typically have a maximal work capacity of a quarter to half normal (Vissing

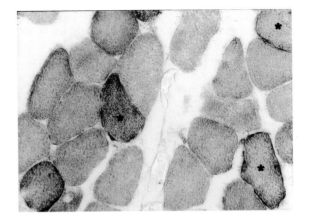

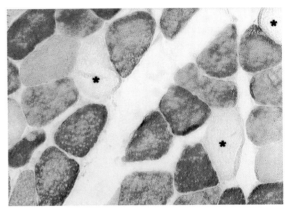

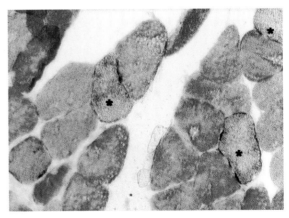

Figure 14.2 — Serial section of skeletal musculature from a patient with a mtDNA deletion from base number 7,177 to 13,767. The heteroplasmy of this deletion was 45% in muscle. Top picture shows ragged red fibres (asterixes) in SDH staining. In the middle picture, muscle is stained for COX, and here the ragged red fibres in the SDH stain are COX-negative. Verification of COX-negativity can be further visualized in the combined COX/SDH-stain shown in the bottom picture, where the COX-negative fibres are counter stained by the SDH and therefore turn blue.

et al 1996, Haller and Vissing 1999). Exaggerated lactic acidosis in exercise is a feature of mitochondrial myopathies (Vissing et al 1996), and, as apparent from Figure 14.3, this may be a distinguishing feature of patients with severe exercise intolerance. However, the overall sensitivity and specificity of the test is low (60–75%; Dandurand et al 1995, Siciliano et al 1996, 1999, Finsterer et al 1998, Dysgaard Jensen et al 2001). Interestingly, the work capacity is correlated closely with the degree of heteroplasmy, but not with the mutation type (Dysgaard Jensen et al 2001). Impaired systemic oxygen extraction during cycle exercise is also a typical feature of mitochondrial muscle OXPHOS defects (Haller et al 1989, 1991, Vissing et al 1996).

Magnetic resonance imaging (MRI) and phosphorous spectroscopy (^{31}P-MRS)

With ^{31}P-MRS, the content of skeletal muscle inorganic phosphate (P_i) and phosphocreatine (PCr) can be monitored at rest and during exercise. Muscle pH can be estimated from the distance between the P_i and PCr peaks (Taylor et al 1983). In mitochondrial myopathy, the normal resting PCR/P_i ratio of about 10, is often decreased to about half (Arnold et al 1984, 1985, Vissing et al 2001). In contrast to findings during cycle exercise, lactate accumulation and

thus exaggerated acidification of working muscle in patients with mitochondrial myopathy is not a common feature (Arnold et al 1984, 1985), although it may occur in patients with high resting plasma lactate levels (Vissing et al 1998a). The essentially normal pH response to exercise in muscle probably is related to an enhanced lactate extrusion capacity of muscle in these conditions (Arnold et al 1985). Mitochondrial myopathy may be associated with an accelerated depletion of PCr in exercise (Taylor et al 1994), and PCr recovery after exercise may be delayed (Arnold et al 1984, 1985) as an indicator of impaired oxidative capacity. Like the cycle test, however, ^{31}P-MRS investigations are not sufficiently sensitivity to exclude a diagnosis of mitochondrial myopathy, and they are associated with great costs, limited accessibility and the demand for skilled personnel.

MRI of skeletal muscle has not been used routinely in mitochondrial myopathies, although patients have occassionally been reported to show dystrophic changes on muscle biopsy (Vissing et al 1998b). It appears that a large number of patients with mitochondrial myopathy, particularly those with CPEO, have marked fat infiltration on skeletal muscle MRI, resembling what is seen in muscular dystrophies (Fleckenstein et al 1992, Olsen et al 2001).

Near infrared spectroscopy (NIRS)

NIRS is still an experimental technique, but it is potentially a promising tool to detect disorders of muscle OXPHOS. With two light-emitting diodes (760 nm and 850 nm to detect deoxyhaemoglobin and oxyhaemoglobin, respectively) placed on the skin over working muscle, the method can detect the changes in oxy- and deoxyhaemoglobin levels in muscle. NIRS can detect impaired deoxygenation in the working muscle of mitochondrial myopathy patients compared with healthy subjects (Bank and Chance 1994, 1997, Abe et al 1997, Van Beekvelt et al 1999), but the NIRS technic can not distinguish between patients with mitochondrial myopathy and McArdle disease (Bank and Chance 1994, 1997), a condition also associated with impaired OXPHOS (Vissing et al 1992).

Forearm exercise test

A forearm exercise test has recently been developed to diagnose mitochondrial myopathies (Dysgaard Jensen et al 2000). In contrast to the classical ischaemic forearm exercise test used to diagnose glycolytic disorders of muscle metabolism, the test for mitochondrial myopathy uses an aerobic exercise protocol. Furthermore, oxygen saturation, and not lactate

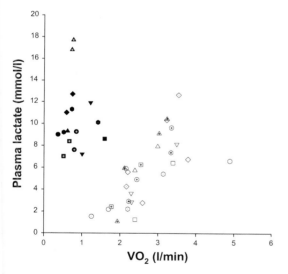

Figure 14.3—Relationship between plasma lactate and oxygen uptake in mitochondrial myopathy patients with severe to moderate exercise intolerance (VO_{2max} between 9 and 26 ml min^{-1} kg^{-1}), and a group of healthy, sedentary, age-matched control subjects (VO_{2max} between 33 and 54 ml min^{-1} kg^{-1}). Patients are shown in black symbols and controls in open symbols. Each symbol represents a person. When two symbols are present for one person, they represent values at submaximal and maximal exercise, respectively.

and ammonia, is measured in venous effluent blood. Impaired oxygen desaturation of venous effluent blood appears to be a simple, specific and sensitive diagnostic tool to recognize mitochondrial myopathies with (Dysgaard Jensen et al 2000).

Other diagnostic procedures for mitochondrial myopathy
Electromyography (EMG) is largely non-informative when trying to establish a diagnosis of mitochondrial myopathy. EMG findings are either normal, show myopathic features or neurogenic changes in the few cases associated with neuropathy. However, none of these findings are specific for mitochondrial myopathy.

Before the era of genetic analysis for pathogenic mtDNA mutations started in 1988, biochemical determination of activities of the five respiratory enzyme complexes was the prime method to establish a molecular diagnosis of disturbed OXPHOS. Today this analysis is particularly useful to guide the direction of genetic investigations. In mutations of mtDNA-encoded subunits of complex I and complexes III–V, enzyme complex activities may conclusively demonstrate which mitochondrial genes should be sequenced for mutations.

Creatine kinase (CK) levels in plasma are generally normal between bouts of physical exertion (Petty et al 1986). However, in all mitochondrial myopathies, CK may be elevated after exercise, particularly in cases associated with mtDNA cytochrome *b* mutations (Andreu et al 1999a, 1999b) and primary coenzyme Q10 deficiency (Sobreira et al 1997). Resting plasma lactate is often elevated in mitochondrial myopathies (Vissing et al 2001). However, elevated plasma lactate may also be seen in β-oxidation defects and in HIV patients treated with antiretroviral drugs. CFS lactate may also be elevated, as well as CSF protein in KSS.

Treatment of mitochondrial myopathies

At present there is no effective treatment of mitochondrial myopathies. An exception appears to be Q10 treatment of the rare primary coenzyme Q10 deficiency (Sobreira et al 1997). Supportive drug therapy is important to control epilepsy or diabetes. Surgical treatment of ptosis is often necessary, particularly in cases of CPEO. In infants, dialysis and bicarbonate treatment may correct severe lactic acidosis. Anecdotal reports have reported beneficial effects of lowering of

lactate by dichloroacetate treatment (Burlina et al 1993, Taivassalo et al 1996, Kimura et al 1997, Saitoh et al 1998), but in adult patients with mitochondrial myopathy, a controlled trial of dichloroacetate did not improve exercise tolerance or muscle OXPHOS (Vissing et al 2001). Creatine treatment of mitochondrial myopathies has no significant clinical effect (Tarnopolsky et al 1997). More than a hundred anecdotal reports have claimed beneficial effects of treatment with a variety of vitamins involved in mitochondrial metabolism, but long-term controlled studies have all been negative (Bresolin et al 1991, Matthews et al 1993). Aerobic training may be a promising therapy for patients with mitochondrial myopathy (Taivassalo et al 1998), but an increase in the heteroplasmy in muscle with training warrants further studies (Taivassalo et al 2000). An interesting observation is that satellite cells in some mitochondrial myopathies preferentially have wild-type mtDNA although the muscle may have a high level of mutated mtDNA. In such patients, muscle regeneration after muscle injury induced by muscle biopsy, injection of myotoxic agents or eccentric exercise has shown absence of mutant mtDNA and restoration of COX activity in the regenerated muscle fibres (Clark et al 1997, Shoubridge et al 1997, Taivassalo et al 1999). Inherent to the complex genetics of mitochondrial diseases, the approach to gene therapy in these conditions must be different from conventional nuclear gene therapy, at least for mtDNA mutations. Selective inhibition of replication of mutated mtDNA after delivery of peptide nucleic acids designed to block mutated mtDNA gives hope for future effective and specific treatment of mitochondrial myopathies (Taylor et al 1997).

References

Abe K, Matsuo Y, Kadekawa J, Inoue S, Yanagihara T. (1997) Measurement of tissue oxygen consumption in patients with mitochondrial myopathy by non-invasive tissue oximetry. *Neurology* 49: 837–841.

Anderson S, Bankier AT, Barrell BG, et al. (1981) Sequence and organization of the human mitochondrial genome. *Science* 290: 447–465.

Andreu AL, Hanna MG, Reichmann H, et al. (1999a) Exercise intolerance due to mutations in the cytochrome b gene of mitochondrial DNA. *N Engl J Med* 341(14): 1037–1044.

Andreu AL, Tanji K, Bruno C, et al. (1999b) Exercise intolerance due to a nonsense mutation in the mtDNA ND4 gene. *Ann Neurol* 45: 820–823.

Arenas J, Campos Y, Ribacoba R, et al. (1998) Complex I defect in muscle from patients with Huntington's disease. *Ann Neurol* 43: 397–400.

Arnold DL, Matthews PM, Radda GK. (1984) Metabolic recovery after exercise and the asessment of mitochondrial function in vivo in human skeletal muscle by means of ^{31}P NMR. *Magn Reson Med* 1: 307–315.

Arnold DL, Taylor DJ, Radda GK. (1985) Investigation of human mitochondrial myopathies by phosphorous magnetic resonance spectroscopy. *Ann Neurol* 18: 189–196.

Ballinger SW, Shoffner JM, Hedaya EV, et al. (1992) Maternally transmitted diabetes and deafness associated with a 10.4 Kb mitochondrial DNA deletion. *Nature Genet* 58: 963–970.

Bank W, Chance B. (1994) An oxidative defect in metabolic myopathies: diagnosis by non-invasive tissue oxymetry. *Ann Neurol* 36: 830–837.

Bank W, Chance B. (1997) Diagnosis of defects in oxidative muscle metabolism by non-invasive tissue oximetry. *Mol Cell Biochem* 174: 7–10.

Bourgeron T, Rustin P, Chretien D, et al. (1995) Mutation of a nuclear succinate dehydrogenase gene results in mitochondrial respiratory chain deficiency. *Nat Genet* 11: 144–149.

Bresolin N, Doriguzzi C, Ponzetto C, et al. (1991) Ubidecarenone in the treatment of mitochondrial myopathies: a multi-center double-blind trial. *J Neurol Sci* 147: 542–548.

Burlina AB, Milanesi O, Biban P, et al. (1993) Beneficial effect of sodium dichloroacetate in muscle cytochrome C oxidase deficiency. *Eur J Pediatr* 152: 537–541.

Chen XY, Prosser R, Simonetti S, Sadlock J, Jagiello G, Schon EA. (1995) Rearranged mitochondrial genomes are present in human oocytes. *Am J Hum Genet* 57: 239–247.

Chinnery PF, Howell N, Lightowlers RN, Turnbull DM. (1997a) Molecular pathology of MELAS and MERRF–The relationship between mutation load and clinical phenotypes. *Brain* 120: 1713–1721.

Chinnery PF, Johnson MA, Taylor RW, Lightowlers RN, Turnbull DM. (1997b) A novel mitochondrial tRNA phenylalanine mutation presenting with acute rhabdomyolysis. *Ann Neurol* 41: 408–410.

Clark KM, Bindoff LA, Lightowlers RN, et al. (1997) Reversal of a mitochondrial DNA defect in human skeletal muscle. *Nature Genet* 16: 222–224.

Collins S, Dennett X, Byrne E. (1995) Contrasting histochemical features of various mitochondrial syndromes. *Acta Neurol Scand* 91: 287–293.

Dandurand RJ, Matthews PM, Arnold AL, Eidelman DH. (1995) Mitochondrial disease: Pulmonary function, exercise performance, and blood lactate levels. *Chest* 108: 182–189.

Drugge U, Holmberg M, Holmgren G, Almay BG, Linderholm H. (1995) Hereditary myopathy with lactic acidosis, succinate dehydrogenase and aconitase deficiency in northern Sweden: a genealogical study. *J Med Genet* 32: 344–347.

Dunbar DR, Moonie PA, Davidson D, Roberts R, Holt IJ. (1993) Maternally transmitted partial direct tandem duplication of mitochondrial DNA associated with diabetes mellitus. *Hum Mol Genet* 2: 1619–1624.

Dysgaard Jensen T, Kazemi P, Skomorowska E, Vissing J. (2000) A diagnostic forearm test for mitochondrial myopathy. *Eur J Neurol* 7 (Suppl. 3): 50.

Dysgaard Jensen T, Olsen DB, Schwartz M, Vissing J. (2001) Correlation between heteroplasmy and physiologic exercise responses in mitochondrial myopathies. *J Neurol Sci* 187(Suppl 1): 114.

Finsterer J, Shorny S, Capek J, et al. (1998) Lactate stress test in the diagnosis of mitochondrial myopathy. *J Neurol Sci* 159(2): 176–180.

Fleckenstein JL, Haller RG, Girson MS, Peshock RM. (1992) Focal muscle lesions in mitochondrial myopathy: MR imaging evaluation. *J Magn Reson Imaging* (supp) 2: 121.

Giles RE, Blanc H, Cann HM, Wallace DC. (1980) Maternal inheritance of human mitochondrial DNA. *Proc Natl Acad Sci USA* 77(11): 6715–6719.

Gray MW, Burger G, Lang BF. (1999) Mitochondrial evolution. *Science* 283: 1476–1481.

Gyllensten U, Wharton D, Josefsson A, Wilson AC. (1991) Paternal inheritance of mitochondrial DNA in mice. *Nature* 352: 255–257.

Hall RE, Henriksson KG, Lewis SF, Haller RG, Kennaway NG. (1993) Mitochondrial myopathy with succinate dehydrogenase and aconitase deficiency: abnormalities of several iron-sulfur proteins. *J Clin Invest* 92: 2660–2666.

Haller RG, Vissing J. (1999) Circulatory regulation in muscle disease. In: Saltin B, Boushel R, Secher N, Mitchel JH (eds). *Exercise and Circulation in Health and Disease*. Champaign, Illinois: Human Kinetics Publishers, pp. 271–282.

Haller RG, Henriksson KG, Jorfeldt L, et al. (1991) Deficiency of skeletal muscle succinate dehydrogenase and aconitase: Pathophysiology of exercise in a novel human muscle oxidative defect. *J Clin Invest* 88: 1197–1206.

Haller RG, Lewis SF, Estabrook RW, DiMauro S, Servidei S, Foster DW. (1989) Exercise intolerance, lactic acidosis, and abnormal cardiopulmonary regulation in exercise associated with adult skeletal muscle cytochrome *c* oxidase deficiency. *J Clin Invest* 84: 155–161.

Hasegawa H, Matsuoka T, Goto Y, Nonaka I. (1991) Strongly succinate dehydrogenase-reactive vessels of muscles from patients with mitochondrial myopathy, encephalopathy, lactic acidosis, and stroke-like episodes. *Ann Neurol* 29: 601–605.

Hayashi JI, Ohta S, Kikuchi A, Takemitsu M, Goto Y-I, Nonaka I. (1991) Introduction of disease-related mitochondrial DNA deletions into HeLa cells lacking mitochondrial DNA results in mitochondrial dysfunction. *Proc Natl Acad Sci USA* 88: 10614–10618.

Hirano M, Silvestri G, Blake DM, et al. (1994) Mitochondrial neurogastrointestinal encephalomyopathy (MNGIE): Clinical, biochemical, and genetic features of an autosomal recessive mitochondrial disorder. *Neurology* 44: 721–727.

Holt IJ, Harding AE, Morgan-Hughes JA. (1988) Deletions of mitochondrial DNA in patients with mitochondrial myopathies. *Nature* 331: 717–719.

Karadimas CL, Greenstein P, Sue CM, et al. (2000) Recurrent myoglobinuria due to a nonsense mutation in the COX I gene of mitochondrial DNA. *Neurology* 55(5): 644–649.

Kaukonen J, Zeviani M, Comi GP, Piscaglia MG, Peltonen L, Suomalainen A. (1999) A third locus predisposing to multiple deletions of mtDNA in autosomal dominant progressive external ophthalmoplegia. *Am J Hum Genet* 65(1): 256–261.

Kaukonen JA, Amati P, Suomalainen A, et al. (1996) An autosomal locus predisposing to multiple deletions of mtDNA on chromosome 3p. *Am J Hum Genet* 58: 763–769.

Keightley JA, Hoffbuhr KC, Burton MD, et al. (1996) A microdeletion in cytochrome c oxidase (COX) subunit III associated with COX deficiency and recurrent myoglobinuria. *Nat Genet* 12: 410–416.

Kimura S, Ohtuki N, Tanaka M, Takeshita S. (1997) Clinical and radiologic improvements in mitochondrial encephalomyelopathy following sodium dichloroacetate therapy. *Brain Dev* 19: 535–540.

Koroshetz WJ, Jenkins BG, Rosen BR, Beal MF. (1997) Energy metabolism defects in Huntington's disease and effects of coenzyme Q_{10}. *Ann Neurol* 41: 160–165.

Leonard JV, Schapira AHV. (2000a) Mitochondrial respiratory chain disorders II: neurodegenerative disorders and nuclear gene defects. *Lancet* 355: 389–394.

Lodi R, Taylor DJ, Tabrizi SJ, et al. (1997) In vivo skeletal muscle mitochondrial function in Leber's hereditary optic neuropathy assessed by ^{31}P magnetic resonance spectroscopy. *Ann Neurol* 42(4): 573–579.

Lodi R, Cooper JM, Bradley JL, et al. (1999) Deficit of in vivo mitochondrial ATP production in patients with Friedreich's ataxia. *Proc Natl Acad Sci USA* 96: 11492–11495.

Loeffen J, Smeitink J, Triepels R, et al. (1998) The first nuclear-encoded complex I mutation in a patient with Leigh syndrome. *Am J Hum Genet* 63: 1598–1608.

Luft R, Ikkos D, Palmieri G, Ernster L, Afzelius B. (1962) A case of severe hypermetabolism of nonthyroid origin with a defect in the maintenance of mitochondrial respiratory control: a correlated clinical, biochemical, and morphological study. *J Clin Invest* 41: 1776–1804.

Manfredi G, Thyagarajan D, Papadopoulou L, Pallotti F, Schon EA. (1997a) The fate of human sperm-derived mtDNA in somatic cells. *Am J Hum Genet* 61: 953–960.

Manfredi G, Vu T, Bonilla E, et al. (1997b) Association of myopathy with large-scale mitochondrial DNA duplications and deletions: which is pathogenic? *Ann Neurol* 42: 180–188.

Matthews PM, Ford B, Dandurand RJ, et al. (1993) Coenzyme Q10 with multiple vitamins is generally ineffective in treatment of mitochondrial disease. *Neurology* 43: 884–890.

Nass S, Nass MMK. (1963) Intramitochondrial fibers with DNA characteristics. *J Cell Biol* 19: 593–629.

Nishino I, Spinazzola A, Papadimitriou A, et al. (2000) Mitochondrial neurogastrointestinal encephalomyopathy: An autosomal recessive disorder due to thymidine phosphorylase mutations. *Ann Neurol* 47: 792–800.

Nishino I, Spinazzola A, Hirano M. (1999) Thymidine phosphorylase gene mutations in MNGIE, a human mitochondrial disorder. *Science* 283: 689–692.

Ogasahara S, Engel AG, Frens D, Mack D. (1989) Muscle coenzyme Q deficiency in familial mitochondrial encephalomyopathy. *Proc Nat Acad Sci USA* 86: 2379–2382.

Olsen DB, Langkilde A, Vissing J. (2001) Muscle fat infiltration is a common finding in patients with mitochondrial myopathy: An MRI study. *J Neurol Sci* 187(Suppl 1): 1113.

Papadimitriou A, Comi GP, Hadjigeorgiou GM, et al. (1998) Partial depletion and multiple deletions of muscle mtDNA in familial MNGIE syndrome. *Neurology* 51: 1086–1092.

Papadopoulou LC, Sue CM, Davidson MM, et al. (1999) Fatal infantile cardioencephalomyopathy with COX deficiency and mutations in SCO2, a COX assembly gene. *Nat Genet* 23: 333–337.

Petty RK, Harding AE, Morgan-Hughes JA. (1986) The clinical features of mitochondrial myopathy. *Brain* 109: 915–938.

Rötig A, Bessis JL, Romero N, et al. (1992) Maternally inherited duplication of the mitochondrial genome in a syndrome of proximal tubulopathy, diabetes mellitus, and cerebellar ataxia. *Am J Hum Genet* 50: 364–370.

Rötig A, Cormier V, Blache S, et al. (1990) Pearson marrow-pancreas syndrome. A multisystem mitochondrial disorder of infancy. *J Clin Invest* 86: 1601–1608.

Rowland LP, Blake DM, Hirano M, et al. (1991) Clinical syndromes associated with ragged red fibres. *Rev Neurol* (Paris) 147: 467–473.

Saitoh S, Momoi MY, Yamagata T, Mori Y, Imai M. (1998) Effects of dichloroacetate in three patients with MELAS. *Neurology* 50: 531–534.

Santorelli FM, Shanske S, Macaya A, DeVivo DC, DiMauro S. (1993) The mutation at nt 8993 of mitochondrial DNA is a common cause of Leigh's syndrome. *Ann Neurol* 34: 827–834.

Saraste M. (1999) Oxidative phosphorylation at the *fin de siècle*. *Science* 283: 1488–1493.

Schapira AHV. (2000) Mitochondrial disorders. *Curr Opin Neurol* 13: 527–532.

Schuelke M, Smeitink J, Mariman E, et al. (1999) Mutant NDUFV1 subunit of mitochondrial complex I causes leukodystrophy and myoclonic epilepsy. *Nat Genet* 21: 260–261.

Servidei S. (2000) Mitochondrial encephalomyopathies: gene mutation. *Neuromusc Disord* 10: X–XV.

Shoubridge EA, Johns T, Karpati G. (1997) Complete restoration of a wild-type mtDNA genotype in regenerating muscle fibres in a patient with a tRNA point mutation and mitochondrial encephalomyopathy. *Hum Mol Genet* 6: 2239–2241.

Siciliano G, Rossi B, Manca L, et al. (1996) Residual muscle cytochrome c oxidase activity accounts for submaximal exercise lactate threshold in chronic progressive external ophthalmoplegia. *Muscle Nerve* 9(3): 342–349.

Siciliano G, Renna M, Manca LM, et al. (1999) The relationship of plasma catecholamine and lactate during anaerobic threshold exercise in mitochondrial myopathies. *Neuromuscular disorders* 9: 411–416.

Sobreira C, Hirano M, Shanske S, et al. (1997) Mitochondrial encephalomyopathy with coenzyme Q10 deficiency. *Neurology* 48: 1238–1243.

Suomalainen A, Kaukonen J, Amati P, et al. (1995) An autosomal locus predisposing to deletions of mitochondrial DNA. *Nature Genet* 9: 146–151.

Taivassalo T, Matthews PM, De Stefano N, et al. (1996) Combined aerobic training and dichloroacetate improve exercise capacity and indices of aerobic metabolism in muscle cytochrome oxidase deficiency. *Neurology* 47: 529–534.

Taivassalo T, De Stefano N, Argov Z, et al. (1998) Effects of aerobic training in patients with mitochondrial myopathies. *Neurology* 50: 1055–1060.

Taivassalo T, Shoubridge E, Kennaway N, DiMauro S, Haller RG. (2000) Aerobic conditioning in mitochondrial myopathies: Physiological, biochemical and genetic effects. *Neurology* 54(supply 3): A331.

Taivassalo T, Fu K, Johns T, Arnold D, Karpati G, Shoubridge EA. (1999) Gene shifting: a novel therapy for mitochondrial myopathy. *Hum Mol Genet* 8: 1047–1052.

Tarnopolsky MA, Roy BD, MacDonald JR. (1997) A randomized, controlled trial of creatine monohydrate in patients with mitochondrial cytopathies. *Muscle Nerve* 20: 1502–1509.

Taylor DJ, Kemp GJ, Radda GK. (1994) Bioenergetics of skeletal muscle in mitochondrial myopathy. *J Neurol Sci* 127: 198–206.

Taylor DJ, Borc PJ, Styles P, Gadia DG, Radda GK. (1983) Bioenergetics of intact human muscle. A ^{31}P nuclear magnetic resonance study. *Mol Biol Med* 1: 77–94.

Taylor RW, Chinnery PF, Turnbull DM, Lightowlers RN. (1997) Selective inhibition of mutant human mitochondrial DNA replication *in vitro* by peptide nucleic acids. *Nature Genet* 15: 212–215.

Tiranti V, Hoertnagel K, Carrozzo R, et al. (1998) Mutations of SURF-1 in Leigh disease associated with cytochrome c oxidase deficiency. *Am J Hum Genet* 63: 1609–1621.

Triepels RH, van den Heuvel LP, Loeffen JLP, et al. (1999) Leigh syndrome associated with a mutation in the NDUFS7 (PSST) nuclear encoded subunit of complex I. *Ann Neurol* 45: 787–790.

Uziel G, Moroni I, Lamantea E, et al. (1997) Mitochondrial disease associated with the T8993G mutation of the mitochondrial ATPase 6 gene: a clinical, biochemical and molecular study in six families. *J Neurol Neurosurg Psych* 63: 16–22.

Van Beekvelt MC, Colier WN, Wevers RA, Van Engelen BG. (1999) Quantitative measurement of oxygen consumption and forearm blood flow in patients with mitochondrial myopathies. *Adv Exp Med Biol* 471: 313–319.

Van den Heuvel L, Ruitenbeek W, Smeets R, et al. (1998) Demonstration of a new pathogenic mutation in human complex I deficiency: a 5-bp duplication in the nuclear gene encoding the 18-kD (AQDQ) subunit. *Am J Hum Genet* 62: 262–268.

Vissing J, Galbo H, Haller RG. (1996) Exercise fuel mobilization in mitochondrial myopathy: A metabolic dilemma. *Ann Neurol* 40: 655–662.

Vissing J, Gansted U, Quistorff B. (2001) Exercise intolerance in mitochondrial myopathy is not related to lactic acidosis. *Ann Neurol* 49: 672–676.

Vissing J, Lewis SF, Galbo H, Haller RG. (1992) Effect of deficient muscular glycogenolysis on extramuscular fuel production in exercise. *J Appl Physiol* 72(5): 1773–1779.

Vissing J, Salamon MB, Arlien-Søborg P, et al. (1998b) A new mitochondrial tRNA[Met] gene mutation in a patient with dystrophic muscle and exercise intolerance. *Neurology* 50: 1875–1878.

Vissing J, Vissing S, MacLean DA, Saltin B, Quistorff B, Haller RG. (1998a) Sympathetic activation in exercise is not dependent on muscle acidosis: Direct evidence from studies in metabolic myopathies. *J Clin Invest* 101(8): 1654–1660.

Wallace DC. (1999) Mitochondrial diseases in man and mouse. *Science* 283: 1482–1488.

Wallace DC, Singh G, Lott MT et al. (1988) Mitochondrial DNA mutation associated with Leber's hereditary optic neuropathy. *Science* 242: 1427–1430.

Wibrand F, Ravn K, Schwartz M, Rosenberg T, Horn N, Vissing J. (2001) Multisystem disorder associated with a missense mutation in the mitochondrial cytochrome *b* gene. *Ann Neurol*; In press.

Yang D, Oyaizu Y, Oyaizu H, Olsen GJ, Woese CR. (1985) Mitochondrial origins. *Proc Natl Acad Sci USA* 82(13): 4443–4447.

Zhu Z, Yao J, Johns T, et al. (1998) SURF1, encoding a factor involved in the biogenesis of cytochrome c oxidase, is mutated in Leigh syndrome. *Nat Genet* 20(4): 337–343.

15

Myopathies involving glycogen and carbohydrate metabolism

Claudio Bruno

Introduction

Metabolic myopathies are clinical disorders in which defects of adenosine triphosphate (ATP) production causes muscle dysfunction. A review of muscle metabolism is beyond the scope of this chapter and readers are referred to other reviews for further details (DiMauro and Tsujino 1994, DiMauro et al 1997). Nevertheless, a brief description of the biochemical pathways supporting the energy requirement of skeletal muscle is necessary to understand the symptoms of patients with metabolic myopathies.

Skeletal muscle is highly energy-dependent and, therefore, vulnerable to disorders of energy metabolism. The hydrolysis of ATP to adenosine diphosphate (ADP) and inorganic phosphate (P_i) is the immediate and essential source of energy for contraction and relaxation of skeletal muscle. In order to regenerate ATP, skeletal muscle utilizes different energy-producing reactions (high-energy phosphate compounds, glucose and glycogen, and free fatty acids (FFAs)), through different metabolic pathways (oxidative phosphorylation, anaerobic glycolysis, and the creatine kinase (CK) reaction). Resting muscle utilizes predominantly FFA (Felig and Wahren 1975), whereas, in working muscle, the type, intensity, and duration of exercise dictate the choice of the bioenergetic pathway (Essen 1978, Haller and Bertocci 1994).

Anaerobic glycolysis and the CK reaction, the major anaerobic sources of ADP phosphorylation, are important fuel sources in ischaemic or *isometric* exercise, when muscle blood flow and oxygen delivery to exercising muscles are interrupted or reduced; or during extremely intense physical activity, when the energy demand is above the anaerobic threshold.

During the *isotonic* form of exercise, such as walking or running, ATP is regenerated during the first several minutes by high-energy phosphate compounds. Subsequently, the amount of energy derived from carbohydrate oxidation increases and glycogen becomes the most important fuel. With prolonged exercise, glucose and glycogen stores are depleted, and glycolysis switches to fatty acid metabolism. After longer period of exercise, FFAs are the predominant sources of ATP. The final common pathway for ATP production is the mitochondrial respiratory chain (oxidative phosphorylation; Fig. 15.1).

Defects in biochemical pathways of ATP production cause clinical disorders characterized by muscle symptoms, and in particular, the specific energy-producing pathway that is altered determines the type of exercise that will cause symptoms. For example, defects of glycolysis will be evident after short intervals of moderate to intense exercise, while fatty acid metabolism disorders will cause symptoms after prolonged exercise.

This chapter will review those disorders of glycogen and carbohydrate metabolism (glycogenoses) affecting skeletal muscle alone, or in combination with other tissues (Fig. 15.2). These disorders—three enzyme defects affecting non-lysosomal glycogenolysis and one affecting lysosomal glycogenolysis, six affecting glycolysis and one affecting glycogen-synthase—have been classified by *roman numerals* in order of their discovery.

Glycogenoses cause two main clinical syndromes (DiMauro and Tsujino 1994).

1. Exercise intolerance, with cramps, and myoglobinuria, and elevated serum CK levels, generally associated with defects of glycogenolysis (phosphorylase kinase and myophosphorylase deficiencies)

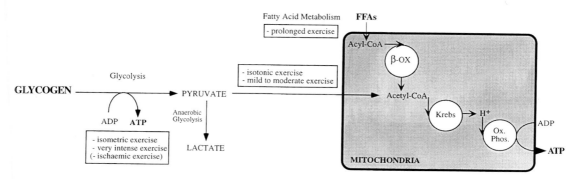

Figure 15.1—Schematic representation of the main bioenergetic pathways utilized by skeletal muscle during exercise (FFAS, free fatty acids; β-OX, β-oxidation; Ox. Phos., oxidative phosphorylation; ADP, adenosine diphosphate; ATP, adenosine triphosphate).

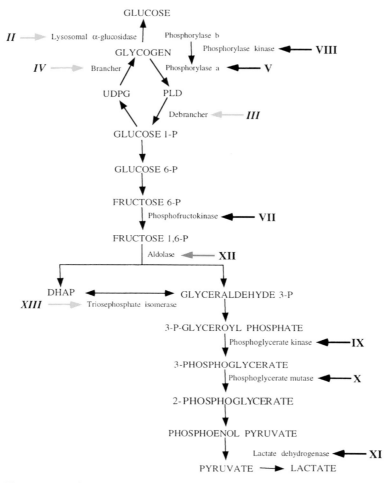

Figure 15.2— Schematic representation of glycogen metabolism and glycolysis. Roman numerals indicate the site of identification enzyme defects. Black arrows indicate glycogenoses associated with exercise intolerance, cramps, and myoglobinuria; grey arrows indicate glycogenoses causing weakness (UDPG, uridine diphosphate glucose; PLD, phosphorylase-limit dextrin; DHAP, dihydroxyacetone phosphate; -P, phosphorylated).

and glycolysis (phosphofructokinase, phosphoglycerate kinase, phosphoglycerate mutase and lactate dehydrogenase deficiencies).

2. Progressive weakness involving limb and trunk muscles, characteristic of defects in the glycogeno-synthetic pathway (brancher enzyme deficiency) and in the lysosomal glycogenolytic system (acid maltase deficiency).

However, there are some exceptions:

• Defects of debrancher, a glycogenolytic enzyme, causes weakness rather than cramps and myoglobinuria.

• Patients with myophosphorylase and phosphofructokinase deficiency often develop fixed weakness later in life.

• Some patients with myophosphorylase, phosphorylase kinase and phosphofructokinase deficiency presents with weakness, without cramps and myoglobinuria.

All glycogenoses are autosomal recessive, except phosphoglycerate kinase, which is X-linked, and phosphorylase kinase, which may be either. All of the genes encoding these enzymes have been cloned, their chromosomes have been localized and many molecular genetic defects have been identified (Table 15.1).

Table 15.1 — Enzymes of glycogen metabolism and glycolysis: tissue specific isozymes, subunit composition and chromosomal assignment

Enzyme defect	Type	Eponymus	Symbol	Inherit.	Subunit/isozyme[b]	Chromosome	References
α-Glucosidase	II	Acid maltase def. Pompe disease (infantile form)	GGA	AR[a]	–	17q23-q25	Hirschhorn 1997
Debrancher	III	Cori disease Forbes disease Limit dextrinosis	AGL	AR	–	1p21	Bao et al 1996a
Brancher	IV	Andersen disease Amylopectinosis	GBE	AR	–	3p12	Thon et al 1993, Bao et al 1996b
Phosphorylase	V	McArdle disease	PYG-M	AR	M L B	11q13 14 10,20	Tsujino et al 1993a, Kubish et al 1998
Phosphofructo-kinase	VII	Tarui disease	PFK-M	AR	M P L	1cen-q32 10p 21q22.3	Nakajima et al 1995, Raben et al 1995a
Phosphorylase kinase	VIII	–	PhK-A1	X-linked AR	α (M) α (L) β γ (M) γ (T)	Xq12-13 Xp22.2-22.1 16q12-13	Wehner et al 1994
Phosphoglycerate kinase	IX	–	PGK-1 PGK-2	X-linked AR	A	Xq13 19	Tsujino et al 1995a
Phosphoglycerate mutase	X	–	PGAM-2	AR	M B	7p13-12.3 10q25	Tsujino et al 1995b
Lactate dehydrogenase	XI	–	LDH-A	AR	M H	11p15.4 12	Kanno and Maekawa 1995
Aldolase	XII	–	ALDO-A	AR	–	16q22-24	Kreuder et al 1996
Triosephosphate isomerase	XIII	–	TPI	AR	–	12p13	Bardosi et al 1990

[a]AR, autosomal recessive
[b]M, muscle; L, liver; B, brain; P, platelets; T, testis; H, heart

The main clinical, laboratory and morphological characteristics of the glycogenoses are summarized in Table 15.2.

In the last decade, the activities of two enzymes of the glycolytic pathway, whose defects have been reported in red blood cells (aldolase A and triosephosphate isomerase), have also been found to be decreased in muscle in two patients with myopathy.

Aldolase A deficiency presents as proximal muscle wasting and weakness together with episodic exacerbation, but no myoglobinuria, and a normal muscle biopsy. This phenotype fits between the two clinical syndromes described earlier. By contrast, the patient with triosephosphate isomerase deficiency had severe muscle weakness, hypotonia, and muscle glycogen storage, and so belongs to the second group.

A brief description of these two new forms of muscle glycogenoses is given at the end of the chapter.

Table 15.2 — Clinical, laboratory and morphological characteristics of muscle glycogenoses

Enzyme defect	Clinical features	Other tissues/other diseases	Resting CK	EMG	FIET	Muscle morphology
Myophosphorylase	Exercise intolerance Myalgia and cramps Myoglobinuria Fixed weakness (late-onset)	None	Increase	Normal or myophatic	No rise in venous lactate	Subsarcolemmal PAS-positive deposits of glycogen, less marked between myofibrills. E.M.: accumulation of normal-looking glycogen under the sarcolemmal and between myofibrills
Phosphofructokinase	Exercise intolerance Myalgia and cramps Myoglobinuria Fixed weakness (late-onset)	RBC: Haemolytic anaemia Skin: jaundice Rheum: gouty arthritis Gut: gastric ulcer	Increase	Myophatic (irritative features)	No rise in venous lactate	Subsarcolemmal PAS-positive deposits of glycogen. Abnormal polysaccharide PAS-positive non-diastase digestible. E.M.: accumulation of normal-looking glycogen under the sarcolemmal. Granular and filamentous material.
Phosphorylase kinase	Exercise intolerance Myalgia and cramps Weakness Myoglobinuria	Liver: Hepatopathy Heart: Cardiopathy	Variable increase	Myopathic	Normal or low rise in venous lactate	Normal or subsarcolemmal PAS-positive deposits of glycogen
Phosphoglycerate kinase	Exercise intolerance Myalgia and cramps Myoglobinuria	RBC: Haemolytic anaemia CNS: seizures mental retardation	Variable increase	Normal	No or low rise in venous lactate	Mild, diffuse PAS-positive deposits of glycogen
Phosphoglycerate mutase	Exercise intolerance Myalgia and cramps Myoglobinuria	None	Increase	Normal	Low rise in venous lactate	Normal or diffuse/patchy PAS-positive deposits of glycogen
Lactate dehydrogenase	Exercise intolerance Myalgia and cramps Myoglobinuria	Skin: acroerythema	Variable increase	ND	Low rise in venous lactate Increase rise in pyruvate	Non-specific myopathic changes
Aldolase	Exercise intolerance, weakness (febrile attacks)	RBC: Haemolytic anaemia	Normal	Normal	ND	Variable fibre size. E.M.: electron-dense accumulation of lipids
Triosephosphate isomerase	Hypotonia Weakness	RBC: Haemolytic anaemia CNS: mental retardation	Normal	Myopathic	ND	Scattered deposits of PAS-positive material. E.M.: increase of glycogen under the sarcolemma
Debrancher	Infancy: hypotonia, weakness Adulthood: distal and proximal weakness	Liver: Hepatomegaly Heart: Cardiopathy Metab: Hypoglycaemia Endocr: Growth failure	Increase	Myophatic	No or low rise in venous lactate	PAS-positive material diastase digestible, under the sarcolemma, and between myofibrils E.M.: free and normal glycogen particles
Brancher	Congenital: hypotonia Childhood: prox. weakness Adulthood: prox. weakness	Liver: Hepatic failure Heart: Cardiopathy	Variable increase	Myopathic (myotonic discharges)	Normal rise in venous lactate	Abnormal polysaccharide PAS-positive partially diastase digestible. E.M.: granular and filamentous material
α-Glucosidase	Infancy: progr. weakness, severe hypotonia	Heart: Cardiomegaly Liver: Hepatomegaly	Increase	Myopathic (myotonic discharges)	Normal rise in venous lactate	PAS-positive material diastase digestible, acid phosphatase positive E.M.: free glycogen in cytoplasm and within lysosomes
	Childhood: progr. weakness Adulthood: progr. weakness	None	Variable increase	Myophatic or normal		

FIET, Forearm ischaemic exercise test; PAS, Periodic Acid–Schiff reaction; E.M., Electron microscopy; RBC, Red blood cells; ND, no data; CNS, central nervous system

Forearm ischaemic exercise test

The forearm ischaemic exercise test (FIET) is a useful tool for corroborating the diagnosis of defects in the glycogenolytic/glycolytic pathways (Fig. 15.3). The test measures basal and post-exercise venous lactate and ammonia levels. A commonly followed protocol is the one described by DiMauro and Bresolin (1986; Table 15.3). In normal adults, lactate increases 3- to 5-fold over baseline with a peak at 1 to 2 min post-exercise, whereas ammonia increases 5- to 10-fold. Patients with myophosphorylase, phosphofructokinase, or distal glycolytic enzyme deficiency, generally

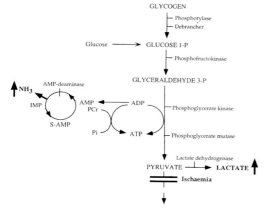

Figure 15.3—Metabolic consequences of forearm ischaemic exercise test (AMP, adenosine monophosphate; ADP, adenosine diphosphate; ATP, adenosine triphosphate; PCr, phosphocreatine; Pi, inorganic phosphate; NH$_3$, ammonia; IMP, inosine-5'-monophosphate; S-AMP, adenylosuccinate).

Table 15.3— Forearm ichaemic exercise test (Protocol according to DiMauro and Bresolin, 1986)

1. Explain the procedure to the patient.
2. Insert an indwelling sterile needle into the patient's antecubital vein. Collect a basal sample of blood for lactate and ammonia measurement.
3. Place a sphygmomanometer cuff above the patient's elbow and inflate above the systolic blood pressure.
4. The patient starts to squeeze another rolled-up sphygamomanometer cuff, trying to push the mercury column to the top, for 1 min.
5. After 1 min of exercise, deflate the blood pressure cuff. If the patient develops a cramp, immediately stop the exercise and deflate the cuff.
6. Withdraw blood samples at 1, 3, 6, and 10 min, after exercise. Keep on ice and sent for lactate and ammonia measurement.

show no or low (less than 1.5-fold) increase in lactate and exaggerated rises in ammonia level (DiMauro and Bresolin 1986). A normal lactate response with impaired ammonia production is characteristic of myoadenylate deaminase deficiency (Fishbein et al 1978).

However, the test has some limitations. The rise of venous lactate depends on the subject's ability and willingness to exercise vigorously. The simultaneous measurement of ammonia levels is, therefore, important in order to confirm the adequate effort of the patient. Furthermore, affected individuals can develop muscle cramping and prolonged contractures during exercise (Meinck et al 1982), and they should immediately stop to reduce the risk of muscle necrosis. Because of these reasons, the test is rarely performed in children. However, a simple modification of the protocol, inflating the sphygmomanometer cuff to the mean arterial pressure (semi-ischaemic test), gave reliable results in children older than 10 years of age (Bruno et al 1998a).

Defects of glycogenolysis

Phosphorylase kinase deficiency

Phosphorylase kinase (PhK) is a multimeric protein composed of four different subunits, α and β (regulatory), γ (catalytic), and δ (identical to calmodulin) (DiMauro and Tsujino 1994, Chen YT and Burchell 1995). Two isoforms are known for subunit α (muscle and liver, α_M and α_L) (Davidson et al 1992) and for subunit γ (muscle and testis, γ_M and γ_T) (Calalb et al 1992). The α_M and α_L genes are both on the X chromosome, while the β, γ_M, and γ_T genes are autosomal (Chen YT and Burchell 1995).

PhK deficiency (glycogenosis type VIII) is associated with four different phenotypes, on the basis of the tissue involvement (liver, muscle, liver and muscle, heart), and mode of inheritance (X-linked or autosomal) (DiMauro and Tsujino 1994).

Isolated myopathy due to PhK deficiency, inherited as an autosomal recessive or as an X-linked trait, has been reported in about 20 cases (Wilkinson et al 1994). The clinical picture is characterized by exercise intolerance, with cramps, myalgia and weakness of exercising muscle. Myoglobinuria after strenuous exercise has been described in less than 50% of cases. Onset is usually in childhood or adolescence. In most patients serum CK is variable increased. The FIET was normal in eight patients studied, and showed a slight rise in venous lactate in three (DiMauro and Tsujino

1994). Electromyography (EMG) can be normal or show non-specific myopathic changes. Muscle biopsy may be normal or show subsarcolemmal accumulation of glycogen. PhK activity in muscle homogenate is absent or markedly decreased (DiMauro and Tsujino 1994).

Human cDNA for the muscle isoform of the PhK α- and γ-subunits, and the human gene encoding the β-subunit have been cloned and sequenced (Wullrich et al 1993, Wehner and Kilimann 1995, Wullrich-Schmoll and Kilimann 1996). To date, only two molecular defects have been identified in the myopathic variant of PhK deficiency, both in the α_M gene (Wehner et al 1994, Bruno et al 1998b).

Phosphorylase deficiency

Human phosphorylase has three mammalian isozymes: muscle, liver and brain, encoded by different genes on different chromosomes (Lebo et al 1984, Newgard et al 1986, Newgard et al 1988). Normal adult human muscle expresses only the muscle isozyme (myophosphorylase), while heart and brain express, in different amount, both the brain and the muscle isoforms (Bresolin et al 1983, DiMauro and Tsujino 1994). In muscle, phosphorylase exists as two forms: a more active, phosphorylated *a* form and a less active, dephosphorylated *b* form.

Muscle phosphorylase deficiency (glycogenosis type V) is characterized by exercise intolerance with premature fatigue, myalgia and cramps. Symptoms usually occur during brief and intense exercise (pushing or lifting heavy objects), or during sustained, but less intense exercise (climbing stairs; DiMauro and Tsujino 1994). Most patients experience the so-called "second-wind" phenomenon: if they rest briefly at the onset of symptoms, they can continue exercising. Myoglobinuria is present in around 50% of the patients; of these, another half develop renal failure. Onset of symptoms usually starts in childhood, but cramps and myoglobinuria develop later in life, and the diagnosis is frequently established in adulthood.

Atypical presentations of McArdle's disease include: a mild form with excessive tiredness and poor stamina (DiMauro and Tsujino 1994); a late-onset form manifesting with fixed weakness in the fifth to sixth decade, without cramps or myoglobinuria (Engel WK et al 1963); a fatal infantile form characterized by weakness, severe respiratory insufficiency and early death (DiMauro and Hartlage 1978, Milstein et al 1989); a case of congenital myopathy in a 4-year-old boy with mental retardation (Cornelio et al 1983).

In addition to the clinical phenotype, the diagnosis is based on laboratory tests (increase resting serum CK, flat venous lactate response to ischaemic exercise, myopathic EMG) and muscle biopsy (subsarcolemmal PAS-positive glycogen deposits and phosphorylase deficiency, documented histochemically and biochemically).

The myophosphorylase gene has been cloned, sequenced (Burke et al 1987) and assigned to chromosome 11q13 (Lebo et al 1984), and the genomic structure has been recently revised (Kubish et al 1998). Molecular genetic analyses have identified around 20 mutations in the myophosphorylase gene from different countries (Tsujino et al 1993a, Bruno et al 1999a).

Debranching deficiency

Debranching enzyme is a monomeric protein with two independent catalytic activities: transferase and α-glucosidase.

Debrancher deficiency (glycogenosis type III) commonly presents as a childhood-onset liver disease with hepatomegaly, growth failure, fasting hypoglycaemia, and infrequently hypoglycaemic seizures (Chen YT and Burchell 1995). Liver symptoms improve with age and, around puberty, there is a frequent inclination to a spontaneous resolution.

Progressive myopathy, neuropathy and cardiomyopathy are often overshadowed, in children, by liver disease, and become the predominant features in adulthood (DiMauro et al 1979, Coleman et al 1992, Lee et al 1997).

Most patients have disease involving both liver and muscle (type IIIa), and around 15% of the patients have only liver involvement (type IIIb) (Chen YT and Burchell 1995). Selective absence of one of the two catalytic activities, glucosidase (type IIIc) or transferase (type IIId), has been reported (Ding et al 1990).

Myopathy tends to present in the third to fourth decades of life, with slowly progressive weakness and muscle wasting. In these patients serum CK is elevated, EMG is myopathic and may show fibrillations. Nerve conduction velocities can be decreased (Chen YT and Burchell 1995).

Muscle biopsy shows numerous PAS-positive vacuoles that are diastase digestible and are located under the sarcolemma and between myofibrils. Ultrastructurally, they appear as collections of free and apparently normal glycogen particles.

The gene for human debrancher enzyme has been cloned, sequenced (Yang et al 1992, Bao et al 1996a) and assigned to chromosome 1p21 (Yang-Feng et al

1992). Different mutations have been identified in Caucasian, Jewish and Japanese patients (Chen YT and Burchell 1995, Parvari et al 1997).

Defects of glycolysis

Phosphofructokinase deficiency

Phosphofructokinase (PFK) is a tetrameric enzyme composed of three distinct subunits—muscle (M), liver (L) and platelets (P)—which are variably expressed in different tissues (Vora 1982). Mature human muscle exclusively contains the M isoform, while erythrocytes express both the M and L subunits.

In the typical form of PFK deficiency (glycogenosis type VII), there is a total lack of activity in muscle and partial enzyme deficiency in erythrocytes. The clinical presentation is indistinguishable from myophosphorylase deficiency, and it is characterized by intolerance to vigorous exercise, with cramps, and myoglobinuria (Tarui et al 1965, Rowland et al 1986, DiMauro and Tsujino 1994). However, PFK deficiency presents also with haemolytic anaemia, jaundice, gouty arthritis and gastric ulcer (Nakajima et al 1995, Nakagawa et al 1995).

Atypical clinical presentations include haemolytic anaemia without myopathy, late-onset fixed weakness (Hays et al 1981, Danon et al 1988) and severe and often fatal infantile myopathy sometimes associated with encephalopathy (Guibaud et al 1978, Danon et al 1981, Servidei et al 1986, Amit et al 1992).

In patients with typical muscle disease, laboratory investigations reveal elevated levels of serum CK, bilirubin, uric acid, and reticulocytosis. EMG shows myopathic pattern with irritative features.

Muscle biopsy shows accumulation of subsarcolemmal and intermyofibrillar glycogen. A specific stain for PFK allows the histochemical diagnosis (Bonilla and Schotland 1970) that can be confirmed biochemically in muscle homogenate. However, in some cases, there is an abnormal polysaccharide, which stains intensely with PAS, but is not digested by diastase (Agamanolis et al 1980, Hays et al 1981, Danon et al 1988). Ultrastructurally, this abnormal glycogen appears as granular and filamentous material, similar to that in branching enzyme deficiency.

The gene encoding subunit M has been assigned to chromosome 1 (Vora et al 1982), and its full-length cDNA and the structure of genomic DNA have been reported (Nakajima et al 1987, Yamasaki et al 1991). Several pathogenic mutations have been founded in patients from United States, Europe and Japan (Raben et al 1995a).

Phosphoglycerate kinase deficiency

Human phosphoglycerate kinase (PGK) is a monomeric enzyme encoded by a single gene located on chromosome Xq13 and is ubiquitously expressed (Chen SH et al 1971). A testicular tissue-specific isozyme (PGK2) is on chromosome 19 (Willard et al 1985).

Since the first report in 1968 (Kraus et al 1968), PGK deficiency has been identified in more than 20 patients with haemolytic anaemia, central nervous system (CNS) dysfunction, or myopathy (Tsujino et al 1995a). The three features occur with similar frequencies, and the coexistence of all in the same patient has been reported only once.

Primary pure myopathy associated with PGK deficiency has been reported in four patients (Rosa et al 1982, DiMauro et al 1983, Tonin et al 1993): one had myopathy and haemolytic anaemia (Fujii et al 1992), and in the other three the myopathy was associated with CNS dysfunction (Sugie et al 1989, Tsujino et al 1994a). All these patients were intolerant to vigorous exercise, and had cramps and myoglobinuria. Resting serum CK was inconsistently increased. FIET caused no venous lactate increase in two patients, and an inadequate rise in one. EMG was normal. Muscle biopsy showed mildly, diffuse increase of PAS-positive material.

The complete amino acid, cDNA, and genomic sequences have been reported (Huang et al 1980, Michelson et al 1983, 1985), and molecular genetic defects have been identified in around 10 patients: only two of them had myopathy (Tsujino et al 1995a).

Phosphoglycerate mutase deficiency

Human phosphoglycerate mutase (PGAM) is a dimeric enzyme containing, in different tissues, different proportions of a slow-migrating muscle isozyme (MM), a fast-migrating brain isozyme (BB) and an intermediate hybrid form (MB). Normal mature muscle contains predominantly the MM homodymer (Omenn and Cheung 1974).

PGAM deficiency (glycogenosis type X) has been reported so far in 12 patients: ten were African Americans (Tsujino et al 1995b), one Italian (Vita et al 1990) and one Japanese (Kawashima et al 1996). All had intolerance to intense exercise, with myalgia and cramps, and five of them had recurrent myoglobinuria. Serum CK was increased. FIET revealed low venous lactate response, but not absence. The muscle biopsy was normal in most of the patients, but in some showed a diffuse or patchy glycogen accumulation.

PGAM activity in muscle ranged from 2 to 6% of the normal mean (Tsujino et al 1995b).

The full-length cDNA encoding the M subunit has been cloned (Shanske et al 1987), and the entire gene encoding PGAM-M has been isolated, sequenced (Tsujino et al 1989) and mapped to chromosome 7p12-7p13 (Edwards et al 1989, Castella-Escola et al 1990). Four mutations in the PGAM-M gene have been described so far: two in African American families (Tsujino et al 1993b), one in an Italian family (Toscano et al 1996) and one in a Japanese family (Hadjigeorgiou et al 1999).

At least in two families, clinical and morphological manifestations occurred in subjects who were heterozygous for PGAM-M mutations.

Lactate dehydrogenase deficiency

Lactate dehydrogenase (LDH) is a tetrameric enzyme composed, in different tissues, of different proportions of three subunits: LDH-M (or A), which predominates in muscle, LDH-H (or B), which predominates in heart, and LDH-C, expressed only in mature testis and sperm (Markert et al 1975).

LDH-M deficiency (glycogenosis type XI) has been documented in six Japanese families (Kanno et al 1980, 1988, Maekawa et al 1990, 1991, 1994) and in four Caucasian patients (Nazzari and Crovato 1992, Tsujino et al 1994b). The clinical features of this disorder are similar to those of other glycogenoses, resulting from a partial or complete block of glycolysis (DiMauro and Tsujino 1994). Some peculiar laboratory and clinical characteristics, however, could be useful for a direct diagnostic approach:

- during an episodes of myoglobinuria, the high levels of serum CK contrast with the low levels of serum LDH
- FIET causes a poor rise of lactate, but an increased rise of pyruvate
- a typical skin eruption has been observed in some patients (Yoshikuni et al 1986, Takayasu et al 1991, Nazzari and Crovato 1992).

Muscle biopsy shows a non-specific myopathy (Tsujino et al 1994b) and biochemical study of muscle homogenate reveals a deficit of LDH activity.

The sequence of the LDH-M cDNA (Tsujibo et al 1985) and the organization of the chromosomal gene (Chung et al 1985) have been reported, and the gene has been assigned to chromosome 11p15.4 (Scrable et al 1990). Genomic analysis has shown the heterogeneities of the mutations causing this disease (Kanno and Maekawa 1995).

Defects of glycogenosynthesis

Brancher deficiency

Glycogen brancher enzyme (GBE) deficiency (glycogenosis type IV) is commonly characterized by progressive liver cirrhosis leading to hepatic failure and death in early childhood (DiMauro and Tsujino 1994, Chen YT and Burchell 1995). A second clinical presentation involves the neuromuscular system, and can be divided on the basis of age at onset as follows:

1. a congenital form, with hypotonia, muscle wasting, neuronal involvement, cardiomyopathy and death in infancy (Zellweger et al 1972, van Noort et al 1993, Tang et al 1994)

2. a childhood form characterized by cardiopathy (Servidei et al 1987) or myopathy (Reusche et al 1992)

3. an adult form, presenting as myopathy (Bornemann et al 1996) or as diffuse central and peripheral nervous system dysfunction (adult polyglucosan body disease; APBD) (Lossos et al 1991, Bruno et al 1993).

In patients with myopathy, serum CK is variable increase, EMG shows myopathic features, and FIET reveals a normal rise of venous lactate.

In muscle, deposits of a basophilic, intensely PAS-positive material are only partially digested by diastase. Electron microscopy reveals, in association with normal glycogen granules, abnormal storage material consisting of filamentous and finely granular amylopectin-like material (DiMauro and Tsujino 1994, Chen YT and Burchell 1995). This abnormal polysaccharide has been found also in skin, liver, heart and the CNS, but the amount varies in different tissue.

Human GBE is a monomeric enzyme encoded by a single gene, which has been cloned, sequenced and assigned to chromosome 3p12 (Thon et al 1993). Different mutations in the GBE gene in patients with different clinical forms have been reported (Bao et al 1996b, Bruno et al 1999b).

Defects of lysosomal glycogenolysis

Acid α-glucosidase deficiency

Acid α-glucosidase, a lysosomal enzyme involved in

carbohydrate metabolism, catalyzes the hydrolysis of α-1,4 and α-1,6 linkages in glycogen, maltose and isomaltose. The enzyme deficiency results in intra-lysosomal accumulation of normal glycogen in several tissues (Hirschhorn 1997).

Acid α-glucosidase (glycogenosis type II, acid maltase deficiency, AMD), results in two clinical syndromes, based on age of onset and severity of the disease:

1. a generalized and lethal disease of early infancy (Pompe disease; Pompe 1932)

2. a milder neuromuscular disorder beginning in childhood or adulthood (Hers 1963, Engel AG et al 1973).

Pompe disease presents at birth or within the first weeks or months of age, and it is characterized by massive deposition of glycogen in the liver, heart and skeletal muscle. Severe hypotonia and weakness are associated with macroglossia, hepatomegaly and cardiomegaly. Cardiac or respiratory failures lead to death before the second year of age. In the childhood form, there is a delay in the onset of walking with slow and progressive weakness of limb girdle and trunk muscle. Respiratory failure causes death in the second or third decade. There is generally no cardiomegaly (Matsuishi et al 1984). The adult phenotype begins in the third or fourth decade, without visceral organ involvement, and is characterized by proximal muscle weakness and frequent respiratory insufficiency due to diaphragmatic involvement (Karpati et al 1977).

Acid α-glucosidase is virtually absent (infantile form) or markedly reduced (juvenile and adult form) in all tissues. Serum CK is elevated, but it can be normal in the adult form. EMG shows a myopathic pattern in all forms, with fibrillations and myotonic discharges.

Muscle biopsy shows a vacuolar myopathy most prominent in the infantile form. The vacuoles are lysosomes filled with PAS-positive diastase-digestible material, which stains intensely for acid phosphatase. Glycogen content is increased up to 10-fold. Electron microscopy shows the presence of glycogen both within lysosomes and free in cytoplasm.

The gene for acid α-glucosidase has been mapped to chromosome 17q21-q23 (Solomon and Barker 1989), and the cDNA and the genomic sequence have been identified (Martiniuk et al 1986, Hoefsloot et al 1990). Mutation studies have revealed the genetic heterogeneity of this disease (Engel AG and Hirschhorn 1994, Raben et al 1995b, Reuser et al 1995, Hirschhorn 1997).

Other defects of glycolysis involving skeletal muscle

Triosephosphate isomerase deficiency

An 8-year-old girl had chronic haemolytic anaemia, severe muscle weakness, hypotonia and moderate mental retardation from early infancy (Bardosi et al 1990). Erythrocyte enzyme screening showed reduced triosephosphate isomerase (TPI) activity. Serum CK was normal and EMG demonstrated myopathic features. Muscle biopsy revealed TPI activity to be histochemically undetectable and less than 10% of normal by biochemical analysis. Morphology studies revealed scattered deposits of PAS-positive material. Ultrastructural studies revealed an increased amount of cytoplasmic glycogen in the subsarcolemmal and interfibrillary regions of muscle (Bardosi et al 1990).

Aldolase A deficiency

A 4.5-year-old boy presented with episodes of exercise intolerance and weakness following attacks of febrile illness. The clinical picture was also characterized by haemolytic anaemia and by slight motor development delay. The highest serum CK level was 6480 U/l (normal: less than 60 U/l), but no myoglobinuria was described. Muscle biopsy was morphologically normal, but it showed a severe defect of aldolase activity (4% of normal) by biochemical analysis. Molecular genetic analysis revealed a homozygous point mutation in a highly conserved region of the aldolase A gene (Kreuder et al 1996).

Acknowledgement

I am grateful to my mentor, Dr Salvatore DiMauro, for his advice and encouragement.

References

Agamanolis DP, Askari AD, DiMauro S, et al. (1980) Muscle phosphofructokinase deficiency: two cases with unusual polysaccharide accumulation and immunologically active enzyme protein. *Muscle Nerve* 3: 456–467.

Amit R, Bashan N, Abarbanel JM, Shapira Y, Sofer S, Moser S. (1992) Fatal familial infantile glycogen storage disease: multisystem phosphofructokinase deficiency. *Muscle Nerve* 15: 455–458.

Bao Y, Dawson TL, Chen YT. (1996a) Human glycogen debranching enzyme gene (AGL): complete structural organization and characterization of the 5′ flanking region. *Genomics* 38: 155–165.

Bao Y, Kishnani P, Wu J-Y, Chen YT. (1996b) Hepatic and neuromuscular forms of glycogen storage disease type IV caused by mutations in the same glycogen-branching enzyme gene. *J Clin Invest* 97: 941–948.

Bardosi A, Eber SW, Hendrys M, Pekrun A. (1990) Myopathy with altered mitochondria due to a triosephosphate isomerase (TPI) deficiency. *Acta Neuropathol* 79: 387–394.

Bonilla E, Schotland DL. (1970) Histochemical diagnosis of muscle phosphofructokinase deficiency. *Arch Neurol* 22: 8–12.

Bornemann A, Besser R, Shin YS, Goebel HH. (1996) A mild adult myopathic variant of type IV glycogenosis. *Neuromusc Dis* 6: 95–99.

Bresolin N, Miranda AF, Jacobson MP, Lee JH, Capilupi T, DiMauro S. (1983) Phosphorylase isoenzymes and human brain. *Neurochem Pathol* 1: 171–178.

Bruno C, Servidei S, Shanske S, et al. (1993) Glycogen branching enzyme deficiency in adult polyglucosan body disease. *Ann Neurol* 33: 88–93.

Bruno C, Bado M, Minetti C, Cordone G. (1998a) Forearm semi-ischemic exercise test in pediatric patients. *J Child Neurol* 13: 288–290.

Bruno C, Manfredi G, Andreu AL, et al. (1998b) A splice junction mutation in the α_M gene of phosphorylase kinase (PhK) in a patient with myopathy. *Biochem Byophys Res Comm* 249: 648–651.

Bruno C, Lofberg M, Tamburino L, et al. (1999a) Molecular characterization of McArdle's in two large Finnish families. *J Neurol Sci* 165: 121–125.

Bruno C, DiRocco M, Doria Lamba L, et al. (1999b) A novel missense mutation in the glycogen branching enzyme gene in a child with myopathy and hepatopathy. *Neuromusc Dis* in press.

Burke J, Hwang P, Anderson L, Lebo R, Gorin F, Fletterick R. (1987) Intron/exon structure of the human gene for the muscle isozyme of glycogen phosphorylase. *Protein* 2: 177–187.

Calalb MB, Fox DT, Hanks SK. (1992) Molecular cloning and enzymatic analysis of the rat homolog of PhK-gamma T, an isoform of phosphorylase kinase catalytic subunit. *J Biol Chem* 267: 1455–1463.

Castella-Escola J, Mattei MG, Ojcius DM, Passage E, Valentin C, Cohen-Solal. (1990) In situ mapping of the muscle-specific form of phosphoglycerate mutase gene to human chromosome 7p12–7p13. *Hum Genet* 84: 210–212.

Chen SH, Malcolm LA, Yoshida A, Giblett E. (1971) Phosphoglycerate kinase: an X-linked polymorphism in man. *Am J Hum Genet* 23: 87–91.

Chen YT, Burchell A. (1995) Glycogen storage disease. In: Scriver CR, Beaudet AL, Sly WS, Valle D, eds. *The metabolic and molecular bases of inherited disease.* 7th ed, vol I. New York: McGraw-Hill, pp. 935–965.

Chung F-Z, Tsujibo H, Bhattacharyya U, Sharief FS, Li SS. (1985) Genomic organization of human lactate dehydrogenase-A gene. *Biochem J* 231: 537–541.

Coleman RA, Winter HS, Wolf B, Gilchrist JM, Chen YT. (1992) Glycogen storage disease type III (glycogen debranching enzyme deficiency): correlation of biochemical defects with myopathy and cardiomyopathy. *Ann Int Med* 116: 896–900.

Cornelio F, Bresolin N, DiMauro S, Mora M, Balestrini MR. (1983) Congenital myopathy due to phosphorylase deficiency. *Neurology* 33: 1383–1385.

Danon MJ, Carpenter S, Manaligod JR, Schliselfeld. (1981) Fatal infantile glycogen storage disease: deficiency of phosphofructokinase and phosphorylase b kinase. *Neurology* 311303–1307.

Danon MJ, Servidei S, DiMauro S, Vora S. (1988) Late-onset muscle phosphofructokinase deficiency. *Neurology* 38: 956–960.

Davidson JJ, Ozcelik T, Hamacher C, Willems PJ, Francke U, Kilimann MW. (1992) cDNA cloning of a liver isoform of the phosphorylase kinase alpha subunit and mapping of the gene to Xp22.2–p22.1, the region of human X-linked liver glycogenosis. *Proc Natl Acad Sci USA* 89: 2096–2100.

DiMauro S, Hartlage P. (1978) Fatal infantile form of muscle phosphorylase deficiency. *Neurology* 28: 1124–1129.

DiMauro S, Geoffrey B, Hartwig GB, et al. (1979) Debrancher deficiency: neuromuscular disorder in 5 adults. *Ann Neurol* 5: 422–436.

DiMauro S, Dalakas M, Miranda AF. (1983) Phosphoglycerate kinase deficiency: another cause of recurrent myoglobinuria. *Ann Neurol* 13: 11–19.

DiMauro S, Bresolin N. (1986) Phosphorylase deficiency. In: Engel AG, Banker BQ, eds. *Myology.* 1st ed, vol 2. New York: McGraw-Hill, pp. 1585–1601.

DiMauro S, Tsujino S. (1994) Nonlysosomal glycogenoses. In: Engel AG, Franzini-Armstrong C, eds. *Myology.* 2nd ed, vol 2. New York: McGraw-Hill, pp. 1554–1576.

DiMauro S, Servidei S, Tsujino S. (1997) Disorders of carbohydrate metabolism: glycogen storage disease. In: Rosemberg RN, Prusiner SB, DiMauro S, Barchi RL, eds. *The molecular and genetic basis of neurological disease.* 2nd ed. Boston: Butterworth-Heinemann, pp. 201–235.

Ding JH, DeBarsy T, Brown BI, Coleman RA, Chen YT. (1990) Immunoblot analysis of glycogen debranching enzyme in different subtypes of glycogen storage disease type III. *J Pediatr* 116: 95–100.

Edwards YH, Sakoda S, Schon EA, Povey S. (1989) The gene for human muscle-specific phosphoglycerate mutase, PGAM2, mapped to chromosome 7 by polymerase chain reaction. *Genomics* 5: 948–951.

Engel AG, Gomez MR, Seybold ME, Lambert EH. (1973) The spectrum and diagnosis of acid maltase deficiency. *Neurology* 23: 95–106.

Engel AG, Hirschhorn R. (1994) In: Engel AG, Franzini-Armstrong C, eds. *Myology.* 2nd ed, vol 2. New York: McGraw-Hill, pp. 1533–1553.

Engel WK, Eyerman EL, Williams HE. (1963) Late-onset type of skeletal-muscle phosphorylase deficiency. A new familial variety with completely and partial affected subjects. *N Engl J Med* 268: 135–137.

Essen B. (1978) Glycogen depletion of different types in human skeletal muscle with prolonged heavy exercise. *Acta Physiol Scand* 107: 257–261.

Felig P, Wahren J. (1975) Fuel homeostasis in exercise. *N Engl J Med* 293: 1078–1084.

Fishbein WN, Armbrustmacher VW, Griffin JL. (1978) Myoadenylate deaminase deficiency: a new disease of muscle. *Science* 200: 545–548.

Fujii H, Kanno H, Hirono A, Shiomura T, Miwa S. (1992) A single amino acid substitution (157 Gly to Val) in a phosphoglycerate kinase variant (PGK Shizuoka) associated with chronic hemolysis and myoglobinuria. *Blood* 79: 1582–1585.

Guibaud P, Carrier H, Mathieu M, et al. (1978) Observation familiale de dystrophie musculaire congenitale par deficit en phosphofructokinase. *Arch Fr Pediatr* 35: 1105–1115.

Hadjigeorgiou GM, Kawashima N, Bruno C, et al. (1999) Manifesting heterozygotes in a Japanese family with a novel mutation in the muscle-specific phosphoglycerate mutase (PGAM-M) gene. *Neuromusc Dis.*

Haller RG, Bertocci LA. (1994) Exercise evaluation of metabolic myopathies. In: Engel AG, Franzini-Armstrong C, eds. *Myology.* 2nd ed, vol 1. New York: McGraw-Hill, pp. 807–821.

Hays AP, Hallett M, Delfs J, et al. (1981) Muscle phosphofructokinase deficiency: abnormal polysaccharide in a case of late-onset myopathy. *Neurology* 31: 1077–1086.

Hers HG. (1963) Alpha-glucosidase deficiency in generalized glycogen-storage disease (Pompe's disease). *Biochem J* 86: 11–16.

Hirschhorn R. (1997) Glycogen storage disease type II: acid α-glucosidase (acid maltase) deficiency. In: Scriver CR, Beaudet AL, Sly WS, Valle D, eds. *The metabolic and molecular bases of inherited disease.* 7th ed, vol II. New York: McGraw-Hill, pp. 2443–2464.

Hoefsloot LH, Hoogeveen-Westerveld M, Reuser AJJ, Oostra BA. (1990) Characterization of the human lysosomal alpha glucosidase gene. *Biochem J* 272: 493–497.

Huang IY, Rubinfien E, Yoshida A. (1980) Complete amino acid sequence of human phosphoglycerate kinase: isolation and amino acid sequence of tryptic peptides. *J Biol Chem* 255: 6408–6411.

Kanno T, Sudo K, Takeuchi I, et al. (1980) Hereditary deficiency of lactate dehydrogenase M-subunit. *Clin Chim Acta* 108: 267–276.

Kanno T, Sudo K, Maekawa M, Nishimura Y, Ukita M, Fukutake K. (1988) Lactate dehydrogenase M-subunit deficiency: a new type of hereditary exertional myopathy. *Clin Chim Acta* 173: 89–98.

Kanno T, Maekawa M. (1995) Lactate dehydrogenase M-subunit deficiencies: clinical features, metabolic background, and genetic heterogeneities. *Muscle Nerve Suppl* 3: S54–S60.

Karpati G, Carpenter S, Eisen A, Aube M, DiMauro S. (1977) The adult form of acid maltase (alpha-1,4-glucosidase) deficiency. *Ann Neurol* 1: 276–280.

Kawashima N, Mishima I, Shindo R, et al. (1996) Partial deficiency of phosphoglycerate mutase with diabetic polyneuropathy: the first Japanese patient. *Intern Med* 35: 799–802.

Kraus AP, Langston MF, Lynch BL. (1968) Red cell phosphoglycerate kinase deficiency; a new case of nonspherocytic hemolytic anemia. *Biochem Biophys Res Comm* 30: 173–177.

Kreuder J, Borkhardt A, Repp R, et al. (1996) Inherited metabolic myopathy and hemolysis due to a mutation in aldolase A. *N Engl J Med* 334: 1100–1104.

Kubish C, Wicklein EM, Jentsch TJ. (1998) Molecular diagnosis of McArdle disease: revised genomic structure of the myophosphorylase gene and identification of a novel mutation. *Hum Mutat* 12: 27–32.

Lebo RV, Gorin F, Fletterick RJ, et al. (1984) High-resolution chromosome sorting and DNA spot-blot analysis assign McArdle's syndrome to chromosome 11. *Science* 225: 57–59.

Lee PJ, Deanfield JE, Burch M, Baig K, McKenna NJ, Leonard JV. (1997) Comparison of the functional significance of the left ventricular hypertrophy in hypertrophic cardiomyopathy and glycogenoses type III. *Am J Cardiol* 76: 834–838.

Lossos A, Barash V, Soffer D, et al. (1991) Hereditary branching enzyme dysfunction in adult polyglucosan body disease. *Ann Neurol* 30: 655–662.

Maekawa M, Sudo K, Li SS-L, Kanno T. (1990) Molecular characterization of genetic mutations in human lactate dehydrogenase-A (M) deficiency. *Biochem Biophys Res Comm* 168: 677–682.

Maekawa M, Sudo K, Li SS-L, Kanno T. (1991) Analysis of genetic mutations in human lactate dehydrogenase A (M) deficiency using DNA conformation polymorphism in combination with polyacrylamide gradient gel and silver staining. *Biochem Biophys Res Comm* 180: 1083–1090.

Maekawa M, Sudo K, Kanno T, et al. (1994) A novel deletion mutation of lactate dehydrogenase A (M) gene in the fifth family with the enzyme deficiency. *Hum Mol Genet* 3: 825–826.

Markert CL, Shaklee JM, Whitt GS. (1975) Evolution of a gene: multiple genes for LDH isozymes provide a model of the evolution of gene structure, function, and regulation. *Science* 189: 102–114.

Martiniuk F, Mehler M, Pellicer A, et al. (1986) Isolation of a cDNA for human acid-alpha-glucosidase and detection of genetic heterogeneity for mRNA in three alpha-glucosidase-deficient patients. *Proc Natl Acad Sci USA* 83: 9641–9644.

Matsuishi T, Yoshino M, Terasawa K, Nonaka I. (1984) Childhood acid maltase deficiency. A clinical, biochemical and morphological study of three patients. *Arch Neurol* 41: 47–52.

Meinck HM, Goebel HH, Rumpf KW, Kaiser H, Neumann P. (1982) Is the forearm ischemic work-test hazardous to McArdle patients? *J Neurol Neurosurg Psychiatry* 45: 1144–1146.

Michelson AM, Markham AF, Orkin SH. (1983) Isolation and DNA sequence of a full-length cDNA clone for human X chromosome-encoded phosphoglycerate kinase. *Proc Natl Acad Sci USA* 80: 472–476.

Michelson AM, Blake CCF, Evans ST, Orkin SH. (1985) Structure of the human phosphoglycerate kinase gene and the intron-mediated evolution and dispersal of the nucleotide-binding domain. *Proc Natl Acad Sci USA* 82: 6965–6969.

Milstein JM, Herron TM, Haas JE. (1989) Fatal infantile phosphorylase deficiency. *J Child Neurol* 4: 186–188.

Nakagawa C, Mineo I, Kaido M, et al. (1995) A new variant case of muscle phosphofructokinase deficiency, coexisting with gastric ulcer, gouty arthritis, and increase hemolysis. *Muscle Nerve Suppl* 3: S39–S44.

Nakajima H, Noguchi T, Yamasaki T, Kono N, Tanaka T, Tarui S. (1987) Cloning of human muscle phosphofructokinase cDNA. *FEBS Lett* 223: 113–116.

Nakajima H, Hamaguchi T, Yamasaki T, Tarui S. (1995) Phosphofructokinase deficiency: recent advances in molecular biology. *Muscle Nerve Suppl* 3: S28–S34.

Nazzari G, Crovato F. (1992) Annually recurring acroerythema and hereditary lactate dehydrogenase M-subunit deficiency. *J Am Acad Dermatol* 27: 262–263.

Newgard CB, Nakano K, Hwang PK, Fletterick RJ. (1986) Sequence analysis of the cDNA encoding human liver glycogen phosphorylase reveals tissue-specific codon usage. *Proc Natl Acad Sci USA* 83: 8132–8136.

Newgard CB, Littman DR, van Genderen C, Fletterick RJ. (1988) Human brain glycogen phosphorylase: cloning, sequence analysis, chromosomal mapping, tissue expression, and comparison with the human liver and muscle isozymes. *J Biol Chem* 263: 3850–3857.

Omenn GS, Cheung J. (1974) Phosphoglycerate mutase: isoenzyme marker for tissue differention in man. *Am J Hum Genet* 26: 393–399.

Parvari R, Moses S, Shen J, Hershkovitz E, Lerner A, Chen YT. (1997) A single-base deletion in the 3'-coding region of glycogen-debranching enzyme is prevalent in glycogen storage disease type IIIA in a population of North African Jewish patients. *Eur J Hum Genet* 5: 266–270.

Pompe JC. (1932) Over idiopathische hypertrophic van het hart. *Ned Tojdschr Geneesk* 76: 304–311.

Raben N, Sherman JB, Adams E, Nakajima H, Argov Z, Plotz P. (1995a) Various classes of mutations in patients with phosphofructokinase deficiency (Tarui's disease). *Muscle Nerve Suppl* 3: S35–S38.

Raben N, Nichols RC, Boerkoel C, Plotz P. (1995b) Genetic defects in patients with glycogenosis type II (acid maltase deficiency). *Muscle Nerve Suppl* 3: S70–S74.

Reusche E, Aksu F, Goebel HH, Shin YS, Yokota T, Reichmann H. (1992) A mild juvenile variant of type IV glycogenosis. *Brain Dev* 14: 36–43.

Reuser AJJ, Kroos MA, Hermans MMP, et al. (1995) Glycogenosys type II (Acid maltase deficiency). *Muscle Nerve Suppl* 3: S61–S69.

Rosa R, George C, Fardeau M, Calvin MC, Rapin M, Rosa J. (1982) A new case of phosphoglycerate kinase deficiency: PGK Creteil associated with rhabdomyolysis and lacking hemolytic anemia. *Blood* 60: 84–91.

Rowland LP, DiMauro S, Layzer RB. (1986) Phosphofructokinase deficiency. In: Engel AG, Banker BQ, eds. *Myology.* 1st ed, vol 2. New York: McGraw-Hill, pp. 1603–1617.

Scrable HJ, Johnson DK, Rinchik EM, Cavenee WK. (1990) Rhabdomyosarcoma-associated locus and MYOD1 are syntenic but separate loci on the short arm of human chromosome 11. *Proc Natl Acad Sci USA* 87: 2182–2186.

Servidei S, Bonilla E, Diedrich RG, et al. (1986) Fatal infantile form of muscle phosphofructokinase deficiency. *Neurology* 36: 1465–1470.

Servidei S, Riepe RE, Langston C, et al. (1987) Severe cardiopathy in branching enzyme deficiency. *J Pediatr* 11: 51–56.

Shanske S, Sakoda S, Hermodson MA, DiMauro S, Schon EA. (1987) Isolation of a cDNA encoding the muscle-specific subunit of human phosphoglycerate mutase. *J Biol Chem* 262: 14612–14617.

Solomon E, Barker DF. (1989) Report of the committee on the genetic constitution of chromosome 17. *Cytogenet Cell Genet* 51: 319–337.

Sugie H, Sugie Y, Nishida M, et al. (1989) Recurrent myoglobinuria in a child with mental retardation: phosphoglycerate kinase deficiency. *J Child Neurol* 4: 95–99.

Tang TT, Segura AD, Chen YT. (1994) Neonatal hypotonia and cardiomyopathy secondary to type IV glycogenosis. *Acta Neuropathol* 87: 531–536.

Takayasu S, Fujivara S, Waki T. (1991) Hereditary lactate dehydrogenase M-subunit deficiency: lactate dehydrogenase activity in skin lesions and in hair follicles. *J Am Acad Dermatol* 24: 339–342.

Tarui S, Okuno G, Ikura Y, Tanaka T, Suda M, Nishikawa M. (1965) Phosphofructokinase deficiency in skeletal muscle: a new type of glycogenosis. *Biochem Biophys Res Comm* 19: 517–523.

Thon VJ, Khalil M, Cannon JF. (1993) Isolation of human glycogen branching enzyme cDNAs by screening complementation in yeast. *J Biol Chem* 268: 7509–7513.

Tonin P, Shanske S, Miranda AF, et al. (1993) Phosphoglycerate kinase deficiency: biochemical and molecular genetic studies in a new myopathic variant (PGK Alberta). *Neurology* 43: 387–391.

Toscano A, Tsujino S, Vita G, Shanske S, Messina C, DiMauro S. (1996) Molecular basis of muscle phosphoglycerate mutase (PGAM-M) deficiency in the Italian kindred. *Muscle Nerve* 19: 1134–1137.

Tsujibo H, Tiano HF, Li SS-L. (1985) Nucleotide sequences of the cDNA and an intronless pseudogene for human lactate dehydrogenase-A isozyme. *Eur J Biochem* 147: 9–15.

Tsujino S, Sakoda S, Mizuno R, et al. (1989) Structure of the gene encoding the muscle-specific subunit of human phosphoglycerate mutase. *J Biol Chem* 264: 15334–15337.

Tsujino S, Shanske S, DiMauro S. (1993a) Molecular genetic heterogeneity of myophosphorylase deficiency (McArdle's disease). *N Engl J Med* 329: 241–245.

Tsujino S, Shanske S, Sakoda S, Fenichel G, DiMauro S. (1993b) The molecular genetic basis of muscle phosphoglycerate mutase (PGAM) deficiency. *Am J Human Genet* 52: 472–477.

Tsujino S, Tonin P, Shanske S, et al. (1994a) A splice junction mutation in a new myopathic variant of phosphoglycerate kinase deficiency (PGK North Carolina). *Ann Neurol* 35: 349–353.

Tsujino S, Shanske S, Brownell AKW, Haller RG, DiMauro S. (1994b) Molecular genetic studies of muscle lactate dehydrogenase deficiency in white patients. *Ann Neurol* 36: 661–665.

Tsujino S, Shanske S, DiMauro S. (1995a) Molecular genetic heterogeneity of phosphoglycerate kinase (PGK) deficiency. *Muscle Nerve Suppl* 3: S45–S49.

Tsujino S, Shanske S, Sakoda S, Toscano A, DiMauro S. (1995b) Molecular genetic studies in muscle phosphoglycerate mutase (PGAM-M) deficiency. *Muscle Nerve Suppl* 3: S50–S53.

Van Noort G, Straks W, van Diggelen OP, Hennekam RCM. (1993) A congenital variant of glycogenosis type IV. *Pediatr Pathol* 13: 685–698.

Vita G, Toscano A, Bresolin N, et al. (1990) Muscle phosphoglycerate mutase (PGAM) deficiency in the first Caucasian patient. *Neurology* 40: 297 (abstract).

Vora S. (1982) Isozymes: isozymes of phosphofructokinase. *Curr Top Biol Med Res* 6: 119–167.

Vora S, Hong F, Olender E. (1982) Isolation of a cDNA for human muscle 6-phosphofructokinase. *Biochem Biophys Res Comm* 135: 615–621.

Wehner M, Clemens PR, Engel AG, Kilimann MW. (1994) Human muscle glycogenosis due to phosphorylase kinase deficiency associated with a nonsense mutation in the muscle isoform of the alpha subunit. *Hum Mol Genet* 3: 1983–1987.

Wehner M, Kilimann MW. (1995) Human cDNA encoding the muscle isoform of the phosphorylase kinase gamma subunit (PHKG1). *Hum Genet* 96: 616–618.

Willard HF, Goss SJ, Holmes MT, Munroe DL. (1985) Regional localization of the phosphoglycerate kinase gene and pseudogene on the human X chromosome and assignment of a related DNA sequence to chromosome 19. *Hum Genet* 71: 138–143.

Wilkinson DA, Tonin P, Shanske S, Lombes A, Carlson GM, DiMauro S. (1994) Clinical and biochemical features of 10 adult patients with muscle phosphorylase kinase deficiency. *Neurology* 44: 461–466.

Wullrich A, Hamacher C, Schneider A, Kilimann MW. (1993) The multiphosphorylation domain of the phosphorylase kinase alpha M and alpha L subunits is a hotspot of differential mRNA processing and of molecular evolution. *J Biol Chem* 268: 23208–23214.

Wullrich-Schmoll A, Kilimann MW. (1996) Structure of the human gene encoding the phosphorylase kinase beta subunit (PHKB). *Eur J Biochem* 238: 374–380.

Yamasaki T, Nakajima H, Kono N, et al. (1991) Structure of the entire human muscle phosphofructokinase-encoding gene: a two promoter system. *Gene* 104: 277–282.

Yang BZ, Ding JH, Enghild JJ, Bao Y, Chen YT. (1992) Molecular cloning and nucleotide sequence of cDNA encoding human muscle glycogen debranching enzyme. *J Biol Chem* 267: 9294–9299.

Yang-Feng TL, Zheng K, Yu J, Yang BZ, Chen YT, Kao FT. (1992) Assignment of the human glycogen debrancher gene to chromosome 1p21. *Genomics* 13: 931–934.

Yoshikuni K, Tagami H, Yamada M, Sudo K, Kanno T. (1986) Erythematosquamous skin lesions in hereditary lactate dehydrogenase M-subunit deficiency. *Arch Dermatol* 122: 1420–1424.

Zellweger H, Mueller S, Ionanescu V, Schochet SS, McCormick WF. (1972) Glycogenosis IV: a new cause of infantile hypotonia. *J Pediatr* 80: 842–844.

16

Neuromuscular aspects of fatigue associated with physical exertion

William J. Kraemer, Jeff S. Volek, Brandon K. Doan,
Robbin B. Wickham and Robert U. Newton

Introduction

Muscular fatigue is the inability to do work or maintain power over a desired period of time. Physical fitness and age can impact these capabilities. Figure 16.1 shows the power output over 60 s in anaerobically fit and untrained men in maintenance of cycle power output. Age, physical fitness, disease state, and/or inherent genetic predisposition can all affect the ability to produce muscular force over time. In Figure 16.1 it can be observed that the fit subjects are better able to maintain a higher level of power output, especially over the last 20 s of the 60 s maximal cycle test. The fatigue involved with this task is also dependent upon the ability to tolerate dramatic acid–base disruption paramount to performance of such tasks. As will become obvious in this chapter, fatigue is a multifactorial phenomenon, which makes the concept of "fatigue" dependent upon the specific context of task, its demands, and the inherent capabilities of an individual.

Every individual will have limits in the ability to perform work. With this comes the question in one form or another "What limits our capacity to perform work? or What causes fatigue?" Virtually all organisms experience some form of fatigue as a result of every day demands, and under unusual circumstances of stress (planned or unplanned) more extreme physical demands and fatigue can result.

A brief historical view of fatigue

Historically, fatigue has been defined many different ways. Early work by scientists in the field of psycho-

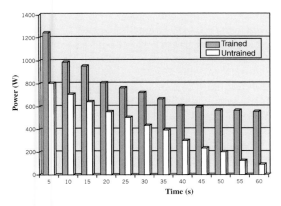

Figure 16.1 — Power output in a maximal cycle exercise task performed with no pacing by anaerobic-trained athletes (n = 15) and untrained men (n = 15). The power output (W) was significantly (p < 0.05) higher at all time points (unpublished data from Dr Kraemer's laboratory).

logy described fatigue in terms of three basic aspects: work decrement, physiological effects and feelings of weariness (Bartley and Chute 1947). Such descriptions contributed to a theory that fatigue may be an "early warning sign" against physiological damage if physical work was continued (Bartley and Chute 1947). A more quantitative definition of fatigue has been the inability to maintain force output leading to reductions in physical performance (Simonson 1971, Asmussen 1979, Edwards 1983). Further operational definitions also included the inability to maintain power output (Edwards 1983, Fitts 1994). Power output remains a crucial aspect of physical performance, even in everyday activities, as time can become an important component of successful performance. As seen in Figure 16.1, the ability of a trained anaerobic athlete to produce greater power and maintain it at a higher level under conditions of anaerobic acidosis allows the athlete a distinct advantage in such performances. To a certain extent physical conditioning allows an individual to improve their ability to fight a specific form of fatigue using specific conditioning programmes related to the needs of the task (Kraemer et al 1995a).

Mosso was one of the pioneers in human fatigue research in the 1890s. He studied individual fatigue curves, and he speculated that all fatigue was of nervous origin. By the mid 1900s, however, experiments with individual muscles revealed peripheral as well as central mechanisms of fatigue, leading to controversy that continued into the present day (Ikai et al 1967, Bigland-Ritchie et al 1978, Edwards 1983, Enoka and Stuart 1992). What has fuelled this controversy is again the multifactorial origin of fatigue in addition to its specificity to the task. Fatigue is a complex phenomenon, and, despite being a highly researched topic, it remains far from being understood as a general phenomenon (Fitts 1994). Perhaps more importantly, fatigue has been shown to depend greatly on the characteristics of the stimulus including variations in the type, intensity and duration of activity. The late Professor Lawrence Henderson of the famed Harvard University "Fatigue Lab" once said, "The beauty of it is that business leaders, engineers, physiologists, and the general public will all agree about the importance of fatigue in spite of the fact that there is no agreement about what the word is supposed to mean" (Simonson 1971).

Fatigue and a reduction in performance

Fatigue may be described best as a reduction in performance capacity due to the inability to maintain the necessary force or power output during a given time period (Asmussen 1979, Kirkendall 1990, McLeser 1997). As was alluded to above, the events that contribute to local muscular fatigue are of central and/or peripheral origins. Scientists have debated as to whether central or peripheral factors play the larger role in muscle fatigue. Merton (1954) attributed the decline in muscular performance to changes in the muscle itself. Krnjevic and Miledi (1958) and Stephens and Taylor (1972), however, proposed neuromuscular transmission as the primary culprit in the development of muscle fatigue. Neuromuscular transmission includes everything from the release of the neurotransmitter from the nerve ending to the neurotransmitter binding at the postsynaptic sarcolemma (Deschenes et al 1994b). In addition, Deschenes et al (1993) had shown that the neuromuscular junction was differentially adaptive to higher and lower intensity types of exercise training. Using the rat model, the investigators showed that physical conditioning at higher intensities of exercise, alters the neuromuscular junction with increases in neurotransmitter concentrations, gutter surface area, and amount of neural branching. Thus, the ability to address the neurological demands of an exercise stimulus involves adaptive changes, with training, in morphological structures in the nervous system.

Central fatigue versus peripheral fatigue theories

Central fatigue results from a decline in motor drive (i.e., nervous system) or lack of motivation (psychological effects). This may be associated with decreased excitatory input to the motor cortex, decreased firing rates from the motor cortex to the lower motor neuron and/or decreased alpha motor neuron excitability (Merton 1954, Bigland-Ritchie et al 1978). Conversely, peripheral fatigue results from alterations in the neuromuscular junction, muscle cell membrane, T-tubules, sarcoplasmic reticulum (calcium release and uptake) or pH (Westerblad et al 1991, Sahlin 1992, McLeser 1997). Other peripheral factors include uncoupling of excitation and contraction, changes in the contractile mechanism, lack of metabolic substrate availability, and failure to adequately clear metabolic by-products (Fitts 1994). In addition, changes in the acid–base status (i.e., increases in concentrations of lactate and hydrogen ions) also contribute to fatigue

and reduction in power output, but they can also be responsible for stimulating repair signals (i.e., increases in concentrations of growth hormone) following the exercise stress (Gordon et al 1994).

Despite the historical controversies, it is now generally accepted that central and peripheral factors may contribute to fatigue in varying degrees depending on the activity characteristics. Thus, fatigue may originate anywhere along the neuromuscular system, from the brain down to the contractile units in the activated muscles themselves. Ultimately, the intensity and duration of the exercise (Green 1997, McLeser 1997), type of muscle action performed (Tesch et al 1990), environmental conditions (Roberts and Smith 1989, Gordon et al 1994) and the fitness level of the individual (Roberts and Smith 1989) will influence the magnitude and timing of fatigue.

Influence of muscle fibre types

The muscle fibre type also plays a role in the development of muscle fatigue. In the untrained state Type IIX fibres (also called IIB) have well developed sarcoplasmic reticulum (SR) and high ATPase activity, but relatively lower oxidative capacity. Therefore, Type IIX fibres fatigue rapidly and they are highly dependent on ATP availability via the glycolytic energy pathway. A lack of substrate availability could reduce the intracellular concentration of the phosphagen, phosphocreatine (PCr), thus limiting the regeneration of ATP. The importance of this fatigue process has been indirectly supported with the recent efficacy of "creatine" supplementation to offset this type of phosphagen-related fatigue processes in Type II muscle fibres during repetitive high intensity exercise challenges (for reviews see Volek and Kraemer 1996, Kraemer and Volek 1999).

Interestingly, there is a transition of myosin-ATPase muscle fibre subtypes going from Type IIX to IIA/X to Type IIA muscle fibres with the activation of motor units as a result of exercise training (Staron et al 1994, Kraemer et al 1995b). In fact, few if any Type IIX fibres remain in a biopsy sample after 12 or more weeks of training (Adams et al 1993, Kraemer et al 1995b). The enhanced ability for performance capabilities in a variety of high-intensity fatigue-related tasks (e.g., strength, repeated muscle actions) has been shown to be associated with these changes (Staron et al 1994, Kraemer et al 1995b). This may be due to the greater plasticity (i.e., functional abilities, improved structures) of the motor units to produce force and recover more quickly (e.g., increased oxidative capacity) with enhanced enzyme and structural improvements in the contractile unit. The concept of enhanced quality and quantity of proteins (e.g., changes in myosin heavy chain proteins, more myofibrillar proteins, increased enzyme concentrations) as a result of physical conditioning presents an interesting case for the role of peripheral fatigue in work tasks. In addition, Staron et al (1994) have shown that many of these changes in muscle (e.g., ATPase fibre changes) occur within several workouts, making the rapid plasticity of the muscle paramount in responding to physical work demands and the associated fatigue. Figure 16.2 demonstrates the rapid changes that occur with heavy resistance training in the myosin-ATPase Type IIB fibre subtype (Staron et al 1994). Within the first week after only two training sessions, significant changes were demonstrated.

Type I (slow oxidative, SO) fibres have greater mitochondrial content and less developed SR, and upon activation they rely for the most part on oxidative energy pathways to supply energy via ATP. They do not produce the magnitude of force that the Type II muscle fibres can produce, but because of both quicker neurological recovery capabilities and aerobic

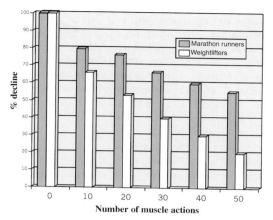

Figure 16.3 — Percentage decline from peak torque over 50 muscle actions for isokinetic concentric knee extensor muscle actions at $180°\ s^{-1}$ in marathon runners (n = 8) compared with weightlifters (n = 10). Weightlifters had significantly ($p < 0.05$) higher peak torque than marathon runners but percentage decline at each time point was significantly greater for the wrestlers (unpublished data from Dr Kraemer's laboratory).

energy-related functions, they can produce or maintain force at lower levels without as great a drop off. Figure 16.3 shows the comparison of marathon runners with Olympic-style weightlifters in repetitive concentric isokinetic knee extensions at $180°\ s^{-1}$ (Kraemer, unpublished observations). The Olympic-style weightlifters were capable of producing greater peak torque and torque values for each of the concentric muscle actions, but the percentage decline is significantly greater for the weightlifters over the 50 isokinetic knee extension muscle actions. The overt physical performance differences in these two athletic groups is most likely reflective of the inherent differences in muscle fibre type and training adaptations. This is also consistent with the differences in inherent single fibre or isolated muscle preparations between fast and slow twitch muscles. These characteristics confer greater resistance to maximal effort fatigue on Type I than on Type II muscle fibres.

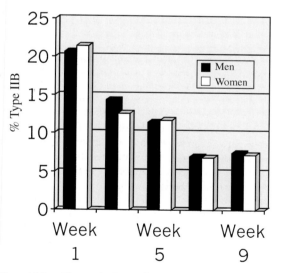

Figure 16.2 — Changes in the % of myosin ATPase Type IIB muscle fibre subtypes. Over the short term training program the percentage of Type IIB muscle fibres were significantly reduced with dramatic changes taking place in the first two weeks. The shift from the Type IIB fibre type toward Type IIA has been shown to occur due to activation of the motor unites with heavy resistance. As the muscle fibres are stimulated with exercise as shift in the isoform from Type IIB towards hybrids (Type IIaB, Type IIAB) occur workouts (adapted from Staron et al 1994).

Influence of the type of exercise challenge

The type of exercise plays a role in the magnitude and rate of development of fatigue. Different types of muscle actions will produce a decidedly different pattern of fatigue, as the type of force and power development is dependent upon the exercise modality (Knuttgen and Kraemer 1987). The type of exercise also configures the dimensional challenges of the physical and psychological stress. Exercise efforts can range from a single maximal effort in lifting a weight (e.g., one repetition maximum in the Olympic Clean & Jerk) to a sprint (e.g., 100 m, 200 m sprints) to an ultra-endurance event (e.g., marathon or ultra-marathon). In addition, a host of different combinations can be seen in sports and manual labour jobs. Here again we see that the sources of fatigue are potentially multifactorial in nature, and they can change over time leading to the concept of a "composite index" for overall fatigue during a day of work or sporting event (Kraemer et al 2000). No changes can be observed in physical performance, but increased perception of effort and fatigue is associated with the test (Kraemer et al 2000). Greater exercise intensity typically requires higher frequency of muscle actions along with the controlled sequences of motor units firing. Failure to propagate the action potential or delayed release of Ca^{2+} from the SR may contribute to development of fatigue in this type of exercise. Reliance on glycolytic pathways for energy production can lead to an increase in intracellular lactate, H+ and phosphate (P_i), which have been shown to decrease peak force development (Donaldson and Hermansen 1978, Fabiato and Fabiato 1978, Hermansen 1979, Nosek et al 1987). During prolonged submaximal exercise, aerobic processes fuel the cell by utilizing fat and carbohydrate energy substrates with some energy coming from protein. With endurance exercise, factors that may contribute to fatigue include depletion of energy substrates such as muscle glycogen stores and/or low blood glucose. In addition, the inability to optimally metabolize fat stores as an energy source for a longer period of time, prior to switching over to carbohydrate metabolism, has also been implicated in the rate of fatigue development in maintaining a higher percentage of maximal oxygen consumption for optimal performance (Maresh et al 1989).

The basic breakdown of functional components of the muscle is important to the understanding of muscle actions. Muscle tissue consists of two principle components:

1. the contractile component including the proteins that cause the muscle to produce force (i.e., actin and myosin proteins in myofibrils)

2. the non-contractile components (e.g., titin), including a series elastic component and a parallel elastic component, made up of proteins that do not contribute to the direct production of force but that can store elastic energy and maintain the structure of muscle. The primary non-contractile components are the muscle tendon, the connective tissue sheath and the sarcolemma.

The typical function of a skeletal muscle is to produce force through a joint involving eccentric (lengthening) muscle activity using gravity versus concentric (shortening) muscle activity against the force of gravity. In activated muscle, the contractile components shorten and thus stretch the elastic components in the cross-bridges, connective tissue and tendons. During concentric and eccentric muscle activity, motor units are recruited to develop force between bony attachments of muscle via cross-bridge interactions of actin and myosin filaments. Several types of muscle actions exist as well.

Isometric muscle activity

Isometric muscle activity is a state of muscle action in which there is no change in muscle length (Knuttgen and Kraemer 1987). The muscle itself does not produce enough force against mass to cause movement. This form of training has been shown to cause increases in strength, but it is related to the number of repetitions performed, the intensity of the muscle activity, and the frequency of training. The amount of force developed is directly related to the number of cross-bridge attachments. Although the amount of external work is normally calculated from the force multiplied by the distance, isometric muscle activity requires no mechanical work, but energy turnover is still required for cross-bridge interaction and, therefore, fatigue results from repetitive isometric exercise.

Concentric muscle activity

During concentric muscle activity, the contractile component shortens while stretching the series elastic component (Knuttgen and Kraemer 1987). A concentric muscle action is a dynamic activity in which force generation brings the bony attachments closer together.

The myosin heads must constantly adjust to actin sites at different inter-filament distances depending upon the rate of movement and the force during active muscle states. The power generated in repetitive movement cycles may include a variable time delay or recovery period as the muscle is returned to a starting position prior to an additional concentric muscle action. The potential power capability of muscle during concentric muscle activity depends upon a dynamic interaction between neural recruitment, muscle excitation-coupling process, and metabolic sources of ATP production.

Eccentric muscle activity

Eccentric muscle action involves muscular activity in which the muscle is forcibly lengthened. Elongation of the muscle is controlled by the activity of contractile components, stretching of the parallel elastic component, and the series elastic component during eccentric action.

The main contribution of net force during an eccentric muscle action is generated by the elastic components rather than the contractile components. Thus, maximum force produced by eccentric muscle action will be greater than that of concentric muscle action for a given muscle because of the increased internal muscle force production. During eccentric muscle activity, the muscle is lengthening, which stretches the non-contractile tissue.

Eccentric muscle activity involves physiological properties of muscle which maintain force during the stretch–shortening cycle. For muscle actions involving a combination of concentric and eccentric activity, eccentric action will typically precede the concentric activity during movement.

The greatest amount of force that can be developed is with an eccentric muscle action at high velocity. This maximal force declines with concentric muscle activity at a high velocity. Bigland and Lippold (1954) first studied electromyographic (EMG) muscular activity, and they found a linear relationship to the force exerted during voluntary isometric activity. Electrical activity in the muscle at a constant velocity of shortening or lengthening is directly proportional to the force. During lengthening, the correlation of this slope declines indicating that the degree of muscle activity required to produce a given force is less when the muscle is lengthened than when shortened at the same velocity. Cavagna et al (1975) also suggested more efficient usage of chemical energy by the contractile component that has been previously stretched. Thus, during eccentric muscle activity, potential energy stored in the elastic components of the muscle can result in greater mechanical efficiency and enhance the peak torque production during accelerated movement.

While the general trend observed in the classic force velocity curve typically holds true, it is interesting to note that the magnitude of such differences in force production between the concentric and eccentric muscle actions for force production is a function of many different variables including the tests conditions (voluntary vs involuntary), in vivo vs in vitro testing, joint tested, and mode of testing (e.g., isokinetic). For example, in voluntary human movements of the knee joint the magnitude of differences in torque values from fast eccentric velocities to slow concentric torque values may not show the magnitude of differences observed in force velocity curves created in the laboratory with stimulation of isolated muscle preparations.

Central fatigue

Central fatigue refers to one of three different phenomena: decreased excitatory input to the motor cortex, decreased excitatory drive to the lower motor neuron, or decreased excitability of the motor neuron itself. Prior to the 1950s, scientists believed the motor cortex was incapable of activating all motor units during a voluntary maximal contraction. In 1954, however, two independent laboratories reported force outputs equal to those generated during supramaximal electrical stimulation during voluntary contraction of the adductor pollicis muscle (Bigland and Lippold 1954, Merton 1954). Highly motivated subjects could even maintain full activation in the presence of fatigue during sustained maximal contraction up to 3 min (Merton 1954).

Interestingly, during long-duration activity requiring submaximal muscle actions, subjects were unable to generate maximal force output voluntarily as indicated by an increase in the force output when a supramaximal burst of electrical stimulation was superimposed on the voluntary maximal contraction (Bigland-Ritchie et al 1978). Therefore, decline in motor drive may indeed play a role in the decrements in performance during prolonged activity. Additionally, during prolonged activity the rate of motor neuron firing declines proportional to the decline in maximal force-generating capacity (Deschenes et al 1994a). High-frequency stimulation results in a more rapid decline in force production, thus, it is obvious that the firing rate is modulated to prolong the onset of fatigue. The CNS regulates motor neuron drive to maintain force output as the contractile properties of the motor unit change via an unknown mechanism.

Peripheral fatigue

Excitation–contraction coupling

Evidence that the mechanism of fatigue development involves excitation–contraction coupling is twofold. First, contraction and relaxation times are prolonged in whole muscle as well as single fibre preparations in the fatigued state (Gordon et al 1990, Thompson et al 1992). Also, the rate of tension development and the maximal shortening velocity are reduced in the fatigued state (Burst 1964, Fitts and Holloszy 1978, Edman and Mattiazzi 1981).

Failure to transmit the rapidly arriving neuronal signal to the interior of the cell has been termed high-frequency fatigue. High-frequency fatigue has been attributed to an inability to restore the electrochemical gradient across the sarcolemma prior to arrival of the next neural impulse (Clausen and Nielsen 1994). With the loss of K^+ from the interior of the cell, the cell becomes hyperpolarized making it more difficult to bring the transmembrane potential to the threshold necessary to elicit an action potential. The SR could also play a role in fatigue. Although one cannot directly measure $[Ca^{2+}]$ in the muscle fibre during repetitive activity, in vitro experiments with intact single fibres have demonstrated decreased force corresponding to decreased cytosolic $[Ca^{2+}]$ (Allen et al 1995). Reduced $[Ca^{2+}]$ may result from reduced release of Ca^{2+} from the SR. Other evidence pointing to the involvement of the SR and $[Ca^{2+}]$ in fatigue includes depressed Ca^{2+} uptake and lower Ca^{2+} ATPase activity during high intensity activity leading to reduced Ca^{2+} in the SR lumen.

Another potential explanation of the reduced force output observed with fatigue is a reduced sensitivity to Ca^{2+} by the myofibrillar apparatus. If a higher $[Ca^{2+}]$ is required to cause the conformational change in the tropomyosin that will reveal the binding sites on the actin filament, force production will decline (Fitts 1994, Allen et al 1995). The rate of cross-bridge cycling depends on myosin-ATPase activity. During intense activity, reduced myosin-ATPase activity has been shown.

Sarcolemma end T-tubule action potential

Some proportion of fatigue effects may result from alterations in membrane excitability caused by exercise-induced increases in $[K^+]$. Early studies reported no decrease in the sarcolemma action potential amplitude recorded from surface electrodes (Merton 1954). More recent studies have found reduced EMG amplitude in conjunction with a reduction in muscle force. However, what is important is whether or not changes in the amplitude of the action potential have a significant impact on force production. Sandow stated that the action potential might decrease with no effect on force production, providing evidence of an action-potential safety factor. However, if the action potential is a limiting factor, the T-tubule is the next possible location for response to fatigue.

The T-tubules allow propagation of the action potential from the sarcolemma into the muscle fibre (Huxley 1971). It found slower muscle-fibre repolarization following a decrease in extracellular $[K^+]$, which led to determination of the idea that the late afterpotential following tetanus was caused by K^+ accumulation in T-tubules. However, it is unclear whether the T-tubular ionic environment changes with fatigue. Several studies indicate varying concentrations of Na^+, Ca^{2+} and K^+ ions within the T-tubules in fatigued muscle (Fitts 1994).

Stretch–shortening cycle and fatigue

Several investigations on fatigue have examined stretch–shortening cycle movements. The stretch–shortening cycle is a movement sequence that is very common in human and animal motion. There is a counter movement during which the muscles involved are first stretched and then shortened to accelerate the body or limb. This sequence results in 18–20% greater impulse during the concentric phase, which enhances performance compared with a purely concentric movement (Bosco et al 1982). There are several mechanisms proposed to explain this effect (Walshe et al 1998) one of which is the storage and recovery of elastic strain energy. Although this mechanism is not a primary factor in single efforts, such as jumping or throwing, it has a major contribution to energy efficiency over repeated cycles, such as occurs during walking and running. Investigation by Avela and Komi (1998) revealed that the decreased muscle performance associated with prolonged stretch–shortening cycle movements is not only a result of central or peripheral fatigue but also of impairment of the ability to utilize stiffness-related elastic energy. They found that fatigue induced a decrease in maximal stretch–shortening cycle performance, a decreased short latency stretch-reflex sensitivity and a reduced eccentric stiffness of the muscle. Additionally, subjects with a greater percentage of fast-twitch fibres have been shown to use a greater percentage of elastic energy than subjects with a higher proportion of slow-twitch fibres. Fatigue of the fast-twitch fibres may decrease the rate of cross-bridge attachment–detachment cycle, allowing a longer relative time period for re-use of stored elastic energy and, thus, reducing the amount of energy recovered (Bosco et al 1986).

Metabolic by-products

At exercise intensities greater than 70% of VO_{2max}, glycolytic activity is high, as is the production of lactic acid and subsequently H^+ (Roberts and Smith 1989, Gordon et al 1994). Tesch et al (1978) and Karlsson et al (1975) have reported decreased force output in proportion to rising lactate and H^+ concentrations. In particular, highly-glycolytic fast-twitch muscle fibres (Type IIx) appear most affected (Tesch et al 1978, 1990). Several mechanisms have been proposed that may partially explain these effects. A decrease in muscle pH may indirectly alter uptake and release of Ca^{2+} by the SR (Nakamaru and Scwartz 1972, Williams et al 1998), reduce Ca^{2+} affinity for troponin (Fabiato and Fabiato 1978), inhibit phosphofructokinase, limit energy supply and exacerbate the high concentrations of inorganic phosphate (McLeser 1997). In addition, lactate itself may depress force production by inhibiting Ca^{2+} release from the SR (Spangenburg et al 1998).

The role of lactic acid in muscle fatigue is not necessarily direct; it is in fact the breakdown products of lactic acid that may disrupt muscle activity. Lactic acid is known to increase in the exercising skeletal muscle during intense exercise (>85% VO_{2max}) and intermittent maximal exercise. Lactic acid is quickly broken down into lactate and H^+, which are then removed from the muscle via transporters and either electrostatic gradients or various buffering compounds, respectively. The build-up of H^+ reduces the local pH of the muscle resulting in a more acidic environment in which certain enzymes, essential to muscle contraction, may fail to function properly. More significant, H^+ ions are theorized to interfere spatially (i.e., get in the way) with the basic skeletal muscle contraction mechanism by occupying the Ca^{2+} binding site on troponin, thereby reducing the ability of muscle to contract. Studies using intermittent maximal exercise have shown reduced force production and peak power output during exercise with concomitant high H^+ concentrations (Gordon et al 1994, Kraemer et al 1995).

Fatigue following concentric versus eccentric exercise

The mode of muscle action influences the fatigue pattern observed during physical activity. Concentric muscle actions show greater force decline when compared with eccentric muscle actions (Gray and Chandler 1989, Tesch et al 1990, Bilcheck et al 1993). Such increased magnitude of force loss during concentric contraction has been attributed to the greater motor unit recruitment needed to produce a given force (Rodgers and Berger 1974) with a concomitant increase in substrate utilization (Knuttgen et al 1971).

The onset of fatigue is also delayed during eccentric muscle actions. Studies have reported no change in eccentric force production during isokinetic testing, while concentric force declined 34–48% (Gray and Chandler 1989, Tesch et al 1990, Bilcheck et al 1993). The series elastic components within the muscle store energy when the muscle is lengthened, and thus they may facilitate maintenance of force during eccentric contractions despite a decline in concentric force (Tesch et al 1990). In addition, the velocity of the exercise plays an important role in the development of fatigue. Komi and Viitasalo (1977) reported larger declines in force over a series of eccentric contractions during slow-velocity isokinetic testing. In addition, high force exercise of the same total work has been shown to produce greater concentrations of blood lactate (Bush et al 1999). Peripheral mechanisms have been implicated in the decline in force with eccentric exercise because the declines in force are not accompanied by changes in integrated electromyography (IEMG) (Tesch et al 1990).

It appears that the same mechanisms that allow greater force production during eccentric contractions also ameliorate the development of fatigue during eccentric contractions. Since relative intensity of an eccentric contraction is reduced compared with concentric contraction, ATP use, the rate of cross-bridge cycling, and production of metabolic by-products (H^+, P_i, lactate and ADP) are decreased (Knuttgen et al 1971, Rodgers and Berger 1974, Tesch et al 1990). Therefore, a greater exercise intensity is necessary to induce fatigue during eccentric activity. Motor units with Type II muscle fibres were found to be preferentially recruited during eccentric training at maximal levels (Friden et al 1983). The biomechanical troponin structure in the Type II muscle fibres may be able to generate an increased rate of Ca^{2+} uptake due to the enlargement of the SR. Thus, the rate of uptake by the Ca^{2+} by the sarcoplasmic reticulum via the Ca^{2+}-ATPase pump may be faster in the Type II fibre.

However, high level of eccentric force results in a significant amount of muscle tissue damage following the acute effort (Clarkson and Tremblay 1988, Clarkson and Sayers 1999).

Overtraining: a model for chronic fatigue

Fatigue not only takes place in the acute sense of performance but also it can be developed chronically as well. A model for this inability to produce the same maximal force or power output can be seen with "overtraining". Overtraining is a reduction in performance that ultimately represents a chronic level of fatigue. The most common mistake made in training related to this type of fatigue is likely related to the "rate of progression". If mechanical and chemical loads are created that damage the fundamental morphological structures involved with the adaptational changes (e.g., increased muscle size) required for improved performance, overtraining can occur rapidly. The morphological damage of vital structures results in a decrease in performance. Thus, acute overtraining can be related to acute tissue damage and the inability to adequately repair over time. Overtraining could arise from mistakes in exercise prescription for physical conditioning.

High force production overtraining models

It must be realized that only a few studies have been performed that have been able to examine various types of overtraining models in the laboratory. Furthermore, the intentional improper programming needed to create a chronic fatigue related to performance has not been easily accomplished in the laboratory environment. A few comments as it relates to fatigue are instructive in order to see that the performance of too much work, or rapid changes in intensity or volume of exercise, can create the type of chronic fatigue related to physical conditioning.

In a study by Callister et al (1990) it was first demonstrated that anaerobic training may present a different set of symptoms than endurance overtraining studies. The investigator in this study increased the volume of resistance training, run training, and practice in U.S. national level judo athletes over a six week programme, and the expected increases in resting heart rate or blood pressure (halter-monitored) did not occur. What these investigators observed were significantly decreased performances in a set of 300 m sprint performance times and decreases in isokinetic force production. Furthermore, the resistance training performed was not effective in showing any signs of enhancing maximal strength (i.e., one repetition maximum; 1 RM) performances, thus, indicating a type of chronic fatigue had set in.

In two studies by Fry et al (1994a, 1994b), it also becomes obvious that, in order to create a successful intensity-specific overtraining protocol for the laboratory, certain factors were needed that would create a reduction in performance or chronic fatigue. In the first attempt (Fry et al 1994a), the importance of rest on the development of an intensity-specific overtraining model was discovered. Recreationally strength-trained men performed, after warm-up, eight sets of machine-squats at 95% of 1 RM. In this protocol Sunday was utilized for rest after 6 days of overtraining. No reduction in the 1 RM performance was observed. What did result were non-specific performance decrements in isolated knee joint isokinetic torque production at $60°\,s^{-1}$, and increases in sprint times and agility speed to the non-dominant side. Therefore, it was discovered that the body protects the high force production of the 1 RM and the use of one day of rest appeared to enhance the toleration of the short-term protocol. Thus, the importance of rest and recovery, as programmed into the theoretical development of periodization of training models, was shown in this study to be a vital principle to effective training to avoid chronic fatigue. In fact, more than one day's rest may be needed to eliminate peripheral sources of fatigue, and the decrements in peripheral performances loom as caution that something was still being negatively affected by the overtraining protocol utilized in this investigation.

In the second study by Fry et al (1994b), the one day of rest was eliminated in the overtraining protocol and each subject was expected after warm-up sets to lift 10 sets of their 1 RM with a short rest between sets. This resulted in a significant decrease (>4.5 kg) in the 1 RM in 73% of the subjects. Chronic fatigue was produced in the laboratory model. The time-course of the physiological development of an overtraining condition or chronic fatigue condition is highly dependent upon individual responses and genetic endowment. While follow-up was not done, it was apparent that intensity-related overtraining would be difficult to carry on for extended periods of time because of the localized stress on the thigh musculature and knee joint. Nevertheless, this study showed that a relatively low volume exercise stress, but one with a high (100%+) relative intensity load, can cause chronic fatigue with associated reductions in physical performance.

The development of this intensity-overtraining model in the laboratory provided the first model to study this type of chronic fatigue or overtraining under controlled conditions. This allowed us to evaluate associated changes in the neuroendocrinological and neuromuscular environments in order to search for potential markers and mechanisms of action. Surprisingly, the neuroendocrine pattern did not follow what might have been expected from prior knowledge of the endurance overtraining studies (e.g., no decreases in resting testosterone or increases in resting cortisol were commonly observed). In fact, it might be theorized that the neuroendocrine responses were first line responses to fight the overtraining stress created by the exercise. Therefore, it might be speculated that in the initial stages of overtraining the body engages all of the potential repair processes it can to offset the extreme physical demands. If unable to cope with the alarm responses of the overtraining stressor of the body, and consistent with Selye's model of distress (1976), a reduction in the anabolic hormone and an increase catabolic hormone response will occur. Therefore, in high force and intensity-related overtraining or overreaching, a suppressed testosterone and elevated cortisol endocrine profile may actually follow the negative response in performance as a result of the inability of the endocrine system to obviate the physiological maladaptation associated with inappropriate exercise stimuli.

Fatigue interventions

Local muscular fatigue involves a series of protective mechanisms that decrease force production in response to intense muscle activity. The loss of force, although potentially necessary to limit muscular injury, is undesirable during certain situations (e.g., sport competition, physical working capacity on the job). As such, the scientific and medical communities have sought to elucidate the potential causes of fatigue so that interventions that may help maintain or improve physical performance could be implemented. For the most part physical conditioning programmes that may help limit the magnitude of fatigue have been classically instrumental in eliciting adaptations which improve the body's physical capacity to produce greater force for longer periods of time at lower perceptual efforts.

Meeting the demands of exercise stress

How much success an individual will have in meeting the challenges of the exercise stress, or in delaying the effects of various fatigue processes, will depend upon what psychological and physiological strategies the individual has available to them (Patton et al 1990). While physical training can impact the magnitude and enhance the individual's inherent abilities, it cannot effect changes at the gene level. Acutely, it is well known that not all individuals will show the same pattern of fatigue with a specific exercise task; this is related to genetic inheritance. The optimization of this ability is enhanced by training to better meet the demands. Similarly, as seen with overtraining, not all individuals are affected by a singular physical stress. In the extreme events and work tasks, such as a marathon race, if an elite performance level is set (e.g., 2 h 8 min for men or 2 h 20 min for women) only a limited number of individuals possess the myriad of physiological and psychological strategies needed to meet that elite physical challenge. A combination of factors would need to be present to fight the exercise-induced stress fatigue that would limit such performances. Consequently, fibre type, body mass, economy of running style, psychological toughness, heart size, etc. would all need to work together in order for an individual to run at that pace for just over 2 h. In the study by Patton et al (1990) it was realized that a discrete factor such as fibre type did not play that much of a role in power production when no performance level was set. In fact in the general population, body mass was the most predictive of maximal lower-body power output. Just as fatigue can come from a combined number of sources, so do the strategies that help to offset fatigue. Nevertheless, one must have the innate capabilities to meet a physical challenge presented.

Summary

Neuromuscular fatigue is characterized by the inability to maintain force production resulting in decrements in physical performance. For decades, athletes, coaches, medical practitioners and research scientists have sought to elucidate the potential causes of fatigue so that interventions that may help maintain or improve physical performance could be implemented. Such quests for a physiological basis of fatigue have led to the well-documented central and peripheral factor theories. Centrally-mediated fatigue has traditionally been described as fatigue resulting from reduced or altered sensory input or motor output within the central nervous system. On the other hand, peripheral fatigue may result from altered transmission or excitation of the peripheral neuromuscular components (e.g., neuromuscular junction, muscle cell membrane, contractile proteins) or changes in metabolic processes.

References

Adams GR, Hather BM, Baldwin KM, Dudley GA. (1993) Skeletal muscle myosin heavy chain composition and resistance training. *J Appl Physiol* 74(2): 911–915.

Allen DG, Lannergren J, Westerblad H. (1995) Muscle cell function during prolonged activity: Cellular mechanisms of fatigue. *Exp Physiol* 80: 497–527.

Asmussen E. (1979) Muscle fatigue. *Med Sci Sports Exerc* 11: 313–321.

Avela J, Komi PV. (1998) Interaction between muscle stiffness and stretch reflex sensitivity after long-term stretch-shortening cycle exercise. *Muscle Nerve* 21(9): 1224–1227.

Bartley SH, Chute E. (1947) *Fatigue and Impairment in Man.* New York: McGraw-Hill.

Bigland B, Lippold OCJ. (1954) Motor unit activity in the voluntary contractions of human muscle. *J Physiol Lond* 125: 322–335.

Bigland-Ritchie B, Jones DA, Hosking GP, Edwards RHT. (1978) Central and peripheral fatigue in sustained maximum voluntary contractions of human quadriceps muscle. *Clin Sci Mol Med* 54: 609–614.

Bigland-Ritchie B, Furbush F, Woods JJ. (1986) Fatigue of intermittent submaximal voluntary contractions: central and peripheral factors. *J Appl Physiol* 61: 421–429.

Bilcheck HM, Kraemer WJ, Maresh C, Zito MA. (1993) The effects of isokinetic fatigue on recovery of maximal isokinetic concentric and eccentric strength in women. *J Strength Cond Res* 7(1): 43–50.

Bosco C, Viitasalo JT, Komi PV, Luhtanen P. (1982) Combined effect of elastic energy and myoelectrical potentiation during stretch-shortening cycle exercise. *Acta Physiol Scand* 114: 557–565.

Bosco C, Tihanyi J, Latteri F, Fekete G, Apor P, Rusko H. (1986) The effect of fatigue of store and re-use of elastic energy in slow and fast types of human skeletal muscle. *Acta Physiol Scand* 128(1): 109–117.

Burst M. (1964) Changes in contractility of frog muscle due to fatigue and inhibitors. *Am J Physiol* 206: 1043–1048.

Bush JA, Kraemer WJ, Mastro AM, et al. (1999) Exercise and recovery responses of adrenal medullary neurohormones to heavy resistance exercise. *Med Sci Sports Exerc* 31(4): 554–559.

Callister R, Callister RJ, Fleck SJ, Dudley GA. (1990) Physiological and performance responses to overtraining in elite judo athletes. *Med Sci Sports Exerc* 22(6): 816–824.

Cavagna G, Citterio J, Juaimi P. (1975) The additional mechanical energy delivered by the contractile component of a previously stretched muscle. *J Physiol* 251: 65.

Clarkson PM, Sayers SP. (1999) Etiology of exercise-induced muscle damage. *Can J Appl Physiol* 24: 234–248.

Clarkson PM, Tremblay I. (1988) Exercise induced muscle damage, repair, and adaptation in humans. *J Appl Physiol* 65: 1–6.

Clausen T, Nielsen OB. (1994) The Na^+, K^+ pump and muscle contractility. *Acta Physiol Scand* 152: 365–373.

Deschenes MR, Maresh CM, Crivello JF, Armstrong LE, Kraemer WJ, Covault J. (1993) The effects of exercise training of different intensities on neuromuscular junction morphology. *J Neurocytol* 22: 603–615.

Deschenes MR, Covault J, Kraemer WJ, Maresh CM. (1994a) The neuromuscular junction: Muscle fibre type differences, plasticity and adaptability to increased and decreased activity. *Sports Med* 17(6): 358–372.

Deschenes MR, Maresh CM, Kraemer WJ. (1994b) The neuromuscular junction: Structure, function, and its role in the excitation of muscle. *J Strength Cond Res* 8(2): 103–109.

Donaldson SK, Hermansen L. (1978) Differential, direct effects of H^+ and Ca^{2+} activated force of skinned fibres from the soleus, cardiac and adductor magnus muscle of rabbits. *Pfleugers Arch* 376: 55–65.

Edman KAP, Mattiazzi AR. (1981) Effects of fatigue and altered pH on isometric force and velocity of shortening at zero load in frog muscle fibres. *J Muscle Res Cell Motil* 2: 321–334.

Edwards RHT. (1983) Biochemical bases of fatigue in exercise performance: catastrophe theory of muscular fatigue. In: *Biochemistry of Exercise* (Knuttgen HG, ed.). Champaign, IL: Human Kinetics pp 3–28.

Emery L, Sitler M, Ryan J. (1994) Mode of action and angular velocity fatigue response of the hamstrings and quadriceps. *Isokinetic Exerc Sci* 4: 91–95.

Enoka RM, Stuart DG. (1992) Neurobiology of muscle fatigue. *J Appl Physiol* 72: 1631–1648.

Fabiato A, Fabiato F. (1978) Effects of pH on the myofilaments and the sarcoplasmic reticulum of skinned cells from cardiac and skeletal muscles. *J Physiol Lond* 276: 233–255.

Fitts RH, Holloszy JO. (1978) Effects of fatigue and recovery on contractile properties of frog muscle. *J Appl Physiol* 45: 899–902.

Fitts RH, Kim DH, Witzmann FA. (1981) The development of fatigue during high intensity and endurance exercise. In: *Exercise in Health and Disease* (Nagle NJ, Montoye HJ, eds). Thomas Press, Springfield, IL, pp. 118–135.

Fitts RH. (1994) Cellular mechanisms of muscle fatigue. *Physiol Reviews* 74(1): 49–94.

Friden J, Sergec J, Sjostrom M, Ekblom B. (1983) Adaptive response in human skeletal muscle to prolonged eccentric training. *Int J Sports Med* 4: 17–183.

Fry AC, Kraemer WJ, Lynch JM, Triplett NT, Koziris LP. (1994a) Does short-term near-maximal intensity machine resistance training induce overtraining. *J Stren Cond Res* 8(3): 188–191.

Fry AC, Kraemer WJ, Van Borselen F, et al. (1994b) Performance decrements with high-intensity resistance exercise overtraining. *Med Sci Sports Exerc* 26(9): 1165–1173.

Gordon SE, Kraemer WJ, Vos NH, Lynch JM, Knuttgen HG. (1994) Effect of acid-base balance on the growth hormone response to acute, high-intensity cycle exercise. *J Appl Physiol* 76(2): 821–829.

Gordon DA, Enoka RM, Karst GM, Stuart DG. (1990) Force development and relaxation in single motor units in adult cats during a standard fatigue test. *J Physiol Lond* 421: 583–594.

Gordon SE, Kraemer WJ, Vos NH, Lynch JM, Knuttgen HG. (1994) Effect of acid-base balance on the growth hormone response to acute, high-intensity cycle exercise. *J Appl Physiol* 76(2): 821–829.

Gray J, Chandler J. (1989) Percent decline in peak torque production during repeated concentric and eccentric contractions of the quadricepts femoris muscle. *J Orthop Sports Phys Ther* 6: 309–314.

Green HJ. (1997) Mechanisms of muscle fatigue in intense exercise. *J Sports Sci* 15: 247–256.

Hermansen L. (1979) Effects of acidosis on skeletal muscle performance during maximal exercise in man. *Bull Eur Physiopathol Respir* 15: 229–238.

Huxley HE. (1971) Structural changes during muscle contraction. *Biochem J* 124(4): 85.

Ikai M. (1967) Nippon Seingaku Zasshi 29(9): 517–522.

Karlsson J, Bonde-Petersen F, Henriksson F, Knuttgen H. (1975) Effects of previous exercise with arms or legs on metabolism and performance in exhaustive exercise. *J Appl Physiol* 38: 763–767.

Kellis E, Baltzopoulos V. (1995) Isokinetic eccentric exercise. *Sports Med* 19: 202–222.

Kirkendall DT. (1990) Mechanisms of peripheral fatigue. *Med Sci Sports Exerc* 22: 444–449.

Knuttgen H, Bonde-Peterson F, Klausen K. (1971) Oxygen uptake and heart rate response to exercise performed with concentric and eccentric muscle contractions. *Med Sci Sports Exerc* 3: 1–5.

Knuttgen HG, Kraemer WJ. (1987) Terminology and measurement in exercise performance. *J Appl Sport Sci Res* 1: 1–10.

Komi PV, Viitasalo JT. (1977) Changes in motor unit activity and metabolism in human skeletal muscle during and after repeated eccentric and concentric contractions. *Acta Physiol Scand* 100: 246–254.

Kraemer WJ, Gordon SE, Lynch JM, Pop M, Clark KL. (1995a) Effects of multibuffer supplementation on acid-base balance and 2,3 diphosphoglycerate following repetitive anaerobic exercise. *Intl J Sport Nutri* 5: 300–314.

Kraemer WJ, Patton J, Gordon SE, Harman EA, Deschenes MR, Reynolds K, Newton RU, Triplett NT, Dziados JE. (1995b) Compatibility of high intensity strength and

endurance training on hormonal and skeletal muscle adaptations. *J Appl Physiol* 78(3): 976–989.

Kraemer WJ, Piorkowski PA, Bush JA, et al. (2000) The effects of NCAA division 1 intercollegiate competitive tennis match play on recovery of physical performance in women. *J Strength Cond Res* 14(3): 265–327.

Kraemer WJ, Volek JS. (1999) Creatine Supplementation: Its Role in Human Performance. In: *Clinics in Sports Medicine* (Wheeler KB, Lombardo JA, eds.) 18(3): 651–666.

Krnjevic K, Miledi R. (1958) Failure of neuromuscular propagation in rats. *J Physiol Lond* 140: 440–461.

Maresh CM, Allison TG, Noble BJ, Drash A, Kraemer WJ. (1989) Substrate and hormone responses to exercise following a marathon run. *Intl J Sports Med* 10(2): 101–106.

McLeser JR. (1997) Muscle contraction and fatigue. The role of adenosine 5′-diphosphate and inorganic phosphate. *Sports Med* 23: 287–305.

Merton PA. (1954) Voluntary strength and fatigue. *J Physiol Lond* 123: 553–564.

Nakamaru Y, Scwartz A. (1972) The influence of hydrogen ion concentration on calcium binding and release by skeletal muscle sarcoplasmic reticulum. *J Gen Physiol* 59: 22–32.

Nosek TM, Fender KY, Godt RE. (1987) It is deprotonated inorganic phosphate that depresses force in skinned skeletal muscle fibres. *Science* 236: 191–193.

Patton JF, Kraemer WJ, Knuttgen HG, Harman EA. (1990) Factors in maximal power production and in exercise endurance relative to maximal power. *Eur J Appl Physiol* 60: 222–227.

Roberts D, Smith DJ. (1989) Biochemical aspects of peripheral muscle fatigue: a review. *Sports Med* 7: 125–138.

Rodgers K, Berger P. (1974) Motor unit involvement and tension during maximal, voluntary concentric, eccentric, and isometric contractions on elbow flexors. *Med Sci Sports Exerc* 8: 253–259.

Sahlin K. (1992) Metabolic factors in fatigue. *Sports Med* 13: 99–107.

Selye H. (1976) *The Stress of Life*. New York: McGraw-Hill.

Simonson E. (1971) *Physiology of Work Capacity and Fatigue*. Springfield, IL: Thomas.

Spangenburg EE, Ward CW, Williams JH. (1998) Effects of lactate on force production by mouse EDL muscle: implications for the development of fatigue. *Can J Physiol Pharmacol* 76: 642–648.

Staron RS, Karapondo DL, Kraemer WJ, et al. (1994) Skeletal muscle adaptations during the early phase of heavy-resistance training in men and women. *J Appl Physiol* 76(3): 1247–1255.

Stephens JA, Taylor A. (1972) Fatigue of maintained voluntary muscle contraction in man. *J Physiol Lond* 220: 1–18.

Tesch P, Sjodin B, Thorstensson A, Karlsson J. (1978) Muscle fatigue and its relation to lactate accumulation and LDH activity in man. *Acta Physiol Scand* 103: 413–420.

Tesch PA, Dudley GA, Duvoisin MR, Hather BM, Harris RT. (1990) Force and EMG signal patterns during repeated bouts of concentric or eccentric muscle actions. *Acta Physiol Scand* 138: 238–271.

Thompson LV, Balog EM, Riley DA, Fitts RH. (1992) Muscle fatigue in frog semitendinosis: alterations in contractile function. *Am J Physiol* 262: C1500–C1506.

Verdonck A, Frobose I, Hardelauf U, Guttge C. (1994) Contraction patterns during isokinetic eccentric and concentric contractions after anterior cruciate ligament injury. *Int J Sports Med* 15 (suppl.): S60–S63.

Volek JS, Kraemer WJ. (1996) Creatine supplementation: Its effect on human muscular performance and body composition. *J Strength Cond Res* 10 (3): 200–210.

Walshe AD, Wilson GJ, Ettema GJ. (1998) Stretch-shorten cycle compared with isometric preload: contributions to enhanced muscular performance. *J Appl Physiol* 84(1): 97–106.

Westerblad H, Lee JA, Lannergren J, Allen DG. (1991) Cellular mechanisms of fatigue in skeletal muscle. *Am J Physiol* 261: C195–C209.

Williams JH, Ward CW, Spangenburg EE, Nelson RM. (1998) Functional aspects of skeletal muscle contractile apparatus and sarcoplasmic reticulum after fatigue. *J Appl Physiol* 85: 619–626.

17

Alcoholic myopathy

Alistair Paice

Introduction

Alcohol is a serious health concern. In the USA alone it is estimated that 175 million people consume some sort of alcohol, and 10 million people have some sort of drinking problem (Snyder and Lader 1986). The simplest cure is abstinence, but this cannot be the sole aim for health management. Indeed, the same could be said of smoking and lung cancer, or sunbathing and skin cancer, but the results still have to be dealt with. In this chapter, I will give an overview of alcohol and the detrimental health considerations associated with its consumption. I will then focus on one particular pathological aspect—myopathy. I shall also mention two areas where research in this field is progressing—ribosomal alterations and apoptosis.

Definition and extent of ethanol misuse

The definition of excessive alcohol intakes varies with cultural, geographical and ethical factors. Daily intakes of greater than 150 g ethanol are often considered excessive because of the greater risk of dependence (Kendell 1979). However, 80 g ethanol per day may cause organ damage and some workers use this value. Women are more susceptible to liver damage from ethanol than men, so the corresponding figure for women would be closer to 60 g ethanol.

There are many explanations as to why individuals drink excessive amounts of alcohol. People often drink for social reasons – to counter loneliness or boredom, or because they like the taste or the effect. Alcoholism is thought to develop from the combined effects of psychological or biological vulnerability and of opportunity (Prescott et al 1994).

Agarwal (1996) reviews genetic determinants of alcoholism and alcohol abuse. Approaches used to investigate the influence of hereditary factors in alcoholism include family studies, twin studies, adoption studies and studies of high-risk groups. Family studies of the relatives of alcoholics have shown that rates of alcoholism are consistently higher than would be expected in the general population. Regardless of the nature of the population studied, an alcoholic is more likely to have a mother, father or a distant relative who is an alcoholic.

Twin studies have shown that there is some degree of genetic predisposition to alcoholism. For example, between monozygotic (MZ) and dizygotic (DZ) twins significant differences were found in concordance rates for alcohol misuse (74% vs 58%) and alcohol dependence (59% vs 36%).

Adoption studies have provided considerable evidence that alcoholism is genetically linked, especially in males. Devor and Cloninger (1989) showed that when adopted-away sons of an alcoholic parent were compared with siblings raised by the alcoholic biological parent, both groups had similar rates of alcoholism. However, studies in female adoptees did not produce similar results (Agarwal 1996).

Systemic effects of alcohol misuse

Chronic alcohol consumption has an association with increased morbidity from acute and chronic infection (Dal Nogare 1991). For example, chronic ethanol administration induced immunosuppression in mice sufficient to permit pulmonary infection with *Pneumocystis carnii* (D'Souza et al 1995). The effects of alcohol ingestion on the immune system are broad-ranging (MacGregor 1985).

Alcohol has been implicated in various cancers. Squamous cell carcinomas of the mouth, oral pharynx, larynx and oesophagus have been linked to alcohol consumption in multiple studies (Thomas 1995). The combined effects of smoking and alcohol are additive and probably mutiplicative, suggesting biological synergism (Andre et al 1995). Carstensen et al (1990) suggested that alcohol increases the risk of rectal cancer. In Japan, alcohol is a common risk factor for sigmoid colonic and rectal adenomas (Honjo et al 1995).

Alcohol also has effects on the hormonal system. Light to moderate drinking in men and women who are generally healthy is linked with enhanced insulin-mediated glucose uptake. There are lower plasma insulin and glucose levels in response to a given oral glucose load, and higher plasma high-density lipoprotein (HDL) levels (Facchini et al 1994). It has been proposed that the lower risk of coronary heart disease in this category of drinkers may be a result of changes in the HDL/LDL profile, although Emerson et al (1995) disputes this.

Organ-specific effects of alcohol abuse

Excessive ethanol consumption causes liver damage. Approximately 10% of chronic alcoholic patients with a history of 10 or more years of daily ingestion of 125 g ethanol showed histological evidence of cirrhosis. An increase in the incidence of cirrhosis is discernible when daily ethanol consumption exceeds 40 g/day (Lieber 1996). The incidence of hepatic damage is the result of the central role of the liver in blood alcohol metabolism. Over 90% of the ethanol absorbed is metabolized in the liver, and ethanol can cause up to 90% of the liver's normal metabolic substrates to be displaced (Lieber 1996). Three main pathways have been proposed for ethanol metabolism in the liver:

- the alcohol dehydrogenase (ADH) pathway
- via peroxisomal catalase
- the microsomal ethanol oxidizing system (MEOS).

All three pathways yield highly toxic acetaldehyde.

Alcohol consumption impairs the cognitive ability of the human brain. This is essentially a response to acute over-consumption. For example, a recent American study found that out of 168 fatally injured truck drivers involved in accidents in eight states over a one-year period, 13% had blood alcohol concentrations that would have impaired their judgement (Crouch et al 1993).

Alcohol is a teratogen. Fetal alcohol syndrome (FAS), predominantly characterized by fetal growth retardation, cardiac defects, mental retardation and limb abnormalities (Geva et al 1994), was identified in 1973. Ouellette et al (1977) showed that in one hospital 32% of infants born to heavy drinkers had congenital abnormalities, compared with 14% in the moderate drinking group and 9% in the abstinence group.

Alcohol has been linked to gastritis, or inflammation of the superficial gastric mucosa (Kumar and Clark 1996). It has been proposed that *Helicobacter pylori* bacteria in the stomach may be one of the causes (Salmela et al 1994).

Alcohol-induced myopathy

Approximately 50% of chronic alcohol misusers have a skeletal muscle myopathy characterized by a preferential decrease in the diameter of Type II skeletal muscle fibres (fast-twitch, anaerobic fibres that utilize glycolytic metabolism; Preedy et al 1994b). Type I fibres (slow twitch, aerobic, oxidative metabolism) are not overtly affected. Inflammation and fibrosis are not involved in the myopathy, and there is no evidence of direct neurological involvement or of liver disease (Preedy et al 1994b). Hypercortisolism is not responsible for the myopathy (Duane and Peters 1987). Alcohol-induced myopathy is also found in the hearts of ethanol misusers (Richardson et al 1986, Rubin and Urbano-Marquez 1994), with differing

responses to acute and chronic dosing (Preedy and Peters 1990c). Alcohol is toxic to both skeletal and cardiac muscle in humans in a dose-dependent manner (Urbano-Marquez et al 1989).

Rodent models have been developed to study the effects of ethanol on skeletal muscle (Preedy and Peters 1990a). In the rat model of chronic alcoholic myopathy, animals fed ethanol for 6 weeks showed the preferential protein loss in Type II fibres characteristic of the clinical condition. Strict pair-feeding regimes ensured changes were caused by the ethanol (and/or derived metabolites or metabolic changes) rather than malnutrition (Preedy et al 1989).

Effects of acute ethanol ingestion on skeletal muscle

Ethanol acutely inhibits glucose-stimulated glycogen deposition in the rat skeletal muscle, with specific targeting of the oxidative muscle (Xu et al 1993). Use of 4-methylpyrazole (an inhibitor of alcohol dehydrogenase) and disulfiram (an inhibitor of acetaldehyde dehydrogenase) shows that the ethanol molecule itself, and not a metabolite such as acetaldehyde, mediated the effect in glycogen metabolism. Acute ethanol dosing also disturbs basal and insulin-induced glucose utilization in rat skeletal muscles and heart (Spolarics et al 1994).

Protein synthesis was reduced in rat skeletal muscle 2.5 h after injection with an acute bolus of 75 mmol ethanol/kg body weight (Tiernan and Ward 1986). The reduction was approximately 30%, with Type II fibres showing a greater change than Type I (Preedy and Peters 1988a). These changes affected sarcoplasmic, stromal and myofibrillar protein fractions equally. Part of this effect was almost certainly a result of the toxicity of the acetaldehyde produced by ethanol metabolism, but ethanol itself seemed to have an independent inhibitory effect (Preedy et al 1992).

Effects of chronic ethanol ingestion on skeletal muscle

The targeting of Type II fibres by ethanol implicates anaerobic glycolytic pathway lesions in the myopathy. To investigate glycolytic deficiency in this condition,

Trouce et al (1990) assayed the activity of all the glycolytic enzymes. They found that the activities of aldolase, pyruvate kinase and lactate dehydrogenase were significantly reduced. Glycolytic insufficiency might explain why the Type II fibres undergo specific atrophy. In human muscle biopsies from chronic alcoholics, there was a reduction in the pyruvate kinase activity before the first signs of myopathy appeared (Vernet et al 1995). Haida et al (1998) found that chronic alcoholics with severe neurological symptoms had an abnormality in aerobic metabolism caused by muscle mitochondrial dysfunction.

Martin and Peters (1985) used urinary 3-methylhistidine/creatinine ratios to ascertain whether muscle protein breakdown was altered in chronic alcoholic patients, compared with non-myopathic alcoholics. There was a significant decrease in muscle breakdown. However, the tissue activities of a Ca^{2+}-induced protease were similar in both groups.

About 5% of chronic alcoholic patients present with frank rhabdomyolysis, defined as an injury to the sarcolemma of skeletal muscles resulting in leakage of muscle components in to the blood and urine (Knockel 1993). Damage to the sarcolemma causes increased sodium permeability facilitating cytosolic Ca^{2+} accumulation and causing cellular injury. The cellular sodium pumps respond by increasing Na^+ extrusion and hyperpolarizing the transmembrane potential (E_m). Once membrane injury has advanced, the cell contents escape and the E_m falls.

The sarcoplasmic reticulum from alcoholic rats was leakier to Ca^{2+} and can store less of this ion (Tsuyoshi 1985). In addition, the sarcoplasmic reticulum of the alcoholic rats was more disordered than the control rats, even when alcohol was not present (Tsuyoshi et al 1985). This may have affected the contractility of muscles in chronic alcoholics.

Some of the effects of chronic ethanol abuse on the muscle could be nutritional. The antioxidants serum α-tocopherol and selenium are low in myopathic alcoholics (Ward and Peters 1992). This implies that ethanol-induced damage to skeletal muscle may partly result from the deleterious effects of reactive oxygen species (Garcia-Bunuel 1984). However, it is not known whether the serum α-tocopherol and selenium deficiencies in myopathic alcoholics are caused by the effects of the alcoholism or the cause of it. In addition, more recent work has shown no change in serum and muscle levels of the antioxidants α-tocopherol, ascorbic acid and retinol in chronic alcoholic patients (Fernandez-Sola et al 1998).

The expression of the acetylcholine receptor α-subunit messenger RNA (mRNA) in the rat soleus muscles of chronic ethanol-fed animals was significantly reduced by 39% (Held et al 1991). This was presumably regulated at the transcriptional and/or post-transcriptional level and could explain some of the muscle weakness seen in chronic alcoholics, due to dysfunction of the neuromuscular junctions.

Protein, RNA and DNA contents and protein synthesis were reduced in rat muscles treated with chronic ethanol dosing (Preedy and Peters 1988b). The effects were greatest in Type II fibres compared with the Type I fibres. In the gastrocnemius, which represents skeletal musculature as a whole, Marway et al (1990) found that RNA was reduced to a greater extent than proteins. After six weeks, RNA content decreased by 35% whereas protein content decreased by 27%. One possible explanation for the reduction in RNA is an increase in RNase activity (Reilly et al 1998). Protein synthesis fell by between 15 and 30% (Preedy and Peters 1990b). It is possible that the reduction of RNA in the skeletal muscle, indicative of a similar reduction in ribosomal RNA (rRNA), is the cause of impaired protein synthesis in alcoholic myopathy (Preedy et al 1991).

The ribosome as a target of ethanol

The ribosome is a key organelle in protein synthesis. It keeps the growing end of the polypeptide chain aligned with the mRNA molecule in such a way that each successive codon in the mRNA engages with a transfer RNA (tRNA) molecule (Alberts et al 1995). The ribosome is a major cellular component—in bacteria ribosomal protein makes up about 10% of total protein mass, and in eukaryotes much of the RNA in the cell is ribosomal. Gunning et al (1981) calculated that in the rat gastrocnemius muscle 65.5% of total cellular RNA is ribosomal, whilst the figure for heart is 71.3%. Ribosomes can be dissociated into two subunits, each with one major rRNA component and many different protein molecules. There may also be smaller RNA molecules in the larger subunits. The structural components of the rat liver cytoplasmic ribosome are summarized in Table 17.1. Ethanol has been shown to change the properties of ribosomes in other tissues. Pinazo-Duran et al (1993) demonstrated that both pre- and post-natal ethanol exposure causes a reduction of the number of ribosomes in the rat optic nerve. In hepatocytes, ethanol redistributed ribosomes from polysomes to smaller ribosomal aggregates, showing an inhibitory action on peptide chain

Table 17.1—The characteristics of a typical eukaryotic ribosome

Characteristic	Whole ribosome	Subunits	
		Small subunit	Large subunit
Sedimentation rate	80S	40S	60S
Mass (kDa)	4220	1400	2820
Major RNAs		18S, 1874 bases	28S, 4718 bases
Minor RNAs		7.8S, 160 bases	
		5S, 120 bases	
RNA mass (kDa)	2520	700	1820
Proportion of total mass that is RNA (%)	60	50	65
Number of polypeptides	72	33	49
Protein mass (kDa)	1700	700	1000
Proportion of total mass that is protein (%)	40	50	35

initiation (Harbitz et al 1984). The formation and recycling of ^{35}S-Met-tRNA-40S complexes was also inhibited. The ribosomal subunits isolated from the brains of rats maintained on a chronic ethanol diet seem to have problems in reassociating (Tewari et al 1980).

There are no in vivo studies to see whether this is a factor in the development of alcohol-induced skeletal muscle myopathy.

Coleman and Cunningham (1991) have examined the biochemical properties of the ribosomes from the mitochondria of rats chronically fed ethanol. Liver mitochondria from ethanol-fed rats display an impaired ability to synthesize protein in vitro. No specific changes were found in the mRNAs and rRNAs associated with ribosomes, but the number of active ribosomes was reduced by 55% in the ethanol-fed rats (Coleman and Cunningham 1991). In addition, the number of whole ribosomes present was reduced by 32% in the mitochondria of ethanol-fed rats. However, the ability of ribosomes to function in poly(U)-directed phenylalanine polymerization was not affected by ethanol consumption. Therefore, ethanol appears to have reduced the number competent ribosomes in liver mitochondria, without affecting their functional ability. Cahill et al (1996) used sucrose density gradients to determine differences in the sedimentation rates of mitochondrial ribosomes from control and ethanol-fed rats. Ribosomes from control rats moved further down the gradient, indicating that ethanol ribosomes had a lower weight (Cahill et al 1996). Ribosomes from ethanol-fed rats were also unstable, as less were present as the intact monosome

on the gradients (Cahill et al 1996). These changes could be causing the reduction in protein synthesis seen in the liver mitochondria of ethanol-fed rats.

Ethanol and apoptosis

Apoptosis is an active process requiring protein synthesis and specific endonucleolytic cleavage of cellular DNA that physiologically adjusts and maintains cell populations (Hoffman and Liebermann 1994, Stewart 1994). Apoptosis is observed in normal physiological conditions and in cell turnover during embryogenesis and the homeostasis of normal tissue such as mammary glands (Duvall and Wyllie 1986). It also occurs in pathological states such as atherosclerosis (Han et al 1995), oncogenesis and tumour homeostasis (Stewart 1994) and in response to cytotoxic drugs and irradiation (Alison and Sarraf 1992). Apoptosis shows both morphological and biochemical characteristics. It is genetically controlled, energy dependent and involves single cells, and it is not associated with an inflammatory reaction (Gerschenson and Rotello 1992). It differs from necrosis, which is a pathological response that occurs as a result of extreme environmental traumas such as severe hypoxia, hyperthermia and viral infections, resulting in direct plasma membrane damage, or blocked ATP synthesis (Alison and Sarraf 1992).

Ethanol has been shown to induce apoptosis in several cell types. For example, chronic ethanol feeding of rats caused a five-fold increase in apoptosis in hepatocytes compared with pair-fed controls (Baroni et al 1994). In vitro, ethanol increased apoptotic cell death of thymocytes (Ewald and Shao 1993, Wang and Spitzer 1997). Possible mechanisms include enhancing tumour necrosis factor (TNF-α) expression (Slomiany et al 1997) or a reduction in the anti-apoptotic action of insulin-like growth factor-1 receptor (IGF-IR; Cui et al 1997). Acetaldehyde, the by-product of alcohol dehydrogenase also induced apoptosis in vitro in Chinese Hamster Ovary cells (Zimmerman et al 1995). It seems likely that ethanol can induce apoptosis in muscle cells as well. Indeed, in many metabolic and degenerative muscle diseases cells die with no overt inflammatory response, and apoptosis is the logical mechanism (Stangel et al 1996). For example, DNA fragmentation is increased in the skeletal muscle nuclei of patients with mitochondrial myopathies (Monici et al 1998). Tews et al (1997) showed that muscle fibres in infantile spinal muscular atrophy have nuclei that undergo apoptosis. Interestingly, proteins targeted by anti-Fas antibody are found in Type II muscle fibres of patients with several muscular disorders (Yamada et al 1995). Anti-Fas antibody has been reported to induce apoptosis. The fact that Type II muscle fibres are preferentially targeted in alcohol-induced skeletal muscle myopathy may implicate apoptosis in alcohol-induced myopathy.

Conclusions

Alcohol is a poison that has detrimental effects on many tissues. In moderation, these effects are minimal. However, one of the tissues damaged by excess alcohol consumption is skeletal muscle. Amongst the present avenues of research are changes in the muscle ribosomes, or apoptosis as a result of either the ethanol itself or the toxic metabolite acetaldehyde.

References

Agarwal DP. (1996) Racial/ethnic and gender differences in alcohol use and misuse. Alcohol Misuse – a European perspective. Harwood Academic Publishers, pp. 23–40.

Alberts B, Bray D, Lewis J, Raff M, Roberts K, Watson JD. (1995) *Molecular Biology of the Cell*. New York: Garland Publishing, pp. 305–309.

Alison MR, Sarraf CE. (1992) Apoptosis: a gene-directed programme of cell death. *J Royal Coll Physicians London* 26: 25–35.

Andre K, Schraub S, Mercier M, Bontemps P. (1995) Role of alcohol and tobacco in the aetiology of head and neck cancer: A case-control study in the Doubs region of France. *Eur J Cancer Part B: Oral Oncol* 31: 301–309.

Baroni GS, Marucci L, Benedetti A, Mancini R, Jezequel A-M, Orlandi F. (1994) Chronic ethanol feeding increases apoptosis and cell proliferation in rat liver. *J Hepatol* 20: 508–513.

Cahill A, Baio DL, Ivester P, Cunningham CC. (1996) Differential effects of chronic ethanol consumption on hepatic mitochondrial and cytoplasmic ribosomes. *Alcoholism Clin Exp Res* 20: 1362–1367.

Carstensen JM, Bygren LO, Hatschek T. (1990) Cancer incidence among Swedish brewery workers. *Int J Cancer* 45: 393–396.

Coleman WB, Cunningham CC. (1991) Effect of chronic ethanol consumption on hepatic mitochondrial transcription and translation. *Biochim Biophys Acta* 1058: 178–186.

Crouch DJ, Birky MM, Gust SW, et al. (1993) The prevalence of drugs and alcohol in fatally-injured truck drivers. *J Forens Sci* 38: 1342–1353.

Cui SJ, Tewari M, Schneider T, Rubin R. (1997) Ethanol promotes cell death by inhibition of the insulin-like growth factor I receptor. *Alcoholism Clin Exp Res* 21: 1121–1127.

Dal Nogare AR. (1991) Septic shock. *Am J Med Sci* 302: 50–65.

Devor EJ, Cloninger CR. (1989) Genetics of alcoholism. *Annu Rev Genet* 23: 19–36.

D'Souza NB, Mandujano JF, Nelson S, Summer WR, Shellito JE. (1995) Alcohol ingestion impairs host defences predisposing otherwise healthy mice to Pneumocystis-carnii infection. *Alcoholism Clin Exp Res* 19: 1219–1225.

Duane P, Peters TJ. (1987) Glucocorticoid status in chronic alcoholics with and without skeletal muscle myopathy. *Clin Sci* 73: 601–603.

Duvall E, Wyllie AH. (1986) Death and the cell. *Immunol Today* 7: 115–119.

Emerson EE, Manaves V, Singer T, Tabesh M. (1995) Chronic alcohol feeding inhibits athersclerosis in c57BL/6 hyperlipidemic mice. *Am J Pathol* 147: 1749–1758.

Ewald SJ, Shao H. (1993) Ethanol increases apoptotic cell death of thymocytes in vitro. *Alcoholism Clin Exp Res* 17: 359–365.

Facchini F, Chen Y-DI, Reaven GR. (1994) Light-to-moderate alcohol intake is associated with enhanced insulin sensitivity. *Diabetes Care* 17: 115–119.

Fernandez-Sola J, Villegas E, Nicolas JM, et al. (1998) Serum and muscle levels of alpha-tocopherol, ascorbic acid and retinol are normal in chronic alcoholic myopathy. *Alcoholism Clin Exp Res* 22: 422–427.

Garcia-Bunuel L. (1984) Lipid peroxidation in alcoholic myopathy and cardiomyopathy. *Med Hypoth* 13: 217–231.

Gerschenson LE, Rotello RJ. (1992) Apoptosis: a different type of cell death. *FASEB J* 6: 2450–2455.

Geva D, Goldschmidt L, Stoffer D, Day NL. (1994) A longitudinal analysis of prenatal alcohol exposure on growth. *Alcoholism Clin Exp Res* 6: 1124–1129.

Gunning PW, Shooter EM, Austin A, Jeffrey PL. (1981) Differential and coordinate regulation of eukaryotic small molecular weight RNAs. *J Biol Chem* 256: 6663–6669.

Haida M, Yazaki K, Kurita D, Shinohara Y. (1998) Mitochondrial dysfunction of human muscle in chronic alcoholism detected by using 31P-magnetic resonance spectroscopy and near-infrared light absorption. *Alcoholism Clin Exp Res* 22: 108S–110S.

Han DKM, Haudenschild CC, Hong MK, Tinkle BT, Leon MB, Liau G. (1995) Evidence for apoptosis in human atherogenesis and in a rat vascular injury model. *Am J Pathol* 147: 267–277.

Harbitz I, Wallin B, Hauge JG, Morland J. (1984) Effect of ethanol metabolism on initiation of protein synthesis in rat hepatocytes. *Biochem Pharmacol* 33: 3465–3470.

Held IR, Sayers ST, McLane JA. (1991) Acetylcholine receptor gene expression in skeletal muscle of chronic ethanol-fed rats. *Alcohol* 9: 79–82.

Hoffman B, Liebermann DA. (1994) Molecular controls of apoptosis: differentiation/growth arrest primary response genes, proto-oncogenes, and tumor suppressor genes as positive and negative modulators. *Oncogene* 9: 1807–1812.

Honjo S, Kono S, Shinchi K, et al. (1995) The relation of smoking, alcohol-use and obesity to risk of sigmoid colon and rectal adenomas. *Japan J Cancer Res* 86: 1019–1026.

Kendell RE. (1979) Alcoholism: a medical or a political problem? *Br Med J* 121: 367–371.

Knockel JP. (1993) Mechanisms of rhabdomyolysis. *Curr Opin Rheumatol* 5: 725–731.

Kumar P, Clark M. (1996) *Clinical Medicine*. Philadelphia W. B. Saunders Publishers, pp. 189–191.

Lieber CS. (1996) The metabolism of alcohol and its implication for the pathogenesis of disease. Alcohol and the gastrointestinal tract. New York: CRC Press, pp. 19–40.

MacGregor RR. (1985) Alcohol and immune defence. *J Am Med Assoc* 256: 1474–1479.

Martin FC, Peters TJ. (1985) Assessment in vitro and in vivo of muscle degradation in chronic skeletal muscle myopathy of alcoholism. *Clin Sci* 68: 693–700.

Marway JS, Preedy VR, Peters TJ. (1990) Experimental alcoholic skeletal muscle myopathy is characterised by a rapid and sustained decrease in muscle RNA content. *Alcohol Alcoholism* 25: 401–406.

Monici MC, Toscano A, Girlanda P, Aguennouz M, Musumeci O, Vita G. (1998) Apoptosis in metabolic myopathies. *Neuroreport* 9(10): 2431–2435.

Ouellette EM, Rosett HL, Rosman NP, Weiner L. (1977) Adverse effects on offspring of maternal alcohol abuse during pregnancy. *N Engl J Med* 297: 528–530.

Pinazo-Duran MD, Renau-Piqueras J, Guerri C. (1993) Developmental changes in the optic nerve related to ethanol consumption in pregnant rats: analysis of the ethanol-exposed optic nerve. *Teratology* 48: 305–322.

Preedy VR, Keating JW, Peters TJ. (1992) The acute effects of ethanol and acetaldehyde on the rates of protein synthesis in type I and type II fibre-rich skeletal muscles of the rat. *Alcohol Alcoholism* 27: 241–251.

Preedy VR, Marway JS, Peters TJ. (1989) Use of the Lieber-DeCarli liquid feeding regime with specific reference to the effects of ethanol on rat skeletal muscle RNA. *Alcohol Alcoholism* 24: 439–445.

Preedy VR, Peters TJ. (1988a) Acute effects of ethanol on protein synthesis in different muscles and muscle protein fractions of the rat. *Clin Sci* 74: 461–466.

Preedy VR, Peters TJ. (1988b) The effect of chronic ethanol ingestion on protein metabolism in type-I- and type-II-fibre-rich skeletal muscles in the rat. *Biochem J* 254: 631–639.

Preedy VR, Peters TJ. (1990a) Alcohol and skeletal muscle disease. *Alcohol Alcoholism* 25: 177–187.

Preedy VR, Peters TJ. (1990c) The acute and chronic effects of ethanol on cardiac muscle protein synthesis in the rat in vivo. *Alcohol* 7: 97–102.

Preedy VR, Peters TJ, Patel VB, Miell JP. (1994b) Chronic alcoholic myopathy: transcription and translational alterations. *FASEB J* 8: 1146–1151.

Preedy VR, Siddiq T, Cook E, Black D, Palmer TN, Peters TJ. (1991) Alcohol and protein turnover. In: Palmer TN. (ed.) *Alcoholism: A molecular perspective*. New York: Plenum Press, pp. 253–273.

Prescott CA, Hewitt JK, Heath AC, Truet KR, Neale MC, Eaves LJ. (1994) Environmental and genetic influences on alcohol in a volunteer study of older twins. *J Studies Alcohol* 55: 18–33.

Reilly ME, Erylmaz EI, Amir A, Peters TJ, Preedy VR. (1998) Skeletal muscle ribonuclease activities in chronically ethanol-treated rats. *Alcoholism Clin Exp Res* 22: 876–883.

Richardson PJ, Wodak AD, Atkinson L, Saunders JB, Jewitt DE. (1986) Relation between alcohol intake, myocardial enzyme activity, and myocardial function in dilated cardiomyopathy. Evidence for the concept of alcohol induced heart muscle disease. *Br Heart J* 56: 165–170.

Rubin E, Urbano-Marquez A. (1994) Alcoholic cardiomyopathy. *Alcoholism Clin Exp Res* 18: 111–114.

Salmela KS, Salaspuro M, Gentry RT, et al. (1994) Helicobacter infection and gastric ethanol metabolism. *Alcoholism Clin Exp Res* 18: 1294–1299.

Slomiany BL, Piotriwski J, Slomiany A. (1997) Chronic ethanol ingestion enhances tumor necrosis factor-alpha expression and salivary gland apoptosis. *Alcoholism Clin Exp Res* 21: 1530–1533.

Snyder SHS, Lader MH. (1986) The History of Alcohol Use. In: *Alcohol and Alcoholism*. London: Burke Publishing, pp. 15–21.

Spolarics Z, Bagby GJ, Pekala PH, Dobrescu C, Skrepnik N, Spitzer JJ. (1994) Acute ethanol administration attenuates insulin-mediated glucose use by skeletal muscle. *Am J Physiol Endocrinol Metab* 267: E886–E891.

Stangel M, Zettl UK, Mix E, et al. (1996) H_2O_2 and nitric oxide-mediated oxidative stress induce apoptosis in rat skeletal muscle myoblasts. *J Neuropathol Exp Neurol* 55: 36–43.

Stewart BW. (1994) Mechanisms of Apoptosis: Integration of Genetic, Biochemical, and Cellular Indicators. *J Nat Cancer Inst* 86: 1286–1296.

Tewari S, Sweeney FM, Fleming EW. (1980) Ethanol-induced changes in properties of rat brain ribosomes. *Neurochem Res* 5: 1025–1035.

Tews DS, Goebel HH, Meinck HM. (1997) DNA-fragmentation and apoptosis-related proteins of muscle cells in motor neurone disorders. *Acta Neurol Scand* 96: 380–386.

Thomas DB. (1995) Alcohol as a cause of cancer. *Env Health Perspectives* 103: 153–160.

Tiernan JM, Ward LC. (1986) Acute effects of ethanol on protein synthesis in the rat. *Alcohol Alcoholism* 21: 171–179.

Trouce I, Byrne E, Dennett X. (1990) Biochemical and morphological studies of skeletal muscle in experimental chronic alcoholic myopathy. *Acta Neurol Scand* 82: 386–391.

Tsuyoshi OS. (1985) Chronic ethanol ingestion alters the calcium permeability of sarcoplasmic reticulum of rat skeletal muscle. *Membrane Biochem* 6: 33–47.

Tsuyoshi OS, Waring AJ, Fang SRG. (1985) Sarcoplasmic reticulum membrane of rat skeletal muscle is disordered with chronic ethanol ingestion. *Membrane Biochem* 6: 49–63.

Urbano-Marquez A, Estruch R, Navarro-Lopez F, Grau JM, Mont L, Rubin E. (1989) The effect of alcoholism on skeletal and cardiac muscle. *N Engl J Med* 15: 409–415.

Vernet M, Cadefau JA, Balague A, Grau JM, Urbano-Marquez A, Cusso R. (1995) Effect of chronic alcoholism on human muscle glycogen and glucose metabolism. *Alcoholism Clin Exp Res* 19: 1295–1299.

Wang JF, Spitzer JJ. (1997) Alcohol-induced thymocyte apoptosis is accompanied by impaired mitochondrial function. *Alcohol* 14: 99–105.

Ward RJ, Peters TJ. (1992) The antioxidant status in patients with either alcohol-induced liver damage or myopathy. *Alcohol Alcoholism* 27: 359–365.

Xu D, Heng JKM, Palmer TN. (1993) The mechanism(s) of alcohol-induced impairment in glycogen synthesis in oxidative skeletal muscles. *Biochem Mol Biol Int* 30: 169–176.

Yamada H, Nakgawa M, Higuchi I, Ohkubo R, Osame M. (1995) Type II muscle fibres are stained by anti-Fas antibody. *J Neurol Sci* 134: 115–118.

Zimmerman BT, Crawford GD, Dahl R, Simon FR, Mapoles JE. (1995) Mechanisms of acetaldehyde-mediated growth inhibition: delayed cell cycle progression and induction of apoptosis. *Alcoholism Clin Exp Res* 19: 434–440.

18

HIV myopathy: pathology, diagnosis and treatment

Shehzad Basaria and Adrian Dobs

Introduction

Neuromuscular disorders are frequent complications of human immunodeficiency virus type-1 (HIV). The involvement of skeletal muscle can occur at all stages of HIV infection. In about 15% of patients with HIV, myopathy is the presenting manifestation and it has been estimated that 50% of all aquired immune deficiency syndrome (AIDS) patients will develop some kind of myopathy during the course of their illness. In the early reports on neurological disorders in patients with HIV infection, more attention was given to central nervous system (CNS) disorders rather than focusing on muscular pathology, which was considered infrequent. In 1987, zidovudine (AZT) was introduced for the treatment of AIDS. Soon after its introduction it was observed that patients receiving AZT reported myalgias and muscle weakness (Dalakas et al 1990). That lowered the threshold among neurologists to perform muscle biopsies in such cases, thus expanding our understanding of muscle pathology in AIDS patients. Many experts also believe that the AIDS wasting syndrome is a form of myopathy since these patients have disproportionately higher wasting of lean body mass (LBM) than fat mass (Simpson et al 1990). In this chapter we will review the various etiologies of AIDS myopathy and the treatment modalities directed towards each cause with special emphasis on anabolic treatment to improve LBM.

Classification

As mentioned above, neurologic disorders are common in patients with HIV. As a result the involvement of spine and peripheral nerves can result in neurogenic myopathy (disuse atrophy). However, in this chapter we will only focus on primary muscular myopathies. Primary muscular diseases in HIV patients can be divided into six categories (Table 18.1).

Pathology

Pure HIV related myopathy

The word "pure" means that this myopathy is primarily a result of HIV infection itself and not caused by drugs, tumours or opportunistic infections. This type of myopathy is much less common than AZT myopathy. This group comprises two different types of myopathies: Polymyositis and Nemaline (rod) myopathy.

HIV polymyositis

The clinical and histological features of HIV polymyositis is similar to polymyositis in patients who are seronegative for HIV (Illa et al 1991). The hallmarks of biopsy specimens from these patients include necrotic myofibres, mononuclear cell infiltration of fascicles and non-necrotic myofibres (Fig. 18.1). Immunohistologically, activated CD8 cells have been identified in the majority of these myofibres (Illa et al 1991). Occasionally, granulomatous myositis with giant cell infiltration of the muscles has been noticed (Bailey et al 1987). The mechanism by which HIV causes muscle damage is not clear. Many attempts to identify the virus particle in muscle fibres, including the use of polymerase chain reaction (PCR) on muscle cultures, have failed (Leon-Monzon et al 1993). However, in a past report, a particle was seen by electron microscopy in muscle endomysium, which was considered to be HIV (Nordstrom et al 1989). In

Table 18.1—HIV related myopathies

Classification of myopathies	Histological features
1. Pure HIV myopathy	
a) polymyositis	Mononuclear infiltrate, CD8 cells
b) nemaline rod myopathy	Rod bodies in centre of myofibres
2. AZT myopathy	AZT fibres, Ultrastructural mitochondrial changes, Increased COX activity
3. Myopathy caused by oppurtunistic infections	*S. aureus, T. gondii, C. neoformans*
4. Myopathy caused by tumour infiltration	Lymphomas, Kaposi's Sarcoma
5. Myopathy caused by vasculitides	Capillaritis resembling Polyarteritis nodosa, Henoch-Schonlein purpura, cryoglobulinaemia
6. Myopathy caused by AIDS wasting syndrome (AIDS cachexia)	Diffuse atrophy, ultrastructural mitochondrial changes, no inflammation

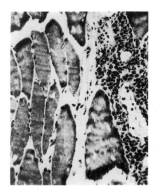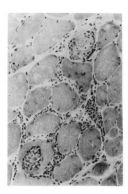

Figure 18.1 — HIV polymyositis. Transverse and oblique sections of muscle biopsy from a patient showing perivascular and endomysial infiltration of mononuclear cells. (Adapted from Dalakas MC, Pezeshkpour GH 1988 with permission.)

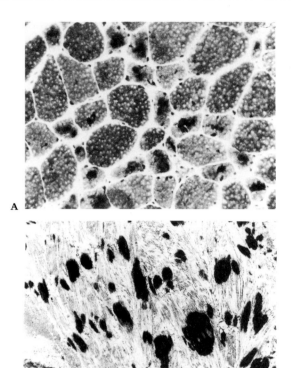

Figure 18.2 — Nemaline "rod" myopathy. **A** Transverse section of a muscle biopsy from a HIV positive patient showing numerous nemaline bodies. **B** Electron micrograph from the same patient showing rods. (Adapted from Dalakas MC, Pezeshkpour GH 1988 with permission.)

another report viral antigens were detected in the endomysium (and not the myofibres; Hantai et al 1991). However, it appears that the involvement of the non-necrotic myofibres away from the centre of inflammation suggests that HIV does not directly involve the muscles but may be doing so through various cytokines.

Nemaline (rod) myopathy

Although most of the clinical features of this entity are shared by other types of HIV myopathies, many patients with rod myopathy have no myalgia (Dwyer et al 1992). Histologically, there are no inflammatory infiltrates nor any necrotic fibres. There is atrophy of myofibres with intracytoplasmic collections of rod bodies in the centre of the fibres (Fig. 18.2). Although a definite aetiology of this myopathy is unclear, a few patients respond to prednisone, making autoimmune mechanism the most likely cause.

AZT myopathy

Since the introduction of AZT, this group comprises the majority of the cases of HIV myopathy. However, in 1991, low doses AZT were introduced, which resulted in some decline in these cases. This myopathy is a reversible mitochondrial myopathy resulting from high cumulative doses of AZT. The evidence of mitochondrial toxicity is evident from the evidence of depletion of mitochondrial DNA in AZT treated patients (Arnaudo et al 1991). Though clinically similar to pure HIV polymyositis, the histological hallmark of AZT myopathy is the presence of ragged-red fibres, which are atrophic and contain cytoplasmic inclusions (Mhiri et al 1991). These fibres are more popularly known as "AZT fibres" (Fig. 18.3; Dalakas et al 1990). Although other mitochondrial myopathies also show ragged-red fibres, AZT fibres are more ragged and smaller. The number of ragged fibres correlates with the severity of myopathy (Dalakas et al 1990). Patients in whom muscle biopsy specimens showed >8% of AZT fibres had more severe myopathy. The presence of inflammation, and failure of some patients to improve after withholding AZT, supports the evidence that other immunological factors may be involved along with direct effects of AZT on muscles (Dalakas et al 1990). Since a subset of patients receiving AZT may have inflammatory processes suggesting polymyositis on biopsy specimens, tests have been developed to correctly distinguish AZT myopathy from polymyositis. The most success achieved in this regard is by checking for histochemical reaction of

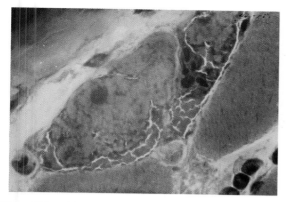

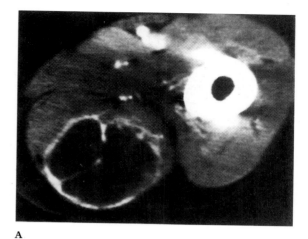

Figure 18.3 — AZT myopathy. Two ragged-red fibres (AZT fibres) seen in a transverse frozen section of muscle biopsy stained with Gomori trichrome.

A

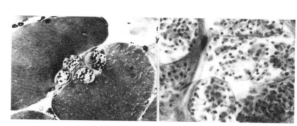

B

muscle biopsy specimens with cytochrome c oxidase (COX) activity (Chariot et al 1993). Since COX is encoded by mitochondrial DNA, patients with myopathy due to AZT show deficiency of this enzyme. All of the patients with AZT-induced myopathy show COX deficiency compared with no subjects with other types of myopathy (Chariot et al 1993). The demonstration of the cytokine interleukin-1 (IL-1) mRNA in AZT fibres suggest that this myopathy may be related to the proteolytic effects of IL-1 on myofibres (Gherardi et al 1994). The IL-1 mRNA is not found in other HIV myopathies. The majority of patients improve when AZT is discontinued (Dalakas et al 1990).

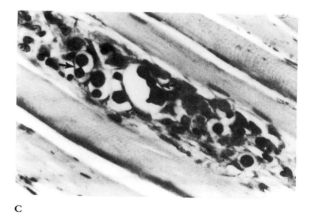

C

Myopathy due to opportunistic infections

Although rare, many opportunistic organisms have been reported to invade muscle tissue in AIDS patients. The most common among these is *Staphylococcus aureus*, which causes pyomyositis, accounting for 90% of the cases (Fig. 18.4a; Al-Tawfiq et al 2000). Thigh and lower leg are the most common sites of infection, and bilateral involvement is more common compared with pyomyositis in HIV negative patients. Surgical excision or needle aspiration is needed for effective therapy, along with intravenous antibiotics. Other bacterial organisms causing pyomyositis in HIV-positive patients include *Salmonella* species, *Streptococcus* species, *Escherichia coli*, *Citrobacter freundii* and *Pseudomonas aeruginosa*.

Toxoplasma gondii infection is the second most common organism, usually affecting patients with end-stage AIDS with low CD4 cell counts who have

Figure 18.4 — Oppurtunistic myopathy. **A** CT scan of the left thigh of a patient with AIDS showing abscess formation. S. aureus was isolated from the lesion. **B** Toxoplasma cysts in muscle fibres in a HIV positive patient. **C** Cryptococcus species within the necrotic muscle fibres. The arrows show the typical budding patterns of these organisms.

evidence of multiple organ involvement with the organism (Gherardi et al 1992). These patients usually present with fever, headache (encephalitis), and multi-organ failure. In one series, muscle toxoplasmosis was found in 4% of muscle biopsy specimens (Gherardi et al 1992). The organism, if found within the muscle fibres, is in the form of solitary cyst or clumps of cysts (Fig. 18.4b). There is often inflammation, necrosis and vacuolization of myocytes. Since these cysts may be found in those parts of muscle tissue free of any inflammation, direct toxicity due to toxoplasmosis is debated, and the possibility of immunological involvement is suggested.

Cryptococcus neoformans also results in a necrotizing myopathy (Wrzolek et al 1990). This organism is also found in capillaries supplying the muscles (Fig. 18.4c). It appears that, by blocking the capillaries, the organism causes an initial ischaemic damage and then invades the muscle tissue. Other conditions involving muscles in HIV patients include Cytomegalovirus and *Microbacterium avium intracellulare* infection, and microsporidiosis.

Myopathy due to tumour infiltration

Lymphomas are the most common tumours involving the muscle tissue in HIV patients. However, considering the increased frequency of CNS lymphomas and others in AIDS patients, the muscle involvement is relatively infrequent. These patients present with fever and a growing muscle mass (Chevalier et al 1993). Histologically, the tumour cells destroy the myocytes, resulting in inflammation. Kaposi's sarcoma can also invade muscle tissue (Gherardi and Goebel 1993).

Myopathy due to vasculitides

A wide spectrum of inflammatory vasculitides can be seen in patients with AIDS. These patients are found to have deposits of complement in the capillaries, and in some the process is severe leading to necrotizing vasculitis as seen in polyarteritis nodosa (Gherardi et al 1993). Cytokines, particularly IL-1, have been implicated in this process. The vasculitis in these patients can resemble that of Henoch–Schonlein purpura, polyarteritis nodosa, hypersensitivity vasculitis and vasculitis due to cryoglobulinaemia.

Myopathy due to AIDS wasting syndrome (AIDS cachexia)

Many experts believe that AIDS wasting syndrome (AWS) is a type of myopathy since these patients lose more LBM compared with fat mass, as determined by their total body potassium levels (Kotler et al 1985). Loss of LBM in HIV patients is also directly related to morbidity and mortality (Kotler et al 1989). In sub-Saharan Africa, AIDS is known as "Slim Disease" because of severe wasting in these subjects. In 1987, Center for Disease Control (CDC Atlanta, Georgia, USA) defined the criteria for the diagnosis of AWS: weight loss of >10% of baseline weight in combination with either chronic diarrhoea for at least 30 days or chronic weakness and fever of at least 30 days duration (in the absence of a concurrent condition responsible for these manifestations).

Muscle biopsy specimens from AWS patients show diffuse atrophy and mild ultrastructural mitochondrial changes without significant inflammation (Belec et al 1992). Cytokines like IL-6, IL-1β and tumour necrosis factor α (TNFα) have been implicated in the process (Grunfeld and Feingold 1992). In contrast to other types of myopathies, which require specific treatment such as withdrawal of an offending drug or treatment of a particular infection, there is no specific therapy available for this type of myopathy. Therefore, AWS myopathy has been the target of a variety of anabolic agents in many studies designed to improve LBM. These studies are discussed later.

Clinical presentation of patients with myopathies

Clinical presentation in patients with HIV myopathy, from whatever cause, is similar, and there is a considerable overlap. However, there are a few unique characteristics of some of these myopathies depending upon the aetiology. Generally, patients with pure HIV polymyositis present with diffuse myalgias that predominantly affect the thigh (Simpson et al 1993). The proximal muscles of the upper and lower limbs are most affected. Symptoms include difficulty in raising arms above the head, difficulty rising from the chair without support and problems in climbing stairs. This weakness usually starts in the lower extremities and slowly involves the proximal muscles of the upper extremities. The involvement is symmetrical. Neck flexors can also be involved (Simpson et al 1990). In the majority of the cases, the weakness progresses slowly. However, there have been reports of several cases presenting with rhabdomyolysis in whom the symptoms are acute or subacute (Chariot et al 1994). Medications, opportunistic infections and HIV itself have been reported to result in rhabdomyolysis. These patients present with myalgias and fever along with weakness (Chariot et al 1994).

Patients with nemaline (rod) myopathy have involvement of the same muscle groups, however, myalgias are usually absent in these subjects.

Patients with muscular toxoplasmosis are usually sick patients with advanced disease and low CD4 counts and evidence of disease in other organs (Gherardi et al 1992). These patients present with fever, asthenia, weight loss, myalgias and proximal myopathy. They may also have seizures due to cerebral involvement. Myopathy caused by AZT presents with similar features to those of patients with polymyositis: fever, bacteraemia, severe pain at the site of involvement (usually thighs), and sometimes a tender mass may be present with *S. aureus* pyomyositis.

Serum creatine kinase (CPK) levels are elevated in most of the patients with HIV myopathy. However, there is no cut-off level that may help in determining the type of myopathy. The levels may be elevated over a wide range, ranging from 2–3 fold the upper normal limit to a thousand-fold elevation (Simpson et al 1993). The levels of CPK do not correlate with the degree of weakness. Patients with rhabdomyolysis, as expected, have higher elevations of CPK and myoglobin.

Treatment of HIV myopathies

Treatment of HIV myopathies should be directed towards the specific aetiology. Many of these myopathies resolve upon withdrawal of the offending agent (AZT) or treatment of an opportunistic infection or surgical removal of tumours. In this section we will not focus on the treatment of opportunistic infections and tumours. However, some reports in the literature suggest that AZT myopathy does not always resolve on removal of the drug (Simpson et al 1993). Many anabolic agents have been used in various trials to treat AWS, since its treatment also results in an increase in LBM and muscle strength and, hence, improvement in myopathy. Furthermore, these agents may be used in the future to treat any of the aforementioned HIV myopathies if specific treatment does not result in any significant improvement. In this section we will focus on agents used to date to treat myopathies. Briefly, we will also discuss the experience with the use of steroids in treating HIV myopathies, especially polymyositis and AZT myopathy.

Glucocorticoids

No randomized prospective trials have been conducted to study the effectiveness of glucocorticoids in the treatment of HIV myopathy. The only information regarding these agents is available through anecdotal case reports and series in which glucocorticoids were used for the treatment of pure HIV myopathy and AZT myopathy. Amongst the different types of HIV myopathy, these two types may theoretically benefit most from these drugs because of the autoimmune process implicated in their pathogenesis. However, the results have been mixed. In one of the largest series reported by Simpson et al (1993), seven patients with polymyositis with increasing weakness and problems with ambulation were started on Prednisone 60 mg/day and the dose was adjusted depending on the response of the patients. All subjects showed reduction in CPK values with improvement in weakness. On the contrary, those patients with polymyositis who were weak but did not receive Prednisone for one reason or the other, continued to have progressive weakness. In another series, two out of five patients with pure HIV myopathy improved on Prednisone, one did not respond, one worsened, and one improved on non-steroidal anti-inflammatory drugs (NSAIDs; Dalakas et al 1990). Although these reports show the benefit of glucocorticoids in pure HIV myopathy, this therapy has its risks in an immunocompromised population. Cases of severe myelopathy and cryptococcal meningitis have been reported as a consequence of Prednisone therapy (Simpson et al 1990, 1993). In the same series by Simpson et al, three patients with AZT myopathy who did not improve on withdrawal of AZT were treated with Prednisone (Simpson et al 1993). All the patients showed improvement in muscle weakness. Similarly, Dalakas et al (1990) also showed improvement in all four patients with AZT myopathy started on Prednisone with doses ranging between 40 and 60 mg/day. Two of these patients showed improvement despite continuing AZT treatment. These reports indicate that glucocorticoids may be helpful in patients belonging to these two classes of myopathy, but they may be associated with side-effects.

Based on Dalakas' treatment plan (Dalakas et al 1990) we recommend that patients with these two types of myopathies initially be started on NSAIDs. If the patient fails to respond, AZT should be discontinued for 4–6 weeks. If patient then improves, AZT should be withheld and treatment with another nucleoside analogue should be initiated. However, if AZT withdrawal does not improve symptoms, AZT should be re-introduced in combination with Prednisone at a dose of 40–60 mg/day. Dose modification should be done in response to treatment.

Clinical trials of other immunosuppressants and plasma-pheresis for the treatment of AZT and pure HIV myopathies need to be done.

Appetite stimulants

The rationale for using anabolic agents in patients with myopathies, particularly AWS, is to increase LBM since a decline in fat-free mass is associated with increased mortality (Kotler et al 1989). Since loss of LBM also includes loss of muscle mass, this decline contributes to the development of myopathy. The use of appetite stimulants like Megestrol Acetate (megace) and Dronabinol to increase LBM have not been met with good success. Although megace does increase weight in these patients, most of the weight gain is in the form of fat mass (Oster et al 1994, Von Roenn et al 1994). Furthermore, megace also exhibits gluco-corticoid activity and, therefore, it may cause muscle catabolism. Dronabinol has failed to produce weight gain in clinical trials (Beal et al 1995, Timpone et al 1997). Although appetite stimulants have failed in this endeavour, four types of treatment modalities have shown promise in the treatment of AWS. These are: nutritional supplementation, testosterone therapy, androgenic anabolic agents, and growth hormone therapy.

Nutritional support

It is important to emphasize that nutritionally based therapies have resulted in an increase in body weight and body cell mass in patients with AWS, and they should form the cornerstone in the management of patients with AWS myopathy. Patients with AIDS who are stable have a high resting energy expenditure, which is further increased if these patients become infected (Grunfeld and Feingold 1992). Therefore, it is important for these patients to maintain adequate caloric intake. In a clinical trial where patients with AWS were randomized to total parenteral nutrition (TPN) or dietary counselling for 8 weeks, patients in the former group gained 8 kg compared with the group on dietary counselling who lost 3 kg (Melchior et al 1996). Similarly, body cell mass increased with the use of TPN in another study (Kotler et al 1990). Glutamine supplementation in these patients has also resulted in an increase in weight due to an increase in body cell mass (Clark et al 2000). These data suggest that adequate nutritional supplementation should be the initial step in the management of patients with AWS myopathy.

Testosterone

Hypogonadism is a common occurrence in patients with AIDS: about 50% of men with AIDS are hypogonadal (Dobs et al 1988). In the same study it was observed that 44% of patients with AIDS related complex (ARC), a stage before frank AIDS, were also hypogonadal. The majority of these patients have central hypogonadism, which may be related to malnutrition, chronic illness or therapy with megace. However, 25% of these patients have primary hypogonadism, which may be related to the HIV infection itself, malignant infiltration or opportunistic infections (Chabon et al 1987, Grinspoon et al 1996). Drugs like ketoconazole and gangcyclovir also inhibit testicular testosterone production (Pont et al 1982, Chachoua et al 1987).

It has been clearly established that loss of muscle mass in patients with AWS is inversely related to serum androgen levels (Grinspoon et al 1996). A number of clinical trials have been performed in HIV patients with various forms and doses of testosterone preparations in an attempt to promote weight gain and increase LBM. Most of these trials are summarized in Table 18.2. A critical review of these trials suggests that in general testosterone therapy does produce an increase in LBM and should be attempted in patients with AWS.

Anabolic androgenic steroids

These agents are orally administered and, although debatable, possess more anabolic rather than androgenic activity; they are specially designed to promote LBM. Oxandrolone has been the most studied agent in this group. In one study, 15 mg/day of this agent increased weight (+2.04 kg) in HIV patients compared with placebo (Berger et al 1996). Poles et al (1995) in their study used Oxandrolone at a dose of 10 mg twice daily and showed a total weight gain of 5.85 kg with body cell mass corresponding to more than 3 kg of this increase. In another study, Oxandrolone at a dose of 20 mg/day, produced nitrogen retention and an increase in muscle strength in patients with HIV-related weight loss (Strawford et al 1999). Nandrolone decanoate, another agent of this class, has been shown to increase weight and LBM in HIV wasting (Bucher et al 1996, Gold et al 1996). Oxymetholone also produced weight gain of 8.2 kg in patients with AWS compared with the placebo group which lost 1.8 kg. These studies suggest that androgenic anabolic steroids are of benefit in patients with AWS, and they may alleviate myopathy.

Table 18.2 — Trials of testosterone therapy in HIV wasting

Author	Treatment	Outcome measures	Result
Wagner et al 1998 (n=19, uncontrolled, 3 months)	i.m. testosterone 400 mg biweekly	Sexual function Quality of life Weight	89% increase 71% increase 2.3 kg increase
Jeantils et al 1993 (uncontrolled, 2 months)	Testosterone undecanoate 40 mg PO TID	Weight gain	8 kg increase
Coodley and Coodley 1997 (n=40, placebo controlled, 3 months)	Testosterone i.m. 200 mg biweekly	Quality of life Weight gain Muscle strength	$p=0.03$ NS $p=0.08$
Dobs et al 1988 (n=130, placebo controlled, 3 months)	Testosterone patch on scrotum, 5 mg daily	Sexual function Quality of life Weight gain	NS $p=0.07$ NS
Bhasin et al 1998 (n=41, placebo controlled, 3 months)	Non-scrotal testosterone patch, 5 mg daily	Weight gain Lean body mass Emotional stability	NS +1.35 kg ($p=0.0254$) $p=0.01$
Grinspoon et al 1998a (placebo controlled, 3 months)	Testosterone enanthate 300 mg q3 wk i.m.	Weight Lean body mass Quality of life	NS +1.9 kg ($p=0.041$) $p=0.04$
Strawford et al 1999 (n=24, placebo controlled, 4 months)	Testosterone enenthate 100 mg/wk all patients, randomized to oxandrolone 20 mg/day	Nitrogen balance Lean body mass Body weight Muscle strength	$p=0.05$ +6.9 kg ($p=0.005$) $p=0.05$ Upper body $p=0.02$ Lower body $p=0.05$
Bhasin et al 2000 (n=61, placebo controlled, 4 months)	Testosterone enanthate (T) 100 mg/wk i.m. with and without exercise (ex)	Body weight Lean body mass Muscle strength	+2.6 kg(T)/2.2 kg(ex) +2.3 kg(T)/2.6 kg(T+ex) $p=<0.001$

PO = per oral (by mouth), TID = three times a day, 300 mg q3 wk = 300 mg every 3 weeks

Growth hormone

Growth hormone (GH) is an anabolic peptide hormone which, if deficient, results in loss of LBM and muscle strength (Baum et al 1996). In men with HIV-associated wasting, there is an acquired resistance to GH that is demonstrated by increased GH pulse frequency and decreased IGF-1 production (Grinspoon et al 1998b). This is a result of down regulation of IGF-1 receptor and defective post-receptor signalling, which improves on nutritional repletion and reversal of wasting (Maiter et al 1989). In a randomized placebo-controlled trial of GH at a dose of 0.1 mg/kg body weight per day for 12 weeks, patients with AWS who received GH experienced a significant increase in LBM (3.0 kg) compared with the placebo group, which lost 0.1 kg (Schambelan et al 1996). Patients in the GH group also had a greater increase in exercise tolerance, which indirectly indicates increased muscular strength. Another study found that GH at 1.4 mg/day for 12 weeks also resulted in an increase in upper and lower body strength (Waters et al 1996). In this study, recombinant human IGF-1 administration also increased LBM. Although more trials are required, GH certainly holds promise for patients with AWS myopathy.

Conclusion and recommendations

Patients with HIV experience a wide variety of neuromuscular disorders. Pure HIV myopathy and AZT myopathy are the most common among the primary myopathic disorders, and they are difficult to distinguish pathologically. Treatment with glucocorticoids has resulted in beneficial responses in some patients with these myopathies. The role of plasmapheresis needs further evaluation. Patients who develop AZT myopathy do respond to AZT withdrawal. Tumour infiltration, opportunistic infections and vasculitic processes can also result in disabling myopathy. Myopathy associated with AWS is common, and this should be treated aggressively since loss of LBM is related to high mortality. Appetite stimulants do not improve myopathy since they only increase fat mass. Nutritional supplementation and testosterone therapy have shown success in the treatment of AWS myopathy. Androgenic anabolic agents, specially oxandrolone, have also produced positive results. Other anabolic agents and GH should be evaluated further for the treatment of AWS myopathy.

We recommend that appropriate nutritional therapy should be the cornerstone of treatment for the patients who present with AWS myopathy. Resistance exercises may also be beneficial. If a man is hypogonadal, he should be started on testosterone replacement therapy. Body weight and LBM should be evaluated at that time. Therapy should be continued if there is an improvement in weight and LBM. If testosterone therapy fails, oxandrolone therapy should be initiated for 16 weeks. Failure of oxandrolone should be followed by GH therapy. Until more research becomes available regarding the efficacy of GH and other anabolic agents, testosterone and oxandrolone should be the major anabolic agents used in the treatment of AWS myopathy.

References

Al-Tawfiq JA, Sarosi GA, Cushing HE. (2000) Pyomyositis in the acquired immunodeficiency syndrome. *South Med J* 93(3): 330–334.

Arnaudo E, Dalakas M, Shanske S, Moraes CT, DiMauro S, Schon EA. (1991) Depletion of muscle mitochondrial DNA in AIDS patients with zidovudine-induced myopathy. *Lancet* 337(8740): 508–510.

Bailey RO, Turok DI, Jaufmann BP, Singh JK. (1987) Myositis and acquired immunodeficiency syndrome. *Hum Pathol* 18(7): 749–751.

Baum HB, Biller BM, Finkelstein JS, et al. (1996) Effects of physiologic growth hormone therapy on bone density and body composition in patients with adult-onset growth hormone deficiency. A randomized, placebo-controlled trial. *Ann Intern Med* 125(11): 883–890.

Beal JE, Olson R, Laubenstein L, et al. (1995) Dronabinol as a treatment for anorexia associated with weight loss in patients with AIDS. *J Pain Symptom Manage* 10(2): 89–97.

Belec L, Mhiri C, DiCostanzo B, Gherardi R. (1992) The HIV wasting syndrome. *Muscle Nerve* 15(7): 856–857.

Berger JR, Pall L, Hall CD, Simpson DM, Berry PS, Dudley R. (1996) Oxandrolone in AIDS-wasting myopathy. *AIDS* 10(14): 1657–1662.

Bhasin S, Sorer TW, Asbel-seth N, et al. (1998) Effects of testosterone replacement with a nongenital transdermal system, androderm, in human immunodeficiency virus-infected me with low testosterone levels. *J Clin Endocrinol Metab* 83(9): 3155–3162.

Bhasin S, Storer TW, Javanbakht M, et al. (2000) Testosterone replacement and resistance exercise in HIV-infected men with weight loss and low testosterone levels. *JAMA* 283(6): 763–770.

Bucher G, Berger DS, Fields-Gardner C, Jones R, Reiter WM. (1996) A prospective study on the safety and effect of nandrolone decanoate in HIV positive patients. *Int Conf AIDS* 11: 26 (abstract # Mo.B. 423).

Chabon AB, Stenger RJ, Grabstald H. (1987) Histopathology of testis in acquired immune deficiency syndrome. *Urology* 29(6): 658–663.

Chachoua A, Dieterich D, Krasinski K, et al. (1987) 9-(1,3-Dihydroxy-2-propoxymethyl)guanine (ganciclovir) in the treatment of cytomegalovirus gastrointestinal disease with the acquired immunodeficiency syndrome. *Ann Intern Med* 107(2): 133–137.

Chariot P, Monnet I, Gherardi R. (1993) Cytochrome c oxidase reaction improves histopathological assessment of zidovudine myopathy. *Ann Neurol* 34(4): 561–565.

Chariot P, Ruet E, Authier FJ, Levy Y, Gherardi R. (1994) Acute rhabdomyolysis in patients infected by human immunodeficiency virus. *Neurology* 44(9): 1692–1696.

Chevalier X, Amoura Z, Viard JP, et al. (1993) Skeletal muscle lymphoma in patients with the acquired immunodeficiency syndrome: a diagnostic challenge. *Arthritis Rheum* 36(3): 426–427.

Clark RH, Feleke G, Din M, et al. (2000) Nutritional treatment for acquired immunodeficiency virus-associated wasting using beta-hydroxy beta-methylbutyrate, glutamine, and arginine: a randomized, double-blind, placebo-controlled study. *J Parenter Enteral Nutr* 24(3): 133–139.

Coodley GO, Coodley MK. (1997) A trial of testosterone therapy for HIV-associated weight loss. *AIDS* 11(11): 1347–1352.

Dalakas MC, Pezeshkpour GH. (1988) Neuromuscular diseases associated with human immuno-deficiency virus infection. *Ann Neurol* 23: S38–S48.

Dalakas MC, Illa I, Pezeshkpour GH, Laukaitis JP, Cohen

B, Griffin JL. (1990) Mitochondrial myopathy caused by long-term zidovudine therapy. *N Engl J Med* 322(16): 1098–1105.

Dobs AS, Cofrancesco J, Nolten WE, et al. (1999) The use of a transscrotal testosterone delivery system in the treatment of patients with weight loss related to human immunodeficiency virus infection. *Am J Med* 107(2): 126–132.

Dobs AS, Dempsey MA, Ladenson PW, Polk BF. (1988) Endocrine disorders in men infected with human immunodeficiency virus. *Am J Med* 84(3 Pt 2): 611–616.

Dwyer BA, Mayer RF, Lee SC. (1992) Progressive nemaline (rod) myopathy as a presentation of human immunodeficiency virus infection. *Arch Neurol* 49(5): 440.

Gherardi R, Baudrimont M, Lionnet F, et al. (1992) Skeletal muscle toxoplasmosis in patients with acquired immunodeficiency syndrome: a clinical and pathological study. *Ann Neurol* 32(4): 535–542.

Gherardi R, Belec L, Mhiri C, et al. (1993) The spectrum of vasculitis in human immunodeficiency virus-infected patients. A clinicopathologic evaluation. *Arthritis Rheum* 36(8): 1164–1174.

Gherardi RK, Florea-Strat A, Fromont G, Poron F, Sabourin JC, Authier J. (1994) Cytokine expression in the muscle of HIV-infected patients: evidence for interleukin-1 alpha accumulation in mitochondria of AZT fibres. *Ann Neurol* 36(5): 752–758.

Gherardi RK, Goebel HH. (1993) Involvement of skeletal muscle. In: *Atlas of the Neuropathology of HIV infection*. Ed. F Gray. Oxford: Oxford University Press, pp. 261–283.

Gold J, High HA, Li Y, et al. (1996) Safety and efficacy of nandrolone decanoate for treatment of wasting in patients with HIV infection. *AIDS* 10(7): 745–752.

Grinspoon S, Corcoran C, Askari H, et al. (1998a) Effects of Androgen administration in men with the AIDS wasting syndrome. *Ann Intern Med* 129: 18–26.

Grinspoon S, Corcoran C, Stanley T, Katznelson L, Klibanski A. (1998b) Effects of androgen administration on the growth hormone–insulin-like growth factor I axis in men with acquired immunodeficiency syndrome wasting. *J Clin Endocrinol Metab* 83(12): 4251–4256.

Grinspoon S, Corcoran C, Lee K, et al. (1996) Loss of lean body and muscle mass correlates with androgen levels in hypogonadal men with acquired immunodeficiency syndrome and wasting. *J Clin Endocrinol Metab* 81(11): 4051–4058.

Grunfeld C, Feingold KR. (1992) Metabolic disturbances and wasting in the acquired immunodeficiency syndrome. *N Engl J Med* 327(5): 329–337.

Hantai D, Fournier JG, Vazeux R, Collin H, Baudrimont M, Fardeau M. (1991) Skeletal muscle involvement in human immunodeficiency virus infection. *Acta Neuropathol (Berl)* 81(5): 496–502.

Illa I, Nath A, Dalakas M. (1991) Immunocytochemical and virological characteristics of HIV-associated inflammatory myopathies: similarities with seronegative polymyositis. *Ann Neurol* 29(5): 474–481.

Jeantils V, Nguyen G, Bacle F, Thomas M, Krivitzky A. (1993) Weight gain under oral testosterone undecanoate in AIDS. *Therapie* 48(1): 71–72.

Kotler DP, Tierney AR, Culpepper-Morgan JA, Wang J, Pierson RN, Jr. (1990) Effect of home total parenteral nutrition on body composition in patients with acquired immunodeficiency syndrome. *J Parenter Enteral Nutr* 14(5): 454–458.

Kotler DP, Tierney AR, Wang J, Pierson RN, Jr. (1989) Magnitude of body-cell-mass depletion and the timing of death from wasting in AIDS. *Am J Clin Nutr* 50(3): 444–447.

Kotler DP, Wang J, Pierson RN. (1985) Body composition studies in patients with the acquired immunodeficiency syndrome. *Am J Clin Nutr* 42(6): 1255–1265.

Leon-Monzon M, Lamperth L, Dalakas MC. (1993) Search for HIV proviral DNA and amplified sequences in the muscle biopsies of patients with HIV polymyositis. *Muscle Nerve* 16(4): 408–413.

Maiter D, Fliesen T, Underwood LE, et al. (1989) Dietary protein restriction decreases insulin-like growth factor I independent of insulin and liver growth hormone binding. *Endocrinology* 124(5): 2604–2611.

Melchior JC, Chastang C, Gelas P, et al. (1996) Efficacy of 2-month total parenteral nutrition in AIDS patients: a controlled randomized prospective trial. The French Multicenter Total Parenteral Nutrition Cooperative Group Study. *AIDS* 10(4): 379–384.

Mhiri C, Baudrimont M, Bonne G, et al. (1991) Zidovudine myopathy: a distinctive disorder associated with mitochondrial dysfunction. *Ann Neurol* 29(6): 606–614.

Nordstrom DM, Petropolis AA, Giorno R, Gates RH, Reddy VB. (1989) Inflammatory myopathy and acquired immunodeficiency syndrome. *Arthritis Rheum* 32(4): 475–479.

Oster MH, Enders SR, Samuels SJ, et al. (1994) Megestrol acetate in patients with AIDS and cachexia. *Ann Intern Med* 121(6): 400–408.

Poles MA, Meller JA, Lin A, et al. (1995) Oxandrolone as a treatment for AIDS-related weight loss and waste. Presented at the *Infectious Disease Society of North America*, San Francisco.

Pont A, Williams PL, Loose DS, et al. (1982) Ketoconazole blocks adrenal steroid synthesis. *Ann Intern Med* 97(3): 370–372.

Schambelan M, Mulligan K, Grunfeld C, et al. (1996) Recombinant human growth hormone in patients with HIV-associated wasting. A randomized, placebo-controlled trial. Serostim Study Group. *Ann Intern Med* 125(11): 873–882.

Simpson DM, Bender AN, Farraye J, Mendelson SG, Wolfe DE. (1990) Human immunodeficiency virus wasting syndrome may represent a treatable myopathy. *Neurology* 40(3 Pt 1): 535–538.

Simpson DM, Citak KA, Godfrey E, Godbold J, Wolfe DE. (1993) Myopathies associated with human immunodeficiency virus and zidovudine: can their effects be distinguished? *Neurology* 43(5): 971–976.

Strawford A, Barbieri T, Van Loan M, et al. (1999) Resistance exercise and supraphysiologic androgen therapy in eugonadal men with HIV-related weight loss: a randomized controlled trial. *JAMA* 281(14): 1282–1290.

Timpone JG, Wright DJ, Li N, et al. (1997) The safety and pharmacokinetics of single-agent and combination therapy with megestrol acetate and dronabinol for the treatment of HIV wasting syndrome. The DATRI 004 Study Group. Division of AIDS Treatment Research Initiative. *AIDS Res Hum Retroviruses* 13(4): 305–315.

Von Roenn JH, Armstrong D, Kotler DP, et al. (1994) Megestrol acetate in patients with AIDS-related cachexia. *Ann Intern Med* 121(6): 393–399.

Wagner GJ, Rabkin JG. (1998) Testosterone therapy for clinical symptoms of hypogonadism in eugonadal men with AIDS. *Int J Std AIDS* 9(1): 41–44.

Waters D, Danska J, Hardy K, et al. (1996) Recombinant human growth hormone, insulin-like growth factor 1, and combination therapy in AIDS-associated wasting. A randomized, double-blind, placebo-controlled trial. *Ann Intern Med* 125(11): 865–872.

Wrzolek MA, Sher JH, Kozlowski PB, Rao C. (1990) Skeletal muscle pathology in AIDS: an autopsy study. *Muscle Nerve* 13(6): 508–515.

19

Myasthenia gravis

Francesca Andreetta and Carlo Antozzi

Introduction

Myasthenia Gravis (MG) is an acquired, organ specific autoimmune disease involving the neuromuscular junction, which is characterized by abnormal weakness and fatigability (Drachman 1994). MG is the best characterized human autoimmune disorder, since the target antigen and pathogenetic mechanisms leading to defective neuromuscular transmission have been identified. MG belongs to a group of autoimmune ion channel diseases, which includes the Lambert–Eaton myasthenic syndrome and acquired neuromyotonia. These disorders share a common pathogenesis mediated by autoantibodies against different ion channels of the neuromuscular junction: antibodies to postsynaptic acetylcholine receptors (anti-AChR Ab) in MG; antibodies to presynaptic voltage-gated calcium channels or potassium channels in the Lambert-Eaton myasthenic syndrome and acquired neuromyotonia (Isaac's syndrome), respectively (Engel 1994, Shillito et al 1995). Moreover, several congenital myasthenic syndromes, which are genetic in nature, have been described (Engel et al 1999). In this review we will focus on the main clinical and pathogenetic features of acquired autoimmune MG.

The neuromuscular junction and the acetylcholine receptor

The neuromuscular junction (NMJ), which is the terminal portion of motor nerve axons that makes contact with the muscle membrane, is the target organ for specific autoantibodies against postsynaptic acetylcholine receptors (AChR) in acquired MG (see Fig. 19.2). The presynaptic membrane is enriched in vesicles containing the neurotransmitter acetylcholine (ACh); the postsynaptic membrane is organized in several junctional folds that expose AChRs on their surface. The propagation of the nerve action potential causes the opening of voltage-gated calcium channels of the presynaptic membrane, leading to an increase in the concentration of cytoplasmic calcium. This in turn causes the fusion of synaptic vesicles with the presynaptic membrane and the consequent release of ACh in the synaptic cleft, which is now able to bind AChRs on the postsynaptic junctional folds and hence propagate the action potential to the muscle surface to promote muscle contraction (Hall and Sanes 1993; Fig. 19.1).

The AChR is a complex pentameric molecule made up of five different subunits arranged around a central ion channel. The stoichiometric ratio of the

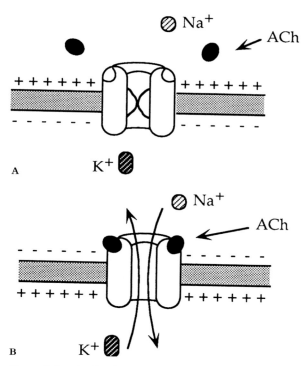

Figure 19.1 — A Closed channel **B** Open channel. Ion channel modification induced by the binding of acetylcholine (ACh) to the acetylcholine receptor (AChR) α-subunit.

five subunits is $\alpha_2\beta\gamma\delta$ in embrionic or denervated muscle and $\alpha_2\beta\epsilon\delta$ in adult muscle. Each α-subunit contains the ACh binding site, located extracellularly, as well as the α-bungarotoxin binding site, a toxin that competes with ACh in binding to the receptor and is, therefore, utilized for immunoprecipitation assays of anti-AChR Ab (Tzartos et al 1991).

Clinical features

The prevalence of MG is between 50 and 125 cases per million population. The incidence peaks around the second or third decade in women and the sixth or seventh decade in men. The clinical hallmarks of MG are weakness and fatigability of skeletal muscles; both tend to increase with repeated exercise and improve with rest, and their degree typically fluctuates from day to day, being usually worse at the end of the day, and varying in their regional distribution. In the majority of patients ptosis and diplopia occur at the onset of the disease; in 15% of patients the symptoms remain restricted to ocular muscles (ocular MG).

However, the great majority of patients show variable degrees of generalized weakness involving trunk and limb muscles; the proximal groups are affected more than distal ones. When bulbar muscle impairment occurs, patients complain of difficulty in chewing and swallowing, nasal voice and dyspnea on exercise or at rest. The severity of the clinical picture may end in a myasthenic crisis, when impairment of respiratory muscles is great enough to require mechanical ventilation. The clinical severity of myasthenia gravis has been graded functionally by the Osserman classification (Osserman and Genkins 1971):

- group I: restricted to ocular muscles
- group IIA: mild generalized disease
- group IIB: severe generalized disease
- group III: acute fulminating disease
- group IV: late severe disease.

MG patients can be subgrouped according to age at onset, human leukocyte antigen (HLA) association and thymic pathology. Early onset MG patients are more frequently women with an hyperplastic thymus; their HLA haplotype shows association with HLA-B8 HLA-B8-DR3. Late onset MG patients, who develop the disease after 40 years, show involuted or atrophic thymuses; the frequency of HLA-B7, -DR2, -DR4 and -DQW8 seems to be increased in this subgroup. On the contrary, Caucasian patients with thymoma-associated MG, usually between 30 and 60 years of age, do not show a clearcut HLA association.

MG shows frequent association with other autoimmune disorders, and among these particularly with thyroid disorders (Grave's disease, thyoiditis, SLE, rheumatoid arthritis). Screening for thyroid function should be always included in the diagnostic protocol for MG patients (Drachman 1994, Engel 1994).

Diagnosis

The diagnosis of acquired MG relies upon clinical, immunological and neurophysiological criteria (Drachman 1994, Engel 1994). The clinical hallmarks are the typical distribution and fluctuation of muscle weakness and fatigability. Diagnostic tests are:

1. anticholinesterase test with edrophonium chloride (Tensilon)

2. repetitive nerve stimulation test

3. anti-AChR Ab immunoprecipitation assay

4. contrast-enhanced computed tomography (CT) scan (or magnetic resonance imaging; MRI) to detect thymic abnormalities.

Anticholinesterase drugs, by inhibiting the activity of acetylcholinesterase, prolong the interaction of ACh with postsynaptic AChRs, thus increasing muscle strength. Typically, the effect of i.v. edrophonium chloride is very rapid (a few seconds) and subsides in about five minutes; attention should be paid to select compromised muscles, which can be easily and objectively tested (e.g., ptosis of the eyelid, overt diplopia, nasal voice). The test is considered positive whenever unequivocal improvement is observed.

The repetitive nerve stimulation test involves the stimulation of a peripheral nerve and recording of the compound muscle action potential (CMAP) from muscle; in MG, a typical decremental response of the CMAP (more than 10%) is considered diagnostic. The test is more informative on involved proximal muscles. The repetitive stimulation should always be performed at both low (3/s) and high rates (50/s) since only the high rates of stimulation allow differentiation between MG and the Lambert–Eaton myasthenic syndrome Lambert–Eaton syndrome shows a decremental response at low rates and a several-fold increase of the response at high rates, which is never observed in MG patients. Single fibre electromyography can be considered in patients with suspected MG and negative laboratory findings; however, it must be remembered that the test has a limited specificity since it can also be positive in disorders of peripheral nerves. The radioimmunoassay for antiAChR Ab, which is specific for MG, employs solubilized AChR labelled with iodinated α-bungarotoxin. The assay is positive in about 95% of patients with generalized MG but only in 50% of patients with pure ocular MG.

Differential diagnosis

The clinical features of MG are usually easily recognizable when they show the typical day to day fluctuation, the characteristic pattern of distribution and response to anticholinesterase drugs. However, several conditions involving either ocular or skeletal muscles must be taken into account in the diagnostic work up for MG (Table 19.1). Diagnostic tests, including neurophysiological, neuroradiological, and muscle biopsy studies can discriminate between these different clinical conditions.

Pathogenesis

MG is an autoimmune disease in which dysfunction of the neuromuscular junction is caused by specific antibodies against the AChR, causing a reduced

Table 19.1—Differential diagnosis of autoimmune myasthenia gravis: other conditions that must be considered

---

Congenital myasthenic syndromes
Lambert–Eaton myasthenic syndrome
Chronic progressive external ophthalmoplegia, mitocondrial myopathy
Oculopharingeal muscular dystrophy
Grave's disease
Lesions of cranial nerves, intracranial compressive lesions
Botulism
Penicillamine-induced myasthenia gravis
Organophosphate intoxication

---

number of functional end-plate AChRs (Engel 1994, Marx et al 1997; Fig. 19.2). Anti-AChR Ab exert their effect through several mechanisms:

- increased turnover of AChRs: autoantibodies are able to reduce the receptor half-life by cross-linking AChRs that are subsequently clustered, internalized by endocitosis, and ultimately more rapidly degraded
- blockade of the ACh binding site
- complement-mediated damage of the post-synaptic membrane of the NMJ, as demonstrated by ultra-structural studies showing deposition of IgG and complement components.

The serum concentration of anti-AChR Ab does not correlate with the severity of the disease; it can be postulated that the functional properties of these antibodies may vary in their interaction with the AChR, probably due to interaction with different epitopes of the receptor molecule and different complement-binding properties. These differences might explain the heterogeneity between patients in their clinical response to the rapid removal of anti-AChR Ab by plasmapheresis.

Anti-AChR Ab represent a heterogeneous population of autoantibodies that interact with different epitopes of the AChR molecule; most of them bind to the extracellular portion of the AChR, and particularly to a limited region identified as the "main immunogenic region" (MIR) of the AChR α-subunit (Tzartos et al 1991). However, the fine specificity of anti-AChR Ab is highly heterogenous, and other epitopes apart from the MIR region can be the target for specific autoantibodies.

About 15% of MG patients with typical clinical features do not have detectable anti-AChR Ab, by immunoprecipitation assay. Several lines of evidence suggested that a plasma factor is able to impair the neuromuscular transmission, as demonstrated by passive transfer studies with plasma of seronegative MG patients, and by inhibition of AChR function on TE671 cells in culture (a rhabdomyosarcoma–derived cell line expressing the fetal form of the AChR). Clinically, seronegative patients may show significant improvement after plasma exchange. Recently, a IgM factor from seronegative MG patients has been reported as able to interfere with the AChR function (Yamamoto et al 1991, Li et al 1996).

In addition to antiAChR Ab, antibodies against other muscle proteins have been detected in MG patients, such as antibodies against actin, myosin, titin, ryanodine receptor and rapsyn (Aarli et al 1998, Agius et al 1998). However, the role of antibodies against non-AChR antigens in the pathogenesis of the disease remains unknown. It is worth noting that the presence of antibodies against titin and ryanodinl receptors correlates with the presence of thymoma.

The autoantibody response in MG is dependent on major histocompatibility complex (MHC) class II restricted T cells. T cell lines specific for the AChR sequence have been raised against human recombinant AChR and most T cells show a Th1 phenotype; however, the possibility of a Th0 phenotype has been recently reported (Zhang 1997, Nagvekar et al 1998). Small overlapping peptides of the AChR subunits have been used to identify T cell epitopes, but the results of these studies have been questioned. Therefore, the information available still does not prove the existence of an immunodominant T cell epitope in the human disease. Moreover, AChR-specific T cells have also been identified in non-myasthenic controls indicating that a lack of tolerance to the AChR is unlikely to be the cause of MG. Further studies are needed to address the issue of AChR-specific autoaggressive T cells, their cytokine profile and ability to help B cells.

The thymus and myasthenia gravis

Thymic abnormalities are found in the majority of myasthenic patients: 70% of cases having thymic hyperplasia; 10%, a neoplastic thymus; and the remainder thymic atrophy. The high frequency of thymic abnormalities strongly suggests its involvement in the pathogenesis of the disease (Melms et al 1988; Hohlfeld and Wekerle 1994, Marx et al 1997).

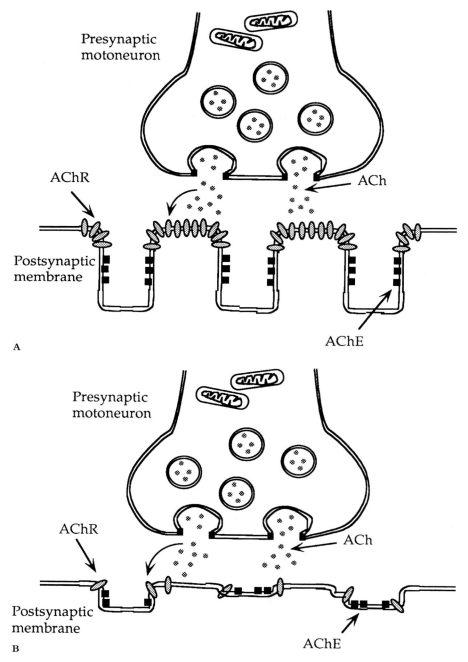

Presynaptic
motoneuron

AChR

Postsynaptic
membrane

ACh

AChE

A

Presynaptic
motoneuron

AChR

ACh

Postsynaptic
membrane

AChE

B

Figure 19.2 — **A** Normal neuromuscular junction **B** Myasthenic neuromuscular junction. Schematic representation of normal (upper panel) and myasthenic (lower panel) neuromuscular junction showing the effect of anti-acetylcholine receptor autoantibodies (ACh, acetylcholine; AChR, acetylcholine receptor; AChE, acetylcholine esterase).

The central point of the intrathymic pathogenesis of MG is the presence of myoid cells within the thymus in either myasthenic or normal subjects (Engel et al 1977). These cells have the ultrastructural and immunohistochemical features of striated muscle cells and express AChR or an AChR-like protein on their surface as shown by mRNA studies, monoclonal antibodies and binding with α-bungarotoxin (Matsumoto et al 1986, Schluep et al 1987, Kaminski et al 1993). The presence of myoid cells within the thymus close to antigen presenting cells and T helper cells creates a microenvironment in which an alteration of the immune regulation can lead to an autoimmune response to the AChR. Therefore, current views favour the hypothesis that, in patients with follicular hyperplasia, an unknown event triggers the abnormal autoimmune response within the thymus, from antigen recognition to autoantibody production; antigen-specific T and B cells can then migrate to peripheral lymphoid organs and perpetuate the autoimmune process. The intrathymic pathogenesis of MG has been also suggested by the observation that SCID mice transplanted with thymic hyperplastic tissue show prolonged synthesis of anti-AChR antibodies, indicating that the thymus contains the tools necessary for the initiation and maintenance of an autoimmune response (Shonbeck et al 1993).

The relationship between MG and thymoma is still under investigation. The majority of patients with thymoma-associated MG do not show histological signs of follicular hyperplasia in their residual thymus. However, thymic epithelial tumours express several potentially myasthenogenic autoantigens such as the AChR, titin, the ryanodine receptor and neuronal antigens (Marx et al 1997). Indeed, most MG patients with thymoma have antibodies to myosin, actin, titin, α-actinin and ryanodine receptor. It is still to be elucidated whether the association between thymoma and antibodies to striated muscle proteins is a primary phenomenon related to the pathogenesis of MG or simply secondary to the tumour. The possibility that antigens expressed by thymic tumours select T cells leading to autoimmunity is still to be confirmed.

Neonatal myasthenia

MG symptoms, particularly respiratory insufficiency and feeding difficulties, can be observed in less than 10% of babies born to myasthenic mothers. The disease, which usually lasts for a few weeks, is a result of passive transplacental transfer of anti-AChR Ab from the mother to the fetus. The disease can be observed also in babies born to mothers without MG symptoms.

Myasthenia gravis and arthrogryposis multiplex congenita

It has been recently reported that, very rarely, MG can be associated with arthrogryposis multiplex congenita, a condition characterized by joint contractures, in utero or evident at birth, frequently associated with several musculoskeletal abnormalities. The disease has been related to maternal antibodies against fetal AChR. It is worth noting that the occurrence of arthrogryposis multiplex congenita is not necessarily associated with MG symptoms in the mother. An animal model of the disease has been recently developed (Jacobson et al 1999).

Treatment

MG is treated with anticholinesterase drugs and by means of generalized immunosuppression with corticosteroids, either alone or associated with immunosuppressive drugs (azathioprine, cyclosporin A, cyclophosphamide) according to the clinical severity of the disease in each patient (Engel 1994). Thymectomy is usually recommended, particularly in young-onset patients. Patients must be operated on according to the classical extended transternal approach (Jaretski 1997). Recently, a new video-thoracoscopic technique, which avoids sternectomy, has been introduced with positive results (Mantegazza et al 1998). Plasmapheresis is very helpful as a short-term measure to overcome a myasthenic crisis (Antozzi et al 1991). Alternatively, high-dose intravenous immunoglobulins can be used (Gajdos et al 1997). Recently, chronic selective IgG immunoadsorption with protein A has been introduced for the long-term management of treatment resistant MG patients (Antozzi et al 1994). A detailed description of therapies available for MG will be considered in a different chapter of this book.

Experimental autoimmune myasthenia gravis

Experiment autoimmune myasthenia gravis (EAMG)

is the animal counterpart of human MG. Chronic EAMG can be induced by immunization with AChR purified from *Torpedo californica* electric organ emulsified with complete Freund's adjuvant (CFA). Several animal species are susceptible to EAMG including rabbits, rats, mice and monkeys; the incidence and severity of the disease varies considerably between different species. These differences are related to MHC background, T cell receptor (TCR) genes and differences in the antibody repertoire. The disease can be easily induced in Lewis rats by one immunization with TAChR. An acute phase begins approximately 7 days after immunization and subsides in a few days; afterwards, experimental animals show clinical signs of the chronic disease 4 to 6 weeks after immunization. Affected animals show muscular weekness, hunched back posture, tremulousness and progressive weight loss. Immunization followed by at least two boosts with TAChR is necessary to develop the disease in the susceptible strain (C57/BL6) of mice. EAMG has also been obtained by passive transfer with policlonal or monoclonal anti-AChR antibodies (Souroujon and Fuchs 1997). The availability of an experimental model of MG proved extremely useful in the investigation of the pathogenesis of MG; a major drawback is that the disease is not spontaneous but must be induced by active immunization with AChR in adjuvant. Nevertheless, the experimental model represents an important tool to investigate new treatment strategies (Drachman 1996). Recently, several studies have been performed in mice (C57/BL6) and rats (Lewis) to investigate new therapeutic strategies. Data available on the structure and immunological recognition of the nicotinic AChR allowed the design of new approaches, potentially able to modulate the autoimmune response in EAMG. Like human MG, EAMG is a T cell-dependent, B cell-mediated disorder. The majority of pathogenic autoantibodies are directed against the MIR of the AChR α-subunit. Moreover, a limited number of epitopes of the AChR are preferentially recognized by T cells in mice and rats. Several strategies have been devised to specifically modulate the experimental disease (Drachman 1996). In recent years, the effect of treatments based on the mucosal delivery of antigens (Weiner 1997) have been investigated also in EAMG in mice and rats. In this regard, EAMG offered the unique opportunity to investigate this approach in a prototypical antibody-mediated disease in which the main antigenic specificities of the AChR, and its recognition by CD4+ T lymphocytes, have been well characterized. Indeed, EAMG has been prevented or treated in rats by the oral and nasal administration of intact purified

TAChR (Okumura et al 1994, Ma et al 1995). The major drawbacks of this approach are the low yield of receptor available after purification, and the high immunogenicity in its native conformation, suggesting the need for more easily available and less immunogenic molecules. Recently, EAMG has been modulated by recombinant fragments of the human AChR α-subunit (Barchan et al 1998); moreover, the disease has been prevented by the administration of synthetic peptides representing immunodominant epitopes of the AChR, confirming that tolerization can be achieved in a T cell-dependent B cell-mediated disease (Karachunski et al 1997, Wu et al 1997). These observations suggest the need for further studies on the cellular and molecular mechanisms underlying the pathogenesis of MG, the prerequisite for an antigen-specific immunotherapeutic approach to the human disease.

References

Aarli J, et al. (1998) Muscle striation antibodies in myasthenia gravis. Diagnostic and functional significance. *Ann NY Acad Sci* 841: 505–515.

Agius MA, et al. (1998) Rapsyn antibodies in myasthenia gravis. *Ann NY Acad Sci* 841: 516–521.

Antozzi C, et al. (1991) A short plasmaexchange protocol is effective in severe myasthenia gravis. *J Neurol* 238: 103–107.

Antozzi C, et al. (1994) Protein-A immunoadsorption in immunosuppression resistant myasthenia gravis. *Lancet* 383: 124.

Barchan D, et al. (1998) Modulation of the anti-acetylcholine receptor response and experimental autoimmune myasthenia gravis by recombinant fragments of the acetylcholine receptor. *Eur J Immunol* 28: 616–624.

Drachman DB. (1994) Myasthenia Gravis. New *Engl J Med* 330: 1797–1810.

Drachman DB. (1996) Immunotherapy in neuromuscular disorders. *Muscle Nerve* 19: 1239–1251.

Engel AG. (1994) Myasthenic syndromes. In: Engel AG, Franzini-Armstrong C, eds. *Myology* 2nd ed. Vol. 2. New York: McGraw-Hill, pp. 1798–1835.

Engel AG, et al. (1999) Congenital myasthenic syndromes: recent advances. *Arch Neurol* 57: 163–167.

Engel WK, et al. (1977) Thymic epithelial cells contains acetylcholine receptor. *Lancet* 1: 1310–1311.

Gajdos P, et al. (1997) Clinical trial of plasmaexchange and high dose intravenous immunoglobulin in myasthenia gravis. *Ann Neurol* 41: 789–796.

Hall ZW, Sanes JR. (1993) Synaptic structure and development: the neuromuscular junction. *Cell* 72: 99–121.

Hohlfeld R, Wekerle H. (1994) The thymus in myasthenia gravis. *Neurol Clin* 12: 331–342.

Jacobson L, et al. (1999) Plasma from human mothers of fetuses with severe arthrogryposis multiplex congenita causes deformities in mice. *J Clin Invest* 103: 1031–1038.

Jaretski A, III. (1997) Thymectomy for myasthenia gravis. Analysis of the controversies regarding technique and results. *Neurology* 48 (Suppl.5): S52–S63.

Kaminski HJ, et al. (1993) Acetylcholine receptor subunit gene expression in thymic tissue. *Muscle Nerve* 16: 1332–1337.

Karachunski PI, et al. (1997) Prevention of experimental myasthenia gravis by nasal administration of synthetic acetylcholine receptor T epitope sequences. *J Clin Invest* 100: 3027–3035.

Li Z, et al. (1996) Modulation of acetylcholine receptor function in TE671 (rhabdomyosarcoma) cells by non-AChR ligands; possible relevance to seronegative myasthenia gravis. *J Neuroimmunol* 64: 179–183.

Ma CG, et al. (1995) Suppression of experimental autoimmune myasthenia gravis by nasal administration of acetylcholine receptor. *J Neuroimmunol* 58: 51–60.

Mamalaki A, Tzartos S, (1994). Nicotinic acetylcholine receptor: structure, function and main immunogenic region. *Adv Neuroimmunol* 4 (4): 339–354.

Mantegazza R, et al. (1998) Video-assisted thoracoscopic extended thymectomy (VATET) in myasthenia gravis. Two-year follow-up in 101 patients and comparison with the transternal approach. *Ann NY Acad Sci* 841: 749–752.

Marx A, et al. (1997) Pathogenesis of myasthenia gravis. *Virchows Arch* 430: 355–364.

Matsumoto J, et al. (1986) Primary culture of human myasthenia gravis thymus: studies of cell morphology, cell proliferation pattern, and localization of α-bungarotoxin binding sites on culture thymic cells. *J Neurol Sci* 75: 121–133.

Melms A, et al. (1988) Thymus in myasthenia gravis. *J Clin Invest* 81: 902–908.

Nagvekar N, et al. (1998) A pathogenetic role for the thymoma in myasthenia gravis. Autosensitization of IL-4 producing T cell clones recognizing extracellular acetylcholine receptor epitopes presented by minority class II isotypes. *J Clin Invest* 101: 2268–2277.

Okumura S, et al. (1994) Oral administration of acetylcholine receptor: effects on experimental autoimmune myasthenia gravis. *Ann Neurol* 36: 704–713.

Osserman KE, Genkins G. (1971) Studies in myasthenia gravis: rewiew of a twenty-year experience in over 1200 patients. *Mt Sinai J Med* 38: 497–537.

Schluep M, et al. (1987). Acetylcholine receptors in human thymic myoid cells in situ: an immunohistological study. *Ann Neurol* 22: 212–222.

Shillito P, et al. (1995) Acquired neuromyotonia: evidence for autoantibodies directed against K+ channels of peripheral nerves. *Ann Neurol* 38: 714–722.

Shonbeck S, et al. (1993) Transplantation of myasthenia gravis thymus to SCID mice. *Ann NY Acad Sci* 681: 66–73.

Souroujon MC, Fuchs S. (1997) Experimental autoimmune myasthenia gravis. In: Lefkovits I, ed. *Immunology methods manual.* Vol. 3. Academic Press: 1764–1773.

Tzartos S, et al. (1991) The main immunogenic region of the acetylcholine receptor. Structure and role in myasthenia gravis. *Autoimmunity* 8: 257–270.

Weiner HL. (1997) Oral tolerance: immune mechanism and treatment of autoimmune diseases. *Immunology Today* 18: 335–343.

Wu B, et al. (1997) Tolerance to a dominant T cell epitope in the acetylcholine receptor molecule induces epitope spread and suppresses murine myasthenia gravis. *J Immunol* 159: 3016–3023.

Yamamoto, et al. (1991) Seronegative myasthenia gravis: a plasmafactor inhibiting agonist-induced receptor function copurifies with IgM. *Ann Neurol* 30: 550–557.

Zhang GX. (1997) Cytokines and the pathogenesis of myasthenia gravis. *Muscle Nerve* 20: 543–551.

20

Effects of scleroderma on skeletal muscle

Jack E. Riggs and Sydney S. Schochet

Introduction

Scleroderma is usually classified into two broad categories: systemic (alternatively known as progressive systemic sclerosis) and localized (morphea or linear scleroderma). The lesions of morphea scleroderma most often appear as circumscribed plaques on the face, truck or extremities. The lesions of linear scleroderma occur predominantly on the anterior scalp or the extremities. Additionally, the CREST syndrome (calcinosis, Raynaud's phenomenon, oesophageal dysmotility, sclerodactyly and telangiectasis) has been considered to represent a limited form of systemic sclerosis. The CREST syndrome is further characterized by an anticentromere pattern of ANA reactivity. Scleroderma is an autoimmune disorder characterized by excessive deposition of collagen. Resultant progressive fibrosis is the pathological hallmark of scleroderma (Jimenez et al 1996). Although skin, lungs, heart and gastrointestinal tract are commonly recognized organ targets of this fibrosis, skeletal muscle is frequently affected in both the systemic and localized forms of scleroderma. Westphal, in 1876, is generally credited with giving the first description of skeletal muscle involvement in scleroderma (Medsger 1979). Reports of scleroderma from the second half of the 19th century and the first half of the 20th century rarely mentioned symptoms referable to skeletal muscle (Medsger 1979). During the last half of the 20th century, however, muscle weakness and/or skeletal myopathy have been increasingly recognized in patients with scleroderma (Medsger et al 1968, Clements et al 1978, Olsen et al 1996).

Clinical features

Clinical skeletal muscle involvement in scleroderma ranges from mild to very severe (Medsger et al 1968, Olsen et al 1996). Easy fatigue and myalgia are the most common muscular symptoms in scleroderma patients. Associated muscle weakness is often proximal and symmetrical in scleroderma. Shoulder girdle and humeral muscles may be particularly prone to display atrophy and weakness in patients with systemic scleroderma (Medsger et al 1968, Thompson et al 1969). In patients with morphea or linear scleroderma, skeletal muscle involvement may be confined to the areas beneath the skin lesions (Schwartz et al 1981, Miike et al 1983). Scleroderma patients with skeletal muscle involvement appear to have an increased risk of cardiac muscle involvement (West et al 1981, Kerr & Spiera 1993, Follansbee et al 1993, Olsen et al 1996).

Cardiac involvement in scleroderma may manifest as atrial and/or ventricular arrhythmias, left ventricular dysfunction with congestive heart failure, cardiac conduction system abnormalities or sudden death. In one large retrospective study, 20% of scleroderma patients with evidence of skeletal myopathy had evidence of cardiac involvement, whereas only 10% of patients without skeletal myopathy had cardiac abnormalities (Follansbee et al 1993). Radionuclide perfusion scintigraphy studies have also demonstrated a high correlation between low perfusion of skeletal and cardiac muscle (Banci et al 1998). Therefore, skeletal muscle abnormalities appear to be an indicator of increased risk of cardiac abnormalities in scleroderma. Based upon the high correlation between skeletal and cardiac muscle involvement, many investigators have suggested that scleroderma patients with evidence of skeletal muscle involvement should be screened for occult cardiac disease (Follansbee et al 1993, Olsen et al 1996). While usually reflecting pulmonary fibrosis, restrictive lung disease in scleroderma can be a result of respiratory muscle weakness (Chausow et al 1984). Extraocular muscle involvement resulting in diplopia has been described in scleroderma (Arnett & Michels 1973, Rush 1981).

Diagnostic studies

Serum levels of muscle enzymes can be elevated in scleroderma patients (Olsen et al 1996). Indeed, a negative correlation between muscle strength and serum creatine kinase levels has been described (Clements et al 1978). Nevertheless, serum creatine kinase may also be normal in scleroderma patients with severe muscle weakness (Olsen et al 1996). Serum aldolase may be elevated in scleroderma patients with normal serum creatine kinase (Clements et al 1978). Serum antinuclear antibodies are frequently present in patients with systemic scleroderma (Jacobsen et al 1998). The anti-U1 ribonuclear protein antinuclear antibody may be correlated with an increased prevalence of skeletal myopathy in scleroderma (Jacobsen et al 1998).

Electromyography in scleroderma patients with skeletal myopathy may show myopathic motor unit potentials and/or fibrillations associated with active myositis (Hausmanowa-Petrusewicz & Kozminska 1961). Scleroderma patients with inflammatory changes in their muscle are more likely to display spontaneous discharges (fibrillations, positive sharp waves and complex repetitive discharges) on electromyography (Ringel et al 1990, Olsen et al 1996).

However, electromyography in scleroderma patients with obvious severe muscle wasting and weakness can also be normal. Continuous myofibre activity, demonstrated on electromyography, has been described in the quadriceps muscle of a 17-year-old boy with linear scleroderma of the overlying skin and subcutaneous tissues (Papadimitriou et al 1998). This muscle hyperexcitability may reflect involvement of motor nerve endings in muscle affected by scleroderma (Papadimitriou et al 1998).

Magnetic resonance imaging (MRI) of skeletal muscle has demonstrated the presence of inflammation, thickened fascia, and fat replacement in scleroderma (King et al 1993, Adams et al 1995). Magnetic resonance spectroscopy demonstrates an elevated ratio of inorganic phosphate to phosphocreatine in skeletal muscle, both at rest and following exercise, indicating inefficient adenosine triphosphate (ATP) generation and/or utilization (King et al 1993, Adams et al 1995).

Pathological features

The typical pathological features of scleroderma skeletal myopathy are fibrosis, capillary thickening, focal inflammation and myofibre atrophy. The fibrosis can vary from mild to severe and affects epimysial (Fig. 20.1), perimysial (Fig. 20.2) and endomysial (Fig. 20.3) connective tissue. Perhaps the most characteristic pathological alteration in scleroderma myopathy is the prominent thickening of capillaries within the muscle (Fig. 20.4) and surrounding connective

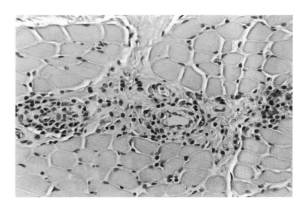

Figure 20.2—Vastus lateralis muscle biopsy specimen from a 9-year-old girl with localized scleroderma. Note the densely fibrotic perimysial connective tissue with perivascular infiltrates of lymphocytes (paraffin embedded section, hematoxylin & eosin, ×230).

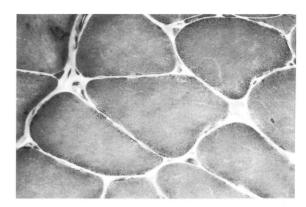

Figure 20.3—Biceps muscle biopsy specimen from a 42-year-old man with scleroderma. Note the mild but widespread endomysial fibrosis (frozen section, modified trichrome, ×450).

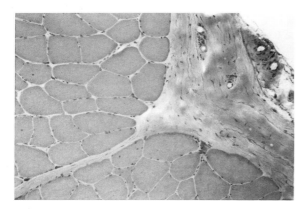

Figure 20.1—Biceps muscle biopsy specimen from a 42-year-old man with scleroderma. The epimysial connective tissue is densely fibrotic. Note also the thickened walls of blood vessels in the epimysial connective tissue (frozen section, hematoxylin & eosin, ×188).

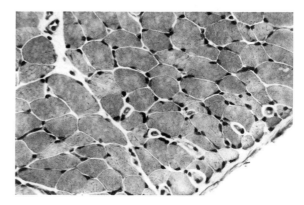

Figure 20.4—Biceps muscle biopsy specimen from a 45-year-old woman with scleroderma. Note the perifascicular myofibre atrophy and the prominent thickening of capillaries within the biopsy specimen (frozen section, hematoxylin & eosin, ×245).

tissue (Fig. 20.5). The focal inflammation seen in scleroderma myopathy is most often perivascular in location (Figs 20.2 and 20.6). The muscle fibre atrophy seen in scleroderma myopathy is often scattered and largely confined to Type II myofibres (Fig. 20.7), but can also be perifascicular involving both major muscle fibre types (Figs 20.4 and 20.8). By electron microscopy, the most distinctive pathological alterations in scleroderma skeletal myopathy are in muscle capillaries that demonstrate endothelial proliferation leading to lumen narrowing and/or obliteration (Michalowski & Kudejko 1966, Russell and Hanna 1988). Skeletal muscle capillary basement membrane abnormalities are most severe in scleroderma patients

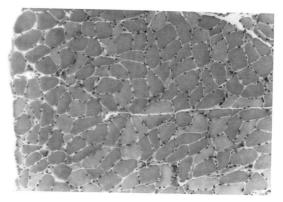

Figure 20.7—Biceps muscle biopsy specimen from a 38-year-old man with scleroderma. Note the numerous atrophic myofibres scattered throughout the biopsy specimen. Fibre typing with ATPase demonstrated that the majority of these atrophic myofibres were type 2 myofibres (frozen section, hematoxylin & eosin, ×188).

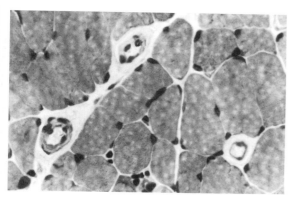

Figure 20.5—Biceps muscle biopsy specimen from a 45-year-old woman with scleroderma. Note the marked thickening of capillaries in the endomysial and perimysial connective tissue (frozen section, hematoxylin & eosin, ×550).

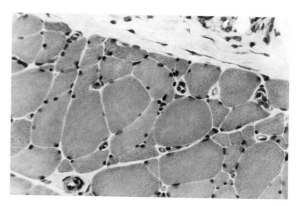

Figure 20.8—Skeletal muscle biopsy specimen from a 61-year-old woman with scleroderma. Note the atrophic muscle fibres adjacent to the fibrotic epimysial connective tissue and scattered within the muscle fascicle (frozen section, hematoxylin & eosin, ×375).

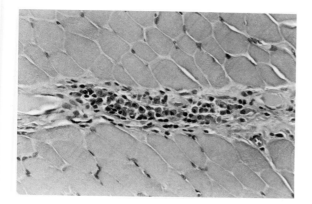

Figure 20.6—Vastus lateralis muscle biopsy specimen from a 9-year-old girl with localized scleroderma. Note the sparsely cellular perimysial connective tissue with inflammatory cells surrounding a blood vessel (paraffin embedded section, hematoxylin & eosin, ×230).

who have the most severe clinical weakness (Russell & Hanna 1983). Although the histological features of scleroderma with myositis resemble those encountered in childhood dermatomyositis, electron microscopy of the capillary endothelial cells does not demonstrate the undulating tubular arrays that are so characteristic of childhood dermatomyositis. Isolated, scattered, angular fibres are frequently encountered in skeletal muscle biopsy specimens of scleroderma myopathy (Fig. 20.9). Calore et al (1995) found angular fibres in five out of six skeletal muscle biopsy specimens from patients with scleroderma. Some of these angular fibres stained positive in the cytoplasm and membrane for neural cell adhesion molecule, a finding indicative of denervation (Calore et at 1995). However, the

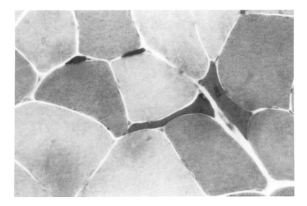

Figure 20.9—Biceps muscle biopsy specimen from a 42-year-old man with scleroderma. Note the angular atrophic denervated myofibres that stain darkly with the non-specific esterase stain (frozen section, non-specific esterase reaction, ×450).

prevalence of a clinically significant generalized peripheral neuropathy in scleroderma patients appears to be relatively low (Ringel et al 1990, Hietaharju et al 1993). Trigeminal sensory neuropathy, however, has been the most frequently described focal neuropathy associated with scleroderma, although histological studies are virtually non-existant. Dyck et al (1997) reported seven patients with peripheral neuropathy among 536 patients with the CREST syndrome. Sural nerve biopsy specimens from four of these patients demonstrated nerve fibre loss and perivascular inflammation; two sural nerve biopsy specimens were suggestive of necrotizing vasculitis, and one specimen was diagnostic of this disease (Dyck et al 1997).

Therapeutic considerations

Controlled clinical trials of therapeutic interventions in scleroderma myopathy have not been performed (Olsen et al 1996). Immunosuppressant agents, such as prednisone, methotrexate azathioprine, and chlorambucil, have been used in the treatment of scleroderma myopathy with only anecdotal success. Extracorporeal photopheresis is a form of immunotherapy that has been used in scleroderma, in which peripheral blood leukocytes are treated with a photosensitizing compound, exposed to ultraviolet irradiation and then reinfused into the patient (Rook et al 1992). Extracorporeal photopheresis has been associated with improved muscle strength, resolution of muscle inflammation seen by magnetic resonance imaging, and improved skeletal muscle utilization and/or generation of high energy phosphate compounds measured by magnetic resonance spectroscopy (Adams et al 1995).

References

Adams LB, Park JH, Olsen NJ, Gardner ES, Hernanz-Schulman M, King LE. (1995) Quantitative evaluation of improvement in muscle weakness in a patient receiving extracorporeal photopheresis for scleroderma: magnetic resonance imaging and magnetic resonance spectroscopy. *J Am Acad Dermatol* 33: 519–522.

Arnett FC, Michels RG. (1973) Inflammatory ocular myopathy in systemic sclerosis (scleroderma). *Arch Intern Med* 132: 740–743.

Banci M, Rinaldi E, Ierardi M, et al. (1998) ⁹⁹ᵐTc SESTAMIBI scintigraphic evaluation of skeletal muscle disease in patients with systemic sclerosis: diagnostic reliability and comparison with cardiac function and perfusion. *Angiology* 49: 641–648.

Calore EE, Cavaliere MJ, Perez NM, Takayasu V, Wakamatsu A, Kiss MH. (1995) Skeletal muscle pathology in systemic sclerosis. *J Rheumatol* 22: 2246–2249.

Chausow AM, Kane T, Levinson D, Szidon JP. (1984) Reversible hypercapnic respiratory insufficiency in scleroderma caused by respiratory muscle weakness. *Am Rev Respir Dis* 130: 130–142.

Clements PJ, Furst DE, Campion DS, et al. (1978) Muscle disease in progressive systemic sclerosis, diagnostic and therapeutic considerations. *Arthritis Rheum* 21: 62–71.

Dyck PJB, Hunder GG, Dyck PJ. (1997) A case-control and nerve biopsy study of CREST multiple mononeuropathy. *Neurology* 49: 1641–1645.

Follansbee WP, Zerbe TR, Medsger TA. (1993) Cardiac and skeletal muscle disease in systemic sclerosis (scleroderma): a high risk association. *Am Heart J* 125: 194–203.

Hausmanowa-Petrusewicz I, Kozminska A. (1961) Electromyographic findings in scleroderma. *Arch Neurol* 4: 281–287.

Hietaharju A, Jaaskelainen S, Kalimo H, Hietarinta M. (1993) Peripheral neuromuscular manifestations in systemic sclerosis (scleroderma). *Muscle Nerve* 16: 1204–1212.

Jacobsen S, Halberg P, Ullman S, et al. (1998) Clinical features and serum antinuclear antibodies in 230 Danish patients with systemic sclerosis. *Br J Rheumatol* 37: 39–45.

Jimenez SA, Hitraya E, Varga J. (1996) Pathogenesis of scleroderma, collagen. *Rheum Dis Clin North Am* 22: 647–674.

Kerr LD, Spiera H. (1993) Myocarditis as a complication in scleroderma patients with myositis. *Clin Cardiol* 16: 895–899.

King LE, Olsen NJ, Puett D, Vital TL, Schulman M, Park JH. (1993) Quantitative evaluation of muscle weakness in scleroderma patients using magnetic resonance imaging and spectroscopy. *Arch Dermatol* 129: 26–247.

Medsger TA. (1979) Progressive systemic sclerosis: skeletal muscle involvement. *Clin Rheum Dis* 5: 103–113.

Medsger TA, Rodnan GP, Moossy J, Vester JW. (1968) Skeletal muscle involvement in progressive systemic sclerosis (scleroderma). *Arthritis Rheum* 11: 554–568.

Michalowski R, Kudejko J. (1966) Electron microscopic observations on skeletal muscle in diffuse scleroderma. *Br J Dermatol* 78: 24–28.

Miike T, Ohtani Y, Hattori S, Ono T, Kageshita T, Matsuda I. (1983) Childhood-type myositis and linear scleroderma. *Neurology* 33: 928–930.

Olsen NJ, King LE, Park JH. (1996) Muscle abnormalities in scleroderma. *Rheum Dis Clin North Am* 22: 783–796.

Papadimitriou A, Chroni E, Anastasopoulos I, Avaramidis I, Hadjigeorgiou G, Koutroumanidis M. (1998) Continuous muscle fiber activity associated with morphea (localized scleroderma). *Neurology* 51: 1763–1764.

Ringel RA, Brick JE, Brick JF, Gutmann L, Riggs JE. (1990) Muscle involvement in scleroderma syndromes. *Arch Intern Med* 150: 2550–2552.

Rook AH, Freundlich B, Jegasothy BV, et al. (1992) Treatment of systemic sclerosis with extracorporeal photochemotherapy. *Arch Dermatol* 128: 337–346.

Rush JA. (1981) Isolated superior oblique paralysis in progressive systemic sclerosis. *Ann Ophthalmol* 13: 217–220.

Russell ML, Hanna WM. (1983) Ultrastructure of muscle microvasculature in progressive systemic sclerosis: relation to clinical weakness. *J Rheumatol* 10: 741–747.

Russell ML, Hanna WM. (1988) Ultrastructural pathology of skeletal muscle in various rheumatic diseases. *J Rheumatol* 15: 445–453.

Schwartz RA, Tedesco AS, Stern LZ, Kaminska AM, Haraldsen JM, Grekin DA. (1981) Myopathy associated with sclerodermal facial hemiatrophy. *Arch Neurol* 38: 592–594.

Thompson JM, Bluestone R, Bywaters EGL, Dorling J, Johnson M. (1969) Skeletal muscle involvement in systemic sclerosis. *Ann Rheum Dis* 28: 281–288.

West SG, Killian PJ, Lawless OJ. (1981) Association of myositis and myocarditis in progressive systemic sclerosis. *Arthritis Rheum* 24: 662–667.

21

Ion channel diseases of skeletal muscle

Rajkumar Rajendram and Timothy J. Peters

Introduction

Ion channels are crucial in the coupling of the action potential (AP) at the neuromuscular junction with the contraction of skeletal muscle. It is, therefore, not surprising that changes in ion channel function manifest as defects of excitation–contraction (EC) coupling. Collectively known as channelopathies, the ion channel mutations in skeletal muscle cause either decreased excitability and muscle paralysis or increased excitability and myotonia or both.

Myotonia appears clinically as delayed relaxation of muscles following either voluntary contraction or direct stimuli such as percussion. This is usually experienced as stiffness, and affected individuals may complain of difficulty releasing handshakes or opening their eyes after squinting in bright sunlight. Unlike cramp, the sustained contraction is usually painless, but some weakness may occur. Myotonia usually diminishes with continued exercise of the muscle over a period of up to 30 min. This "warm-up" phenomenon may be beneficial in overcoming the disability produced by the initial myotonia, although occasional patients with myotonia and notably paramyotonia, show a paradoxical response: myotonia being aggravated by exercise.

Membrane excitability is *enhanced* in myotonic muscles, and voluntary contraction can initiate repetitive discharges that persist for several seconds. The associated electromyographic abnormality is known as the "myotonic run". Classically, the discharge frequency increases and the spike amplitude decreases as the run progresses, producing the "dive-bomber" effect when heard over loudspeakers. These potentials are absent at rest, and they are unaffected by non-depolarizing blockade of neuromuscular junction transmission by, for example, curare, confirming that the myotonia is intrinsic to the muscle fibre.

The periodic paralyses (PP) lie at the other end of the range of muscle excitability. The episodic weakness that the affected individuals complain of is caused by reduced membrane excitability, and it results in paroxysmal muscle paralysis. During attacks of *weakness*, the electromyogram is silent, the membrane is depolarized at −50 to −60 mV (from a normal value of −90 mV), and AP cannot be generated, even by direct galvanic shock.

The majority of the periodic paralyses are due to genetic effects and, in a given pedigree, the plasma potassium (K^+) either rises or falls during paralysis. Periodic paralyses are classified clinically into hyperkalaemic (HyperPP; plasma K^+ >4.5 mM), and hypokalaemic periodic paralyses (HypoPP; plasma K^+

<2.0 mM). The paralysis is episodic and lasts from minutes to hours, but muscle strength is normal between attacks. There is no associated seizure, cardiac arrhythmia, sensory abnormality or alteration of consciousness. In paramyotonia congenita (PMC), paralysis is rare, but myotonia may occur at the onset of weakness or between episodes of paralysis. Thus, an affected individual may experience myotonia because of muscle membrane hyperexcitability at one moment yet weakness due to inexcitability minutes later.

The molecular basis of these diseases was elucidated by cloning cDNAs and testing candidate genes. This established linkage with skeletal muscle voltage-operated ion channels. Mutations were identified in genes for sodium (Na^+), chloride (Cl^-) and calcium (Ca^{2+}) channels (Fontaine et al 1990, Koch et al 1992, Fontaine et al 1994).

Chloride channel myotonias

Myotonia congenita (MC) was first described in 1876 by Thomsen, a physician himself afflicted with the dominant form of the disease. However, the first insights into its pathogenesis were gleaned from studies on goats with a form of congenital myotonia that resembles Thomsen's disease (Bryant 1969). Microelectrode recordings revealed that the membrane resistance of excised muscle fibres from these goats was greatly increased. Variation of the bathing solutions then revealed that the increased resistance resulted from a reduction in Cl^- conductance (G_{Cl}). Further studies led Adrian and Bryant (1974) to propose that the after-potentials were a result of K^+ accumulation in the T tubule, an extracellular space that limits diffusion.

In normal muscle, a prolonged depolarizing current elicits a single AP, but in myotonic muscle causes a series of discharges. Each AP causes K^+ efflux from the sarcoplasm into the T tubule. The G_{Cl}, which is about 70% of resting membrane conductance (−90 mV), normally counteracts the depolarizing effects of the T tubule accumulation of K^+. Absence of the G_{Cl} increases membrane resistance, slowing repolarization after a discharge. Extracellular accumulation of K^+ depolarizes the T tubule by shifting the K^+ equilibrium to a less negative potential. T tubule depolarization opens the voltage-operated sodium channels (VOSC) and, as membrane resistance is increased, even small currents can elicit another AP and cause myotonia (reviewed in Bryant 1979). However, progressive attenuation of the myotonic discharges occurs as K^+ accumulates and the membrane potential approaches a stable depolarized value of -40 mV and the voltage-operated Na^+ channels inactivate. The G_{Cl} of muscle fibres from patients with Thomsen's disease is also reduced (Lipicky et al 1971). Congenital myotonia shows genetic linkage to chromosome 7q35 and the *CLCN1* gene, encoding the major skeletal muscle Cl^- channel (Abdalla et al 1992, Koch et al 1992, Koty et al 1994). More than 30 point mutations and three deletions have been found in *CLCN1* in individual families. The individual mutations, which cause either Thomsen's (dominant) or Becker's (recessive) myo-

tonia congenita (Fig. 21.1), have been summarized by Mäilander et al (1996).

The mechanism by which mutations in the same gene produce either dominant or recessive effects is not known, as the functional domains of Cl^- channels have not been identified. However, Cl^- channel blocking drugs and computer models have revealed that myotonia occurs when 80% of G_{Cl} is blocked. Thus, a 50% reduction in G_{Cl} should result in an asymptomatic carrier state (Barchi 1975, Kwiecinski et al 1988). Mutations which introduce stop codons or frameshifts early in the coding sequence are expected to encode non-functional products. However, in the

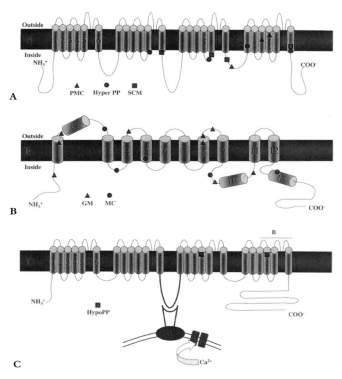

Figure 21.1 — **A** A model of the α-subunit of the skeletal muscle voltage-operated sodium channel (VOSC). The locations of the mutations that cause hyperkalaemic periodic paralysis (Hyper PP), Paramyotonia Congenita (PMC) and Sodium Channel Myotonia (SCM) are indicated (adapted from Cannon 1996). **B** A model of the skeletal muscle chloride channel. The approximate location of mutations reported in the skeletal muscle voltage-dependent chloride channel associated either with dominant (MC) or recessive (GM) myotonia congenita are indicated. Although the secondary and tertiary structures of this channel remain largely unresolved, the model presented here is derived from that of Jentsch et al (1994). The functional channel probably contains four of these monomeric subunits (redrawn and adapted from Barchi 1997). **C** A model of the α-subunit of the skeletal muscle dihydropyridine receptor. The voltage-operated calcium channel shown here shares significant homology with the α-subunit of the VOSC. The sites of the 3 mutations which cause hypokalaemic periodic paralysis are indicated. The skeletal muscle calcium channel is known to interact with the ryanodine receptor (RyR) which resides in the sarcoplasmic reticulum (SR) membrane. The contribution of this channel to the calcium flux across the sarcolemma is small. The depolarization of the membrane is sensed by the channel, which, through an interaction with the RyR causes opening of a calcium slow release channel in the SR. It is the movement of calcium from the SR to the cytosol that causes the contraction of muscle. B indicates the DHP binding site (adapted from Cannon 1996).

presence of a normal allele, a single abnormal allele should be asymptomatic, but could produce disease if both gene copies were affected.

Chloride channels exist as homotetramers in vitro and, in channels containing mixtures of both, affected subunits could affect normal subunits. In this way dominant expression of the disease phenotype could occur. Furthermore, a dominant negative effect has been demonstrated for several MC mutations in vitro using heterologous gene expression in oocyte methodology. Expression of the mutant channel alone produces either no current (Steinmeyer et al 1994) or currents with abnormal kinetics (Pusch et al 1995). Expression of 1:1 ratios of mutant to wild-type channels produces unexpectedly low current levels, suggesting that only those channels containing 3 or 4 wild-type subunits function normally. The stringency of this dominant negative effect may vary with the nature of the mutation.

Sodium channelopathies

Hyperkalaemic PP, PMC and the sodium channel myotonias (SCM) are dominantly inherited traits linked to chromosome 17q23.1-25.3 (Fontaine et al 1990, Ebers et al 1991). This encodes the α-subunit of SkM1 (George et al 1991; see Fig. 21.1), the tetrodotoxin-sensitive, VOSC expressed in skeletal muscle.

Mutations of SkM1 can cause either myotonia or periodic paralysis but do not affect other excitable tissues. Fourteen mutations have been identified in families with HyperPP, PMC or SCM (for review, see Rüdel et al 1993, Barchi 1995). In each case a single nucleotide transversion produces a missense mutation that encodes a substitution at a residue which is highly conserved amongst Na^+ channel α-subunits.

The functional consequences of the mutations have been tested by heterologous expression in mammalian cells (Cannon and Strittmatter 1993, Cummins et al 1993, Chahine et al 1994, Mitrovic et al 1994, Yang et al 1994). The main deficit in each case is impaired channel *inactivation* resulting in persistent currents, slowed decay of the transient current, shift in the voltage-dependence of inactivation, or a combination of these effects. Three mutations arise at a single residue, G1306, in the cytoplasmic link between domains III and IV (Fig. 21.2). Each mutation causes a form of myotonia without significant weakness, but the degree of muscle stiffness correlates with the nature of the amino acid substitution (alanine <valine <glutamate) (Lerche et al 1993).

These genotype–phenotype correlations suggest that each mutation causes a specific change in Na^+ channel function, thereby resulting in unique phenotypes. However, the severity of symptoms varies even between affected members of the same family (McClatchey et al 1992). The severity of these dominantly inherited traits may depend on the relative levels of mutant and wild-type α-subunit mRNA (Zhou et al 1994). Alternatively, allelic variability of other ion channels may influence the consequences of Na^+ channel mutations.

The defects are consistent with ball and chain models of Na^+ channel structure, which propose that rapid inactivation results from occlusion of the pore by a *ball* formed from the cytoplasmic loop (*chain*) linking domains III and IV. Four mutations occur within this chain, and six others lie at the cytoplasmic end of transmembrane segments S5 or S6 in domains II, III or IV. These latter sites may line the mouth of the pore formed by the S5–S6 loop. Thus, at least 10 mutations could disrupt the inactivation particle or its binding. Two mutations occur in an arginine in domain IV (Ptacek et al 1992) in which an alternating sequence of hydrophobic and basic residues (arginine or lysine) is thought to form part of the voltage sensor for channel activation. These mutations also disrupt inactivation without affecting activation, possibly by modifying the coupling of channel opening and inactivation (Chahine et al 1994).

Both theoretical and animal models have demonstrated that the inactivation defect of Na^+ channels can cause either myotonia or paralysis (Cannon and Corey 1993, Cannon et al 1993). Rat skeletal muscle exposed to ATX II, a sea anemone toxin, mimics the inactivation defect in HyperPP. Micromolar concentrations of ATX II toxin disrupt the inactivation comparable to that observed in Na^+ currents from HyperPP myotubules. The resultant small persistent Na^+ current produces myotonia with a tenfold slowing in twitch force relaxation (Cannon and Corey 1993).

Sodium channels are normally closed at resting potential. On depolarization, Na^+ channels open briefly, close, then inactivate. Membrane hyperpolarization restores Na^+ channels to the closed state from which reopening can occur. In HyperPP, Na^+ channels occasionally fail to inactivate, resulting in prolonged opening or bursts of opening and closing throughout the depolarization. Bursts of reopenings occur very rarely (perhaps 1 in 2000 openings) in normal channels (Patlak and Ortiz 1986). However, in HyperPP myotubules failure of inactivation is 20–50 times more common, resulting in a small persistent Na^+ current.

Cannon and Corey (1993) demonstrated that K^+ accumulation in T tubules also contributes to myotonia in muscles with sodium channelopathies. Osmotic disruption of the T tubule electrically uncouples the T tubule from the surface membrane. Long current pulses still elicit repetitive discharges in detubulated fibres exposed to ATX II, because of the resultant defect in Na^+ channel inactivation. However, in the absence of T tubule K^+ accumulation, the membrane does not progressively depolarize with each successive impulse and hence there is no stimulus to trigger after-potentials.

The mechanism by which disrupted inactivation causes myotonia or paralysis has also been studied with muscle fibres simulations (Cannon et al 1993). Consistent with the experimental data, simulations with a small proportion (~2%) of non-inactivating Na^+ channels express myotonic discharges. Slightly higher proportions ($\geq$3%) cause progressive attenuation of myotonic discharges as K^+ accumulates in the T tubule and the membrane potential approaches a stable depolarized value of -40 mV. At this depolarized potential, AP are not elicited by subsequent stimuli as the majority of Na^+ channels (both wild-type and mutant) are inactivated. The muscle fibre is paralysed and inexcitable. The dominant inheritance of HyperPP can be explained by the gain of function (i.e. the partial loss of Na^+ channel inactivation) caused by the mutations. This is sufficient to cause paralysis as normal Na^+ channels inactivate because of membrane depolarization.

Computer modelling has also shown that the predisposition to myotonia or paralysis depends on the type of inactivation defect (Cannon 1996). Simulations with persistent Na^+ currents, as seen in the HyperPP-associated mutations, primarily cause large depolarizing shifts in the resting potential and paralysis. Myotonia occurs only over a narrow range of mild inactivation loss. Conversely, shifts in the voltage-dependence of inactivation, and slowed rates of inactivation, cause myotonic discharges over a wide range of parameter values. This type of inactivation defect occurs with α-subunit mutations found in the myotonic disorders (PMC and SCM). Therefore, the genotype–phenotype correlation of Na^+ channelopathies is probably partly due to the specific inactivation defect caused by each mutation.

Calcium channelopathies

Two major Ca^{2+} channels are expressed in adult skeletal muscle, the dihydropyridine receptor (DHPR) and the ryanodine receptor (RYR1). They are located at the triadic junctions of the T tubules and the sarcoplasmic reticulum (SR), respectively. Mutations causing HypoPP have been identified in the DHPR whilst mutations causing malignant hyperthermia have been identified in both.

Hypokalaemic periodic paralysis is the most prevalent inherited periodic paralysis. It is inherited as autosomal dominant, but an acquired form is also seen in hyperthyroidism, typically in Orientals. However, it is rare with a prevalence of only 1 in 100 000. The symptoms of episodic weakness associated with low plasma K^+ characteristically begin late at night or in the morning, often following large, carbohydrate-rich or salty meals or vigorous exercise the previous day. Paralysis is associated with membrane depolarization and increased resting Na^+ conductance, but this is not affected by tetrodotoxin, a blocker of VOSC (Rüdel et al 1984).

HypoPP is linked to chromosome 1q31-32 which encodes the DHPR α_{1S}-subunit (Fontaine et al 1994). Although DHPR has at least five subunits, the channel-forming α_{1S}-subunit is homologous to the α-subunit of Na^+ channels (Catterall 1992) (compare Fig. 21.1B and Fig. 21.1C). Three mutations have been identified, by sequencing cDNA derived from muscle biopsies from affected individuals, two of which occur at the same site and are homologous to the mutations of the Na^+ channel α-subunit that cause PMC/HyperPP (Boerman et al 1995, Elbaz et al 1995, Fouad et al 1997).

The pathophysiological mechanism linking these channel mutations to the depolarization seen during HypoPP paralytic episodes remains unclear. The DHPR is a voltage-dependent L-type Ca^{2+} channel, but it does not appear to function as an ion-conducting channel in skeletal muscle. The DHPR acts as the voltage sensor for the RYR1, which is not itself voltage dependent. The DHPR is thought to couple T tubule depolarization with RYR1 activation, which releases Ca^{2+} from the SR, initiating contraction (Melzer et al 1995). However, electrical muscle activity, evoked by nerve stimulation, is reduced or even absent during attacks, therefore, a failure of excitation is more likely than a disruption of EC coupling (Engel et al 1965, Links et al 1994). However, the hypokalaemia-induced membrane depolarization observed in excised muscle fibres could inactivate sarcolemmal and T tubular Na^+ channels reducing Ca^{2+} release (Rüdel et al 1984). This could also explain the mechanism by which membrane repolarization by activation of ATP-sensitive K^+ channels, restores force in HypoPP (Grafe et al 1990).

Malignant hyperthermia (MH) is an autosomal

dominant inherited predisposition to an abnormal response following exposure to volatile anaesthetics (e.g. halothane) or depolarizing muscle relaxants (e.g. suxamethonium). Exposure to the triggering agents results in excessive Ca^{2+} release from the SR (Iaizzo et al 1988). Muscle metabolism is greatly increased causing muscle rigidity, hyperthermia, hyperkalaemia, metabolic acidosis and hypoxia. Without immediate treatment, up to 70% of patients die (Gronert 1994). Dantrolene, an inhibitor of Ca^{2+} release from the SR, can halt the development of crises and has reduced mortality to less than 10%.

Point mutations in the intracellular connection between domains III and IV of the DHPR α_{1S}-subunit have also been associated with malignant hyperthermia (Monnier et al 1997), although the significance of this region in EC coupling is not known. In addition, over 20 disease-causing mutations of RYR1 have been identified in humans, emphasizing the functional relationship between the DHPR and the RYR1. All mutations are situated in the N-terminal region of RYR1, which contains the binding sites for various activating ligands (Ca^{2+}, μM; caffeine and ryanodine, nM) and inactivating ligands (Ca^{2+}, $>10\ \mu M$; Mg^{2+}, mM; Meissner 1994). The mutations are thought to alter RYR1 function such that Ca^{2+} can excessively activate the channel at lower levels, and greater Ca^{2+} concentrations are required for inhibition (Mickelson and Louis 1996). Functional characterization of some mutations has revealed increased sensitivity of mutant RYR1 to exogenous ligands (caffeine and halothane) as well as activating levels of Ca^{2+} (Richter et al 1997, Tong et al 1997). Overexpression of a mutant RYR in normal human muscle also increased the Ca^{2+} response during exposure to a triggering agent (Censier et al 1998). A reduced inhibition of Ca^{2+} release by Mg^{2+} has been observed in muscle predisposed to MH (Laver et al 1997) and is thought to be an important role in the pathogenesis of MH.

Treatment of channelopathies

Local anaesthetics—e.g., lidocaine (lignocaine)—and class IB antiarrhythmics (e.g., mexelitine) effectively prevent the muscle stiffness of the Na^+ channelopathies, particularly PMC (Streib 1987). A reduction of stiffness is also seen in the Cl^- channelopathies and myotonic dystrophy (Rüdel et al 1980). The therapeutic effect is due to the use-dependent block of Na^+ channels, which inhibits the final common pathway of the generation of myotonia by preventing repeated firing of action potentials. However, mexiletine does not improve the spontaneous and K^+-induced attacks of weakness typical for HyperPP (Ricker et al 1983). Fortunately, diuretics such as hydrochlorothiazide and acetazolamide decrease the frequency and severity of paralysis by reducing serum K^+ (Ricker et al 1983). Treatment of HypoPP is also non-specific, involving avoidance of precipitating factors, prophylaxis with oral K^+ supplements and acetazolamide.

Summary

Understanding of the ion channel diseases of skeletal muscle has expanded exponentially in recent years. These advances revealed much about the electrophysiology of skeletal muscle contraction and enabled rational application of pharmacological therapies for several channelopathies. However, there is a need for improved pharmacological agents as gene therapy is still many years away and gene screening tests for antenatal diagnosis have not yet been developed.

However, several questions regarding the pathophysiology of the channelopathies remain unanswered. For example, the mechanisms behind the phenotypic expression of mutations located in functionally uncharacterized regions of channel proteins are not known. Furthermore, the relevance of the environmental trigger factors in the episodic expression of symptoms is poorly understood. The answers to these and other questions will probably come with the identification of new disease-causing mutations and characterization of channel function on the molecular level.

References

Abdalla JA, Casley WL, Cousin HK, et al. (1992) Linkage of Thomsen disease to the T-cell-receptor beta (TCRB) locus on chromosome 7q35. *Am J Hum Genet* 51: 579–584.

Adrian RH, Bryant SH. (1974) On the repetitive discharge in myotonic muscle fibres. *J Physiol (Lond)* 240: 505–515.

Barchi RL. (1975) Myotonia. An evaluation of the chloride hypothesis. *Arch Neurol* 32: 175–180.

Barchi RL. (1995) Molecular pathology of the skeletal muscle sodium channel. *Annu Rev Physiol* 57: 355–385.

Barchi RL. (1997) Ion channel mutations and diseases of skeletal muscle. *Neurobiol Dis* 4: 254–264.

Boerman RH, Ophoff RA, Links TP, et al. (1995) Mutation in DHP-receptor $_1$-subunit (CACNL1A3) gene in a Dutch family with hypokalemic periodic paralysis. *J Med Genet* 32: 44–47.

Bryant SH. (1969) Cable properties of external intercostal muscle fibres from myotonic and nonmyotonic goats. *J Physiol (Lond)* 204: 539–550.

Bryant SH. (1979) Myotonia in the goat. *Ann N Y Acad Sci* 317: 314–325.

Cannon SC. (1996) Ion channel defects and abberant excitability in myotonia and periodic paralysis. *TINS* 19: 3–10.

Cannon SC, Brown RH, Jr, Corey DP. (1993) Theoretical reconstruction of myotonia and paralysis caused by incomplete inactivation of sodium channels. *Biophys J* 65: 270–288.

Cannon SC, Corey DP. (1993) Loss of Na^+ channel inactivation by anemone toxin (ATX II) mimics the myotonic state in hyperkalaemic periodic paralysis. *J Physiol (Lond)* 466: 501–520.

Cannon SC, Strittmatter SM. (1993) Functional expression of sodium channel mutations identified in families with periodic paralysis. *Neuron* 10: 317–326.

Catterall WA. (1992) Cellular and molecular biology of voltage-gated sodium channels. *Physiol Rev* 72(Suppl): S15–48.

Censier K, Urwyler A, Zorzato F, Treves S. (1998) Intracellular calcium homeostasis in human primary muscle cells from malignant hyperthermia-susceptible and normal individuals. Effect of overexpression of recombinant wild-type and Arg163Cys mutated ryanodine receptors. *J Clin Invest* 101: 1233–1242.

Chahine M, George AL, Jr, Zhou M, et al. (1994) Sodium channel mutations in paramyotonia congenita uncouple inactivation from activation. *Neuron* 12: 281–294.

Cummins TR, Zhou J, Sigworth FJ, et al. (1993) Functional consequences of a Na^+ channel mutation causing hyperkalemic periodic paralysis. *Neuron* 10: 667–678.

Ebers GC, George AL, Barchi RL, et al. (1991) Paramyotonia congenita and hyperkalemic periodic paralysis are linked to the adult muscle sodium channel gene. *Ann Neurol* 30: 810–816.

Elbaz A, Vale-Santos J, Jurkat-Rott K, et al. (1995) Hypokalemic periodic paralysis (HYPOPP) and the dihydropyridine receptor (CACNL1A3): genotype/phenotype correlations for two predominant mutations and evidence for the absence of a founder effect in 16 caucasian families. *Am J Hum Gen* 56: 374–380.

Engel AG, Lambert EH, Rosevaer JW, Newlon TW. (1965) Clinical and electromyographic studies in a patient with primary hypokalemic periodic paralysis. *Am J Med* 38: 626–640.

Fontaine B, Khurana TS, Hoffman EP, et al. (1990) Hyperkalemic periodic paralysis and the adult muscle sodium channel alpha-subunit gene. *Science* 250: 1000–1002.

Fontaine B, Vale-Santos J, Jurkat-Rott K, et al. (1994) Mapping of the hypokalaemic periodic paralysis (HypoPP) locus to chromosome 1q31-32 in three European families. *Nat Genet* 6: 267–272.

Fouad G, Dalakas M, Servedei S, et al. (1997) Genotype-phenotype correlations of DHP receptor $_1$-subunit gene mutations causing hypokalemic periodic paralysis. *Neuromuscular Disorders* 7: 33–38.

George AL, Jr, Komisarof J, Kallen RG, Barchi RL. (1992) Primary structure of the adult human skeletal muscle voltage-dependent sodium channel. *Ann Neurol* 31: 131–137.

George AL, Jr, Ledbetter DH, Kallen RG, Barchi RL. (1991) Assignment of a human skeletal muscle sodium channel alpha-subunit gene (SCN4A) to 17q23.1–25.3. *Genomics* 9: 555–556.

Grafe P, Quasthoff S, Strupp M, Lehmann-Horn F. (1990) Enhancement of K^+ conductance improves in vitro the contraction force of skeletal muscle in hypokalemic periodic paralysis. *Muscle Nerve* 13: 451–457.

Gronert GA. (1994) Malignant hyperthermia. In: Engel AG, Franzini-Armstrong C, eds. *Myology* 2nd ed. New York: McGraw-Hill, pp. 1661–1678.

Iaizzo PA, Klein W, Lehmann-Horn F. (1988) Fura-2 detected myoplasmic calcium and its correlation with contracture force in skeletal muscle from normal and malignant hyperthermia susceptible pigs. *Pflüger Arch* 411: 648–653.

Jentsch TJ. (1994) Molecular physiology of anion channels. *Curr Opin Cell Biol* 6: 600–606.

Koch MC, Steinmeyer K, Lorenz C. (1992) The skeletal muscle chloride channel in dominant and recessive human myotonia. *Science* 257: 797–800.

Koty PP, Marks HG, Turel A, et al. (1994) Linkage analysis of Thomsen and Becker myotonia families. *Am J Hum Genetics Suppl* 55: A227.

Kwiecinski H, Lehmann-Horn F, Rudel R. (1988) Drug-induced myotonia in human intercostal muscle. *Muscle Nerve* 11: 576–581.

Laver DR, Owen VJ, Junankar PR, Taske NL, Dulhunty AF, Lamb GD. (1997) Reduced inhibitory effect of Mg^{2+} on ryanodine receptor-Ca^{2+} release channels in malignant hyperthermia. *Biophys J* 73: 1913–1924.

Lerche H, Heine R, Pika U, et al. (1993) Human sodium channel myotonia: slowed channel inactivation due to substitutions for a glycine within the III-IV linker. *J Physiol (Lond)* 470: 13–22.

Links TP, Vanderhoeven JH, Zwarts MJ. (1994) Surface EMG and muscle fiber conduction during attacks of hypokalaemic periodic paralysis. *J Neurol Neurosurg Psychiatry* 57: 632–634.

Lipicky RJ, Bryant SH, Salmon JH. (1971) Cable parameters, sodium, potassium, chloride, and water content, and potassium efflux in isolated external intercostal muscle of normal volunteers and patients with myotonia congenita. *J Clin Invest* 50: 2091–2103.

Mäilander V, Heine R, Deymeer F, Lehmann-Horn F. (1996) Novel muscle chloride channels mutations and their effects on heterozygous carriers. *Am J Hum Genetics* 58: 317–324.

McClatchey AI, McKenna-Yasek D, Cros D, et al. (1992) Novel mutations in families with unusual and variable disorders of the skeletal muscle sodium channel. *Nat Genet* 2: 148–152.

Meissner G. (1994) Ryanodine receptor/Ca^{2+} release channels and their regulation by endogenous effectors. *Annu Rev Physiol* 56: 485–508.

Melzer W, Herrmann-Frank A, Lüttgau HC. (1995) The role of Ca^{2+} ions in excitation-contraction coupling of skeletal muscle fibers. *Biochem Biophys Acta* 1241: 59–116.

Mickelson JR, Louis CF. (1996) Malignant hyperthermia: excitation-contraction coupling, Ca^{2+} release channel, and cell Ca^{2+} regulation defects. *Physiol Rev* 76: 537–592.

Mitrovic N, George AL, Jr, Heine R. (1994) K^+-aggravated myotonia: destabilization of the inactivated state of the human muscle Na^+ channel by the V1589M mutation. *J Physiol (Lond)* 478: 395–402.

Monnier N, Procaccio V, Stieglitz S, Lunardi P. (1997) Malignant-hyperthermia susceptibility is associated with a mutation of the α_1-subunit of the human dihydropyridine-sensitive L-type voltage-dependent calcium-channel receptor in skeletal muscle. *Am J Hum Genet* 60: 1316–1325.

Patlak JB, Ortiz M. (1986) Two modes of gating during late Na^+ channel currents in frog sartorius muscle. *J Gen Physiol* 87: 305–326.

Ptacek LJ, George AL, Jr, Barchi RL, et al. (1992) Mutations in an S4 segment of the adult skeletal muscle sodium channel cause paramyotonia congenita. *Neuron* 8: 891–897.

Pusch M, Steinmeyer K, Koch MC, Jentsch TJ. (1995) Mutations in dominant human myotonia congenita drastically alter the coltage dependence of the ClC-1 chloride channel. *Neuron* 15: 1455–1463.

Richter M, Schleithoff L, Deufel T, Lehmann-Horn F, Herrmann-Frank A. (1997) Functional characterization of a distinct ryanodine receptor mutation in human malignant hyperthermia-susceptible muscle. *J Biol Chem* 272: 5256–5260.

Ricker K, Böhlen R, Rohkamm R. (1983) Different effectiveness of tocainide and hydrochlorothiazide in paramyotonia congenita with hyperkalemic episodic paralysis. *Neurology* 33: 1615–1618.

Rüdel R, Dengler R, Ricker K, Haass A, Emser W. (1980) Improved therapy of myotonia with the lidocaine derivative tocainide. *J Neurol* 222: 275–278.

Rüdel R, Lehmann-Horn F, Ricker K, Küther G. (1984) Hypokalemic periodic paralysis: in vitro investigation of muscle fiber membrane parameters. *Muscle Nerve* 7: 110–120.

Rüdel R, Ricker K, Lehmann-Horn F. (1993) Genotype-phenotype correlations in human skeletal muscle sodium channel diseases. *Arch Neurol* 50: 1241–1248.

Steinmeyer K, Lorenz C, Pusch M et al. (1994) Multimeric structure of ClC-1 chloride channel revealed by mutations in dominant myotonia congenita. *EMBO J* 13: 737.

Streib EW. (1987) Paramyotonia congenita: successful treatment with tocainide. Clinical and electrophysiological findings in seven patients. *Muscle Nerve* 10: 155–162.

Thomsen J. (1876) Tonische Krämpfe in willkürlich beweglichen Muskeln in Folge von ererbter psychischer Disposition. *Arch Psychiatrie Nerv* 6: 702–718.

Tong J, Oyamada H, Demaurex N, Grinstein S, McCarthy TV, Maclennan DH. (1997) Caffeine and halothane sensitivity of intracellular Ca^{2+} release is altered by 15 calcium release channel (ryanodine receptor) mutations associated with malignant hyperthermia and/or central core disease. *J Biol Chem* 272: 26332–26339.

Yang N, Ji S, Zhou M, et al. (1994). Sodium channel mutations in paramyotonia congenita exhibit similar biophysical phenotypes in vitro. *Proc Natl Acad Sci USA* 91: 12785–12789.

Zhou J, Spier SJ, Beech J, Hoffman EP. (1994) Pathophysiology of sodium channelopathies: correlation of normal/mutant mRNA ratios with clinical phenotype in dominantly inherited periodic paralysis. *Hum Mol Genet* 3: 1599–1603.

22

Inclusion body myositis

Michael R. Rose and Robert C. Griggs

Introduction

Yunis and Samaha (1971) first coined the term inclusion body myositis (IBM) in 1971 but the first recorded description of the disease was in 1967 when Chou reported an unusual case of "chronic polymyositis" in which muscle biopsy showed inflammatory infiltration with muscle fibres containing basophilic rimmed vacuoles and filamentous cytoplasmic and nuclear inclusions. A readily recognisable clinical phenotype for this condition has emerged, but despite this many patients with IBM continue to have initial mis-diagnoses. Even so, from being an apparently rare entity IBM has now become the commonest acquired myopathy over the age of 50 years and more common than its other inflammatory counterparts such as polymyositis and dermatomyositis. Although the inflammatory component is a prominent histological feature, there are additional features of abnormal protein upregulation and deposition which are probably part of the primary pathological change. IBM is a slowly progressive myopathy that does not appear to respond to current anti-inflammatory or immunosuppressive treatments.

Clinical features

Incidence and prevalence

In the initial published series IBM was found to comprise 17% (Carpenter et al 1978), 28% (Lotz et al 1989) or as high as 30% (Karpati et al 1988) of all cases of inflammatory myopathy. However most myologists report that IBM is far more common than either polymyositis or dermatomyositis comprising as many as 60 or 70% of inflammatory myopathies (Maat-Shieman 1992). IBM is usually of late onset, with more than 80% of cases occurring over the age of 50 years (Lotz et al 1989), although childhood onset has been described (Riggs et al 1989). The male:female ratio is greater than 2:1 contrasting with the female predominance of polymyositis (Carpenter et al 1978, Lotz et al 1989). The vast majority of cases of inclusion body *myositis* are sporadic. Apparently familial cases are most likely to be cases of inclusion body *myopathy,* that is, cases in which there is no inflammation on muscle biopsy (see differential diagnosis below), but there are a small number of case reports of familial, otherwise typical, inclusion body *myositis* (Amato and Shebert 1998, Naumann and Toyka 1999).

Presentation

The first symptom is often one of unprovoked and initially puzzling falls that, on further questioning, prove to be a result of buckling at the knees. This is a manifestation of quadriceps weakness, which may also cause anxiety when descending stairs since this is likely to provoke crumpling at the knees. Sometimes there are other more classical features of proximal lower limb weakness such as difficulty climbing stairs and rising from chairs. Another group of characteristic presenting symptoms are those due to distal weakness in the feet and, more particularly, in the hands. Distal, anterior compartment foot weakness may cause foot drop and tripping. Distal hand weakness characteristically affects the long finger flexors producing symptoms such as golf clubs flying out of a weak hand grip, cases slipping out of the fingers and difficulty with tasks such as pulling up car door lock buttons and turning keys and door handles. Although distal limb involvement can be prominent compared with proximal disease (Carpenter et al 1978) one series showed that while distal weakness occurred in half the cases, it exceeded proximal weakness in only one third (Lotz et al 1989). IBM may, therefore, present with solely proximal weakness creating a wider differential diagnosis (see below).

Examination often shows wasting and weakness of the quadriceps (Fig. 22.1) and forearm flexors with the later causing a very characteristic scooped appearance of the volar aspect of the forearm (Fig. 22.2) and weakness of flexion at the proximal interphalangeal (PIP) and distal interphalangeal (DIP) finger joints. Reflexes, particularly in the lower limbs may be absent, and this may bring to mind alternative diagnoses such as peripheral neuropathy or anterior horn disease. There are no sensory findings attributable to IBM although patients may have age-related loss of vibration sensation. The symptoms and their accompanying signs are often asymmetrical, and they sometimes have a unilateral onset. The asymmetry often persists as the disease progresses.

An additional symptom, sometimes attributed to IBM, is dysphagia. Incidence has been variously reported as "one third" or "up to 60%" (Lotz et al 1989, Lindberg et al 1994). In one series it was reported in 16 out of 19 patients (Houser et al 1998). While the dysphagia can be mild, in a very small number of patients it has either been a severe presenting problem, preceding limb muscle weakness by years, or it becomes a major management problem as the disease

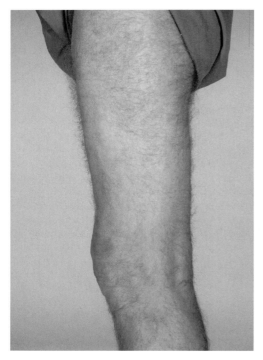

Figure 22.1 — An example of quadriceps wasting in a case of inclusion body myositis.

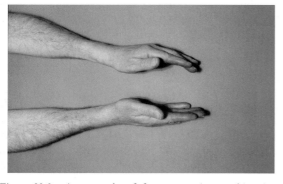

Figure 22.2 — An example of forearm wasting resulting in a "scooped" appearance in a case of inclusion body myositis.

progresses (Wintzen et al 1988, Danon and Friedman 1989, Verma et al 1991, Danon and Friedman 1992, Riminton et al 1993).

There is no ocular involvement with IBM and patients do not complain of facial weakness, but in one third of cases examination shows mild weakness of eyelid or lip closure, which is not a feature of alternative inflammatory myopathies such as polymyositis

and dermatomyositis. There may be neck flexion or extension weakness, with the latter being severe enough to present with dropped head syndrome (Luque et al 1994). Other cranial nerves are spared.

There are no expected general medical findings associated with IBM. Early suggestions of cardiac involvement (Lotz et al 1989) have not been substantiated. Patients have the usual incidence of age related hypertensive or ischaemic cardiac manifestations. Neuromuscular respiratory weakness is a late feature (Lotz et al 1989, Lindberg et al 1994).

Associated diseases

Association with other connective tissue and autoimmune diseases has been described including lupus erythematosus, Sjogren's syndrome, scleroderma, interstitial pneumonitis, psoriasis, sarcoidosis and dermatomyositis (Julien et al 1982, Gutmann et al 1985, Danon et al 1986, Rugiero et al 1998) with an overall incidence of 15% in one series (Lotz et al 1989). Diabetes mellitus occurred in 20% of cases (Lotz et al 1989). There is no association between IBM and malignancy.

Investigations

Blood tests

The erythrocyte sedimentation rate (ESR) is usually normal. Serum creatine kinase levels may be normal or mildly elevated, usually by 2 to 5 times normal but in rare cases up to 12 fold. Myositis associated antibodies are not a feature of IBM and it has been suggested that the presence of Jo1 antibodies excludes IBM (Hengstman et al 1998).

Electromyography

Needle electromyography (EMG) is invariably abnormal. The commonest pattern is similar to that found in polymyositis, consisting of increased insertional activity with fibrillation potentials, positive sharp waves and short duration/small amplitude motor unit potentials (MUPs). In about a third of cases there is a mixture of short duration/small amplitude MUPs and long duration/large amplitude MUPs with a reduced interference pattern; the latter two features have been traditionally regarded as "neurogenic" (Joy et al 1990). This mixed myopathic and "neurogenic" pattern on EMG has been regarded by some as highly specific for IBM (Eisen et al 1983) but others have described it in polymyositis (Mechler 1974, Lotz et al 1989), X-linked humeroperoneal neuromuscular disease (Water et al 1975), familial rimmed vacuolar myopathy sparing the quadriceps (Argov and Yarom 1984), and sporadic distal myopathy (Vaccario et al 1981). A small proportion of patients with S-IBM have a purely "neurogenic" EMG picture of normal or long duration/large amplitude MUPs with a reduced interference pattern. Nerve conduction studies (NCS) can show mild slowing in more than one third of cases, particularly in those with "neurogenic" features on EMG (Lacy et al 1982, Lotz et al 1989, Joy et al 1990). Single fibre EMF (sfEMG) studies can show an increased fibre density and moderately abnormal jitter in severely affected muscles (Eisen et al 1983, Joy et al 1990). The "neurogenic" features seen neurophysiologically as well as histologically (grouped fibre atrophy and small angulated fibres) have generated discussion about whether there is a neurogenic component to IBM. However, the technique of macroEMG shows only myogenic features (Luciano and Dalakas 1997). The EMG "neurogenic" features may all be indicators of the chronicity of a myopathic process, perhaps occurring because regenerating muscle fibres have not yet been reinnervated by nerve (Desmedt and Borenstein 1975). Nerve biopsies in S-IBM have shown mild non-specific reduction in myelinated fibres (Lacy et al 1982, Ringel et al 1987) or a mild axonal neuropathy (Lindberg et al 1990).

Muscle imaging

T_1-weighted magnetic resonance images of the forearms shows marbled brightness of the flexor digitorum profundus in the majority of those with IBM, sometimes preceding detectable weakness of that muscle. Other forearm flexor muscles are less often involved, particularly flexor digitorum superficialis, and the extensors show normal scan appearances (Sekul et al 1997).

Muscle biopsy

Muscle biopsy is essential for a definitive diagnosis of IBM. Histochemical stains show variation in fibre size, with both fibre hypertrophy and atrophy of both fibre types. The atrophic fibres may have an angulated appearance suggestive of denervated fibres. Hypertrophied fibres are more frequently seen in IBM than in other inflammatory myopathies, perhaps reflecting the chronicity of this condition (Verma et al 1992). Fibre type grouping is unusual. There may be an increase in endomysial connective tissue and, in severely affected muscle, replacement of muscle fibres

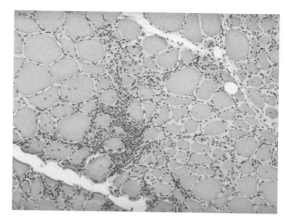

Figure 22.3 — Muscle biopsy of a case of inclusion body myositis. Haematoxylin and eosin stain showing inflammatory infiltrates.

by fat and fibrous tissue. The presence of inflammatory infiltrates is an absolute requirement for the diagnosis of IBM (Fig. 22.3). These are primarily endomysial and predominantly composed of T cells and macrophages. The T cells are $CD4^+$ and $CD8^+$ cells, with the latter often invading non-necrotic muscle fibres (Arahata and Engel 1984, 1988a, b). A key, but not pathognomonic, feature of IBM is the presence of single or multiple rimmed vacuoles 2–15 μm in diameter which can occur in up to 10% of fibres (Carpenter et al 1978). Sometimes the rimmed vacuoles cannot be found despite a diligent search. Rimmed vacuoles are so called because of their granular basophilic (on haematoxylin and eosin) or red (on Gomori trichrome) peripheral staining (Figs 22.4

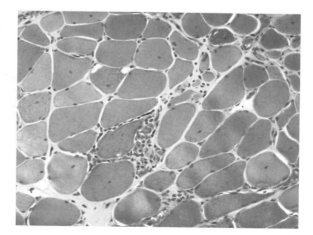

Figure 22.4 — Muscle biopsy of a case of inclusion body myositis. Gomori trichrome stain showing inflammatory infiltrates and rimmed vacuoles.

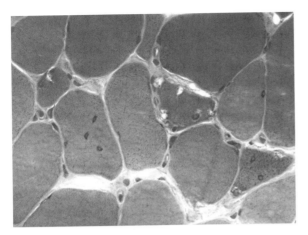

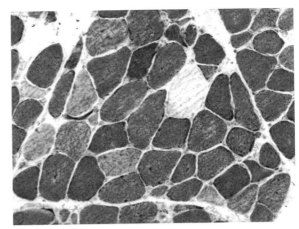

Figure 22.5—Muscle biopsy of a case of inclusion body myositis. Gomori trichrome stain showing close up of vacuoles.

Figure 22.7—Muscle biopsy of a case of inclusion body myositis. Cytochrome oxidase stain showing cytochrome oxidase negative fibres.

and 22.5). These vacuoles do not contain glycogen or lipid, and they do not have the degree of acid phosphatase activity seen in similar vacuoles associated with some drug-induced myopathies and in lysosomal storage diseases such as acid maltase deficiency. Haematoxylin and eosin stain may also show eosinophilic inclusions (Lotz et al 1989). Ragged red fibres representing sub-sarcolemmal accumulations of mitochondria are seen in excess of those expected for this age group, suggesting that the pathogenesis of IBM includes impaired mitochondrial function (Rifai et al 1995; Fig. 22.6). In keeping with this there may be cytochrome oxidase negative fibres (Fig. 22.7). Muscle fibre capillary density is increased, contrasting with the decrease seen in dermatomyositis, and the normal density seen in polymyositis (Carpenter et al 1978). One of the additional muscle biopsy features required for a definite diagnosis of IBM is the demonstration of intracellular amyloid by Congo Red staining or fluorescence techniques (Mendell et al 1991, Askanas et al 1993).

Electron microscopy (EM) shows that the rimmed vacuoles contain amorphous debris and whorls of membranous material. EM may also show the presence of amyloid and various abnormalities of mitochondrial structure. A more specific finding is that of tubulofilaments of 15–18 nm diameter and 1–5 nm in length. These may be intranuclear or cytoplasmic, the latter often in association with the rimmed vacuoles. They may be in random or parallel orientation and in compact or loose groups. They may allow a diagnosis of definite IBM in the absence of any demonstration of amyloid.

Diagnostic criteria

A workshop has published criteria for the diagnosis of IBM based upon a combination of clinical, laboratory and histological data (Table 22.1; Griggs et al 1995). These criteria allow a definite diagnosis of IBM to be made on histological grounds regardless of the clinical phenotype. A definite diagnosis requires the histological evidence of inflammatory infiltrates with the demonstration of either amyloid or tubulofilaments (see above). These criteria also allow for a diagnosis of possible IBM where there is a typical clinical phenotype but an incomplete histological picture.

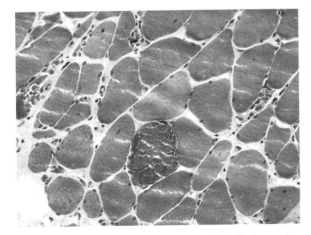

Figure 22.6—Muscle biopsy of a case of inclusion body myositis. Gomori trichrome stain showing ragged red fibre.

Table 22.1 — Diagnosis criteria for inclusion body myositis

I. Characteristic features – inclusion criteria
A. Clinical features
  1. Duration of illness > 6 months
  2. Age of onset > 30 years old
  3. Muscle weakness
    Must affect proximal and distal muscles of arms and legs and Patient must exhibit at least one of the following features:
    a. Finger flexor weakness
    b. Wrist flexor > wrist extensor weakness
    c. Quadriceps muscle weakness (= or < grade 4 MRC)
B. Laboratory features
  1. Serum creatine kinase < 12 times normal
  2. Muscle biopsy
    a. Inflammatory myopathy characterized by mononuclear cell invasion of nonnecrotic muscle fibres
    b. Vacuolared muscle fibres
    c. Either
      (i) Intracellular amyloid deposits (must use fluroescent method of identification before excluding the presence of amyloid) *or*
      (ii) 15 – 18-nm tubulofilaments by electron microscopy
  3. Electromyography must be consistent with features of an inflammatory myopathy (however, long–duration potentials are commonly observed and do not exclude diagnosis of sporadic inclusion body myositis).
C. Family history
  Rarely, inclusion body myositis may be observed in families. This condition is different from hereditary inclusion body myopathy without inflammation. The diagnosis of familial inclusion body myositis requires specific documentation of the inflammatory component by muscle biopsy in addition to vacuolated muscle fibres, intracellular (within muscle fibres) amyloid, and 15-18-nm tubulofilaments.
II. Associated disorders
  Inclusion body myositis occurs with a variety of other, especially immune-mediated conditions. An associated condition does not preclude a diagnosis of inclusion body myositis if diagnostic criteria (below) are fulfilled.
III. Diagnostic criteria for inclusion body myositis
  A. *Definite* inclusion body myositis
    Patients must exhibit all muscle biopsy features including invasion of nonnecrotic fibres by mononuclear cells, vacuolated muscle fibres, and intracellular (within muscle fibres) amyloid deposits or 15-18-nm tubulofilaments. None of the other clinical or laboratory features are mandatory if muscle biopsy features are diagnostic.
  B. *Possible* inclusion body myositis
    If the muscle shows only inflammation (invasion of nonnecrotic muscle fibres by mononuclear cells) *without* other pathological features of inclusion body myositis, then a diagnosis of possible inclusion body myositis can be given of the patent exhibits the characteristic clinical (A1,2,3)and laboratory (B1,3) features.

Differential diagnosis

A particular differential diagnosis of IBM is that of other inflammatory myopathies. Dermatomyositis usually presents acutely or sub-acutely rather than chronically. There is a proximal not distal emphasis to the weakness. There may be associated characteristic cutaneous and other non-muscle features. The muscle pathology reflects the immune complex related vasculopathy that underlies this disease, with peri-vascular B cell containing inflammatory infiltrates, muscle infarction and perifascicular atrophy. There are rare cases of dermatomyositis which, after a disease-free interval, have presented with IBM (McCoy et al 1999). Also described is a case of overlap between IBM and dermatomyositis (Talanin et al 1999). There is no doubt that the literature on polymyositis is contaminated by mis-diagnosed cases of IBM. One has to speculate as to whether reported cases of polymyositis with facial or distal weakness might not be re-diagnosed as IBM nowadays (Hollinrake 1969, Bates et al 1973, Yamane et al 1978, van Kasteren 1979, Sundaram and Ashenhurst 1981, Marconi et al 1982). It is a frequent experience to diagnose IBM when reviewing patients with treatment-resistant polymyositis, and so IBM should always be a suspected diagnosis in such cases. The practical clinical difficulty that may arise is in differentiating a case of evolving IBM that has yet to develop all the characteristic histological features from a case of polymyositis. Upon this distinction may rest the decision of whether to start steroid treatment and the expectation of a response to such treatment. There is no evidence upon which to base a rational decision of what constitutes an adequate trial of immunosuppressive treatment that will determine whether a case of inflammatory myopathy is responsive or not, particularly as late responders have been described (Rose et al 1999). The presence of cytochrome oxidase negative fibres in what appears to be a polymyositis predicts a poor response to steroid treatment but it is not yet clear whether it presages the appearance of IBM (Blume et al 1997).

Alternative differential diagnoses include neurological diseases, including other muscle diseases, which may have distal weakness, and other myopathies associated with rimmed vacuoles on muscle biopsy (Table 22.2). Of the alternative neurological diseases amyotrophic lateral sclerosis/motor neurone disease is worthy of mention since this has obvious prognostic implications. When the needle EMG appears to show only neurogenic features, the distinction between IBM and amyotrophic lateral sclerosis/motor neurone disease requires clinical vigilance with possible recourse to a muscle biopsy.

Management

General

Since IBM generally occurs in an elderly population, it is important to recognise that there may be a variety of symptoms due to coexisting disease that, unlike IBM, may be eminently treatable. Therefore, cardiac and most respiratory symptoms should not be accepted as being caused by IBM, and they should be investigated and treated on their merits. Respiratory symptoms might be associated with IBM if due to aspiration pneumonia in someone with severe dysphagia and impaired cough reflex. Neuromuscular respiratory failure is a late complication in severe cases of IBM. Pain is not a feature of IBM per se, and it may be caused by coexisting arthritis or polymyalgia rheumatica. Arthritic changes in the knees seem particularly

Table 22.2—Differential diagnosis for inclusion body myositis

Inflammatory myopathies
  Polymyositis
  Dermatomyositis
Myopathies with distal weakness
  Myotonic dystrophy
  Distal myopathies
Rimmed vacuolar myopathies
  Familial inclusion body myositis
    Limb girdle muscular dystrophy
    With quadriceps sparing
    With excessive autophagy
    With dystrophin gene abnormality
    With electrical myotonia
    With leukodystrophy
  Distal myopathies
  Oculopharyngeal dystrophies
  Miscellaneous
    Rigid spine
    Post poliomyelitis syndrome
    Neuropathy; amyloid, vasculitic
    Spinal muscular atrophy
Other neuromuscular diseases
  Amyotrophic lateral sclerosis/motor neurone disease
  Multifocal neuropathy with conduction block
  Motor neuropathy

common, and they may relate to instability of the joint induced by quadriceps weakness. Lightweight ankle foot orthoses may benefit foot drop. Unfortunately orthotic devices do not reduce the tendency to falls resulting from quadriceps weakness. One study suggests that resistance muscle strength training does no harm, at least over a 12 week period, and it leads to an increase in dynamic muscle performance; the functional benefit of this is uncertain (Spector et al 1997). Dysphagia in IBM has occasionally been treated with cricoparyngeal myotomy (Danon and Friedman 1989, 1992).

Drug treatment

The prominence of the inflammation in the histology of IBM has led to the assumption that this disease ought to respond to immuno-suppressive or immuno-modulating drugs. Consequently, most of these have been tried (Table 22.3). The recognition that mitochondrial function is specifically impaired in IBM has also resulted in the use of treatments attempting to

Table 22.3— Treatments proposed for inclusion body myositis

Immunosupressive and immunomodulatory
Prednisone (and other corticosteroids)
Cyclophosphamide
Chlorambucil
Azathioprine
Methotrexate
Cyclosporin
Total body irradiation
Leukopheresis
Plasma exchange
Intravenous immune globulin
Mitochondrial
Carnitine
Ubiquinone/CoQ
Anti-oxidants
Vitamin E

boost mitochondrial respiratory chain function (Table 22.3). Anti-oxidants have also been suggested treatment following recognition that markers of oxidative stress are increased on IBM (Yang et al 1996). The literature evidence of whether any of these therapies is efficacious is bedevilled by the scarcity of randomised controlled trials. In some trials the outcome measures that are used to assess the effect of treatment (such as CK values and qualitative, rather than quantitative, strength measures) are suspect. CK values may be reduced by corticosteroid treatment in both inflammatory and non-inflammatory muscle diseases without any other clinical improvement. In natural history studies even quantitative let alone qualitative strength measures may appear to stabilise or "improve" in the short term (Rose et al 1996). In many trials the small numbers of subjects and the short treatment periods render the trial inadequately powered to show even reversal of disease progression let alone slowing or arrest of progression (Griggs and Rose 1998, Rose et al 1999).

Corticosteroids

In the vast majority of cases corticosteroids do not appear to be of any benefit. There are occasional cases reported of "stabilisation" for a period of months but this may just reflect the natural history of the disease (Rose et al 1996). In rare cases improvement has been claimed, but these have been uncontrolled trials and coexisting steroid-responsive disease may not have been excluded. These cases have often only been published in abstract form and subsequent enquiry has established that the improvements have not necessarily been maintained (Griggs and Rose 1998). Two prospective open labelled trials of prednisone showed no benefit. In one of these trials, muscle biopsy following treatment showed a reduction in inflammatory infiltrates but it also showed an increase in the number of rimmed vacuoles and amyloid deposits (Lindberg et al 1994, Barohn 1995).

Cytotoxic drugs

Cytotoxic drugs have usually been added to corticosteroids following failure to respond to steroids alone. The response to cyclophosphamide, chlorambucil, azathioprine, and cyclosporin is unimpressive in the small numbers reported (Griggs and Rose 1998). Methotrexate has been studied in larger numbers with a few showing apparent stabilisation or improvement but the study period has been short (Sayers et al 1992, Joffe et al 1993, Leff et al 1993).

Immuno-modulating therapy

Total body radiation, leukopheresis and plasma exchange have not shown convincing benefit (Kelly et al 1984, 1986, Dau 1987, Miller et al 1992). Initial prospective trials of intravenous immunoglobulin appeared promising, but randomised controlled trials have not substantiated any worthwhile benefit particularly given the expense of this treatment (Soueidan and Dalakas 1993, Dalakas et al 1995, 1997, Walter et al 2000).

Other treatments

There is no sound evidence for the efficacy of treatments designed to increase mitochondrial respiratory chain function such as carnitine or CoQ/ ubiquinone, nor for drugs designed to reduce oxidative stress such as vitamin E (Engel and Askanas 1998).

Prognosis

Prospective, longitudinal studies of the natural history of IBM are needed. In trying to date the progression of this disease one has to bear in mind the uncertainty that may exist over the onset of this insidious disease. Timing progression from the time of diagnosis is inappropriate, particularly as a combination of slow onset and either lack of recognition or mis-diagnosis of this disease by the initial physician may contribute to a delay in final diagnosis that ranges from 4 months to 36 years with an average of 3 years (Sayers et al 1992). Some studies have measured the rate of decline of muscle strength using different and non-comparable methods (Lindberg et al 1994, Rose et al 1996). The clinical experience is that strength does decline inexorably over the years despite attempts at treatment, but there may be periods of short term (months?) natural stabilisation (Rose et al 1996). In one study 10 out of 14 patients required a walking stick 5 years after disease onset and 3 out of 5 surviving 10 years after diagnosis were wheelchair bound (Sekul and Dalakas 1993). Death is usually from co-existing and unrelated disease rather than IBM.

Aetiology

The aetiology of IBM is not known. Any aetiological hypothesis needs to incorporate several distinct features that have been found to occur in IBM including: an inflammatory component, up-regulation of various "alien" (so-called "brain-specific") proteins, mitochondrial abnormalities, evidence for oxidative stress, involvement of heat shock proteins and myonuclear changes. Many of these features are shared with the hereditary inclusion myopathies, raising the possibility of a genetic susceptibility to sporadic IBM. The notable absence of inflammation in the hereditary inclusion body myopathies makes the study of the commonalities and differences in other pathological changes seen in the hereditary inclusion body myopathies compared with those seen in IBM a useful research tool.

Inflammatory changes

Immunohistochemical studies have established that the predominantly endomysial inflammatory infiltrate seen in IBM contains 74% T cells, 24% macrophages and virtually no B cells. The majority of the T cells are CD8$^+$, with some CD3$^+$ and CD4$^+$ cells. Although CD16$^+$ natural killer cells are not seen, 29% of the CD3$^+$ cells express CD57 and in vitro such cells can mediate cytotoxicity, albeit lectin-dependent rather than the spontaneous cytotoxicity of natural killer cells. The CD8$^+$ cells surround and invade non-necrotic muscle fibres, and such invaded fibres are 5.5 times more frequent than necrotic fibres. Both the total number of T cells and the number invaded muscle fibres is higher in IBM than is seen in either polymyositis or dermatomyositis. Just over one third of the invading CD8$^+$ cells and one quarter of the

surrounding but non-invading CD8$^+$ cells express major histocompatibility complex (MHC) class II and CD45RO markers, typical of activated and antigen-primed T cells. Investigation of the T cell receptor repertoire of the infiltrating T cells shows an oligoclonal pattern rearrangement with increased frequency of the V3, V2 and V6 gene families with heterogeneity of the CDR3 domain sequence. This suggests that the T cell response is triggered by a superantigen rather than by a muscle-specific antigen. All the invaded muscle fibres express HLA class I antigen on their surface suggesting a MHC class I restricted cytotoxic cell mediated attack on the fibres.

Examination of cytokine expression in IBM shows prominent expression of interleukins IL-α, IL-β and TGF3 with lesser expression of tumour necrosis factor (TNF) (Lundberg et al 1997, Lundberg and Nyberg 1998). There are two main pathways by which the activated T cells might destroy muscle fibres, and there is evidence for both occurring in IBM. In favour of the perforin-granzyme pathway is the presence of perforin-positive cells in IBM, while in support of activation of the Fas–Fas ligand pathway is the demonstration of Fas in IBM muscle (Orimo et al 1994, Goebels et al 1996, Behrens et al 1997, Fyhr and Oldfors 1998). Both pathways induce apoptosis but no evidence has yet been found for this occurring in IBM so the precise mode by which T cells destroy invaded muscle fibres remains unclear (Schneider et al 1996, Hutchinson 1998).

Up-regulation of alien proteins

Studies of muscle biopsies in IBM have shown the cytoplasmic deposition of a variety of proteins normally only expressed in adult muscle at the neuromuscular junction, including amyloid precursor protein, β-amyloid, ubiquitin, prion protein, apolipoprotein E and presenilin. For amyloid and prion protein, increased levels of the appropriate messenger RNA (mRNA) has been found suggesting that up-regulation of the transcription of these genes has occurred. Hyperphosphorylated tau, not normally seen in muscle, is also present in IBM muscle samples (Askanas et al 1991, 1993, Sarkosi et al 1944, Mirabella et al 1996). In muscle cell culture and in transgenic mice over-expression of amyloid precursor protein can induce a vacuolar abnormality of muscle (Arkanas et al 1994, Fukuchi et al 1998, Jin et al 1998). Transgenic mice over-expressing wild type prion protein become weak, with evidence of a neuropathy and a myopathy albeit without the morphological features seen in IBM (Westaway et al 1994).

Mitochondrial abnormalities

Morphological, biochemical and mitochondrial DNA (mtDNA) defects are a feature of normal aging, but the morphological changes in IBM—namely the ragged red fibres, cytochrome oxidase fibres and ultra-structural mitochondrial abnormalities—are greater than those seen in age matched controls (Oldfors et al 1993, Rifai et al 1995). It has been suggested that the increase in muscle capillary density seen in IBM might be a reaction to defective aerobic metabolism resulting from mitochondrial abnormalities (Carpenter et al 1978). In situ hybridisation studies have shown that the IBM cytochrome negative fibres have accumulated mutant mtDNA containing a deletion, and they have reduced amounts of the wild type mtDNA (Oldfors et al 1993). Southern blotting and polymerase chain reaction techniques in IBM muscle samples show a low level of multiple mtDNA deletions, including the common deletion seen in classical mitochondrial myopathies (Santorelli et al 1996). However, each individual cytochrome oxidase muscle fibre contains mutant mtDNA with only one type of deletion (Oldfors et al 1995). In classical mitochondrial myopathies, mtDNA deletions tend to occur in sites flanked by nucleotide repeat sequences and the same is true for the various deletions seen in IBM (Moslemi et al 1997). This pattern of mutant mtDNA with multiple deletions is similar to that seen in autosomal dominant mitochondrial myopathies with multiple deletions, in which it is likely that the multiple deletions result from a defect in nuclear control of mtDNA replication. It is arguable as to whether the mitochondrial changes in themselves would be sufficient to account for the weakness seen in IBM. The morphological mitochondrial abnormalities seem outweighed by the more likely contributing factors such as the inflammation, muscle fibre necrosis and endomysial fibrosis. Nevertheless, a similar degree of mitochondrial change appears to be sufficient to cause weakness in the classical mitochondrial myopathies.

Myonuclear abnormalities

The precise chemical identity of the intranuclear 15–18 nm tubulofilaments seen in IBM is unknown, but they may be derived from components of the nuclear matrix. It is possible that they have a role in the degradation of myonuclei, which is a feature of IBM, either by space-occupying effect or through more direct mechanisms. The presence in cytoplasm of these same tubulofilaments, particularly in association with the rimmed vacuoles, may be evidence that myonuclear degradation is a particular feature of IBM and that rimmed vacuoles may mark the sites of myonuclear degeneration. The presence within vacuoles of a variety of tubular filaments similar to those seen in myonuclei lends some support to this hypothesis (Karpati and Carpenter 2000). An unidentified protein that binds to single stranded DNA of any sequence structure appears to be the earliest sign of myonuclear abnormality (Nalbantoglu et al 1994). One potential candidate protein might be the nuclear replication protein A, which is up-regulated in IBM and does bind single stranded DNA. However, more myonuclei contain this replication protein A than show single stranded DNA binding, suggesting that a different protein is likely to be involved (Nalbantoglu et al 1994).

Oxidative stress

Neuronal nitric oxide synthetases (nNOS), inducible nitric oxide synthetases (iNOS) and nitrotyrosine are abnormally accumulated in vacuolated fibres of IBM, and they are not seen in other inflammatory myopathies (Yang et al 1996, 1997). These markers of increased oxidative stress might suggest that increased nitric oxide species may contribute to the pathophysiology of IBM. Superoxide dismutase 1 (SOD1) and mRNA for SOD1 are also found in IBM vacuolated muscle fibres, and they may represent an attempt to limit the effects of oxidative stress in IBM (Askanas et al 1996).

Heat shock proteins

One study has shown that there is over-expression of the small heat shock protein αB-crystallin in IBM. Such over-expression was seen in IBM muscle fibres that were structurally abnormal in a variety of ways such as invaded by inflammatory cells, showing amyloid deposits and containing vacuoles. αB-crystallin was also seen in damaged muscle fibres in other muscle diseases. However increased αB-crystallin deposition was seen in healthy looking fibres only in IBM and in two cases of treatment-resistant polymyositis thought to be potential cases of IBM thus suggesting that it might be an early primary pathological event occurring in response to an as yet unidentified biological stress (Banwell and Engel 2000).

Genetic susceptibility

The hereditary inclusion body myopathies show that

many of the pathological features of IBM can arise from genetic mechanisms. As IBM is an inflammatory, possibly autoimmune, myopathy and because it has some association with autoimmune diseases, one group of candidate susceptibility genes would be those thought to play a part in autoimmunity. One such group would be those within the major histocompatibility complex (MHC). Studies have shown an obvious increase in the frequency of DR3A with smaller increases in the frequencies of B8, DR1 and null alleles at the C4A locus in association with IBM (Garlepp et al 1994, Sivakumar et al 1997). The DR3/B8 haplotype is associated with other autoimmune diseases including polymyositis and dermatomyositis. It is also seen with systemic lupus erythematosis, selective IgA deficiency and common variable Ig deficiency, each of which have been described in association with IBM (Yood and Smith 1985, Lindberg et al 1994, Dalakas and Illa 1995).

Another group of candidate susceptibility genes would be those encoding proteins that show abnormal up-regulation in IBM. No mutations of exons 16 and 17 of the amyloid precursor protein gene, such as seen in Alzheimer's disease, have been found in IBM (Garlepp et al 1998). Reports of an increase in the frequency of the homozygosity at codon 129 of the prion protein gene in IBM, such as seen in Creutzfeldt Jacob disease, have been contradictory (Garlepp et al 1998, Lamp et al 1999). The pathogenic similarities between IBM and Alzheimer's disease have also led to several studies of the ε4 variant of the apolipoprotein E gene in IBM since this allele is associated with some hereditary forms of Alzheimer's disease as well as a susceptibility to sporadic Alzheimer's disease. Again the results are contradictory with an increase in the ε4 allele found by some (Garlepp et al 1995) but not by others (Harrington et al 1995, Askanas et al 1996).

Aetiological hypothesis

The main debate regarding any aetiological hypothesis for IBM focuses on the nature of the primary pathological event. Attempts to do this have relied on evidence that the change in question (amyloid deposition, αB-crystallin, etc) is seen in the absence of other pathology. The separate strands of evidence highlighted above can be linked in a variety of ways. One hypothesis is that some viral or other insult in genetically susceptible elderly persons triggers myonuclear degeneration and disturbance of gene function leading to up-regulation of alien proteins, one or more of which triggers the inflammatory response. Disturbed nuclear gene function may lead to impairment of mitochondrial replication, and consequently to the mitochondrial abnormalities found in IBM. Oxidative stress may be induced by the inflammation, and this would exacerbate the mitochondrial abnormalities. An alternative hypothesis places the inflammation at the forefront, suggesting that this is enough in elderly and genetically susceptible individuals to initiate all the changes seen in IBM including vacuoles, mitochondrial abnormalities, oxidative stress and up-regulation of β-amyloid precursor protein via cytokines. The presence of αB-crystallin prior to any other structural change suggests that the initiating stressor event may actually occur much earlier in life, rather than being one to which the elderly are susceptible. Some have argued that the failure of IBM to respond to anti-inflammatory treatment suggests that it is not the primary pathology. However, the prominence of inflammation above all the other pathological changes has been demonstrated by the fact that non-necrotic invaded muscle fibres are far more common than those showing amyloid deposits or other pathology described above (Pruitt et al 1996).

Conclusions

There are three main inter-linking challenges in IBM. Recognition of IBM has improved in the last 5 years but, in many cases, there is still a delay in diagnosis. The lack of good knowledge regarding the early stages of this disease makes it difficult to appreciate the true sequence of the pathological changes. It is also possible that potential treatments have a greater chance of success if applied early in the course of the disease. If treatment serves to arrest or delay disease progression then early diagnosis becomes all the more imperative. There is clearly a need for adequately powered randomised controlled trials of therapy for IBM using robust outcome measures with a sufficient duration of treatment to reasonably answer the question of whether a particular treatment helps or not. To date for most interventions the conclusion is "there is *lack of evidence* for efficacy" rather than "no evidence for efficacy". Such trials are likely to require multicentre involvement in order to obtain the numbers required. Finally, further basic research is needed to clarify the contribution of each of the pathological elements seen in IBM and to place them into a coherent and accurate framework for the pathophysiology of this disease.

References

Amato AA, Shebert RT. (1998) Inclusion body myositis in twins. *Neurology* 51: 598–600.

Arahata K, Engel AG. (1984) Monoclonal antibody analysis of mononuclear cells in myopathies. I: Quantitation of subsets according to diagnosis and sites of accumulation and demonstration and counts of muscle fibers invaded by T cells. *Ann Neurol* 16: 193–208.

Arahata K, Engel AG. (1988a) Monoclonal antibody analysis of mononuclear cells in myopathies. IV: Cell-mediated cytotoxicity and muscle fiber necrosis. *Ann Neurol* 23: 168–173.

Arahata K, Engel AG. (1988b) Monoclonal antibody analysis of mononuclear cells in myopathies V. Identification and quantitation of T8+ cytotoxic and T8+ suppressor cells. *Ann Neurol* 23: 493–499.

Argov Z, Yarom R. (1984) Rimmed vacuole myopathy sparing the quadriceps. *J Neurol Sci* 64: 33–43.

Askanas V, Alvarez RB, Engel WK. (1993) Beta-amyloid precursor epitopes in muscle fibers of inclusion body myositis. *Ann Neurol* 34: 551–560.

Askanas V, Engel WK, Alvarez RB. (1993) Enhanced detection of congo-red-positive amyloid deposits in muscle fibers of inclusion body myositis and brain of Alzheimer's disease using fluorescence technique. *Neurology* 43: 1265–1267.

Askanas V, Engel WK, Mirabella M, et al. (1996) Apolipoprotein E alleles in sporadic inclusion-body myositis and hereditary inclusion-body myopathy. *Ann Neurol* 40: 264–265.

Askanas V, McFerrin J, Alvarez RB, Baque S, Engel WK. (1997) Beta APP gene transfer into cultured human muscle induces inclusion-body myositis aspects. *Neuroreport* 8: 2155–2158.

Askanas V, Sarkozi E, Alvarez RB, McFerrin J, Siddique T, Engel WK. (1996) Superoxide dismutase 1 gene and protein in vacuolated muscle fibers of sporadic inclusion body myositis, hereditary inclusion body myoathy and in cultured human muscle after β-amyloid precursor gene transfer. *Neurology* 46: 487.

Askanas V, Serdaroglu P, Engel WK, Alvarez RB. (1991) Immunolocalization of ubiquitin in muscle biopsies of patients with inclusion body myositis and oculopharyngeal muscular dystrophy. *Neurosci Lett* 130: 73–76.

Banwell BL, Engel AG. (2000) αB-crystallin immunolocalisation yields new insights into inclusion body myositis. *Neurology* 54: 1033–1041.

Barohn RJ, Amato AA, Sahenk Z, Kissel JT, Mendell JR. (1995) Inclusion body myositis: explanation for poor response to immunosuppressive therapy.

Bates D, Stevens JC, Hudgson P. (1973) "Polymyositis" with involvement of facial and distal musculature. One form of the fascioscapulohumeral syndrome? *J Neurol Sci* 19(1): 105–108.

Behrens L, Bender A, Johnson MA, Hohlfeld R. (1997) Cytotoxic mechanisms in inflammatory myopathies. Co-expression of Fas and protective Bcl-2 in muscle fibres and inflammatory cells. *Brain* 120: 929–938.

Blume G, Pestronk A, Frank B, Johns DR. (1997) Polymyositis with cytochrome oxidase negative muscle fibres. Early quadriceps weakness and poor response to immunosuppressive therapy. *Brain* 120: 39–45.

Carpenter S, Karpati G, Heller I, Eisen A. (1978) Inclusion body myositis: a distinct variety of idiopathic inflammatory myopathy. *Neurology*; 28: 8–17.

Chou SM. (1967) Myxovirus like structures in a case of human chronic polymyositis. *Science*; 158: 1453–1455.

Dalakas MC, Dambrosia JM, Sekul EA, Cupler EJ, Sivakumar K. (1995) The efficacy of high dose intravenous immunoglogulin (IVIg) in patients with inclusion body myositis (IBM). *Neurology* 45 (Suppl 4):174S.

Dalakas MC, Illa I. (1995) Common variable immunodeficiency and inclusion body myositis – a distinct myopathy mediated by natural killer cells. *Ann Neurol* 37: 806–810.

Dalakas MC, Sonies B, Dambrosia J, Sekul E, Cupler E, Sivakumar K. (1997) Treatment of inclusion-body myositis with IVIg: a double-blind, placebo-controlled study [see comments]. *Neurology* 48: 712–716.

Danon MJ, Friedman M. (1989) Inclusion body myositis associated with progressive dysphagia: treatment with cricopharyngeal myotomy. *Can J Neurol Sci* 16: 436–438.

Danon MJ, Friedman M. (1992) Inclusion body myositis with cricopharyngeus muscle involvement and severe dysphagia [letter; comment]. *Muscle Nerve* 15: 115.

Danon MJ, Perurena OH, Ronan S, Manaligod JR. (1986) Inclusion body myositis associated with systemic sarcoidosis. *Can J Neurol Sci* 13: 334–336.

Dau PC. (1987) Leukocytapheresis in inclusion body myositis. *J Clin Apheresis* 3: 167–170.

Desmedt JE, Borenstein S. (1975) Relationship of spontaneous fibrillation potentials to muscle fibre segmentation in human muscular dystrophy. *Nature* 258: 531–534.

Eisen A, Berry K, Gibson G. (1983) Inclusion body myositis (IBM): myopathy or neuropathy? *Neurology* 33: 1109–1114.

Engel WK, Askanas V. (1998) Treatment of inclusion body myositis and hereditary inclusion body myopathy with reference to pathogenic mechanisms: personal experience. In: Askanas V, Serratrice G, Engel WK, eds. *Inclusion body myositis and myopathies.* Cambridge: Cambridge University Press, pp 351–382.

Fukuchi K, Pham D, Hart M, Li L, Lindsey JR. (1998) Amyloid-beta deposition in skeletal muscle of transgenic mice: possible model of inclusion body myopathy [see comments]. *Am J Pathol* 153: 1687–1693.

Fyhr IM, Oldfors A. (1998) Upregulation of Fas/Fas ligand in inclusion body myositis. *Ann Neurol* 43: 127–130.

Garlepp MJ, Blechynden L, Tabarias H, Lawson C, van Bockxmeer FM, Mastaglia F. (1998) Genetic factors in sporadic inclusion body myositis. In: Askanas V, Serratrice G, Engel WK, eds. *Inclusion body myositis and myopathies*. Cambridge: Cambridge University Press, pp. 177–188.

Garlepp MJ, Laing B, Zilko PJ, Ollier W, Mastaglia FL. (1994) HLA associations with inclusion body myositis. *Clin Exp Immunol* 98: 40–45.

Garlepp MJ, Tabarias H, van Bockxmeer FM, Zilko PJ, Laing B. (1995) Apolipoprotein E epsilon 4 in inclusion body myositis. *Ann Neurol* 38: 957–959.

Goebels N, Michaelis D, Engelhardt M, et al. (1996) Differential expression of perforin in muscle-infiltrating T cells in polymyositis and dermatomyositis. *J Clin Invest* 97(12): 2905–2910.

Griggs RC, Askanas V, DiMauro S, et al. (1995) Inclusion body myositis and myopathies. *Ann Neurol* 38: 705–713.

Griggs RC, Rose MR. (1998) Evaluation of treatment for sporadic inclusion body myositis. In: Askanas V, Serratrice G, Engel WK, eds. *Inclusion body myositis and myopathies*. Cambridge University Press: 331–350.

Gutmann L, Govindan S, Riggs JE, Schochet SS, Jr. (1985) Inclusion body myositis and Sjogren's syndrome. *Arch Neurol* 42: 1021–1022.

Harrington CR, Anderson JR, Chan KK. (1995) Apolipoprotein E type epsilon 4 allele frequency is not increased in patients with sporadic inclusion body myositis. *Neurosci Lett* 183: 35–38.

Hengstman GJ, van Engelen BG, Badrising UA, van den Hoogen FH, van, Venrooij WJ. (1998) Presence of the anti-Jo-1 autoantibody excludes inclusion body myositis. *Ann Neurol* 44: 423.

Hollinrake K. (1969) Polymyositis presenting as distal muscle weakness. A case report. *J Neurol Sci* 8(3): 479–484.

Houser SN, Calabrese LH, Strome M. (1998) Dysphagia in patients with inclusion body myositis. *Laryngoscope* 108: 1001–1005.

Hutchinson DO. (1998) Inclusion body myositis: abnormal protein accumulation does not trigger apoptosis. *Neurology* 51: 1742–1745.

Jin LW, Hearn MG, Ogburn CE, et al. (1998) Transgenic mice over-expressing the C-99 fragment of betaPP with an alpha-secretase site mutation develop a myopathy similar to human inclusion body myositis [see comments]. *Am J Pathol* 153: 1679–1686.

Joffe MM, Love LA, Leff RL, et al. (1993) Drug therapy of the idiopathic inflammatory myopathies: predictors of response to prednisone, azathioprine, and methotrexate and a comparision of their efficacy. *Am J Med* 94: 379–387.

Joy JL, Oh SJ, Baysal AI. (1990) Electrophysiological spectrum of inclusion body myositis. *Muscle Nerve* 13: 949–951.

Julien J, Vital C, Vallat JM, Lagueny A, Sapina D. (1982) Inclusion body myositis: clinical, biological and ultrastructural study. *J Neurol* 55: 15–24.

Karpati G, Carpenter S, Heller I, Eisen A. (1988) Idiopathic inflammatory myopathies. *Curr Op Neurol Neurosurg* 1: 806–814.

Karpati G, Carpenter S. (2000) Myonuclear abnormalities may play a central role in the pathogenesis of muscle fibre damage in inclusion body myositis. In: Askanas V, Serratrice G, Engel WK, eds. *Inclusion body myositis and myopathies*. Cambridge: Cambridge University Press, pp. 291–296.

Kelly JJ, Jr, Madoc-Jones H, Adelman LS, Andres PL, Munsat TL. (1986) Total body irradiation not effective in inclusion body myositis. *Neurology* 36: 1264–1266.

Kelly JJ, Madoc-Jones H, Adelman L, Munsat TL. (1984) Treatment of refractory polymyositis with total body irradiation. *Neurology* 34 (supp 1): 80.

Lacy JR, Simon DB, Neville HE, Ringel SP. (1982) Inclusion body myositis: electrodiagnostic and nerve biopsy findings. *Neurology* 32 (Suppl 2):A202.

Lampe J, Kitzler H, Walter MC, Lochmuller H, Reichmann H. (1999) Methionine homozygosity at prion gene codon 129 may predispose to sporadic inclusion-body myositis. *Lancet* 353: 465–466.

Leff RL, Miller FW, Hicks J, Fraser DD, Plotz PH. (1993) The treatment of inclusion body myositis: a retrospective review and a randomised prospective trial of immunosuppressive therapy. *Medicine* 72: 225–235.

Lindberg C, Oldfors A, Hedstrom A. (1990) Inclusion body myositis: peripheral nerve involvement. Combined morphological and electrophysiological studies on peripheral nerves. *J Neurol Sci* 99: 327–338.

Lindberg C, Persson LI, Bjorkander J, Oldfors A. (1994) Inclusion body myositis: clinical, morphological, physiological and laboratory findings in 18 cases. *Acta Neurol Scand* 89: 123–131.

Lotz BP, Engel AG, Nishino H, Stevens JC, Litchy WJ. (1989) Inclusion body myositis. Observations in 40 patients. *Brain* 112: 727–747.

Luciano CA, Dalakas MC. (1997) Inclusion body myositis; No evidence for a neurogenic component. *Neurology* 48: 29–33.

Lundberg I, Ulfgren AK, Nyberg P, Andersson U, Klareskog L. (1997) Cytokine production in muscle tissue of patients with idiopathic inflammatory myopathies. *Arthritis Rheumatism* 40: 865–874.

Lundberg IE, Nyberg P. (1998) New developments in the role of cytokines and chemokines in inflammatory myopathies. *Curr Opin Rheumatol* 10: 521–529.

Luque FA, Rosenkilde C, Valsamis M, Danon MJ. (1994) Inclusion body myositis (IBM) presenting as the dropped head syndrome (DHS). *Brain Path* 4: 568.

Maat-Schieman ML, Macfarlane JD, Bots GT, Wintzen AR. (1992) Inclusion body myositis: its relative frequency in elderly people. *Clin Neurol Neurosurg* 94 Suppl: S118–S120.

Marconi G, Ronchi O, Taiuti R. (1982) Polymyositis with severe distal muscular involvement. *Acta Neurol (Napoli)* 4(5): 340–346.

McCoy AL, Bubb MR, Plotz PH, Davis JC. (1999) Inclusion body myositis long after dermatomyositis: a report of two cases. *Clin Exp Rheumatol* 17(2): 235–239.

Mechler F. (1974) Changing electromyographic findings during the chronic course of polymyositis. *J Neurol Sci* 23: 237–242.

Mendell JR, Sahenk Z, Gales T, Paul L. (1991) Amyloid filaments in inclusion body myositis. Novel findings provide insight into nature of filaments. *Arch Neurol* 48: 1229–1234.

Miller FW, Leitman SF, Cronin ME, et al. (1992) Controlled trial of plasma exchange and leukapheresis in polymyositis and dermatomyositis. *N Engl J Med* 326: 1380–1384.

Mirabella M, Alvarez RB, Bilak M, Engel WK, Askanas V. (1996) Difference in expression of phosphorylated tau epitopes between sporadic inclusion-body myositis and hereditary inclusion-body myopathies [see comments]. *J Neuropathol Exp Neurol* 55: 774–786.

Moslemi AR, Lindberg C, Oldfors A. (1997) Analysis of multiple mitochondrial DNA deletions in inclusion body myositis. *Hum Mutat* 10(5): 381–386.

Nalbantoglu J, Karpati G, Carpenter S. (1994) Conspicuous accumulation of a single-stranded DNA binding protein in skeletal muscle fibers in inclusion body myositis. *Am J Pathol* 144: 874–882.

Naumann M, Toyka KV. (1999) Inclusion body myositis in twins. *Neurology* 53: 659.

Oldfors A, Larsson NG, Lindberg C, Holme E. (1993) Mitochondrial DNA deletions in inclusion body myositis. *Brain* 116: 325–336.

Oldors A, Muslemi AR, Fyhr IM, Holme E, Larsson NG, Lindberg C. (1995) Mitochondrial DNA deletions in muscle fibers in inclusion body myositis. *Journal of Neuropathology & Experimental Neurology*; 54: 581–587.

Orimo S, Koga R, Goto K, et al. (1994) Immunohisto-chemical analysis of perforin and granzyme A in inflammatory myopathies. *Neuromuscul Disord* 4(3): 219–226.

Pruitt JN, Showalter CJ, Engel AG. (1996) Sporadic inclusion body myositis: counts of different types of abnormal fibers. *Ann Neurol* 39: 139–143.

Rifai Z, Welle S, Kamp C, Thornton CA. (1995) Ragged red fibers in normal aging and inflammatory myopathy. *Ann Neurol* 37: 24–29.

Riggs JE, Schochet SS, Jr, Gutmann L, Lerfald SC. (1989) Childhood onset inclusion body myositis mimicking limb-girdle muscular dystrophy. *Journal of Child Neurology* 4: 283–285.

Riminton DS, Chambers ST, Parkin PJ, Pollock M, Donaldson IM. (1993) Inclusion body myositis presenting solely as dysphagia. *Neurology* 43(6): 1241–1243.

Ringel SP, Kenny CE, Neville HE, Giorno R, Carry MR. (1987) Spectrum of inclusion body myositis. *Arch Neurol* 44: 1154–1157.

Rose MR, Griggs R, Dalakas M. (1999) Immunotherapy for inclusion body myositis (Protocol for a Cochrane Review). In: *The Cochrane Library [Issue 4]*. Update Software. Ref Type: Electronic Citation

Rose MR, Levin KH, Griggs RC. (1999) The dropped head plus syndrome: quantitation of response to corticosteroids. *Muscle Nerve* 22: 115–118.

Rose MR, McDermott MP, Thomton CA, Palenski G, Griggs RC. (2001) A prospective longitudinal natural history study of inclusion body myositis; implications for clinical trials. *Neurology* 57: 548–550.

Rugiero M, Koffman B, Dalakas MC. (1998) Association of inclusion body myositis with autoimmune diseases and autoantibodies. *Ann Neurol* 38: 333.

Santorelli FM, Sciacco M, Tanji K, et al. (1996) Multiple mitochondrial DNA deletions in sporadic inclusion body myositis: a study of 56 patients. *Ann Neurol* 39: 789–795.

Sarkozi E, Askanas V, Engel WK. (1994) Abnormal accumulation of prion protein mRNA in muscle fibers of patients with sporadic inclusion-body myositis and hereditary inclusion-body myopathy. *Am J Pathol* 145: 1280–1284.

Sayers ME, Chou SM, Calabrese LH. (1992) Inclusion body myositis: analysis of 32 cases. *J Rheumatol* 19: 1385–1389.

Schneider C, Gold R, Dalakas MC, et al. (1996) MHC class I-mediated cytotoxicity does not induce apoptosis in muscle fibers nor in inflammatory T cells: studies in patients with polymyositis, dermatomyositis, and inclusion body myositis. *J Neuropathol Exp Neurol* 55(12): 1205–1209.

Sekul EA, Chow C, Dalakas MC. (1997) Magnetic resonance imaging of the forearm as a diagnostic aid in patients with sporadic inclusion body myositis. *Neurology* 48: 863–866.

Sekul EA, Dalakas MC. (1993) Inclusion body myositis: new concepts. *Seminars Neurol* 13: 256–263.

Sivakumar K, Semino-Mora C, Dalakas MC. (1997) An inflammatory, familial, inclusion body myositis with autoimmune features and a phenotype identical to sporadic inclusion body myositis. Studies in three families. *Brain* 120: 653–661.

Soueidan SA, Dalakas M. (1993) Treatment of inclusion body myositis with high dose intravenous immunoglobulin. *Neurology* 43: 876–879.

Spector SA, Lemmer JT, Koffman BM, et al. (1997) Safety and efficacy of strength training in patients with sporadic inclusion body myositis. *Muscle Nerve* 20: 1242–1248.

Sundaram MB, Ashenhurst EM. (1981) Polymyositis presenting with distal and asymmetrical weakness. *Can J Neurol Sci* 8(2): 147–149.

Talanin NY, Bushore D, Rasberry R, Rudolph T, Tuli M, Friedman-Musicante R. (1999) Dermatomyositis with the features of inclusion body myositis associated with carcinoma of the bladder. *Br J Dermatol* 141(5): 926–930.

Vaccario ML, Scoppetta C, Bracaglia R, Uncini A. (1981) Sporadic distal myopathy. *J Neurol* 224: 291–295.

Van Kasteren BJ. (1979) Polymyositis presenting with chronic progressive distal muscular weakness. *J Neurol Sci* 41(3): 307–310.

Verma A, Bradley WG, Adesina AM, Sofferman R, Pendlebury WW. (1991) Inclusion body myositis with cricopharyngeus muscle involvement and severe dysphagia [see comments]. *Muscle Nerve* 14: 470–473.

Verma A, Bradley WG, Soule NW, et al. (1992) Quantitative morphometric study of muscle in inclusion body myositis. *J Neurol Sci* 112: 192–198.

Walter MC, Lochmuller H, Toepfer M, et al. (2000) High dose immunoglobulin therapy in sporadic inclusion body myositis: a double blind, placebo-controlled study. *J Neurol* 247: 22–28.

Waters DD, Nutter DO, Hopkins LC, Dorney ER. (1975) Cardiac features of an unusual X-linked humeroperoneal neuromuscular disease. *N Engl J Med* 293: 1017–1022.

Westaway D, DeArmond SJ, Cayetano-Canlas J, et al. (1994) Degeneration of skeletal muscle, peripheral nerves, and the central nervous system in transgenic mice overexpressing wild-type prion proteins. *Cell* 76(1): 117–129.

Wintzen AR, Bots GT, de Bakker HM, Hulshof JH, Padberg GW. (1988) Dysphagia in inclusion body myositis. *J Neurol Neurosurg Psychiatry* 51(12): 1542–1545.

Yamane K, Uchigata M, Nozawa T, Tanabe H. (1978) A case of chronic polymyositis with oculo-pharyngo-distal distribution. *Rinsho Shinkeigaku* 18(7): 369–375.

Yang CC, Alvarez RB, Engel WK, Askanas V. (1996) Increase of nitric oxide synthases and nitrotyrosine in inclusion-body myositis. *Neuroreport* 8: 153–158.

Yang CC, Alvarez RB, Engel WK, Askanas V. (1997) Nitric oxide induced oxidative stress in the muscle fibres of hereditary inclusion body myositis and sporadic inclusion body myositis. *Neurology* 48: A331.

Yood RA, Smith TW. (1985) Inclusion body myositis and systemic lupus erythematosus. *J Rheumatol* 12: 568–570.

Yunis EJ, Samaha FJ. (1971) Inclusion body myositis. *Laboratory Investigation* 25: 240–248.

23

Desmin-related disorders

Hans H. Goebel

Introduction

Definition

Desmin-related disorders are myopathies that develop sporadically or in families following autosomal-dominant or recessive modes of inheritance. They may become apparent in children or in adults. Some patients seem to have a single-organ condition, e.g., a myopathy, others a multiorgan disorder affecting the heart or peripheral nerves and the intestine. The pure myopathy may be slowly progressive, but involvement of the heart may represent a fatal condition. The common morphological feature of desmin-related myopathies is a surplus of desmin within muscle fibres.

Normal desmin

Early on, the intermediate filament of the desmin type was also called skeletin (Edström et al 1980). Conversely, it is unfortunate to note that the term desmin is also applied to a completely different compound associated with coagulation of the blood—a dermatan sulphate (Legnani et al 1994) called Desmin 370.

Desmin is a protein of 53 kD composed of some 300 amino acids. The protein forms filaments of the intermediate category belonging to class III, which also comprises vimentin, glial fibrillary acidic protein and peripherin (Goebel 1995). Desmin appears early in myogenesis; it is more intensely expressed in fetal than mature muscle fibres. It forms a network and appears to link sarcomeres at the Z-disk level with the plasma membrane and, thus, it can be immunomorphologically identified both at the Z-disk as well as subsarcolemmally (Fig. 23.1). Desmin is found in skeletal muscle fibres, cardiac myocytes and smooth muscle cells. The respective gene is located on chromosome 2, i.e. 2q35.

In normal muscle cells, desmin filaments are difficult to identify, and at the subsarcolemmal level desmin appears to be present in a non-filamentous form as other sub- and transmembraneous proteins, i.e. dystrophin, utrophin, plectin or sarcoglycans.

There are other intermediate filaments of muscle fibres: vimentin in immature myofibres and nestin, which is prominent in regenerating fibres (Sjöberg et al 1994) and less so in mature muscle fibres, however, it belongs to class VI of intermediate filaments.

Non-specific pathology of desmin

Desmin is abundant in immature muscle fibres including the early stage of myotubes, although ultrastructurally a large amount of desmin does not mean a higher density of desmin intermediate filaments. Regenerating muscle fibres, irrespective of whether they are present in inflammatory, dystrophic or metabolic myopathies, are rich in desmin. Vimentin is sometimes present in myotubes or immature muscle fibres, but it is absent from mature muscle fibres. Certain neuromuscular disorders of early childhood, therefore, display muscle fibres rich in desmin, such as myotubular myopathy, centronuclear myopathy, infantile myotonic dystrophy, and infantile spinal muscular atrophy (Goebel 1995). The regenerating and immature muscle fibres show a uniform enrichment of desmin rather than a focal one. Expression of desmin is also enhanced in neoplastic cells belonging to rhabdomyomas and rhabdomyosarcomas, but also in certain other neoplasms, such as leiomyomas, leiomyosarcomas and malignant mesothelioma (Truong et al 1990).

Denervated muscle fibres have been shown to show a diffuse increase in desmin, but it has not been determined whether this increase is real or only represents selective loss of other proteins in an atrophic muscle fibre, with desmin preserved longer. It has also not been clearly determined whether such small muscle fibres in a neurogenic process actually are those in an early state of reinnervation and, therefore, at the beginning of regeneration as well.

Desmin-related myopathies

Desmin-related myopathies are marked by multifocal accumulation of desmin with an excess both of fila-

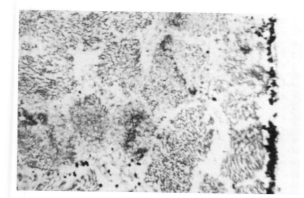

Figure 23.1—Desmin is located beneath the sarcolemma (immunogold technique, × 57 000).

mentous and non-filamentous appearance. This excess was originally documented in conjunction with sarcoplasmic bodies (Edström et al 1980) and cytoplasmic bodies (Osborn and Goebel 1983), seen in respective congenital myopathies. Similar inclusions are spheroid bodies (Goebel et al 1978) and Mallory body–like inclusions (Fidzianska et al 1983). Increase within muscle fibres in a more disseminated, though not diffuse, fashion in granulofilamentous myopathy (Fardeau et al 1978, Rappaport et al 1988) enlarged the spectrum of morphological and nosological conditions. These were variously called desmin-related myopathies (Goebel and Fardeau 1996, Goebel 1997), desminopathies (Vajsar et al 1993, Goebel and Fardeau 1997), desmin myopathy (Ariza et al 1995, Cameron et al 1995) or myopathy with desmin storage (Horowitz and Schmalbruch 1994). The subsequent finding of other proteins in excess, together with desmin, by numerous investigators has accumulated in the more generic term of myofibrillar myopathy (De Bleecker et al 1996), at that time suggesting accumulation of desmin (and other proteins) as a non-specific phenomenon of non-catabolized muscle fibre proteins in certain chronic sporadic and familial myopathies. Recent discoveries of mutations in the desmin gene in a few families with these desmin-related myopathies re-emphasize the nosological role of desmin in these conditions.

Based on diagnostic criteria (Goebel and Fardeau 1997), desminopathies may encompass three broad categories:

Autosomal-dominant granulofilamentous myopathy

Autosomal-dominant granulofilamentous myopathy may start in adulthood (Fardeau et al 1978) and only occasionally in childhood (Vajsar et al 1993). In adults the disease is marked by distal muscle weakness and muscle atrophy, with particular involvement of velopharyngeal muscles whereas eye muscles appear normal. A consistent feature is life-threatening cardiomyopathy (Lobrinus et al 1998), which may abruptly terminate life, perhaps related to chest pain, whilst the myopathy is only slowly progressive. Actually, cardiac abnormalities may precede the myopathy by several years (Goebel et al 1994). Neuropathy (Bertini et al 1991, Sabatelli et al 1992) as well as intestinal malabsorption (Ariza et al 1995) may indicate multiorgan involvement. Creatine kinase (CK) may only be mildly elevated, and the electromyogram may show a myopathic pattern or a mixed myopathic-neurogenic profile.

Inclusion-body type desminopathy

Inclusion-body type desminopathy also largely affects adults (Edström et al 1980, Goebel et al 1997), but occasionally a child (Mizuno et al 1989) or an adolescent (Reed et al 1997) may be affected. Muscle weakness might be more wide-spread, distal in some (Goebel et al 1978), but generalized or proximal in others. More often, respiratory muscles are involved resulting in life-threatening respiratory insufficiency (Jerusalem et al 1979, Chapon et al 1989). Cardiac involvement appears to be the exception (Edström et al 1980). Rarely, a rigid spine is prominent (Reichmann et al 1997). In one family, only elevated CK (hyperCKemia) was present (Prelle et al 1996). The course is usually slowly progressive, but an episode of severe respiratory insufficiency may end a patient's life prematurely. Creatine kinase is only mildy elevated, the electromyogram may show a myopathic pattern, but occasionally neurogenic features have been seen (Goebel et al 1978).

Hyaline/desmin-plaque myopathy

Hyaline/desmin-plaque myopathy. This often rather severe and even fatal muscular condition has been seen at several occasions by Fidzianska, first in Germany (Fidzianska et al 1983), then in Warsaw (Fidzianska et al 1995). The children, some of them siblings, have shown generalized or proximal weakness, severe scoliosis, occasional respiratory failure and facial weakness but no eye involvement. Cardiac involvement is not a feature. Creatine kinase is mildly elevated, electromyography gives a myopathic pattern. Nosological separation of this neuromuscular condition requires confirmation by other investigators or the identification of a genetic profile differing from those mentioned above.

Morphological aspects

As the concept of the desminopathies has evolved from the morphological features forming the basis of the three groups described above, there might, nevertheless, be some overlap especially among the first two groups. Granulofilamentous material is marked by a granular component and filaments which accumulate subsarcolemmally, but also among sarcomeres. Cytoplasmic inclusion bodies, composed also of a granular core and a halo of filaments may co-appear with the granulofilamentous material, or they may form the sole type of inclusion in cytoplasmic body myopathy,

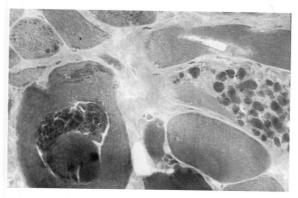

Figure 23.2—Spheroid body aggregate in several muscle fibres (modified trichrome stain, × 550; by courtesy of Dr D'Agostino, Portland (OR), USA).

an early term. Spheroid bodies (Fig. 23.2) show a less distinct separation of the granular and filamentous components (Goebel et al 1978), though occasionally they form large complexes which are then called cytoplasmic–spheroid complexes (Halbig et al 1991).

Granulofilamentous material (Fig. 23.3) and the inclusion bodies have been found so frequently overlapping that it resulted in the new common term "myofibrillar myopathy" (De Bleecker et al 1996, Nakano et al 1996) observed both in sporadic as well as familial cases, although separation of the two types was still acknowledged (Nakano et al 1996). Granulofilamentous material has not only been observed in skeletal muscle fibres, but also in cardiac myocytes (Bertini et al 1991, Ariza et al 1995, Lobrinus et al 1998). Morphologically, cardiac myocytes showed, at the electron microscopic level, features identical to those seen in skeletal muscle fibres (Lobrinus et al 1998).

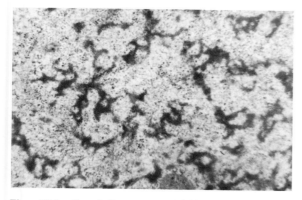

Figure 23.3—Granulofilamentous material in a muscle fibre (× 82 500).

Occasionally, smooth muscle cells have been affected (Ariza et al 1995, Abraham et al 1998), and peripheral axons were enlarged by accumulation of neurofilaments (Bertini et al 1991, Sabatelli et al 1992). While giant axons are a feature of autosomal-recessive giant axonal neuropathy as well as of acquired intoxication by organic solvents, skeletal and cardiac muscles are not affected in these conditions. However, from a separate family afflicted with giant axons (Vogel et al 1985, Goebel et al 1986) displaying giant axons in peripheral nerves of several neuropathy-affected family members, one also had cardiomyopathy.

The inclusions seen within muscle fibres, but not yet shown in cardiac myocytes of the hyaline/desmin plaque type (Fidzianska et al 1995), originally prompted Fidzianska et al (1983) to call them Mallory body-like inclusions because they resembled Mallory bodies of hepatocytes. They also contain filaments, and the term hyaline (Fidzianska et al 1995, De Bleecker et al 1996) appears somewhat inappropriate in view of the separate congenital myopathy with hyaline bodies or hyaline body myopathy (Ceuterick et al 1993, Barohn et al 1994), these hyaline bodies being marked by granular electron-lucent material rich in myosin and myofibrillar ATPase activity, but without filaments.

Additonal features in conjunction with desmin-related inclusions have been the presence of tubulofilamentous profiles (Reichmann et al 1997) as well as coexistence of reducing bodies (Bertini et al 1994, Goebel et al 1995). Whether the coexistence of reducing bodies and cytoplasmic bodies is a mere coincidence or indicates some unexplained relationship of these two types of inclusion bodies—the cytoplasmic bodies thought to be derived from Z-disk material, the reducing body being of still unidentified origin— currently is not clear. However, reducing bodies may occur as a non-specific feature in a number of well-defined neuromuscular conditions other than desminopathies, and reducing body myopathy with cytoplasmic bodies may just belong to this list of neuromuscular conditions.

Immunohistochemical data

In the early 1980s (Osborn and Goebel 1983), desmin was found to be associated with cytoplasmic bodies and this finding has subsequently been confirmed in numerous instances, finally resulting in the term desmin storage myopathy, desmin-related myopathy or desminopathy. Although occasionally desmin could not be identified in conjunction with cytoplasmic bodies by immunohistochemistry (Guimaraes et al 1996), the term desmin myopathy has, nevertheless, been applied (Baeta et al 1996). Inclusions named differently, such as sarcoplasmic bodies (Edström et al 1980) or spheroid bodies have also been shown to contain desmin (Goebel et al 1997). The increased amount of desmin in granulofilamentous myopathy (Figs 23.4 and 23.5) has been found to be abnormally phosphorylated (Rappaport et al 1988). In addition to one desmin component of normal molecular weight (53 KD), a second abnormal desmin component of lower molecular weight (49 kD) has also been identified (Lobrinus et al 1998) indicating either evidence of degradation or of a mutation in the gene for desmin.

Subsequent to the discovery of desmin accumulating in desminopathy, other proteins such as dystrophin (Caron et al 1993, Goebel et al 1994), vimentin (Helliwell et al 1994) and α-B crystallin (Figs 23.6 and 23.7; Goebel et al 1994, 1997, Reed et al 1997), as well as ubiquitin (Goebel et al 1997) have been documented. Finally, De Bleecker et al (1996) succeeded not only in confirming the presence of the wide variety of these proteins but also in demonstrating a considerable number of additional proteins, some quite unusual such as gelsolin, α-antichymotrypsin and proteins of the β-A4-amyloid precursor protein complex (De Bleecker et al 1996).

This large gamut of diversified proteins, accumulating in conjunction with granulofilamentous material and the inclusion bodies, among the desminopathies suggested abnormal degradation of proteins rather than abnormal synthesis. Occasionally, autophagic vacuoles were prominent close to these inclusions, but evidence of true lysosomal activation has not been shown.

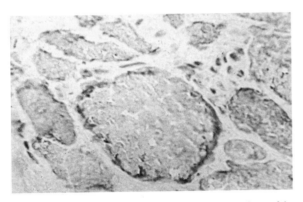

Figure 23.4— Increased amounts of desmin in the periphery of the central muscle fibre, granulofilamentous myopathy (immunoperoxidase preparation, × 900).

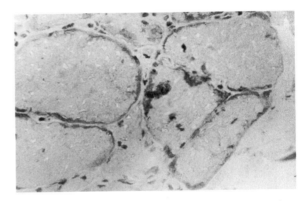

Figure 23.6— Increased amounts of α-B crystallin in the periphery of several muscle fibres (× 680).

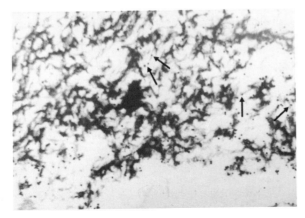

Figure 23.5— Labelling of desmin and its filaments (arrows) of the granulofilamentous material (immunogold technique, × 63 700).

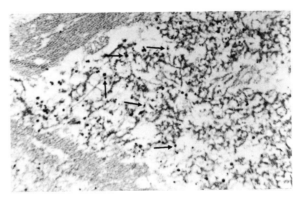

Figure 23.7—Labelling of α-B crystallin in granulofilamentous material including the filamentous component (arrows) (immunogold technique, × 61 880).

It is of interest that the electron microscopic features of the granular and filamentous components of both the granulofilamentous material and the desmin-associated inclusion bodies are similar to other such inclusions in other cell types—e.g. the intraneuronal Lewy bodies in Parkinson's and Lewy body diseases, Rosenthal fibres within neoplastic and non-neoplastic astrocytes (the latter also rich in α-B crystallin), and Mallory bodies in epithelial cells of the liver. Some of these conditions such as Parkinson's disease and alcohol intoxication of the liver are acquired, others hereditary, such as familial Parkinson's disease and giant axonal neuropathy, which is also marked by abundant Rosenthal fibres. Since pathogenesis and morphogenesis of the desminopathic lesions within muscle fibres (as well as the mixed granulofilamentous inclusions in other cell types of the above-named diseases) are still incompletely understood, any further similarities apart from phenomenological aspects remain speculative. However, these non-myofibrillar inclusions, consisting of cell-specific type intermediate filaments and a granular component of unexplained origin also show accumulation of proteins other than the respective intermediate filaments, i.e. α-B crystallin (Lowe et al 1992), and ubiquitin (Trojanowski et al 1998).

Desmin-related genetic abnormalities

The abundant accumulation of diversified proteins in association with the accretion of desmin resulting in the term "myofibrillar myopathy" (De Bleecker et al 1996, Nakano et al 1996) suggested an impaired epiphenomenal degradation of intracellular proteins rather than any gene-related defects.

The generation of a homozygous knock-out mouse model for desmin (Li et al 1996, Milner et al 1996) produced severe, life-shortening cardiopathy, myopathy, and vasculopathy, marked by disruption of muscle fibre architecture (especially of sarcomeres), degeneration of muscle fibres and even necrosis of the heart muscle associated with calcification. Similarly vascular smooth muscle cells showed signs of degeneration. All of this was supposedly based on the absence of desmin and its intracellular network, the absence of which did not hamper development and maturation of muscle fibres, but apparently affected maintenance. However, the cardiomyopathy and myopathy produced in mice without desmin genes are not identical to the human spontaneous desmin-related myopathy

Table 23.1 — Genetic abnormalities in desminopathies

- Linkage to chromosome 12 (Wilhelmsen et al 1996)
- Heterozygous R120G missense mutation in the α-B crystallin gene 7q 21-23 (Vicart et al 1998)
- Missense mutation in desmin gene 2q35 (Brown et al 1995) (Hypertrophic cardiomyopathy)
- Autosomal (heterozygous) A337B mutation in desmin gene 2q35 (Goldfarb et al 1998)
- Compound (heterozygous) A360B and N393I mutations in desmin gene 2q35 (Goldfarb et al 1998)
- Homozygous 7 aminoacid residue deletion in desmin gene 2q35 (Muñoz-Mármol et al 1998)

and cardiomyopathy, and a vasculopathy is hardly ever a component of human desminopathy (Abraham et al 1998). On the contrary, in the human desminopathy there is too much desmin or too many desmin-intermediate filaments within muscle fibres rather than too few or none. Thus, the desmin knock-out mouse has given valuable insight into the physiological role of desmin, but its significance as a model for human desminopathies has not yet convincingly been shown (Capetanaki et al 1997, Li et al 1997, Thornell et al 1997).

This assumption was further supported by the failure to find mutations in the desmin gene in granulofilamentous myopathy (Vicart et al 1996), in which abnormal biochemistry of desmin had been recorded owing to abnormal phosphorylation (Rappaport et al 1988). The presence of one normal 53 kD desmin protein and an additional abnormal 49 kD desmin in the skeletal muscle of a mother and her daughter, both affected by familial cardiomyopathy and distal myopathy of the granulofilamentous type (Lobrinus et al 1998), suggested either a degradation product of desmin or an additional gene-encoded second desmin protein.

In an autosomal-dominant scapuloperoneal muscular dystrophy, which showed cytoplasmic bodies in biopsied muscle specimens, linkage was established to chromosome 12 (Wilhelmsen et al 1996), but no further mutations and no precise relationship to desmin were established. Therefore, whether this represents the first desminopathy marked by a genetic abnormality remains to be seen. Moreover, a family with hypertrophic cardiomyopathy was found to have a missense mutation in the desmin gene (Brown et al 1995), but neither morphology of the disease in the heart muscle nor involvement of the skeletal muscle were reported. The relationship of this family's cardiomyopathy to the desmin-related myopathy and cardiomyopathy also remains unclear as patients suffering from such desmin-related myopathies and cardiomyopathies, although having a cardiomyopathy, were not reported to have the hypertrophic type of cardiomyopathy. Notwithstanding the tenuous relationship of this familial scapuloperoneal muscular dystrophy (Wilhelmsen et al 1996) and this hypertrophic cardiomyopathy (Brown et al 1995) to desmin, they may be components of the diversified spectrum of mutation-related desminopathies.

The genetic spectrum of the desminopathies was further augmented when a missense mutation in the α-B crystallin gene was found in French families with granulofilamentous desmin-related myopathy (Vicart et al 1998), which earlier had been shown not to have a mutation in the desmin gene (Vicart et al 1996). This not only represented the first documentation of a mutation in the α-B crystallin gene as a disease-related phenomenon, but it also showed that mutations have been and should be sought among such associated proteins when the desmin gene appears intact. The observation of a mutation in the α-B crystallin gene in this granulofilamentous desminopathy (Vicart et al 1998) also suggested that other proteins could accumulate due to their related gene mutations. In this family the accumulation of desmin resulting from an associated non-desmin gene-related phenomenon requires explanation of why desmin accumulates when the gene of another protein, in this case α-B crystallin, is faulty. Cultured muscle cells were transfected with this mutated α-B crystallin gene upon which aggregates containing both α-B crystallin and desmin appeared in these transfected myoblast cell lines. This further supported the notion that a mutation in the desmin gene is not necessary to produce gene-related accumulation of desmin.

Finally, it was shown by two independent groups (Goldfarb et al 1998, Muñoz-Mármol et al 1998) that indeed mutations in the desmin gene may also result in human desminopathies. One family with desmin-related myopathy and cardiomyopathy of autosomal-dominant nature had a heterozygous alanine to proline (A337P) mutation conforming to the adult-onset type of desminopathy (Goldfarb et al 1998). Another family showed compound heterozygosity to other mutations, alanine to proline (A360P) and asparagine to isoleucine (N393I), producing an autosomal-recessive childhood type of a more severe desminopathy (Goldfarb et al 1998). These two families, therefore, showed that mutations in the desmin gene may cause both an autosomal-dominant, late-onset desminopathy and an autosomal-recessive early-onset desminopathy, depending on the type of mutation.

Another patient, who had been found to have a desminopathy affecting the skeletal, cardiac and smooth muscle (Ariza et al 1995) was later shown to have a 21 nucleotide deletion in the desmin gene resulting in a truncated desmin protein lacking seven amino acid residues (Muñoz-Mármol et al 1998). This mutation was homozygous and showed that transfecting cells with the mutant gene caused an abnormal structure of clumped desmin material, rather than the regular intracellular network. During development of muscle cells, vimentin had apparently replaced desmin to enable normal development. The desmin-related myopathy was of the granulofilamentous type. Therefore, this ganulofilamentous myopathy appears genetically heterogeneous, i.e., caused by mutations in either the α-B crystallin gene or the desmin gene.

Conclusions

The evolution of our knowledge about the desminopathies has had three different stages:

Stage I: a descriptive stage, when cytoplasmic bodies, spheroid bodies and granulofilamentous material were described by electron microscopy

Stage II: the immunohistochemical association of cytoplasmic and spheroid bodies and granulofilamentous material with desmin—and later with other proteins including α-B crystallin—resulting in the firmly established concept of the desminopathies and the incipient

Stage III: the recent discovery of the mutations in desminopathy-related genes—the desmin and α-B crystallin genes, and perhaps other genes as well.

The absence of a mutation in the desmin gene in the rather large kinship afflicted with spheroid body myopathy (Goebel et al 1997) suggests that other genes responsible for desminopathies await their discovery.

Acknowledgements

The work presented here was supported by the Deutsche Gesellschaft für Muskelkranke e.V., Freiburg/Germany and the European Neuromuscular Center (ENMC), Baarn/The Netherlands.

The antibodies against α-B crystallin were kindly supplied by Prof. A.K. Mayer, Nottingham, U.K. and Dr. J.E. Goldmann, New York City (NY), USA. Margarete Schlie and Irene Warlo provided light and electron microscopic as well as immunomorphological preparations. Walter Meffert helped with photography and Astrid Wöber edited the manuscript.

References

Abraham SC, DeNofrio D, Loh E, et al. (1998) Desmin myopathy involving cardiac, skeletal, and vascular smooth muscle: report of a case with immunoelectron microscopy. *Hum Pathol* 29: 876–882.

Ariza A, Coll J, Fernández-Figueras MT. (1995) Desmin myopathy: a multisystem disorder involving skeletal, cardiac, and smooth muscle. *Hum Pathol* 26: 1032–1037.

Baeta AM, Figarella-Branger D, Bille-Turc F, Lepidi H, Pellissier J-F. (1996) Familial desmin myopathies and cytoplasmic body myopathies. *Acta Neuropathol (Berl)* 92: 499–510.

Barohn RJ, Brumback RA, Mendell JR. (1994) Hyaline body myopathy. *Neuromusc Disord* 4: 257–262.

Bertini E, Bosman C, Ricci E, et al. (1991) Neuromyopathy and restrictive cardiomyopathy with accumulation of intermediate filaments: a clinical, morphological and biochemical study. *Acta Neuropathol (Berl)* 81: 632–640.

Bertini E, Salviati G, Apollo F, et al. (1994) Reducing body myopathy and desmin storage in skeletal muscle: morphological and biochemical findings. *Acta Neuropathol (Berl)* 87: 106–112.

Brown BD, Scheffold T, Rottbauer W, et al. (1995) Intermediate filament desmin gene missense mutation found in a family suffering from hypertrophic cardiomyopathy. *Circulation* 92 (suppl. I): I-233 (abstr)

Cameron CHS, Mirakhur M, Allen IV. (1995) Desmin myopathy with cardiomyopathy. *Acta Neuropathol (Berl)* 89: 560–566.

Capetanaki Y, Milner DJ, Weitzer G. (1997) Desmin in muscle formation and maintenance: knockouts and consequences. *Cell Struct Funct* 22: 103–116.

Caron A, Chapon F, Berthelin C, Viader F, Lechevalier B. (1993) Inclusions in familial cytoplasmic body myopathy are stained by anti-dystrophin antibodies. *Neuromusc Disord* 3: 541–546.

Ceuterick C, Martin J-J, Martens C. (1993) Hyaline bodies in skeletal muscle of a patient with a mild chronic non-progressive congenital myopathy. *Clin Neuropathol* 12: 79–83.

Chapon F, Viader F, Fardeau M. (1989) Myopathie familiale avec inclusions de type «corps cytoplasmiques» (ou «sphéroides») révélée par une insuffisance respiratoire. *Rev Neurol (Paris)* 145: 460–465.

De Bleecker JL, Engel AG, Ertl BB. (1996) Myofibrillar myopathy with abnormal foci of desmin positivity. II. Immunocytochemical analysis reveals accumulation of multiple other proteins. *J Neuropathol Exp Neurol* 55: 563–577.

Edström L, Thornell L-E, Eriksson A. (1980) A new type of hereditary distal myopathy with characteristic sarcoplasmic bodies and intermediate (skeletin) filaments. *J Neurol Sci* 47: 171–190.

Fardeau M, Godet-Guillain J, Tomé FSM. (1978) Une nouvelle affection musculaire familiale, définie par l'accumulation intra-sarco-plasmique d'un matériel granulo-filamentaire dense en microscopie électronique. *Rev Neurol (Paris)* 134: 411–425.

Fidzianska A, Goebel HH, Osborn M, Lenard HG, Osse G, Langenbeck U. (1983) Mallory body-like inclusions in a hereditary congenital neuromuscular disease. *Muscle Nerve* 6: 195–200.

Fidzianska A, Ryniewicz B, Barcikowska M, Goebel HH. (1995) A new familial congenital myopathy in children with desmin and dystrophin reacting plaques. *J Neurol Sci* 131: 88–95.

Goebel HH. (1995) Desmin-related neuromuscular disorders. *Muscle Nerve* 18: 1306–1320.

Goebel HH. (1997) Desmin-related myopathies. *Curr Opin Neurol* 10: 426–429.

Goebel HH. (1998) Congenital myopathies with inclusion bodies: a brief review. *Neuromusc Disord* 8: 162–168.

Goebel HH, Fardeau M. (1995) Desmin in myology. 24th European Neuromuscular Center-sponsored workshop, held November 5–6, 1993, Naarden, The Netherlands. *Neuromusc Disord* 5: 161–166.

Goebel HH, Fardeau M. (1996) Familial desmin-related myopathies and cardiomyopathies – from myopathology to molecular and clinical genetics. *Neuromusc Disord* 6: 383–388.

Goebel HH, Fardeau M. (1997) Desminopathies. In: Emery AEH, ed. *Diagnostic Criteria for Neuromuscular Disorders.* London: Royal Society of Medicine Press, pp. 75–79.

Goebel HH, Muller J, Gillen HW, Merritt AD. (1978) Autosomal dominant "spheroid body myopathy". *Muscle Nerve* 1: 14–26.

Goebel HH, Vogel P, Gabriel M. (1986) Neuropathologic and morphometric studies in hereditary motor and sensory neuropathy type II with neurofilament accumulation. *Ital J Neurol Sci* 7: 325–332.

Goebel HH, Voit T, Warlo I, Jacobs K, Johannsen U, Müller CR. (1994) Immunohistologic and electron microscopic abnormalities of desmin and dystrophin in familial cardiomyopathy and myopathy. *Rev Neurol (Paris)* 150: 452–459.

Goebel HH, Voit T, Schober R. (1995) Combined cytoplasmic body and reducing body myopathy – a mixed congenital myopathy. *J Neuropathol Exp Neurol* 54: 453.

Goebel HH, D'Agostino AN, Wilson J, et al. (1997) Spheroid body myopathy – revisited. *Muscle Nerve* 20: 1127–1136.

Goldfarb LG, Park K-Y, Cervenáková S, et al. (1998) Missense mutations in desmin associated with familial cardiac and skeletal myopathy [letter]. *Nature Genet* 19: 402–403.

Guimaraes A, Rebelo O, Magalhaes M. (1996) Familial cytoplasmic body myopathy. *Neuropathol Appl Neurobiol* 22 (suppl 1): 4 (C 12).

Halbig L, Goebel HH, Hopf HC, Moll R. (1991) Spheroid-cytoplasmic complexes in a congenital myopathy. *Rev Neurol (Paris)* 147: 300–307.

Helliwell TR, Green ART, Green A, Edwards RHT. (1994) Hereditary distal myopathy with granulo-filamentous cytoplasmic inclusions containing desmin, dystrophin and vimentin. *J Neurol Sci* 124: 174–187.

Horowitz SH, Schmalbruch H. (1994) Autosomal dominant distal myopathy with desmin storage: a clinicopathologic and electrophysiologic study of a large kinship. *Muscle Nerve* 17: 151–160.

Jerusalem F, Ludin H, Bischoff A, Hartmann G. (1979) Cytoplasmic body neuromyopathy presenting as respiratory failure and weight loss. *J Neurol Sci* 41: 1–9.

Legnani C, Palareti G, Biagi R, et al. (1994) Acute and chronic effects of a new low molecular weight dermatan sulphate (Desmin 370) on blood coagulation and fibrinolysis in healthy subjects. *Eur J Clin Pharmacol* 47: 247–252.

Li Z, Colucci-Guyon E, Pincon-Raymond M, et al. (1996) Cardiovascular lesions and skeletal myopathy in mice lacking desmin. *Dev Biol* 175: 362–366.

Li Z, Maricskay M, Agbulut O. (1997) Desmin is essential for the tensile strength and integrity of myofibrils but not for myogenic commitment, differentiation, and fusion of skeletal muscle. *J Cell Biol* 139: 129–144.

Lobrinus JA, Janzer RC, Kuntzer T. (1998) Familial cardiomyopathy and distal myopathy with abnormal desmin accumulation and migration. *Neuromusc Disord* 8: 77–86.

Lowe J, McDermott H, Pike I, Spendlove I, Landon M, Mayer RJ. (1992) Alpha-B crystallin expression in non-lenticular tissues and selective presence in ubiquitinated inclusion bodies in human disease. *J Pathol* 166: 61–68.

Milner DJ, Weitzer G, Tran D, Bradley A, Capetanaki Y. (1996) Disruption of muscle architecture and myocardial degeneration in mice lacking desmin. *J Cell Biol* 134: 1255–1270.

Mizuno Y, Nakamura Y, Komiya K. (1989) The spectrum of cytoplasmic body myopathy: report of a congenital severe case. *Brain Dev* 11: 20–25.

Muñoz-Mármol AM, Strasser G, Isamat M, et al. (1998) A dysfunctional desmin mutation in a patient with severe generalized myopathy. *Proc Natl Acad Sci USA* 95: 11312–11317.

Nakano S, Engel AG, Waclawik AJ, Emslie-Smith AM, Busis NA. (1996) Myofibrillar myopathy with abnormal foci of desmin positivity. I. Light and electron microscopy analysis of 10 cases. *J Neuropathol Exp Neurol* 55: 549–562.

Osborn M, Goebel HH. (1983) The cytoplasmic bodies in a congenital myopathy can be stained with antibodies to desmin, the muscle-specific intermediate filament protein. *Acta Neuropathol (Berl)* 62: 149–152.

Prelle A, Rigoletto C, Moggio M, et al. (1996) Asymptomatic familial hyperCKemia associated with desmin accumulation in skeletal muscle. *J Neurol Sci* 140: 132–136.

Rappaport L, Contard F, Samuel JL, et al. (1988) Storage of phosphorylated desmin in a familial myopathy. *FEBS Lett* 231: 421–425.

Reed L, Young J, Goebel HH, Schochet SS. (1997) Congenital cytoplasmic body myopathy: case report. *J Child Neurol* 12: 149–152.

Reichmann H, Goebel HH, Schneider Ch, Toyka KV. (1997) Familial mixed congenital myopathy with rigid spine syndrome. *Muscle Nerve* 20: 411–417.

Sabatelli M, Bertini E, Ricci E, et al. (1992) Peripheral neuropathy with giant axons and cardiomyopathy associated with desmin type intermediate filaments in skeletal muscle. *J Neurol Sci* 109: 1–10.

Sjöberg G, Jiang W-Q, Ringertz NR, Lendahl U, Sejersen T. (1994) Colocalization of nestin and vimentin/desmin in skeletal muscle cells demonstrated by three-dimensional fluorescence digital imaging microscopy. *Exp Cell Res* 214: 447–458.

Thornell L-E, Carlsson L, Mericskay M, Paulin D. (1997) Null mutation in the desmin gene gives rise to a cardiomyopathy. *J Mol Cell Cardiol* 29: 2107–2124.

Trojanowski JQ, Goedert M, Iwatsubo T, Lee VM-Y. (1998) Fatal attractions: abnormal protein aggregation and neuron death in Parkinson's disease and Lewy body dementia. *Cell Death Differentiation* 5: 832–837.

Truong LD, Rangdaeng S, Cagle P, Ro JY, Hawkins H, Font RL. (1990) The diagnostic utility of desmin. *Am J Clin Pathol* 93: 305–314.

Vajsar J, Becker LE, Freedom RM, Murphy EG. (1993) Familial desminopathy: myopathy with accumulation of desmin-type intermediate filaments. *J Neurol Neurosurg Psychiatry* 56: 644–648.

Vicart P, Dupret J-M, Hazan J, et al. (1996) Human desmin gene: cDNA sequence, regional localization and exclusion of the locus in a familial desmin-related myopathy. *Human Genetics* 98: 422–429.

Vicart P, Caron A, Guicheney P, et al. (1998) A missense mutation in the alpha-B crystallin chaperone gene causes a desmin-related myopathy. *Nature Genet* 20: 92–95.

Vogel P, Gabriel M, Goebel HH, Dyck PJ. (1985) Hereditary motor sensory neuropathy type II with neurofilament accumulation: new finding or new disorder? *Ann Neurol* 17: 455–461.

Wilhelmsen KC, Blake DM, Lynch T. (1996) Chromosome 12-linked autosomal dominant scapuloperoneal muscular dystrophy. *Ann Neurol* 39: 507–520.

24

AMP deaminase (myoadenylate deaminase) deficiencys

Manfred Gross

Introduction

Lack of adenosine monophosphate (AMP) deaminase (AMPD; EC 3.5.4.6) activity in skeletal muscle—also called myoadenylate deaminase (MAD) deficiency—is by far the most common muscle enzyme defect in humans. It was first described in humans in 1978 by Fishbein et al in five patients with muscular symptoms. It is found in about 2–3% of all muscle biopsies. Despite this high prevalence, the knowledge about clinical relevance, pathogenesis of symptoms and therapeutic options is still limited.

Biochemical aspects of normal AMP deaminase

AMP deaminase catalyses the deamination of AMP to inosine monophosphate (IMP) with liberation of ammonia (Fig. 24.1). This reaction is part of the purine nucleotide cycle (Lowenstein and Tornheim 1971). AMP can be converted into adenylosuccinate by adenylosuccinate synthetase (EC 6.3.4.4). Adenylosuccinate is reconverted into AMP by the adenylosuccinate lyase or adenylosuccinase (EC 4.3.2.2).

Several functions of AMP deaminase have been assumed. It plays an important role in stabilization of the energy charge during ATP consumption. As part of the purine nucleotide cycle, AMP deaminase is important for purine nucleotide interconversion, the replenishment of citric acid intermediates by formation of fumarate, the deamination of amino acids (aspartate), and the regulation of the activities of phosphofructokinase and phosphorylase b by formation of ammonia and IMP (Sabina et al 1989b). The impor-

tant role of this enzyme is underlined by the fact that AMPD is found in all eukaryotic cells.

AMPD activity differs between various human tissues or cell types. The highest activity is measured in skeletal muscle (Ogasawara et al 1982b). Among human striated muscle, the highest activity is found in white muscle fibres. The activity in red muscle fibres as well as in autonomic innervated muscle is less than half of the activity in white muscle (Meyer and Terjung 1980, Fishbein et al 1984, Fishbein 1986). In cardiac or smooth muscle, as well as in the liver, brain or kidney, the AMPD activity is only a few per cent of the activity found in striated muscle (Fishbein et al 1993).

Tissue and stage specific isoforms of AMPD exist in many eukaryotes (Ogasawara et al 1978, 1982b, Marquetant et al 1987). In humans, there are at least four isoforms encoded by three genes. All native isoforms are tetramers of identical subunits.

The muscle specific isoform of AMPD is also called myoadenylate deaminase (MAD). The other isoforms are the predominant form in liver (L) and the two isoforms found in erythrocytes (E1 and E2) (Ogasawara et al 1982a,b).

Clinical aspects of myoadenylate deaminase deficiency

MAD deficiency exhibits an autosomal recessive pattern of inheritance. The vast majority of homozygous subjects are asymptomatic. The patients with symptomatic MAD deficiency usually suffer from features of a metabolic myopathy mainly with exercise-induced

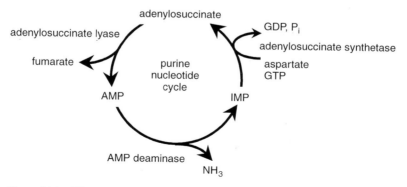

Figure 24.1—The purine nucleotide cycle (AMP, adenosine monophosphate; GDP, guanosine diphosphate; GTP, guanosine triphosphate; IMP, inosine monophosphate; NH₃, ammonia; Pᵢ, inorganic phosphate).

muscle pain, early fatigue and/or cramps. In typical cases, the patient is free of symptoms when not performing muscular exercise. Muscular work first causes myalgia with increasing severity, followed in some patients by muscular cramps. After exercise, the symptoms slowly regress, much slower than in patients with a macroangiopathy. After severe pain, the symptoms can persist even for several days.

All skeletal muscles can be affected such as the muscles of shoulder girdle or even the muscles of the forearm in a patient playing the accordion. Usually, the large muscles of upper arms and legs are the primary sites of ache. Smooth muscles and the heart are not affected.

However, the range of symptoms is very broad. Some patients develop rhabdomyolysis, either single or recurrent episodes. Many patients report arthralgias without clinical hints for arthritis. In some patients, the complaints resemble those of fibromyalgia. Joint-related complaints cannot be directly attributed to MAD deficiency since only skeletal muscle lacks this enzyme activity. Some patients may interpret muscular symptoms as joint problems thus influencing the presentation of the symptoms to the physician, or the association of these symptoms and MAD deficiency may be by coincidence.

Some patients with MAD deficiency suffer from muscle pain even at rest. If these symptoms are provoked by severe exercise and decrease in severity when resting, they may be caused by the enzyme defect. Other patients report muscle ache independent of exercise: not or hardly aggravated by muscular work, not relieved when resting. In these patients, the symptoms can not be explained by MAD deficiency since this enzyme is not active under resting conditions. In these patients, other causes for the complaints must be looked for.

The vast majority of patients suffer from mild symptoms only. Some patients, however, report severe symptoms preventing them from practicing their profession if muscular work is necessary. Even in patients with very severe symptoms, no structural alterations in the myoskeletal systems are found, especially no muscle atrophy or joint destruction. No patient has to use a wheelchair because of MAD deficiency.

The age at onset of symptoms ranges from early childhood to late adulthood. About one in four patients report symptoms first in each of childhood, as teenagers, young adults or in late adulthood (Sabina et al 1989b). There seems to be a correlation between age at onset and severity of symptoms: patients with early onset seem to suffer more from muscle symptoms than those with late onset.

Biochemical aspects of myoadenylate deaminase deficiency

In patients with inherited MAD deficiency, the enzyme defect affects only skeletal muscle. Normal AMPD activity was reported in granulocytes and lymphocytes (Fishbein 1986) as well as in fibroblasts (DiMauro et al 1980) of patients.

The metabolic basis for the development of symptoms in patients with MAD deficiency is not yet clear. In part, the biochemical findings in these patients are contradictory (Sabina et al 1989b, Gross and Gresser 1993). Initially, the myocytes in MAD deficient patients were expected to lose purine nucleotides during exercise. Due to the lack of AMP deaminase activity, the accumulating AMP was assumed to be degraded into adenosine, which is able to permeate rapidly out of the muscle tissue (Sabina et al 1980). However, subsequent studies did not confirm this hypothesis. In contrast, the lack of increase in hypoxanthine plasma level after ischaemic exercise test even became a hallmark of this disorder (Patterson et al 1983).

Instead, the most important biochemical consequence of MAD deficiency seems to be the lack of fumarate production. Fumarate production by the purine nucleotide cycle is sufficient to account for the increase in metabolites of the citric acid cycle during exercise (Aragon and Lowenstein 1980). Therefore, the disruption of the purine nucleotide cycle in MAD deficiency may result in an insufficient activation of the citric acid cycle and, subsequently, insufficient energy production. This hypothesis is supported by the higher increase in lactate plasma level during exercise in patients with MAD deficiency compared with healthy control subjects (Gross et al 1991).

Therapy

In some patients, the oral administration of D-ribose or xylitol can prevent the exercise-induced symptoms (Zöllner et al 1986, Bruyland and Ebinger 1994). Since the administration of xylitol is associated with side-effects, mainly severe increase in serum uric acid level (Heuckenkamp and Zöllner 1972), most experiences were obtained with ribose. Both carbohydrates can enter the pentose phosphate pathway. Ribose is converted into ribose-5-phosphate, which can enter several reactions. After conversion into phosphoribosyl pyrophosphate, it may stimulate both de novo synthesis of purine nucleotides as well as the hypoxanthine-guanine-phosphoribosyl-transerase (HPRT) dependent salvage pathway.

There is evidence that ribose is degraded into lactate via the reactions of the pentose phosphate pathway with formation of ATP. There is a higher increase in serum lactate concentration in patients with MAD deficiency during exercise if the patients are treated with ribose (Gross et al 1991). The energy obtained by this degradation of ribose into lactate may be helpful in compensating for insufficient ATP synthesis in MAD deficiency. However, the symptomatic therapy with ribose is not successful in all patients (Pongratz et al 1987). Despite of several studies on ribose metabolism, this phenomenon, as well as the pharmacological effect of ribose, is not yet fully understood (Gross et al 1989, 1991, Gross and Zöllner 1991).

Genetic basis of myoadenylate deaminase deficiency

The muscle isoform MAD is encoded by the *AMPD1* gene, which is located on chromosome 1 p13-p21 (Kingsmore et al 1990, Sabina et al 1990). It consists of 16 exons. The human liver isoform is encoded by the *AMPD2* gene (Bausch-Jurken et al 1992), and the erythrocyte isoforms E1 and E2 are encoded by the *AMPD3* gene (Mahnke-Zizelman and Sabina 1992, Yamada et al 1992).

In a small percentage of the *AMPD1* transcript, the exon 2 sequence is removed from the mRNA by a process called alternative splicing (Mineo et al 1990, Mineo and Holmes 1991). Since exon 2 consists of 12 nucleotides, alternative splicing does not change the

reading frame. The biochemical significance of this alternative splicing is not yet understood (Morisaki et al 1993, Gross et al 1995). No structural defects in the *AMPD1* gene of patients were detected (Gross et al 1990). Sequencing of the *AMPD1* cDNA of two German patients revealed two mutations for which both patients were homozygous (Morisaki et al 1992). The first mutation (C34-T) at the last nucleotide of exon 2 creates a stop-codon; the second mutation in exon 3 (C143-T) results in the amino acid residue proline48 being replaced by leucine. Since then, 16 other German patients and one Turkish girl with primary MAD deficiency were analysed for both mutations. All of them were homozygous for both mutations (Morisaki et al 1992, Gross 1994b). Therefore, a single mutation accounted for all cases of primary MAD deficiency studied in the past. More recent studies however demonstrated the presence of more than one mutation in the population.

The C34-T mutation creates a stop-codon and, therefore, results in an early stop of protein synthesis after only 11 amino acid residues. This truncated peptide is not catalytically active. The second C143-T mutation would result in an amino acid exchange if the translation had not stopped earlier. The effect of the second mutation on enzyme activity was studied by in vivo protein expression of human MAD cDNA harbouring this mutation. No difference in specific activity could be measured between wild-type and mutant protein (Gross et al 1995).

The mutated cytosine is followed in both mutations by a guanosine. These CG-dinucleotides are hot spots for C-T mutations and therefore account for many of the mutations in other genes as well (Youssoufian et al 1986). However, the fact that the vast majority of patients are homozygous for both mutations may indicate a founder effect in the Caucasian population.

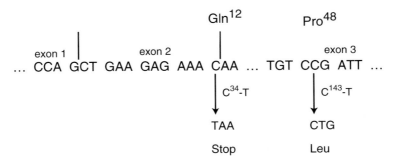

Figure 24.2—Point mutations in the AMPD1 cDNA of patients with myoadenylate deaminase deficiency. Effects of the point mutations C34-T and C143-T on the aminoacid sequence (Gln, glutamine; Leu, leucine; Pro, proline).

Diagnostic techniques

Patients with MAD deficiency produce no or only minimal amounts of ammonia during ischaemic exercise. This phenomenon can be used for screening of patients for MAD deficiency (ischaemic forearm test, Sinkeler et al 1986, Valen et al 1987). To create ischaemic conditions, a sphygmomanometer cuff is inflated above systolic blood pressure around the upper arm. During ischaemia, exercise is performed by opening and closing the fist vigorously for 1–2 min at a rate of 30/min. Immediately after exercise, the cuff is deflated. Blood samples are drawn from the antecubital vein before exercise and at several time points after exercise (e.g. at 0, 2 and 4 min) for determination of ammonia and lactate. The ratio of maximum ammonia increase and maximum lactate increase is normally above 0.7%. In MAD deficient patients, the ratio is below 0.4%.

To prove the diagnosis of MAD deficiency, the activity of this enzyme can be measured in a muscle biopsy. A minimal residual activity is often found, which can be due to expression of *AMD2* or *AMPD3* or alternatively spliced *AMPD1* transcript lacking the exon 2 sequence. Prior to direct measurement of MAD activity, a histochemical staining procedure is usually carried out with the muscle biopsy (Fishbein et al 1978).

Since the vast majority of patients with inherited MAD deficiency is homozygous for one mutation, genetic testing is possible for this disease. The C34-T mutation affects the last nucleotide in exon 2. It destroys the only *Mae*II restriction site in this domain of the *AMPD1* gene. Therefore, this mutation can easily be screened for by polymerase chain reaction (PCR) of exon 2 with the adjacent introns of the *AMPD1* gene followed by *Mae*II restriction analysis.

After incubation with *Mae*II, the restricted PCR product can be size separated by agarose gel electrophoresis. A similar but more convenient method based on a PCR induced restriction site is available (Gross 1994a).

Prevalence

In the first 5 years since the initial report, reports of more than 100 patients with this enzyme defect were published. Screening studies on large numbers of muscle biopsies in Europe and USA revealed a high prevalence of MAD: about 2–3% of all samples (Shumate et al 1979, Fishbein et al 1980, Heffner 1980, Kar and Pearson 1981, Hayes et al 1982, Kelemen et al 1982, Goebel and Bardosi 1987, Mercelis et al 1987).

Several groups of subjects were studied for the frequency of the mutant allele: 59 American Caucasians, 13 Afro-Americans, 106 Japanese (Morisaki et al 1992) and 106 Germans (Gross 1994b) were screened, all subjects were randomly selected. The results are given in Table 24.1.

The frequency of the mutant allele among Caucasian US citizens and Germans matches very well (about 12% of all alleles carry the C34-T mutation). Among 212 Japanese alleles, the mutation could not be detected.

Genotype–phenotype correlation

Based on the allele frequency, about 1.5% of the Caucasian American and German population is expected to be homozygous for the C34-T mutation.

Table 24.1— Frequency of C34-T mutation in the *AMPD1* gene in randomly selected subjects

Population	n	Nucleotide 34			Mutant allele frequency	Expected frequency of homozygous subjects
		C/C	C/T	T/T		
Caucasian US citizens[a]	59	47	10	2	0.119	1.4%
Black US citizens[a]	13	9	3	1	0.192	3.7%
Japanese[a]	106	–	–	0	0	
Germans[b]	106	83	20	3	0.123	1.5%

[a] Data from Morisaki et al 1992
[b] Data from Gross 1994b

Obviously, this frequency is much higher than the prevalence of a metabolic myopathy. Therefore, most homozygous subjects are presumably asymptomatic. This is surprising considering the multiple functions of the purine nucleotide cycle.

One explanation for the presence of homozygous asymptomatic subjects may be alternative splicing of exon 2 of *AMPD1*. As described before, the mutation affects the last nucleotide of exon 2, which is subject to alternative splicing in 0.6–2% of *AMPD1* mRNA (Morisaki et al 1993). In homozygous subjects, alternative splicing would remove the nonsense-mutation and a catalytically active MAD protein could therefore be synthesized since the second C143-T mutation does not affect enzyme activity or protein stability.

Since the mutation C34-T affects the exon–intron boundary of exon 2, it might change the splicing pattern of the mutant allele by changing the 5′ splicing donor site. Therefore, splicing of the mutant allele was studied by transfection of a human *AMPD1* minigene into cultured cells (Morisaki et al 1993). Both in murine myoblasts and myotubes, alternative splicing is promoted by the C34-T mutation.

In MAD deficient patients, there is an even greater *AMPD1* mRNA abundance than in control subjects (Morisaki et al 1993). If anything, the mutation itself increases the proportion of alternatively spliced mRNA. Therefore, homozygous subjects may have more *AMPD1* mRNA lacking the exon 2 sequence. The resulting MAD activity may explain the broad range of severity of symptoms in MAD deficient patients as well as the presence of asymptomatic subjects. However, recent studies on splicing in MAD deficient patients did not support this hypothesis (Gross, manuscript in preparation).

Alternatively, increased expression of *AMPD2* or *AMPD3* could prevent muscular symptoms. There is some evidence for this hypothesis: immunoprecipitation with anti-MAD antibodies removes less than half of the residual activity, and significant amounts of the residual activity can be removed by anti-E1 antibodies (Fishbein et al 1993). Therefore, part of the residual activity might be a result of expression of *AMPD2* or *AMPD3* in skeletal muscle.

Primary and secondary MAD deficiency

In about half of all MAD deficient muscle biopsies, this enzyme defect is the only abnormal finding in the biopsy, besides minor non-specific changes in muscle

structure. In other patients, neuromuscular disorders such as inflammatory and other miscellaneous myopathies, or muscular dystrophies are found in addition to MAD deficiency (Shumate et al 1979, Heffner 1980, Fishbein et al 1980,1981, Kar and Pearson 1981). This type of MAD deficiency associated with another neuromuscular disease is considered to be a secondary or acquired MAD deficiency. In contrast to patients with primary deficiency, the clinical symptoms in secondary forms of MAD deficiency are mainly provoked by the neuromuscular disorder, and they are, therefore, very inhomogeneous.

The differentiation between primary and secondary MAD deficiency is supported by findings that discriminate between both forms. In secondary deficiency, the activities of other muscle enzymes such as creatine kinase and adenylate kinase are also decreased (Fishbein and Armbrustmacher 1984). The decline in MAD activity often parallels the severity of pathologic damage to the muscle cells by the neuromuscular disorder (Kar and Pearson 1973, Fishbein 1986, Nagao et al 1986). The residual MAD activity in primary forms is 1–2% of the normal value at the most, whereas the activity in secondary forms is often above 2% and not immunoreactive with MAD-specific antiserum (Fishbein and Armbrustmacher 1984).

In secondary MAD deficiency, the molecular findings in muscle biopsies are heterogenous. Normal MAD-mRNA abundance was found in patients with denervation and Becker-type dystrophy, whereas reduced transcript abundance of MAD and M-creatine kinase was found in inflammatory myopathies (Sabina et al 1992). The decrease in *AMPD1* transcript abundance parallels the decrease in MAD activity in polymyositis (Sabina et al 1991). These findings support the hypothesis that MAD activity can be reduced as a consequence of inflammatory muscle diseases.

There are various types of MAD deficiency. Primary MAD deficiency is inherited but MAD deficiency can also be a secondary phenomenon in some patients with neuromuscular disorders that reduce expression of muscle genes. There may be a third type of MAD deficiency resulting from the combination of primary MAD deficiency and another neuromuscular disorder by incidence (Verzijl et al 1998, Fishbein 1999). More research is necessary to clarify this.

References

Aragon JJ, Lowenstein JM. (1980) The purine-nucleotide cycle. Comparison of the levels of citric acid cycle intermediates with the operation of the purine nucleotide cycle in rat skeletal muscle during exercise and recovery from exercise. *Eur J Biochem* 110: 371–377.

Bausch-Jurken MT, Mahnke-Zizelman DK, Morisaki T, Sabina RL. (1992) Molecular cloning of AMP deaminase isoform L. Sequence and bacterial expression of human AMPD2 cDNA. *J Biol Chem* 267: 22407–22413.

Bruyland M, Ebinger G. (1994) Beneficial effect of a treatment with xylitol in a patient with myoadenylate deaminase deficiency. *Clin Neuropharmacol* 17: 492–493.

DiMauro S, Miranda AF, Hays AP, et al. (1980) Myoadenylate deaminase deficiency. Muscle biopsy and muscle culture in a patient with gout. *J Neurol Sci* 47: 191–202.

Fishbein WN. (1986) Myoadenylate deaminase deficiency: primary and secondary types. *Toxicol Ind Health* 2: 105–118.

Fishbein WN. (1999) Primary, secondary, and coincidental types of myoadenylate deaminase deficiency. *Ann Neurol* 45: 547–548.

Fishbein WN, Armbrustmacher VW. (1984) Primary and secondary forms of myoadenylate deaminase deficiency (MDD). *Clin Res* 32: 288A.

Fishbein WN, Armbrustmacher VW, Griffin JL. (1978) Myoadenylate deaminase deficiency: a new disease of muscle. *Science* 200: 545–548.

Fishbein WN, Armbrustmacher VW, Griffin JL. (1980) Skeletal muscle adenylate deaminase, adenylate kinase, and creatine kinase in myo-adenylate deaminase deficiency and malignant hyperthermia. *Clin Res* 28: 288A.

Fishbein WN, Armbrustmacher VW, Griffin JL. (1981) Myo-adenylate deaminase deficiency: verification on repeat biopsy, fresh or frozen, and origin of the residual enzyme. *IRCS Med Sci Biochem* 9: 103–104.

Fishbein WN, Armbrustmacher VW, Griffin JL, Davis JI, Foster WD. (1984) Levels of adenylate deaminase, adenylate kinase, and creatine kinase in frozen human muscle biopsy specimens relative to type 1/type 2 fiber distribution: evidence for a carrier state of myoadenylate deaminase deficiency. *Ann Neurol* 15: 271–277.

Fishbein WN, Sabina RL, Ogasawara N, Holmes EW. (1993) Immunological evidence for three isoforms of AMP deaminase (AMPD) in mature skeletal muscle. *Biochim Biophys Acta* 1163: 97–104.

Goebel HH, Bardosi A. (1987) Myoadenylate deaminase deficiency. *Klin Wochenschr* 65: 1023–1033.

Gross M. (1994a) New method for detection of C34-T mutation in the AMPD1 gene causing myoadenylate deaminase deficiency. *Ann Rheum Dis* 53: 353–354.

Gross M. (1994b) *Der MAD-Mangel. Biochemische und molekulargenetische Aspekte des Myoadenylatdesaminase-Mangels*. I. Holzapfel, München, ISBN 3-926098-02-3.

Gross M, Zöllner N. (1991) Serum levels of glucose, insulin and C-peptide during long-term D-ribose administration in man. *Klin Wochenschr* 69: 31–36.

Gross M, Gresser U. (1993) Ergometer exercise in myoadenylate deaminase deficient patients. *Clin Investig* 71: 461–465.

Gross M, Reiter S, Zöllner N. (1989) Metabolism of D-ribose administered continuously to healthy persons and to patients with myoadenylate deaminase deficiency. *Klin Wochenschr* 67: 1205–1213.

Gross M, Morisaki T, Pongratz D, Holmes EW, Zöllner N. (1990) Normal restriction pattern (Hind III) of the myoadenylate deaminase gene in enzyme deficient patients. *Klin Wochenschr* 68: 1084.

Gross M, Kormann B, Zöllner N. (1991) Ribose administration during exercise: Effects on substrates and products of energy metabolism in healthy subjects and a patient with myoadenylate deaminase deficiency. *Klin Wochenschr* 69: 151–155.

Gross M, Morisaki H, Morisaki T, Holmes EW. (1995) Identification of functional domains in AMPD1 by mutational analysis. *Biochem Biophys Res Comm* 205: 1010–1017.

Hayes DJ, Summers BA, Morgan-Hughes JA. (1982) Myoadenylate deaminase deficiency or not? Observations on two brothers with exercise-induced muscle pain. *J Neurol Science* 53: 125–136.

Heffner RR. (1980) Myoadenylate deaminase deficiency. *J Neuropathol Exp Neurol* 39: 360.

Heuckenkamp PU, Zöllner N. (1972) Xylitbilanz während mehrstündiger Infusionen mit konstanten Zufuhrraten bei gesunden Menschen. *Klin Wochenschr* 50: 1063–1065.

Kar NC, Pearson CM. (1973) Muscle adenylic acid deaminase activity. Selective decrease in early-onset Duchenne muscular dystrophy. *Neurology* 23: 478–482.

Kar NC, Pearson CM. (1981) Muscle adenylate deaminase deficiency. Report of six new cases. *Arch Neurol* 38: 279–281.

Kelemen J, Rice DR, Bradley WG, Munsat TL, DiMauro S, Hogan EL. (1982) Familial myoadenylate deaminase deficiency and exertional myalgia. *Neurology* 32: 857–863.

Kingsmore SF, Moseley WS, Watson ML, Sabina RL, Holmes EW, Seldin MF. (1990) Long-range restriction site mapping of a syntenic segment conserved between human chromosome 1 and mouse chromosome 3. *Genomics* 7: 75–83.

Lowenstein J, Tornheim K. (1971) Ammonia production in muscle: the purine nucleotide cycle. *Science* 171: 397–400.

Mahnke-Zizelman DK, Sabina RL. (1992) Cloning of human AMP deaminase isoform E cDNAs. Evidence for a third AMPD gene exhibiting alternatively spliced 5'-exons. *J Biol Chem* 267: 20866–20877.

Marquetant R, Desai NM, Sabina RL, Holmes EW. (1987) Evidence for sequential expression of multiple AMP deaminase isoforms during skeletal muscle development. *Proc Natl Acad Sci USA* 84: 2345–2349.

Mercelis R, Martin JJ, de Barsy T, Van de Berghe G. (1987) Myoadenylate deaminase deficiency: absence of correlation with exercise intolerance in 452 muscle biopsies. *J Neurol* 234: 385–389.

Meyer RA, Terjung RL. (1980) AMP deamination and IMP reanimation in working skeletal muscle. *Am J Physiol* 239: C32–C38.

Mineo I, Clarke PRH, Sabina RL, Holmes EW. (1990) A novel pathway for alternative splicing: identification of an RNA intermediate that generates an alternative 5′ splice donor site not present in the primary transcript of AMPD1. *Mol Cell Biol* 10: 5271–5278.

Mineo I, Holmes EW. (1991) Exon recognition and nucleocytoplasmic partitioning determine AMPD1 alternative transcript production. *Mol Cell Biol* 11: 5356–5363.

Morisaki T, Gross M, Morisaki H, Pongratz D, Zöllner N, Holmes EW. (1992) Molecular basis of AMP deaminase deficiency in skeletal muscle. *Proc Natl Acad Sci USA* 89: 6457–6461.

Morisaki H, Morisaki T, Newby LK, Holmes EW. (1993) Alternative splicing: a mechanism for phenotypic rescue of a common inherited defect. *J Clin Invest* 91: 2275–2280.

Nagao H, Habara S, Morimoto T, et al. (1986) AMP deaminase activity of skeletal muscle in neuromuscular disorders in childhood. Histochemical and biochemical studies. *Neuropediatrics* 17: 193–198.

Ogasawara N, Goto H, Yamada Y, Watanabe T. (1978) Distribution of AMP-deaminase isozymes in rat tissues. *Eur J Biochem* 87: 297–304.

Ogasawara N, Goto H, Yamada Y. (1982a) AMP deaminase isozymes in human blood cells. *J Clin Chem Clin Biochem* 20: 401.

Ogasawara N, Goto H, Yamada Y, Watanabe T, Asano T. (1982b) AMP deaminase isozymes in human tissues. *Biochim Biophys Acta* 714: 298–306.

Patterson VH, Kaiser KK, Brooke MH. (1983) Exercising muscle does not produce hypoxanthine in adenylate deaminase deficiency. *Neurology* 33: 784–786.

Pongratz DE, Reimers CD, Gross M, Paetzke I, Zimmer HG. (1987) Symptomatische Therapie des primären Myoadenylatdeaminase-Mangels sowie der Glykogenose Typ V mit D-Ribose. *Fortschr Myologie* IX: 42.

Sabina RL, Fishbein WN, Pezeshkpour G, Clarke PRH, Holmes EW. (1992) Molecular analysis of the myoadenylate deaminase deficiencies. *Neurology* 42: 170–179.

Sabina RL, Morisaki T, Clarke P, et al. (1990) Characterization of the human and rat myoadenylate deaminase genes. *J Biol Chem* 265: 9423–9433.

Sabina RL, Sulaiman AR, Wortmann RL. (1991) Molecular analysis of acquired myoadenylate deaminase deficiency in polymyositis (idiopathic inflammatory myopathy). *Adv Exp Med Biol* 309B: 203–205.

Sabina RL, Swain JL, Holmes EW. (1989b). Myoadenylate deaminase deficiency. In: Scriver CR, Beaudet AL, Sly WS, Valle D, eds. *The metabolic basis of inherited disease, 6th ed.* New York: McGraw-Hill, pp. 1077–1084.

Sabina RL, Swain JL, Patten BM, Ashizawa T, O'Brien WE, Holmes EW. (1980) Disruption of the purine nucleotide cycle. A potential explanation for muscle dysfunction in myoadenylate deaminase deficiency. *J Clin Invest* 66: 1419–1423.

Shumate J, Kaiser KK, Brooke MH, Carroll JE. (1979) Myoadenylate deaminase deficiency: disease or normal variant? *Neurology* 29: 558.

Sinkeler SP, Wevers RA, Joosten EM, et al. (1986) Improvement of screening in exertional myalgia with a standardized ischemic forearm test. *Muscle Nerve* 9: 731–737.

Valen PA, Nakayama DA, Veum J, Sulaiman AR, Wortmann RL. (1987) Myoadenylate deaminase deficiency and forearm ischemic exercise testing. *Arthritis Rheumatism* 30: 661–668.

Verzijl HAT, van Engelen BG, Luyten JA, et al. (1998) Genetic characteristics of myoadenylate deaminase deficiency. *Ann Neurol* 44: 140–143.

Yamada Y, Goto H, Ogasawara N. (1992) Cloning and nucleotide sequence of the cDNA encoding human erythrocyte-specific AMP deaminase. *Biochim Biophys Acta* 1171: 125–128.

Youssoufian H, Kazazian JJ, Phillips DG, et al. (1986) Recurrent mutations in haemophilia A give evidence for CpG mutation hotspots. *Nature* 324: 380–382.

Zöllner N, Reiter S, Gross M, et al. (1986) Myoadenylate deaminase deficiency: Successful symptomatic therapy by high dose oral administration of ribose. *Klin Wochenschr* 64: 1281–1290.

25

Capillary no-flow

Michael D. Menger and Brigitte Vollmar

Physiology of striated muscle capillary perfusion

Adequate transport of oxygen to tissue is the major prerequisite for the maintenance of organ physiology and function. Apart from the appropriate transendothelial exchange, function of the microcirculation has to guarantee oxygen supply to tissue, and dysfunction of the nutritive microcirculation in distinct diseases, such as ischaemia-reperfusion, shock and sepsis, has to be considered as the determinant for tissue injury and organ failure (Menger et al 1997). The microvasculature includes three major distinct segments: the terminal arterioles, the capillaries, and the postcapillary and collecting venules. Although the arrangement of the microvessels differs markedly between individual tissues, their function is thought to be quite similar: Terminal arterioles control regional blood supply by dilation and constriction, thereby influencing systemic vascular resistance. Capillaries mainly contribute to the exchange of oxygen and other substrates to tissue, and they are, therefore, regarded as the nutritional segment of the microcirculation. Postcapillary and collecting venules drain the blood out of the microcirculation, but they also function as the primary target for inflammatory cell adhesion and invasion.

In striated muscle, capillaries are arranged in parallel to each other and present with frequent interconnections, displaying a ropeladder-like configuration (Fig. 25.1). One terminal arteriole feeds 5–15 capillaries with lengths varying from 200 μm to more than 1500 μm. The capillaries display an intercapillary distance of 10 to 80 μm and individual diameters between 4 and 10 μm (Endrich et al 1980, Lehr et al 1993, Lam et al 1994, Kindig et al 1998). Because of the heterogeneous distribution of capillary length and diameter, the capillary red blood cell velocities vary over a wide range, with values between 0.1 and 3.8 mm/s (Endrich et al 1980, Lehr et al 1993).

In addition, arterioles may not only feed the individual nutritive capillaries, but they may also transport blood directly into postcapillary venules via arteriolovenular shunts. These downstream shunts regularly present with higher flow rates, resulting in preferential distribution of leukocytes into these shunts, and thereby preventing leukocyte-induced capillary obstruction (Ley et al 1989).

Striated muscle capillary leukocyte plugging

Leukocytes, although not activated, may plug capillaries under physiological conditions, resulting in capillary no-flow. Intravital microscopy in spinotrapezius muscle revealed, however, that plugging by leukocytes occurs in only one third of capillary branches, and that the median duration of these pluggings is just 0.12 s, thus only minimally affecting blood flow resistance under physiological conditions (Warnke and Skalak 1992). Activation of leukocytes significantly increases the duration of capillary leukocyte pluggings and, thus, capillary no-flow. This is probably due to increased leukocyte stiffness, and may be the cause for the more than 10-fold increase of microvascular flow resistance (Harris and Skalak 1993a). Interestingly, the plugging of capillaries by leukocytes seems not to depend on cell adhesion mechanisms, as reported for leukocyte adhesion in venules, but it is likely to be related to the leukocyte cytoplasmic viscosity. This is because the prevention of FMLP-induced increase of leukocyte cytoplasmic viscosity by cytochalasin D has been shown to effectively reduce the duration of capillary plugging and, thus, the increase of microvascular resistance (Harris and Skalak 1993b).

Striated muscle capillary recruitment

Recruitment of capillaries that are not perfused under physiological conditions may represent a mechanism of control to appropriately respond to increased metabolic demands. While a variety of reports indicate that capillary recruitment does not exist in brain (Gobel

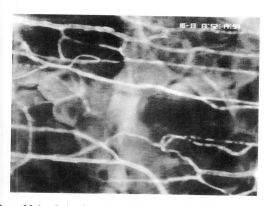

Figure 25.1—Striated muscle capillary network of the m. cutaneus maximus of the hamster as visualized by intravital fluorescence microscopy. The capillaries are arranged in parallel and present with frequent interconnections, displaying a rope-ladder-like configuration. Note the variability in capillary diameters and intercapillary distances (magnification ×200).

et al 1989, Chen et al 1994, Hudetz 1997) and heart (Eliasen and Amtorp 1985, Wahlander et al 1993), there is some evidence that this mechanism is involved in the regulation of microvascular perfusion in skeletal muscle (Honig et al 1980, Klitzman et al 1982). Honig et al (1980) demonstrated, during exercise in dog gracilis muscle, a 7-fold increase in flow and a 1.5- to 3-fold increase in capillary density, the latter reflecting recruitment of capillaries. These results, obtained from freeze-clamped tissue sections, are supported by in vivo observations that demonstrated some increase of capillary density, and thus capillary recruitment, in hamster cremaster muscle during twitch contraction at 1 Hz (Klitzman et al 1982). Furthermore, Segal (1991) reported capillary recruitment in hamster cremaster muscle upon acetylcholine-induced vasodilatation. However, this recruitment of capillaries was dependent on re-establishment of flow in terminal arterioles that were devoid of flow under normal conditions.

In contrast, in vivo microscopic analysis of terminal arterioles and capillaries in tenuissimus muscle of anaesthetized rabbits revealed that all arterioles and capillaries that were perfused during adenosine- or reactive hyperaemia-induced vasodilatation were also found perfused at rest (Oude-Vrielink et al 1987). The authors concluded that in the tenuissimus muscle no recruitment of capillaries occurs in an anatomical sense of the word. Thus, from the present data available in the literature, it cannot definitely be said whether under normal conditions a relevant fraction of capillaries presents with no-flow, being only recruited by increased demands during exercise and hyperaemia.

Striated muscle capillary flowmotion

Capillary flowmotion characterizes cyclic changes of red blood cell velocity with periods of capillary no-flow and periods of normal capillary perfusion. Capillary flowmotion is induced directly by arteriolar vasomotion (Rücker et al 2000), which is defined as spontaneous rhythmic changes of arteriolar diameter (Allegra et al 1993; Fig. 25.2). Fast-wave flowmotion (8–20 cycles/min) is assumed to be related to terminal arterioles (Weiner et al 1989), whereas slow-wave flowmotion (1–5 cycles/min) is thought to be due to the activity of more proximal transverse arterioles (Schmidt et al 1993a). Although the pacemaker of vasomotion and flowmotion is not identified yet, it is well known that these regulatory mechanisms depend on voltage-operated calcium channels, because a variety of studies have demonstrated abrogation of vasomotion/flowmotion by vasoselective calcium

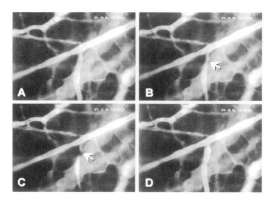

Figure 25.2—Striated muscle arterioles of the m. cutaneus maximus of the hamster, presenting with slow-wave vasomotion. Note the constriction of the transverse arteriole at its bifurcation during the 15-second vasomotion cycle (**B** and **C**, arrows) with a short period of complete shutdown of perfusion (**B**). At the end of the cycle (**D**) arteriolar diameter dimension is restored (magnification ×100).

channel blockers (Colantuoni et al 1984, Goligorsky et al 1995, Rücker et al 2000).

Until the early 1990s, it was suggested that vasomotion and flowmotion represent mainly physiological conditions in a variety of tissues including skeletal muscle (Funk and Intaglietta 1983, Allegra et al 1993). Early studies further indicated that vasomotion and flowmotion are abrogated under pathological conditions such as haemorrhagic shock (Colantuoni et al 1985) and local arterial pressure reduction (Meyer et al 1988, Borgström et al 1990). More recent reports, however, support the view that vasomotion and flowmotion are rarely active during normal perfusion, but that they are induced during conditions of critical perfusion, including fixed-volume haemorrhage (Borgström et al 1992) and local arterial pressure reduction (Schmidt et al 1992). From these reports it was hypothesized that critical perfusion-induced vasomotion and flowmotion compensates locally for inadequate microvascular blood supply (Schmidt et al 1993a). This hypothesis was confirmed by a recent in vivo microscopic study, demonstrating in a rat multi-tissue preparation that, under critical perfusion conditions, arteriolar vasomotion and capillary flowmotion occur only in skeletal muscle but not in periosteum, subcutis and skin, and that the onset of this muscle capillary flowmotion prevents critical perfusion-induced capillary perfusion failure, guaranteeing appropriate tissue oxygenation (Rücker et al 2000). Interestingly, capillary flowmotion in muscle preserved not only capillary perfusion in muscle itself but also the density of perfused capillaries in those adjacent tissues that were not able to elicit the compensatory flowmotion perfusion pattern (Rücker et al 2000).

Pathology of striated muscle capillary perfusion

Distinct pathological conditions, such as haemorrhagic shock, ischaemia-reperfusion and inflammation, are well known to alter capillary perfusion with development of capillary no-flow states, which finally determine the manifestation of organ dysfunction and injury.

Striated muscle capillary no-flow in haemorrhagic shock

Haemorrhage is associated with reduction of arterial blood pressure, and it results in critical perfusion conditions, primarily in peripheral tissues including skeletal muscle. While muscle capillary perfusion failure under critical perfusion conditions with an arterial pressure of 30 to 50 mmHg may be counteracted by capillary flowmotion (Schmidt et al 1993b, Rücker et al 2000), further reduction of blood pressure to values below 30 mmHg is associated with capillary no-flow, as reflected by a significantly reduced capillary density (Rücker et al 2000). Under those conditions microvascular blood flow is characterized by a pronounced heterogeneity in distribution, with normally perfused capillaries also presenting with slow flow or remaining constantly unperfused (Haljamae 1984). The alteration of capillary perfusion consequently results in significant deterioration of capillary oxygen partial pressure (PO$_2$) and, hence, reduction of tissue oxygenation (Kerger et al 1996). The compromise of capillary perfusion is thought to result from capillary luminal narrowing (Mazzoni et al 1989), which is induced in a major part by endothelial cell swelling (Kretschmar and Engelhardt 1994). The endothelial swelling is caused by systemic blood acidosis and not by the low-flow state per se (Mazzoni et al 1994); it may involve Na$^+$-H$^+$-exchange mechanisms, because specific blockade with amiloride analogues completely prevents the shock-induced luminal narrowing of the capillaries (Mazzoni et al 1992).

The elevated hydraulic resistance caused by capillary endothelial swelling (Mazzoni et al 1992) may be further increased by activated leukocytes (Mazzoni et al 1995), which themselves additionally aggravate the shock-associated capillary no-flow syndrome (Bagge et al 1980). The stasis of the leukocytes within the capillaries, however, does not represent irreversible plugging, but rather it is a pressure-related phenomenon, which is not receptor/adhesion molecule dependent, and which is freely reversible with early restoration of perfusion pressure (Hansell et al 1993).

Striated muscle capillary no-flow in ischaemia-reperfusion

Since the early 1990s, a considerable number of experimental studies have demonstrated that both ischaemia and reperfusion contribute to the pathogenesis of organ injury. Moreover, these studies have deduced that the injury caused by reperfusion is different in nature from that caused by ischaemia; it is characterized by the deterioration of the microcirculation, the activation of white blood cells and the action of an array of inflammatory mediators, resulting in a distinct type and pattern of parenchymal and non-parenchymal cell damage, termed "reperfusion injury" (Welbourn et al 1991, Granger and Kubes 1994, Menger et al 1997).

The perfusion of nutritive capillaries guarantees adequate oxygen supply to tissue, and it is therefore of essential importance for organ survival and function. The lack of nutritive capillary perfusion despite reperfusion of the ischaemic tissue (termed capillary no-reflow), first described by Majno et al (1967), must be considered as the most deleterious dysfunction in striated muscle ischaemia/reperfusion, because no-reflow in capillaries results in prolongation of tissue hypoxia during reperfusion, thus, aggravating the ischaemic tissue injury (Menger et al 1989a, 1992a).

Several mechanisms have been suggested to promote the development of postischaemic capillary no-reflow, including intravascular haemoconcentration (Fischer and Ames 1972, Menger et al 1988) and thrombosis (Quiñones-Baldrich et al 1991), swelling of capillary endothelial cells (Gidlöf et al 1987, Hammersen et al 1989), plugging of capillaries by leukocytes (Schmid-Schönbein 1987) and increased extravascular pressure due to interstitial oedema formation (Jerome et al 1993, 1994). Although platelets may adhere to capillary endothelium during postischaemic reperfusion (Fig. 25.3), capillary thrombus formation may not play the major role for the manifestation of capillary no-reflow, because light- and electron-microscopic studies could not confirm platelet or fibrin thrombi, and heparin was not effective to attenuate postischaemic reperfusion

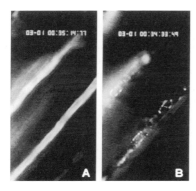

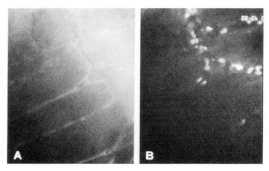

Figure 25.3—Striated muscle capillaries of the semitendinosus muscle of the rat as visualized by intravital microscopy during postischaemic reperfusion. **A** Adequate perfusion as indicated by the appropriate fluorescent staining of intravascular plasma by FITC-dextran 150 000. **B** The same capillaries showing fluorescently stained platelets adherent to the capillary endothelial lining (magnification ×500).

Figure 25.4—Striated muscle capillary network of the m. cutaneus maximus of the hamster draining into a postcapillary venule as visualized by intravital fluorescence microscopy. **A** Individual capillary perfusion deficits as indicated by some lack of FITC-dextran-stained intravascular plasma. **B** The same capillaries with fluorescently stained leukocytes, which selectively adhere in the venules but which do not plug the capillaries. Note the formation of interstitial oedema, as indicated by the leakage of the high molecular weight tracer FITC-dextran 150 000 (bright background) in **A** (magnification ×200).

failure (Strock and Majno 1969). In contrast, impairment of microvascular blood fluidity due to intravascular haemoconcentration, caused by the disruption of the integrity of the endothelial lining (Hammersen et al 1989), may largely contribute to the no-reflow, since lowering of the systemic haematocrit to 30% effectively attenuates capillary perfusion failure (Menger et al 1988). In addition, there is substantial evidence that swelling of capillary endothelial cells is involved in the pathogenesis of no-reflow by elevating hydraulic resistance, and so hindering restoration of capillary blood flow during reperfusion (Menger et al 1989b). Interestingly, the swelling of endothelial cells of skeletal muscle capillaries already occurs during ischaemia, but it is markedly more pronounced after onset of postischaemic reperfusion (Gidlöf et al 1987). The narrowing of the luminal diameter of the capillaries, which results in postischaemic no-reflow, has been suggested to be additionally provoked by active capillary constriction, involving both pericyte function and the action of endothelins (Menger et al 1997). However, this hypothesis remains to be confirmed by appropriate in vivo experiments.

There is major controversy over whether leukocytes may plug capillaries and so induce no-reflow during postischaemic reperfusion. Schmid-Schönbein (1987) proposed that under conditions when capillary perfusion pressure is reduced, and/or elevated levels of inflammatory products are present, granulocytes may become stuck in capillaries. After restoration of perfusion pressure these granulocytes are not removed from the capillary lumen because they adhere to the endothelial surface, thereby contributing to no-

reflow. However, while microvascular reperfusion injury is hallmarked by leukocyte adhesion to the endothelium of postcapillary venules, indicating inflammation (Menger et al 1992b, Jerome et al 1993, 1994), recruitment of leukocytes in capillaries of muscle seems to be a rare event (Fig. 25.4). In fact, Hansell et al (1993) have shown that if stasis of leukocytes in muscle capillaries is observed after ischaemia/reperfusion, this is solely related to decreased perfusion pressure conditions, and it is not a result of adhesive interactions with the capillary endothelium or hindrance of lumenal passage. This finding supports previous observations, demonstrating that stasis of leukocytes in skeletal muscle capillaries depends on local haemodynamics including a critical shear rate threshold (Mayrovitz et al 1987). It also confirms the view that, at least in skeletal muscle, plugging of capillaries by leukocytes is not a significant mechanism of no-reflow.

Apart from the idea that leukocytes plug capillaries, leukocytes adherent to the endothelial lining of postcapillary venules may significantly contribute to the development of capillary no-reflow. Besides capillary perfusion hindrance due to the increase in postcapillary vascular resistance (Korthuis et al 1988), those leukocytes may disrupt the endothelial integrity by releasing cytotoxic mediators, resulting in an increase of microvascular permeability and a shift of fluid to the interstitial space (Menger et al 1992b). Because skeletal muscle is limited in expansion, the formation of interstitial oedema can be accompanied by a rise of interstitial pressure sufficient to produce significant compression of the capillaries (Jerome et al 1993). This view is supported by experiments, demonstrating that the blockade of postischaemic venular leukocyte adhesion (by anti-neutrophil serum or monoclonal antibodies directed against the leukocytic or endothelial adhesion molecules CD18, P-selectin and ICAM-1) effectively abolishes the formation of interstitial oedema (Carden et al 1990) and significantly attenuates the manifestation of capillary no-reflow (Jerome et al 1993, 1994).

Striated capillary no-flow in inflammation and sepsis

The microcirculation of almost all organs, including striated muscle, is a major site of attack during inflammation and sepsis (Hinshaw 1996). Apart from massive accumulation of white blood cells within postcapillary venules (Hoffmann et al 1999), the alteration of nutritive blood perfusion is triggered by a differential arteriolar vasomotor response upon endotoxin challenge with constriction of large arterioles and dilation of terminal feeding vessels (Cryer et al 1988, 1990); this probably involves endothelins, nitric oxide and prostaglandins (Cryer et al 1990, Lübbe et al 1992, Schiffrin 1994). The compromised blood supply to the microvascular bed results in slowing of capillary blood flow and, additionally, in stasis of perfusion, as indicated by a significant decrease of functional capillary density (Lam et al 1994, Hoffmann et al 1999). The marked increase of heterogeneity of capillary perfusion caused by individual capillary no-flow (Lam et al 1994) finally produces significant tissue hypoxia (Gutierrez et al 1991) and muscle dysfunction (Lam et al 1994). While a single bolus injection of endotoxin induces reversible alterations of the microcirculation with a reduction in functional capillary density by 35 to 50% (Lam et al 1994, Hoffmann et al 1999), repeated endotoxin challenges, mimicking the clinical conditions of sepsis, induce a dramatic loss of capillary perfusion of almost 90% (Hoffmann et al 1999), which, indeed, is the determinant for organ failure and fatal outcome.

The mechanisms causing sepsis-induced capillary no-flow are far from being clear. They may include decrease of perfusion pressure, constriction of arterioles with arterio-venous shunting, decrease of deformability of red and white blood cells, and plugging of microvessels with "sludge" (Hinshaw 1996). Whether the activation of the coagulation cascade with disseminated intravascular coagulation (DIC) is involved in sepsis-induced capillary no-flow remains to be determined. Although antithrombin has been shown to effectively reduce endotoxin-induced leukocytic response and capillary perfusion failure, these effects are probably due to the modulation of the cyclo-oxygenase pathway with release of prostaglandins (Hoffmann et al 2000a). In fact, more recent studies brought evidence that hirudin, although improving DIC parameters, even aggravates endotoxin-induced capillary perfusion failure, indicating that the coagulation cascade does not play a major role in the capillary no-flow syndrome triggered by sepsis (Hoffmann et al 2000b).

Conclusion

Although there may be individual capillaries not perfused at rest and recruited during exercise, there is little evidence for permanent or intermittent muscle capillary no-flow caused by leukocyte plugging or capillary flowmotion under physiological conditions. Pathological conditions, such as haemorrhagic shock, ischaemia-reperfusion and sepsis, are associated with significant capillary no-flow, which may determine metabolic dysfunction and tissue injury. The mechanisms provoking this nutritive perfusion failure include endothelial cell swelling, intravascular haemoconcentration, interstitial oedema formation and vasomotor dysfunction, the latter probably involving an endothelin/nitric oxide imbalance. Therapeutic strategies should, therefore, consider these mechanisms, as shown by the effective abrogation of capillary no-flow using hyperosmolar solutions, isovolaemic haemodilution and inhibitors of those mediators that trigger the formation of interstitial oedema.

References

Allegra C, Intaglietta M, Messmer K. (1993) Vasomotion and flowmotion. *Prog Appl Microcirc* 20: 1–88.

Bagge U, Amundson B, Lauritzen C. (1980) White blood cell deformability and plugging of skeletal muscle capillaries in hemorrhagic shock. *Acta Physiol Scand* 108: 159–163.

Borgström P, Lindbom L, Meyer JU, Sjoquist M, Arfors KE, Intaglietta M. (1990) Hemodynamic responses in rabbit tenuissimus muscle arterioles during local reduction in perfusion pressure. *Int J Microcirc Clin Exp* 9: 175–186.

Borgström P, Schmidt JA, Bruttig SP, Intaglietta M, Arfors KE. (1992) Slow-wave flowmotion in rabbit skeletal muscle after acute fixed-volume hemorrhage. *Circ Shock* 36: 57–61.

Carden DL, Smith JK, Korthuis RJ. (1990) Neutrophil-mediated microvascular dysfunction in postischemic canine skeletal muscle. *Circ Res* 66: 1436–1444.

Chen JL, Wei L, Bereczki D, et al. (1994) Virtually unaltered permeability-surface area products imply little capillary recruitment in brain with hypoxia. *Microcirculation* 1: 35–47.

Colantuoni A, Bertuglia S, Intaglietta M. (1984) The effects of alpha- or beta-adrenergic receptor agonists and antagonists and calcium entry blockers on the spontaneous vasomotion. *Microvasc Res* 28: 143–158.

Colantuoni A, Bertuglia S, Intaglietta M. (1985) Microvessel diameter changes during hemorrhagic shock in unanesthetized hamsters. *Microvasc Res* 30: 133–142.

Cryer HM, Garrison RN, Harris PD. (1988) Role of muscle microvasculature during hyperdynamic and hypodynamic phases of endotoxin shock in decerebrate rats. *J Trauma* 28: 312–318.

Cryer HG, Garrison RN, Harris PD, Greenwald BH, Alsip NL. (1990) Prostaglandins mediate skeletal muscle arteriole dilation in hyperdynamic bacteremia. *Am J Physiol* 259: H728–H734.

Eliasen P, Amtorp O. (1985) Absence of capillary recruitment during increased coronary blood flow in the working dog heart. *Acta Physiol Scand* 124: 181–187.

Endrich B, Asaishi K, Götz A, Messmer K. (1980) Technical report – a new chamber technique for microvascular studies in unanesthetized hamsters. *Res Exp Med* 177: 125–134.

Fischer EG, Ames A. (1972) Studies on mechanisms of impairment of cerebral circulation following ischemia: Effect of hemodilution and perfusion pressure. *Stroke* 3: 538–542.

Funk W, Intaglietta M. (1983) Spontaneous arteriolar vasomotion. *Prog Appl Microcirc* 3: 66–82.

Gidlöf A, Lewis DH, Hammersen F. (1987) The effect of prolonged total ischemia on the ultrastructure of human skeletal muscle capillaries. A morphometric analysis. *Int J Microcirc Clin Exp* 7: 67–86.

Gobel U, Klein B, Schrock H, Kuschinsky W. (1989) Lack of capillary recruitment in the brains of awake rats during hypercapnia. *J Cereb Blood Flow Metab* 9: 491–499.

Goligorsky MS, Colflesh D, Gordienko D, Moore LC. (1995) Branching points of renal resistance arteries are enriched in L-type calcium channels and initiate vasoconstriction. *Am J Physiol* 268: F251–F257.

Granger DN, Kubes P. (1994) The microcirculation and inflammation: modulation of leukocyte-endothelial cell adhesion. *J Leukoc Biol* 55: 662–675.

Gutierrez G, Lund N, Palizas F. (1991) Rabbit skeletal muscle PO_2 during hypodynamic sepsis. *Chest* 99: 224–229.

Haljamae H. (1984) Microcirculation and hemorrhagic shock. *Am J Emerg Med* 2: 100–107.

Hammersen F, Barker JH, Gidlöf A, Menger MD, Hammersen E, Messmer K. (1989) The ultrastructure of microvessels and their contents following ischemia and reperfusion. *Prog Appl Microcirc* 13: 1–26.

Hansell P, Borgström P, Arfors KE. (1993) Pressure-related capillary leukostasis following ischemia-reperfusion and hemorrhagic shock. *Am J Physiol* 265: H381–388.

Harris AG, Skalak TC. (1993a) Effects of leukocyte activation on capillary hemodynamics in skeletal muscle. *Am J Physiol* 264: H909–H916.

Harris AG, Skalak TC. (1993b) Leukocyte cytoskeletal structure determines capillary plugging and network resistance. *Am J Physiol* 265: H1670–1675.

Hinshaw LB. (1996) Sepsis/septic shock: participation of the microcirculation: an abbreviated review. *Crit Care Med* 24: 1072–1078.

Hoffmann JN, Vollmar B, Inthorn D, Schildberg FW, Menger MD. (1999) A chronic model for intravital microscopic study of microcirculatory disorders and leukocyte/endothelial cell interaction during normotensive endotoxemia. *Shock* 12: 355–364.

Hoffmann JN, Vollmar B, Inthorn D, Schildberg FW, Menger MD. (2000a) Antithrombin reduces leukocyte adhesion during chronic endotoxemia by modulation of the cyclooxygenase pathway. *Am J Physiol* 279: C98–C107.

Hoffmann JN, Vollmar B, Inthorn D, Schildberg FW, Menger MD. (2000b) The thrombin antagonist hirudin fails to inhibit endotoxin-induced leukocyte-endothelial cell interaction and microvascular perfusion failure. *Shock* 14: 528–534.

Honig CR, Odoroff CL, Frierson JL. (1980) Capillary recruitment in exercise: rate, extent, uniformity, and relation to blood flow. *Am J Physiol* 238: H31–H42.

Hudetz AG. (1997) Blood flow in the cerebral capillary network: a review emphasizing observations with intravital microscopy. *Microcirculation* 4: 233–252.

Jerome SN, Smith CW, Korthuis RJ. (1993) CD18-dependent adherence reactions play an important role in the development of the no-reflow phenomenon. *Am J Physiol* 264: H479–H483.

Jerome SN, Dore M, Paulson JC, Smith CW, Korthuis RJ. (1994) P-selectin and ICAM-1 dependent adherence reactions: role in the genesis of postischemic no-reflow. *Am J Physiol* 266: H1316–H1321.

Kerger H, Saltzman DJ, Menger MD, Messmer K, Intaglietta M. (1996) Systemic and subcutaneous microvascular PO_2 dissociation during 4-h hemorrhagic shock in conscious hamsters. *Am J Physiol* 270: H827–H836.

Kindig CA, Sexton WL, Fedde MR, Poole DC. (1998)

Skeletal muscle microcirculatory structure and hemo-dynamics in diabetes. *Respir Physiol* 111: 163–175.

Klitzman B, Damon DN, Gorczynski RJ, Duling BR. (1982) Augmented tissue oxygen supply during striated muscle contraction in the hamster. Relative contributions of capillary recruitment, functional dilation, and reduced tissue Po$_2$. *Circ Res* 51: 711–721.

Korthuis RJ, Grisham MB, Granger DN. (1988) Leukocyte depletion attenuates vascular injury in postischemic skeletal muscle. *Am J Physiol* 254: H823–H827.

Kretschmar K, Engelhardt T. (1994) Swelling of capillary endothelial cells contributes to traumatic hemorrhagic shock-induced microvascular injury: a morphologic and morphometric analysis. *Int J Microcirc Clin Exp* 14: 45–49.

Lam C, Tyml K, Martin C, Sibbald W. (1994) Micro-vascular perfusion is impaired in a rat model of normoten-sive sepsis. *J Clin Invest* 94: 2077–2083.

Lehr HA, Leunig M, Menger MD, Nolte D, Messmer K. (1993) Dorsal skinfold chamber technique for intravital microscopy in nude mice. *Am J Pathol* 143: 1055–1062.

Ley K, Meyer JU, Intaglietta M, Arfors KE. (1989) Shunting of leukocytes in rabbit tenuissimus muscle. *Am J Physiol* 256: H85–H93.

Lübbe AS, Garrison RN, Cryer HM, Alsip NL, Harris PD. (1992) EDRF as a possible mediator of sepsis-induced arteriolar dilation in skeletal muscle. *Am J Physiol* 262: H880–H887.

Majno G, Ames A III, Chiang J, Wright RL. (1967) No reflow after cerebral ischaemia. *Lancet* 2: 569–570.

Mayrovitz HN, Kang SJ, Herscovici B, Sampsell RN. (1987) Leukocyte adherence initiation in skeletal muscle capillaries and venules. *Microvasc Res* 33: 22–34.

Mazzoni MC, Borgström P, Intaglietta M, Arfors KE. (1989) Lumenal narrowing and endothelial cell swelling in skeletal muscle capillaries during hemorrhagic shock. *Circ Shock* 29: 27–39.

Mazzoni MC, Intaglietta M, Cragoe EJ, Jr, Arfors KE. (1992) Amiloride-sensitive Na$^+$ pathways in capillary endothelial cell swelling during hemorrhagic shock. *J Appl Physiol* 73: 1467–1473.

Mazzoni MC, Cragoe EJ, Jr, Arfors KE. (1994) Systemic blood acidosis in low-flow ischemia induces capillary luminal narrowing. *Int J Microcirc Clin Exp* 14: 144–150.

Mazzoni MC, Borgström P, Warnke KC, Skalak TC, Intaglietta M, Arfors KE. (1995) Mechanisms and impli-cations of capillary endothelial swelling and luminal narrowing in low-flow ischemias. *Int J Microcirc Clin Exp* 15: 265–270.

Menger MD, Sack FU, Barker JH, Feifel G, Messmer K. (1988) Quantitative analysis of microcirculatory disorders after prolonged ischemia in skeletal muscle: Therapeutic effects of prophylactic isovolemic hemodilution. *Res Exp Med* 188: 151–166.

Menger MD, Sack FU, Hammersen F, Messmer K. (1989a) Tissue oxygenation after prolonged ischemia in skeletal muscle: Therapeutic effect of prophylactic isovolemic hemodilution. *Adv Exp Med Biol* 248: 387–395.

Menger MD, Hammersen F, Barker J, Feifel G, Messmer K. (1989b) Ischemia and reperfusion in skeletal muscle: Experiments with tourniquet ischemia in the awake Syrian golden hamster. *Prog Appl Microcirc* 13: 93–108.

Menger MD, Steiner D, Messmer K. (1992a) Microvascular ischemia-reperfusion injury in striated muscle: signifi-cance of "no-reflow". *Am J Physiol* 263: H1892–H1900.

Menger MD, Pelikan S, Steiner D, Messmer K. (1992b) Microvascular ischemia-reperfusion injury in striated muscle: significance of "reflow-paradox". *Am J Physiol* 263: H1901–H1906.

Menger MD, Rücker M, Vollmar B. (1997) Capillary dys-function in striated muscle ischemia/reperfusion: On the mechanisms of capillary "no-reflow". *Shock* 8: 2–7.

Meyer JU, Borgström P, Lindbom L, Intaglietta M. (1988) Vasomotion patterns in skeletal muscle arterioles during changes in arterial pressure. *Microvasc Res* 35: 193–203.

Oude-Vrielink HH, Slaaf DW, Tangelder GJ, Reneman RS. (1987) Does capillary recruitment exist in young rabbit skeletal muscle? *Int J Microcirc Clin Exp* 6: 321–332.

Quiñones-Baldrich WJ, Chervu A, Hernandez JJ, Colburn M, Moore WS. (1991) Skeletal muscle function after ischemia: "No reflow" versus reperfusion injury. *J Surg Res* 51: 5–12.

Rücker M, Strobel O, Vollmar B, Roesken F, Menger MD. (2000) Vasomotion in critically perfused muscle protects adjacent tissue from capillary perfusion failure. *Am J Physiol* 279: H550–H558.

Schiffrin EL. (1994) The endothelium and control of blood vessel function in health and disease. *Clin Invest Med* 17: 602–620.

Schmid-Schönbein GW. (1987) Capillary plugging by granulocytes and the no-reflow phenomenon in the microcirculation. *Fed Proc* 46: 2397–2401.

Schmidt JA, Intaglietta M, Borgström P. (1992) Periodic hemodynamics in skeletal muscle during local arterial pressure reduction. *J Appl Physiol* 73: 1077–1083.

Schmidt JA, Borgström P, Intaglietta M. (1993a) The vascular origin of slow wave flowmotion in skeletal muscle during local hypotension. *Int J Microcirc Clin Exp* 12: 287–297.

Schmidt JA, Borgström P, Bruttig SP, Fronek A, Intaglietta M. (1993b) Vasomotion as a flow-dependent phenome-non. *Prog Appl Microcirc* 20: 34–51.

Segal SS. (1991) Microvascular recruitment in hamster

striated muscle: role for conducted vasodilation. *Am J Physiol* 261: H181–H189.

Strock PE, Majno G. (1969) Microvascular changes in acutely ischemic rat muscle. *Surg Gynecol Obstet* 129: 1213–1224.

Wahlander H, Friberg P, Haraldsson B. (1993) Changes in myocardial capillary diffusion capacity during infusion of vasoactive drugs. *Acta Physiol Scand* 147: 49–58.

Warnke KC, Skalak TC. (1992) Leukocyte plugging in vivo in skeletal muscle arteriolar trees. *Am J Physiol* 262: H1149–H1155.

Weiner RM, Borgström P, Intaglietta M. (1989) Induction of vasomotion by hemorrhagic hypotension in rabbit tenuissimus muscle. *Prog Appl Microcirc* 15: 93–99.

Welbourn CRB, Goldman G, Paterson IS, Valeri CR, Shepro D, Hechtman HB. (1991) Pathophysiology of ischemia reperfusion injury: central role of the neutrophil. *Br J Surg* 78: 651–655.

26

Mechanisms of skeletal muscle pain

Siegfried Mense and Ulrich Hoheisel

Introduction

Muscle pain has several features by which it differs from cutaneous and visceral pain. Subjectively, muscle pain is perceived as aching and cramping; it is difficult to localize and referred to other deep somatic tissues. Objectively, the information from muscle nociceptors appears to be processed differently in the central nervous system. For instance, it has a special relay in the mesencephalon (Keay and Bandler 1993), and it is tonically inhibited by a particular descending pathway (Yu and Mense 1990).

This article deals with peripheral and central nervous mechanisms of muscle pain and tries to draw parallels between data obtained in animal experiments and symptoms in patients. Necessarily, such parallels are speculative.

Peripheral mechanisms

Physiological properties of muscle nociceptors

A nociceptor is a receptive ending that is activated by noxious (tissue threatening, subjectively painful) or potentially noxious stimulation, and it is capable by its response behaviour of distinguishing between innocuous and noxious stimuli. As an additional feature most nociceptors have a high stimulation threshold (for reviews, see Besson and Chaouch 1987, Belmonte and Cervero 1996).

Recordings of the electrical activity of single muscle afferent fibres in various species have shown that, in skeletal muscle, nociceptors (in the sense of the above definition) are present. If tested with natural stimuli (mechanical and chemical), these receptors do not respond to everyday stimuli such as weak local pressure, contractions and stretches within the physiological range but require high intensities of stimulation to be activated (Paintal 1960, Mense and Meyer 1985). Judging from their conduction velocity, most of the nociceptive fibres are unmyelinated or thin myelinated and, therefore, they are likely to terminate in free nerve endings.

Particularly effective stimulants for free nerve endings including nociceptors are endogenous pain-producing substances such as bradykinin (BKN), 5-hydroxytryptamine (5-HT, serotonin) and high concentrations of potassium ions (Franz and Mense 1975, Kumazawa and Mizumura 1977, Kaufman et al 1982). The typical muscle nociceptor responds to both noxious local pressure and injections of BKN, but in animal experiments receptors can also be found that are activated by only one type of noxious stimulation (mechanical or chemical). This finding indicates that different types of nociceptors are present in skeletal muscle, similar to the skin where mechano-, mechano-heat-, and polymodal nociceptors have been reported to exist (Besson and Chaouch 1987).

In microneurographic recordings from muscle nerves in humans, muscle nociceptors with moderate to high mechanical threshold were found that could be activated by i.m. injections of capsaicin, the active ingredient of chilli pepper (Marchettini et al 1996). The behaviour of these receptors was largely identical to that of muscle nociceptors in cat and rat.

Recent data from nociceptors in joints and other tissues have shown that the above-mentioned endogenous agents act on the receptive ending by binding to specific receptor molecules in the membrane of the ending (Kidd et al 1996, Cesare and McNaughton 1997; Fig. 26.1). The composition of the receptor molecules in the membrane changes when the ending is sensitized (i.e. exhibits an increased sensitivity, see below): in normal tissue, BKN activates the ending by binding to the B_2 receptor molecule, while the sensitized ending (e.g. in inflamed tissue) is excited by BKN through B_1 receptors, which are synthesized in the sensitized neurone. Another new aspect of the function of nociceptive free nerve endings is that they possess tetrodotoxin (TTX)-resistant Na^+ channels. This means that in comparison to fibres of other modalities (which can be blocked by TTX) nociceptive fibres are less affected by the neurotoxin TTX.

Morphology and neuropeptide content of muscle nociceptors

To date, no neuropeptide has been found that is specific for sensory fibres from muscle or for muscle nociceptors. Dorsal root ganglion cells projecting in a muscle nerve contain substance P (SP), calcitonin-gene related peptide (CGRP) and somatostatin (SOM), and thus present a neuropeptide pattern similar to that of cutaneous nerves (Molander et al 1987). Of these neuropeptides, SP is of particular interest, because in experiments on fibres from the skin SP has been shown to be predominantly present in nociceptive fibres (Lawson et al 1997). The peptides are released during excitation of the ending, and they influence the chemical milieu of the tissue around the receptor.

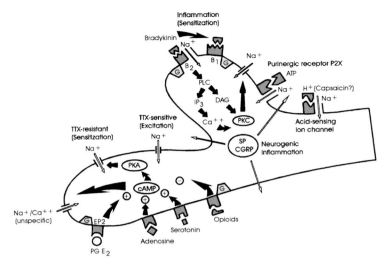

Figure 26.1— Excitation and sensitization of a nociceptive nerve ending. A schematic drawing showing membrane receptor molecules and intracellular events that increase or decrease the sensitivity of the ending. Of clinical importance are the following processes: 1. Sensitization is not an unspecific process but is caused by binding of the sensitizing substances (prostaglandin E_2 (PGE_2), serotonin, adenosine) to specific membrane receptors, which induce intracellular cascades of events that increase the sensitivity of the Na^+ channels. The larger ion currents that flow through the channel proteins of a sensitized ending render the ending more sensitive. 2. Normally, bradykinin excites nociceptors by binding to the B_2 receptor molecule. The sensitized ending is excited by bradykinin binding to the B_1 receptor molecule. The binding of bradykinin to the receptor molecules leads either to a direct influx of cations into the ending, or to the activation of protein kinase C (PKC), which increases the sensitivity of the Na^+ channels to stimulus-induced depolarizations. 3. Nociceptors possess a special type of Na^+ channel in their membrane, the tetrodotoxin (TTX)-resistant Na^+ channel. In the course of sensitization, more TTX-resistant channel protein molecules are synthesized and built into the membrane. (cAMP, cyclic adenosine monophosphate; DAG, diacylglycerol; G, G protein; IP3, inositol triphosphate; PKA, protein kinase A; PLC, phospholipase C. Modified after Kidd et al 1996, Cesare and McNaughton 1997.) More recent data indicate that the B_1 and B_2 receptors do not control Na^+ channels but are both coupled to G proteins.

Interactions between stimulants at the receptive nerve ending

Prostaglandin E_2 (PGE_2) and 5-HT have been shown to enhance the excitatory action of BKN on slowly conducting muscle afferents (Mense 1981). The pain elicited in volunteers by intramuscular injection of a combination of BKN and 5-HT is likewise stronger than that caused by each stimulant alone (Jensen et al 1990). These interactions are probably of great clinical importance, since in damaged tissue the substances are released together.

The concentration of PGE_2 and 5-HT that is required for potentiating the BKN action on muscle receptors is lower than that for exciting the receptive ending. In the beginning of a pathological tissue alteration, when the concentrations of sensitizing agents are increasing, the receptive ending is first sensitized and then excited. This assumption is consistent with the clinical observation that in the course of a pathological alteration the patient first experiences tenderness (due to nociceptor sensitization) and then spontaneous pain (due to nociceptor excitation).

Sensitization of nociceptors as the peripheral neurophysiological basis of tenderness and hyperalgesia

Many of the chemical stimulants increase the mechanical sensitivity of nociceptors. For instance, BKN is capable of sensitizing muscle nociceptors to mechanical stimuli. This process is characterized by a decrease in the mechanical threshold of the receptor, so that it responds to weak pressure stimuli. The sensitized receptor is still connected to nociceptive central nervous pathways and, therefore, it elicits subjective pain when activated by weak mechanical stimulation. This sensitization of muscle nociceptors is the main peripheral mechanism underlying local tenderness and pain upon movement of a pathologically altered muscle. Moreover, the response magnitude of a sensitized nociceptor to noxious stimuli increases. As a stronger pain response to a painful stimulus is defined as hyperalgesia, the sensitization of nociceptors offers a peripheral mechanism for the hyperalgesia of patients with muscle pain.

Pathological alterations of muscle not only sensitize nociceptors but also alter the innervation density of muscle tissue with neuropeptide-containing nerve endings. Experiments on the rat gastrocnemius-soleus (GS) muscle showed that a muscle inflammation of 12 days duration is followed by an increase in innervation density with these fibres. The effect was particularly great in fibres that can be visualized with antibodies to SP (Fig. 26.2); the density of these SP-immuno-reactive fibres increased by a factor of about 2 (Reinert et al 1998). Since many of the SP-immunoreactive fibres are likely to be nociceptors, the increase in innervation density is probably associated with enhanced pain sensations.

Mechanisms of muscle pain at the spinal level

A longer lasting input from nociceptors in skeletal muscle is known to lead to changes in the functional connectivity of sensory dorsal horn neurones. The changes are so marked that the term "lesion-induced functional reorganisation of the dorsal horn" has been used to describe these changes (Hoheisel et al 1994). In animal experiments, such changes occur within a few hours following an experimental muscle lesion. For instance, one of the effects of an acute experimental inflammation of the GS muscle in anaesthetized rats was an expansion of the spinal input region of the muscle nerve, i.e., the population of dorsal horn neu-

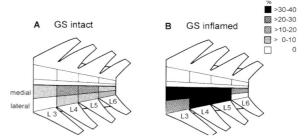

Figure 26.3 — Expansion of the spinal input region of the gastrocnemius-soleus (GS) muscle nerves following induction of a myositis of the GS muscle. The figure shows dorsal views of the lumbar spinal cord of the rat. The spinal dorsal horn in the segments L3-L6 is subdivided into eight regions. In each of the 8 regions the proportion of neurones was determined that could be activated by a standard electrical stimulus to the GS nerves. The different grades of shading indicate the percentage of cells that responded to the standard stimulus. In animals with intact muscle (**A**) the main input area was the medial dorsal horn in the segments L4 and L5. In animals with inflamed muscle (**B**) the population of responding neurones showed a large expansion. This effect was most marked in the lateral dorsal horn and in the segment L3, i.e., in regions that normally do not receive much input from the GS nerves.

rones responding to an electrical standard stimulus applied to the GS muscle nerve grew larger (Hoheisel et al 1994; Fig. 26.3). This effect was most marked in the spinal segment L3, which normally does not receive much input from the GS muscle. In the lateral segment L3, there was a qualitative effect: in animals with intact muscle, not a single neurone responded to input from the GS muscle, but in animals with inflamed muscle more than 20% did. Probably, the synaptic connections between these neurones and muscle afferents have become more efficient in myositis animals. The higher synaptic efficacy can result either from changes in the synapses themselves, or from hyperexcitability of the spinal neurones (central sensitization). Actually, in myositis animals the neurones were hyperexcitable because the cells' responses to noxious stimuli were larger. In patients, this hyperexcitability probably causes more pain in response to a noxious stimulus (i.e. hyperalgesia).

A possible explanation for the myositis-induced expansion of the responding neurone population is given in Fig. 26.4. It shows that in the spinal cord many ineffective (silent) synapses are present, which may become effective under the influence of a nociceptive input from muscle. The lesion-induced expansion of the input region of the GS muscle nerve may underly the spread and referral that is so typical of muscle pain.

In order to find out which neurotransmitters are responsible for the myositis-induced increase in

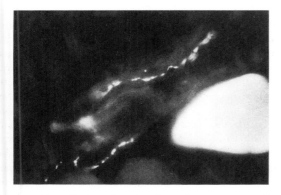

Figure 26.2 — Histological section from the rat gastrocnemius-soleus muscle showing two free nerve endings that are immunoreactive for the neuropeptide substance P (SP). The endings exhibit the typical appearance of pearls on a string, the "pearls" being expansions of the axon that contain the neuropeptide. The neuropeptide was visualized using fluorescent antibodies to SP. The large pale structure to the lower right is a cross-sectioned single muscle cell.

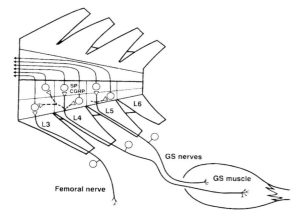

Figure 26.4—Hypothetical explanation of the expansion of the input region of the gastrocnemius-soleus (GS) nerves shown in Figure 26.3. The basic assumption is that dorsal horn neurones have two types of functional connections with the body periphery: 1. connections that are synaptically highly effective and always functional (open); these are drawn as solid lines. From the GS muscle they run to the medial dorsal horn in L4 and L5; 2. connections of low synaptic efficacy, which normally are not open. These "silent" connections are drawn as dashed lines. When the muscle is inflamed, the silent (ineffective) connections become effective, and thus the input from the GS muscle can activate more neurones in the segment L3 and in lateral L4 and L5.

excitability, the spinal cord was treated with solutions that contained one of the following antagonists or blockers:

1. antagonists to the neurokinin-1 receptor (the main receptor for SP)

2. antagonists to the N-methyl-D-aspartate (NMDA) receptor (one of the glutamate receptors)

3. antagonists to the AMPA/kainate receptor (the so-called non-NMDA glutamate receptors)

4. blockers of the nitric oxide synthase (NOS), the enzyme that synthesizes NO.

Spinal administration of the neurokinin and NMDA receptor antagonists during the development of the myositis prevented the hyperexcitability, whereas blocking of the nitric oxide (NO) synthesis was ineffective in this regard. These data suggest that both neurokinin and NMDA receptors are involved in the myositis-induced hyperexcitability of dorsal horn cells, and that the synthesis of NO is not of importance for these changes.

In contrast, the background activity of dorsal horn neurones (i.e. electrical activity in the absence of intentional stimulation) appears to depend strongly on the release of NO in the spinal cord (Hoheisel et al

1995). A block of the NOS led to a highly significant increase in background activity without affecting the excitability of the dorsal horn neurones. These data suggest that normally nitric oxide (NO) is continuously released in the dorsal horn and inhibits the background discharge of the neurones. The background activity is of clinical importance because it is probably responsible for spontaneous pain and dysaesthesia.

Myositis patients complain of hyperalgesia and hyperaesthesia as well as of spontaneous pain and dysaesthesia (DeVere and Bradley 1975, Ansell 1984). Under the assumption that hyperalgesia is at least partly caused by increased central nervous excitability, and spontaneous pain by increased background activity, the present data suggest that hyperalgesia is mediated by activation of neurokinin and NMDA receptors, whereas spontaneous pain is caused by other processes (e.g. reduced spinal release of NO).

These functional changes in the behaviour of dorsal horn neurones are neuroplastic because they are likely to outlast the peripheral lesion. Neuroplastic changes have to be considered as an important step in the transition from acute to chronic pain because they can persist under unfavourable circumstances. Another step in the direction of chronic pain is lesion-induced metabolic change in sensory spinal neurones. Such changes have been studied in cells that are capable of synthesizing NO.

The NO-synthesizing cells can be visualized with the histochemical diaphorase reaction or immunohistochemically with antibodies to NOS. Figure 26.5 shows the effects of an experimental myositis on the number of diaphorase-positive neurones in the superficial dorsal horn. Tissue sections from animals with an acute myositis (8 h duration) showed a significant increase, whereas sections from animals with a subacute myositis (12 day duration) a significant decrease in the number of cells with diaphorase activity. Apparently, the afferent input from inflamed muscle can increase or decrease the diaphorase activity in dorsal horn cells depending on the extent and duration of the lesion. The cell system of NO-synthesizing neurones behaves like a sensor for peripheral lesions, and, by influencing the background activity of nociceptive neurones, it is likely to determine spontaneous pain in patients (Callsen-Cencic et al 1999).

The last step in the transition from acute to chronic muscle pain involves morphological changes in the circuitry of the spinal dorsal horn. These changes consist of sprouting of the spinal terminals of afferent fibres and of new formation and broadening of synaptic contacts. Through these structural alterations, the functional changes become permanent, and the func-

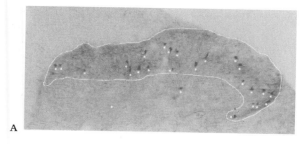

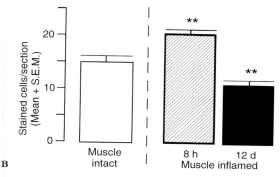

Figure 26.5—Effect of afferent input from muscle on the number of diaphorase-stained spinal neurones. **A** Intact muscle; the white line marks the superficial dorsal horn in which the cell counts were made. Each diaphorase-positive cell is marked by a white asterisk. **B** Number of diaphorase-positive neurones in animals with intact muscle (open bar), acute myositis (8 h, hatched bar), and subacute myositis (12 days, filled bar). ★★, $p < 0.01$; comparison with "muscle intact".

tion of the spinal cord is persistently altered. In our animal model, the first signs of structural changes in the spinal dorsal horn could be detected a few hours after induction of the myositis.

In patients, the development of lesion-induced structural changes in the dorsal horn may take longer than in the rat, but it is highly probable that they do occur also in humans in response to longer lasting muscle pain. When structural changes in the spinal cord are present, treatment of muscle pain can not be expected to have immediate success because the alterations in spinal circuitry take time to return to normal. Therefore, an important principle in the treatment of muscle pain is to abolish the nociceptive input from muscle to the spinal cord as early as possible to prevent lesion-induced spinal alterations.

References

Ansell BM. (1984) *Inflammatory disorders of muscle. Clinics in Rheumatic Diseases.* London: Saunders.

Belmonte C, Cervero F. (1996) *Neurobiology of Nociceptors.* Oxford: Oxford University Press.

Besson JM, Chaouch A. (1987) Peripheral and spinal mechanisms of nociception. *Physiol Rev* 67: 67–186.

Callsen-Cencic P, Hoheisel U, Kaske A, Mense S, Tenschert S. (1999) The controversy about spinal neuronal nitric oxide synthase: under which conditions is it up- or downregulated? *Cell Tissue Res* 295: 183–194.

Cesare P, McNaughton P. (1997) Peripheral pain mechanisms. *Curr Opin Neurobiol* 7: 493–499.

De Vere R, Bradley WG. (1975) Polymyositis: its presentation, morbidity and mortality. *Brain* 98: 637–666.

Franz M, Mense S. (1975) Muscle receptors with group IV afferent fibres responding to application of bradykinin. *Brain Res* 92: 369–383.

Hoheisel U, Koch K, Mense S. (1994) Functional reorganisation in the rat dorsal horn during an experimental myositis. *Pain* 59: 111–118.

Hoheisel U, Sander B, Mense S. (1995) Blockade of nitric oxide synthase differentially influences background activity and electrical excitability in rat dorsal horn neurones. *Neurosci Lett* 188: 143–146.

Hoheisel U, Sander B, Mense S. (1997) Myositis-induced functional reorganisation of the rat dorsal horn: effects of spinal superfusion with antagonists to neurokinin and glutamate receptors. *Pain* 69: 219–230.

Jensen K, Tuxen C, Pedersen-Bjergaard U, Jansen I, Edvinsson L, Olesen J. (1990) Pain and tenderness in human temporal muscle induced by bradykinin and 5-hydroxytryptamine. *Peptides* 11: 1127–1132.

Kaufman MP, Iwamoto GA, Longhurst JC, Mitchell JH. (1982) Effects of capsaicin and bradykinin on afferent fibers with endings in skeletal muscle. *Circ Res* 50: 133–139.

Keay KA, Bandler R. (1993) Deep and superficial noxious stimulation increases Fos-like immunoreactivity in different regions of the midbrain periaqueductal grey of the rat. *Neurosci Lett* 154: 23–26.

Kidd BL, Morris VH, Urban L. (1996) Pathophysiology of joint pain. *Ann Rheum Dis* 55: 276–283.

Kumazawa T, Mizumura K. (1977) Thin-fibre receptors responding to mechanical, chemical and thermal stimulation in the skeletal muscle of the dog. *J Physiol* 273: 179–194.

Lawson SN, Crepps BA, Perl ER. (1997) Relationship of substance P to afferent characteristics of dorsal root ganglion neurones in guinea-pig. *J Physiol* 505: 177–191.

Marchettini P, Simone DA, Caputi G, Ochoa JL. (1996) Pain from excitation of identified muscle nociceptors in humans. *Brain Res* 740: 109–116.

Mense S. (1981) Sensitization of group IV muscle receptors to bradykinin by 5-hydroxytryptamine and prostaglandin E$_2$. *Brain Res* 225: 95–105.

Mense S, Meyer H. (1985) Different types of slowly conducting afferent units in cat skeletal muscle and tendon. *J Physiol* 363: 403–417.

Molander C, Ygge I, Dalsgaard C-J. (1987) Substance P-, somatostatin-, and calcitonin gene-related peptide-like immunoreactivity and fluoride resistant acid phosphatase-activity in relation to retrogradely labeled cutaneous, muscular and visceral primary sensory neurones in the rat. *Neurosci Lett* 74: 37–42.

Paintal AS. (1960) Functional analysis of group III afferent fibres of mammalian muscles. *J Physiol* 152: 250–270.

Reinert A, Kaske A, Mense S. (1998) Inflammation-induced increase in the density of neuropeptide-immunoreactive nerve endings in rat skeletal muscle. *Exp Brain Res* 121: 174–180.

Yu XM, Mense S. (1990) Response properties and descending control of rat dorsal horn neurones with deep receptive fields. *Neurosci* 39: 823–831.

27

Skeletal muscle and cytokines in sepsis and severe injury

John E. Rectenwald and Lyle L. Moldawer

Clinical significance

The catabolic response in skeletal muscle to sepsis and severe injury is one of the most pronounced metabolic changes seen within the human body (Hill and Hill 1998; Fig. 27.1). Skeletal muscle comprises the major protein pool within the body, and it appears to be a primary site for this stimulated proteolysis. Most septic or severely injured patients experience an increase in resting energy expenditure on the order of 5–60% depending on the magnitude of injury. This hyper-metabolic response results in whole body protein breakdown primarily due to elevated muscle proteolysis of myofibrillar proteins. This is evidenced by net release of protein from muscle (Rosenblatt et al

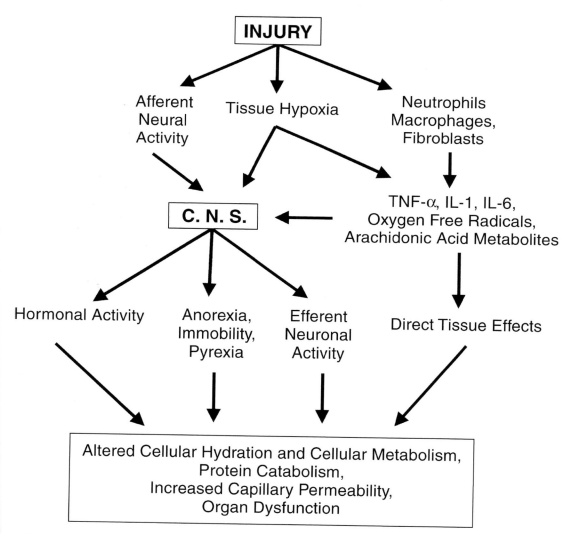

Figure 27.1—Schematic representation of the complex neuroendocrine and inflammatory response to sepsis and severe injury. Injury initiates a cascade of afferent neuronal activity, tissue hypoxia, and stimulation of inflammatory mediators. These events stimulate the central nervous system (C.N.S.) to coordinate the response from peripheral tissues such as the liver, skeletal muscle, and gut. The end results are changes in metabolism, cellular kinetics, tissue permeability, and organ dysfunction. (Modified from Hill AG and Hill GL. (1998) Metabolic response to severe injury. *Br J Surgery* 85: 884–890.)

1983) and enhanced urinary 3-methylhistidine excretion (Long et al 1981), although reduced protein synthesis and inhibited amino acid transport may possibly contribute to the overall protein loss in septic or injured muscle.

The result of muscle proteolysis in patients undergoing severe physiological stress is the peripheral release of free amino acids, specifically alanine and glutamine. Most of these released amino acids are taken up and utilized by the liver in the process of gluconeogenesis and acute-phase protein synthesis. Other amino acids released from muscle protein, such as glutamine, are essential for normal function of enterocytes and cells of the immune system.

Muscle catabolism and release of amino acids may play a beneficial role in the short term survival of the severely injured patient by providing necessary amino acids for vital functions. However, prolonged and unchecked muscle breakdown may be maladaptive and lead to respiratory weakness and difficulty weaning from ventilatory support, as well as muscle atrophy and difficulty ambulating after sepsis has resolved. It is estimated that nearly one fifth of the body's stores of protein can be lost in the first three weeks, the majority of which occurs in the first 10 days. Furthermore, two thirds of the total amount of protein lost comes from skeletal muscle (Hill and Hill 1998).

The neuroendocrine axis

Of the many components that influence the metabolic response to injury in muscle, the role of both stress hormones and peripheral nerves was first elucidated. Early studies showed an attenuated nitrogen loss in adrenalectomized rats, compared with controls, undergoing femoral shaft fracture injury (Hill and Hill 1998). This data suggested an important role for stress hormones, such as catecholamines and glucocorticoids, in muscle's metabolic response to injury. Administration of exogenous glucocorticoids in humans has been shown to result in an increase in muscle protein degradation, particularly myofibrillar proteins (Darmaun et al 1988). Data on healthy men have shown that infusion of catecholamines, glucocorticoids and glucagon results in metabolic alterations qualitatively similar to those seen in injured patients (Bessey et al 1984, Darmaun et al 1988). Treatment of septic muscle with RU 38486, a glucocorticoid receptor antagonist, significantly decreased but did not eliminate sepsis-induced muscle proteolysis in septic rats (Hall-Angeras et al 1991). In the same experiment, decreased protein synthesis was not affected by RU 38486 arguing that

other mechanisms are involved in muscle proteolysis in sepsis. Similarly, in another study done on healthy human volunteers that included an etiocholanolone (a naturally occurring pyrogen) control arm, the data suggested that both inflammatory and endocrine processes are needed to manifest the complete host response to severe injury and sepsis (Watters et al 1986).

Early work demonstrated the importance of the peripheral nervous system on the early endocrine response to injury. Anaesthetized dogs undergoing hindlimb disarticulation sparing the femoral artery, vein and sciatic nerve responded to injury in the enervated, but severed limb, with an acute increase in glucocorticoid secretion as would be expected in a normal animal (Egdahl 1959). However, if the sciatic nerve was severed and the femoral artery and vein left intact subsequent trauma to the limb did not evoke a glucocorticoid response arguing that peripheral nerve function is important to the metabolic response to injury (Egdahl 1959).

The neuroendocrine response to surgery has been found to be primarily limited to 24 h, but the increased nitrogen output is not maximal for several days after the initial perioperative period, suggesting that other factors may mediate the muscle proteolysis in response to severe injury or sepsis (Cuthbertson 1964). Proinflammatory cytokines, in addition to neuroendocrine response, have been found to regulate muscle proteolysis during sepsis.

Pathways of muscle proteolysis in sepsis and injury

Specific mechanisms of muscle proteolysis in severe injury, burns and sepsis have recently been reviewed (Hasselgren 1999a, 1999b). Intracellular protein breakdown during sepsis and severe injury is regulated by several distinct proteolytic pathways. Injury-induced muscle proteolysis may occur by three separate mechanisms: lysosomal, calcium-dependent and energy-dependent ubiquitin–proteasome mechanisms. In general, it is believed that the lysosomal pathway accounts for the degradation of more long-lived proteins and membrane proteins and that the energy (ATP) dependent ubiquitin–proteasome pathway is responsible for proteolysis of abnormal proteins, short-lived proteins and myofibrillar proteins (Hasselgren 1995).

The ubiquitin–proteasome pathway involves both energy-dependent protein breakdown and conjugation of these protein substrates with multiple molecules of ubiquitin before degradation. Ubiquitination of proteins is regulated by multiple enzymes: an activating enzyme (E1), a ubiquitin conjugating enzyme (E2, specifically E2$_{14k}$) and a ubiquitin protein ligase (E3α). Ubiquinated proteins are then recognized by the 26S proteolytic complex and, after binding and unfolding, the ubiquinated protein is funnelled through the 20S proteasome (the catalytic core of the 26S proteasome) and degraded (Fig. 27.2).

The importance of the energy-dependent ubiquitin–proteasome pathway in sepsis-induced proteolysis is supported by data from extensor digitorum longus muscle obtained from septic rats that was incubated in the presence of lysosomal or calcium-independent protein degradation inhibitors or in energy-depleting media (Tiao et al 1994). The results from this caecal ligation and puncture model suggested that sepsis-induced muscle proteolysis is primarily a non-lysosomal, calcium-independent but energy-dependent process (Tiao et al 1994). The majority of protein released from the septic rat muscle appeared to be of myofibrillar origin, as measure by 3-methylhistidine release and urinary excretion. In this same experiment

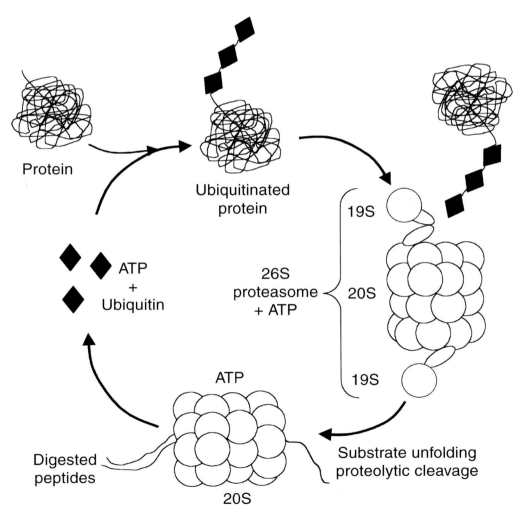

Figure 27.2 — Simplified schematic representation of the ubiquitin-dependent proteolytic pathway. (Modified from Hasselgren and Fischer 1997.)

gene expression of ubiquitin and the total amount of ubiquinated proteins were elevated in septic muscles, as determined by Northern and Western analysis respectively, suggesting that ubiquitin-dependent proteolysis participates in muscle catabolism in sepsis.

Evidence of increased expression of other components of the ubiquitin–proteasome pathway in sepsis-induced proteolysis are increased as well. mRNA and proteolytic activity levels for subunits of the 20S proteasome have also been noted to be increased in septic muscle of humans. In a small study on humans, mRNA levels for ubiquitin and a 20S proteasome subunit (HC3) were found to be elevated in muscle tissue approximately 3–4 fold in septic patients, by Northern blot analysis, compared with controls. Although urine cortisol levels were slightly elevated in the septic patients, the difference was not significant when compared with control patients (Tiao et al 1997a).

Similar results concerning muscle proteolysis were obtained in a different rodent model of sepsis involving intravenous infusion of live *Escherichia coli*. Interestingly, this study found that, in addition to ubiquitin-dependent muscle breakdown, activation of calcium-dependent and lysosomal systems may also be important for regulation of proteolysis during the late and chronic phases of endotoxin-induced sepsis (Voisin et al 1996). Although the ubiquitin-dependent mechanism of proteolysis appears to be the major regulator of muscle proteolysis, recent evidence points to an integral role for the calcium-dependent, ubiquitin energy-independent process in muscle proteolysis (Fagan et al 1996, Hasselgren 1999b). Early events in sepsis-related muscle breakdown may be a calcium-dependent, calpain-mediated release of myofilaments from the Z-disks.

Furthermore, muscle protein breakdown can be almost completely reversed when septic rat muscle is treated in vitro with N-acetyl-L-leucinyl-L-leucinal-L-norleucinal (LLnL), a peptide aldehyde that reversibly blocks the chymotryptic and peptidylglutamyl activities of the proteasome (Hobler et al 1998). Lactacystin, a more specific proteasome blocker than LLnL that does not inhibit some calpains and cathepsins, inhibited myofibrillar and total proteolysis in septic muscle (Hobler et al 1998). Similar data were produced using a more active form of lactacystin, lactacystin β-lactone, in burned rats (Fang et al 1998).

Differences in fast- and slow-twitch muscle have also emphasized the importance of the energy-dependent ubiquitin–proteasome pathway in sepsis and burn-induced muscle protein breakdown. White, fast-twitch muscle (the extensor digitorum longus muscle)

in burned or septic rats had significant amounts of muscle proteolysis in addition to elevated levels of mRNA for ubiquitin and several proteasome subunits. Only minor amounts of proteolysis and slightly elevated levels of mRNA for ubiquitin and proteasomes occurred in the red, slow-twitch muscle (soleus muscle) of these same rats (Tiao et al 1997b).

Therefore, the energy-dependent, ubiquitin–proteasome pathway appears to be the predominant pathway of muscle proteolysis in sepsis and burn injury. Data suggest that the lysosomal and calcium-dependent pathways play a less significant role in muscle protein breakdown during severe injury. The major mediators of these processes have not been sufficiently identified but they may include glucocorticoids and numerous cytokines.

Cytokines

In general, proinflammatory cytokines are regulatory proteins released primarily from inflammatory cells that serve to activate the innate and acquired immune systems. Although cytokines generally act locally in a paracrine fashion, elevated systemic levels of cytokines have been noted in the plasma of septic and injured patients (Fischer and Hasselgren 1991). Pro-inflammatory cytokines such as tumour necrosis factor (TNF-α), and interleukins 1 and 6 (IL-1, IL-6) participate in the regulation of protein metabolism during sepsis and severe injury (Table 27.1). Injection of these cytokines into healthy humans or animals has been shown to induce metabolic changes similar to sepsis, suggesting that these cytokines may be capable of functioning as endocrine hormones as well (Starnes et al 1988, Fischer and Hasselgren 1991, Hasselgren 1995).

In vitro experiments in isolated hepatocytes have suggested that a combination of IL-1, IL-6, interferon β₂, and TNF-α are required to induce the complete acute phase response initiated by severe injury or sepsis. Glucocorticoids have been found to augment the acute phase response when administered concurrently with cytokines, but they do not affect hepatic acute phase synthesis when administered alone (Baumann et al 1987). Cytokines appear to play a role in the hepatic acute phase response in sepsis and trauma, but what role, if any, do they play in muscle proteolysis associated with these illnesses?

TNF-α has already been shown to induce a catabolic state when infused into animals and humans in a dose-dependent fashion. TNF-α causes enhanced energy expenditure, increased hepatic gluconeogenesis, and whole body proteolysis and lipolysis (Tracey et

Table 27.1 – Cytokine sources and their metabolic effects in severe injury and sepsis

Cytokine	Source	Biological effects
Tumor necrosis factor-α	Monocytes/macrophages Fibroblasts Vascular smooth muscle cells	Increases energy expenditure Induces gluconeogenesis Induces proteolysis Induces lipolysis
Interleukin-1	Monocytes/macrophages Fibroblasts Vascular smooth muscle cells Endothelial cells	Induces proteolysis Decreases IGF-1 activity Activates ubiquitin proteolysis?
Interleukin-6	Monocytes/macrophages Fibroblasts Keratinocytes Endothelial cells	Induces acute phase response Induces proteolysis Increases activity of the 26S proteasome Increases lysosomal proteolysis

al 1988, Fong et al 1989, Hill and Hill 1998). IL-1 at higher concentrations stimulates production of mediators that cause many biologic effects such as fever, hypotension, inflammation and proteolysis (Dinarello 1991, Zamir et al 1993, Dinarello 1996). In addition, TNF-α and IL-1 appear to act synergistically in sepsis and severe injury. In rabbits, infusion of TNF-α and IL-1 together results in greater metabolic effects than infusion of either cytokine alone (Tredget et al 1988).

Interleukin-1α and IL-1β have been shown to participate in the regulation of muscle proteolysis in several studies (Attaix et al 1994). IL-1α, when administered chronically in rats, is found to induce muscle proteolysis and reduce myofibrillar protein mRNA levels (Fong et al 1989). In another separate experiment IL-1α given intraperitoneally in divided doses over 16 h was found to stimulate myofibrillar muscle protein breakdown (Zamir et al 1993). Additionally, studies in the rat found that the catabolic effect of TNF-α on muscle was augmented by infusion of IL-1β (Flores et al 1989). IL-1 administration was not found to affect muscle protein synthesis. Furthermore, septic and endotoxemic rats treated with an IL-1 receptor antagonist (IL-1ra) decreased the amount of muscle proteolysis induced in a rat model of caecal ligation and puncture (Zamir et al 1994) and after exposure to endotoxin (Zamir et al 1992). The presence of IL-1 detected in nerve fibres within the central nervous system innervating the hypothalamus argues that IL-1 is integral to the process of injury-induced proteolysis. In fact, chronic exogenous intrathecal IL-1 administration in rats

results in catabolism that is not mediated by glucocorticoids (Hill et al 1996).

However, data from human studies suggest that IL-1 induction alone is not sufficient to induce the muscle proteolysis directly. Healthy male subjects given intramuscular etiocholanolone (an exogenous inducer of IL-1) daily for 3 days did not exhibit elevated levels of counter-regulatory hormones, but they did have increased plasma activity of IL-1. These subjects failed to show altered protein metabolism as evidenced by nitrogen balance, ^{15}N turnover, and forearm flux of alanine and glutamine (Watters et al 1985).

Another cytokine, IL-6, is well known to induce acute phase protein synthesis in the liver, but its role in muscle proteolysis induced by sepsis and severe injury is less well understood. It is known, however, that intraperitoneal administration (two doses of 125 μg/kg) of IL-6 to rats resulted in increased myofibrillar protein breakdown as measured by release of 3-methylhistidine in incubated rat muscle. In the same experiment, muscle incubated with IL-6 in vitro did not increase muscle proteolysis, arguing that IL-6 does not have a direct effect on skeletal muscle (Hasselgren 1995). In one other study, using transgenic mice over-expressing human IL-6, the gastrocnemius muscles of these transgenic mice became atrophic by 16 weeks of age despite significant increases in body weight (Tsujinaka et al 1995). Therefore, IL-6 appears to indeed play some role in muscle proteolysis secondary to injury.

Overall, the consensus of the data suggests that

cytokines such as TNF-α, IL-1 and IL-6 appear to regulate muscle proteolysis in vivo, however, experimental evidence that these cytokines effect muscle protein breakdown in vitro is controversial. Some investigators have noted little to no muscle proteolysis caused by direct administration of TNF-α or IL-1 systemically on skeletal muscle (Moldawer et al 1987, Kettelhut and Goldberg 1988, Hasselgren 1995). In contrast, the systemic infusion of TNF-α and IL-1 concurrently with ^{14}C-leucine in the rat over 6 h resulted in increased muscle protein breakdown, as measured by the dilution of the free radioactive leucine pool in muscle tissue (Flores et al 1989).

The exact cellular mechanisms of cytokine-induced muscle proteolysis are currently not well understood. It is known that the half-life of long-lived proteins in a myotubule cell culture system was shortened by the addition of 100 units/ml of recombinant human IL-6. IL-6 administered in this experiment also increased the activity of the 26S proteasome by 31.5%, cathepsin B by 53.5%, and cathepsins B+L by 21.3%, suggesting that IL-6 may induce muscle protein breakdown through these mediators (Ebisui et al 1995). In this same cell culture system, administration of 1000 units/ml of recombinant human TNF-α *prolonged* the half-life of long-lived proteins and reduced the protease activities of the 20S proteasome by 27.1%, cathepsin B by 61.6% and cathepsins B+L by 54.9% (Ebisui et al 1995). IL-6 may induce proteolysis by activating both the non-lysosomal proteasome and lysosomal (cathepsins) proteolytic pathways. The role of TNF-α in this process is still unclear.

Data obtained from muscle biopsies in patients (Ebisui et al 1995) who have suffered severe traumatic head injury support these findings. Measured mRNA levels for the lysosomal pathway (cathepsin D, m-calpain), and the ubiquitin–proteasome pathway (ubiquitin, ubiquitin-conjugating enzyme E2 and the proteasome subunits) were elevated in these patients, all of which were in negative nitrogen balance with increased rates of whole body and myofibrillar protein breakdown. Significantly elevated serum levels of IL-1β and IL-6, but not TNF-α, were also noted in these patients, suggesting that these cytokines may contribute to the activation of the ubiquitin proteolytic pathway in head injured patients (Mansoor et al 1996).

The concept that cytokines may induce muscle protein breakdown through some mediator other than glucocorticoids has been proposed, and this is highly plausible. There are theories involving cytokine induction and muscle proteolysis through the inhibition of anabolic substances within muscle, such as insulin-like growth factor-1 (IGF-1) (Hasselgren 1995). TNF-α has been shown to block the anabolic effects of IGF-1 in chondrocytes (Lazarus et al 1993), however, conclusive evidence that a similar TNF-α effect occurs in skeletal muscle is lacking.

Evidence that IL-1 influences IGF-1 function in sepsis is more conclusive. Rats with chronic abdominal sepsis given IL-1ra continuously over 5 days had lower plasma, liver and gastrocnemius muscle concentrations of IGF-1 than saline-treated controls. Additionally, IL-1ra treatment prevented the sepsis-induced increase in IGF-1 in the blood and liver of septic rats. IGFBP-1 (insulin-like growth factor binding protein) levels were not attenuated in the muscle of septic rats and the rate of gastrocnemius muscle protein synthesis in vivo was decreased. Overall, systemic administration of IL-1ra appears to prevent a decrease in the IGF-1 content of septic muscle, and this response was associated with an enhanced rate of protein synthesis (Lang et al 1996). The effect of IL-1 on septic muscle may be mediated in part by it's effects on the central nervous system (Lang et al 1998).

Conclusion

Sepsis and severe injury evoke a complex metabolic response that stimulates significant metabolic changes in the host. One of the most dramatic is the whole body mobilization of proteins from skeletal muscle. The proteins released by skeletal muscle are used in the liver for gluconeogenesis and as fuel for the cells of the immune system and gut. While this process is felt to be advantageous in the short term, after injury or the beginning of sepsis, prolonged and unchecked skeletal muscle proteolysis leads to muscle wasting, ventilator dependence and ultimately death. A better understanding of the mechanisms and signalling processes of muscle protein breakdown, including the pathways of proteolysis, has obvious importance in the care and management of septic and severely injured patients. Although great strides have been made in understanding the role of glucocorticoids and cytokine regulation of this process, much remains to be understood in this complex process.

References

Attaix D, Taillandier D, Temparis S, et al. (1994) Regulation of ATP-ubiquitin-dependent proteolysis in muscle wasting. *Reprod Nutr Dev* 34: 583–597.

Baumann H, Richards C, Gauldie J. (1987) Interaction among hepatocyte-stimulating factors, interleukin 1, and glucocorticoids for regulation of acute phase plasma proteins in human hepatoma (HepG2) cells. *J Immunol* 139: 4122–4128.

Bessey PQ, Watters JM, Aoki TT, Wilmore DW. (1984) Combined hormonal infusion simulates the metabolic response to injury. *Ann Surg* 200: 264–281.

Cuthbertson DP. (1964) Physical injury and its effects on protein metabolism. In: *Mammalian Protein Metabolism*. 2. New York: Academic Press, pp. 373–414.

Darmaun D, Matthews DE, Bier DM. (1988) Physiological hypercortisolemia increases proteolysis, glutamine, and alanine production. *Am J Physiol* 255: E366–E373.

Dinarello CA. (1991) Interleukin-1 and interleukin-1 antagonism. *Blood* 77: 1627–1652.

Dinarello CA. (1996) Biologic basis for interleukin-1 in disease. *Blood* 87: 2095–2147.

Ebisui C, Tsujinaka T, Morimoto T, et al. (1995) Interleukin-6 induces proteolysis by activating intracellular proteases (cathepsins B and L, proteasome) in C2C12 myotubes. *Clin Sci (Colch)* 89: 431–439.

Egdahl RH. (1959) Pituitary-adrenal response following trauma to the isolated leg. *Surgery* 46: 9–21.

Fagan JM, Ganguly M, Tiao G, Fischer JE, Hasselgren PO. (1996) Sepsis increases oxidatively damaged proteins in skeletal muscle. *Arch Surg* 131: 1326–1331.

Fang CH, Wang JJ, Hobler S, Li BG, Fischer JE, Hasselgren PO. (1998) Proteasome blockers inhibit protein breakdown in skeletal muscle after burn injury in rats. *Clin Sci (Colch)* 95: 225–233.

Fischer JE, Hasselgren PO. (1991) Cytokines and glucocorticoids in the regulation of the "hepato-skeletal muscle axis" in sepsis. *Am J Surg* 161: 266–271.

Flores EA, Bistrian BR, Pomposelli JJ, Dinarello CA, Blackburn GL, Istfan NW. (1989) Infusion of tumor necrosis factor/cachectin promotes muscle catabolism in the rat. A synergistic effect with interleukin 1. *J Clin Invest* 83: 1614–1622.

Fong Y, Moldawer LL, Marano M, et al. (1989) Cachectin/TNF or IL-1 alpha induces cachexia with redistribution of body proteins. *Am J Physiol* 256: R659–R665.

Hall-Angeras M, Angeras U, Zamir O, Hasselgren PO, Fischer JE. (1991) Effect of the glucocorticoid receptor antagonist RU 38486 on muscle protein breakdown in sepsis. *Surgery* 109: 468–473.

Hasselgren PO. (1995) Muscle protein metabolism during sepsis. *Biochem Soc Trans* 23: 1019–1025.

Hasselgren PO, Fischer JE. (1997) The Ubiquitin-Proteosome Pathway. Ann Surgery 225(3): 307–316.

Hasselgren PO. (1999a) Pathways of muscle protein breakdown in injury and sepsis. *Curr Opin Clin Nutr Metab Care* 2: 155–160.

Hasselgren PO. (1999b) Role of the ubiquitin-proteasome pathway in sepsis-induced muscle catabolism. *Mol Biol Rep* 26: 71–76.

Hill AG, Hill GL. (1998) Metabolic response to severe injury. *Br J Surg* 85: 884–890.

Hill AG, Jacobson L, Gonzalez J, Rounds J, Majzoub JA, Wilmore DW. (1996) Chronic central nervous system exposure to interleukin-1 beta causes catabolism in the rat. *Am J Physiol* 271: R1142–R1148.

Hobler SC, Tiao G, Fischer JE, Monaco J, Hasselgren PO. (1998) Sepsis-induced increase in muscle proteolysis is blocked by specific proteasome inhibitors. *Am J Physiol* 274: R30–R37.

Kettelhut IC, Goldberg AL. (1988) Tumor necrosis factor can induce fever in rats without activating protein breakdown in muscle or lipolysis in adipose tissue. *J Clin Invest* 81: 1384–1389.

Lang CH, Fan J, Cooney R, Vary TC. (1996) IL-1 receptor antagonist attenuates sepsis-induced alterations in the IGF system and protein synthesis. *Am J Physiol* 270: E430–E437.

Lang CH, Fan J, Wojnar MM, Vary TC, Cooney R. (1998) Role of central IL-1 in regulating peripheral IGF-I during endotoxemia and sepsis. *Am J Physiol* 274: R956–R962.

Lazarus DD, Moldawer LL, Lowry SF. (1993) Insulin-like growth factor-1 activity is inhibited by interleukin-1 alpha, tumor necrosis factor-alpha, and interleukin-6. *Lymphokine Cytokine Res* 12: 219–223.

Long CL, Birkhahn RH, Geiger JW, Betts JE, Schiller WR, Blakemore WS. (1981) Urinary excretion of 3-methylhistidine: an assessment of muscle protein catabolism in adult normal subjects and during malnutrition, sepsis, and skeletal trauma. *Metabolism* 30: 765–776.

Mansoor O, Beaufrere B, Boirie Y, et al. (1996) Increased mRNA levels for components of the lysosomal, Ca2+-activated, and ATP-ubiquitin-dependent proteolytic pathways in skeletal muscle from head trauma patients. *Proc Natl Acad Sci USA* 93: 2714–2718.

Moldawer LL, Svaninger G, Gelin J, Lundholm KG. (1987) Interleukin 1 and tumor necrosis factor do not regulate protein balance in skeletal muscle. *Am J Physiol* 253: C766–C773.

Rosenblatt S, Clowes GHJ, George BC, Hirsch E, Lindberg B. (1983) Exchange of amino acids by muscle and liver in sepsis. *Arch Surg* 118: 167–175.

Starnes HFJ, Warren RS, Jeevanandam M, et al. (1988) Tumor necrosis factor and the acute metabolic response to tissue injury in man. *J Clin Invest* 82: 1321–1325.

Tiao G, Fagan JM, Samuels N, et al. (1994) Sepsis stimulates nonlysosomal, energy-dependent proteolysis and increases ubiquitin mRNA levels in rat skeletal muscle. *J Clin Invest* 94: 2255–2264.

Tiao G, Hobler S, Wang JJ, et al. (1997a) Sepsis is associated with increased mRNAs of the ubiquitin-proteasome proteolytic pathway in human skeletal muscle. *J Clin Invest* 99: 163–168.

Tiao G, Lieberman M, Fischer JE, Hasselgren PO. (1997b) Intracellular regulation of protein degradation during sepsis is different in fast- and slow-twitch muscle. *Am J Physiol* 272: R849–R856.

Tracey KJ, Wei H, Manogue KR, et al. (1988). Cachectin/tumor necrosis factor induces cachexia, anemia, and inflammation. *J Exp Med* 167: 1211–1227.

Tredget EE, Yu YM, Zhong S, et al. (1988) Role of interleukin 1 and tumor necrosis factor on energy metabolism in rabbits. *Am J Physiol* 255: E760–E768.

Tsujinaka T, Ebisui C, Fujita J, et al. (1995) Muscle undergoes atrophy in association with increase of lysosomal cathepsin activity in interleukin-6 transgenic mouse. *Biochem Biophys Res Commun* 207: 168–174.

Voisin L, Breuille D, Combaret L, et al. (1996) Muscle wasting in a rat model of long-lasting sepsis results from the activation of lysosomal, Ca2+-activated, and ubiquitin-proteasome proteolytic pathways. *J Clin Invest* 97: 1610–1617.

Watters JM, Bessey PQ, Dinarello CA, Wolff SM, Wilmore DW. (1985) The induction of interleukin-1 in humans and its metabolic effects. *Surgery* 98: 298–306.

Watters JM, Bessey PQ, Dinarello CA, Wolff SM, Wilmore DW. (1986) Both inflammatory and endocrine mediators stimulate host responses to sepsis. *Arch Surg* 121: 179–190.

Zamir O, Hasselgren PO, O'Brien W, Thompson RC, Fischer JE. (1992) Muscle protein breakdown during endotoxemia in rats and after treatment with interleukin-1 receptor antagonist (IL-1ra). *Ann.Surg* 216: 381–385.

Zamir O, Hasselgren PO, von AD, Fischer JE. (1993) In vivo administration of interleukin-1 alpha induces muscle proteolysis in normal and adrenalectomized rats. *Metabolism* 42: 204–208.

Zamir O, O'Brien W, Thompson R, Bloedow DC, Fischer JE, Hasselgren PO. (1994) Reduced muscle protein breakdown in septic rats following treatment with interleukin-1 receptor antagonist. *Int J Biochem* 26: 943–950.

28

Skeletal muscle infections

John D. Urschel

Introduction

Skeletal muscle infections may be classified into four major categories: bacterial pyomyositis, viral myositis, parasitic myositis, and necrotizing soft tissue infections. Necrotizing soft tissue infections are the most clinically important of these skeletal muscle infections, and the majority of this chapter is devoted to them.

Bacterial pyomyositis (tropical pyomyositis)

Pyomyositis is an acute bacterial infection of skeletal muscle that is usually caused by *Staphylococcus aureus* (Levin et al 1971, Das et al 1996). A localized abscess develops within a skeletal muscle. It may be primary (spontaneously occurring) or secondary to a penetrating injury or contiguous anatomic infection. However, the term pyomyositis usually implies primary pyomyositis, and, since most cases occur in the tropics, the term tropical pyomyositis is often used to denote this clinical scenario. The presumed pathogenesis of pyomyositis involves a staphylococcal bacteremia in the setting of non-penetrating muscle trauma or strain. Pyomyositis occurs more commonly in children than in adults. The major muscles of the lower extremity and the gluteal muscles are typically affected. Occasionally an abdominal muscle can be involved, and, therefore, pyomyositis is an important entity to consider in the differential diagnosis of acute abdominal conditions in tropical regions.

Patients typically present with pain, tenderness and oedema of the involved muscle group. Fever and leukocytosis are common, but profound systemic sepsis is usually only seen in neglected cases. The abscess is easy to overlook in the early stages, but eventually skin erythema and fluctuance make the diagnosis more obvious. Needle aspiration, or operative incision and drainage, will confirm the diagnosis. The treatment is adequate drainage (surgical or percutaneous) combined with antibiotic therapy directed against *Staphylococcus aureus* (the responsible organism in 95% of cases). The outcome is almost uniformly favourable if appropriate diagnostic and treatment guidelines are followed (Levin et al 1971, Das et al 1996).

Pyomyositis has occurred in non-tropical regions, but it is exceptionally rare (Gibson et al 1984, Das et al 1996). Although *Stapylococcus aureus* is the usual cause, a wide variety of bacteria have also been responsible for non-tropical pyomyositis. In contrast to necrotizing soft tissue infections, pyomyositis is characterized by a localized infectious process (abscess), conventional purulence (pus), lack of surrounding tissue necrosis, and a favourable response to simple incisional drainage.

Viral myositis

Myalgia is a prominent symptom of many systemic viral infections, but pathologic examination of muscle tissue in these circumstances is generally lacking. Influenza occasionally causes profound myalgia and muscle weakness (Mejlszenkier et al 1973). Of the few muscle biopsies reported in this setting, most show non-specific inflammation. However, there are reports of viral isolation from muscle (Kessler et al 1980). This supports the notion that viral illnesses may cause true skeletal muscle infection, as opposed to an immunologic reaction in muscle. Human immunodeficiency virus (HIV) myopathies can result from both HIV infection and its treatment (Ch.18).

Parasitic myositis

Trichinosis is the commonest cause of parasitic myositis in man. It is caused by eating poorly cooked pork or carnivore meat containing cysts of *Trichinella spiralis* (Liu and Weller 1994). Many mild cases of trichinosis are self-limiting, but deaths from myocardial involvement, encephalitis or pneumonia do occur. Larvae migrate from the gut to skeletal muscle where they provoke an intense local and systemic inflammatory response. Myalgia and muscle weakness develop, along with systemic reactions to the migrating larvae. Fever and eosinophilia are common. Muscles of the head and neck region are commonly affected. Extraocular muscle involvement may manifest itself as periorbital oedema. Serologic testing usually provides a diagnosis, but occasionally muscle biopsy is needed. This shows encysted *Trichenella spiralis* larvae and non-specific myositis. Fortunately, most patients eventually recover with supportive measures and rest. Mebendazole is effective in the enteric stages of infection, but it is probably not effective in eradicating larvae encysted in muscle. Corticosteroids may be useful for severe myositis.

Necrotizing soft tissue infections involving skeletal muscle

Overview

Necrotizing soft tissue infections are a highly lethal group of infections that require early and aggressive surgical debridement (Sutherland and Meyer 1994, Chapnick and Abter 1996, Urschel et al 1997). These infections may occur in almost any anatomic area, but they most frequently involve the abdomen, perineum and lower extremities. Surgery and trauma are common aetiologies, but in some cases the aetiology remains uncertain (Janevicius et al 1982, Freischlag et al 1985). Immunocompromised patients, especially those with diabetes, are more likely to develop necrotizing infections. Although a great deal of attention has been directed toward classifying these infections by bacteriological features or layers of tissue involved, it is useful to view necrotizing infections as a spectrum of clinical conditions with similar pathophysiological features and common treatment principles (Dellinger 1981, Kaiser and Cerra 1981, Urschel et al 1997).

Clinical features of necrotizing soft tissue infections include wound pain, crepitus, foul watery wound discharge, skin blistering and rapid progression to septic shock (Green et al 1996, Chapnick and Abter 1996). The external appearance of the skin wound may initially belie the magnitude of the necrotizing infection beneath it; this contributes to diagnostic delay. Soft tissue gas, detected clinically or radiologically, is a classic sign, but its absence does not exclude the presence of a necrotizing infection (Elliot et al 1996). This common misconception is also responsible for delayed diagnosis in some cases. The infection spreads rapidly through the soft tissue planes, and it produces severe systemic sepsis. Progression to septic shock, multiple organ failure and death ensues if aggressive treatment is not instituted immediately. Even with timely and skilled treatment, mortality of necrotizing soft tissue infections is 15–50% (Sutherland and Meyer 1994, Chapnick and Abter 1996, Elliot et al 1996).

Some necrotizing infections are caused by single organisms. Myonecrosis (gas gangrene) from *Clostridium* infection and necrotizing fasciitis from group A *Streptococcus* are two classic examples of single organism necrotizing infection. However, most necrotizing soft tissue infections are caused by a mixture of aerobic and anaerobic bacteria that act synergistically to cause fulminant infection (Giuliano et al 1977, File and Tan 1995). Organisms commonly identified include aerobic and anaerobic streptococci, coagulase-negative and coagulase-positive staphylococci, facultative and aerobic gram-negative rods, *Bacteroides* species, and *Clostridium* species (Giuliano et al 1977, Elliot et al 1996). Facultative organisms lower the oxidation–reduction potential of the wound microenvironment, and promote favourable conditions for the growth of anaerobes. Anaerobes interfere with host phagocyte function, and thereby facilitate the proliferation of aerobic bacteria (Rotstein et al 1985). Several bacteria, such as *Bacteroides fragilis*, produce β-lactamase enzymes that interfere with antibiotic activity.

Bacterial necrotoxins, such as those produced by *Clostridium perfringens* and *Streptococcus pyogenes*, cause tissue necrosis (Chapnick and Abter 1996). In addition, the infectious process activates the coagulation system, which in turn produces local vascular thrombosis and infarction. Bacterial heparinase production contributes to this process. As the infection progresses, pressure increases within the soft tissues causing further impairment of blood supply (File and Tan 1995).

The diagnosis of necrotizing soft tissue infections is usually made at the time of surgical exploration. Securing a diagnosis non-invasively is very difficult; this contributes to diagnostic delay and the ultimate demise of many patients (Sutherland and Meyer 1994, Low and McGeer 1998). The clinical presentation is often mistaken for simple cellulitis. However, pain in the affected region and systemic toxicity are more pronounced than would be expected in simple cellulitis (Bisno and Stevens 1996). Despite recommendations for the diagnostic use of computed tomography (CT) and magnetic resonance imaging (MRI) studies in these infections (Loh et al 1997, Wysoki et al 1997), the best diagnostic strategy is to perform surgical exploration when clinical features raise the possibility of necrotizing soft tissue infection (McHenry et al 1995, Majeski and Majeski 1997). Initially, diagnostic surgical exploration can be very limited in scope; small incisions under local anaesthesia serve to establish the presence or absence of fascial and muscle necrosis. Frozen section examination of tissue specimens will establish the diagnosis if the gross findings at surgical exploration leave any doubt (Stamenkovic and Lew 1984, Majeski and Majeski 1997). Although limited surgical interventions are appropriate for diagnostic purposes, there is no role for conservative surgical treatment strategies (Urschel et al 1997).

Treatment of necrotizing soft tissue infections entails early surgical debridement, fluid resuscitation, antibiotics and general cardiorespiratory supportive care to maintain vital organ function (Table 28.1; Gozal et al 1986, Bosshardt et al 1996). After diagnostic delay, the most common pitfall in treatment is inadequacy of surgical debridement. Debridement should be early and aggressive; all necrotic tissue must be excised (Urschel et al 1993, McHenry et al 1995). "Incision and drainage" approaches are not appropriate. These infections are characterized by necrotic tissue and watery drainage, as opposed to the viable tissue and pus that typify localized bacterial abscesses.

Table 28.1— Management principles for necrotizing soft tissue infections

Clinical suspicion
Early surgical exploration
Aggressive and repetitive debridement
Antibiotics
Cardiopulmonary support
Nutritional support
Hyperbaric oxygen (if available)

Repeat debridement, sometimes on a daily basis, should be done until the local infectious process has been arrested (Rea and Wyrick 1970, Pessa and Howard 1985). After sepsis is controlled, coverage of the wound is usually obtained by skin grafting.

Intravenous fluid resuscitation, mechanical ventilation and inotropic support are instituted according to established principles for managing septic shock. These principles are reviewed elsewhere (Edwards 1993, Demling et al 1994, Dunn 1994). Nutritional support is instituted after urgent resuscitation and debridement are carried out. Antibiotic coverage should be broad spectrum, and anaerobic coverage is essential. Many antibiotic combinations are acceptable. Usually penicillin (or a cephalosporin), anaerobic coverage (clindamycin or metronidazole), and Gram-negative coverage (aminoglycoside, 3rd generation cephalosporin, or ciprofloxacin) are used together (Chapnick and Abter 1996). Antimicrobial therapy of life-threatening surgical infections has recently been reviewed in detail elsewhere (Shands 1993, Solomkin and Miyagawa 1994, File and Tan 1995). Antibiotics are modified after gram stains and culture reports become available. In addition, the information gained during surgical exploration (tissues involved with necrotic process) also points to one of several specific clinical–bacteriologic entities that are reviewed below.

Hyperbaric oxygen therapy has an uncertain role in the management of necrotizing soft tissue infections. Some studies suggest a survival benefit (Gozal et al 1986, Riseman et al 1990, Brown et al 1994), but others do not (Darke et al 1977, Pessa and Howard 1985). Survival from Clostridial myonecrosis is probably improved by hyperbaric oxygen therapy (Jackson and Waddell 1973, Darke et al 1977). For other types of necrotizing soft tissue infection, hyperbaric oxygen therapy may hasten local wound healing and closure (Riseman et al 1990, Elliott et al 1996). Most investigators agree on one point; hyperbaric oxygen therapy

is not as important as urgent surgical intervention. Debridement should take priority over patient transfer to a hyperbaric oxygen facility.

Despite aggressive therapy, the mortality of necrotizing soft tissue infections remains high (15–50%; Chapnick and Abter 1996). Factors associated with increased mortality include extent of soft tissue involvement, delay in diagnosis, inadequate debridement, advanced age and truncal involvement (Rea and Wyrick 1970, Pessa and Howard 1985, Bosshardt et al 1996). Chest wall involvement is particularly ominous: survival is rare (Urschel et al 1997, Hammainen and Kostiainen 1998).

Specific syndromes

Many authors have stressed the importance of a unified approach to necrotizing soft tissue infections (Dellinger 1981, Kaiser and Cerra 1981, Urschel et al 1997). The initial diagnostic and management approach is similar for all of the entities within the spectrum of necrotizing soft tissue infections. Previous complex classification schemes were not relevant for the initial care of patients; confused clinicians were left without practical management algorithms (Sutherland and Meyer 1994). Nevertheless, there are several distinct clinical–bacteriological entities that should be recognized (Table 28.2). After initial treatment has been instituted, subtle differences in management for the various specific syndromes become important (Giuliano et al 1977, Low and McGeer 1998). However, it is worth reiterating that the broad general principles of diagnosis and treatment outlined above are undoubtedly more important than the specifics discussed below. Three of the major necrotizing soft tissue infections will be reviewed: necrotizing fasciitis type I (polymicrobial), necrotizing fasciitis type II (group A streptococcal), and Clostridial myonecrosis (gas gangrene). Finally, several other non-clostridial myonecrosis entities will be briefly described.

Necrotizing fasciitis type I (polymicrobial)

Necrotizing fasciitis usually occurs after trauma or surgery (Wilson 1952, Green et al 1996). In type I, the subcutaneous fat and fascia overlying muscle are prominently involved, but in the late stages extension occurs into the muscle tissue itself. Anaerobes and facultative bacteria act synergistically to cause tissue destruction. The clinical pace of disease is usually somewhat slower than that seen with type II (streptococcal) necrotizing fasciitis and clostridial myonecrosis, but its overall severity and lethality should not be

Table 28.2—Necrotizing soft tissue infections – major clinical entities

Infection	Predisposing factors	Bacteriology	Dominant features	Management
Necrotizing fasciitis type I (polymicrobial)	Surgery, trauma, diabetes mellitus	Anaerobes, Gram-negative aerobic bacilli	Necrosis of fat and fascia, may have gas	Debridement, broad spectrum antibiotics, intensive care support
Necrotizing fasciitis type II (group A streptococcal)	Surgery, minor trauma, varicella	*Streptococcus pyogenes*	Rapidly progressing necrosis of multiple tissue layers, no gas, shock	Debridement, Penicillin & clindamycin, intensive care support
Clostridial myonecrosis (gas gangrene)	Trauma, surgery, spontaneous (cancer)	Clostridial species	Fulminant myonecrosis, Prominent gas formation	Debridement, Penicillin & clindamycin, intensive care support, hyperbaric oxygen

underestimated. Clinicians often mistake it for simple wound cellulitis, but severe pain and systemic toxicity are out of proportion to that expected with cellulitis. The diagnosis is easily established by making a small skin incision and passing a haemostat or probe through the subcutaneous tissues (Wilson 1952). In necrotizing fasciitis the subcutaneous and fascial layers lack resistance to this manoeuvre, a feature that indicates widespread tissue necrosis underneath seemingly viable skin. Gas may or may not be present in the soft tissues. Histology of affected tissues shows widespread necrosis of subcutaneous fat and fascia, with relative sparing of muscle. An acute inflammatory reaction, with many polymorphonuclear cells, is seen. Thrombosis of blood vessels and abundant bacteria are other typical histologic findings. Aggressive surgical debridement is the key to successful treatment.

Necrotizing fasciitis may occur in the perineum. This type of infection is usually secondary to urogenital or anorectal infections. It is termed Fournier's gangrene (Clayton et al 1990). Patients usually have a predisposing systemic illness, such as diabetes mellitus. Another distinct form of necrotizing fasciitis is that caused by salt water contamination of an otherwise minor skin wound. *Vibrio* species are responsible. The affected patients usually suffer from a predisposing condition, such as chronic liver disease. This form of necrotizing fasciitis is highly lethal (Howard and Bennett 1993).

Necrotizing fasciitis type II (group A streptococcal)

This type of necrotizing soft tissue infection is caused by virulent subtypes of *Streptococcus pyogenes* (Bisno and Stevens 1996, Low and McGeer 1998). The occurrence of outbreaks of streptococcal necrotizing fasciitis has set it apart from related infections, and captured the public's attention. It has gained considerable recent attention in the lay press where the bacteria is often referred to as "flesh-eating bacteria." The incidence of this infection seems to have increased since the early 1980s, but this could simply reflect improvements in diagnosis and reporting (Chapnick and Abter 1996). Alternatively, there is some evidence to suggest a true increase in incidence (Cleary et al 1992). It could be the result of an evolutionary trend towards greater organism virulence in the setting of a more immunologically naïve population (Cleary et al 1992, Low and McGeer 1998). The presence of the M1 and M3 proteins is associated with virulent infection. Most of the general features of necrotizing soft tissue infections apply to this particular entity, but the presence of gas in tissues is unusual. There are some other unique aspects of this condition that warrant further discussion.

Two specific predisposing factors are varicella infection and the use of non-steroidal anti-inflammatory drugs (NSAIDs). Although necrotizing fasciitis is rare in children, almost half of cases occur in the setting of varicella (Kaul et al 1997). NSAIDs may attenuate host immune responses and, therefore, they may predispose to, and adversely effect the outcome of, streptococcal necrotizing fasciitis (Brun-Buisson et al 1985, Bisno and Stevens 1996). However, some investigators have failed to find an increased incidence or severity of streptococcal necrotizing fasciitis in patients using NSAIDs (Choo et al 1997, Kaul et al 1997). Another distinct feature of this form of necrotizing fasciitis is its frequent association with streptococcal toxic shock syndrome (Stevens et al 1989). This syndrome is similar to that originally described for staphylococcal infections. Its features include a high fever, early onset of shock, multiple organ failure and a very high mortality rate. Approximately 50% of patients with streptococcal toxic shock syndrome have streptococcal necrotizing fasciitis as the initiating infection.

Treatment of type II necrotizing fasciitis is generally in keeping with the principles outlined above. Once the diagnosis has been established penicillin combined with clindamycin replaces the previous broad spectrum empiric antimicrobial therapy. The combination of clindamycin and penicillin appears to be superior to the traditional treatment with penicillin alone (Bisno and Stevens 1996). Finally, there is some evidence to support the use of intravenous immunoglobulin as an immunomodulator in this condition (Kaul et al 1997).

Clostridial myonecrosis (gas gangrene)

Clostridial myonecrosis is a distinct necrotizing infection of skeletal muscle (Altemeier and Fullen 1971, Hart et al 1983). As the older term gas gangrene suggests, muscle necrosis and gas production are prominent features of this illness. Most cases arise in the setting of recent surgery or trauma, but some arise spontaneously. *Clostridium perfringens* (formerly *C. welchii*) is the most common causative organism. This anaerobic Gram-positive spore-forming bacillus is widely distributed in soil, and it can be found within the gastrointestinal tract of animals and humans. The organism produces over 10 different exotoxins of which the α-toxin is the most important (McDonel 1980). The α-toxin hydrolyses cell membranes. It causes tissue necrosis, inactivates leukocytes and haemolyses red blood cells. In addition, the α-toxin has direct cardiodepressive effects.

The pathologic features of clostridial myonecrosis are very dramatic. Grossly, there is obvious release of gas upon surgically entering the involved muscle compartment. The muscle is oedematous, pale or grey, and it does not bleed or contract when cut. Unlike the other necrotizing infections described above, clostridial myonecrosis shows very little inflammation on histologic examination. This lack of inflammatory host response goes along with the classic fulminant clinical course of clostridial myonecrosis. The infection rapidly advances, often over a matter of hours.

Surgical debridement and antibiotics are the mainstays of treatment. As for necrotizing infections caused by group A streptococci, clindamycin combined with penicillin is preferable to penicillin alone (Chapnick

and Abter 1996). Hyperbaric oxygen is of greater benefit for clostridial myonecrosis than it is for other necrotizing infections (Shupak et al 1984, Rudge 1993). This is logical, since clostridial myonecrosis is a monomicrobial anaerobic infection. After aggressive debridement and stabilization, hyperbaric oxygen therapy should be instituted if available. It inhibits clostridial growth and arrests α-toxin production (Kindwall 1992).

Spontaneously occurring clostridial myonecrosis is usually caused by *Clostridium septicum* (Kornbluth et al 1989). The organism spreads to muscle haematogenously from a small break in the normal gastrointestinal mucosal barrier. It usually occurs in patients suffering from either colon cancer or leukaemia.

Other non-clostridial myonecrosis entities

Anaerobic streptococcal myonecrosis is a necrotizing infection of the skeletal muscle that clinically resembles clostridial myonecrosis (Chambers et al 1974, Swartz 1995). Compared with clostridial myonecrosis, the pace of this infectious process is slower and gas production is not as marked. Anaerobic streptococcal myonecrosis is a polymicrobial infection. General treatment principles of necrotizing soft tissue infections are applicable.

Aeromonas hydrophilia is a facultatively anaerobic, Gram-negative bacillus, which causes a fulminant myonecrosis (Heckerling et al 1983, Hennessy et al 1988). The rapidity of the infectious process is similar to that of clostridial myonecrosis, but gas production is not a consistent feature. The infection usually occurs in the setting of penetrating freshwater trauma. Aggressive surgical debridement and antibiotic coverage for Gram-negative rods are the essential features of treatment.

References

Altemeier WA, Fullen WD. (1971) Prevention and treatment of gas gangrene. *JAMA* 217: 806–813.

Bisno AL, Stevens DL. (1996) Streptococcal infections of skin and soft tissues. *N Engl J Med* 334: 240–245.

Bosshardt TL, Henderson VJ, Organ CH, Jr. (1996) Necrotizing soft-tissue infections. *Arch Surg* 131: 846–852.

Brown DR, Davis NL, Lepawsky M, et al. (1994) A multicenter review of the treatment of major truncal necrotizing infections with and without hyperbaric oxygen therapy. *Am J Surg* 167: 485–489.

Brun-Buisson CJ, Saada M, Trunet P, et al. (1985) Haemolytic streptococcal gangrene and non-steroidal anti-inflammatory drugs. *Br Med J* 290: 1786.

Chambers CH, Bond GF, Morris JH. (1974) Synergistic necrotizing myositis complicating vascular injury. *J Trauma* 14: 980–984.

Chapnick EK, Abter EI. (1996) Necrotizing soft-tissue infections. *Infect Dis Clin North Am* 10: 835–855.

Choo PW, Donahue JG, Platt R. (1997) Ibuprofen and skin and soft tissue superinfections in children with varicella. *Ann Epidemiol* 7: 440–445.

Clayton MD, Fowler JE, Jr, Sharifi R, et al. (1990) Causes, presentation and survival of 57 patients with necrotizing fasciitis of the male genitalia. *Surg Gynecol Obstet* 170: 49–55.

Cleary PP, Kaplan EL, Handley JP, et al. (1992) Clonal basis for resurgence of serious Streptococcus pyogenes disease in the 1980's. *Lancet* 339: 518–521.

Darke SG, King AM, Slack WK. (1977) Gas gangrene and related infection: classification, clinical features and aetiology, management and mortality. A report of 88 cases. *Br J Surg* 64: 104–112.

Das I, Jayatunga AP, Symonds JM. (1996) Pyomyositis: an unusual infection due to Staphylococcus aureus. *J R Coll Surg Edinb* 41: 182–183.

Dellinger EP. (1981) Severe necrotizing soft-tissue infections: Multiple disease entities requiring a common approach. *JAMA* 246: 1717–1721.

Demling RH, Lalonde C, Ikegami K. (1994) Physiologic support of the septic patient. *Surg Clin North Am* 74: 637–658.

Dunn DL. (1994) Gram-negative bacterial sepsis and sepsis syndrome. *Surg Clin North Am* 74: 621–635.

Edwards JD. (1993) Management of septic shock. *Br Med J* 306: 1661–1664.

Elliott DC, Kufera JA, Myers RAM. (1996) Necrotizing soft tissue infections: risk factors for mortality and strategies for management. *Ann Surg* 224: 672–683.

File TM, Jr, Tan JS. (1995) Treatment of skin and soft-tissue infections. *Am J Surg* 169(suppl): 27S–33S.

Freischlag JA, Ajalat G, Busuttil RW. (1985) Treatment of necrotizing soft tissue infections: the need for a new approach. *Am J Surg* 149: 751–755.

Gibson RK, Rosenthal SJ, Lukert BP. (1984) Pyomyositis: increasing recognition in temperate climates. *Am J Med* 77: 768–772.

Giuliano A, Lewis F, Hadley K, Blaisdell FW. (1977) Bacteriology of necrotizing fasciitis. *Am J Surg* 134: 52–57.

Gozal D, Ziser A, Shupak A, et al. (1986) Necrotizing fasciitis. *Arch Surg* 121: 233–235.

Green RJ, Dafoe DC, Raffin TA. (1996) Necrotizing fasciitis. *Chest* 110: 219–229.

Hammainen P, Kostiainen S. (1998) Postoperative necrotizing chest-wall infection. *Scand Cardiovasc J* 32: 243–245.

Hart GB, Lamb RC, Strauss MB. (1983) Gas gangrene. *J Trauma* 23: 991–1000.

Heckerling PS, Stine TM, Pottage JC, Jr, et al. (1983) Aeromonas hydrophilia myonecrosis and gas gangrene in a nonimmunocompromised host. *Arch Intern Med* 143: 2005–2007.

Hennessy MJ, Ballon-Landa GR, Jones JW, et al. (1988) Aeromonas hydrophilia gas gangrene: A case report of management with surgery and hyperbaric oxygenation. *Orthopedics* 1: 289–293.

Howard RJ, Bennett NT. (1993) Infections caused by halophilic marine Vibrio bacteria. *Ann Surg* 217: 525–531.

Jackson RW, Waddell JP. (1973) Hyperbaric oxygen in the management of clostridial myonecrosis (gas gangrene). *Clin Orthop* 96: 271–276.

Janevicius RV, Hann SE, Batt MD. (1982) Necrotizing fasciitis. *Surg Gynecol Obstet* 154: 97–102.

Kaiser RE, Cerra FB. (1981) Progressive necrotizing surgical infections: A unified approach. *J Trauma* 21: 349–355.

Kaul R, McGeer A, Low DE, et al. (1997) Population-based surveillance for group A streptococcal necrotizing fasciitis: clinical features, prognostic indicators and microbiologic analysis of 77 cases. *Am J Med* 103: 18–24.

Kessler HA, Trenholme GM, Harris AA, et al. (1980) Acute myopathy associated with influenza A/Texas/1/77 infection. Isolation of virus from a muscle biopsy specimen. *JAMA* 243: 461–462.

Kindwall EP. (1992) Uses of hyperbaric oxygen therapy in the 1990s. *Cleve Clin J Med* 59: 517–528.

Kornbluth AA, Danzig JB, Bernstein LH. (1989) Clostridium septicum infection and associated malignancy. *Medicine* 68: 30–37.

Levin MJ, Gardner P, Waldvogel FA. (1971) An unusual infection due to Staphylococcus aureus. *N Engl J Med* 284: 196–198.

Liu LX, Weller PF. (1994) Trichinosis and tissue nematodes. In: Isselbacher KJ, Braunwald E, Wilson JD, et al. ed. *Harrison's principles of internal medicine. 13th ed.* New York: McGraw-Hill, pp. 914–916.

Loh NN, Chien IY, Cheung LP, et al. (1997) Deep fascial hyperintensity in soft-tissue abnormalities as revealed by T-2 weighted MR imaging. *Am J Roentgenol* 168: 1301–1304.

Low DE, McGeer A. (1998) Skin and soft tissue infection: necrotizing fasciitis. *Curr Opin Infect Dis* 11: 119–123.

Majeski J, Majeski E. (1997) Necrotizing fasciitis: improved survival with early recognition by tissue biopsy and aggressive surgical treatment. *South Med J* 90: 1065–1068.

McDonel JL. (1980) *Clostridium perfringens* toxins (type A, B, C, D, E). *Pharmacol Ther* 10: 617–655.

McHenry CR, Piotrowski JJ, Petrinic D, et al. (1995) Determinants of mortality for necrotizing soft-tissue infections. *Ann Surg* 221: 558–565.

Mejlszenkier JD, Safran AP, Healy JJ, et al. (1973) The myositis of influenza. *Arch Neurol* 29: 441–443.

Pessa ME, Howard RJ. (1985) Necrotizing fasciitis. *Surg Gynecol Obstet* 161: 357–361.

Rea WJ, Wyrick WJ. (1970) Necrotizing fasciitis. *Ann Surg* 172: 957–964.

Riseman JA, Zamboni WA, Curtis A, et al. (1990) Hyperbaric oxygen therapy for necrotizing fasciitis reduces mortality and the need for debridements. *Surgery* 108: 847–850.

Rotstein OD, Pruett TL, Simmons RL. (1985) Mechanisms of microbial synergy in polymicrobial surgical infections. *Rev Infect Dis* 7: 151–170.

Rudge FW. (1993) The role of hyperbaric oxygenation in the treatment of clostridial myonecrosis. *Military Med* 158: 80–83.

Shands JW, Jr. (1993) Empiric antibiotic therapy of abdominal sepsis and serious perioperative infections. *Surg Clin North Am* 73: 291–306.

Shupak A, Halpern P, Ziser A, et al. (1984) Hyperbaric oxygen therapy for gas gangrene casualties in the Lebanon War, 1982. *Isr J Med Sci* 20: 323–326.

Solomkin JS, Miyagawa CI. (1994) Principles of antibiotic therapy. *Surg Clin North Am* 74: 497–517.

Stamenkovic I, Lew PD. (1984) Early recognition of potentially fatal necrotizing fasciitis: the use of frozen section biopsy. *N Engl J Med* 310: 1689–1693.

Stevens DL, Tanner MH, Winship J, et al. (1989) Severe group A streptococcal infections associated with a toxic shock-like syndrome and scarlet fever toxin A. *N Engl J Med* 321: 1–7.

Sutherland ME, Meyer AA. (1994) Necrotizing soft-tissue infections. *Surg Clin North Am* 74: 591–607.

Swartz MN. (1995) Myositis. In: Mandell GL, Bennett JE, Dolin R, eds. *Principles and practice of infectious diseases. 4th ed.* New York: Churchill Livingstone, pp. 929–936.

Urschel JD, Horan TA, Unruh HW. (1993) Necrotizing chest wall infection. *Comp Surg* 12: 37–43.

Urschel JD, Takita H, Antkowiak JG. (1997) Necrotizing soft tissue infections of the chest wall. *Ann Thorac Surg* 64: 276–279.

Wilson B. (1952) Necrotizing fasciitis. *Am Surg* 18: 416–431.

Wysoki MG, Santora TA, Shah RM, et al. (1997) Necrotizing fasciitis: CT characteristics. *Radiology* 203: 859–863.

29

Skeletal muscle in liver disease

Shinzo Kato, Shohei Ohnishi, Hajime Yamazaki and Hiromasa Ishii

Introduction

Until recently, little attention has been paid to skeletal muscle by hepatologists. For example, muscle cramps, which are recognized as common symptoms in patients with cirrhosis, were often ignored. However, in the mid 1980s, Konikoff and Theodor (1986) reported that 88% of cirrhotic patients had muscle cramps in calf muscles, which were characterized by severe pain. These symptoms occurred several times a week, mainly at rest or during sleep, and they lasted for a few minutes. Subsequently, there were few articles on musculoskeletal problems in liver disease, and muscle cramps were usually not referred to (Asherson and Hughes 1991, van den Bogaerde and Beynon 1999). However, muscle function or physical fitness becomes more important, when the patient's quality of life is taken into account, for the subsequent management of chronic liver disease. The assessment of skeletal muscle strength and capacity of physical exercise in patients with liver disease is a difficult problem to address in clinical practice. In this chapter, we will focus on recent advances in the pathogenesis of muscle disorders in liver disease.

It has been noted that there is a close metabolic relationship between skeletal muscle and liver—sharing pathways or intermediate metabolites, such as glucose utilization and ammonia metabolism—and both of these tissues rely on, or compensate for, each other. The interaction of liver and muscle in the regulation of metabolism of carbohydrate, fat and protein has been reviewed elsewhere (Hellerstein and Munro 1994). It may be of interest to point out that oriental traditional medicine has already described the relationship between liver and muscle in Su wen, the first volume of the Huang di nei jiing, written around BC 2nd century in China (Anonymous, 2nd Century BC). Without knowledge of metabolic interactions, but from subjective symptoms and physical findings, they indicated that there was a close relationship between skeletal muscle and liver (Anonymous, 2nd Century BC). Over two thousand years later, these suppositions have been confirmed, and it has been reported that liver disease influences muscle volume and strength, and that musculoskeletal problems affect quality of life measures in patients with chronic liver diseases (Thuluvath and Triger 1994, Caregaro et al 1996, Tarter et al 1997, Beyer et al 1999).

Muscle volume and strength in patients with liver disease

In cirrhotic patients, muscle volume and strength is reduced irrespective of its aetiology (Thuluvath and Triger 1994, Caregaro et al 1996). Protein calorie malnutrition occurs in alcoholic patients with liver disease (Mendenhall et al 1995), and both chronic and acute alcohol administration or exposure causes a reduction in skeletal muscle protein synthesis, which may contribute to the pathogenic mechanism of altered muscle function in alcoholic liver disease (Preedy et al 1999). However, malnutrition is also found in patients with non-alcoholic liver cirrhosis. The prevalence and severity of protein and energy malnutrition have been assessed in patients with cirrhosis, and found to be comparable in alcoholic and viral cirrhosis (Thuluvath and Triger 1994, Caregaro et al 1996). Energy malnutrition, defined as triceps skinfold thickness (TSF) and/or midarm muscle circumference (MAMC) below the 5th percentile of standard values, was found in 34% of the patients with liver cirrhosis. Patients below the 5th percentile for MAMC and/or TSF showed lower survival rates compared with patients above the 5th percentile (Caregaro et al 1996). The malnutrition in cirrhotic patients correlates well with the clinical severity of the liver disease, but not with its aetiology (Caregaro et al 1996).

Alcoholics with cirrhosis have reduced measures of isokinetic muscle strength in both eccentric and concentric muscle movements compared with normal controls. This is not different from non-alcoholic cirrhotics (Tarter et al 1997), suggesting that cirrhosis rather than alcoholism per se or poor intake of food is responsible for the muscle weakness. Patients with cirrhosis have a smaller lean body mass than controls, and lower nutritional protein status than alcoholics without cirrhosis (Estruch et al 1993). Lean body mass correlates with muscle weakness in cirrhotics (Andersen et al 1998). These data suggest that reductions in muscle volume and strength in cirrhotic patients are related to malfunction or metabolic disturbances in the liver.

Exercise in patients with cirrhosis

Bed rest or restriction of physical activity has previously been recommended for the management of patients with chronic liver disease. However, it may cause muscle atrophy, which is often found in cirrhotics, as stated above. It is now assumed that patients with well-compensated chronic liver disease should be advised to engage in physical exercise as it may improve their feeling of well being (Kawase et al 1993, Ritland et al 1983, Courneya and Friedenreich 1999). Further, maintenance of muscle volume and function may be beneficial to compensate for reduced hepatic function in the metabolism of carbohydrate, amino acids or ammonia. However, there is an essential need to know whether physical exercise really improves the physical condition of patients with cirrhosis, and how much exercise can be recommended to patients at different stages of liver diseases.

Impairment of insulin sensitivity, and the failure to compensate for it by an increase in insulin secretion, both contribute to the development of glucose intolerance or diabetes in cirrhotic patients (Petrides 1994). Physical exercise is expected to have beneficial effects on glucose metabolism. However, single bouts of moderate exercise increase insulin sensitivity only during euglycaemia, but not during the more physiological condition of hyperglycaemia (Petrides et al 1997). This suggests that a single bout of exercise may not have beneficial effects in cirrhotics.

Furthermore, excessive exercise may be detrimental. Plasma levels of ammonia become higher during and after physical exercise, and the return to baseline level of plasma ammonia during rest is delayed in patients with well-compensated liver disease (Dietrich et al 1990). This suggests that cirrhotic patients with subclinical hepatic encephalopathy may be more prone to the development of hepatic coma by strenuous exercise. Moderate physical exercise also results in a marked impairment in the renal function of only those patients with ascites with concomitant activation of rennin-aldosterone and sympathetic nervous system (Salo et al 1997). Therefore, bed rest is recommended to cirrhotic patients with ascites who respond poorly to diuretics, but patients with moderate sodium retention may perform moderate physical exercise without any negative influence on renal function (Salo et al 1997).

Cirrhotic patients with portal hypertension should be aware of the potential risks of bleeding during moderate to severe exercise. Changes of portal pressure have been estimated by hepatic venous pressure gradients (HVPG), the difference between wedged hepatic venous pressure (WHVP) and free hepatic venous pressure (FHVP). Moderate exercise increases portal pressure, which may therefore increase the risk of variceal bleeding (Garcia-Pagàn et al 1996).

Since moderate physical exercise has no detrimental effects on renal function in cirrhotic patients with ascites with no or mild activation of renin-aldosterone and sympathetic nervous system (Salo et al 1997), moderate exercise can be recommended to patients with well-compensated liver disease without oesophageal varices. Further studies are needed to evaluate the beneficial and detrimental effects of exercise. This should be coupled with measures defining the optimum intensity and duration of exercise, and the severity of liver disease and its complications.

Muscle problems after liver transplantation

Musculoskeletal problems disturb the quality of life in patients who undergo orthotopic liver transplantation (OLT). Nicholas et al (1994) reported that 37% of OLT patients noted some extremity weakness, and 18% noted pain in an extremity. Although general endurance was markedly improved after OLT, employment ratios fell from 87% to 60%. The presence of musculoskeletal symptoms, marital status and duration of liver disease were associated with the employment ratio. Persons with no musculoskeletal system problems were 7.8 times more likely to be working post-transplant compared with subjects with musculoskeletal problems (Nicholas et al 1994). Belle et al (1997) examined the quality of life of 346 adults before and 1 year after liver transplantation from three clinical centers in the USA. Although the largest number of patients were distressed by fatigue and muscle weakness, both before transplantation and 1 year after surgery, they were no longer limited at follow-up, whereas 58% of the patients were prevented by their disease from going to work or school before surgery.

Hussaini et al (1998) assessed changes in body composition after transplantation using dual energy X-ray absorptiometry and total body potassium. After liver transplantation there was an initial fall in body weight due to a loss of lean mass. Lean mass did not recover after transplantation, although there was an increase in fat mass (Hussaini et al 1998). They also investigated risk factors for the decline in lean mass after OLT, and found a positive correlation between the fall in lean mass and cumulative dose of steroids administered at 2–5 months, and length of hospital stay after transplantation. A hypercatabolic post-transplant state, immobility, lack of exercise and steroid induced catabolism of muscle may have been responsible for this (Hussaini et al 1998).

Exercise programmes after OLT are important strategies to improve quality of life measures and morbidity. Beyer et al (1999) reported preoperative physical fitness, and muscle strength after OLT, was 40–50% less than expected in the age-matched general population. Post-OLT, all patients underwent a supervised exercise programme for 8 to 24 weeks, and showed a significant increase in physical performance after OLT. One-year post surgery, general health was improved and perceived as "excellent" or "good" in all patients. This suggests that a supervised post-OLT exercise programme may improve physical fitness, muscle strength and functional performance in individuals with chronic liver disease (Beyer et al 1999).

Muscle cramps in patients with cirrhosis

Muscle cramps are painful and involuntary contractions (occurring at rest and/or during sleep), and now recognized as common symptoms in liver cirrhosis (Konikoff and Theodor 1986, Kobayashi et al 1992, Abrams et al 1996). Although not life threatening, these symptoms affect quality of life measures. Chronic muscle cramps are more common in patients with cirrhosis (52%), compared with patients with chronic hepatitis (7.5%) or congestive heart failure (20%). Weekly or daily cramps have been reported in 22% of patients with liver cirrhosis (Abrams et al 1996). The prevalence of cramps is related to the duration of cirrhosis and the severity of liver dysfunction. Presence of ascites, low values of mean arterial pressure and high values of plasma renin activity are independent predictive factors for the occurrence of cramps (Angeli et al 1996). Factors such as age, gender, alcoholic liver disease, electrolytes and diuretic use are similar among cirrhotic patients with and without cramps (Abrams et al 1996).

For the treatment of muscle cramps in cirrhotics, weekly infusion of human albumin may be effective (Angeli et al 1996). Quinine is widely used for idiopathic leg cramps, but it may have serious side-effects and should be avoided in patients with liver disease (Mandal et al 1995, Farver and Lavin 1999). Niuche-shen-qi-wan (TJ-107; herbal medicine) is currently used with safety in Japan for the treatment of muscle cramps in cirrhotics (Motoo et al 1997). Taurine (Matsuzaki et al 1993, Yamamoto 1994, 1996) or zinc sulphate (Kugelmas 2000) may also be beneficial for muscle cramps in cirrhotics. Further research is necessary to develop safe and effective treatment for this condition.

Conclusion

Musculoskeletal problems in liver disease are common. There is a fundamental need to pay more attention to muscle in patients with chronic liver disease and to improve their muscle strength and their quality of life for life-long periods. However, further work is needed to evaluate the necessary strength and duration of suitable exercise regimens and to determine beneficial and detrimental effects.

References

Abrams GA, Concato J, Fallon MB. (1996) Muscle cramps in patients with cirrhosis. *Am J Gastroenterol* 91: 1363–1366.

Andersen H, Borre M, Jakobsen J, et al. (1998) Decreased muscle strength in patients with alcoholic liver cirrhosis in relation to nutritional status, alcohol abstinence, liver function, and neuropathy. *Hepatology* 27: 1200–1206.

Angeli P, Albino G, Carraro P, et al. (1996) Cirrhosis and muscle cramps: evidence of a causal relationship. *Hepatology* 23: 264–273.

Anonymous. (BC 2nd Century) Huang di nei jing: (The yellow emperor's canon of internal medicine) Su Wen (The first volume of the Huang di nei jing) In English Nathan Sivin (1993) "Huang ti nei ching" In: Michael Loewe, editor. *Early Chinese Texts: A Bibliographical Guide, vol. 2, Early China Special Monograph Series.* Berkeley, CA: Society for the Study of Early China, Institute of East Asian Studies, University of California, Berkeley.

Asherson RA, Hughes GRV. (1991) Musculoskeletal problems in liver disease. In: McIntyre NM, Benhamou JP, Bircher J, et al. eds. *Oxford Textbook of Hepatology.* Oxford: Oxford Medical Publications, pp. 1260–1263.

Belle SH, Porayko MK, Hoofnagle JH, et al. (1997) Changes in quality of life after liver transplantation among adults. National Institute of Diabetes and Digestive and Kidney Diseases (NIDDK) Liver Transplantation Database (LTD). *Liver Transpl Surg* 3: 93–104.

Beyer N, Aadahl M, Strange B, et al. (1999) Improved physical performance after orthotopic liver transplantation. *Liver Transpl Surg* 5: 301–309.

Caregaro L, Alberino F, Amodio P, et al. (1996) Malnutrition in alcoholic and virus-related cirrhosis. *Am J Clin Nutr* 63: 602–609.

Courneya KS, Friedenreich CM. (1999) Physical exercise and quality of life following cancer diagnosis: a literature review. *Ann Behav Med* 21: 171–179.

Dietrich R, Bachmann C, Lauterburg BH. (1990) Exercised-induced hyperammmonenia in patients with compensated chronic liver disease. *Scand J Gastroenterol* 25: 329–334.

Estruch R, Nicolas JM, Villegas E, et al. (1993) Relationship between ethanol-related diseases and nutritional status in chronically alcoholic men. *Alcohol Alcohol* 28: 543–550.

Farver DK, Lavin MN. (1999) Quinine-induced hepatotoxicity. *Ann Pharmacother* 33: 32–34.

Garcia-Pagàn JC, Santos C, Barbera JA, et al. (1996) Physical exercise increases portal pressure in patients with cirrhosis and portal hypertension. *Gastroenterology* 111: 1300–1306.

Hellerstein MK, Munro HN. (1994) Interaction of liver, muscle, and adipose tissue in the regulation of metabolism in response to nutritional and other factors. In: Arias IM, Boyer JL, Fausto N, et al. eds. *The Liver Biology and Pathobiology*. 3rd ed. New York: Raven Press, pp. 1169–1191.

Hussaini SH, Soo S, Stewart SP, et al. (1998) Risk factors for loss of lean body mass after liver transplantation. *Appl Radiat Isot* 49: 663–664.

Kawase K, Yoshida T, Moriwaki H, et al. (1993) Effect of physical training on clinical and laboratory parameters in patients with compensated liver cirrhosis. *Acta hepatologica Japonica* 34: 950–959.

Kobayashi Y, Kawasaki T, Yoshimi T, et al. (1992) Muscle cramps in chronic liver diseases and treatment with antispastic agent. *Dig Dis Sci* 37: 1145–1146.

Konikoff F, Theodor E. (1986) Painful muscle cramps. A symptom of liver cirrhosis? *J Clin Gastroenterol* 8: 669–672.

Kugelmas M. (2000) Preliminary observation: oral zinc sulfate replacement is effective in treating muscle cramps in cirrhotic patients. *J Am Coll Nutr* 19: 13–15.

Mandal AK, Abernathy T, Nelluri SN, et al. (1995) Is quinine effective and safe in leg cramps? *J Clin Pharmacol* 35: 588–593.

Matsuzaki Y, Tanaka N, Osuga T. (1993) Is taurine effective for treatment of painful muscle cramps in liver cirrhosis? *Am J Gastroenterol* 88: 1466–1467.

Mendenhall C, Roselle GA, Gartside P, et al. (1995) Relationship of protein calorie malnutrition to alcoholic liver disease: a reexamination of data from two Veterans Administration Cooperative Studies. *Alcohol Clin Exp Res* 19: 635–641.

Motoo Y, Taga H, Yamaguchi Y, et al. (1997) Effect of niuche-shen-qi-wan on painful muscle cramps in patients with liver cirrhosis: a preliminary report. *Am J Chin Med* 25: 97–102.

Nicholas JJ, Oleske D, Robinson LR, et al. (1994) The quality of life after orthotopic liver transplantation: an analysis of 166 cases. *Arch Phys Med Rehabil* 75: 431–435.

Petrides AS. (1994) Liver disease and diabetes mellitus. *Diabetes Rev* 2: 1–18.

Petrides AS, Matthews DE, Esser U. (1997) Effect of moderate exercise on insulin sensitivity and substrate metabolism during post-exercise recovery in cirrhosis. *Hepatology* 26: 972–979.

Preedy VR, Reilly ME, Patel VB, et al. (1999) Protein metabolism in alcoholism: effects on specific tissues and the whole body. *Nutrition* 15: 604–608.

Ritland S, Petlund CF, Knudsen T, et al. (1983) Improvement of physical capacity after long-term training in patients with chronic active hepatitis. *Scand J Gastroenterol* 18: 1083–1087.

Salo J, Gervara M, Fernandez-Espararach G, et al. (1997) Impairment of renal function during moderate physical exercise in cirrhotic patients with ascites: relationship with the activity of neurohormonal systems. *Hepatology* 25: 1338–1342.

Tarter RE, Panzak G, Switala J, et al. (1997) Isokinetic muscle strength and its association with neuropsychological capacity in cirrhotic alcoholics. *Alcohol Clin Exp Res* 21: 191–196.

Thuluvath PJ, Triger DR. (1994) Evaluation of nutritional status by using anthropometry in adults with alcoholic and nonalcoholic liver disease. *Am J Clin Nutr* 60: 269–273.

Van den Bogaerde J, Beynon HLC. (1999) Musculoskeletal problems in liver disease. In: McIntyre NM, Benhamou JP, Bircher J, et al. eds. *Oxford Textbook of Hepatology*. Oxford: Oxford Medical Publications, pp. 1260–1263.

Yamamoto S. (1994) Oral taurine therapy for painful muscle cramp in liver cirrhosis. *Am J Gastroenterol* 89: 457–458.

Yamamoto S. (1996) Plasma taurine in liver cirrhosis with painful muscle cramps. *Adv Exp Med Biol* 403(-HD-): 597–600.

30

Free radical mediated injury
in skeletal muscle

David Mantle

Introduction

Free radicals are highly reactive, transient chemical species characterized by the presence of unpaired electrons (conventionally denoted by a point suffix). In biological systems, free radicals may be centred on oxygen, carbon or sulphur atoms. Most research has focused on oxygen centred radicals, with the hydroxyl ($OH^\bullet$) and superoxide ($O_2^{-\bullet}$) radicals considered to be the most physiologically important primary tissue damaging free radical species. Other important radicals derived from these primary species include the peroxyl ($RO_2^\bullet$) and alkoxyl ($RO^\bullet$) species. Hydrogen peroxide (H_2O_2) is also capable of inducing tissue damage directly, but it is not classed as a free radical since it does not contain unpaired electrons; these species ($OH^\bullet$, $O_2^{-\bullet}$, $RO_2^\bullet$, $RO^\bullet$, H_2O_2) are, therefore, conveniently classed as reactive oxygen species (ROS; Cheeseman and Slater 1993).

In relatively few instances, free radicals may perform beneficial functions, e.g. $O_2^{-\bullet}$ generation during phagocytic activation and nitric oxide ($NO^\bullet$) in the regulation of vascular tone. In general however, free radicals are unwanted by-products of normal aerobic cellular metabolism, with the potential to damage the various intracellular organelles and components (nucleic acids, lipids and proteins) on which normal cell function depends. Free radical reactions are characterized by induction, propagation and termination phases (of particular importance in the peroxidation of the lipid components of cell membranes). The $OH^\bullet$ radical is the most oxidizing (reactive) free radical species (estimated half-life in the nanosecond range) found in biological systems, reacting indiscriminately with most biomolecular targets at near diffusion-controlled rates, and capable of causing extensive damage within a small radius of the site of production. Compared with $OH^\bullet$, $O_2^{-\bullet}$ is a less damaging free radical species, with the potential for greater discrimination in biomolecular targeting (half-life approx. 10 μsec); $O_2^{-\bullet}$ can also react rapidly with $NO^\bullet$ to form peroxynitrite, a potentially damaging species which can generate $OH^\bullet$ radicals. Hydrogen peroxide has the capacity to oxidise intracellular components directly, although it is a relatively unreactive species compared with the above (half-life in the order of minutes), and it is able to diffuse between and within cells, and cross cell membranes. The main significance of H_2O_2 is as a source of $OH^\bullet$, via reaction with transition metal ions (as described in the following section). Nucleic acids, lipids and proteins are attacked by $OH^\bullet$, whereas $O_2^{-\bullet}$ and H_2O_2 do not attack DNA or initiate lipid per-

oxidation. Proteins are susceptible to attack by all ROS species, either by oxidation of essential sulph-hydryl (SH) groups, or other chemical modifications of the constituent amino acids (Del Maestro 1980).

Sources of reactive oxygen species

The principal source of ROS generation in vivo results from leakage of electrons from the mitochondrial respiratory chain (i.e., from intermediate electron carriers onto molecular oxygen) during oxidative metabolism to generate ATP (Chance et al 1979), a process of particular importance in skeletal muscle, given the unique requirement and ability of this tissue to undertake rapid changes in oxygen flux and energy supply during contraction. It has been estimated that 3–5% of total electron flux results in the formation of ROS, which in a typical human (even at rest) corresponds to the production of approximately 2 Kg $O_2^{-\bullet}$ per annum (Chance et al 1979). Additionally, $O_2^{-\bullet}$ generation results from the action of specific enzymes (principally oxidases) during the metabolism of purines (xanthine oxidases), catecholamines (monoamine oxidase), prostanoids (lipoxygenase) and xenobiotics (cytochrome P_{450}). The generation of ROS via the above reactions may be exacerbated by such factors as failure of Ca^{2+} homeostasis, following trauma or ischaemia. The main source of $OH^\bullet$ generation is the interaction of H_2O_2 with transition metal ions (normally sequestered by binding proteins in vivo) such as Fe^{2+} or Cu^{2+} (Fenton reaction), as well as via the Fe^{2+} catalysed reaction between H_2O_2 and $O_2^{-\bullet}$ (Haber–Weiss reaction). Hydroxyl radicals are also generated from peroxynitrite (which rapidly disproportionates at physiological pH), which is in turn rapidly formed via reaction between $NO^\bullet$ and $O_2^{-\bullet}$ under appropriate stoichiometric conditions. Hydrogen peroxide is formed via the dismutation of $O_2^{-\bullet}$ catalysed by the enzyme superoxide dismutase, and it is also produced via the action of several other oxidase enzymes (e.g. amino acid oxidases). Nitric oxide ($NO^\bullet$) is synthesised from the amino acid L-arginine by the enzyme nitric oxide synthase in endothelial cells (as a regulator of vascular tone), as well as in many other cell types (where it may act as a second messenger, readily diffusing through cell membranes). In contracting skeletal muscle, sarcolemmal-associated nitric oxide synthase may regulate sarcolemmal depolarization, as well as vasodilatation in response to exercise (via a cGMP mediated pathway). The total body generation of NO$^\bullet$ is appreciable, of the order of 1 mmol/day based on quantitation of NO_2^- and NO_3^- (end products of NO$^\bullet$ oxidation) in plasma (Wennmalm et al 1994). As well as the above, activated phagocytes are capable of generating $O_2^{-\bullet}$, H_2O_2 and NO$^\bullet$ species (as well as hypochlorous acid, HOCl), all of which may contribute to tissue injury during inflammation. In addition, ROS may amplify the inflammation process by upregulation of various species involved in the inflammatory response, particularly via activation of the nuclear transcription factor NFKβ, which in turn upregulates pro-inflammatory cytokines and leukocyte adhesion molecules. There is evidence that NO$^\bullet$ may act as a messenger for cell fusion in chick embryonic myoblasts, and that NFKβ-dependent expression of nitric oxide synthase (NOS) is an important step in myoblast membrane fusion (Lee et al 1997).

Antioxidants

Cells are protected from free radical induced damage by a variety of endogenous radical scavenging proteins, enzymes and chemical (water or lipid soluble) compounds. These include metal ion sequestering proteins such as transferrin (Fe^{2+}) or ceruloplasmin (Cu^{2+}), and ROS metabolizing enzymes such as superoxide dismutase ($O_2^{-\bullet}$), catalase and glutathione peroxidase (H_2O_2); the latter seleno-enzyme forms part of a self regenerating cycle involving reduced/oxidized glutathione and the enzyme glutathione reductase. Glutathione peroxidase and superoxide dismutase occur in both mitochondrial and cytoplasmic isoforms. As well as biothiols such as glutathione, other important antioxidant compounds include α-tocopherol (vitamin E), ascorbic acid (vitamin C), uric acid, and the histidine-containing dipeptides carnosine and anserine (Buettner 1993). The contribution of α-tocopherol, ascorbic acid (and the enzymic cofactor selenium; Se) to the oxidative stability of muscle is largely influenced by diet. The tissue concentrations of carnosine and anserine are less affected by diet; their levels vary widely with species and muscle type (Chan and Decker 1994). Muscle tissues with a high oxidative capacity (slow-twitch muscles) have higher antioxidant levels than those with a lower oxygen demand (fast-twitch muscles), therefore Type I fibres contain higher activities of superoxide dismutase, catalase and glutathione peroxidase than Type II fibres (Assayama et al 1986). However in relative terms, the antioxidant capacity of skeletal muscle is amongst the lowest of the various tissues within the body (which may be a

reflection of the comparatively low resting oxygen demand of this tissue), although muscle tissue can show remarkable adaptive increases in antioxidant capacity in response to sustained exercise. In addition to the above, a number of plant-derived dietary antioxidant compounds such as carotenoids and flavonoids have also been identified (Bors et al 1996). There are also a number of enzymic mechanisms to salvage and repair oxidative damage to nucleic acids and proteins; these may be of particular importance in counteracting oxidative damage caused by the OH$^\bullet$ radical, which may not be efficiently scavenged by antioxidants because of its high reactivity with potential biomolecular targets.

Measurement of reactive oxygen species

Because of their high reactivity (second order rate constants approx. 10^6–10^9 M^{-1} s^{-1}) and short half-lives (10^{-9}–10^{-4} s), direct analysis of ROS (especially in humans) is extremely difficult (Jackson et al 1984, Halliwell and Grootveld 1987). The only technique capable of direct analysis of ROS is that of electron spin resonance (ESR) spectroscopy, which is normally used in conjunction with chemical compounds (typically nitrone derivatives) known as spin trapping agents, which produce longer lived radicals with distinctive ESR spectra. Phenyl-N-tert-butylnitrone (PBN) and 5,5-dimethyl-1-pyroline-N-oxide (DMPO) are used in the identification and quantification of OH$^\bullet$ and $O_2^{-\bullet}$ respectively (Knecht and Mason 1993). Because of the low steady-state concentrations of ROS formed in tissues, this technique suffers from relatively poor sensitivity, and there are also ethical considerations precluding the administration of potentially toxic spin trapping agents to patients. An alternative approach has been described to measure OH$^\bullet$ levels in vivo, based on its reaction with salicylate, which is less toxic than other spin traps, and reacts rapidly with OH$^\bullet$ to form stable products. One of the main products formed is dihydroxybenzoic acid (DHBA), which does not occur endogenously in biological systems, and which can be quantitated via high performance liquid chromatography (HPLC) with electrochemical detection.

Another approach to quantification of ROS is based on the indirect analysis of ROS damage products in tissues, resulting from oxidative attack on nucleic acids, lipids and proteins (Reznick and Packer 1994). Oxidative damage to DNA is typically quantified by measurement of the marker 8-OH-guanosine in tissues or urine via HPLC with electrochemical detection (Okamura et al 1997). Malondialdehyde and 4-hydroxynonenol (end products of the peroxidation of polyunsaturated fatty acids) are used as markers to assess ROS-induced lipid peroxidation. The most common assay procedure for measurement of these compounds has relied on the derivitization reaction obtained by boiling the sample with acidified thiobaribuic acid; this methodology is now known to be subject to artefact (Marshall et al 1985). Quantification of lipid peroxidation via measurement of diene conjugation in tissues or urine is regarded as a similarly non-specific and unreliable methodology. Lipid peroxides are now quantified via HPLC with electrochemical detection, either directly or following reaction with thiobarbituric acid (Reznick and Packer 1994).

The measurement of oxidized nucleic acids has been of particular value in investigating the role of ROS in malignant disease (Shigenaga et al 1990) and lipid peroxidation in the pathogenesis of cardiovascular disease and degenerative disorders of the central nervous system (CNS) (Hall et al 1990). However, because of the unique structure of skeletal muscle tissue, measurement of protein oxidative damage is arguably of greatest relevance to research into the role of ROS in muscle disorders. Oxidative damage by ROS to proteins induces a variety of structural modifications (Giulivi and Davies 1993), the most extensively studied being the formation of carbonyl groups in amino acid residues (especially proline, arginine, lysine and threonine), which can be quantified via reaction with 2,4-dinitrophenylhydrazine to form a yellow protein hydrazone adduct. The quantification of carbonyl groups by this method is considered to be a reliable hallmark of oxidative damage to proteins, providing appropriate practical precautions (e.g., removal of nucleic acids from samples) are taken into account. Protein carbonyl levels can be measured by a colourimetric assay procedure (for determination of total protein oxidation (Reznick and Packer 1994), or by immunoblotting analysis using commercially available monoclonal antibodies to 2,4-dinitrophenylhydrazine (for identification of oxidative damage to individual proteins; Levine et al 1994). Experiments in vitro, based on exposure of normal muscle tissue sections to $OH^\bullet$ or $O_2^{-\bullet}$ radicals generated via ^{60}Co gamma irradiation (with subsequent analysis of target protein damage via histochemical, immunocytochemical and electron microscopical techniques), have shown evidence for the differential susceptibility of muscle proteins to oxidative damage. Mitochondria and mitochondrial associated proteins appeared to be

particularly susceptible to oxidative damage, and it was speculated that this may represent the principal initial route of free radical induced damage within muscle tissue (Haycock et al 1996a).

Levels of $NO^\bullet$ have been determined by both direct (electrochemical, ESR spectroscopy) and indirect (measurement of NO_2^- or NO_3^- oxidation product levels) methods. Oxidative damage to proteins by $NO^\bullet$ results in the formation of nitrotyrosine, which can be quantified via HPLC with electrochemical detection, or immunologically using commercial antibodies against nitrotyrosine. In addition, NOS can be measured via analysis of mRNA (Northern blotting, in situ hybridization, polymerase chain reaction), DNA analysis (Southern blotting, polymerase chain reaction) or protein analysis (Western blotting, immunocytochemistry) (MacAllister and Vallance 1996). Another indirect method of quantifying ROS activity is by measurement of changes in tissue antioxidant levels, either as total antioxidant capacity or as the activity of individual antioxidant enzymes or chemical compounds. Decreases in antioxidant levels, for example, following surgically-induced ischaemia reperfusion injury, have been interpreted as an indirect measure of ROS production (Khaira et al 1996). Alternatively, moderate increases in ROS generation may result in adaptive increases in antioxidant levels (e.g., following exercise training).

Cellular damage resulting from an imbalance between the free radical generating and scavenging systems described above (oxidative stress) has been implicated in the pathogenesis of a variety of disorders, including diseases of muscle (Halliwell and Gutteridge 1990) as reviewed in the following sections.

Reactive oxygen species in normal muscle contraction

There is increasing evidence that ROS are produced during strenuous skeletal muscle contraction (resulting from increased O_2 consumption and mitochondrial electron transport flux), and that they may contribute to the development of muscle fatigue via modulation of contractile function. Data supporting this hypothesis include:

- direct (ESR spectroscopy) and indirect (markers of lipid and protein oxidation or altered antioxidant capacity) evidence for increased ROS production in contracting muscle

- evidence that ROS scavenging compounds reduce the development of muscle fatigue
- evidence that pharmacological or dietary depletion of muscle antioxidant capacity increases the degree of muscle fatigue after exercise.

Much of the research in this area has utilized the rat diaphragm muscle (in vivo or in vitro) as a model system for electrophysiological and biochemical studies. Rats subjected to severe inspiratory resistive loading show increased production of ROS (associated with respiratory failure) as demonstrated directly by ESR spectroscopy analysis (Borzone et al 1994). Diaphragmatic fatigue in rats induced by electrical stimulation or mechanical ventilation showed a subsequent inverse relation between the reduction in contractile force (approx. 60%) and increase in the levels of 2, 3- and 2, 5-dihydroxybenzoate, suggesting diaphragmatic fatigue is related to the generation of $OH^\bullet$ (Hasegawa et al 1997). In cats, an increase in $OH^\bullet$ production in vivo during intermittent static contraction of the triceps surae muscles has been demonstrated, quantitated by formation of ortho, meta and para tyrosines formed by the reaction between $OH^\bullet$ and phenylalanine (administered prior to contraction). The rate of tyrosine production increased in proportion to the percentage maximum muscle tension developed, showing that significant free radical production can occur before the onset of fatigue. Pre-treatment with deferoxamine or dimethyl urea decreased the rate of formation of tyrosines during and after contraction (O'Neill et al 1996). Induction of diaphragmatic fatigue (via electrical stimulation) in rats resulted in increased generation of $O_2^{-\bullet}$, as measured via interaction with cytochrome c in the perfusate, which correlated with the reduction (approx. 90%) in contractile force; this stimulation-induced increase in $O_2^{-\bullet}$ was blocked in the presence of added superoxide dismutase (Kolbeck et al 1997). In rats subjected to resistive breathing exercise, there was a reduction in contractile function, increase in lipid peroxidation and decrease in reduced/oxidized glutathione ratio in diaphragms from vitamin E deficient rats compared with controls (Anzueto et al 1993). Infusion of a free radical generating solution (iron/ADP complex) into rat diaphragm showed a reduction in contractility, which was largely prevented by concomitant infusion of superoxide dismutase (Nashawati et al 1993). Although the precise cellular mechanisms by which ROS may alter the force-generating capacity of muscle remain to be elucidated, specific interactions with contractile proteins, sarcoplasmic reticulum associated ATPases/Ca^{2+} pumps, and mitochondrial

proteins have been suggested. Significantly greater force production was observed in rat diaphragm strips (fatigued via electrical stimulation) following inclusion of the disulphide reducing agent dithiothreitol (DTT, approx. 1 mM) in the perfusing fluid, suggesting that downregulation of force production during fatigue may result from ROS-induced oxidation of SH groups on key contractile proteins (Diaz et al 1998). Sustained contractile activity, resulting from prolonged (4 day) electrical stimulation of rabbit fast-twitch muscle caused partial (50% reduction) inactivation of sarcoplasmic reticulum associated Ca^{2+} ATPase; although markers of lipid peroxidation and SH group levels were unaltered, protein carbonyl groups were increased by about 50% in sarcoplasmic reticulum from stimulated muscles. Immunoblotting analysis with anti-dinitrophenyl hydrazine and anti-nitrotyrosine antibodies revealed strong labelling of the Ca^{2+} ATPase, indicating that inactivation of the enzyme results from protein oxidation and peroxynitrite-mediated tyrosine nitration (Klebl et al 1998). A link between strenuous physical exercise, oxidative stress and perturbation of K^+ homeostasis has also been reported; in muscle derived cells treated with t-butyl hydroperoxide (TBA; as a source of ROS) the inward K^+ transport system was particularly sensitive to oxidative exposure (Sen et al 1995). In addition to the intracellular generation of ROS described above, there is evidence that contractile stimulation of isolated diaphragm muscle fibres results in the release of $O_2^{-\bullet}$ (measured via reaction with cytochrome c) into the extracellular space (Reid et al 1992).

Reactive oxygen species and exercise training/antioxidant supplementation

There is evidence that trained individuals (human or animal) have an advantage, compared with untrained individuals, in resisting the effects of oxidative stress induced muscle fatigue, resulting from adaptive increases in the overall antioxidant capacity and/or specific antioxidant enzymes (Dekkers et al 1996). Thus in rats, treadmill endurance training improved the ability of diaphragm muscle to resist exercise-induced oxidative stress via upregulation of antioxidant enzymes. There was also evidence from this study that acute exercise may cause oxidative damage in rat diaphragm by activation of the inflammatory pathway (via measurement of interleukin 1), and that endurance training may minimize such acute exercise-induced oxidative stress (Ohishi et al 1997). Exhaustive running exercise in rats results in increased levels of lipid peroxidation in heart and skeletal muscles (with a corresponding increase in creatine kinase efflux into serum), with the generation of peroxidation products persisting in the latter tissue for a relatively long time after exercise. Endurance training decreased the susceptibility of tissues to oxidative damage by ROS, the effect being more pronounced in muscle tissue than in liver (Frakiewicz-Jozko et al 1996). Exhaustive swimming exercise training also increased levels of antioxidant enzymes/antioxidant capacity in muscle, with a corresponding reduction in muscle tissue damage assessed via sarcoplasmic reticulum integrity and lipid peroxidation levels (Venditti and Meo 1997).

In humans, jump training resulted in increased levels of antioxidant enzymes in muscle tissue (but not in blood), with a corresponding decrease in muscle-derived creatine kinase efflux, compared with untrained controls; however muscle lipid peroxidation levels were not significantly different in the trained and untrained groups (Ortenblad et al 1997). Intermittent sprint cycle training (over several weeks) has been shown (via muscle biopsy) to increase the levels of muscle antioxidant enzymes (Hellsten et al 1996). Although participation in events such as long distance triathlons would be expected to generate ROS, because of the large consumption of oxygen, there was no evidence for oxidative damage in muscle tissue (quantified by efflux of lipid peroxidation markers, and reduced/oxidized glutathione ratios, in blood) in trained triathletes after competition (Margaritis et al 1997).

There is also evidence that manipulation of endogenous or exogenous (dietary) antioxidants may reduce exercise-induced fatigue and muscle damage associated with increased ROS generation. Supplementation with vitamin E reduced muscle membrane disruption (as assessed by creatine kinase efflux) resulting from increased ROS production (determined as plasma malondialdehyde) associated with high intensity resistance exercise in weight trained males, compared with placebo (McBride et al 1998). Exhaustive cycling exercise in male subjects resulted in a 70% decrease in muscle urate levels, with a corresponding threefold increase in allantoin levels. The concentration of urate in muscle rapidly (within 3 min) reverted to resting levels after exercise, although levels of allantoin in muscle and plasma remained elevated during recovery. These data support the importance of urate

as a free radical scavenger in vivo in preventing exercise induced muscle injury (Hellsten et al 1997).

In rats, swimming exercise resulted in oxidative stress (quantified via measurement of lipid peroxidation and reduced/oxidized glutathione ratio) in several tissues, including muscle; the level of oxidative stress was significantly reduced by prior administration of indolamines such as melatonin (Hara et al 1997). Finally, there is evidence that dietary magnesium deficiency in rats enhances free radical production and tissue damage in skeletal muscle. Swelling of mitochondria and disorganization of the sarcoplasmic reticulum were evident (from electron microscopy) with corresponding increases in $OH^\bullet$ radicals (via ESR/spin trapping) and lipid peroxidation products (TBA reactive substances), and decreased levels of SH groups (compared with controls) (Rock et al 1995).

Reactive oxygen species and muscular dystrophy

Duchenne and Becker muscular dystrophies (DMD and BMD) are X-linked (p21 region) degenerative disorders of human skeletal muscle, resulting from genetic mutations causing altered expression (quantity and/or molecular size) of dystrophin (Hoffman et al 1987), a 427 kDa protein which links actin filaments within the muscle cell to a complex of plasma membrane associated glycoproteins (Ervasti and Campbell 1993). In general terms, the milder BMD clinical phenotype is associated with mutations that maintain an open reading frame in the dystrophin gene, producing a truncated, partially functional protein. In DMD, where the clinical phenotype is more severe, the genetic reading frame is completely disrupted (Koenig et al 1988). While the absence of dystrophin is generally believed to weaken the muscle cell membrane, resulting in contractile-induced cellular damage, the precise degenerative mechanism causing necrosis and muscle wastage is currently unknown. Research directed towards patient therapy has been based mainly on gene/myoblast transfer therapy (Mulligan 1993). Unfortunately, technical difficulties have continued to limit the effectiveness of these techniques (Morgan 1994), and it is, therefore, of value to develop novel pharmacologically-based alternative therapeutic strategies. To develop such strategies on a rational basis, it is necessary to have some understanding of the factors that underly the process of dystrophic muscle degeneration. In this regard, it has been suggested that ROS may contribute to the pathogenesis of muscular dystrophy (Murphy and Kehrer 1989). A potential role for ROS in the latter disorder was first indicated following the recognition of a form of muscular dystrophy in animals induced by nutritional deficiencies of vitamin E and/or selenium (Bradley and Fell 1980). More recently, excessive production of ROS resulting from proteolytic activation of the xanthine dehydrogenase/xanthine oxidase system (following increased cell membrane permeability and altered intracellular Ca^{2+} homeostasis) has been suggested (Austin 1990). Direct experimental confirmation of such hypotheses is difficult because of the technical problems involved in the identification and quantification of ROS in tissues in vivo, as outlined above. Much of the previous research into the potential role of ROS in the pathogenesis of muscular dystrophy has, therefore, been based on indirect methods that quantify ROS damage products in tissues from human or animal model systems. A number of problems have become apparent in the interpretation of such data, on which the hypothesis of ROS involvement in muscular dystrophy was based. These include:

- the choice of unsuitable animal models, with little relevance to the human form of muscular dystrophy (Muzuno 1998)
- the quantification of ROS induced damage by measurement of lipid peroxidation products via the thiobarbituric acid reaction, the methodology of which is now known to be subject to artefact (Marshall et al 1985)
- changes in antioxidant levels in muscle or blood of DMD patients reported variously to show increased, decreased or unchanged levels (Austin et al 1992)
- the use of non-specific markers of oxidative stress, such as the quantification of oxidized biomolecules via increased chemiluminescence in urine (Lissi et al 1994).

However several lines of evidence obtained recently suggest that oxidative stress and free radical mediated injury may lead to muscle necrosis in muscular dystrophy. Using myotube cultures from normal and dystrophin deficient (mdx) mice, the susceptibilities of cells to different metabolic stresses in vitro has been determined. Dystrophin deficient cells were more susceptible to ROS-induced injury compared with normal cells, but the two populations were equally susceptible to other forms of metabolic stress. This differential response appeared to be specifically related to dystrophin expression, since undifferentiated myoblasts (which do not express dystrophin) from normal and mdx mice were equally sensitive to oxidative stress

(Rando et al 1998). In addition, mdx mice have been shown to have significantly increased levels of the $OH^\bullet$ tissue damage biomarker o-tyrosine compared with controls (although mitochondrial enzyme activities measured in muscle homogenates were not impaired; Hauser et al 1995). Therefore, the absence of dystrophin appears to render muscle specifically more susceptible to ROS induced injury.

Further data in support of the hypothesis for ROS involvement in muscle cell damage in DMD have recently been reported; levels of protein carbonyl in quadriceps muscle biopsy were significantly increased (2.1-fold) in tissue from DMD cases compared with controls, indicating that cellular proteins present in DMD muscle are present in a quantitatively more oxidized state (Haycock et al 1996b). A subsequent investigation based on immunoblotting analysis of quadriceps muscle biopsy tissue from DMD, BMD and control cases, using commercially available monoclonal antibody against dinitrophenylhydrazine has been reported; this study showed that most structural and contractile proteins, whether in normal or pathological tissue, contain perhaps a surprisingly high proportion of oxidized protein. However, a heavily oxidized protein species with a molecular mass of about 125 kDa was identified in DMD/BMD tissue, which was completely absent (or present in very low levels) in control tissue. The intensity of the latter immunoreactive band was less in muscle from BMD cases compared with DMD samples, suggesting a correlation between the immunoblotting intensity of this oxidized protein species and the overall clinical severity of the muscle disease. It was not possible to assign an identity to the above species based on molecular mass alone, but, using N-terminal sequencing, an amino acid sequence corresponding to myosin was identified, indicating that the 125 kDa immunoreactive protein is a heavily oxidized form of myosin (Haycock et al 1998). The question as to why myosin should be particularly susceptible to ROS-induced oxidative damage in dystrophic muscle, and what role such damage may play in the disease process, remains to be determined.

In this regard, the recent finding of the absence of NOS in DMD or mdx muscle is of note. Nitric oxide synthase is normally present in the sarcolemma of fast-twitch fibres, associated with dystrophin protein (via a Gly LeuGly Phe (GLGF) protein associated motif present near the enzymic N-terminus that anchors the latter into the cell membrane), and it is responsible for the generation of $NO^\bullet$ (Bredt 1996). In addition to its useful physiological roles, $NO^\bullet$ is generally regarded as a potentially damaging species (as noted above). However, investigations using NONOates as physiologically relevant sources of $NO^\bullet$ now suggest that $NO^\bullet$ may have protective effects against the damaging action of ROS, i.e., that $NO^\bullet$ at low concentrations protects against toxicity by $O_2^-{}^\bullet$, H_2O_2 and alkyl peroxides, and that NONOates protect cultured cells against H_2O_2 and alkyl hydroperoxide mediated toxicity (Wink et al 1995). The novel $NO^\bullet$ releasing drug C87-375 prevents $O_2^-{}^\bullet$ formation during stretch induced programmed myocyte cell death (Cheng et al 1995). It is possible, therefore, that $NO^\bullet$ may have a role in preventing oxidative damage in normal muscle, and that absence of dystrophin and NOS in dystrophic muscle results in increased oxidative damage. There have been reports indicating a possible increase in oxidative stress in patients with myotonic dystrophy. In these patients, levels of free radicals in blood (assessed via ESR spectroscopy using DMPO spintrap) and serum lipid peroxide levels were increased relative to controls, with corresponding reductions in some serum antioxidants (vitamin E, coenzyme Q_{10}, selenium; Ihara et al 1995). However, there is as yet no obvious link between possible ROS involvement in the disease process and the known gene defect responsible for myotonic dystrophy, which codes for a protein kinase putatively responsible for modulation of Na^+ channels in skeletal muscle (Mounsey et al 1995).

Therapeutic trials of antioxidants in muscle disease

Since the 1970's, a number of therapeutic trials of antioxidants have been carried out in DMD and BMD patients, including vitamin E and/or selenium (Edwards et al 1984, Gamstorp et al 1986, Jackson et al 1989), allopurinol (Griffiths et al 1985), coenzyme Q_{10} (Folkers and Simonsen 1995) and superoxide dismutase (SOD; Stern et al 1982). No beneficial effects were demonstrated in any of the above trials, controlled in accordance with previous recommendations (Dubowitz and Heckmatt 1980). In particular, exogenous administration of SOD or catalase (orally or via injection) is unlikely to prove of benefit, given the lack of absorption from the gut (Greenwald 1990) and the circulatory half-lives of 8 and 20 min respectively; however, conjugation with polythylene glycol or albumin has been shown to increase bioavailability of these enzymes (Radak et al 1996).

It is of note that 21 aminosteroid-related compounds (lazeroids) have recently been shown to promote myogenesis in cultured cells, which is thought to be mediated via scavenging of ROS (Vernier et al 1995). Both vitamin E derived U83836E and glucocorticoid derived U74389P enhanced myogenesis of dystrophin deficient cultures, as determined by the number of myotubes, and levels of myosin light chain, α-actin and acetylcholine receptors (Metzinger et al 1994). The potential of these compounds in the treatment of DMD and BMD remains to be determined.

Free radicals and muscle ischaemia–reperfusion injury

Muscle ischaemia may occur as a result of vascular insufficiency, following trauma or during surgery, and may result in serious tissue injury (in some cases necessitating amputation) as well as the possibility of multi-organ involvement (particularly remote organ injury to the lungs, liver and gut). Direct evidence that ROS are formed during ischaemia–reperfusion of skeletal muscle has been obtained via ESR spectroscopy/spin trapping, using reduced rectoris femoris muscle flap as a microsurgical model system in the rat (De Santis and Pinelli 1994). The generation of $OH^\bullet$ in vivo has also been demonstrated in a rat hind limb model of ischaemia–reperfusion injury, using 4-hydroxybenzoate as a radical trap, with quantitation of the hydroxylation product 3,4-dihydroxybenzoate (3,4-DHBA) via HPLC with electrochemical detection. Perfusion with cross-linked haemoglobin-SOD-catalase reduced $OH^\bullet$ generation in this model system (D'Agnillo and Chang 1997). Postischaemic infusion of phosphoenolpyruvate and ATP significantly reduced ischaemia–reperfusion injury in rabbit skeletal muscle. This protective effect is most likely to be a result of supplementation of intracellular ATP stores, rather than inhibition of $O_2^-{}^\bullet$ from infiltrating neutrophils (Hickey et al 1995). Sarcoplasmic reticulum vesicles isolated from rabbit skeletal muscle were exposed to $OH^\bullet$ (generated by reaction between H_2O_2 and Fe^{2+}); data obtained suggest $OH^\bullet$ denatures $Ca^{2+}ATPase$ by directly attacking the ATP binding site, and therefore, occupation of the active site by ATP protects against $OH^\bullet$ induced loss of enzymatic activity and Ca^{2+} transport. The depletion of ATP that occurs during ischaemia may enhance the toxic effect of $OH^\bullet$ at the time of reperfusion (Xu et al 1997). Reperfusion injury in isolated rabbit hind limb muscle is at least partially mediated by polymorphonuclear leukocytes. Free radical scavengers such as SOD and catalase reduce leukocyte dependent injury, suggesting oxygen derived free radicals are mediators of tissue injury and/or involved in the interaction between leukocytes and the microvascular system (Oredsson et al 1995). The 21 aminosteroid-related lazeroid compounds have been shown to limit ischaemic injury in muscle tissue. The mechanism of action is uncertain, but it may include scavenging of lipid peroxyradicals, iron binding or direct membrane interaction. High grade partial ischaemia of skeletal muscle was associated with iron delocalization, which persisted on reperfusion. Each compound investigated (U74500A and U74389F) achieved a similar membrane protecting effect, despite lack of iron binding by U74389F, suggesting direct interaction with the cell membrane (Fantini et al 1996). Pre-treatment with the lazeroid U74006F can effectively decrease the rise of vascular resistance and preserve contractile function of rat muscle following ischaemia-reperfusion (Korompilas et al 1997). In skeletal muscle reperfusion injury in rabbits, administration of lazeroid U74389G significantly decreased reperfusion muscle necrosis; the beneficial effects were observed whether the lazeroid was administered prior to ischaemia or prior to reperfusion, and they were independent of leukocyte sequestration (Hoballah et al 1996).

References

Anzueto A, Andrade FH, Maxwell LC, Levine SM, Lawrance RA, Jenkinson SG. (1993) Diaphragmatic function after resistive breathing in vitamin E deficient rats. *J Appl Physiol* 74: 267–271.

Assayama K, Dettbarn WD, Burr IM. (1986) Differential effects of denervation on free radical scavenging enzymes in slow and fast muscle of the rat. *J Neurochem* 46: 604–609.

Austin L. (1990) How the lack of dystrophin may upset calcium regulation and lead to oxidative damage. In: Kakulas BA, Mastaglia FL, eds. *Pathogenesis and therapy of Duchenne and Becker muscular dystrophy*. New York: Raven Press, pp. 69–82.

Austin L, di Niese M, McGregor A, Arthur H, Gurusinghe A, Gould MK. (1992) Potential oxyradical damage and energy status in individual fibres from degenerative muscle diseases. *Neuromusc Disord* 75: 27–33.

Bors W, Heller W, Michel C, Steffmaier K. (1996) Flavonoids and polyphenols: chemistry and biology. In: Cadenas E, Packer L, eds. *Handbook of antioxidants*. New York: Marcel Dekker, pp. 409–466.

Borzone G, Zhao B, Merola AJ, Berliner L, Clanton TL. (1994) Detection of free radicals by electron spin resonance in rat diaphragm after resistive loading. *J Appl Physiol* 7: 812–818.

Bradley R, Fell BF. (1980) Myopathies in animals. In: Walton JN ed. *Disorders of voluntary muscle, 3rd edition*. London: Churchill-Livingston, pp. 824–872.

Bredt DS. (1996) Targeting nitric oxide to its targets. *Proc Soc Exper Biol Med* 211: 41–48.

Buettner GR. (1993) The pecking order of free radicals and antioxidants: lipid peroxidation, α-tocopherol and ascorbate. *Arch Biochem Biophys* 300: 535–543.

Chan KM, Dekker EA. (1994) Endogenous skeletal muscle antioxidants. *Crit Rev Food Sci Nutr* 34: 403–426.

Chance B, Sies H, Boveris A. (1979) Hydroperoxide metabolism in mammalian organs. *Physiol Rev* 59: 527–605.

Cheeseman KH, Slater TF. (1993) An introduction to free radical biochemistry. *Br Med Bull* 49: 481–493.

Cheng W, Li B, Kajstura J, et al. (1995) Stretch induced programmed myocyte cell death. *J Clin Invest* 96: 2247–2259.

D'Agnillo F, Chang TM. (1997) Reduction of hydroxyl radical generation in a rat hindlimb model of ischaemia reperfusion injury using cross-linked haemoglobin-superoxide dismutase-catalase. *Art Cells Blood Sub Immobil Biotech* 25: 163–180.

Dekkers JC, van Doornen LJ, Kemper HC. (1996) The role of antioxidant vitamins and enzymes in the prevention of exercise induced muscle damage. *Sports Med* 21: 213–238.

Del Maestro RL. (1980) An approach to free radicals in medicine and biology. *Acta Physiol Scand* 492: 153–168.

De Santis G, Pinelli M. (1994) Microsurgical model of ischemia reperfusion in rat muscle: evidence of free radical formation by spin trapping. *Microsurg* 15: 655–659.

Diaz PT, Costanza MJ, Wright VP, Julian MW, Diaz JA, Clanton TL. (1998) Dithiothreitol improves recovery from in vitro diaphragm fatigue. *Med Sci Sports Exercise* 30: 421–426.

Dubowitz V, Heckmatt JZ. (1980) Management of muscular dystrophy. *Br Med Bull* 36: 139–144.

Edwards RHT, Jones DA, Jackson MJ. (1984) An approach to treatment trials in muscular dystrophy with particular reference to agents influencing free radical damage. *Med Biol* 62: 143–147.

Ervasti JM, Campbell KP. (1993) A role for the dystrophin glycoprotein complex as a transmembrane link between laminin and actin. *J Cell Biol* 122: 809–823.

Fantini GA, Kirschner RE, Chiao JJ. (1996) Reperfusion injury of post ischemic skeletal muscle is attenuated by the 21 aminosteroids U-74389F and U74500A independent of iron binding. *Surgery* 120: 859–865.

Folkers K, Simonsen R. (1995) Two successful double blind trials with coenzyme Q$_{10}$ on muscular dystrophies and neurogenic atrophies. *Biochim Biophys Acta* 1271: 281–286.

Frakiewicz-Jozko A, Faff J, Sierddzan-Gabelska. (1996) Changes in concentrations of tissue free radical marker and serum creatine kinase during the post exercise period in rats. *Eur J Appl Physiol Occupat Physiol* 74: 470–474.

Gamstorp I, Gustavson KH, Helstrom O, Nordgren B. (1986) A trial of selenium and vitamin E in boys with muscular dystrophy. *J Child Neurol* 1: 211–214.

Giulivi C, Davies KJA. (1993) Dityrosine and tyrosine oxidation products are endogenous markers for selective proteolysis of oxidatively modified red blood cell haemoglobin by proteasomes. *J Biol Chem* 268: 8752–8759.

Greenwald RA. (1990) Superoxide dismutase and catalase as therapeutic agents for human diseases: a critical review. *Free Rad Biol Med* 8: 201–209.

Griffiths RD, Cady EB, Edwards RHT, Wilkie DR. (1985) Muscle energy metabolism in Duchenne dystrophy studied by ^{31}P nmr: controlled trials show no effect of allopurinol. *Muscle Nerve* 8: 760–767.

Hall ED, Braughler JM, McCall JM. (1990) Role of oxygen radicals in stroke: effects of 21 aminosteroids (lazeroids). A novel class of antioxidants. *Prog Clin Biol Res* 361: 351–362.

Halliwell B, Grootveld M. (1987) The measurement of free radical reactions in humans. Some thoughts for future experimentation. *FEBS Lett* 213: 9–14.

Halliwell B, Gutteridge JMC. (1990) Role of free radicals and metal ions in human disease: an overview. *Methods Enzymol* 186: 1–85.

Hara M, Iigo M, Ontani R, Suzuki T, Reiter RJ, Hirata K. (1997) Administration of melatonin and related indoles prevents exercise induced cellular oxidative changes in rats. *Biol Sig* 6: 90–100.

Hasegawa A, Suzuki S, Matsumoto Y, Okobo T. (1997) In vivo fatiguing contraction of rat diaphragm produces hydroxyl radicals. *Free Rad Biol Med* 22: 349–354.

Hauser E, Hoger H, Bittner R, Widhalm K, Herknerk K, Lubec G. (1995) Oxyradical damage and mitochondrial enzyme activities in the mdx mouse. *Neuropaed* 26: 260–262.

Haycock JW, Jones P, Harris JB, Mantle D. (1996a) Differential susceptibility of human skeletal muscle proteins to free radical induced oxidative damage: a histochemical, immunocytochemical and electron microscopical study in vitro. *Acta Neuropath* 92: 331–340.

Haycock JW, McNeil S, Jones P, Harris JB, Mantle D. (1996b) Oxidative damage to muscle protein in Duchenne muscular dystrophy. *Neuroreport* 8: 357–361.

Haycock JW, McNeil S, Mantle D. (1998) Differential protein oxidation in Duchenne and Becker muscular dystrophy. *Neuroreport* 9: 2201–2207.

Hellsten Y, Apple FS, Sjodin B. (1996) Effect of sprint cycle training on activities of antioxidant enzymes in human skeletal muscle. *J Appl Physiol* 81: 1484–1487.

Hellsten Y, Tullson PC, Richter EA, Bangsbo J. (1997) Oxidation of urate in human skeletal muscle during exercise. *Free Rad Biol Med* 22: 169–174.

Hoballah JJ, Mohan CR, Schipper PH, Chalmers RT, Corson JD. (1996) Effects of the lazeroid U74389G (21 aminosteroid) on skeletal muscle reperfusion injury in rabbits. *Int Angiol* 15: 61–66.

Hoffmann EP, Brown RH, Kunkel LM. (1987) Dystrophin, the protein product of the Duchenne muscular dystrophy locus. *Cell* 51: 919–928.

Hickey MJ, Knight KR, Hurley JV, Lepore DA. (1995) Phosphoenol pyruvate/ATP enhances post-ischemic survival of skeletal muscle. *J Reconstruct Microsurg* 11: 415–422.

Ihara Y, Mori T, Namba A, Nobukini K, Sato K, Miyata S. (1995) Free radicals, lipid peroxides and antioxidants in blood of patients with myotonic dystrophy. *J Neurol* 242: 119–122.

Jackson MJ, Jones DA, Edwards RHT. (1984) Techniques for studying free radical damage in muscular dystrophy. *Med Biol* 62: 135–138.

Jackson MJ, Coakley J, Stokes M, Edwards RHT, Oster O. (1989) Selenium metabolism and supplementation in patients with Duchenne muscular dystrophy. *Neurol* 39: 655–659.

Khaira HS, Maxwell SRJ, Thomason H, Thorpe GHG, Green MA, Shearman CP. (1996) Antioxidant depletion during aortic aneurysm repair. *Br J Surg* 83: 401–403.

Klebl BM, Ayoub AT, Peite D. (1998) Protein oxidation, tyrosine nitration and inactivation of sarcoplasmic reticulum Ca^{2+}ATPase in low frequency stimulated rabbit muscle. *FEBS Lett* 422: 381–384.

Knecht KT, Mason RP. (1993) In vivo spin trapping of xenobiotic free radical metabolites. *Arch Biochem Biophys* 303: 185–194.

Koenig M, Monaco AP, Kunkel LM. (1988) The complete sequence of dystrophin predicts a rod shaped cytoskeletal protein. *Cell* 53: 219–228.

Kolbeck RC, She ZW, Callachan LA, Nosek TM. (1997) Increased superoxide production during fatigue in the perfused rat diaphragm. *Am J Respir Crit Care Med* 156: 140–145.

Korompilas AV, Chen LE, Seaber AV, Urbaniak JR. (1997) Studies of ischaemia reperfusion injury in skeletal muscle: efficacy of 21 amino steroids on microcirculation and muscle contraction after an extended period of warm ischemia. *J Orthopaed Res* 15: 512–518.

Lee KH, Kim DG, Shin NY, et al. (1997) NF Kappa β dependent expression of nitric oxide synthase is required for membrane fusion of chick embryonic myoblasts. *Biochem J* 324: 237–242.

Levine RL, Williams JA, Stadtman ER, Schacter E. (1994) Carbonyl assays for determination of oxidatively modified proteins. *Methods Enzymol* 233: 346–357.

Lissi EA, Salim Hanna M, Videla LA. (1994) Spontaneous urinary visible luminescence: characteristics and modification by oxidative stress related conditions. *Braz J Med Biol Res* 27: 1491–1505.

Macallister RJ, Vallance P. (1996) The L-arginine: nitric oxide pathway in the human cardiovascular system. *J Intl Fed Clin Chem* 8: 152–158.

Margaritis I, Tessier F, Richard MJ, Marconnet P. (1997) No evidence of oxidative stress after a triathlon race in highly trained competitors. *Intl J Sports Med* 18: 186–190.

Marshall PJ, Warso MA, Lands WE. (1985) Selective micro-determination of lipid peroxides. *Anal Biochem* 145: 192–199.

McBride JM, Kraemer WJ, Triplett-McBride T, Sebastianelli W. (1998) Effect of resistance exercise on free radical production. *Med Sci Sports Ex* 30: 67–72.

Metzinger L, Passaquin AC, Vernier A, Thiriet N, Warter JM, Poindron P. (1994) Lazeroids enhance skeletal myogenesis in primary cultures of dystrophin deficient mdx mice. *J Neurol Sci* 126: 138–145.

Morgan JE. (1994) Cell and gene therapy in Duchenne muscular dystrophy. *Hum Gene Therap* 5: 165–173.

Mounsey JP, Xu P, John JE, et al. (1995) Modulation of skeletal muscle sodium channels by human myotonin protein kinase. *J Clin Invest* 95: 2379–2384.

Mulligan RC. (1993) The basic science of gene therapy. *Science* 260: 926–932.

Murphy ME, Kehrer JP. (1989) Oxidation state of tissue thiol groups and content of protein carbonyl groups in chickens with inherited muscular dystrophy. *Biochem J* 260: 359–364.

Muzuno KOY. (1998) Pathogenesis of progressive muscular dystrophy: studies on free radical metabolism in an animal model. *Acta Nurol Scand* 77: 108–114.

Nashawati E, Dimarco A, Supinski G. (1993) Effects produced by infusion of a free radical generating solution into the diaphragm. *Am Rev Respir Dis* 147: 60–65.

Ohishi S, Kizaki T, Ookawara T, et al. (1997) Endurance training improves the resistance of rat diaphragm to exercise induced oxidative stress. *Am J Respir Crit Care Med* 156: 1579–1585.

Okamura K, Doi T, Hamada K. (1997) Effect of repeated exercise on urinary 8-hydroxydeoxyguanosine excretion in humans. *Free Rad Res* 26: 507–514.

O'Neill CA, Stebbins CL, Bonigut S, Halliwell B, Longhurst JC. (1996) Production of hydroxyl radicals in contracting skeletal muscle of cats. *J Appl Physiol* 81: 1197–1206.

Oredsson S, Quarfordt P, Plate G. (1995) Polymorpho-nuclear leukocytes increase reperfusion injury in skeletal muscle. *Int Angiol* 14: 80–88.

Ortenblad N, Madsenk D, Jurhuus MS. (1997) Antioxidant status and lipid peroxidation after short term maximal exercise in trained and untrained humans. *Am J Physiol* 272: 258–263.

Radak Z, Asano K, Inoue M, et al. (1996) Superoxide dis-mutase derivative prevents oxidative damage in liver and kidney of rats induced by exhausting exercise. *Eur J Appl Physiol Occup Physiol* 72: 189–194.

Rando TA, Disatnik MH, Yu Y, Franco A. (1998) Muscle cells from mdx mice have an increased susceptibility to oxidative stress. *Neuromusc Dis* 8: 14–21.

Reid MB, Shoj T, Moody MR, Entman ML. (1992) Reactive oxygen in skeletal muscle. Extracellular release of free radicals. *J Appl Physiol* 73: 1805–1809.

Reznick AZ, Packer L. (1994) Oxidative damage to proteins: spectrophotometric method for carbonyl assay. *Methods Enzymol* 233: 357–363.

Reznick AZ, Packer L, Sen CK. (1998) Strategies to assess oxidative stress. In: Reznick AZ, ed. *Oxidative stress in skeletal muscle*. Basel: Birhauser Verlag, pp. 43–58.

Rock E, Astier C, Lab C, et al. (1995) Dietary magnesium deficiency in rats enhances free radical production in skeletal muscle. *J Nutr* 125: 1205–1210.

Sen CK, Kolosova I, Hanninen O, Orlov SN. (1995) Inward potassium transport systems in skeletal muscle derived cells are highly sensitive to oxidant exposure. *Free Rad Biol Med* 18: 795–800.

Shigenaga MK, Park JW, Cundy KC, Gimeno CJ, Ames BN. (1990) In vivo oxidative DNA damage: measurement of 8-hydroxy-2-deoxyguanosine in DNA and urine by HPLC with electrochemical detection. *Methods Enzymol* 186: 521–530.

Stern LZ, Ringel SP, Ziter FA, et al. (1982) Drug trial of superoxide dismutase in Duchenne muscular dystrophy. *Arch neurol* 39: 342–346.

Vendilti P, DiMeo S. (1997) Effect of training on antioxidant capacity, tissue damage and endurance of adult male rats. *Intl J Sports Med* 18: 497–502.

Vernier A, Metzinger L, Warter JM, Poindron P, Passaquin AC. (1995) Antioxidant lazeroids enhance differentiation of C2 skeletal muscle cells. *Neurosci Lett* 186: 179–180.

Wennmalm A, Benthin G, Jungersten L, Edlund A, Petersson AS. (1994) Nitric oxide formation in man as reflected by plasma levels of nitrate, with special focus on kinetics, confounding factors and response to immuno-logical challenge. In: Moncada S, Feelish M, Busse R, Higgs EA, eds. *The biology of nitric oxide*. Oxford: Portland Press, pp. 474–476.

Wink DA, Cook JA, Pacelli R, Liebmann J, Krishna MC, Mitchell JB. (1995) Nitric oxide (NO) protects against cellular damage by reactive oxygen species. *Toxicol Lett* 82: 221–226.

Xu KY, Zweier JL, Becker LC. (1997) Hydroxyl radical inhibits sarcoplasmic reticulum Ca^{2+}ATPase function by direct attack on the ATP binding site. *Circ Res* 80: 76–81.

31

Histochemical staining techniques for examination of skeletal muscle

Yoshihiro Sato

Introduction

The diagnosis of neuromuscular disease rests on determination of clinical features, electromyographic assessment, and histologic and histochemical examination of a muscle biopsy specimen. The muscle biopsy should be performed only after making a preliminary diagnosis from clinical information, such as patterns and tempo of occurrence of weakness and wasting. Skeletal muscle abnormalities and dysfunction can arise from many causes. Therefore, a definite diagnosis requires histochemical analysis to confirm diseases such as distal myopathy with rimmed vacuole formation, nemaline myopathy, central core disease, myotubular myopathy, glycogen storage disease or mitochondrial myopathy. In addition, histochemical analysis of atrophic muscle can help to elucidate the pathogenesis of a specific disease.

Cryostat sections

Cryostat sections are used for histochemical analysis. The portion of the specimen intended for cryostat sectioning is mounted on a cork chuck in a transverse orientation, embedded in 10% (w/v) tragacanth gum, and frozen in isopentane previously cooled by immersion in liquid nitrogen. At a temperature of −196°C, isopentane has a slightly syrupy consistency. If liquid nitrogen is unavailable, the specimen can be frozen in a slurry of dry ice and isopentane at −70°C, a technique routinely used by the author. The disadvantage of this method is ice-crystal formation in the tissue that markedly degrades the quality of the frozen section unless special care is taken. To minimize ice-crystal artefacts, the chuck with the mounted specimen should be immersed in the dry ice/isopentane slurry suddenly and moved rapidly from side to side once bubbling from the slurry has become constant. The specimen can then be enclosed in a vinyl wrapper and stored at −70°C until sectioning.

Many specimens can be sectioned at a cryostat temperature of −20°C, but those with abundant fatty tissue are easier to section at −22°C.

For routine studies in the author's laboratory 18 successive cryostat sections are picked up on 18 coverslips. To assure identical orientation of the sections on the coverslips, care is taken that the upper border of each section is directed toward the upper edge of each coverslip. For the nine basic stains or reactions, 18 coverslips are mounted on nine glass slides (two coverslips per slide). Among these, haematoxylin and eosin (H and E), modified Gomori trichrome, and

nicotinamide adenosine dinucleotide (NADH)-tetrazolium reductase stains are essential for routine diagnosis of almost all neuromuscular diseases.

Histological stains

The two stains the author uses routinely are H and E, and modified Gomori trichrome (Engel and Cunningham 1963). Both stains are useful for observing the morphology of muscle fibres, non-contractile elements such as blood vessels, connective tissue, adipose tissue, cell nuclei and abnormal structures in the muscle fibres such as ragged-red fibres or nemaline rods.

H and E staining

1. Stain sections in filtered Harris haematoxylin (available commercially, or see below) for 10 min at room temperature.

2. Wash in three changes of tap water for 10 min for each change.

3. Place in 1% eosin for 30 s to 1 min at room temperature.

4. Dehydrate rapidly in ascending alcohol concentrations 70%, 80%, 95% and 100% (w/v) in that sequence.

5. Clear in xylene for 1 min and mount in Entellan New (E. Merck).

Since some commercially available Harris haematoxylin is of poor quality, making up one's own solution in advance is of advantage, as follows: Mix 50% (v/v) alcohol (300 ml), Al $NH_4(SO_4)_2 \cdot (12H_2O$ (0.9 g) and haematoxylin (1.5 g). Add 1.8 g mercuric chloride while boiling the solution for 20 min. After cooling, let the solution stand at room temperature overnight. For each use, mix 10 ml of this solution and 40 ml of saturated Al $NH_4(SO_4)_2 \cdot (12H_2O$ solution.

H and E staining is the fundamental technique used to assess skeletal muscle morphology, and it rapidly demonstrates many abnormalities such as neurogenic atrophy, inflammation of muscle, vasculitis, fibre splitting, fibre necrosis, degeneration and regeneration, opaque fibres and other findings.

Modified Gomori trichrome (Engel and Cunningham 1963)

1. Place sections in filtered Harris haematoxylin for 10 min.

2. Rinse in tap water.

3. Stain in the following Gomori solution for 10 min at room temperature:
chromotrope 2R (0.6 g)
fast green FCF (0.3 g)
phosphotungstic acid (0.6 g)
glacial acetic acid (1 ml)
distilled water (100 ml).
The pH of the solution should be adjusted to 3.4 with 1.0 M NaOH.

4. Dip sections in 0.2% (v/v) acetic acid three times, each for 1 min.

5. Dehydrate through ascending alcohol concentrations 70%, 80%, 95% and 100% (w/v) in that sequence to xylene, and mount in Permount (Fisher Scientific Inc.).

The Gomori solution should be made fresh every 2 weeks. The quality of the stain depends largely on the purity of the Chromotrope 2R and fast green FCF.

Trichrome-stained sections depict a membranous intermyofibrillar network composed of mitochondria and sarcoplasmic reticulum. Trichrome staining is essential for making a diagnosis of mitochondrial myopathy (ragged-red fibres; Fig. 31.1) and nemaline myopathy, and for identifying rimmed vacuoles, or cytoplasmic bodies. Additionally, grouped atrophy or small angulated fibres can be seen in trichrome-stained specimens (Fig. 31.2).

Routine histochemical stains

Nicotinamide adenosine dinucleotide NADH-tetrazolium reductase (Nachlas et al 1958)

1. Prepare 15 ml of incubation mixture from stock solutions as follows:
NADH (50 mg in 200 ml of distilled water); 2.1 ml;
nitroblue tetrazolium (NBT), 0.2% (w/v); 7.5 ml;
phosphate buffer (0.2 M; pH adjusted to 7.2–7.4); 3 ml;
saline; 2.4 ml.
Incubate sections in the mixture for 30–40 min at 37°C.

2. Rinse in distilled water.

3. Dry at room temperature.

4. Mount in glycerine gelatin (Sigma).

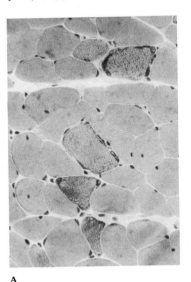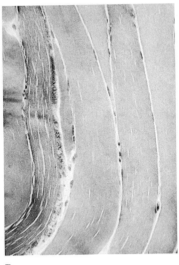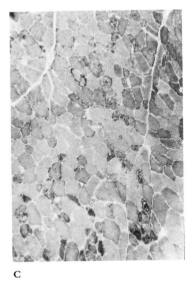

A   B   C

Figure 31.1 — Mitochondrial abnormalities observed with trichrome staining. **A** Increased membranous material occurs beneath the sarcolemma, with varying amounts of this material accumulating between myofibrils (ragged-red fibres) in a patient with acute stroke manifesting respiratory failure (×100; Sato et al 1996). **B** Longitudinal section of ragged-red fibres (×100). **C** Many ragged-red fibres from a patient with the disease entity of mitochondrial myopathy, encephalopathy, lactic acidosis and strokelike episodes (MELAS) in a specimen obtained after 15 years of symptoms. Some fibres show relatively pale staining, and some are vacuolated (×25).

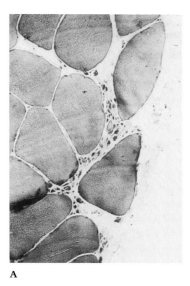 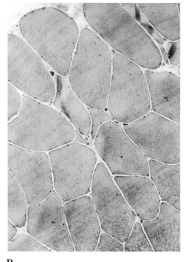

A   B

Figure 31.2—Small fibres showing grouped atrophy (**A**) and small angulated fibre (**B**) in tricrome-stained sections (×100).

The intermyofibrillar network, seen in specimens stained for oxidative enzyme reactions such as NADH-tetrazolium reductase, normally has a uniform, regularly ordered reticular appearance throughout individual muscle fibres. In some abnormal situations, Type I fibres (see adenosine triphosphate, below) show whorling of the intermyofibrillar network resembling the eddying current of a stream. This pattern is associated with areas that do not react with oxidative enzymes, presenting a moth-eaten appearance (Brook and Engel 1966). The abnormal areas are pleomorphic and variable in size, extending for varying distances along the long axis of the muscle fibre. Large numbers of moth-eaten fibres commonly occur in myopathies such as facioscapulohumeral dystrophy, limb girdle dystrophy, oculopharyngeal dystrophy and malignant hyperthermia. The distribution of mitochondria in individual fibres can be inferred from the oxidative enzyme reaction (Fig. 31.3); zones of decreased enzyme activity lack these organelles (Fig. 31.4).

Adenosine triphosphatase (ATPase; Guth and Samaha 1970)

The pH of the preincubation solution is very important in distinguishing between Type I and Type II fibres. The optimal pH should be determined in each laboratory. The ideal pH for routine (alkaline) ATPase staining lies within a narrow range from 10.3 to 10.8

with slightly higher pHs giving better results in winter. In the author's laboratory pH 10.7 is used. The best pHs for acidic ATPase staining range from 4.5 to 4.6, and from 4.2 to 4.35. The ATPase protocol is performed at room temperature for all steps.

1. Preincubation.
   A. Alkaline (routine) reaction. Incubate sections at room temperature for 15 min in a solution:
   0.1 M sodium barbital (4 ml);
   0.18 M calcium chloride (4 ml); and
   distilled water (12 ml).
   The pH should be adjusted to 10.3 to 10.8.

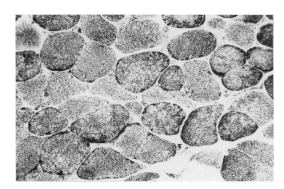

Figure 31.3—NADH dehydrogenase. Many Type I fibres show focal increases of oxidative enzyme activity in subsarcolemmal areas and focally decreased activity within muscle fibres. Acute respiratory failure due to stroke (×40; Sato et al 1996).

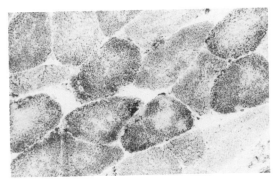

Figure 31.4—Multiple foci of decreased oxidative enzyme activity can be seen in both Type I and II muscle fibres. Chronic respiratory failure due to pulmonary emphysema. NADH dehydrogenase (×100; Sato et al 1997a).

B. Acidic reaction (pH 4.5 to 4.6). Incubate sections at room temperature for 5 min in a solution combining the following:
barbital acetate solution (sodium acetate, 1.94 g; sodium barbital, 2.94 g; and distilled water, 100 ml); 51 ml
0.1 M HCL; 10 ml
distilled water; 8 ml.
The pH should be adjusted to 4.5 to 4.6.
C. Acidic reaction (pH 4.2 to 4.35). Incubate sections at room temperature for 5 min in a solution combining the following:
barbital acetate solution (see B above); 5 ml
0.1 M HCL; 10 ml
distilled water; 8 ml.
The pH should be adjusted to 4.2 to 4.35.

2. Rinse (required following acidic preincubation only). Rinse continuously for 1 min in the following solution (D1):
0.1 M sodium barbital; 4 ml
0.18 M calcium chloride; 2 ml
distilled water; 14 ml.
The pH should be adjusted to 9.4.
D1 solution may be prepared in bulk as follows:
Mix 0.1 M sodium barbital, 80 ml; 0.18 M calcium chloride, 40 ml; and distilled water, 280 ml.

3. Incubate sections at room temperature for 45 min in D2 solution:
0.1 M sodium barbital; 4 ml
0.18 M calcium chloride; 2 ml
distilled water; 12 ml
ATP disodium salt; 50 mg.
D2 solution may be prepared in bulk as follows:
Mix 0.1 M sodium barbital, 80 ml; 0.18 M cal-

cium chloride, 40 ml; ATP disodium salt, 100 mg/40 ml; and distilled water, 280 ml.

4. Rinse three times in 1% (w/v) calcium chloride solution, allowing 2 min per rinse.

5. Incubate in 2% (w/v) calcium chloride solution for 2 min.

6. Washing in tap water for 5–7 min.

7. Rinse three times in 0.01 M sodium barbital, allowing 2 min per rinse.

8. Place sections in 4 ml yellow ammonium sulphide/40 ml distilled water for 3 min.

9. Dehydration.
A. For pH 4.2-preincubated sections, place in 1% (w/v) eosin for 1 min and then dehydrate.
B. For pH 4.5- and 10.7-preincubated sections, dehydrate completely for 10 min.

10. Clear in xylene and mount in canada balsum.

The routine (alkaline) ATPase reaction takes place in myofibrils; the intermyofibrillar network appears to dissolve out of the tissue section at a certain stage of processing. Thus, on examination of an individual fibre, the myofibrils are separated by an unstained zone representing the intermyofibrillar network. In examining the muscle section as a whole, clear differentiation can be made two fibre types. In the routine reaction, Type I fibres are more lightly stained and the Type II fibres are more heavily stained. Further, Type II fibres fall into two subtypes: Type IIA fibres are unstained in the reaction at pH 4.5, and Type IIB fibres are unstained at pH 4.2. The above three fibre types occur in roughly equal proportions in a pattern that rarely varies. However, certain muscles have relatively individual characteristics. For instance, the anterior tibial muscles include more Type I fibres than Type II fibres. In other muscles (deltoid, triceps and vastus lateralis) Type II fibres are more abundant in superficial regions than in deeper regions (Johnson et al 1973). The normal ratio of Type I to Type II fibres in sites frequently biopsied, such as superficial triceps, biceps or vastus lateralis, is approximately 1:2, and these two types of fibres show a checkerboard distribution pattern.

Fibres of a given histochemical type may be preferentially involved or preferentially degenerate when a disease selectively or predominantly affects muscle fibres of that type. Disease involvement of both fibre types also may interfere with the normal mosaic pattern of fibre type distribution. Selective Type I fibre atrophy is relatively uncommon, but it can occur in

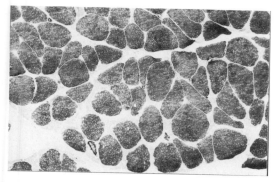

Figure 31.5—Adenosine triphosphatase staining at pH 4.3. Severe selective Type II atrophy can be seen. Anorexia nervosa (×50; Sato et al 1997b).

carnitine deficiency myopathy, rheumatoid arthritis, myotonic dystrophy, myotubular myopathy, nemaline myopathy and congenital fibre type disproportion. Selective Type II fibre atrophy has been shown to occur in association with disuse secondary to chronic respiratory failure (Sato et al 1997a), anorexia nervosa (Fig. 31.5; Sato et al 1997b), or prolonged bedrest. In myopathies with tubular aggregates, type 2 fibres are particular likely to contain large collections of tubules.

The checkerboard pattern of fibre types also is altered when denervated muscle is reinnervated by branching from intact distal axons supplying neighbouring motor units, resulting in enlargement of individual motor units. Consequently, since reinnervated fibres acquire the characteristics of their new motor unit, an increased number of fibres of a single type appear immediately adjacent to each other. Such a histochemical change, termed fibre type grouping, provides a means of early recognition of disorders involving denervation of muscle (Fig. 31.6).

An abnormality that may on occasion be mistaken for atrophy and hypertrophy is an increase in variability of fibre size, which results in widening of the distribution curve for fibre diameter even though the mean fibre diameter may remain within normal limits. This change is frequent in myopathic diseases.

Acid phosphatase (Barka and Anderson 1962)

1. Make solution 1 as follows:
   Gradually heat a mixture of pararosaniline hydrochloride (2 g) and 2N HCl (50 ml), allowing it to cool to room temperature.
   Filter the solution.
   Add 0.8 ml of 4% $NaNO_2$ to 0.8 ml of the filtrate.
   Adjust pH 4.7 to 5.0.

2. Make solution 2 by combining 1 ml of a previously made solution of naphthol AS-B1 (50 mg of acid

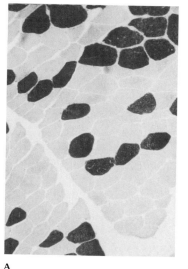

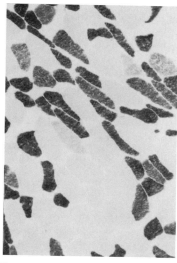

A   B

Figure 31.6—Adenosine triphosphatase at pH 4.3. The normal checkerboard mosaic of histochemical fibre types becomes disturbed, when increased numbers of fibres of a single type appear immediately adjacent to each other. Such grouping is seen in reinnervation following atrophy of both fibre types (**A**) or of only Type II fibres with secondary to disuse (**B**) (×50; Sato et al 1997a).

phosphate in 5 ml of N, N-dimethyl formamide) with 5 ml of veronal acetate buffer ($3H_2O$ sodium acetate, 9.7 g; sodium barbital, 14.7 g; and distilled water, 500 ml) and 14 ml of distilled water. Adjust the pH to 4.7 to 5.0.

3. Mix solutions 1 and 2 for 2 min.

4. Incubate sections in the mixed solution for 60 min at 37°C.

5. Wash in distilled water for 3 min.

6. Incubate with 2% methyl green for 3 min. Repeat for a total of three incubations.

7. Dehydrate rapidly in an ascending series of alcohol concentrations 70%, 80%, 95%, and 100% (w/v) in that sequence.

8. Clear in xylene and mount in Permount.

The acid phosphatase reaction detects increased lysosomal enzyme activity, as in the vacuolar myopathy of acid maltase deficiency, where an intense reaction for acid phosphatase is seen in vacuoles.

Phosphorylase (Takeuchi 1958)

1. Incubate sections at 37°C for 30 to 60 min a medium containing:
   0.1 M sodium acetate buffer (pH 5.6, 15 ml)
   adenosine monophosphate (sodium salt, 15 mg)
   glucose-1-phosphate (75 mg)
   0.2 M sodium fluoride (1.9 ml)
   Soluble insulin (40 μ/Ml; 0.01 ml)
   glycogen (1.5 mg)
   distilled water (9.4 ml)
   polyvinylpyrrolidone (1.4 g),
   pH adjusted to 5.7.

2. Rinse in distilled water.

3. Place in 10% (w/v) Lugol's iodine (lugol solution, 100 ml and potassium iodine solution 1 l) solution for 1 min.

4. Mount in glycerine.

The colour will fade rapidly within a few days upon storage. Absent staining for phosphorylase in a specimen is essential for diagnosis of McArdle's disease (deficiency of myophosphorylase).

Periodic Acid-Schiff (PAS; Dubowitz and Brooke 1973)

1. Fix in Carnoy's fixative (absolute alcohol, 300 ml;

chloroform, 150 ml; glacial acetic acid, 50 ml) for 10 min at room temperature.

2. Wash in tap water for 5 min.

3. Place in 1% periodic acid for 5 min.

4. Wash in distilled water for 5 min.

5. Place in Schiff's reagent (commercially available) for 15 min at room temperature.

6. Wash in tap water for 10 min.

7. Dehydrate in ascending alcohols.

8. Clear in xylene and mount in Permount.

The glycogen content of the fibres can be estimated by PAS staining, making it useful for diagnosis of glycogen storage diseases such as Pompe's disease, MacArdle's disease and Tarui's disease, as well as debranching enzyme deficiency.

Oil red O (Dubowitz and Brooke 1973)

1. Prepare a saturated solution of oil red O in isopropyl alcohol. Filter the solution and dilute 6 ml of it with 4 ml distilled water.

2. Stain the tissue section in this solution for 30 min at room temperature.

3. Wash in tap water.

4. Mount the sections in glycerine gel.

The glycerine gel can be placed on the section easily only when the gel is sufficiently warm. If the gel is too warm, however, the fat within the section will melt, producing artefacts.

In normal muscle, Type I fibres contain more lipid droplets than Type II fibres. In lipid-storage myopathies such as carnitine deficiency, many lipid droplets are seen with oil red O staining. This finding also may occur in some mitochondrial myopathies such as cytochrome c oxidase deficiency.

Additional histochemical stains

Additional histochemical stains described in the present section are useful to assess activity of specific enzymes such as phosphorylase, phosphofructokinase, cytochrome *c* oxidase, lactate dehydrogenase and AMP deaminase.

Phosphofructokinase (Bonilla and Schotland 1970)

1. Incubate at 37°C for 60 min in a medium made by mixing the following:
   20 mM sodium arsenate (pH 7.0, 12.5 ml)
   10 mM fructose-6-phosphate (5 ml)
   10 mM diphosphopyridine nucleotide (NAD, 2.5 ml)
   10 mM ATP sodium salt (2.5 ml)
   40 mM magnesium sulphate (0.6 ml)
   Nitroblue tetorazolium (10 mg)
   distilled water to give 25 ml of solution.
   Before incubation the pH should be adjusted to 7.0.

2. Wash in tap water.

3. Mount sections in glycerine jelly.

In Tarui's disease (type VII glycogenosis), a muscle biopsy specimen will show no phosphofructokinase activity.

Cytochrome c oxidase (Seligman et al 1968)

1. Prepare a solution by mixing:
   0.1 M acetate buffer (14 ml)
   1% (w/v) $MnCl_2$ (1.5 ml)
   3,3′-diaminobenzidine tetrahydrochloride (DAB, 30 mg)
   0.1% (v/v) H_2O_2 (0.15 ml).
   Adjust the pH to 5.5±0.03 and filter the solution.

2. Incubate sections at 37°C for 1–4 h in the above solution.

3. Wash sections in distilled water.

4. Incubate for 5 min in 1% (w/v) $CuSO_4$ at room temperature.

5. Wash sections in distilled water.

6. Dry sections at room temperature.

7. Mount in glycerine gel.

A defect in cytochrome c oxidase has been demonstrated in muscle biopsy specimens from children with generalized weakness, lactic acidosis, abnormal muscle mitochondria and the de Toni–Fanconi–Debré syndrome. Excessive numbers of mitochondria and amounts of lipid and glycogen, as well as markedly reduced cytochrome c oxidase activity, are demonstrated. Biochemical studies are needed to confirm an isolated defect of cytochrome c oxidase activity.

Adenosine monophosphate (AMP) deaminase (Fishbein et al 1980)

1. Prepare a solution as follows:
   Nitroblue tetrazolium (15 mg)
   AMP•$3H_2O$ (6 mg)
   distilled water (14 ml)
   After dissolving the solution, add 3 M KCL (1 ml) and adjust the pH to 6.1 using 0.1 N NaOH. Then add dithiothreitol (8 mg).

2. Incubate sections at room temperature for 1 h in the above solution.

3. Wash in 50 ml of 150 mM KCl/1.5 mM citrate (pH 6.0).

4. Dry at room temperature.

5. Mount the sections in glycerine gel.

This stain permits screening of muscle biopsy specimens for deficiency of adenylate deaminase. The diagnosis should be suspected when the ratio of blood ammonia to lactate is abnormal following ischaemic exercise. Most patients with reduced enzyme activity in muscle tissues can be identified by reduction or absence of adenylate deaminase staining. The prevalence of histochemically proven deficiency is 1.5% of all muscle biopsies.

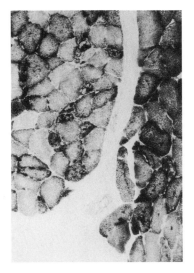

Figure 31.7— Succinate dehydrogenase (SDH). Many fibres show ragged-red clumps. However, strongly SDH-reactive blood vessels (SSV) are not seen. Mitochondrial myopathy, encephalopathy, lactic acidosis and strokelike episodes (MELAS; ×50).

Table 31.1— Further stains applicable to cryostat sections of muscle

Substance or structure	Stains or reactions
Calcific minerals	Alizarin red, von Kossa stain
Amyloid	Congo red, sirus red, crystal violet
Acid mucins	Alcian blue at pH 2.6
Glycolipid, mucins	Periodic acid-Schiff after diastase digestion
Lipid material:	
Neutral fats and phospholipids	Sudan black B
Phospholipids, neutral fats, cholesterol	Osmium tetroxide-α-naphthylamine reaction
Acidic lipids	Nile blue sulphate
Cholesteryl esters	Perchloric acid-naphthoquinone

Modified from Engel A. (1986) Myology. New York: MacGraw-Hill.

Succinate dehydrogenase (SDH; Nichlas et al 1957)

1. Incubate at 37°C for 60 min in the following solution:

   0.2 M sodium succinate (10 ml)
   0.2 M phosphate buffer (pH 7.2 to 7.6, 10 ml)
   Nitroblue tetrazolium (20 mg).

2. Extract sections in acetone (60%, 90%, 60%).

3. Wash in distilled water.

4. Mount in glycerine gel.

In 90% of cases of the entity of mitochondrial myopathy, encephalopathy, lactic acidosis and stroke-like episodes (MELAS), which usually involves a mitochondrial DNA mutation at position 3243, muscle biopsy specimens show strongly SDH-reactive blood vessels (SSV; Goto et al 1992). This abnormality, reflecting increased numbers of mitochondria in smooth muscle cells of muscular arteries, is an important finding in MELAS in addition to ragged-red fibres.

Table 31.1 lists still more stains that may at times be useful in the study of cryostat sections (Engel 1986).

Acknowledgments

The author would like to thank Professor Kotaro Oizumi (First Department of Internal Medicine, Kurume University School of Medicine) for his assistance in drafting the manuscript.

References

Barka T, Anderson PJ. (1962) Histochemical methods for acid phosphatase using hexazonium pararosalin as coupler. *J Histochem Cytochem* 10: 741–744.

Bonilla E, Schotland DL. (1970) Histochemical diagnosis of muscle phosphofructokinase deficiency. *Arch Neurol* 22: 8–13.

Brook MH, Engel WK. (1966) The histologic diagnosis of neuromuscular diseases: a review of 79 biopsies. *Arch Phy Med Rehabil* 47: 99–121.

Dubobitz V, Brook MH. (1973) *Histological and histochemical stains and reactions: Muscle biopsy: A modern approach.* London: Saunders.

Engel WK, Cunningham GC. (1963) Rapid examination of muscle tissue. An improved trichrome method for fresh-frozen biopsy sections. *Neurology* 13: 919.

Engel AG, Banker BQ (eds). (1986) The muscle biopsy. In: *Myology.* New York: MacGraw-Hill.

Fishbein WN, Griffin JL, Armbrustmacher VW. (1980) Stain for skeletal muscle adenylate deaminase: An effective tetrazolium stain for frozen biopsy specimens. *Arch Path Lab Med* 104: 462–466.

Goto Y, Horai S, Matsuoka T, et al. (1992) Mitochondrial myopathy, encephalopathy, lactic acidosis, and stroke-like episodes (MELAS): A correlative study of the clinical features and mitochondrial DNA mutation. *Neurology* 42: 545–550.

Guth L, Samaha FJ. (1970) Procedure for the histochemical demonstration of actomyosin. ATPase. *Exp Neurol* 28: 340–365.

Nachlas MM, Walker DG, Seligman AM. (1958) A histochemical method for the demonstration of diphosphopridine nucleotide diaphorase. *J Biophys Biochem Cytol* 4: 29–33.

Nachlas MM, Tsou K-C, de Souza E, Cheng C-S, Seligman AM. (1957) Cytochemical demonstration of succinic dehydrogenase by the use of a new p–nitro-phenyl substituted ditetrazole. *J Histochem Cytochem* 5: 420–426.

Johnson MA, Polgar J, Leightman D, Pippelton D. (1973) Data on the distribution of fiber types in thirty-six human muscles. An autopsy study. *J Neurol Sci* 18: 111–121.

Sato Y, Honda Y, Oizumi K, et al. (1996) Morphological and histochemical study of nonhemiplegic muscle in acute stroke patients manifesting respiratory failure. *Eur Neurol* 36: 13–19.

Sato Y, Asoh T, Honda Y, Fujimatsu Y, Higuchi I, Oizumi K. (1997a) Morphologic and histochemical evaluation of muscle in patients with chronic pulmonary emphysema manifesting generalized emaciation. *Eur Neurol* 37: 116–121.

Sato Y, Fujimatsu Y, Honda Y, Higuchi I. (1997b) Type 2 fiber atrophy in anorexia nervosa. *Neurol Med (Tokyo)* 46: 434–436.

Seligman AM, Karnovsky MJ, Wasserkrug HL, Hanker JS. (1968) Non-droplet ultrastructural demonstration of cytochrome oxidase activity with polymerising osmiophilic reagant, diaminobenzidine (DAB). *J Cell Biol* 38: 1–9.

Takeuchi T. (1958) Histochemical demonstration of branching enzyme (amylo-1,4→1,6-transglucosidase) in animal tissues. *J Histochem Cytochem* 6: 208–211.

32

Immunohistochemical methods for examining skeletal muscle

Setsuko Nakanishi

Introduction

Immunohistochemistry is a branch of histochemistry that demonstrates the localization of a protein by means of a specific immunoreaction between an antigen in the tissues and an antibody. Histochemistry has an important role in the diagnosis and pathology of skeletal muscle diseases. It is expected that the importance of immunohistochemical studies of molecules expressed in skeletal muscle will continue to increase. The ensuing chapter comments briefly on some aspects of immunohistochemistry and uses the detection of ryanodine receptors in skeletal muscle as an example to show some standard procedures.

Preparation of tissue sections

One of the requirements of histochemistry is that the substance of interest is fixed in the tissues without displacing it from its native location. Immunohistochemistry has two additional requirements for the fixation of tissues: the antigen should retain antigenicity, and it should remain accessible to the antibody. The main class of antibodies is the γ-immunoglobulins. The molecular weight of these proteins is about 150 kD and the diameter is about 10 nm. If the epitope localizes on the surface of the tissue section, the antibody reacts with the antigen without a problem, but the quantity of the antigen present on the surface of the section may be much less than that inside the section. Consequently the fixed tissue has to have spaces through which the antibody molecules can easily move to react with the antigen. This means that strong cross-linking reagents such as glutaraldehyde should be avoided, or should be used in a low concentration (0.1–0.25% (v/v)), in the fixative.

In general, skeletal muscle from a biopsy is rapidly frozen without fixation, and sections cut with a cryostat are used for histochemistry. To perform immunohistochemistry, cryostat sections from unfixed frozen tissues need to be fixed. After a section is cut by a cryostat and mounted on a glass slide, it is air-dried with a hair dryer for about 1 min and immersed in a cooled fixative such as 4% (w/v) paraformaldehyde or acetone for 10 min. After washing in phosphate-buffered saline (PBS) or Tris base/saline (TBS), the section is ready for immunohistochemistry. A fresh-frozen cryostat section post-fixed with acetone or ethanol is prone to give the greatest degree of non-specific staining (Pearse 1980). This is discussed later, in the section on reducing non-specific staining.

After the skeletal muscle is dissected, it is pinned to a support to prevent it from shrinking and then immersed in the fixative. After fixation and washing with buffer solution, the tissue is placed in a sucrose solution (20% (w/v) sucrose in 0.1 M phosphate buffer, pH 7.4) for cryoprotection. When the tissue sinks to the bottom of the container, it is ready for rapid freezing.

If a small animal is used, one can fix the whole body by transcardiac perfusion. This enables the examination of a wide range of skeletal muscles. Bouin's, Zamboni's and Carnoy's fixatives contain coagulating reagents such as picric acid or acetic acid. If one of these fixatives is used for transcardiac perfusion, the blood must first be evacuated by perfusion with saline.

The choice of the fixative depends on the antigen and the antibody. The first choice should be 4% (w/v) paraformaldehyde-based fixative. This fixative is suitable for protein antigens. For glycoprotein antigens, periodate-lysine-paraformaldehyde (PLP) fixative (McLean and Nakane 1974) is another choice. Bouin's fixative and Zamboni's fixative are useful for polypeptides because they contain picric acid, which acts as a rapid penetrating reagent. Some antibodies may require acetone or ethanol as a fixative, but these fixatives may cause diffusion of the antigen. After fixation, the tissues should be washed with buffer or buffered saline to prevent the loss of antigenicity by excess fixation and to prevent non-specific reactions between the antibody and tissue components.

The quality of a frozen tissue largely depends on the speed at which it is frozen. It is better to freeze the tissue with continuous agitation in a solution of isopentane cooled with liquid nitrogen. If the tissue is embedded in an embedding medium, Tissue-Tek II O.C.T. compound (Baxter), plastic moulds should be avoided. In this case, a mould can be prepared with aluminium foil by hand. The frozen tissues can be stocked in a well sealed container or bag for 1 year or more. After cutting off a few sections, the frozen tissue block can be stored for continuous use if the surface of the block is wrapped with aluminium foil without a dead space. Unprotected tissues will become desiccated in a freezer.

The quality of the section is also important. To keep the tissue section on the slide during the procedure, the surface of the slide needs an appropriate coating. The most practical reagent for coating is a gelatin chrome-alum solution. If the antigens are still reactive after treatment at elevated temperature, one can embed fixed tissues in paraffin. Paraffin sections give better morphology and lower background staining than cryostat sections.

The antibodies

Characterization and maintenance

Another important factor in determining the results of immunohistochemistry is the quality of the antibody. It is necessary to use a good antibody under well controlled conditions to obtain consistent results. The non-specificity and background staining of the antibody should be as low as possible.

If a commercially purchased antibody is used, most of the information necessary for immunohistochemistry may be found in the data sheet. To prevent bacterial decomposition, addition of sodium azide to a concentration of about 0.1% (w/v) is necessary and freezing of an aliquot quantity is advisable. Repeated freezing and thawing should be avoided.

If it is not clear whether an antibody can be used for immunohistochemistry, different fixation methods (post-fixed section from fresh-frozen tissue or prefixed tissue), different fixatives and different sectioning techniques (cryostat section or paraffin section) should be examined. Western blotting can be used to characterize an antibody, but usually it can not detect the specificity of an antibody because the antigen may have been denatured. This is especially true in the case of monoclonal antibodies.

In immunohistochemistry, monoclonal antibodies do not always provide useful results. Instead, polyclonal antibodies are often more suitable and more useful for detecting antigens in tissue sections. Since a monoclonal antibody recognizes only a single epitope, if this epitope is modified by fixation or is not physically accessible to the monoclonal antibody in the tissue section, there will be no immunohistochemical reaction. In addition, if the same epitope exists in another molecule, the monoclonal antibody may also recognize that molecule. Monoclonal antibodies often lose their activity when they are conjugated with any molecule for labelling. It is possible that a monoclonal antibody that reacts with purified antigen would not react with a fixed antigen.

Determination of the proper concentration

The concentration of antibody in the working solution should be carefully determined by a series of dilutions. Finding the proper dilution of antibody is critically important for obtaining the specific localization of an antigen with minimum background staining.

Control of the specificity of the reaction

It is necessary to control the specificity of the immunohistochemical reaction. A negative control should be done by incubating an adjacent section with preimmune serum or immunoglobulins (Igs) at the same concentration as the antibody. If the isotype of the antibody is known, an isotype that is the same as that of the antibody should be used as a negative control. An antibody against a different antigen can be used as a negative control. Incubation without a primary antibody (i.e., incubation with only the buffer solution) is a control but not a sufficient one.

If there is no staining on the section, the use of a positive control can help to troubleshoot the basic procedures.

If a good quantity of antigen is available, the antibody can be reacted with an excess quantity of antigen and after centrifugation (10 000 g, 1 h) the supernatant can be reacted with the tissue section. After absorption the staining may become weak.

Visualization of immunoreactive sites in the tissue section

The so-called direct method uses a labelled antibody. Labelling of an antibody usually results in the lowering of its activity, and it is a time-consuming procedure. In the so-called indirect method, the use of a labelled secondary antibody eliminates the necessity of labelling the primary antibody, but the increase in the number of steps in the immunohistochemical procedures increases the problems of non-specific background staining.

Commonly used labels of secondary antibodies today are fluorescent molecules, horseradish peroxidase (HRP) and biotin. Fluorescent labelling has an advantage in that it gives fine images with high signal-to-noise ratios, but the images are not permanent. It is necessary to take pictures of the results before the fluorescence fades.

HRP can be visualized with an excellent substrate introduced by Graham and Karnovsky (1966), 3, 3'-

diaminobenzidine hydrochloride (DAB). DAB produces brown precipitates in the tissue with so little diffusion that it is barely visible under the electron microscope. The brown colour can be intensified by adding 0.01 M imidazole (Trojanowski et al 1983). The visualization of biotin-labelled secondary antibody needs a further reaction with avidin-biotinylated peroxidase complex (ABC). One molecule of avidin has four binding sites for biotin, and the binding of avidin and biotin is specific and irreversible. This enables the so-called ABC method to amplify the reaction (Hsu et al 1981). A disadvantage of this method is that the complex is large, and it can cause steric hindrance.

Reduction of background staining

Non-specific staining must be reduced as much as possible to increase the strength of the signal compared with the background. However, blocking of non-specific staining is not simple because many factors are involved, and they are sometimes difficult to control. The first thing to try is to dilute the antibody. Lowering the concentration of the antibody gives a better signal-to-noise ratio. Although the causes of non-specific staining vary from tissue to tissue, the most important thing to block is non-specific binding of antibody to tissue components. If an HRP-labelled antibody or the ABC method is used, it is also important to block endogenous molecules, such as biotin, and enzymes, such as peroxidase or alkaline phosphatase.

Non-specific binding of antibodies to tissue sections is considered to be due to free aldehyde groups introduced by aldehyde-based fixatives and hydrophobic or ionic interactions between proteins. Free aldehyde groups can be blocked by saturation with Tris-glycine before incubation with the antibody. Hydrophobic or ionic interactions may cause non-specific binding of antibodies, which can be eliminated by elevating the concentration of salt in the washing buffer (0.15–0.2 M) or by using a non-ionic detergent such as Triton X-100 or Tween-20 at a low concentration (e.g., 0.1% (v/v)) in the washing buffer. Addition of such detergents in the working solution of the primary antibody should be avoided as the antigenicity of some antigens is destroyed by detergent.

Irrelevant proteins can be effective blocking agents. Normal serum is thought to prevent non-specific binding of antibodies via the Fc receptor and complement receptors in tissue sections. Although such non-specific binding generally occurs to a lesser extent in paraffin-embedded sections, incubation with normal serum is recommended. Addition of normal serum and bovine serum albumin (BSA) to a diluent of the primary antibody can be effective if a highly diluted antibody is used.

Endogenous Igs in tissue sections are thought to be a cause of non-specific staining. This is especially a problem for the immunohistochemistry of mouse tissues when using murine monoclonal antibodies. The presence of endogenous Igs in intercellular spaces makes it difficult to detect antigens localized on or near the cell surface or in the extracellular matrix. These homologous Igs are also recognized by the secondary antibody, which makes it difficult to distinguish the specific binding sites from non-specific staining. Recently a method to overcome this problem was developed for the study of dystrophin in cryostat sections of fibres from mdx mice (the mouse homologue of Duchenne muscular dystrophy; Lu and Partridge 1998). The authors found that non-specific binding mainly results from the binding of both Fab and Fc of the secondary antibody to tissue Igs and other components and proposed the use of unpurified papain-digested secondary anti-mouse Igs enriched with the Fc fragment of the same Igs. It should be kept in mind that Fc receptors are mainly a problem in living cells and frozen sections, rather than in fixed tissues (Sternberger 1985).

Endogenous peroxidase activities can be blocked by incubating the sections with hydrogen peroxide (H_2O_2) in methanol. Endogenous alkaline phosphatase activity can be blocked by adding 5 mM of levamisole to the substrate solution.

Biotin is a coenzyme of carboxylases and the muscle tissues are rich in endogenous biotin (Kirkeby et al 1993). Since endogenous biotin is generally decomposed by aldehyde fixatives, blocking is not necessary in aldehyde-fixed paraffin sections, but fresh-frozen cryostat sections postfixed with acetone or ethanol may need blocking. Biotin-dependent carboxylases are present in the mitochondria and cytoplasm of muscular tissues. Endogenous biotin can be blocked by incubating sections with 0.1–0.01% (w/v) avidin solution followed by PBS washing and incubation with 0.01–0.001% (w/v) biotin solution.

In the case of immunofluorescence, there is the problem of autofluorescence. This is thought to be caused by reactions between aldehyde fixatives and certain endogenous molecules. These reactions may be reduced by doing the procedures at 4°C in the dark.

Interpretation of the results

If there is staining in a tissue section, careful examination with the different controls mentioned above is necessary to determine whether the results are specific or not.

If there is no staining, tissue preparation and other procedures should be reexamined. If fresh-frozen tissue sections that were postfixed with acetone or 4% (w/v) paraformaldehyde give no staining, the antibody used may not be suitable for immunohistochemistry. In any case, the interpretation of immunohistochemistry must be done with great care.

Immunohistochemical localization of ryanodine receptors in skeletal muscle

The ryanodine receptors are intracellular Ca^{2+} channel proteins that mediate Ca^{2+}-induced Ca^{2+} release. The localization of ryanodine receptors has been demonstrated in the junctional terminal cisternae of the sarcoplasmic reticulum by immunofluorescence (Yuan et al 1991). Figure 32.1 shows the localization of ryanodine receptors in murine anterior tibial muscle by using polyclonal antibodies raised against a synthetic peptide corresponding to parts of both skeletal and cardiac muscle rabbit ryanodine receptors. These antibodies have been characterized (Kuwajima et al 1992, Nakanishi et al 1992). Mice were fixed by transcardiac perfusion with Bouin's fixative or Carnoy's fixative and 6 μm-thick paraffin sections were processed using the ABC method. Tissue sections prepared by both fixatives demonstrated that ryanodine receptors may localize not only in junctional terminal cisternae but also in non-junctional sarcoplasmic reticulum.

General procedure

As a precautionary measure, the incubations of the sections on the slides should be done in a moist chamber. Care should be taken not to dry out the sections during the steps as dried sections are prone to nonspecific staining. NaN_3 should not be present in the solutions for HRP because it inhibits HRP activity.

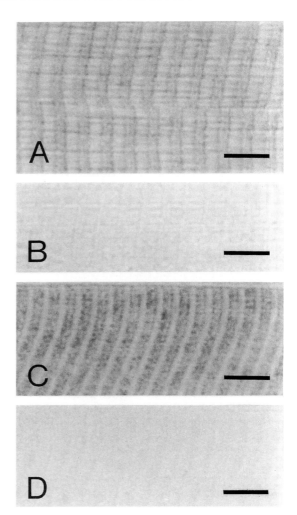

Figure 32.1—Localization of ryanodine receptors in the anterior tibial muscle of mouse, fixed by Bouin's fixative (**A**, **B**) and by Carnoy's fixative (**C**, **D**). Part of the interface between the A- and I-bands is stained. Moderate staining is also found in the I-bands. Control sections remain unstained (**B**, **D**). Bar, 5 μm.

1. If O.C.T.-compound-embedded cryostat sections are used, wash the slides three times for 5 min each in TBS to eliminate the O.C.T.-compound. If paraffin-embedded sections are used, deparaffinize and bring sections to water.

2. Incubate the slides in a solution of 0.3% (v/v) H_2O_2 in methanol for 20 min at room temperature.

3. Wash the slides three times for 5 min each in TBS.

4. Blot round edges of sections. Apply a solution of

5% (v/v) normal serum of the animal used for production of the secondary antibody onto the section. Incubate for 20 min at room temperature.

5. Blot round sections, apply a solution of the primary antibody or appropriate control and incubate for 2 h at room temperature or at 4°C overnight.

6. After blotting round sections, wash the slides five times for 5 min each in TBS.

7. Blot round sections, apply a solution of secondary antibody and incubate for 1 h at room temperature.

8. Wash the slides three times for 5 min each in TBS.

9. Blot round sections, apply a solution of ABC prepared at least 30 min before use. Incubate the slides for 30 min at room temperature.

10. Wash the slides three times for 5 min each in TBS.

11. Apply a substrate solution containing DAB/H_2O_2 and incubate at room temperature. Examine the slide under the microscope at low magnification (4× or 10×).

12. Wash the slides in running tap water to stop HRP activity.

13. Counterstain the slides with methyl green solution.

14. Wash the slides again in running tap water, dehydrate and embed in permanent mounting medium.

For fluorescent–labelled antibodies, embed the section in aqueous mounting medium containing an anti-fading reagent and store the slides at −20°C.

Preparation of reagents

Fixative: 4% (w/v) paraformaldehyde in 0.1 M phosphate buffer, pH 7.4

Paraformaldehyde fixative should be prepared soon before use because, when stored, paraformaldehyde polymerizes and loses its strength.

1. Heat 40 ml of water to 60–70°C and dissolve 4 g of paraformaldehyde. It can be dissolved completely by adding one or two drops of 40% (w/v) NaOH. Cool the solution to room temperature.

2. Adjust the volume to 50 ml with distilled water and add 50 ml of 0.2 M phosphate buffer, pH 7.4.

3. If this fixative is used for transcardiac perfusion, it must be filtered through Whatman No. 1 filter paper.

Coating of slides: 0.1% (w/v) gelatin and 0.01% (w/v) chrome alum

If the tissue sections need a greater degree of adhesion, the concentration of gelatin and chrome alum can be increased.

1. Put the pre-cleaned glass slides in racks and soak them in absolute ethanol overnight.

2. Dry the slides in an oven at 60–70°C and cool to room temperature.

3. Dissolve 200 mg of gelatin in 200 ml of distilled water and allow the solution to cool at room temperature.

4. Dissolve 20 mg of chromium (III) potassium sulphate in the gelatin solution.

5. Dip the racks of slides in the gelatin chrome alum solution for a few seconds.

6. Place the racks of slides in a 50–60°C oven until they are dry.

7. Store the slides in dust-free slide boxes.

Tris-glycine: 0.1 M glycine

1. Dissolve 750 mg of glycine in 100 ml of distilled water.

2. Adjust the pH to 7.2–7.4 by adding 30–40 μl of 1 M Tris base.

3. Store at room temperature.

PBS: 0.1 M phosphate buffer, pH 7.4, 0.9% (w/v) NaCl

1. Make a 0.2 M solution of NaH_2HO_4 and a 0.2 M solution of Na_2HPO_4.

2. Make a pH 7.4 buffer by adding the appropriate amounts of the two solutions and then dilute with an equal amount of water.

3. Add NaCl to a final concentration of 0.9%.

4. Store at 4°C up to 1 month. Add 0.01% NaN_3 or thimerosal for longer periods.

TBS: 20 mM Tris-HCl, pH 7.5, 150 mM NaCl

1. To prepare 10 × TBS, make 0.2 M Tris by dissolving 24.2 g of Tris base in 1 l of distilled water and 0.2 M of HCl by dissolving 16.7 ml of concentrated HCl and adjusting to 1 l with distilled water.

2. Adjust the pH by mixing 0.2 M Tris and 0.2 M HCl to pH 7.5.

3. Add NaCl to a final concentration of 1.5 M.

4. Store at room temperature.

5. Dilute 1/10 with distilled water to make a working solution.

Antibody diluent: 2% (v/v) normal serum, 0.1 mg/ml BSA in PBS or TBS

1. Prepare a 10 × BSA solution of 1 mg/ml in distilled water and divide into 1 ml aliquots. Store at −20°C.

2. To make 10 ml of antibody diluent, mix 1 ml of 10 × BSA, 0.2 ml of normal serum and 8.8 ml of PBS or TBS.

5 × DAB stock solution

Note that DAB is a carcinogen and should be handled with great care.

1. Prepare a solution of DAB at a concentration of 5 mg/ml in distilled water.

2. Divide into 1 ml aliquots.

3. Store at −20°C in a container that protects it from the light.

DAB working solution: 0.1% (w/v) DAB, 0.024% (v/v) H_2O_2 in 0.05 M Tris-HCl, pH 7.6

This solution should be prepared just before use in a cleaned container. If a working solution becomes tainted, it must be discarded.

1. Bring a frozen 5 × DAB solution to room temperature.

2. Add 2 ml of 0.1 M Tris-HCl, pH 7.6 and 2 ml of distilled water to make 5 ml of working solution.

3. Add 4 μl of 30% (v/v) H_2O_2.

4. If desired, dissolve 3.4 mg of imidazole at a final concentration of 0.024% (w/v).

Veronal acetate buffered 1% (w/v) methyl green solution, pH 4.0

1. Dissolve 0.55 g of sodium acetate and 0.83 g of barbital sodium in 140 ml of distilled water.

2. Add 60 ml of 0.1 N HCl.

3. Dissolve 2.0 g of methyl green in this solution.

4. Filter with Whatman No. 1 paper.

References

Graham RC, Jr, Karnovsky MJ. (1966) The early stages of absorption of injected horseradish peroxidase in the proximal tubules of mouse kidney: ultrastructural cytochemistry by a new technique. *J Histochem Cytochem* 14: 291–302.

Hsu SM, Raine L, Fanger H. (1981) The use of avidin-biotin-peroxidase complex (ABC) in immunoperoxidase technique: A comparison between ABC and unlabeled antibody (PAP) procedures. *J Histochem Cytochem* 29: 577–580.

Kirkeby S, Moe D, Bog-Hansen TC, van Noorden CJF. (1993) Biotin carboxylases in mitochondria and the cytosol from skeletal and cardiac muscle as detected by avidin binding. *Histochemistry* 100: 415–421.

Kuwajima G, Futatsugi A, Niinobe M, Nakanishi S, Mikoshiba K. (1992). Two types of ryanodine receptors in mouse brain; skeletal muscle type exclusively in Purkinje cells and cardiac muscle type in various neurons. *Neuron* 9: 1133–1142.

Lu QL, Partridge TA. (1998) A new blocking method for application of murine monoclonal antibody to mouse tissue sections. *J Histochem Cytochem* 46: 977–983.

McLean IW, Nakane PK. (1974) Periodate-lysine-paraformaldehyde fixative. A new fixative for immunoelectron microscopy. *J Histochem Cytochem* 22: 1077–1083.

Nakanishi S, Kuwajima G, Mikoshiba K. (1992) Immunohistochemical localization of ryanodine receptors in mouse central nervous system. *Neurosci Res* 15: 130–142.

Pearse AGE. (1980) *Histochemistry Theoretical and Applied, 4th ed*. Edinburgh: Churchill Livingstone.

Sternberger LA. (1985) *Immunocytochemistry. 3rd ed*. New York: John Wiley & Sons.

Trojanowsky JQ, Obrocka MA, Lee VMY. (1983) A comparison of eight different chromogen protocols for the demonstration of immunoreactive neurofilaments or glial filaments in rat cerebellum using the peroxidase-antiperoxidase method and monoclonal antibodies. *J Histochem Cytochem* 31: 1217–1223.

Yuan S, Arnold W, Jorgensen AO. (1991) Biogenesis of transverse tubules and triads: immunolocalization of the 1,4-dihydropyridine receptor, TS28, and the ryanodine receptor in rabbit skeletal muscle developing in situ. *J Cell Biol* 112: 289–301.

33

Methods for examinations of antibodies in skeletal muscle disease

Renato Mantegazza, Fulvio Baggi, Pia Bernasconi

Introduction

The neuromuscular junction (NMJ) and the muscle tissue are a target of immune-mediated reactions, mostly antibodies. The antibodies may be of pathogenic and/or diagnostic value and we will discuss later the principal diseases in which these autoantibodies have a role, the main methods for their detection, and their significance in clinical neuroimmunology.

The NMJ is a highly specialized structure (see Fig. 33.1) characterized by a presynaptic portion, the ending of a motor nerve, and a postsynaptic portion, which is the muscle area through which the signals for muscle contraction are triggered (reviewed in Engel 1994a). The motor nerve ending, devoid of myelin sheath, sprouts on the muscle plasmalemma with small "buttons" in close contact with the postsynaptic infoldings; on top of these clefts acetylcholine receptors (AChRs) are densely packaged. The sub-synaptic space is filled with basal lamina and acetylcholin-esterase. Neuromuscular transmission is a complex event involving the sequential activation of different ion channels:

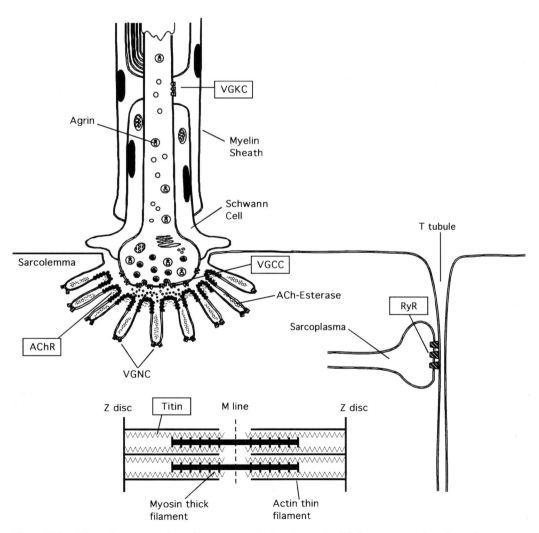

Figure 33.1—Schematic representation of a neuromuscular junction, a simplified sarcomere and triad muscle structure. Diagram not to scale. The autoantigen targets of autoimmune attack are boxed (VGKC, voltage-gated potassium channel; VGCC, voltage-gated calcium channel; AChR, acetylcholine receptor; RyR, ryanodin receptor).

1. Depolarization of the nerve terminal causes opening of voltage-gated Ca^{++} channels which induce a localized release of acetylcholine (ACh) into the synaptic space

2. ACh binding to AChRs opens their cation channels and induces a Na^+ flux into muscle cells

3. The local depolarization of the plasmalemma opens voltage-gated Na^+ channels, which induce a depolarization wave along the membrane

4. The generalized depolarization of muscle plasmalemma activates voltage-gated Ca^{++} channels, localized on the transverse tubules, to induce release of Ca^{++} from the sarcoplasmic reticulum (e.g. ryanodin receptor) into the cytosol; the sudden increase of cytosolic Ca^{++} causes the myofibrils to contract.

A perturbation in these mechanisms leads to muscle weakness and fatigability. Some of the ion channels and muscle proteins (on the cytoskeleton or in the sarcoplasmic reticulum), previously described, are the target of an antibody-mediated attack in autoimmune diseases of the NMJ.

The muscle autoimmune diseases that we will consider in this chapter are:

• Myasthenia gravis (MG), associated or not with thymoma
• Lambert–Eaton syndrome (LEMS), associated or not with cancer
• Acquired neuromyotonia (NMT)
• Inflammatory myopathies (IM).

Myasthenia gravis

Myasthenia gravis is an autoimmune disease caused by the presence of antibodies (Abs) directed against the nicotinic AChRs present at the NMJ (reviewed in Drachman 1994). The binding of these Abs leads to a loss of functional AChRs, which impairs neuromuscular signal transmission and thus leads to characteristic myasthenic symptoms. Anti-AChR Abs exert their action via three different modalities, which are not mutually exclusive:

• by binding and complement fixation
• by binding and inducing an accelerated AChR turn-over on the NMJ
• by a direct blocking activity on the AChR opening.

Anti-AChR Abs are detected in about 85% of MG patients. The anti-AChR Abs are polyclonal and heterogeneous (Lindstrom et al 1976, Vincent and Newsom-Davis 1985), and the majority of them are directed against a small region called the main immunogenic region (Tzartos et al 1986). Some MG patients (approximately 10–15%) have no detectable anti-AChR Abs, although they do respond to immunosuppressive treatment and plasmapheresis; they are defined as "seronegative" MG (Yamamoto et al 1991, Li et al 1996). No correlation is observed between anti-AChR antibody titres and muscle weakness between patients, probably reflecting Ab heterogeneity, while on the contrary, there is a good correlation between antibody titre and muscle weakness in individual MG patients. Receptor antibody titres tend to rise several weeks before exacerbations in patients with established MG. Consequently, serial measurements of AChR Abs can be useful in monitoring disease progression as well as effects of treatment (Mantegazza et al 1988, Antozzi et al 1994). The disease prevalence is about 5–9 per 10^5, and there is evidence of heterogeneity of disease expression, that probably reflects different aetiologic mechanisms. Electromyography (EMG) of MG patients is characterized by a reduction in the muscle action potential (MAP) after repetitive stimulation at low frequency (3–5 Hz): a positive test is seen in about 75% of patients (Mantegazza et al 1990). MG is more severe in patients with thymoma compared with those who have non-neoplastic MG. Most MG patients with thymoma have autoantibodies to components of striated muscle such as titin and ryanodin receptor (RyR) (Mygland et al 1992, Gautel et al 1993). Titin is a 2800 kD protein that comprises 10% of the myofibrillar mass and is involved in the elastic recoil of muscle (see Fig. 33.1). RyR is the calcium release channel of the sarcoplasmic reticulum involved in the mechanism of excitation–contraction coupling in striated muscle (see Fig. 33.1). Antibodies against titin and RyR are considered as markers for thymoma. Moreover, the presence of anti-titin and anti-RyR Abs in MG with thymoma suggests that these antigens may have a pathogenetic role in association with neoplastic transformation of thymus. Evaluation of autoimmunity to titin and RyR might help in the pre-surgical screening of MG patients (Baggi et al 1998). Since the anti-AChR assay is used for the diagnosis and management of the disease, the determination of AChR Abs in serum must be highly specific and very sensitive. Serum Abs that bind AChR are then measured using immunoprecipitation assays in which nicotinic AChRs from skeletal muscle are specifically labelled with $[^{125}I]$-α-Bungarotoxin(-α-BuTx). Human muscle AChR is present in two isoforms, with differences in their electrophysiologic properties and antigenic determinants. AChR from adult innervated muscle (adult subtype) is composed of α_2, β, δ and ε-subunits, while in fetal and denervated muscles the ε-subunit is not transcribed and it is replaced by the γ subunit (fetal subtype). Since MG is a disease of adulthood, the mature AChR subtype from normal human muscle should represent the best preparation for diagnostic anti-AChR assays. However, although most of MG patients have antibodies against this antigen, high-titre sera bind equally well either fetal AChR and adult AChR (Vincent and Newsom-Davis 1982, Gotti et al 1984). The most used antigen preparation for measuring anti-AChR Abs is a solubilized AChR from ischaemic (partially denervated) limb muscle from amputations, which contains a mix of innervated and denervated AChR. To overcome the difficulties in obtaining amputated leg muscle, a myogenic cell line (TE671) was engineered to produce the adult form of AChR (by stable transfection of the ε-gene of AChR) in parallel to the fetal AChR (Beeson et al 1996) and used as a source of antigen best replacing muscle tissue for antigen preparation in the MG diagnostic assays (Somnier 1994).

Several laboratories have developed non-radioactive methods for assaying anti-AChR Abs, using preparations of AChR from different origin (human or fetal calf muscles) or with differences in the antigen preparations (Voltz et al 1991); efforts have been made to develop enzyme-linked immunosorbant assays (ELISA), either directly coating AChR onto the plates or using monoclonal Abs against different AChR subunits (Kawanami et al 1984, Hofstad et al 1992, Gotti et al 1997). However, these methods are cumbersome and time-consuming, and so not reliable for a screening assay.

Preparation of acetylcholine receptor crude extract

Human muscle from amputated limb is stored at −70°C. It is cleaned of connective tissue and homogenized in two volumes of 0.1 M phosphate buffer, pH 7.4, with protease inhibitors. After centrifugation, the membrane pellets are resuspended in 0.02 M phosphate buffer, pH 7.4, containing 2% Triton X100, for AChR solubilization and incubated for 2 h at room temperature, or overnight at 4°C. After centrifugation, the supernatant is filtered to remove fat material and stored at 4°C until use. As a protease inhibitor, phenylmethyl sulphonylfluoride (PMSF) should be used throughout all passages in order to minimize AChR degradation and loss of activity.

Acetylcholine receptor assay

50–100 µl of AChR crude extract are incubated with $[^{125}I]$-α-BuTx (1nM) for 4 h at room temperature; then the labelled extract is applied to presoaked DE81 filter disks and washed with 0.02 M phosphate buffer, pH 7.4, containing 0.1% Triton X100. The disks are counted and results are expressed as pmol toxin binding sites/ml extract. Duplicates of extract are preincubated with unlabelled α-BuTx before addition of $[^{125}I]$-α-BuTx (aspecific counts) and the corresponding counts are substracted.

Anti-AChR Abs assay

A standard amount of $[^{125}I]$-α-BuTx labelled AChR (20–50 fmol, usually labelled to 80% saturation) is incubated with standard dilution of MG serum (from 0.1 to 5 µl) in a final volume to 100 µl overnight at 4°C. During this time, autoantibodies present in the patient's serum attach to the labelled receptors. The resulting immune complexes are then precipitated by adding anti-human IgG secondary antibody (generally from rabbit or goat) and incubated for further 2–4 h at room temperature. The precipitates are pelleted, washed three times with 0.02 M phosphate buffer, pH 7.4, 0.1% Triton X100, and counted. The amount of radioactivity is directly proportional to the concentration of AChR autoantibodies present in the sample. Values are normally expressed as nmol $[^{125}I]$-α-BuTx binding sites/L serum (or nM). Positive (one high titre and one low titre) and negative controls are routinely performed each time, and any laboratory must have its own negative control group, since normal individuals sometimes have a very low level of anti-AChR Abs (usually below 0.2 nmol/L). Samples are considered to be positive when their titre is above 0.5 nmol/L and values between 0.2–0.5 nmol/L are designed equivocal and a newer serum sample should be tested.

Anti-titin and anti-ryanodine receptor antibody detection

Anti-titin Abs are assayed by an ELISA method using the MGT–30 recombinant fragment of titin. MG and control sera are diluted 1:200 in phosphate-buffered saline (PBS). A large group of healthy donors is tested in order to determine the cut-off value, defined as mean optical density (OD) value + 3 standard deviations (SD). Anti-RyR Abs are assayed by Western-blot analysis. RyR is isolated from rabbit skeletal muscle, loaded on sodium dodecyl sulphate polyacrylamide-gel electrophoresis (SDS-PAGE) and transferred on to nitrocellulose sheets. The membranes are incubated with sera diluted 1:50 for 2 h, washed with PBS-Tween 20 (0.05%) and incubated with peroxidase-conjugated rabbit anti-human IgG (1:500) for the detection of human IgG reacting with RyR band.

Lambert–Eaton syndrome

LEMS is a myasthenic syndrome in which Abs to the voltage-gated calcium channels (VGCC) are found (Sher et al 1989, Engel 1994b, Lang et al 1998). Although symptoms may overlap with those of MG, a clinical diagnosis is usually made on the basis of a relative sparing of extraocular symptoms and absence or reduction of tendon reflexes, which may reappear after voluntary contraction. EMG shows typically a small MAP that increases in amplitude after voluntary contraction or after high frequency stimulation (50 Hz). Characteristically various autonomic symptoms may be present. In about 50% of cases, cancer may be associated with LEMS: small cell lung carcinoma (SCLC) is the most frequently associated tumour, though others may be associated. VGCCs are localized in the active-zone particles on the presynaptic portion of the NMJ. In normal subjects freeze-fracture electron microscopy analysis of the active-zone particles shows a double parallel row pattern arrangement; the latter is altered in LEMS patients with a marked reduction of the active-zone particles (Fukunaga et al 1982). Fukuoka et al (1987) localized IgG to the sites of active-zones by immunohistochemistry. VGCC are expressed on SCLC and are sensitive to LEMS Abs by inducing a reduction of Ca^{++} influx. Four classes of VGCCs (T, N, L and P type) have been distinguished. These channels can be specifically labelled by means of toxins from venoms of two different marine snails (ω-Ctx MVIIC from *Conus magus* and ω-Ctx GVIA *Conus geographicus*) or spider (ω-Aga from *Agelenopsis aperta*). These toxins bind with high affinity to VGCCs, and their iodinated form allows the use of these toxin–antigen complexes in a soluble radioimmunological assay for the detection of anti-VGCCs antibodies in LEMS patients (Leys et al 1991).

In LEMS patient autoantibodies against N-type and P-/Q-type VGCCs are detected. The latter autoantigen seems more directly involved in the neurotransmitter release at the NMJ. Antibodies against N-type are present in 44–52% of LEMS patients, whereas those against the P-/Q-type of VGCC are present in 92% of clinically definite LEMS patients (Motomura et al 1995).

Acquired neuromyotonia

Acquired neuromyotonia (Isaacs' syndrome) is a human disorder characterized by hyperexcitable motor nerves and sometimes by central abnormalities (Isaacs 1961); it is associated with Abs to voltage-gated potassium channels (VGKC) that interfere with potassium channel function resulting in neuronal hyperactivity (Hart et al 1997, Vincent et al 1998). This condition may be associated with thymoma and, in some cases, anti-AChR Abs are present. The candidate antigen is a neuronal shaker-related VGKC and in particular its (α-subunit which is present in different subtypes (KCNA1–6). The cDNA of the genes encoding VGKC subunits have been cloned and expressed in Xenopus oocytes; the expressed α-chains can be used as target for detecting autoantibodies by immunohistochemistry on frozen sections of oocytes. Moreover, α-dendrotoxin (α-Dtx) is a specific ligand for some of the VGKC subtypes, and the iodinated form of α-Dtx ([^{125}I]-α-Dtx) can also be used for labelling VGKCs in an immunoprecipitation assay for the detection of antibodies against KCNA6 channels. Comparing results between the molecular immunohistochemical assay and the radioimmunological assay, Hart et al (1997) were able to detect antibodies to human brain VGKCs in all of 12 neuromyotonia patients and in none of 18 control subjects.

Inflammatory myopathies

Inflammatory myopathies (IM) are an heterogeneous group of muscle disease, characterized by muscle degeneration mediated by inflammatory mechanisms (Engel et al 1994c, Dalakas 1995, Mantegazza et al 1997). Three major forms can be found: dermatomyositis (DM), polymyositis (PM) and inclusion body myositis (IBM). The three forms share some pathological alterations, such as muscle fibres at various stages of necrosis and regeneration, proliferation of connective tissue within muscle tissue, presence of mononuclear cells at perimysial, perivascular and endomysial sites, but the main difference is that PM and IBM are T cell mediated whereas DM is considered an antibody mediated disease. The mechanisms by which the autoimmune attack is triggered and the putative autoantigen are still unknown. PM and DM are often associated with malignancies and other immune-mediated diseases such as systemic lupus erythematosus (SLE), Sjögren's syndrome, scleroderma, mixed connective tissue disease (overlap syndromes). Some authors identify an antisynthetase syndrome, in which patients are positive to different transfer RNA (tRNA) synthetase antibodies (Miller 1993, Targoff 1993a); nevertheless, it is not yet clear whether this group of patients is clinically different from patients with overlap syndromes.

In IM, several autoantibodies can be detected in serum of affected patients: 60–80% of DM and PM patients are positive for serum autoantibodies against intracellular proteins (Targoff 1992). The principal antibodies tested, and useful for differential diagnosis, are against the following (see Table 33.1):

- true antinuclear antigens (ANA)
- extractable nuclear antigens (ENA) (Smith, Sm; n-ribonucleoprotein, RNP; systemic sclerosis-related anti-topoisomerase I, Scl-70; anti-aminoacyl-tRNA synthetase, PM-1)
- cytoplasmic antigens (SS-A/Ro; SS-B/La)

Antibodies against five different aminoacyl-tRNA synthetases can be detected. Histidyl-tRNA synthetase (anti Jo-1), glycyl-tRNA synthetase (anti EJ), isoleucyl-tRNA synthetase (anti OJ), threonyl-tRNA synthetase (anti PL-7), alanyl-tRNA synthetase (PL-12). These antibodies are usually present in a subgroup of IM patients with interstitial lung disease, arthritis and Raynaud's phenomenon (Hirakata et al 1999), and they act to inhibit the aminoacylation of their respective tRNAs. The correlation between certain forms of myositis and the production of these antibodies is still unknown. It has been hypothesized that they are induced by the interaction of the synthetase with picornaviral RNA (Targoff et al 1993b).

Anti-Jo-1 Abs bind to histidyl-transfer RNA synthetase (HRS), recognizing a small number of epitopes crucial for molecule activity. Since HRS is important in protein assembly, the HRS inhibition (intracytoplasmatic binding and enzyme inhibition in vivo) may potentially contribute to the pathogenesis of autoimmune muscle damage in IM (Mathews and Bernstein 1983). Anti-Jo-1 antibodies can be found in a clinically distinct subgroup of PM and DM patients (Table 33.1) and in 15% of patients with myositis associated with connective tissue disease (Nishikai and Reichlin 1980, Biswas et al 1987, Shi et al 1991). Moreover, anti-Jo-1 positivity is strongly associated with DR3, DRw52 and DQA1*0501 human leukocyte antigen (HLA) haplotypes (Love et al 1991, Miller 1993). Although it is not clear whether anti-Jo-1 Abs are pathogenetic, they are closely related to factors (i.e., T cells or cytokines) responsible for the progression of the disease. In fact, anti-Jo-1 antibody titre (primarily of IgG_1 isotype) varies according to the disease activity; patients with myositis become antibody negative when the disease remits after treatment, suggesting that the timing of antibody screening is very important as it must be performed during a period of active disease and before therapy. The restricted isotype resembles that of other autoimmune disorders as MG or SLE, suggesting that T lymphocytes are important in Ab production and regulation, and that this production is antigen-driven (Miller et al 1990). Rutjes et al (1997) demonstrated that anti-Jo-1 Abs are frequently associated with Abs against the Ro52 protein; in fact of 112 IM patients tested 21% were anti-Jo-1 positive and among them 58% were also positive for anti-Ro52 with no cross-reactivity between the two Abs. More recently Frank et al

Table 33.1—Myositis specific antibodies

Autoantibody (antigen)	Presence in PM/DM (%)[a]
Antisynthetases	25–33
Anti-Jo-1 (histidyl-transfer RNA synthetase)	20
Anti-PL-7 (threonyl-transfer RNA synthetase)	3
Anti-PL-12 (alanyl-transfer RNA synthetase)	3
Anti-OJ (isoleucyl-transfer RNA synthetase and synthetase complex)	1
Anti-EJ (glycyl-transfer RNA synthetase)	1
Anti-Mi-2 (nuclear helicase)	15–20 (in DM)
Anti-PM-Scl (nuclear/nucleolar protein complex)	5–10

[a]Percentages are for all polymyositis/dermatomyositis patients (PM/DM)

(1999) reported that the presence of anti-Ro52 Abs can be associated not only with anti-Jo-1, but also with anti-SRP (anti-signal recognition particle) and anti-PM-Scl Abs which are absent, or occur infrequently, in patients positive for anti-Mi-2, anti-Scl-70 or anti-centromere Abs, suggesting that anti-Ro52 are produced by a particular group of IM patients, and they could be used to discriminate between IM patients.

Anti-PL-7 and anti-PL-12 antibodies are present in 3% of PM/DM patients, while anti-EJ and anti-OJ antibodies are detected in 1% of patients (Table 33.1).

Anti-SRP Abs can be detected in about 4% of PM patients. They are usually associated with a severe refractory disease, myalgias, increased palpitations and higher death rates (Love et al 1991). SRP are composed of six proteins that promote translocation of newly synthesized polypeptides into the endoplasmic reticulum. Anti-SRP antibody positivity was associated with DR5, DRw52, and DQA1*0301 HLA haplotypes.

Antibodies anti Mi-2 are associated exclusively with DM (Targoff and Reichlin 1985; Love et al 1991) and are found in 15-20% of the DM patients; patients positive for anti Mi-2 antibodies have florid cutaneous manifestations but they do not show the typical constellation of findings usually associated with the antisynthetase syndrome as interstitial lung disease, arthritis or Raynaud's phenomenon (Love et al 1991). Antibodies anti Mi-2 react with a nuclear antigen, absent from the cytoplasm and the nucleoli (Targoff and Reichlin 1985). Studies on anti Mi-2 reactivity showed that all anti Mi-2 sera recognized a cDNA clone encoding a portion of the Mi-2 240 kD protein. The analysis of the protein revealed the presence of a zinc-finger motifs, proline-rich regions and charged regions, suggesting that Mi-2 is involved in DNA processing, regulation of transcription or other cellular processes (Ge et al 1995).

Other autoantibodies that can be detected in myositis (anti-U1RNP or anti Ro/SSA), with a low percentage of positivity, are indicative of an autoimmune disease but not of a myositis-specific disorder (Targoff et al 1997).

For testing antibodies anti PM-Scl the epitope analysis of the PM-Scl 100 kD protein, the major antigen of the PM-Scl complex, revealed that a peptide (aa 226-246), localized in the N-terminal half of the 100 kD protein within the active region, is useful for antibody detection by ELISA (Ge et al 1996).

ELISA, immunoprecipitation or immunoblot can detect antibodies. For determination of anti-ENA and anti-ANA antibodies by ELISA commercial kits are available. Recently, anti PL-12 and anti Jo-1 antibodies have been tested by ELISA using recombinant proteins (Garcia-Lozano et al 1998, Nishikai et al 1998) with a 95% of sensitivity and 100% of specificity. Immunodiffusion, and ELISA have tested six autoantibodies (Sm, RNP, SSA/Ro, SSB/La, Scl-70, Jo-1). All three methods revealed antibodies in serum of 36/53 patients with connective tissue disease but the immunoblot was more sensitive in detecting anti RNP and anti-SSB/La, while ELISA was more accurate for detection of anti-SSA/Ro antibodies. The authors suggest that these two methods combined were highly sensitive and specific (Bridges et al 1997).

References

Antozzi C, Berta E, Confalonieri P, Zuffi M, Cornelio F, Mantegazza R. (1994) Protein-A adsorption is effective in immunosuppression resistant myasthenia gravis. *Lancet* 343: 124.

Baggi F, Andreetta F, Antozzi C, et al. (1998) Anti-titin and anti-ryanodine receptor antibodies in myasthenia gravis patients with thymoma. *Ann NY Acad Sci* 841: 538–541.

Beeson D, Jacobson L, Newsom-Davis J, Vincent A. (1996) A transfected human muscle cell line expressing the adult subtype of the human muscle acetylcholine receptor for diagnostic assays in myasthenia gravis. *Neurology* 47: 1552–1555.

Biswas T, Miller FW, Takagaki Y, Plotz PH. (1987) An enzyme-linked immunosorbent assay for the detection and quantitation of anti-Jo-1 antibody in human serum. *J Immunol Methods* 98: 243–248.

Bridges AJ, Lorden TE, Havighurst TC. (1997) Autoantibody testing for connective tissue diseases. Comparison of immunodiffusion, immunoblot, and enzyme immunoassay. *Am J Clin Pathol* 108: 406–410.

Dalakas MC. (1995) Immunopathogenesis of inflammatory myopathies. *Ann Neurol* 37: 74–86.

Drachman D. (1994) Myasthenia gravis. *N Engl J Med* 330: 1797–1810.

Engel AG. (1994a) The neuromuscular junction. In: Engel AG, Franzini-Armstrong C, eds. *Myology*. *2nd ed*. New York: McGraw-Hill, pp. 261–302.

Engel AG. (1994b) Myasthenic syndromes. In: Engel AG, Franzini-Armstrong C, eds. *Myology*. *2nd ed*. New York: McGraw-Hill, pp. 1798–1835.

Engel AG, Hohlfeld R, Banker BQ. (1994c) The polymyositis and dermatomyositis syndromes. In: Engel AG, Franzini-Armstrong C, eds. *Myology*. *2nd ed*. New York: McGraw-Hill, pp. 1335–1383.

Frank MB, McCubbin V, Trieu E, Wu Y, Isenberg DA,

Targoff IN. (1999) The association of anti-Ro52 auto-antibodies with myositis and scleroderma autoantibodies. *J Autoimmun* 12: 137–142.

Fukunaga H, Engel AG, Osame M, Lambert EH. (1982) Paucity and disorganization of presynaptic membrane active zones in the Lambert-Eaton myasthenic syndrome. *Muscle Nerve* 5: 686–697.

Fukuoka T, Engel AG, Lang B, Newsom-Davis J, Vincent A. (1987) Lambert-Eaton myasthenic syndrome: II. Immunoelectron microscopy localization of IgG at the mouse end-plate. *Ann Neurol* 22: 200–211.

Garcia-Lozano JR, Gonzalez-Escribano MF, Rodriguez R, et al. (1998) Detection of anti-PL-12 autoantibodies by ELISA using a recombinant antigen; study of the immunoreactive region. *Clin Exp Immunol* 114: 161–165.

Gautel M, Lakey A, Barlow DP, et al. (1993) Titin auto-antibodies in myasthenia gravis: identification of a major immunogenic region of titin. *Neurology* 43: 1581–1585.

Ge Q, Nilasena DS, O'Brien CA, Frank MB, Targoff IN. (1995) Molecular analysis of a major antigenic region of the 240-kD protein of Mi-2 autoantigen. *J Clin Invest* 96: 1730–1737.

Ge Q, Wu Y, James JA, Targoff IN. (1996) Epitope analysis of the major reactive region of the 100-kd protein of PM-Scl autoantigen. *Arthritis Rheum* 39: 1588–1595.

Gotti C, Mantegazza R, Clementi F. (1984) New antigen for antibody detection in myasthenia gravis. *Neurology* 34: 374–377.

Gotti C, Balestra B, Mantegazza R, Tzartos S, Moretti M, Clementi F. (1997) Detection of antibody classes and subpopulations in myasthenia gravis patients using a non radioactive enzyme immunoassay. *Muscle Nerve* 20: 800–808.

Hart IK, Waters C, Vincent A, et al. (1997) Autoantibodies detected to expressed K+ channels are implicated in neuromyotonia (Isaac's syndrome). *Ann Neurol* 41: 238–246.

Hirakata M, Suwa A, Nagai S, et al. (1999) Anti-KS: identi-fication of autoantibodies to asparaginyl-transfer RNA synthetase associated with interstitial lung disease. *J Immunol* 62: 2315–2320.

Hofstad H, Ulvestad E, Gilhus NE, Matre R, Aarli JA. (1992) Myasthenia gravis muscle antibodies examined by ELISA: IgG and IgM antibodies characterize different patient subgroups. *Acta Neurol Scand* 85: 233–238.

Isaacs H. (1961) A syndrome of continuous muscle-fibre activity. *J Neurol Neurosurg Psychiatry* 24: 319–325.

Kawanami S, Tsuji R, Oda K. (1984) Enzyme-linked immunosorbent assay for antibody against the nicotinic acetylcholine receptor in human myasthenia gravis. *Ann Neurol* 15: 195–200.

Lang B, Waterman S, Pinto A, et al. (1998) The role of autoantibodies in Lambert-Eaton myasthenic syndrome. *Ann NY Acad Sci* 841: 596–605.

Leys K, Lang B, Johnson I, Newsom-Davis J. (1991) Calcium channel autoantibodies in the Lambert-Eaton myasthenic syndrome. *Ann Neurol* 29: 307–314.

Li Z, Forester N, Vincent A. (1996) Modulation of acetyl-choline receptor function in TE671 (rhabdomyosarcoma) cells by non-AChR ligands: a role in seronegative myas-thenia gravis? *J Neuroimmunol* 64: 179–183.

Lindstrom JM, Seybold ME, Lennon VA, Whittingham S, Duane DD. (1976) Antibody to acetylcholine receptor in myasthenia gravis. *Neurology* 26: 1054–1059.

Love LA, Leff RL, Fraser DD, et al. (1991) A new approach to the classification of idiopathic inflammatory myopathy: myositis-specific autoantibodies define useful homoge-neous patient groups. *Medicine* 70: 360–374.

Mantegazza R, Antozzi C, Pelucchetti D, Sghirlanzoni A, Cornelio F. (1988) Azathioprine as a single drug or in combination with steroids in the treatment of myasthenia gravis. *J Neurol* 235: 449–453.

Mantegazza R, Beghi E, Pareyson D, et al. (1990) A multi-centre follow-up study of 1152 patients with Myasthenia Gravis in Italy. *J Neurol* 237: 339–344.

Mantegazza R, Bernasconi P, Confalonieri P, Cornelio F. (1997) Inflammatory myopathies and systemic disorders: A review of immunopathogenetic mechanisms and clini-cal features. *J Neurol* 244: 277–287.

Mathews MB, Bernstein RM. (1983) Myositis autoantibody inhibits histidyl-tRNA synthetase: a model for autoim-munity. *Nature* 304: 177–179.

Miller FW, Twitty SA, Biswas T, Plotz PH. (1990) Origin and regulation of a disease-specific autoantibody response. Antigenic epitopes, spectrotype stability, and isotype restriction of anti-Jo-1 autoantibodies. *J Clin Invest* 85: 468–475.

Miller FW. (1993) Myositis-specific autoantibodies. Touch-stones for understanding the inflammatory myopathies. *JAMA* 270: 1846–1849.

Motomura M, Johnson I, Lang B, Vincent A, Newsom-Davis J. (1995) An improved diagnostic assay for Lambert-Eaton myasthenic syndrome. *J Neurol Neurosurg Psychiatry* 58: 85–87.

Mygland A, Tysnes OB, Aarli JA, Flood PR, Gilhus NE. (1992) Myasthenia gravis patients with a thymoma have antibodies against a high molecular weight protein in sarcoplasmic reticulum. *J Neuroimmunol* 37: 1–7.

Nishikai M, Reichlin M. (1980) Heterogeneity of precipi-tating antibodies in polymyositis and dermatomyositis: characterization of the Jo-1 antibody system. *Arthritis Rheum* 23: 881–888.

Nishikai M, Ohya K, Kosaka M, Akiya K, Tojo T. (1998) Anti-Jo-1 antibodies in polymyositis or dermatomyositis: evaluation by ELISA using recombinant fusion protein Jo-1 as antigen. *Br J Rheumatol* 37: 357–361.

Rutjes SA, Vree Egberts WT, Jongen P, Van Den Hoogen F, Pruijn GJ, Van Venrooij WJ. (1997) Anti-Ro52 antibodies frequently co-occur with anti-Jo-1 antibodies in sera from patients with idiopathic inflammatory myopathy. *Clin Exp Immunol* 109: 32–40.

Sher E, Gotti C, Canal N, et al. (1989) Specificity of calcium channel autoantibodies in Lambert-Eaton myasthenic syndrome. *Lancet* 2: 640–643.

Shi MH, Tsui FW, Rubin LA. (1991) Cellular localization of the target structures recognized by the anti-Jo-1 antibody: immunofluorescence studies on cultured human myoblasts. *J Rheumatol* 18: 252–258.

Somnier FE. (1994) Anti-acetylcholine receptor (AChR) antibodies measurement in myasthenia gravis: The use of cell line TE671 as a source of AChR antigen. *J Neuroimmunol* 51: 63–68.

Targoff IN, Reichlin M. (1985) The association between Mi-2 antibodies and dermatomyositis. *Arthritis Rheum* 28: 796–803.

Targoff IN. (1992) Autoantibodies in polymyositis. *Rheum Dis Clin North Am* 18: 455–482.

Targoff IN. (1993a) Humoral immunity in polymyositis/dermatomyositis. *J Invest Dermatol* 100: 116S–123S.

Targoff IN, Trieu EP, Miller FW. (1993b) Reaction of anti-OJ autoantibodies with components of the multi-enzyme complex of aminoacyl-tRNA synthetases in addition to isoleucyl-tRNA synthetase. *J Clin Invest* 91: 2556–2564.

Targoff IN, Miller FW, Medsger TA, Oddis CV. (1997) Classification criteria for the idiopathic inflammatory myopathies. *Curr Opin Rheumatol* 9: 527–535.

Tzartos S, Langeberg L, Hochschwender S, Swanson L, Lindstrom J. (1986) Characterization of monoclonal antibodies to denatured Torpedo and to native calf acetylcholine receptors: species, subunit and region specificity. *J Neuroimmunol* 10: 235–253.

Vincent A, Newsom-Davis J. (1982) Acetylcholine receptor characteristics in myasthenia gravis. I. Patients with generalised myasthenia or disease restricted to ocular muscle. *Clin Exp Immunol* 49: 257–265.

Vincent A, Newsom-Davis J. (1985) Acetylcholine receptor antibody as a diagnostic test for myasthenia gravis: results in 153 validated cases and 2967 diagnostic assays. *J Neurol Neurosurg Psychiatry* 48: 1246–1252.

Vincent A, Jacobson L, Plested P, et al. (1998) Antibodies affecting ion channel function in acquired neuromyotonia, in seropositive and seronegative myasthenia gravis, and in antibody-mediated arthrogryposis multiplex congenita. *Ann NY Acad Sci* 841: 482–496.

Voltz R, Hohlfeld R, Fateh-Moghadam A, et al. (1991) Myasthenia gravis: measurement of anti-AChR autoantibodies using cell line TE671. *Neurology* 41: 1836–1838.

Yamamoto T, Vincent A, Ciulla T, Lang B, Johnson I, Newsom-Davis J. (1991) Seronegative myasthenia gravis patient: a plasma factor inhibiting agonist-induced acetylcholine receptor function copurifies with IgM. *Ann Neurol* 30: 550–557.

34

Electron microscopic methods for examination of skeletal muscle

Yoshihiro Wakayama

Introduction

Most diseased muscles show morphological changes that can be detected by light microscope. However, electron microscopic examination is useful in the diagnosis of several muscle diseases (Table 34.1). In the interpretation of ultrastructural muscle pathology, the investigators must exercise the greatest caution, since artefacts are apt to occur in the various processes, such as biopsy and clamping of muscle specimens, fixation, dehydration, mounting, staining and sectioning. For example, swelling of the sarcoplasmic reticulum or mitochondria often occurs as a result of fixation, caused by hypotonic fixative. The aims of this Chapter are to describe some specific details on preparing muscle for electron microscopy and to show the general structural damage that is discernible at the electron microscopic level. In addition, immunoelectron microscopic techniques are also described for the investigation of normal and diseased muscles at the molecular level.

Table 34.1— Myopathies in which electron microscopic examination are useful for diagnosis

Rimmed vacuolar distal myopathy
Inclusion body myositis
Congenital myopathies
Central core disease
Mitochondrial myopathy
Nemaline myopathy
Multicore disease
Zebra body myopathy
Fingerprint body myopathy
Vacuolar myopathies
Glycogen storage disease
Lipid storage disease
Hypokalaemic myopathy
Periodic paralysis
Viral myositis
Others
Cytoplasmic body myopathy
Myopathy with tubular aggregates etc

Preparation of muscle samples for diagnostic electron microscopy

Fixation of muscle samples

To avoid the hypercontraction of biopsied muscle fibres, the muscle fibre bundle to be excised should be put in a U-shaped muscle clamp and the excised muscles immersed in chilled (4°C) 4% (w/v) paraformaldehyde solution in 0.1 M phosphate buffer (pH 7.4) for 1 h. The diameter of muscle bundle to be excised should be about 0.5 cm in order to obtain good fixation. Solutions of 2.5% (w/v) glutaraldehyde in 0.1 M phosphate buffer (pH 7.4) or 4% (w/v) paraformaldehyde in 0.1 M phosphate buffer (pH 7.4) are usually used as fixatives. Glutaraldehyde and paraformaldehyde have two and one aldehyde moieties, respectively, and the antigenicity of muscle samples will disappear if glutaraldehyde solution is used as a fixative. Therefore, paraformaldehyde is used for immunoelectron microscopic examinations. The temperature of the fixative is also important: the preferable temperature is 0–4°C, and this temperature should be maintained during the fixation in order to avoid artefacts during the preparation. In our experience, the osmolarity of the fixative solution seems to be adequate for muscle samples, with no addition of adjusting substance, providing the original fixative is diluted in 0.1 M phosphate buffer (pH 7.4). However, this applies to muscle fixation only, and not to other tissues. The pH of final diluted fixative should also be adjusted to 7.4. Before postfixation by 1 or 2% (w/v) O_5O_4 aqueous solution, the fixed muscle samples should be washed three times in phosphate buffered saline (PBS) and cut into small pieces (about 1 mm thick and 2 mm long) for simple ultrastructural examinations.

Pre-embedding immunolabelling methods

For pre-embedding immunoelectron microscopy, the paraformaldehyde-fixed and washed muscle samples are frozen in liquid–nitrogen-cooled isopentane and the specimens cut into thin sections in a cryostat and washed in PBS. This process is essential for the good immersion of antibodies deep into the myofibre interior. For the thin sectioning of samples, the direction in which the myofibres run is important. To eliminate nonspecific reactions, the slices are incubated for 30 min at room temperature in PBS containing 5% (w/v) preimmune serum of the secondary antibody generated in an animal such as goat or donkey. For immunolabelling experiments, the diluted primary antibody is applied to the sections at 4°C for 24 h. In multiple labelling experiments, several diluted antibodies in appropriate combinations are mixed and applied together; however, each primary antibody should be generated in different animals such as mouse, rabbit and sheep. After labelling, the specimens should be washed thoroughly in PBS. The diluted secondary antibody or antibodies are then applied to the sections at 4°C for 24 h. For multiple labelling, different sized gold particles of the colloidal-gold-conjugated secondary antibodies should be used for each respective primary antibody. Control sections are prepared by incubating the muscle sections in diluted preimmune or normal serum from the same type of animal that produced primary antibody. In general, smaller gold particles can penetrate deep into the myofibre interior, but in some studies, the immunoperoxidase method for electron microscopy has been used, because substrates such as peroxidase are much better for penetration deep into the myofibre interior. However, the multiple labelling experiment is difficult using this peroxidase method.

Post fixation, dehydration and embedding

The specimens, with or without immunolabelling of pre-embedded samples, are post fixed in chilled 1 or 2% (w/v) OsO_4 aqueous solution for 1 hour. The specimens are dehydrated in an ascending series of ethanol (example: 30%, 50%, 70%, 80%, 90%, 95%, 100%; each process for 5 min), propylene oxide (twice, each for 5 min) and propylene oxide : resine (1:1 for several hours) and then embedded in resin. In this dehydration process, the water component should be eliminated from the specimens completely, otherwise polymerization would be incomplete. In addition, attention should be paid to the direction of the muscle fibres when the muscle blocks are put into resin. The muscle samples for simple ultrastructural examination and immunoelectron microscopy are then cut into ultrathin sections, and put onto grids. Ultrathin sections for simple ultrastructural examination are stained doubly with uranyl acetate and lead citrate and examined; those for immunoelectron microscopy are examined with or without staining.

Post-embedding immunolabelling methods

Another method for immunolabelling is the post-embedding method. After embedding the materials in plastic and cutting the resin with muscle samples into ultrathin sections with an ultramicrotome, the sections on the grids are stained with primary and secondary antibodies. For this method, the temperature of resin polymerization is important, since the antigenicity of the muscle samples will disappear if the temperature is too high. Recently new resins, such as LR white, have become available that are able to polymerize in low temperature. The other method is to obtain cryo-ultrathin sections for subsequent immunoelectron microscopy. Chemically fixed or unfixed muscle samples are cut into ultrathin sections in a cryo-ultra-microtome, and the sections are put onto grids and stained as for the post-embedding methods. In general, the signal density of the muscle samples are denser with the post-embedding methods. Control sections are prepared by staining the muscle sections in diluted preimmune serum or in normal serum from the same type of animal that generated the primary antibody.

Artefacts occurring in the preparation of muscle samples

Artefacts can occur at every stage of sample preparation (Carpenter and Karpati 1984). Table 34.2 summarizes the artefacts that are prone to occur.

Table 34.2 — Artefacts that are prone to occur during sample preparation

Process	Type of artefact
1 Biopsy and clamping of muscle specimen	• Hypercontraction • Slow fixation of too large samples
2. Fixation	• Vacuolation of cell organelles such as mitochondria and sarcoplasmic reticulum due to hypotonic fixative • Shrinkage of cell and its organelles due to hypertonic fixative
3. Dehydration	• Drying of specimens
4. Inappropriate mounting resin	• Dot like precipitates
5. Staining	• Precipitates
6. Sectioning	• Chatter or knife marks

Ultrastructural changes of muscle fibres in diseased muscles

Table 34.1 includes the muscle diseases in which electron microscopic examination is useful for diagnosis. The ultrastructural changes of myofibres in some of these myopathies are illustrated below.

Rimmed vacuolar distal myopathy

The myofibre with rimmed vacuole contains granular materials as seen by light microscopy (Nonaka et al 1981). In these myofibres, positive staining for acid phosphatase (Wakayama and Shibuya 1985) and cathepsin is seen (Jimi et al 1992). Figure 34.1A and B show electron micrographs of the rimmed vacuole, and the granular material seen by light microscopy is the membranous whorl structured material considered to be secondary lysosomes.

Inclusion body myositis

The biopsied muscle contains rimmed vacuoles where electron microscopic examination shows the presence of secondary lysosomes (Fig. 34.1C) and intranuclear and/or cytoplasmic filamentous inclusions (Fig. 34.1C, D). The filamentous structures in the higher power view measure about 10 nm in diameter (Fig. 34.1D), and they were previously thought to be viral particles (Chou 1967). However, recent studies provide evidence for the accumulation of several proteins such as prion (Sarkozi et al 1994) and β-amyloid precursor protein (Askanas and Engel 1998) in myofibres with inclusions.

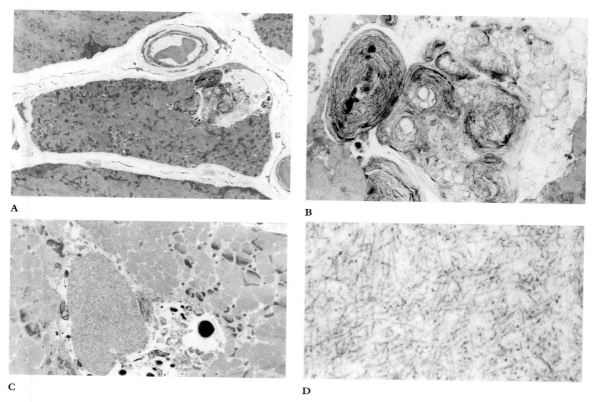

A

B

C

D

Figure 34.1—Electron micrographs showing rimmed vacuoles (**A, B**) and inclusion bodies (**C, D**) at low (**A, C**) and high (**B, D**) magnification (Magnification: **A** × 2000; **B** × 8600; **C** × 4200; **D** × 43 300).
Lower (Fig. A) and higher (Fig. B) power electron micrographs show the myofibre with a rimmed vacuole in which the vacuole contains many membranous whorls. Electron micrograph with lower magnification (Fig. C) reveals the presence of intracytoplasmic filamentous inclusions and membranous materials or electron dense secondary lysosomes in a myofibres of a patient with inclusion body myositis. The higher power view of the filamentous structure measured about 10 nm in diameter (Fig. D).

Congenital myopathies

Central core disease

The central cores can be defined by applying a number of staining techniques to the cryostat sections. In particular, the absence or decrease in the activities of oxidative enzymes such as succinate dehydrogenase or nicotinamide adenine dinucleotide dehydrogenase (NADH) is observed in the core area. This contrasts markedly with the normal oxidative enzyme activity in the surrounding muscle fibre. Electron microscopically, the core contains no mitochondria, or fewer than normal, disorganized myofilaments and Z bands, and a disoriented transverse tubular system (Fig. 34.2A).

Multicore disease

Light microscopic finding of multicore fibres displays tiny foci of pallor within the muscle fibres. These foci are more easily recognized in longitudinal sections, in which a loss of cross-striations is seen. In the majority of multicore fibres, there are multiple lesions which are smaller than the affected fibres of central core disease. In addition the multicore does not extend the whole length of the myofibre, differing from the finding of central core fibres. Electron microscopy of the affected foci shows the absence, or reduced number, of mitochondria. In some of the cores, the Z band material is clumped (Fig. 34.2B), the longitudinal filaments are disoriented and the transverse tubular system runs longitudinally (Fig. 34.2C).

Mitochondrial myopathy

The clinical manifestations of mitochondrial (encephalo)myopathy contain diverse signs and symptoms such as muscle atrophy, weakness, external ophthalmoplegia, headache, stroke-like episodes and myoclonus epilepsy (Morgan-Hughes 1986). The mode of mitochondrial DNA abnormalities may differ in individual cases, for example, mitochondrial DNA deletions or point mutations. However, muscle biopsies of these patients show the rather unique feature of the presence of ragged red fibres light microscopically. At an ultrastructural level, the mitochondria are typically embedded in the space between the myofilaments (Fig. 34.3A) or in glycogen-rich sarcoplasm where the

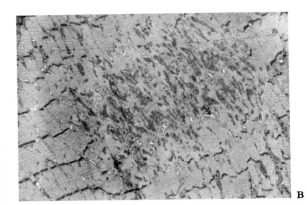

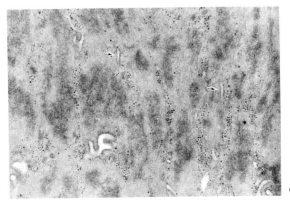

Figure 34.2—Electron micrographs showing myofibres with central cores and multicores. **A** The lower part of the electron micrograph shows a myofibre with a central core, with no or less numerous mitochondria, disorganized myofilaments and Z bands, and a disorientated transverse tubular system (arrow). **B** A lower magnification view of a multicore fibre, where the streaming of Z band material can be seen at the centre of the figure. **C** A higher magnification view of the multicore portion, where the transverse tubular system often runs longitudinally (arrows) and mitochondria are not observed in the core area (Magnification: **A** ×6300; **B** × 4300; **C** × 17 300).

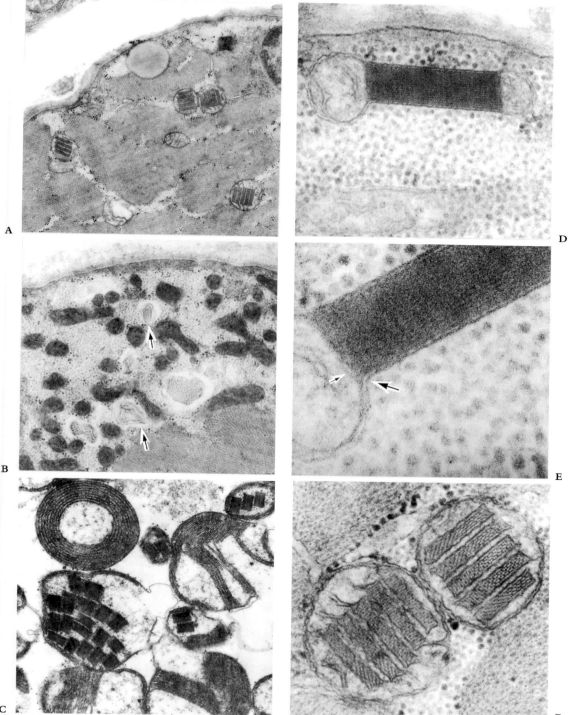

Figure 34.3—Electron micrographs showing mitochondria in mitochondrial myopathy. The mitochondria are typically embedded in the space between the myofilaments (**A**) or in glycogen-rich sarcoplasm, where the membranous whorls are often observed (arrows in **B**). Individual mitochondria are often elongated and enlarged, and they contain proliferated cristae which are distorted or concentrically arranged (**C, D**). The most common form of intramitochondrial inclusion body is the "parking lot" paracrystalline form, which is either located between the outer (large arrow) and inner (small arrow) mitochondrial membranes (**E**) or within the cristae (**F**) (Magnification: A ×13 300; **B** ×19 900; **C** ×33 700; **D** ×66 400; **E** ×32 800; F ×66 400).

membranous whorls are often observed (Fig. 34.3B), and exhibit a variety of alterations in their fine structure. Individual mitochondria are often elongated and enlarged, and may contain proliferated cristae which are distorted or concentrically arranged (Figs 34.3C,D). Among different forms of intramitochondrial inclusion bodies, the most common form is the "parking lot" paracrystalline inclusion which is either located between the outer and inner mitochondrial membranes or within the cristae (Figs 3E,F). Electron cytochemistry of crystalline inclusions demonstrate that the inclusions are non-functional (Bonilla et al 1975).

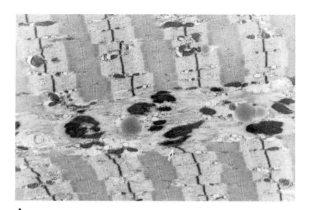

A

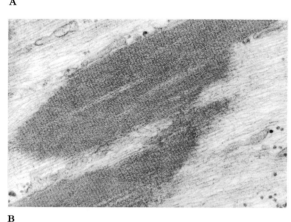

B

Figure 34.4—Electron micrographs showing nemaline bodies. **A** The lower power magnification electron micrograph displays the electron dense nemaline bodies that can be detected between the myofilaments, and the continuity of nemaline body with Z band is noted in some instances (arrow). **B** At higher magnification, the nemaline bodies are continuous with thin filaments and disclose periodic lines parallel and perpendicular to the long axis (Magnification: **A** ×5000; **B** ×43 100).

Nemaline myopathy

The term nemaline myopathy is derived from the Greek "nema" which means threadlike. Therefore, the myofibres with nemaline myopathy exhibit, light microscopically, threadlike intrasarcoplasmic inclusion bodies especially in Gomori trichrome stained sections. These intrasarcoplasmic inclusions tend to appear in Type I, red fibres. The ultrastructural features consist of the accumulation of nemaline bodies, which often show continuity with the enlarged and streamed Z disks (Fig. 34.4A). Normal Z disks in Type I, red fibres are usually thicker than those in type II, white fibres, and this may have something to do with the appearance of nemaline bodies in Type I myofibres. Low-magnification electron micrography shows electron dense nemaline bodies, which can be detected either under the sarcolemma or between the myofilaments (Fig. 34.4A). At higher magnification, the nemaline bodies can be seen to be continuous with the thin filaments and disclose periodic lines parallel and perpendicular to the long axis (Fig. 34.4B).

Zebra body myopathy

Zebra bodies are also called leptomeres and are more easily identified in extraocular muscles or developing and regenerating myotubes (Lake and Wilson 1975, Wakayama et al 1980). They consist of dense striae linked with fine filaments and the striae are 0.15 to 0.2 μm length apart (Fig. 34.5). The density of striae is similar to that of Z disks.

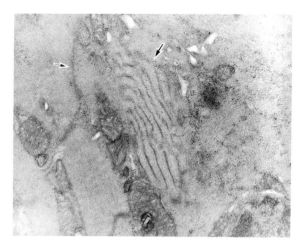

Figure 34.5—Electron micrograph showing zebra bodies. A zebra body (large arrow) can be observed, which consists of dense striae linked with fine filaments and the striae are spaced 0.15 to 0.2 μm apart. The density of striae is similar to that of Z lines (small arrow). Magnification ×16 700.

Fingerprint body myopathy

In fingerprint body myopathy, similar staining properties to the myofibrils with the stains of hematoxylin eosin and Gomori-trichrome are observed (Engel et al 1972). At the electron microscopic level, the pathological area is composed of convoluted lamellae arranged in a fingerprint pattern (Fig. 34.6).

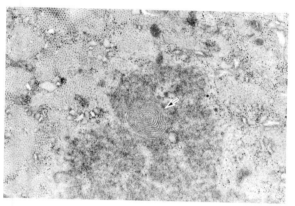

A

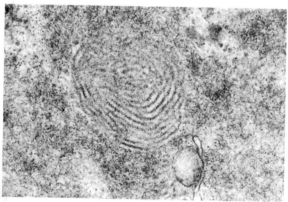

B

Figure 34.6—Electron micrographs showing fingerprint bodies. Low magnification electron micrograph (**A**) illustrates the existence of Z materials, and the fingerprint body is noted at the centre of the figure (arrow). The fingerprint body consists of sawtooth-like projections at higher magnification (**B**). (Magnification **A** ×17 000; **B** ×52 900).

Ultrastructural localization of myopathy–related molecules in skeletal myofibres

Application of single and double immunogold labelling methods

Dystrophin is the 427 kDa protein product of the Duchenne muscular dystrophy gene (Hoffman et al 1987, Koening et al 1988). The procedures for localizing the dystrophin molecule in normal skeletal myofibres were performed as described earlier. The dystrophin is localized at the inside surface of muscle plasma membrane (Fig. 34.7A) and the sarcoplasmic side of vesicular structures near the muscle plasma membrane. The signals of dystrophin molecules were denser in costameric structures. Double immunogold labelling electron microscopy was performed with the primary antibody combinations of α_1-syntrophin and dystrophin, and α_1-syntrophin and β-spectrin in normal skeletal myofibres. All these molecules were present at the inside surface of normal muscle plasma membrane and the sarcoplasmic side of vesicular structures and mitochondria near muscle plasma membranes (Wakayama et al 1999, Cullen et al 1990, Samitt and Bonilla 1990, Byers et al 1991, Wakayama and Shibuya 1991, Wakayama et al 1997). The close association of signals of α_1-syntrophin and dystrophin, and α_1-syntrophin and β-spectrin was observed as doublets of different sized gold particles. The frequency of doublets with the antibody combination of α_1-syntrophin and dystrophin was higher than that with α_1-syntrophin and β-spectrin (Fig. 34.7A, B; Wakayama et al 1997).

Application of triple immunogold labelling methods

Triple immunogold labelling electron microscopy was conducted with the primary antibody combinations against α-, β- and γ-sarcoglycans. The epitope signals of α-, β- and γ-sarcoglycans were located at the muscle plasma membranes of normal skeletal myofibres. The close association of two epitope signals was more frequently observed than that of all three epitope signals in the normal skeletal myofibres (Fig. 34.7C; Wakayama et al 1999).

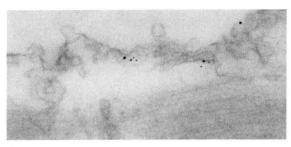

A

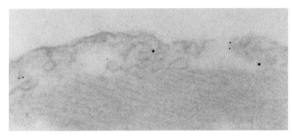

B

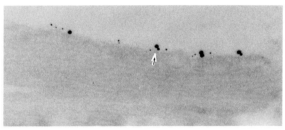

C

Figure 34.7— Examples of double and triple immunogold labelling. **A** Electron micrographs of the myofibre surfaces which have been **A** double labelled with the primary antibodies to α_1-syntrophin (5 nm gold) dystrophin (10 nm), **B** double labelled with antibodies to α_1-syntrophin (5 nm gold) and β-spectrin (10 nm gold) and **C** triple labelled with primary antibodies to α-, β- and γ-sarcoglycans. (Magnification: **A**, **B**, **C** ×71 300).

Conclusion

Electron microscopic techniques for diagnosis and investigation are described in this chapter as well as some examples of the pathological alterations of skeletal muscle fibres in several muscle diseases. Also included were materials pertaining to dystrophin and its associated proteins such as α_1-syntrophin and α-, β- and γ-sarcoglycans. Electron microscopic methods are an important tool in the investigation of the molecular pathophysiology of the muscle diseases as well as the diagnosis of myopathies.

References

Askanas V, Engel WK. (1998) Sporadic inclusion-body myositis and hereditary inclusion-body myopathies: current concepts of diagnosis and pathogenesis. *Curr Opin Rheumatol* 10: 530–542.

Bonilla E, Schotland DL, DiMauro S, Aldover B. (1975) Electron cytochemistry of crystalline inclusions in human skeletal muscle mitochondria. *J Ultrastruct Res* 51: 404–408.

Byers TJ, Kunkel LM, Watkins SC. (1991) The subcellular distribution of dystrophin in mouse skeletal, cardiac, and smooth muscle. *J Cell Biol* 115: 411–421.

Carpenter S, Karpati G. (1984) *Pathology of the skeletal muscle*. *1st ed*. New York: Churchill Livingstone.

Chou SM. (1967) Myxovirus-like structures in a case of human chronic polymyositis. *Science* 158: 1453–1455.

Cullen MJ, Walsh J, Nicholson LV, Harris JB. (1990) Vitrastructural localization of dystrophin in human muscle by using gold immunolabelling. *Proc R Soc Lond B Biol Sci* 240: 197–210.

Engel AG, Angelini C, Gomez MR. (1972) Fingerprint body myopathy, a newly recognized congenital muscle disease. *Mayo Clin Proc* 47: 377–388.

Hoffman EP, Brown RH Jr, Kunkel LM. (1987) Dystrophin: the protein product of the Duchenne muscular dystrophy locus. *Cell* 51: 919–928.

Jimi T, Satoh Y, Takeda A, Shibuya S, Wakayama Y, Sugita K. (1992) Strong immunoreactivity of cathepsin L at the site of rimmed vacuoles in diseased muscles. *Brain* 115: 249–260.

Koening M, Monaco AP, Kunkel LM. (1988) The complete sequence of dystrophin predicts a rod-shaped cytoskeletal protein. *Cell* 53: 219–226.

Lake BD, Wilson J. (1975) Zebra body myopathy. Clinical, histochemical and ultrastructural studies. *J Neurol Sci* 24: 437–446.

Morgan-Hughes JA. (1986) The mitochondrial myopathies. In: Engel AG, Banker BQ, eds. *Myology*. *Vol. 2*. New York: McGraw-Hill, pp. 1709–1743.

Nonaka I, Sunohara N, Ishiura S, Satoyoshi E. (1981) Familial distal myopathy with rimmed vacuole and lamellar (myeloid) body formation. *J Neurol Sci* 51: 141–155.

Samitt CE, Bonilla E. (1990) Immunocytochemical study of dystrophin at the myotendinous junction. *Muscle Nerve* 13: 493–500.

Sarkozi E, Askanas V, Engel WK. (1994) Abnormal accumulation of prion protein mRNA in muscle fibres of patients with sporadic inclusion-body myositis and hereditary inclusion-body myopathy. *Am J Pathol* 145: 1280–1284.

Wakayama Y, Schotland DL, Bonilla E. (1980). Transplantation of human skeletal muscle to nude mice: a sequential morphologic study. *Neurology* 30: 740–748.

Wakayama Y, Shibuya S. (1985) Vitrastructural localization of acid phosphatase in myofibre of rimmed vacuole distal myopathy. *J Clin Elect Microsc* 18: 588–589.

Wakayama Y, Shibuya S. (1991) Gold–labelled dystrophin molecule in muscle plasmalemma of mdx control mice as seen by electron microscopy of deep etching replica. *Acta Neuropathol* 82: 178–184.

Wakayama Y, Inoue M, Murahashi M, et al. (1997) Ultrastructural localization of α_1-syntrophin and neuronal nitric oxide synthase in normal skeletal myofibre, and their relation to each other and to dystrophin. *Acta Neuropathol* 94: 455–464.

Wakayama Y, Inoue M, Kojima H, et al. (1999) Ultrastructural localization of α-, β- and γ-sarcoglycan and their mutual relations, and relation to dystrophin, β-dystroglycan and β-spectrin in normal skeletal myofibre. *Acta Neuropathol* 97: 288–296.

Watkins SC, Hoffman EP, Slayter HS, Kunkel LM. (1988) Immunoelectron microscopic localization of dystrophin in myofibres. *Nature* 333: 863–866.

35

Muscle pain evoked by intraneural stimulation and recording from sympathetic and sensory muscle nerves

Paolo Marchettini and Antonio Barbieri

Introduction

The technique of microneurography was pioneered in the late 1960s by Vallbo and Hagbarth (1968, Hagbarth and Vallbo 1969) who fulfilled the dream of Adrian (1931) "to read between the receptor and the brain". A productive school of outstanding fellows in Sweden, and later abroad, exploited this elegant and powerful, yet time demanding and invasive, method to describe the physiological and pathophysiological behaviour of the entire spectrum of nerve fibres in peripheral sensory and motor nerves (Wall and McMahon 1985, Burke 1997). The first recordings were of large myelinated afferents from cutaneous low-threshold mechanoreceptors (Johansson 1978, Johansson and Vallbo 1979, 1983) and muscle spindles (Vallbo 1974, Hagbarth et al 1975, Burke et al 1978, 1979). This was followed by the recording of the massive spontaneous and reflex sympathetic activity (Vallbo et al 1979, Delius et al 1972a, 1972b) and, in the early 1970s, of isolated unmyelinated sympathetic (Hallin & Torebjörk 1974) and cutaneous nociceptive fibres (Torebjörk 1974, Torebjörk & Hallin 1974). Torebjörk and Ochoa later added the option of micro-stimulating single sensory fibres, opening the field to the correlation of cognitive perception and axonal activity at a unitary level (Torebjörk and Ochoa, 1980, 1983, 1990, Ochoa and Torebjörk 1983).

The correlation of unitary activity involving characterised low- and high-threshold cutaneous receptors and sensation evoked by the electrical stimulation of their isolated axons facilitated an extensive exploration of the physiological correlation between touch, thermal perception and pain evoked by stimulation of the skin (Vallbo 1981, Torebjörk and Ochoa 1983, Ochoa and Torebjörk 1983, 1989). Intraneural stimulation evokes paraesthesiae, occasionally even unitary paraesthesiae, that are felt as isolated tapping (in the case of low-threshold mechanoreceptors with large myelinated fibre stimulation; Ochoa and Torebjörk 1983, Torebjörk and Ochoa 1983), or well localised stinging (mechano-nociceptors with small myelinated afferents) or burning (polymodal mechano-heat nociceptors with unmyelinated afferents; Torebjörk et al 1987, Ochoa and Torebjörk 1989). By taking advantage of such an intraneurally evoked sensation physiologists have been able to guide the intraneural microelectrode within the cutaneous nerve fascicles in search of units corresponding to well-defined cutaneous territories. This technique has been used widely in studying experimental pain in human volunteers and clinical paraesthesiae and pain in human patients (Ochoa and Torebjörk 1980, Nyström and Hagbarth

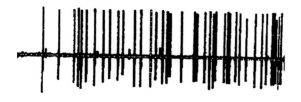

Figure 35.1— **A** Sustained ectopic discharge of a single afferent unit at slightly irregular frequency (mean frequency = 32.8 Hz). **B** Repetitive bursting discharge of a single afferent unit. Note a significant increase in firing rate during mechanical stimulation of the cutaneous receptive field (thick bars) followed by transient suppression of the ongoing discharge. Bar = 100 ms. (Reproduced with permission from Campero et al 1998.)

1981, Ochoa 1982, Ochoa et al 1982, 1985, 1987, 1991, 1993, Nordin et al 1984, Burke and Applegate 1989, Marchettini and Ochoa 1994, Campero et al 1998; Fig. 35.1).

Experimental work

Intraneural recording allowed the pioneers of microneurography to prove that the peripheral nerve fascicles that innervate muscles are well segregated from those involved in cutaneous innervation. The continuous intermingling of fibres that, on the basis of histological observations, Sunderland (1945) described in different fascicles was not replicated by physiological recordings (Vallbo et al 1979). This specific anatomical selectivity of cutaneous and muscle fascicular innervation was used by Hagbarth et al (1972) to describe the different characteristics of skin sympathetic activity (SSA) and muscle sympathetic activity (MSA; Delius et al 1972a), recorded from fascicles innervating either skin or muscle. MSA was described in great detail, showing it to be quite different from

SSA in regulating systemic blood pressure in response to stress, exercise and changes in body position (e.g. moving from lying to standing) (Delius et al 1972a). Microneurographic studies on humans have shown that MSA discharges can be provoked by manoeuvres that decrease carotid sinus activity and, conversely, are inhibited by stimulation of the carotid sinus (Delius et al 1972b). Anaesthesia of the glossopharyngeal and vagus nerves increases MSA and abolishes physiological cardiac rhythmicity, transforming MSA activity into irregular discharges similar to SSA. MSA modification by vagal block proves that MSA rhythmicity is mediated by cardiac inhibitory input and it is not an intrinsic characteristic of the central sympathetic drive (Fagius et al 1985). This is relevant to the interpretation of sympathetic hyperactivity in demyelinating neuropathies such as the Guillain Barré syndrome (Fagius et al 1985). In systemic hypertension (Mark 1990, Anderson et al 1989) MSA, not SSA, is increased. In fact the increase in MSA is not caused by the arterial baroreceptors becoming less inhibitory, but rather by a presumed heightened central nervous system drive (Mark 1990). Increase in MSA shows a significantly positive correlation with age in both hypertensive and normotensive subjects (Yamada et al 1989). Note that in pathological conditions with orthostatic hypotension, or with generalised sympathetic failure, tonic MSA discharge, or reflexively-evoked response, may be abnormally reduced (Dotson et al 1990; Fig. 35.2).

Intraneural stimulation of muscle nerve fascicles evokes a sensation peculiar to muscle, quite different from the sensation referred to skin. The only afferents that can be found in both cutaneous and muscle nerve fascicles, and that evoke the same sensation when stimulated, are large fibre afferents supplying the joints (Macefield et al 1990, Gandevia et al 1992). Such units, mostly recorded in cutaneous fascicles, produce a sensation of joint distortion (twisting or flexing) corresponding to the complex multiaxial responsiveness of the supplied receptor (Gandevia et al 1992). The stimulation of large sensory afferents from spindle receptors, both isolated and as fibre groups, usually evokes no conscious sensation (Macefield et al 1990, Gandevia et al 1992). Only on one occasion did the stimulation of a spindle afferent supplying intrinsic muscles of the hand evoke a cognitive perception, the sensation being described as that normally associated with muscle lengthening (Gandevia et al 1992). Considering that selective stimulation of the spindle receptors through vibratory stimuli and complete cutaneous anaesthesia evokes the sensation of movement (Gandevia et al 1992), it seems surprising that

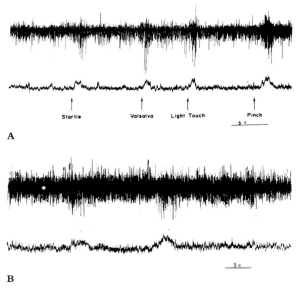

A

B

Figure 35.2— **A** Microneurographic recording of skin sympathetic neural activity in a normal subject. Reflexly induced sympathetic afferent activity occurs in response to various manoeuvres, such as startle, Valsalva, and light touch and pinch delivered outside the cutaneous receptive field for the fascicle. The discriminated (top tracing) and integrated (bottom tracing) neurograms are shown. **B** Microneurographic recoding of spontaneously occuring bursts of multiunit sympathetic efferent neural discharges are marked by asterisks. The sympathetic activity is not responsive to manoeuvres that normally influence skin sympathetic efferent neural output, such as startle, Valsalva manoeuvre, and cold water immersion of the feet. The discriminated (top tracing) and integrated (bottom tracing) neurograms are shown. (Reproduced with permission from Dotson et al 1990.)

there is no evocable sensation from the direct stimulation of the spindle afferent fibres. In fact the large myelinated afferents from muscle, most of which are from spindle afferents, are well represented in the cortex, as witnessed by the cortical response evoked by electrical stimulation of entire nerve fascicles supplying muscle (Gandevia et al 1984, 1988).

There could also be an apparent absence of conscious perception, simply resulting from the inadequacy of intraneural stimulation to produce the proper spatial–temporal summation or coding pattern required to evoke conscious perception from spindle afferent units. Gandevia et al summarised their observations on this subject by stating: "the discharge of spindle afferents appears to be insufficient to elicit the sensations attributed to the discharge of a population of them", and also: "psychophysical studies suggest that the number and discharge frequency of spindle afferents influence the perceived velocity of illusory movements" (Gandevia 1985, Gandevia et al 1992).

The most peculiar sensation evoked by the stimulation of nerve muscle fascicles is that of deep, cramp-like pain (Torebjörk et al 1984, Marchettini et al 1990). Nordin et al (1986) microrecorded and microstimulated the facial nerve that has neither spindle afferent activity nor sympathetic efferent discharges, and they found that such stimulation could evoke a sensation of deep pain in the cheek, a pain recalling that felt in the muscles of the limbs. Ochoa and Torebjörk were particularly puzzled by the muscle pain evoked by intraneural stimulation; together with Schady they evoked muscle pain by stimulating median nerve fascicles that innervate only muscle (Torebjörk et al 1984). They noted that in some cases the pain, originally projected distally from the point of stimulation and localised in the muscular territory innervated by the stimulated fascicle, spreads proximally as the intensity of the stimulation is increased. Curiously the proximal spread involves muscular territory not innervated by the stimulated fascicle, and not even innervated by the median nerve (Torebjörk et al 1984). Furthermore, the quality of the pain evoked by the stimulation of fascicles innervating muscle is different from cutaneous pain, evoked by the same technique, in cutaneous nerve fascicles. This "muscle pain" is not one of burning, nor is it associated with a stinging sensation or paraesthesiae; it has a typical "muscle quality", being cramp-like, not well-localised and deep (Torebjörk et al 1984). The experiments of pain evoked by "muscle nerve fascicle" stimulation recall early human experiments on muscle pain sensation at the beginning of the 1930s and 1940s (Lewis 1932, 1942, Kellgren 1937–38, 1939).

In 1932 Lewis observed that the injection of substances into muscle provokes a pain of a quality similar to ischaemic pain. He concluded that the pain quality provoked in somatic structures depends more on the structure stimulated than on the nature of the stimulus (Lewis 1932, 1942). Kellgren pursued the studies on muscle pain, injecting saline solution into muscle or fascia while the skin was anaesthetised with lidocaine (Kellgren 1937–8, 1939). Kellgren found that when muscle pain is very intense it extends over areas larger than the one injected, spreading along limbs in a fashion that recalls the distribution of radicular territories. Interestingly the author noted that such territories are not like the radicular territories described by Foerster (1933), who obtained cutaneous vasodilatation antidromically by stimulating cutaneous sensory fibres, nor are they like the dermatomes connected with radicular Herpes Zoster distribution reported by Head and Campbell (1900). Kellgren (1937–8) stated that muscle pain is not as well localised

as pain originating from the skin, and the greater the intensity of the pain the less accurate was its localisation. This implies that the cortical localisation function of muscle pain may be modulated by the intensity of the stimulus; however, this has been interpreted generically as a demonstration that muscle pain is not well localised. In 1967, Hockaday and Whitty repeated the experimental saline injections into spinal ligaments and paraspinal muscles to study deep referred pain, and they gave further support to Lewis and Kellgren's conclusions, without emphasising the correlation existing between the intensity of muscle pain and the progressive worsening of its localisation.

Intrafascicular stimulation of muscle nerves was extended to study the ulnar nerve territories (Marchettini et al 1990). The findings were similar to those reported for the median nerve, the distribution of pain being in a lower radicular distribution (C8-T1). This "radicular" distribution does not match the cutaneous territory of C8-T1, it rather resembles the territory of motor innervation (Fig. 35.3). The stimulation of cutaneous nerve fascicles at very strong

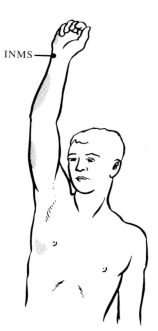

Figure 35.3—Areas of the body where painful sensations may be referred during strong intraneural stimulation at wrist level of single ulnar nerve fascicles supplying hand muscles. Muscle pain was projected most commonly to distal muscles in the hand. Proximally referred pain was localized most commonly to ulnar forearm and less frequently to posterior upper arm, lateral chest wall and scapular region (not shown). INMS, intraneural muscle fascicle stimulation. (Reproduced with permission from Marchettini et al 1990.)

intensities in that study was done to explore whether the projection of pain depends in any way on a temporal and spatial summation of the stimulus, or on the quality of the receptive field (muscular versus cutaneous). Despite very high current intensities (up to 20 V, with 400 s duration) and the duration of the stimuli (up to 15 min), the cutaneous pain, unlike that of muscle, remained confined to the territory of the stimulated nerve (Marchettini et al 1990).

Using the technique of microneurography to stimulate and record, carefully checking the area of projected sensation while applying varying intensities of pressure, led to the identification of muscle sensory afferents with the physiological characteristics of noci-

ceptors (Marchettini 1993, Simone et al 1994, Marchettini et al 1996; Fig. 35.4). The conduction rate of these afferents is in the range of Group III (small myelinated, conducting at 3.1–13.5 m/s) and Group IV (unmyelinated, conducting at 0.6–1.9 m/s). All these units adapt slowly and have a moderate/high threshold to mechanical stimuli. Interestingly their threshold for mechanical stimuli may, in some cases, be below the threshold for pain. On the other hand, electrical stimulation of these slowly-conducting muscle afferents provoked only pain. Despite the common belief that muscle pain is poorly localised, the painful muscle sensation evoked by single nociceptor stimulation was localised, with fair accuracy, to

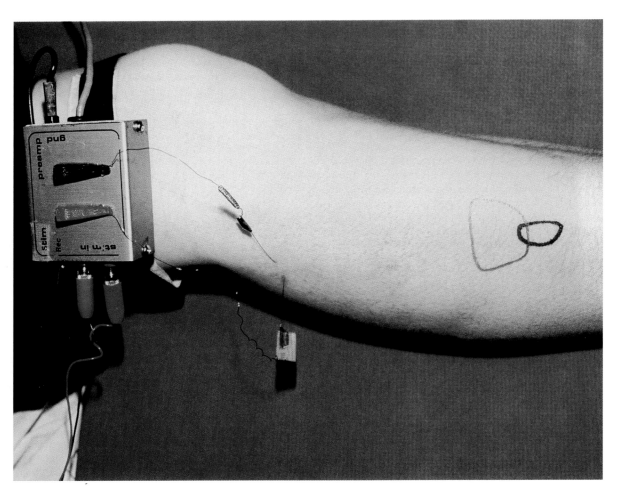

Figure 35.4—General setup to search for and identify muscle nociceptors. The preamplifier is attached behind the knee. A microelectrode (distal) was inserted into the common peroneal nerve and a reference electrode (proximal) was inserted into subcutaneous tissue nearby. The area outlined in red represents the projection of deep pain to underlying muscle during intraneural microstimulation (INMS) at threshold for pain sensation. The area outlined in black represents the mechanosensitive receptive field (RF) of a Group IV nociceptor with conduction velocity of 1.9 m/s. (Reproduced with permission from Simone et al 1994.)

the area where a high-threshold receptor was identified. The initial area of projected pain was rather small (3.2 ± 0.84 mm^2 for Group III, 4.7 ± 1.03 mm^2 for Group IV), but maintaining a constant stimulus intensity caused the area of projected pain to expand progressively (Simone et al 1994, Marchettini et al 1996). These units responded to capsaicin—an agent that induces pain when injected into muscle and that selectively excites human mechano-heat nociceptors, but no other cutaneous receptors, when applied to the skin (Marchettini et al 1996).

The human experiments on muscle pain obtained with intraneural recordings, and the identification of the characteristics of receptor response of muscle nociceptors, resulted in data akin to that from animal studies. In 1943, Lloyd, studying nerve afferents from muscle, identified different fibre populations, and proposed the classification of muscle sensory afferents separately from cutaneous afferents, putting them into four conduction velocity-based groups. The fastest large myelinated fibres, in the A range, were defined as groups I and II, the small myelinated fibres with conduction in the A range as group III and the slowest unmyelinated C fibres as Group IV. In 1960, Paintal recorded Group III afferents with functional characteristics of nociceptors, and the following year Iggo (1961) observed the response of unmyelinated afferent fibres to stimulation of endings within mammalian skeletal muscle. The anatomical demonstration that free nerve endings exist in the skeletal muscle of the cat came in 1969 (Stacey 1969). Mense and co-workers in Germany described in great detail the functional characteristics (in cats) of receptors that respond to chemicals and are mainly innervated by Group IV afferents, but also by Group III (Mense and Schmidt 1974, Franz and Mense 1975, Hertel et al 1976, Hiss and Mense 1976). In 1977, Kumazawa and Mizumura demonstrated the response of thin fibre afferents following mechanical, chemical and thermal stimulation of the skeletal muscle of the dog. They considered these units with slowly adapting behaviour as nociceptors, although some responded to low intensity mechanical stimuli that would certainly not provoke pain in humans. The information acquired by this body of research was summarised by Mense in 1986: a rich network of receptors innervated by small myelinated (Group III) and unmyelinated (Group IV) fibres supplies muscles. The majority of these afferents show:

- increased response to progressively increasing the intensity of stimulation, and modification in threshold following injection of sensitising inflammatory agents or repeated activation

- response to inflammatory agents (like bradychinin) known to produce pain in humans
- increased response under ischaemic conditions
- decreased response to inflammatory agents following application of anti-inflammatory drugs (aspirin).

Such mechanosensitive units adapt slowly with variable thresholds; the majority have a high threshold although some have a low–medium threshold (Mense 1986). Based on all the above characteristics, small afferents from muscle can be classified as nociceptors. Units with such characteristics project to laminae I and V of the dorsal horn (Mense and Craig 1988).

Clinical considerations

Nociceptor activation

Muscle nociceptors are mechanosensitive, and they may be sensitised by hypoxia and inflammatory agents. Experts on muscle disease are well aware that muscle pain in the clinic is a puzzling symptom that is not related to the severity of muscle damage. Devastating primary muscle disease, like Duchenne dystrophy, is in no way painful; pain in polymiositis may be absent or moderate. On the contrary unusual muscle effort may cause intense pain in healthy subjects (Mills et al 1982, Rowland 1985, Edwards 1990). Therefore, it is likely that the sensory apparatus encoding muscle pain is close to the muscle cell, but that it is not activated by primary muscle cell damage; such activity is a result of changes in the chemical environment surrounding muscle tissue, or stimulation of the fascia (Marchettini 1993). Muscle nociceptors are activated by mechanical stimuli (Mense 1986, Simone et al 1994, Marchettini et al 1996) and it has been demonstrated that hypoxia lowers their threshold (Mense 1986). Additionally, several inflammatory agents have been shown to reduce the muscle nociceptor threshold in animals (Mense and Schmidt 1974) and humans (Marchettini et al 1996). On the basis of these observations the apparent discrepancy between muscle pain and muscle tissue injury may be reconciled. Diseases that affect muscle cells from within do not cause increased pressure on nociceptors and thus cause no pain. Intense exercise of untrained muscle may lead to a sensitisation of nociceptors, lasting many hours. This could explain pain and soreness that persist for days after unusual muscle effort in hypoxic conditions and that are peculiarly increased or evoked by movement. By analogy, inflammation of muscular tissue and injection of substances into muscle also cause pain through chemical or mechanical stimulation. In general, it could be said that muscle pain is a symptom originating from the structures surrounding muscle, rather than from the muscle tissue itself.

Symptoms of neuropathy

Muscle nociceptors are innervated by small myelinated and unmyelinated fibres, and muscle pain can be reproduced by intraneural stimulation. Most physicians would easily recognise from the words "pins and needles, tingling, burning" the cutaneous symptoms of a sensory neuropathy (Ochoa 1982, Ochoa et al 1987, 1991, Ochoa and Marchettini 1993). Few physicians would so readily recognise that deep pressure and cramp-like pain may also be symptoms of peripheral neuropathy. Polyneuropathies may produce muscle pain when small myelinated or unmyelinated fibres are involved. For the symptoms to be present, it is, of course, necessary that abnormal activity be produced in diseased nerve afferents from muscle, as is the case for a spectrum of positive neuropathic symptoms (Ochoa 1982, Ochoa and Marchettini 1993). Patients who complain of neuropathic muscle pain usually localise it in the calf muscles. The reason for these favoured muscles, midway as opposed to distal, is not clear: perhaps within the population of distal axons, sensory afferents from other deep tissues prevail, and thus distal axonopathy is perceived generically as deep pain; or calf muscles have a greater muscle nociceptor density and preferential cortical localisation (Marchettini 1993, Marchettini and Ochoa 1994). Calf pain is frequent in polyneuropathy, and it is usually considered a neuropathic symptom when associated with other signs and symptoms of polyneuropathy, as in diabetic or porphyric neuropathy (Ridley 1984). Muscle pain is less well identified as a neuropathic sensory disorder when it appears in isolation, as is the case in restless legs syndrome (Ekbom 1970).

Proximally referred pain

Muscle pain may be proximally referred. Experiments with intraneural stimulation have shown that when a sensory fascicle innervating muscle is appropriately stimulated, the only symptoms may be deep pain in the innervated territory and proximally referred pains (Torebjörk et al 1984, Marchettini et al 1990). Entrapment median neuropathy at the wrist is a common condition and carpal tunnel release is a frequent intervention. Peripheral nerve clinicians and surgeons quickly recognise the arm and shoulder pain that is relieved by carpal tunnel surgery, knowing it to be a proximally referred symptom of median nerve entrapment (Golding 1968, Kummel and Zazanis 1973). Less well known is that deep pain in the scapular area may be a symptom of ulnar nerve entrapment at the elbow, or cervical root compression (Marchettini 1993); the only symptom of lumbar or sacral radiculopathy might be deep pain in the lower limb. This misleading "neuropathic muscle pain" also pertains to thoracic roots and may mimic angina (Lindhal and Hamberg 1981). Thus, localised muscle pain can be a valuable symptom in identifying focal nerve or root entrapment, even in the absence of motor deficit and cutaneous sensory abnormalities (Marchettini and Ochoa 1994). The radicular representation of deep pain from muscles, tendons and bones (Inman and Saunders 1944) is a likely explanation for the discrepancy in classic dermatome charts (Head and Campbell 1900, Foerster 1933, Keegan and Garrett 1948, Marchettini 1993). Pain territories delineated by intraneural microstimulation could, in a way, be considered charts of the "sensory myotome" and they could be advantageously incorporated into clinical criteria for the diagnosis of pain caused by radiculopathy (Marchettini and Ochoa 1994).

References

Adrian ED. (1931) The messages in sensory nerve fibres and their interpretation. *Proc R Soc B* 109: 1–18.

Anderson EA, Sinkey CA, Lawton WJ, Mark AL. (1989) Elevated sympathetic nerve activity in borderline hypertensive humans. Evidence from direct intraneural recordings. *Hyperten* 14: 177–183.

Burke D. (1997) Unit identification, sampling bias and technical issues in microneurographic recordings from muscle spindle afferents. *J Neurosc Meth* 74: 137–144.

Burke D, Applegate C. (1989) Paraesthesie and hypaesthesiae following prolonged high frequency stimulation of cutaneous afferents. *Brain* 112: 913–929.

Burke D, Hagbarth KE, Löfstedt L. (1978) Muscle spindle activity in man during shortening and lengthening contractions. *J Physiol* 277: 131–142.

Burke D, Skuse NF, Stuart DG. (1979) The regularity of muscle spindle discharge in man. *J Physiol* 291: 277–290.

Campero M, Serra J, Marchettini P, Ochoa JL. (1998) Ectopic impulse generation and autoexcitation in single myelinated afferent fibers in patients with peripheral neuropathy and positive sensory symptoms. *Muscle Nerve* 21: 1661–1667.

Delius W, Hagbarth K-E, Hongell A, Wallin BG. (1972a)

General characteristics of sympathetic activity in human muscle nerves. *Acta Physiol Scand* 84: 65–81.

Delius W, Hagbarth KE, Hongell A, Wallin BG. (1972b) Manoeuvres affecting sympathetic outflow in human muscle nerves. *Acta Physiol Scand* 84: 82–94.

Dotson R, Ochoa J, Marchettini P, Cline M. (1990) Sympathetic Neural Outflow directly recorded in patients with primary autonomic failure: clinical observations, microneurography and hystopathology. *Neurology* 40: 1079–1085.

Edwards RHT. (1990) Pathophysiology of muscle pain. In: Lipton S et al, eds. *Advances in pain therapy Vol 13*. New York: Raven Press, pp. 157–163.

Ekbom KA. (1970) Restless legs. In: Vinken PJ, Bruyn GW, eds. *Handbook of clinical Neurology. Vol 8*. Amsterdam: North Holland, pp. 311–320.

Fagius J, Wallin BG, Sundlof G, Nerhed C, Englesson S. (1985) Sympathetic outflow in man after anaesthesia of the glossopharyngeal and vagus nerves. *Brain* 108: 423–438.

Foerster O. (1933) The dermatomes in man. *Brain* 56: 1–39.

Franz M, Mense S. (1975) Muscle receptors with group IV afferent fibres responding to application of bradychinin. *Brain Res* 92: 369–383.

Gandevia SC. (1985) Illusory movements produced by electrical stimulation of low-threshold muscle afferents from the hand. *Brain* 108: 965–981.

Gandevia SC, Burke D. (1988) Projection to the cerebral cortex from proximal and distal muscles in the human upper limb. *Brain* 111: 389–403.

Gandevia SC, Burke D, McKeon B. (1984) The projection of muscle afferents from the hand to cerebral cortex in man. *Brain* 107: 1–13.

Gandevia SC, McCIoskey DI, Burke D. (1992) Kinaesthetic signals and muscle contraction. *Trends Neurosci* 5: 62–65.

Golding DN. (1968) Brachial neuralgia and the carpal tunnel syndrome. *Br Med J* 3: 803–812.

Hagbarth KE, Hallin RG, Hongell A, Torebjörk HE, Wallin BG. (1972) General characteristics of sympathetic activity in human skin nerves. *Acta Physiol Scand* 84: 164–176.

Hagbarth KE, Vallbo ÅB. (1969) Single unit recordings from muscle nerves in human subjects. *Acta Physiol Scand* 76: 321–334.

Hagbarth KE, Wallin BG, Löfstedt L. (1975) Muscle spindle activity in man during voluntary fast alternating movements. *J Neurol Neurosurg Psych* 38: 625–635.

Hallin RG, Torebjörk HE. (1974) Single unit sympathetic activity in human skin nerves during rest and various manoeuvres. *Acta Physiol Scand* 92: 303–317.

Head H, Campbell AW. (1900) The pathology of herpes zoster and its bearing on sensory localization. *Brain* 23: 23–523.

Hertel HC, Howaldt B, Mense S. (1976) Responses of group IV and group III muscle afferents to thermal stimuli. *Brain Res* 113: 201–205.

Hiss E, Mense S. (1976) Evidence for the existence of different receptor sites for algesic agents at the endings of muscular Group IV afferent units. *Pflügers Arch Ges Physiol* 362: 141–146.

Hockaday JM, Whitty CWM. (1967) Patterns of referred pain in the normal subject. *Brain* 40: 481–496.

Iggo A. (1961) Non-myelinated afferent fibers from mammalian skeletal muscle. *J Physiol* 155: 52–53.

Inman VT, Saunders JB deCM. (1944) Referred pain from skeletal structures. *J Nerv Ment Dis* 99: 660–667.

Johansson RS. (1978) Tactile sensibility in the human hand receptive field characteristics of mechanoreceptive units in the glabrous skin areas. *J Physiol* 281: 101–123.

Johansson RS, Vallbo ÅB. (1979) Tactile sensibility in the human hand: relative and absolute densities of four types of mechanoreceptive units in the glabrous skin. *J Physiol* 286: 283–300.

Johansson RS, Vallbo ÅB. (1983) Tactile sensory coding in the glabrous skin of the human hand. *Trends Neurosci* 6: 27–32.

Keegan JJ, Garrett FD. (1948) The segmental distribution of the cutaneous nerves in the limbs of man. *Anat Rec* 102: 409–443.

Kellgren JH. (1937–8) Observations on referred pain arising from muscle. *Clin Sci* 3: 175–190.

Kellgren JH. (1939) On the distribution of pain arising from deep structures, with charts of segmental pain areas. *Clin Sci* 4: 35–46.

Kumazawa T, Mizumura K. (1977) Thin-fibre receptors responding to mechanical, chemical, and thermal stimulation in the skeletal muscle of the dog. *J Physiol* 273: 179–194.

Kummel BM, Zazanis GA. (1973) Shoulder pain as the presenting complaint in carpal tunnel syndrome. *Clin Orthop* 92: 227–230.

Lewis T. (1932) Pain in muscular ischemia. *Arch Int Med* 49: 713–727.

Lewis T. (1942) *Vascular disorders of the limb, described for practitioners and students*. Reprint 1981. London: MacMillan, pp. 40–41, 96–103, 120–121.

Lindhal O, Hamberg J. (1981) Angina pectoris symptoms caused by thoracic spine disorders. Neuroanatomical considerations. *Acta Med Scand* 644: 81–83.

Lloyd DPC. (1943) Neuron patterns controlling transmission of ipsilateral hindlimb reflexes in cat. *J Neurophysiol* 6: 293–315.

Macefield G, Gandevia SC, Burke D. (1990) Perceptual responses to microstimulation of single afferents innervating the joints, muscles and skin of the human hand. *J Physiol* 429: 113–129.

Marchettini P. (1993) Muscle pain: animal and human experimental and clinical studies. *Muscle Nerve* 16: 1033–1039.

Marchettini P, Ochoa JL. (1994) The clinical implications of referred muscle pain sensation. *Am Pain Soc J* 3: 10–12.

Marchettini P, Cline M, Ochoa J. (1990) Innervation territories for touch and pain afferents of single fascicles of the human ulnar nerve. *Brain* 113: 1491–1500.

Marchettini P, Simone D, Caputi G, Ochoa J. (1996) Slowly conducting high threshold mechanoreceptors microrecorded from human striated muscle. Receptor responses, axonal conduction velocity and projected pain. *Brain Res* 740: 109–116.

Mark AL. (1990) Regulation of sympathetic nerve activity in mild human hypertension. *J Hyperten* 8: 67–75.

Mense S. (1986) Slowly conducting afferent fibers from deep tissues: neurobiological properties and central nervous actions. *Prog Sens Physiol* 6: 139–219.

Mense S, Schmidt RF. (1974) Activation of group IV afferent units from muscle by algesic agents. *Brain Res* 109: 402–406.

Mense S, Craig AD Jr. (1988) Spinal and supraspinal terminations of primary afferent fibers from the gastrocnemius-soleus muscle in the cat. *Neurosci* 26: 1023–1035.

Mills KR, Newham DJ, Edwards RHT. (1982) Force, contraction frequency and energy metabolism as determinants of ischemic muscle pain. *Pain* 14: 149–154.

Nordin M, Nyström B, Wallin U, Hagbarth KE. (1984) Ectopic sensory discharges and paresthesiae in patients with disorders of peripheral nerves, dorsal roots and dorsal columns. *Pain* 20: 231–245.

Nordin M, Hagbarth KE, Thomander L, Wallin U. (1986) Microelectrode recordings from the facial nerve in man. *Acta Physiol Scand* 128: 379–387.

Nyström B, Hagbarth KE. (1981) Microelectrode recordings from transected nerves in amputees with phantom limb pain. *Neurosci Lett* 27: 211–216.

Ochoa J. (1982) Pain in local nerve lesions. In: Ochoa J, Culp WJ, eds. *Abnormal nerves and muscles as impulse generators*. New York: Oxford Univ Press 28: 568–587.

Ochoa J, Marchettini P. (1993) Painful polyneuropathic sensory syndromes. In: Vecchiet L, Albe-Fessard A, Lindblom U, eds. *New Trends in Referred Pain and Hyperalgesia*. Amsterdam: Elsevier, pp. 319–328.

Ochoa J, Torebjörk E. (1980) Paraesthesiae from ectopic impulse generation in human sensory nerves. *Brain* 103: 835–853.

Ochoa J, Torebjörk E. (1983) Sensations evoked by intraneural microstimulation of single mechanoreceptor units innervating the human hand. *J Physiol* 342: 633–654.

Ochoa J, Torebjörk E. (1989) Sensation evoked by intraneural microstimulation of C nociceptors fibers in human skin nerves. *J Physiol* 415: 583–599.

Ochoa J, Torebjörk E, Culp WJ, Schady W. (1982) Abnormal spontaneous activity in single sensory nerve fibers in humans. *Muscle Nerve* 5: 74–77.

Ochoa J, Torebjörk E, Marchettini P, Sivak M. (1985) Mechanism of Neuropathic Pain – Cumulative Observations, new Experiments and further Speculation. In: Fields H, Dubner R, Cervero F, eds. *Advances in Pain Research and Therapy*. New York: Raven Press, pp. 431–450.

Ochoa J, Cline M, Dotson R, Marchettini P. (1987) Pain and paresthesias provoked mechanically in human cervical root entrapment (sign of Spurling). Single sensory unit antidromic recording of ectopic, bursting, propagated nerve impulse activity. In: Pubols LM, Sessle BJ, eds. *Effects of injury on trigeminal and spinal somatosensory systems*. New York: Alan R. Liss, pp. 389–397.

Ochoa J, Marchettini P, Cline M. (1991) Lessons from human research on the pathophysiology of neuropathic pains in limbs. In: Parry W, ed. *Management of Pain in the Hand and Wrist*. Edinburgh: Churchill Livingstone, pp. 28–33.

Ochoa JL, Yarnitsky D, Marchettini P, Dotson R, Cline M. (1993) Interactions between sympathetic vasoconstrictor outflow and C nociceptor-induced antidromic vasodilatation. *Pain* 54: 191–196.

Paintal AS. (1960) Functional analysis of group III afferent fibres of mammalian muscles. *J Physiol* 152: 250–270.

Ridley A. (1984) Porphyric neuropathy. In: Dyck PJ, Thomas PK, Lambert EH, Bunge R, eds. *Peripheral neuropathy. Vol 2*. Philadelphia: Saunders Co 72: 1704–1716.

Rowland LP. (1985) Cramps, spasm and muscle stiffness. *Rev Neurol* 141: 261–273.

Simone DA, Marchettini P, Caputi G, Ochoa JL. (1994) Identification of muscle afferents subserving sensation of deep pain in humans. *J Neurophys* 72: 883–889.

Stacey MJ. (1969) Free nerve endings in skeletal muscle of the cat. *J Anat* 105: 231–254.

Sunderland S. (1945) The intraneural topography of the radial, median and ulnar nerves. *Brain* 68: 243–299.

Torebjörk HE. (1974) Afferent C units responding to mechanical, thermal and chemical stimuli in human nonglabrous skin. *Acta Physiol Scand* 92: 374–390.

Torebjörk HE, Hallin RG. (1974) Identification of afferent C units in intact human skin nerves. *Brain Res* 67: 387–403.

Torebjörk E, Ochoa J. (1980) Specific sensations evoked by activity in single identified sensory units in man. *Acta Physiol Scand* 110: 445–447.

Torebjörk HE, Ochoa J. (1983) Selective stimulation of sensory units in man. *Adv Pain Res Ther* 5: 99–104.

Torebjörk HE, Ochoa JL. (1990) New method to identify nociceptor units innervating glabrous skin of the human hand. *Exp Brain Res* 81: 509–514.

Torebjörk E, Vallbo ÅB, Ochoa JL. (1987). Intraneural microstimulation in man: Its relation to specificity of tactile sensations. *Brain* 110: 1509–1529.

Torebjörk HE, Ochoa JL, Schady W. (1984) Referred pain from intraneural stimulation of muscle fascicles in the median nerve. *Pain* 18: 145–156.

Vallbo ÅB. (1974) Afferent discharges from human muscle spindles in noncontracting muscles. Steady state impulse frequency as a function of joint angle. *Acta Physiol Scand* 90: 303–318.

Vallbo ÅB. (1981) Sensation evoked from the glabrous skin of the human hand by electrical stimulation of unitary mechanosensitive afferents. *Brain Res* 215: 359–363.

Vallbo ÅB, Hagbarth KE. (1968) Activity from skin mechanoreceptors recoded percutaneously in awake human subjects. *Exp Neurol* 21: 270–289.

Vallbo ÅB, Hagbarth KE, Torebjörk E, Wallin BG. (1979) Somatosensory, proprioceptive and sympathetic activity in human peripheral nerves. *Physiol Rev* 59: 919–957.

Wall PD, McMahon SB. (1985) Microneurography and its relation to perceived sensation. A critical review. *Pain* 21: 209–229.

Yamada Y, Miyajima E, Tochikubo O, Matsukawa T, Ishii M. (1989) Age-related changes in muscle sympathetic nerve activity in essential hypertension. *Hypertens* 13: 870–877.

36

Skeletal muscle biopsy techniques: practice and procedures

Amyn M. Rojiani, Fernando Vale

Introduction

The accurate diagnosis of neuromuscular disease often requires a muscle biopsy in addition to clinical evaluation. Muscle biopsies may be performed for a variety of disorders, either to assess primary muscle disease or to determine the secondary involvement of skeletal muscle as part of systemic processes. Primary disorders in which a muscle biopsy may yield helpful information include various myopathies including the range of dystrophinopathies and congenital myopathies, as well as metabolic disorders. Skeletal muscle biopsy may also prove to be a valuable aid in the diagnosis of certain systemic conditions including vasculitides and connective tissue disorders. Additionally, the muscle biopsy will serve to distinguish conditions that are primarily neurogenic in origin as opposed to myopathic conditions, a situation in which there is often some overlap in clinical findings. It must be recognized that while the muscle biopsy may provide significant clues and often the correct diagnosis, it nonetheless serves as an adjunct to various other investigations in the diagnostic evaluation process. These include complete clinical evaluation of the patient, electromyography and nerve conduction studies, various other laboratory tests such as serum levels of muscle enzymes, inflammatory and other markers that may be elevated in connective tissue diseases.

Typically, the muscle biopsy is evaluated on hematoxylin and eosin stained sections derived from formalin-fixed, paraffin-embedded tissue. Histologic examination of the tissue and histochemical assessment of various enzymes is also performed on cryostat sections in the cross-sectional plane. Specialized techniques such as electron microscopy for ultrastructural analysis require tissue specifically fixed for this purpose in glutaraldehyde, and finally enzymatic and molecular genetic analysis is best performed on flash-frozen specimens.

Biopsy site selection

Before embarking on the muscle biopsy procedure itself, a number of factors must be considered and implemented to ensure the maximum clinical benefit from this invasive procedure. Communication with the consulting physician, usually a neuropathologist, who will actually evaluate the specimen is critical. This will facilitate the determination of specimen size, and it will permit the consulting laboratory to receive and handle the specimen appropriately. For example, in certain myopathies a larger portion of the tissue may need to be made available for molecular genetic studies, whereas in most inflammatory situations a better yield may be obtained from processing more tissue in paraffin for routine histology. The selection of the site for the muscle biopsy is equally important. It is imperative that the biopsy sample be representative of the disease, however, it should not be obtained from a site that is severely affected. Severe atrophy and fibrosis with infiltration of the muscle by fat, so-called "end stage muscle", will impair the ability to obtain an accurate diagnosis. Similarly, a muscle site that has been subjected to previous trauma, such as that induced by intramuscular injections, electromyography needles, etc., should be avoided. The histopathologic changes that are associated with such trauma including necrosis of fibres, inflammatory infiltrates and regenerative changes could make pathologic evaluation difficult and often incorrect.

The biopsy should be obtained from the belly of the muscle and at a reasonable distance from the myotendinous junction. The site of tendinous insertion of the muscle results in marked variability in myofibre diameter, increased numbers of internalized or centrally placed nuclei and extensive fibrous bands that may suggest myopathic changes. The muscles typically selected for biopsy include the quadriceps femoris in the anterior thigh, gastrocnemius muscle of the lower extremity, biceps brachii in the arm or the deltoid muscle in the shoulder. The primary reason for selecting one of these sites, in addition to the criteria mentioned above, is the fact that these sites are well characterized with regard to normal morphometric and biochemical parameters. Clearly, if the condition involves a specific area as in a neoplasm or a focal inflammatory process then the affected muscle, if not necrotic or severely atrophic, should be targeted. Occasionally, when only distal muscle involvement is clinically detected or if proximal muscles are very severely affected then smaller muscles such as the extensor carpi radialis or the anterior tibial muscle may be useful alternatives. Under these circumstances, however, one must be aware of the variability in fibre type from these various groups in order to accurately interpret the pathology. The issues of site selection and specimen handling are of paramount importance if the biopsy is to yield satisfactory diagnostic results (Bossen 1984, Carpenter and Karpati 1984, Dubowitz 1985, Engel 1994).

Open or needle biopsy?

Muscle biopsies may be performed either as percutaneous needle biopsies or as open biopsies. The choice of procedure must be based on the amount of tissue required for accurate assessment. For example, in certain metabolic conditions where enzyme studies and molecular genetic analysis must be performed in concert with histologic studies an open biopsy may be preferable. Similarly, for evaluation of inflammatory myopathy where the process may be patchy or focal, an open biopsy may have a better yield. Other obvious advantages of an open biopsy include the ability to obtain a relatively large sample that can be oriented along the length of the fibres, as well as the ability to visualize the field and obtain haemostasis. The limitations of this procedure include the need for anaesthesia, an increased risk of infection and the residual surgical scar. The percutaneous needle biopsy, in contrast, can be performed as an outpatient or office procedure, and it has minimal risk of infection. The limited anaesthesia remains its most distinctive advantage as well as the relative speed with which the specimen is obtained and the small excisional scar that results. Additionally, multiple sites may be sampled within the same muscle. The single most significant disadvantage is the limited specimen that is obtained and the difficulty encountered in orienting the specimen in a manner that permits evaluation in cross-section.

There have been many studies that have compared the needle biopsy with the open biopsy with regards to the orientation of the specimen and also the fact that the needle biopsy does not permit the specimen to be held at resting length. Fukuyama and Suzuki (1981) reported on 33 simultaneously obtained needle and open biopsies. They did not find any significant histological or histochemical difference between the two types of specimens. In a methodical study, Blomstrand and Ekblom (1982) investigated fibre type determination in human skeletal muscle using the needle biopsy technique. They found that the variation between duplicate biopsies taken by needle biopsy was 6.2% when fibre type determination was evaluated. In their study, increased numbers of fibres did not reduce the calculated variability, confirming that open biopsy did not have any significant advantage over needle biopsy in this respect. In an evaluation of 379 muscle biopsies obtained by a modified Bergstrom technique, Mubarak et al (1992) determined that the size and quality of muscle samples obtained were sufficient to yield an accurate diagnosis in 98.4% of the patients biopsied. In the remaining 1.6% of cases, which were hypotonic infants, open biopsies were necessary because of marked muscle atrophy. No difficulties in interpretation were encountered, and the diagnosis was made in all per-

cutaneous samples. Complications were rare and included one superficial haematoma that resolved without additional treatment, and there were no infections. The utilization of this procedure and their results have been described by various authors. In all of these studies there were no major complications reported and in the vast majority (>85%) of cases adequate tissue was obtained for diagnosis (Nicols et al 1968, Edwards et al 1973, 1980, 1983, Fukuyama and Suzuki 1981, Mubarak et al 1992, Heckmatt et al 1984, Mahon et al 1984). Reports describing the inadequacy of needle biopsy specimens in providing sufficient and appropriate tissue for accurate diagnosis are infrequent. In our opinion both specimen types have proven to be satisfactory, and it is often the clinical situation and experience with one technique versus the other that becomes the deciding factor when making the choice between procedures.

Surgical procedure

Open biopsy

Following aseptic procedures, the selected area is draped in the usual fashion. A linear skin incision is made after injection with local anaesthetic. Care should be taken to avoid injecting the medication directly into the muscle fibres. The biopsy incision should always be longitudinal on extremities (Fig. 36.1). Haemostasis is meticulously maintained and bleeding vessels are ligated rather than electro-coagulated to avoid cautery damage to the biopsied tissue. After exposing the muscle, using sharp, atraumatic dissection, a section of muscle that measures at least 1.5 cm in length is dissected free from the rest of the fibres. The surgically resected specimen must be maintained in an isometric state, and this is achieved by use of a muscle clamp (Berman 1985; Fig. 36.2). The muscle clamp prevents the undesirable shrinking artefact that results from excision of the specimen and immersion into fixative. It is important to remove the specimen in a way that permits orientation along the long axis of the muscle, as both cross- and longitudinal sections of the muscle are necessary for accurate diagnositic evaluation. The resected surgical specimen would then be within the confines of the muscle clamp and typically measures about 1.5 cm in length and about 0.8 cm in diameter. If a large muscle is biopsied, such as the vastus lateralis, then an additional similar sized sample may also be obtained for further studies.

The need for the use of a muscle clamp to obtain the biopsy has been questioned on multiple occasions.

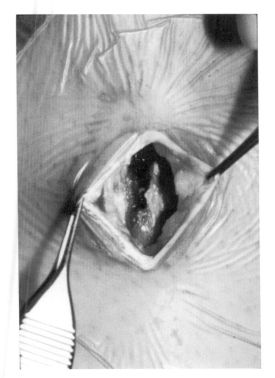

Figure 36.1—A longitudinally oriented incision is made, usually on the lower extremity. The specimen is removed after haemostasis is secured by ligation rather than electrocoagulation.

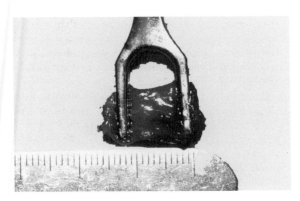

Figure 36.2—The biopsy specimen may be obtained in a muscle clamp, thereby maintaining the muscle in an isometric state. It should measure approximately 1.5 cm in length.

Additionally the application of the muscle biopsy clamp is more difficult in the paediatric patient and often without significant advantage. Alternatively, sutures using 3-0 silk may be applied to either end of the specimen with surgical resection just beyond the suture sites on either side. The resected specimen is

then gently stretched along a wooden applicator stick. This method results in less trauma to the specimen and better histologic preservation.

Percutaneous needle biopsy technique

The second approach to muscle biopsy is a percutaneous needle biopsy, usually performed under local anaesthesia, occasionally supplemented with a sedative. The technique, initially described by Bergstrom in 1962, involves sampling of skeletal muscle using a cylindrical conically tipped trocar with an inner cutting sleeve. While the Bergstrom needle is by far the most widely used, other similar instruments are also available. These include the Tru-cut needle, similar to that used for renal and liver biopsies, which has been used in children (Curless and Nelson 1975, Fukuyama and Suzuki 1981) and the University College Hospital muscle biopsy needle (Young et 1978). A semi-open technique using alligator-type forceps through a small incision has also been reported (Henriksson 1979). After the area is prepared in the usual fashion, the skin is infiltrated with local anaesthetic. It is important to ensure that the site to be biopsied is not directly injected with anaesthetic, as this would traumatize the biopsy specimen. A number 11 scalpel blade is used to make a small stab wound in the skin and fascia. The Bergstrom needle is then inserted into the muscle at an oblique angle (Fig. 36.3). The specimen is obtained by compressing the cutting needle into the trocar. Once the specimen is cut, the needle is removed from the muscle and the specimen is extracted from the chamber using a fine needle. A 10 ml syringe with an i.v. catheter may be connected to the biopsy needle. The application of gentle suction results in the muscle specimen being pulled into the cutting chamber where it is then easily cut (Mubarak et al 1982). The specimen is then removed from within the cutting needle as described above. This process can be repeated multiple times. The skin is sutured using a subcuticular layer of reabsorbable sutures followed by placement of Steristrips. The patient is then allowed to ambulate as desired.

The biopsy specimen

Once the specimen has been obtained, either by a needle biopsy or by open procedure, it must immediately be placed on saline-moistened gauze and rapidly transported to the neuropathology laboratory. It is important that the specimen not be divided up into multiple segments in the surgical suite as this may hamper proper orientation of the specimen at the time

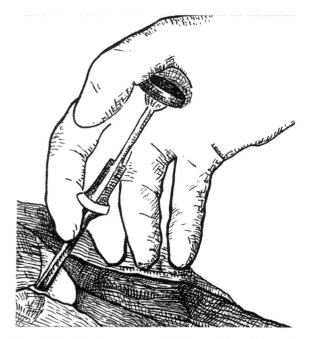

Figure 36.3—The Bergstrom needle, illustrated here, is inserted into the muscle at an angle, through a small stab wound made with a scalpel. The cutting needle is depressed into the trocar, incising the muscle, which is removed from the barrel when the needle is withdrawn.

of tissue processing. If significant delay between surgery and receipt of the specimen in the laboratory is anticipated, then the specimen should be maintained at 4°C, either on ice or refrigerated; however, it should not be allowed to freeze. Further processing of the specimen in the laboratory is described in subsequent chapters.

References

Bergstrom J. (1962) Muscle electrolytes in man: determination by neutron activation analysis in needle biopsy specimens: a study in normal subjects, kidney patients, and patients with chronic diarrhea. *Scand J Clin Lab Invest* 14 (suppl 68): 1–110.

Bergstrom J. (1975) Percutaneous needle biopsy of skeletal muscle in physiological and clinical research. *Scan J Clin Lab Invest* 35: 609-616.

Berman AT, Garbarino JL, Rosenberg H, Heiman-Patterson T, Bosacco SJ, Weiss AA. (1985) Muscle biopsy: Proper surgical Technique. *Clin Orthoped Related Res* 198: 240–243.

Blomstrand E, Ekblom B. (1982) The needle biopsy technique for fibre type determination in human skeletal muscle – a methodological study. *Acta Phylol Scand* 116: 437–442.

Bossen EH. (1984) Collection and preparation of the muscle biopsy. In: Heffner RR, ed. *Muscle Pathology*. New York, NY: Churchill Livingstone, pp. 11–14.

Carpenter S, Karpati G. (1984) *Pathology of Skeletal Muscle*. New York, NY: Churchill Livingstone:

Curless RG, Nelson MB. (1975) Congenital fiber type disproportion in identical twins. *Ann Neurol 2*: 455

DiLiberti JH, D'Agnostino AN, Cole G. (1985) Needle muscle biopsy in infants and children. *J Pediatr* 103: 566–570.

Dubowitz V. (1985) *Muscle Biopsy. A Practical Approach*. *2nd ed*. London, England: Bailliere Tindall, pp. 3–18.

Edwards RHT, Lewis PD, Maunder C, Pearse AGE. (1973) Percutaneous needle biopsy in the diagnosis of muscle diseases. *Lancet* 3: 1070–1071.

Edwards RHT, Young A, Wiles M. (1980) Needle biopsy of skeletal muscle in the diagnosis of myopathy and the clinical study of muscle function and repair. *N Engl J Med* 302: 261–271.

Edwards RHT, Round JM, Jones DA. (1983) Needle biopsy of skeletal muscle: a review of 10 years' experience. *Muscle Nerve* 6: 678–683.

Engel AG. (1994) The Muscle Biopsy. In: Engel AG, Franzini-Armstrong C, eds. *Myology: Basic and Clinical*. *2nd edition*. New York: McGraw-Hill, pp. 822–831.

Fukuyama Y, Suzuki Y. (1981) Percutaneous needle biopsy in the diagnosis of neuromuscular disorders in children. *Brain Dev* 3: 277–287.

Heckmatt JZ, Moosa A, Hutson C, Maunder-Sewry CA, Dubowitz V. (1984) Diagnostic needle muscle biopsy: a practical and reliable alternative to open biopsy. *Arch Dis Child* 59: 528–532.

Henriksson KG. (1979) Semi-open muscle biopsy technique: a simple outpatient procedure. *Acta Neurol Scand* 59: 317–323.

Mahon M, Toma A, Willan PLT, Bagnall KM. (1984) Variability of histochemical and morphometric data from needle biopsy specimens of human quadriceps femoris muscle. *J Neurol Sci* 63: 85–100.

Mubarak SJ, Chambers HG, Wenger DR. (1992) Percutaneous muscle biopsy in the diagnosis of neuromuscular disease. *J Pediatr Orthopaedics* 12: 191–196.

Nicols BL, Hazlewood CF, Barnes DJ. (1968) Percutaneous needle biopsy of quadriceps muscle: potassium analysis in normal children. *J Pediatr* 72: 840–852.

Pearl GS, Ghatak NR. (1995) Muscle biopsy. *Arch Pathol Lab Med* 119: 303–306.

Young A, Wiles CM, Edwards RHT. (1978) University College Hospital muscle-biopsy needle. *Lancet* 8: 1285.

37

Electromyography

Mohammed Ferdjallah and Jacqueline J. Wertsch

Introduction

Electromyography (EMG) testing reflects the complex function of the motor system, which consists of upper and lower motor neurones, the neuromuscular junction and the muscle. Knowledge of the physiologic mechanisms underlying normal muscle contraction is paramount to understanding various abnormalities that characterize disorders of the motor system. Multiple factors such as muscular properties, the electrical specifications of the electrodes and the recording apparatus can significantly affect EMG recordings. EMG physiologic data is most useful in the context of the overall clinical picture. Electromyography should be considered as an extension of the history and physical examination (Hausmanowa-Petrusewicz et al 1967, Basmajian and De Luca 1985).

Electromyographic instrumentation

Instrumentation for EMG recording includes a signal acquisition system with audio and visual displays, which contains amplification and filtering stages suitable for EMG processing with minimum noise and artefacts (Barry 1991). Characteristics such as signal to noise ratio, gain, common mode rejection ratio, input impedance and bandwidth are standardized in most EMG instruments today. There are several types of electrodes that are currently used for the detection of EMG signals: concentric needles, monopolar needles, single fibre EMG (SFEMG) needles, macro EMG needles, surface electrodes and kinesiologic fine wire electrodes (Dorfmann et al 1985).

Anatomy and physiology of skeletal muscle

Functional anatomy

Individual muscle fibres consist of clusters of individual myofibrils which in turn consist of aggregates of myosin and actin filaments (Fig. 37.1). The sarcomere is a single anatomic unit consisting of overlapping myosin and actin filaments from one Z line to the next Z line in the muscle. The sarcomere comprises of I bands containing only actin, H bands containing only myosin, and A bands where myosin overlaps the actin fibres (Huxley 1953). The actin filament is a thin fibre whereas the myosin filament is a much thicker fila-

ment. Muscle fibres can be divided into three broad categories based on appearance, speed of contraction, and fatigability (Eberstein and Goodgold 1968). Slow twitch muscles take more than 35 ms to complete a depolarization/repolarization cycle and are reddish in appearance. Type I fast twitch fatigue resistant muscles are pale in appearance and, like the slow twitch muscles have a considerable ability for aerobic metabolism. Type II fast twitch fatigable muscles take less than 35 ms to complete a twitch cycle and are whitish in appearance. The morphological differentiation of the fibre type is determined by the type of motor nerve that activates it. Most muscles contain a mixture of fast and slow twitch fibres (Johnson et al 1973). In general, Type I fibres are smaller in size, produce less tension, and tend to maintain a tonic repetitive discharge. Type II fibres have a low reflex threshold, and they respond reflexively with short burst patterns.

The motor unit

The motor unit consists of a neuron cell body, its axon, the neuromuscular junction and the muscle fibres it innervates. The number of muscle fibres per motor unit (innervation ratio) varies in human muscles (McComas et al 1971). The lower motor axon branches to the muscle fibres at the motor end-plate, creating neuromuscular junction (Fig. 37.2). In adulthood each muscle fibre usually has only one end-plate, and it is innervated by one branch of a motor axon. The motor nerve fibre loses the myelin sheath at the nerve terminals. At the junctional region between the nerve ending and end-plate, Schwann cells are absent (Buchthal and Schmalbruch 1980).

Electrophysiology of skeletal muscle

At rest, the transmembrane potential of the muscle fibre (-90 mV) results from an unequal ionic distribution across the membrane of potassium (K^+), sodium (Na^+) and chloride (Cl^-) (Catterall 1995). At rest, the presynaptic ending spontaneously releases acetylcholine (ACh) molecules, which migrate into the junctional cleft and generate miniature end-plate potentials (MEPPs; Wiederholt 1970). Depolarization of the presynaptic ending at the axon terminal triggers an influx of calcium (Ca^{2+}), initiating the (Ca^{2+}) dependent release of large amount of ACh which gives rise to a non-propagated end-plate potential (EPP). When the EPP exceeds the excitability threshold of the

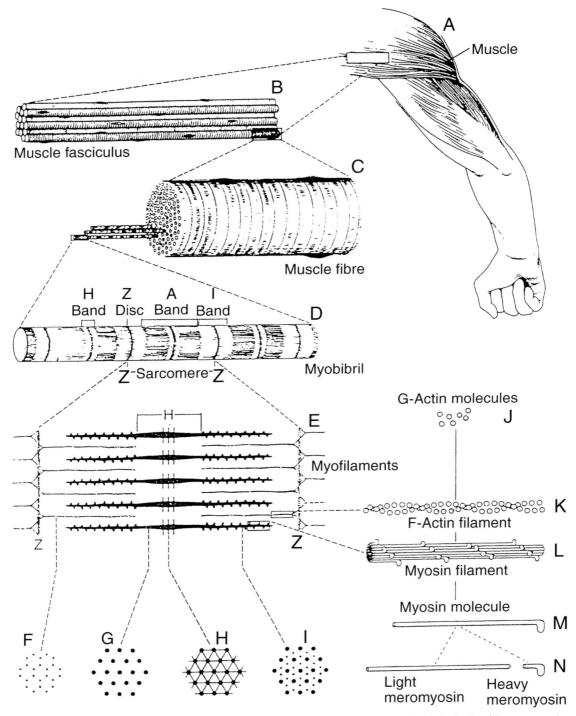

Figure 37.1—Organization of skeletal muscle from the gross (**A**) to the molecular (**J, K, L, M, N**) level. **F, G, H** and **I** are cross–sections of the level indicated. (Adapted from Guyton and Hall: Textbook of Medical Physiology. Ninth Edition, Philadelphia, W. B. Saunders Company 1996. Modified after Fawcett: Bloom and Fawcett: A Textbook of Histology. Twelfth Edition, New York, Chapman & Hall, 1994, with permission.)

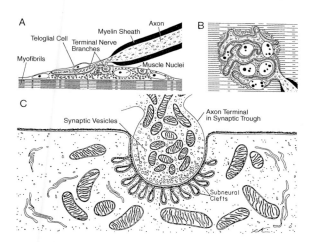

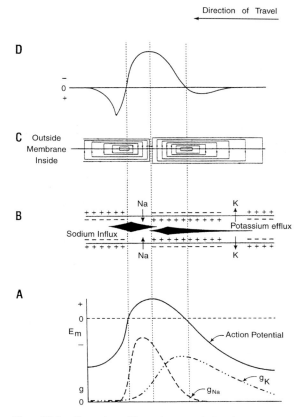

Figure 37.2—Illustration of different views of the neuromuscular junction. **A** A longitudinal section through the end-plate. **B** A surface view of the end-plate. **C** An electron micrographic appearance of the contact point between one of the axon terminals and the muscle fibre membrane. (Adapted from Fawcett: Bloom and Fawcett: A Textbook of Histology. Twelfth Edition, New York, Chapman & Hall, 1994, with permission.)

muscle cell, an action potential propagates and activates the contractile elements of the muscle fibre (Fig. 37.3). The action potential propagates bidirectionally along the fibre at 3–5 m/s along the muscle membrane. Because the branching nerve fibres vary in their length and diameter, the nerve action potential reaches the motor end-plates at different times, resulting in an asynchronous activation of the muscle fibres belonging to a motor unit. Different motor units may overlap their territories. The action potentials from each of the muscle fibres spatially and temporally summate to form a motor unit action potential (Daube 1978). The spread of action potential from the motor end-plate to the transverse tubules initiates muscle contraction (Weber and Murray 1973). The electrical activity of the muscle fibre activates different structures within the fibre. The transverse tubules lie at the junctions of the A and I bands and contain extracellular fluid. The longitudinal tubule or sarcoplasmic reticulum, surrounds the myofibrils of a muscle fibre (Fig. 37.4). The propagated action potentials cross the muscle fibres through the transverse tubules to come into contact with the terminal of the longitudinal tubules. The action potential initiates the release of Ca^{2+} from the longitudinal tubules into the sarcoplasm of the myofilaments, and triggers the formation of bridges between thin and thick filaments (Chandler et al 1976). Sliding of thin filaments against thick filaments results in contraction of the myofibril. At the end of the muscle action potential, the longitudinal

Figure 37.3—Illustration of dynamic events during the propagation of muscle action potential. **A** The increase in sodium (g_{Na}) and potassium (g_K) conduction gives arise to an intracellular action potential. **B** Within the associated region of transmembrane ion flow voltage-dependent ion gates open. **C** The opening of sodium gates generates local circuit currents. **D** The monophasic intracellular action potential and its associated dynamic events give arise to an extracellular triphasic signal muscle action potential. (Adapted from Dumitru D: Electrodiagnostic Medicine: Philadelphia, Hanley and Belfus, Inc., 1994, with permission.)

tubules rapidly withdraw Ca^{2+} and lower its concentration in the sarcoplasm (Fig. 37.5). The myofibres relax and break the bridges between filaments.

Needle electromyography

There are four main categories of physiologic information gathered during the electromyographic examination (Daube 1991):

1. Insertional activity

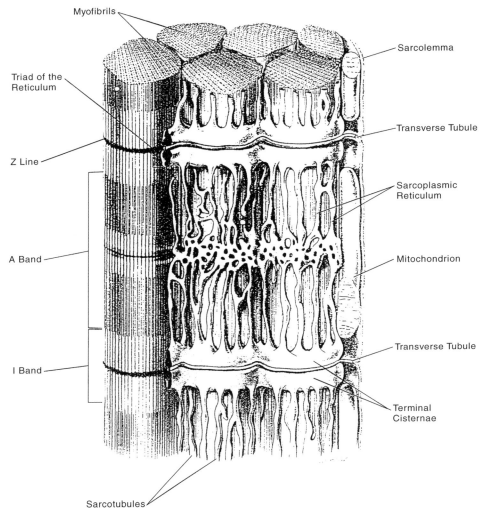

Figure 37.4— Illustration of the various subcomponents of a frog muscle tissue, which has only one T tubule per sarcomere located at the Z line. Mammalian muscle tissue has two T tubules per sarcomere, which align with the A/I bands as opposed to the Z line. (Adapted from Fawcett: Bloom and Fawcett: A Textbook of Histology. Twelfth Edition, New York, Chapman & Hall, 1994, with permission.)

2. Spontaneous activity

3. Motor unit action potential morphology and stability

4. Motor unit action potential recruitment.

Insertional activity

A muscle is electrically silent at rest. Insertion of a needle electrode into the muscle gives rise to brief bursts of electrical activity (Kugelberg and Petersen 1949). It appears as positive or negative high frequency spikes in a cluster (Fig. 37.6). This burst of electrical activity (insertional activity) lasts as long as the needle is moved. It is characterized as normal, decreased or increased. Traditionally, decreased insertional activity is seen when there has been loss of muscle cells and replacement by fibrous tissue. Increased insertional activity suggests increased muscle cell membrane irritability, which can be a result of denervation, myopathy, local trauma or inflammatory or metabolic processes.

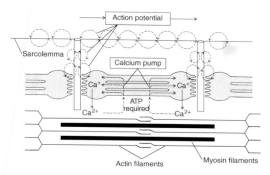

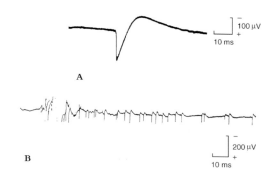

Figure 37.5—Illustration of excitation-contraction coupling and sarcoplasmic calcium release. The propagating action potential into the T tubule system, carries the impulse into the muscle and causes the release of Ca^{2+} from the sarcoplasmic reticulum and the re-uptake of the Ca^{2+} by a calcium pump. (Adapted from Guyton and Hall: Textbook of Medical Physiology. Ninth Edition, Philadelphia, W. B Saunders Company, 1996, with permission.)

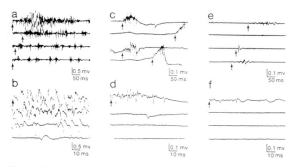

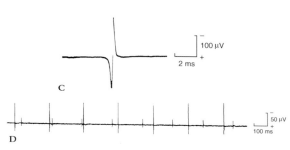

Figure 37.6—Insertional activities. Increased insertional activity from the first dorsal interosseus of a subject with tardy ulnar palsy (**A** & **B**). Normal insertional activity from tibialis anterior of a normal subject (**C** & **D**). Decreased insertional activity from fibrotic deltoid of a subject with severe dermatomyositis (**E** & **F**). (Adapted from Kimura J: Electrodiagnosis in Diseases of Nerve and Muscle: Principles and Practice. Second Edition, Philadelphia, F. A. Davis Company, 1989, with permission.)

Spontaneous activity

Normally the muscle cell does not depolarize unless there is an impulse that crosses the neuromuscular junction. Spontaneous activity refers to the abnormal, "spontaneous" depolarization of a muscle cell (Buchthal and Rosenfalck 1966, Brown and Varkey 1981). There are many types of spontaneous potentials depending on the generator of the impulse. If the generator is a single muscle cell, it is called a spontaneous single muscle fibre potential (SSMFP). The SSMFP can appear as either a spike or a positive wave. Traditionally the spikes were called fibrillation potentials

Figure 37.7—Fibrillation potentials. Samples of a positive sharp waveform (**A**), train of positive sharp waveforms (**B**), a spike waveform (**C**) and a train of spike waveforms (**D**). (Adapted from Dumitru D: Electrodiagnostic Medicine: Philadelphia, Hanley & Belfus, Inc., 1994. Modified and adapted from material submitted by members of the AAEE, with permission.)

(fibs) and the positive waves were referred to as positive sharp waves (PSW). However, more recently it has been recognized that the generator for both fibs and PSW is the single muscle cell, so the term SSMFP is preferred to accurately portray the generator of this type of spontaneous potential (Fig. 37.7; Dumitru 1996).

Other types of spontaneous potentials include fasciculation potentials (Richardson 1954, Wettstein 1979), myokymic discharges (Gutmann 1991), complex repetitive discharges, neuromyotonia and myotonic discharges (Fig. 37.8; Tobergsen et al 1996). Each type of spontaneous potential represents different generators and has different pathophysiologic significance (Heckmann and Ludin 1982). Spontaneous activity provides an unequivocal sign of abnormality, and it is one of the most useful findings in clinical electromyography. When found in disorders of the lower motor neurone, the distribution of spontaneous potentials can aid in localization of lesions of the spinal cord, root, plexus or peripheral nerve.

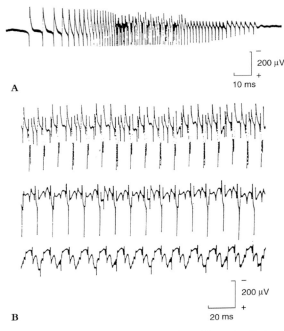

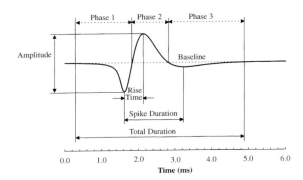

Figure 37.9—Illustration of a single motor unit action potential with various characteristics that can be measured during clinical evolution.

Figure 37.8—Spontaneous depolarization. Myotonic discharge sample (**A**). Complex repetitive discharge sample (**B**). (Adapted from Dumitru D: Electrodiagnostic Medicine. Philadelphia, Hanley & Belfus Inc., 1994, Modified and adapted from material submitted by members of the AAEE with permission.)

Motor unit action potential

The motor unit physiology depends on the innervation ratio, fibre density, propagation velocity and integrity of neuromuscular transmission (Stalberg and Antoni 1980). The shape of a motor unit action potential (MUAP) reflects the spatial relationship between the needle and individual muscle fibres located near the tip of the recording needle electrode. Thus, a new profile for the same motor unit will be introduced by a slight repositioning of the electrode (Van Dijl et al 1995). The distance between the tip of the needle electrode and the discharging motor unit is estimated by the rise time, which is measured as the time lag from the initial positive peak to the subsequent negative peak. In addition, other variables, such as the resistance and capacitance of the intervening tissue (volume conductor) (Dumitru and DeLisa 1991), intramuscular temperature (Denys 1991), the type of needle electrode and the instrumentation setup, affect the profile of the motor unit potential. A distant unit has a greater rise time because the volume conductor acts as a low frequency filter. The synchrony among individual muscle fibres is indicated by the duration,

which is the time from the initial takeoff to the return to the baseline. Generators away from the electrode contribute to the ends of the MUAP, and thus a slight shift in the needle position does not significantly influence the duration (Fig. 37.9) (Buchthal et al 1954).

Morphology and stability

Every time a motor unit fires, the resultant MUAP should look the same. Motor units normally discharge with successive nearly identical potentials. Lack of MUAP stability always implies pathophysiologic process (Trojaborg 1978). In defective neuromuscular transmission, the amplitude of a repetitively firing unit may fluctuate or decrease steadily, suggesting intermittent blocking of individual muscle fibres within the unit. Other sources of unstable MUAP morphology include motor neuron diseases, neuropathies or myopathies (Hilfiker and Meyer 1984, Wilbourn 1993).

Increased amplitude and duration of MUAPs generally suggest disorders of the lower motor neurone, such as motor neurone disease, polimyelitis and syringomyelia, or diseases of the peripheral nerve, such as chronic neuropathy and reinnervation after nerve injury (Petajan 1974). Increased amplitude suggests greater muscle fibre density due to the sprouting fibres within the territory of the surviving axon. In myopathic disorders, short, small amplitude polyphasic MUAPs can be seen (Fig. 37.10; Dorfman et al 1989).

Motor unit action potential recruitment

Motor units are recruited in an orderly, predictable pattern. In the early days of clinical electromyography, interference patterns were subjectively assessed. There are problems with both false positive and false negative

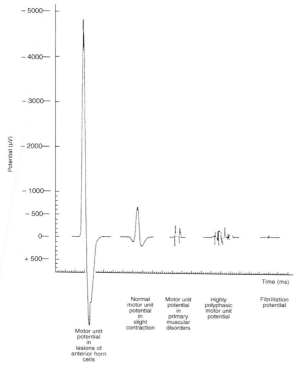

Potential (μV)

Time (ms)

Motor unit potential in lesions of anterior horn cells

Normal motor unit potential in slight contraction

Motor unit potential in primary muscular disorders

Highly polyphasic motor unit potential

Fibrillation potential

Figure 37.10— Illustration of relative average durations and amplitudes of various electric potentials observed in human muscles and neuromuscular disorders. (Adapted from Daube JR: AAEM Minimonograph # 11: Needle Examination in Clinical Electromyography. Muscle & Nerve 1991; 14: 685–700, with permission.)

assessments using interference patterns so the clinical use of this method is discourage. Instead the electromyographer now looks at specific recruitment information such as onset frequency, recruitment frequency, recruitment ratio, rank order and temporal and spatial summation (Petajan 1991). Based on the size principle of Hennemen, it is known that the initially recruited MUAP will be small and the subsequent MUAPs will be progressively bigger (Ertas et al 1995). Attention to this rank order can be very useful to detect earlier myopathic process. The onset frequency in human skeletal extremity muscle is about 5–7 Hz with recruitment frequency about 10–12 Hz. The calculated recruitment ratio should be about 5.

Single fibre and macro electromyography

SFEMG is used to determine the fibre density and the electromyographic jitter. SFEMG records potential discharges from individual muscle cells (Fig. 37.11). An increase in fibre density usually indicates the presence of fibre sprouting, although fibre density increases slowly with age (Stalberg and Thiele 1975). The jitter represents the variability of the inter-potential interval between single muscle fibres belonging to the same motor unit (Ekstedt et al 1974, Salmi 1983). In contrast to conventional needle EMG or SFEMG, macro EMG uses an electrode with a greater recording surface, and it provides information about the whole motor unit (Fig. 37.12; Chan and Hsu 1991). The factors that determine the characteristics of macro EMG include number of fibres, fibre diameter, endplate scatter, pattern of nerve branching, motor unit territory and electrode position.

SFEMG can detect disturbances of neuromuscular transmission (Keesey 1989). Disorders associated with abnormal SFEMG include degenerative processes of the anterior horn cell and tetanus (Stalberg et al 1975). Progressive fibre sprouting, seen in spinal muscular atrophy, shows the highest fibre density among motor neurone diseases. Clinical studies have revealed an inverse relationship between muscle strength and fibre density. Rapidly progressive diseases such as myotrophic lateral sclerosis show increased jitter and blocking. Disorders of the peripheral nerves also show increased jitter, occasional blocking and increased fibre density. Normal muscles show increased jitter in 5% of recorded pairs of potentials (Stalberg et al 1971). Increased jitter or blocking is regarded as evidence of defective neuromuscular transmission (Fig. 37.12). Dystrophic muscle in general shows increase in fibre density and jitter (Hilton-Brown et al 1985). As a result of fibre loss, fibre regeneration and reinnervation, a motor unit may undergo a structural remodelling (Jaber 1991). Macro EMG studies show normal diameter of motor units with no signs of abnormal volume conduction.

Surface electromyography

Surface EMG provides indirect means for the study of muscular functions during biofeedback training, activities of sports or daily living, and in pathologic states of musculoskeleton or neuromuscular systems. Surface EMG has been processed in several ways to enhance and facilitate its interpretation. Spectral analysis methods are used to assess fatigue patterns during function. Parameters such as mean frequency and median frequency have been proven to provide

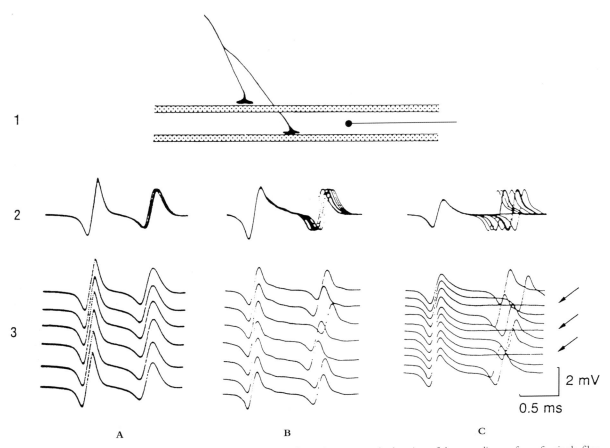

2 mV

0.5 ms

A   B   C

Figure 37.11—Illustration of single fibre electromyographic recordings. **1** represents the location of the recording surface of a single fibre electrode between two muscle fibres innervated by the same motor neurone. **2** and **3** represent consecutive potential discharges in superimposed and raster displays respectively. **A**, **B** and **C** represent normal jitter, increased jitter and decreased jitter, respectively, recorded from the extensor digitorum communis of a patient with myasthenia gravis. (Adapted from Dumitru D: Electrodiagnostic Medicine. Philadelphia, Hanley & Belfus Inc., 1994, Modified and adapted from material submitted by members of the AAEE, with permission.)

information regarding muscular fatigue. Surface EMG shows interference patterns, which depend upon the type of muscle contraction. Isometric contractions are muscle contractions in which a constant muscle length is maintained, and surface EMG recordings are typically greatest under isometric testing conditions. Concentric contractions occur when the muscle shortens, whereas eccentric contractions occur when the muscle lengthens. Surface EMG recruitment patterns may differ in an open versus closed kinetic chain: in an open kinetic chain, the distal segment is free to move; in a closed kinetic chain, the distal segment is fixed. Surface EMG recruitment patterns are typically greater under closed kinetic chain conditions. Surface EMG may identify the relative amount of muscular effort used during various activities, but it

does not specify the actual force responsible for the muscular activity. For instance, isometric and eccentric contractions may have the same EMG quantification outputs. Moreover the faster a muscle contracts, the less force can be generated for the same effort. During maximum efforts at any speed the EMG is relatively constant, even though the forces differ (Osternig et al 1984). Nonetheless, surface EMG offers valuable information concerning the timing of muscular activity and its relative intensity (Patla et al 1982).

Detection and processing

EMG signals generated by muscle fibres propagate through muscles and layers of tissue (Gath and Stalberg 1977). Signals detected by the recording elec-

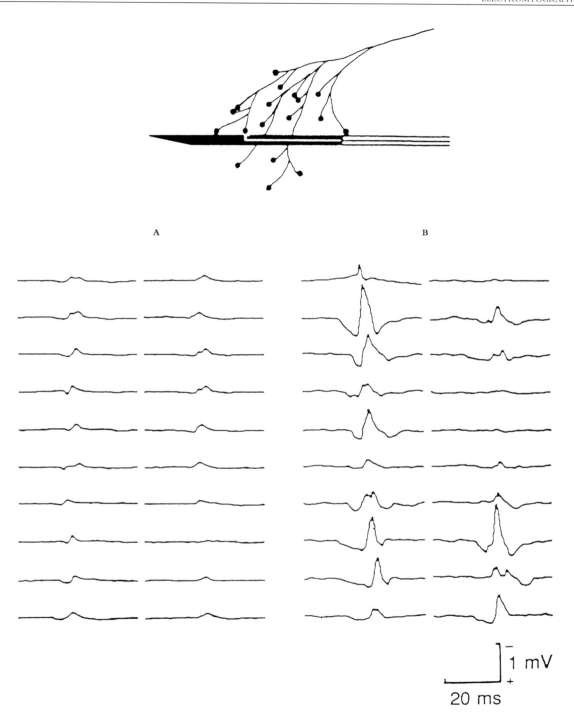

A

B

1 mV

20 ms

Figure 37.12 — Illustration of macroelectromyographic recordings. The top diagram represents the location of the recording surface of the macroelectromyographic needle in the vicinity of muscle fibres innervated by the same motor neurone. **A** Recordings from a healthy subject. **B** Recordings from a patient with amyotrophic lateral sclerosis. (Adapted from Dumitru D: Electrodiagnostic Medicine. Philadelphia, Hanley & Belfus, Inc., 1994, Modified and adapted from material submitted by members of the AAEE, with permission.)

trodes may be erroneously interpreted as generated by muscle fibres within the sampling field of the electrode. Cross-talk is due to volume conduction dispersion effect on the EMG signal and action potentials on their way to the electrode site (De Luca and Merletti 1988). The surface EMG signal detected should be considered as a summation of filtered signals resulting from a number of concurrently active motor units generating volume conducted currents and associated potential fields. Nonetheless, there are available techniques, such as high pass filtering and double differentiation, for improving the selectivity of EMG recordings. The double differential technique allows the cancellation of signals simultaneously present at every electrode couple. Other methods, such as smaller electrode surface area and reduced bipolar spacing, may reduce cross-talk by limiting the range of electrode pick up. Quantification of EMG is a multi-task signal-processing procedure requiring wave rectification, linear envelope or moving average, and integration of the rectified EMG signal (Fig. 37.13; Harris and Wertsch 1994). The linear envelope, obtained by filtering the rectified EMG signal with a low pass filter, is useful in assessing the time of onsets and cessation of muscular activity. For relative effort estimation of the processed EMG data, a normalization method is required to accommodate the individual variation in muscle fibre anatomy and alignment and the number of motor units detected by the

electrode sampling field (Yang and Winter 1984). Although timing of muscular electrical activity can be determined directly from the raw EMG signals, defining the exact onset and cessation points of the muscular electrical activity interval remains a subjective decision (DiFabio 1987).

Clinical assessment using surface electromyography

Unlike other types of EMG, surface evaluation of neuromuscular system is much broader and more generic. The use of surface EMG in the clinical assessment of various syndromes examines how muscular energy is used during movement. Often, several channels are monitored to study the right and left aspect of two opposing muscles. The surface EMG record can be examined for amplitude, frequency content and timing. Differences in the symmetry of surface EMG patterns could help to explain patterns of symmetry or asymmetry in movement. Evaluation of muscular timing issues is complex, and it usually requires examination of multiple muscles under various conditions, such as agonist/antagonist and reciprocation versus co-contraction. Movement and muscular timing are affected by muscular fatigue. The effects of muscle fatigue are associated with inadequate perfusion of the tissue, the depletion of energy sources and the buildup of metabolites in the muscular tissue. During fatigue and prior to muscular failure, surface EMG patterns

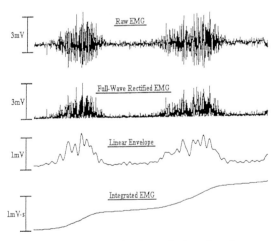

Figure 37.13 — Illustration of analysis of gait surface electromyography (EMG) data. The top row shows typical raw bipolar surface EMG. The second row shows the results of full-wave rectification (absolute value) of the signal. The third and fourth rows show the results of linear envelope (moving average) and integrated processing of the rectified EMG signal. (Adapted from Harris GF, Wertsch JJ: Review Article: Procedures for Gait Analysis. Arch Phy Med Rehabil 1994; 75: 216–225, with permission.)

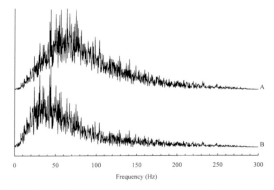

Figure 37.14 — Illustration of the spectral content of surface electromyography (EMG) signals during the assessment of muscular fatigue. Normalized frequency spectrum of surface EMG signal after the 1st second of contraction (**A**) and after the 59th second of contraction (**B**). Notice the spectral shift toward lower frequencies indicating muscular fatigue.

show an increased amplitude associated with synchronization of the motor unit pools and a reduction of the mean and median frequencies of its spectral energy (Fig. 37.14; Merletti et al 1990, 1991). The amount of force generated by a muscle depends upon the resting length of the muscle (Inbar et al 1987). The contraction velocity of a muscle also affects the amount of tension or force that a muscle produces. The speed at which a muscle can contract is limited by the rate of cross-bridging between myosin and actin fibres at the cellular level.

References

Barry DT. (1991) AAEM minimonograph # 36: Basic concepts of electricity and electronics in clinical electromyography. *Muscle Nerve* 14: 937–946.

Basmajian JV, De Luca CJ. (1985) *Muscle alive 5th ed.* Baltimore: Williams & Wilkins.

Brown WF, Varkey GP. (1981) The origin of spontaneous electrical activity at the end plate zone. *Ann Neurol* 10: 557–560.

Buchthal F, Guld C, Rosenfalck P. (1954) Action potential parameters in normal human muscle and their dependence on physical variables. *Acta Physiol Scand* 32: 200–218.

Buchthal F, Rosenfalck P. (1966) Spontaneous electrical activity of human muscle. *Electroencephalogr Clin Neurolphysiol* 20: 321–336.

Buchthal F, Schmalbruch H. (1980) Motor unit of mammalian muscle. *Physiol Rev* 60: 90–142.

Catterall WA. (1995) Structure and function of voltage-gated ion channels. *Ann Rev Biochem* 64: 493–531.

Chan RC, Hsu TC. (1991) Quantitative comparison of motor unit potential parameters between monopolar and concentric needles. *Muscle Nerve* 14: 1028–1032.

Chandler WK, Rakowski RF, Schneider MF. (1976) A non-linear voltage dependent charge movement in frog skeletal muscle. *J Physiol (Lond)* 254: 245–283.

Daube JR. (1978) The description of motor unit potentials in electromyography. *Neurology* 28: 623–625.

Daube JR. (1991) AAEM minimonograph # 11: Needle examination in clinical electromyography. *Muscle Nerve* 14: 685–700.

De Luca CJ, Merletti R. (1988) Surface myoelectric signal cross-talk among muscle of the leg. *Electroenceph Clin Neurophysiol* 69: 568–575.

Denys EH. (1991) AAEM minimonograph # 14: The influence of temperature in clinical neurophysiology. *Muscle Nerve* 14: 795–811.

DiFabio PP. (1987) Reliability of computerized surface electromyography for determining the onset of muscular activity. *Physical Therapy* 67(1): 43–48.

Dorfmann LD, McGill KC, Cummins KL. (1985) Electrical properties of commercial concentric EMG electrodes. *Muscle Nerve* 8: 1–8.

Dorfmann LD, Howard JE, McGill KC. (1989) Motor unit firing rates and firing rate variability in the detection of neuromuscular disorders. *Electroenceph Clin Neurophysiol* 73: 215–224.

Dumitru D. (1996) Single muscle fiber discharges (insertional activity, end-plate potentials, positive sharp waves, and fibrillation potentials): A unifying proposal. *Muscle Nerve* 19: 221–226.

Dumitru D, DeLisa JA. (1991) AAEM minimonograph # 10: Volume conduction. *Muscle Nerve* 14: 605–634.

Eberstein A, Goodgold J. (1968) Slow and fast twitch fibers in human skeletal muscle. *Am J Physiol* 215: 535–541.

Ekstedt J, Nilsson G, Stalberg E. (1974) Calculation of the electromyography jitter. *J Neurol Neurosurg Psychiatry* 37: 526–539.

Ertas M, Stalberg E, Falck B. (1995) Can the size principle be detected in conventional EMG recordings? *Muscle Nerve* 18: 435–439.

Gath I, Stalberg E. (1977) On the volume conduction in human skeletal muscle: In situ measurements. *Electroencephalogr Clin Neurophysiol* 43: 106–110.

Gutmann L. (1991) AAEM minimonograph # 37: Facial and limb myokymia. *Muscle Nerve* 14: 1043–1049.

Harris GF, Wertsch JJ. (1994) Procedures for gait analysis. *Arch Phys Med Rehabil* 75: 216–225.

Hausmanowa-Petrusewicz I, Emeryk B, Wasowicz B, Kopec A. (1967) Electromyography in neuromuscular diagnostics. *Electromyography* 7: 203–225.

Heckmann R, Ludin HP. (1982) Differentiation of spontaneous activity from normal and denervated skeletal muscle. *J Neurol Neurosurg Psychiatry* 45: 331–336.

Hilfiker P, Meyer M. (1984) Normal and myopathic propagation of surface motor unit action potentials. *Electroencephalogr Clin Neurophysiol* 57: 21–31.

Hilton-Brown P, Stalberg E, Trontelj J, Mihelin M. (1985) Causes of the increased fiber density in muscular dystrophies studied with single fiber EMG during electrical stimulation. *Muscle Nerve* 8: 383–388.

Huxley HE. (1953) Electron microscope studies of the organization of the filaments in striated muscle. *Biochem Biophys Acta* 12: 387–394.

Inbar GF, Allin J, Kranz H. (1987) Surface EMG spectral changes with muscle length. *Med Biol Eng Computing* 25: 683–689.

Jaber JF. (1991) Concentric macro electromyography. *Muscle Nerve* 14: 820–825.

Johnson MA, Polgar J, Weightman D, Appleton D. (1973) Data on the distribution of fiber types in thirty six human muscles: An autopsy study. *J Neurol Sci* 18: 111–129.

Keesey JC. (1989) AAEM minimonograph # 33: Electrodiagnostic approach to defects of neuromuscular transmission. *Muscle Nerve* 12: 613–626.

Kugelberg E, Petersen I. (1949) Insertion activity in electromyography. *J Neurol Neurosurg Psychiatry* 12: 268–273.

McComas AJ, Fawcett PRW, Campbell MJ, Sics REP. (1971) Electrophysiological estimation of the number of motor units within a human muscle. *J Neurol Neurosurg Psychiatry* 34: 121–131.

Merletti R, Knaflitz M, De Luca CJ. (1990) Myoelectric manifestations of fatigue in voluntary and electrically elicited contractions. *J Appl Physiol* 69: 1810–1820.

Merletti R, Lo Conte LR, Orizio C. (1991) Indices of muscle fatigue. *J Electromyography Kinesiology* 1: 20–33.

Osternig LR, Hamill J, Corcos DM, Lander J. (1984) Electromyographic patterns accompanying isokinetic exercise under varying speed and sequencing conditions. *Am J Physical Med* 63(6): 289–297.

Patla AE, Hudgins BS, Parker PA. (1982) Myoelectric signal as a quantitative measure of muscle mechanical output. *Med Biol Eng Computing* 20: 319–328.

Petajan JH. (1974) Clinical electromyographic studies of diseases of the motor unit. *Electroencephalogr Clin Neurophysiol* 36: 395–401.

Petajan JH. (1991) AAEM minimonograph # 3: Motor unit recruitment. *Muscle Nerve* 14: 489–502.

Richardson AT. (1954) Muscle fasciculation. *Arch Phys Med Rehabil* 35: 281–286.

Salmi T. (1983) A duration matching method for the measurement of jitter in single fiber EMG. *Electroencephalogr Clin Neurophysiol* 56: 515–520.

Stalberg E, Antoni L. (1980) Electrophysiological cross section of the motor unit. *J Neurol Neurosurg Psychiatry* 43: 469–474.

Stalberg E, Ekstedt J, Broman A. (1971) The electromyographic jitter in normal human muscles. *Electroencephalogr Clin Neurophysiol* 31: 429–438.

Stalberg E, Schwartz MS, Trontelj JV. (1975) Single fiber electromyography in various processes affecting the anterior horn cell. *J Neurol Sci* 24: 403–415.

Stalberg E, Thiele B. (1975) Motor unit fiber density in the extensor digitorum communis muscle: Single fiber electromyographic study in normal subjects at different ages. *J Neurol Neurosurg Psychiatry* 38: 874–880.

Torbergsen T, Stalberg E, Brautaset NJ. (1996) Generator sites for spontaneous activity in neuromyotonia. An EMG study. *Electroencephalogr Clin Neurophysiol* 101: 69–78.

Trojaborg W. (1978) Early electrophysiologic changes in conduction block. *Muscle Nerve* 1: 400–403.

Van Dijl JG, Tjon-A-Tsien A, Van der Kamp W. (1995) CMAP variability as a function of electrode site and size. *Muscle Nerve* 18: 68–73.

Weber A, Murray JM. (1973) Molecular control mechanisms in muscle contractions. *Physiol Rev* 53: 612–673.

Wettstein A. (1979) The origin of fasciculation in motorneuron disease. *Ann Neurol* 5: 295–300.

Wiederholt WC. (1970) "End plate noise" in electromyography. *Neurology* 20: 214–224.

Wilbourn AJ. (1993) The electrodiagnostic examination with myopathies. *J Clin Neurophysiol* 10: 132–148.

Yang JF, Winter DA. (1984) Electromyographic amplitude normalization methods: improving their sensitivity as diagnostic tools in gait analysis. *Arch Phys Med Rehabil* 65: 517–512.

38

Magnetic resonance imaging of muscle pathology

David A. Bluemke and Shaifali Kaushik

Introduction

Magnetic resonance imaging (MRI) has revolutionized non-invasive soft tissue imaging, particularly for muscle. Its ability to detect and characterize muscle and bone marrow abnormalities has made it an important modality in the evaluation of musculoskeletal systems. It is superior to other modalities in determining not only the soft tissue lesions, and characterizing their contents and extent, but also the involvement of osseous and extraosseous structures such as neurovascular bundles.

Magnetic resonance imaging techniques

We will limit our descriptions to most commonly used sequences and algorithms. Detailed information about these sequences can be obtained from any standard MRI text. These protocols may be altered according to clinical need and area imaged.

Radio-frequency coils

The choice of radio-frequency (rf) coils depends upon the anatomic region needing to be imaged. For larger body area coverage, the body coil is found to be useful. Phased array coils are available in receive-only mode, have high signal to noise ratios and can cover a relatively large field of view.

Signal intensity

Signal intensity is the amplitude of a radiowave, emitted by a tissue. In MR terminology a bright/white area on an image is called hyperintense and low signal area is referred to as hypointense. A number of factors determine the signal intensity (darkness or brightness): inherent characteristics of a particular tissue (T1 and T2 relaxation times, proton density, flow) and operator controlled factors (pulse repetition time (TR), echo delay time (TE), and inversion time (T1)). A brief description of some of these terminology is provided.

T1 (spin–lattice/longitudinal) relaxation time

After transmitting rf energy into a patient, the protons resonate and then loose the energy as they return to their resting equilibrium state. T1 is a time constant of an exponential process during which energy is transferred from the resonating hydrogen nuclei to the environment (lattice). T1 depends upon the tissue composition, structure and the environment. The nuclei and electrons in the environment of the resonating protons create fluctuations in the local magnetic fields, which are responsible for the energy dissipation/transfer. Fluctuations near the Larmor frequency facilitate quick energy transfer from the protons to the lattice and these tissues known to have short T1 relaxation time, appearing bright on T1 weighted sequence. Conversely, tissues with rapidly moving molecules such as water have magnetic fluctuations occurring at a high frequency, making less efficient dissipations of energy to the lattice resulting in a long T1 relaxation time and appearing dark on T1 weighted sequence.

T2 (Spin–spin/transverse) relaxation time

T2 is a time constant of exponential energy decay caused by local magnetic heterogeneities in the local magnetic field due to chemical composition. Different tissues have different T2 relaxation times. Pure liquids (e.g. water) have long T2 relaxation times appearing very bright on a T2 weighted sequence. Impure liquids or fluids with cellular components have relatively shorter T2, having various degrees of signal brightness on a T2 weighted sequence.

Proton density

Proton density refers to the number of mobile hydrogen nuclei, excited/spinning from the application of a radio-frequency pulse. The number of mobile protons depends upon the water and lipid contents of the biologic tissues. Tissues with a small number of mobile protons (e.g., cortical bone, gas) appear dark on MRI sequences.

Pulse sequences

Spin echo

Spin echo sequences may be acquired as a single echo, multiple echoes or fast spin echoes. Spin echo images can be obtained with T1, T2 or proton density weighting. The time between successive excitation pulses for a particular slice is called TR (repetition time). TE (echo time) refers to the time between the excitation pulse to the echo maximum.

Fast (Turbo) spin echo (FSE) is the most frequently used MRI technique in which an excitation pulse (90°) is followed by one or more 180° rf pulses. Every spin echo needs a 180° rf pulse for its production. A gradient pulse of opposite polarity is applied to refocus the protons. Rapid acquisition with relaxation enhanced (RARE) technique is the basis of fast spin echo. Multiple 180° pulses are used to generate multiple echoes. Different TEs and gradient pulses are used for each echo.

Inversion recovery sequence

An inversion recovery sequence (IR) is a variation of spin echo sequences in which an additional 180° radio-frequency pulse is applied prior to the excitation pulse; this inverts proton magnetization. Inversion time (TI) is the time delay between the 180° inversion pulse and the excitation pulse. TR times are usually long for IR sequences as sufficient time is required for maximum T1 relaxation between rf pulses. IR sequence does not depend on uniform field homogeneity, and it can be used for small body parts or off-centre imaging or at low field magnet strengths, where homogeneous fat suppression can be a challenge. Limitations of this sequence include reduced signal to noise ratio, long scan time and magnetic and radio-frequency field related heterogeneities. IR, however, is particularly useful in musculoskeletal imaging in the detection of marrow and muscle abnormalities including oedema, infection or tumour.

Gradient echo sequence

In gradient echo sequence and its variations, gradient reversal instead of 180° rf pulse is used to refocus the protons. Imaging gradients dephase the protons. The gradient is reversed and an echo is produced when a second gradient pulse of the opposite polarity but similar direction and magnitude is applied. Absence of the 180° rf pulse allows more imaging slices to be acquired for the same TR when compared with spin

echo sequence. Gradient echo also has less rf power deposition into the patient, compared with spin echo. However, magnetic susceptibility artefacts are also more pronounced for the same reason. Spoiled gradient echo is a frequently used type of gradient echo sequence, and it is fairly suitable for T1 weighting in the abdominal and musculoskeletal imaging in multiple planes with intravenous gadolinium administration. This technique relies upon relatively long TR (140 ms), combined with short TE times (4.5 ms at 1.5 T) and excitation angles between 60°–90°.

In general, gradient echo T1 weighting is obtained using large excitation angles (up to 80°), short TR (100–150 ms) and short TE (10 ms). Proton density weighted images are produced using small excitation angles (15° to 20°), relatively long TR (500 ms) and short TE (10 ms). T2* weighted images require similar excitation angles and TR but with a longer TE (25 ms). For spoiled gradient echo, TE determines the amount of T2* than T2 contrast.

Muscle imaging

We have found the following protocol useful in muscle imaging: Coronal and/or sagittal FSE T2 fat saturated or inversion recovery (Fig. 38.1) sequences to define the extent of the lesion with axial FSE T2 fat saturated or IR to evaluate signal intensity (tumour, trauma, oedema, haemorrhage). Axial T1 images are then acquired to detect muscle anatomy, architecture and better visualize myotendinous junction, tendons and ligaments. T1 images are also used for the detection of haemorrhage and to characterize fatty lesions.

Table 38.1 — Relative magnetic resonance imaging signal intensities for some tissues

	T1 weighted	T2 weighted
Cortical bone	Low	Low
Tendons, ligaments	Low	Low
Muscle	Intermediate	Low
Fat	High	High/Intermediate
Soft tissue tumours	Low/Intermediate	High
Osteoid matrix	Low	Low
Cartilage matrix	Intermediate	High
Haemorrhage (variable):		
Acute	Intermediate	Low
Early subacute	High	Low
Late subacute	High	High
Chronic	High	High with low rim

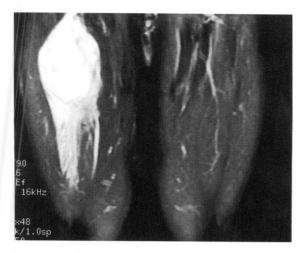

Figure 38.1 — Coronal inversion recovery (STIR) sequence is good for outlining the cranio-caudal extent of the tumour (hyperintense mass).

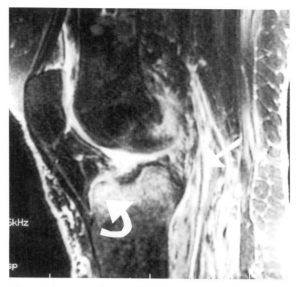

Figure 38.2 — Knee: Sagittal T2 FSE sequence with fat saturation. Gastrocnemius muscle strain is seen as oedema haemorrhage in between the muscle fibres (straight arrow). Ruptured anterior cruciate ligament (non-visualization of ACL) and bone bruise (curved arrow) are also noted.

Exercise related muscle changes

Transient increased T2 muscle signal after exercise is a well known phenomenon (Fleckenstein et al 1988,1989a, Fisher et al 1990, Shellock et al 1991a, de Kerviler et al 1991). It is apparent for only 10–30 min after stopping the exercise (Fisher et al 1990) and thought to be related to increased water content and circulatory changes without a well understood underlying mechanism (Fleckenstein et al 1988, Fisher et al 1990, Shellock et al 1991a, de Kerviler et al 1991, Morvan et al 1992, Fleckenstein et al 1992).

Muscle injuries

Most muscle injuries are sports related, and they may occur with intense exercise in unaccustomed individuals (Shellock et al 1991b). The patient presents with acute pain during exercise which does not resolve (Fleckenstein et al 1989b). MRI shows increased T2 signal in the affected muscle. This is thought to represent oedema and/or haemorrhage, which may appear focal or mass like in some cases (DeSmet 1993). In some cases, the muscle may have a rim of high T2 signal, similar to perifascial fluid (Fleckenstein et al 1989c). First degree muscle strain is a stretch injury (Fig. 38.2), second degree is partial tear and third degree is compatible with complete rupture (Zarins and Ciullo 1983). All of these are readily detected and characterized by MRI. Partial muscle tears are manifested by abnormal muscle and perifascial fluid, findings similar to muscle strain. However, there is

often an associated area of muscle attenuation and a surrounding focal zone of increased signal intensity (Greco et al 1991). Acute complete muscle tears can be difficult to diagnose in the presence of large amounts of haemorrhage, oedema or spasm, which are often associated with such injuries (Hernandez et al 1992). MRI of myotendinous strain (Palmer et al 1999) in athletes is valuable in demonstrating the exact site and severity of strain, which is crucial information for surgical planning and prognosis.

Delayed onset muscle soreness

Delayed onset muscle soreness (DOMS) is a separate entity from acute exertional strain injuries (Noonan and Garrett 1992). This postexertional syndrome is characterized by muscle soreness, swelling and joint swelling. The symptoms typically begin several hours after exercise, peak at 2–5 days and often disappear in 7–10 days. MRI displays an increased T2 muscle signal, which correlates best with muscle injury at 48 h (Nurenberg et al 1992).

Compartment syndrome

Oedema or haemorrhage within the confines of closed fascial planes (Fig. 38.3) leading to abnormally high

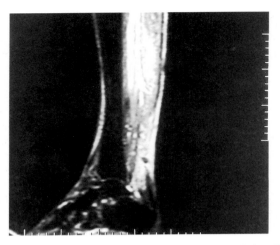

Figure 38.3—Sagittal inversion recovery sequence through the calf region. Posterior compartment muscle oedema and haemorrhage resulting in compartment syndrome. A complete tear of Achilles tendon is noted at the myotendinous junction.

pressure and severed circulation is known as compartment syndrome. This entity requires differentiation from deep venous thrombosis, and this may be achieved by MRI or ultrasound.

Muscle infarction

Focal muscle infarctions are reported in diabetic patients with severe multiorgan involvement (Banker and Chester 1973, Levinsohn and Bryan 1979, Chester CS 1986, Lauro et al 1991, Barohn and Kissel 1992, Nunez-Hoyo et al 1993). This entity most commonly involves the anterior thigh with common contralateral recurrence. Quadriceps, thigh adductors, hamstrings and calf muscles are most commonly involved in decreasing order of frequency. Patients usually complain of abrupt onset of severe pain, tenderness and swelling, and there is often a palpable mass without history of trauma. The patients are usually afebrile and have a normal or mildly elevated white blood cell count and creatine kinase level. The underlying pathogenesis of diabetic muscle infarction is thought to be microvascular disease (arteriosclerosis obliterans) in diabetes mellitus (Banker and Chester 1973). On MRI, fluid sensitive (STIR or FSE T2 fat saturated) sequences demonstrate muscle, perifascial and subcutaneous oedema in affected muscle groups. However, imaging findings in diabetic muscle infarction are non-specific and characteristic clinical presentation is necessary for diagnosis, as well as exclusion of other conditions mimicking this entity (myositis,

osteomyelitis, abscess, fascitis, thrombophlebitis, haematoma, neoplasm, ruptured Baker's cyst, diabetic amyotrophy, exertional muscle rupture).

Rhabdomyolysis

Muscle injury as a result of various aetiologies (trauma, systemic metabolic abnormalities, metabolic disorders linked with inherited deficiency of glycolytic enzymes such as McArdle's disease or from other causes) may cause rhabdomyolysis, resulting in release of cell contents into the extracellular fluid and plasma (Lamminen et al 1989, Fleckenstein et al 1989b, 1991a; Fleckenstein and Shellock 1991). Non-specific muscle oedema is seen in involved muscles on STIR or T2 weighted sequences on MRI. Painful muscle contractures and increased serum creatine kinase are common findings in rhabdomyolysis related to metabolic myopathies. MRI findings of muscle oedema, atrophy and fatty infiltration in combination are often considered to be indications of myopathic or neurogenic disorders (Fleckenstein and Shellock 1991, Fleckenstein et al 1991a).

Congenital muscle diseases

MRI specificity is limited in diagnosing congenital myopathies and inherited muscular dystrophies. The presence of focal and symmetric muscle oedema-like patterns on MRI followed by fatty replacement in appropriate clinical setting should raise the suspicion of Duchenne's or Becker's muscular dystrophy. MRI can be helpful in defining specific muscle group atrophy and suggesting particular diseases in unsuspected cases. For example, extraocular muscle atrophy can be seen in oculopharyngeal muscular dystrophy, parascapular muscle atrophy is seen in facioscapulohumeral muscular dystrophy and humeroperoneal distribution of muscle atrophy is characteristic of Emery–Dreifuss muscular dystrophy.

Congenital myopathies show shortening of T1 relaxation times of muscle related to fatty infiltration. Involvement of selective muscle and sparing of certain muscle groups is noted in different congenital myopathies and muscular dystrophies.

Some myopathies are characterized by myotonias or abnormal muscle relaxation after contraction. Decreased muscle thickness (tibialis anterior, rectus femoris, vastus intermedius, triceps brachii and sternocleidomastoid muscles) and increased subcutaneous fat are seen in myotonic dystrophy (the most common degenerative myopathy affecting adults). With disease progression, the medial and lateral head of the gastrocnemius and soleus muscles as well as the spine extensor muscles show similar changes, with significant sparing of sartorius and gracilis muscles. Although similar muscle groups can be affected in spinal muscular atrophies, muscle atrophy is diffuse and generalized without focal sparing of any groups, although certain muscle groups may be more involved by the disease than others (Suput et al 1993). Paradoxically, MRI in patients with congenital myotonia shows muscle hypertrophy without signal abnormalities (Reimers and Vogl 1996).

Denervation injury

Afferent nerve injury results in an abnormal muscle signal in the affected group. Although variable in the acute phase, afferent nerve injury is frequently demonstrated as prolonged tissue T1 and T2 values in the subacute phase (1 to 12 months; Fleckenstein et al 1993), and it is thought to be related to an increase in extracellular fluid (Shabas et al 1987, Polak et al 1988, Frostick et al 1992).

Inflammatory myopathies

Abnormal muscle signals in inflammatory myopathies such as polymyositis, dermatomyositis, scleroderma, sarcoidosis and inclusion body myositis, are those of non-specific muscle oedema on T2 weighted (Fig. 38.4), and they are dark to isointense with muscle on T1 sequences in acute disease (Hernandez et al 1993, Reimers et al 1994). With disease progression and chronicity, fatty replacement is seen with the presence of increased T1 signal between the affected muscle fibres.

Muscle infection

MRI is frequently utilized in the diagnosis and differentiation of pyomyositis, abscess and necrotizing fasciitis. The last two conditions require surgical drainage or debridement.

Pyomyositis, previously reported in the tropics and in temperate climates, has been noticed with increasing incidence in human immunodeficiency virus (HIV) infected patients. Other risk factors include diabetes mellitus, prolonged steroid use, certain haematologic and connective tissue diseases (Rodgers et al 1993, Belsky et al 1994, Gordon et al 1995). MRI shows enlargement and increased T2 signal within involved muscles (Gordon et al 1995). The T1 signal of affected muscles may also be increased. Involved muscle enhancement is noted on gadolinium-enhanced images (Fig. 38.5).

Abscesses appear as well defined areas, dark on T1 and bright on T2 weighted sequences, often with a relatively hyperintense rim on T1. The rim shows evidence of gadolinium enhancement with lack of central enhancement in the abscess (Fig. 38.4).

MRI of necrotizing fasciitis shows an increased T2 signal in the involved muscles and fascial planes (perifascial fluid; Rahmouni et al 1994).

Bacillary angiomatosis, an infectious entity seen in patients with acquired immunodeficiency syndrome (AIDS), shows increased T2 MRI signal in affected muscles with flow voids compatible with small vessels. Intense Gadolinium-enhancement of vascular tissue is suggested (Moore et al 1995).

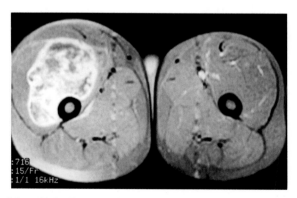

Figure 38.5—Pyomyositis. Heterogeneous areas of rim and central enhancement in the infected right thigh muscle (vastus intermedius) on a T1 weighted axial image post intravenous gadolinium administration.

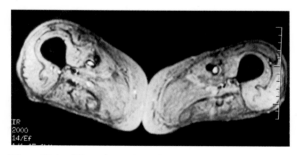

Figure 38.4—Bilateral muscle oedema is seen as diffuse muscle hyperintensity on the axial IR images through the thigh region in a patient with dermatomyositis.

Muscle haemorrhage

Muscle injury can lead to interstitial haemorrhage within connective tissues or a focal collection of blood (haematoma) within or in between muscle fibres. The affected muscle is often increased in size and displays variable MRI signal intensity depending upon the duration of blood products. In the early acute phase, haemorrhage is isointense with muscle on T1 weighted sequences and bright on T2 or STIR sequences (Fig. 38.6). During the early subacute stage, the haematoma has a heterogeneous signal with T1 shortening (hyperintense on T1 pulse sequence areas), attributable to intracellular methaemoglobin (oxidative denaturation of haemoglobin). The T1 signal increases for up to 90 hours after the injury. T2 shortening (low T2 signal) results from deoxyhaemoglobin within intact red blood cells. In the late subacute stage, methaemoglobin becomes extracellular, appearing hyperintense on T1 and T2 weighted sequences. With chronic haematoma, there is low T1 and bright T2 signal. A low signal intensity rim is present due to haemosiderin. There is a significant overlap between signal characteristics of muscle haemorrhages, which do not always follow the above described classic pattern of haematomas in other tissues.

Interstitial haemorrhage appears low on T1 and high on T2 signal in the acute stage. A high T2 signal with interstitial haemorrhage shows little, if any, change over time. This is a less understood phenomenon, thought by some investigators to be secondary to associated muscle oedema and/or inflammatory changes.

Muscle tumours

MRI is superior to other imaging modalities in diagnosing soft tissue tumours and defining their osseous extent. Plain radiographs may provide further information about the nature of the tumour matrix or soft tissues and, therefore, they should always be obtained and correlated with MRI findings in the evaluation of bone involvement. Although highly sensitive, MRI does not have equally high specificity in differentiating benign from malignant masses. Certain MRI features can be suggestive of malignancy: irregular tumour margins, heterogeneous signal, surrounding marrow or soft tissue oedema/mass (Figs 38.7, 38.8). Pathologic fracture or neurovascular bundle involvement (Fig. 38.9) also suggest malignancy. There is an overlap of these findings in benign lesions, and the differentiation could be difficult at times based on imaging criteria alone.

Miscelleneous conditions

MRI is the modality of choice for recognition of congenital muscle variants, accessory muscles and postoperative reconstructive anatomy, which may often simulate a soft tissue mass. Accessory muscles

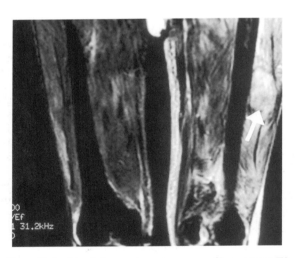

Figure 38.6—Muscle haemorrhage: large areas of hyperintense T2 signal predominantly in the left vastus lateralis muscle in a patient on anticoagulant treatment. Corresponding T1 image showed bright signal (not included). Focal mass like area (arrow) requires differentiation from a soft tissue tumour and needs to be followed up to complete resolution.

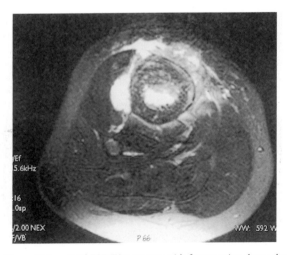

Figure 38.7—Axial FSE T2 sequence with fat saturation shows the bone marrow and peri-osseous soft tissue tumour (extensor digitorum muscle) involvement as hyperintense signal in a patient with Ewing's sarcoma.

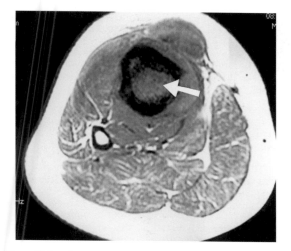

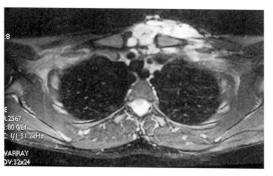

Figure 38.10—Axial T2 FSE image: A multilobulated bright mass in the left sternoclavicular joint region extends into the anterior mediastinum. Corresponding gradient sequence (not included) showed the vascular nature of the lesion, confirming the diagnosis of hemangioma.

Figure 38.8—Corresponding T1 axial image of the same patient (as in Figure 38.7) shows the tibial tumour to be of low signal (arrow) compared to the bright normal fatty marrow in the fibula.

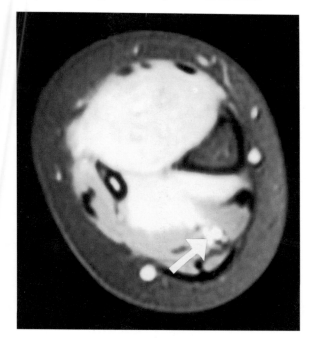

Figure 38.9—Axial T1 weighted gadolinium enhanced fat saturated image through the patient's right calf shows a large enhancing tumour involving the anterior and posterior tibial muscles and reasching in close proximity of posterior tibial artery and vein (arrow).

display normal muscle signal on all pulse sequences. Accessory soleus (Paul et al 1991) is the most commonly described muscle in this normal variant group. However, there have been reports of accessory hand muscles (e.g extensor digitorum manus brevis;

Anderson et al 1995) and accessory semimembranosus muscle.

Myositis ossificans is a benign mass with progressive ossification often related to previous trauma. Diagnostic clue lies in the radiographic evidence of progressive maturation from a tender soft-tissue mass-like abnormality into an ossified mass with relatively lucent centre and calcified periphery. MRI and biopsy can often be misleading, mimicking a malignancy. Observation and radiographic correlation are crucial (Kransdorf et al 1991).

Haemangioma and arteriovenous malformations are benign lesions made up of vascular channels, septae, fat and may contain phleboliths, thrombosed vascular segments (haemangioma) or large tangle of vessels (arteriovenous malformation). Haemangioma are isointense with muscle on T1 weighted sequence, may contain bright foci (fat) and show a hyperintense signal on T2 weighted sequence (Fig. 38.10) with scattered dark signal foci representing phleboliths or thrombosed vascular channels. Arteriovenous malformations have low T1 and T2 flow void areas corresponding to rapidly flowing blood in vascular channels.

In summary, MRI is an excellent and sensitive modality for soft tissue imaging. Current research in spectroscopy and functional imaging will further advance the diagnostic potential of MRI.

References

Anderson MW, Benedetti P, Walter J, Steinberg DR. (1995) MR appearance of the extensor digitorum manus brevis muscle: A pseudotumor of the hand. *AJR* 164: 1477–1479.

Banker BQ, Chester CS. (1973) Infarction of thigh muscle in the diabetic patient. *Neurology* 23: 667–677.

Barohn RJ, Kissel JR. (1992) Case of the month: Painful thigh mass in a young woman: diabetic muscle infarction. *Muscle Nerve* 15: 850–855.

Belsky DS, Teates CD, Hartman ML. (1994) Case report; Diabetes mellitus as a predisposing factor in the development of pyomyositis. *Am J Med Sci* 308: 251–254.

Chester CS, Banker BQ. (1986) Focal infarction of muscle in diabetics. *Diabetes Care* 9: 623–630.

de Kerviler E, Leroy-Willig A, Jehenson P, Duboc D, Eymard B, Syrota A. (1991) Exercise-induced muscle modifications: study of healthy subjects and patients with metabolic myopathies with MR imaging and P-31 spectroscopy. *Radiology* 181: 259–264.

DeSmet A. (1993) Magnetic resonance findings in skeletal muscle tears. *Skeletal Radiol* 22: 479–484.

Fisher MJ, Meyer RA, Adams GR, Foley JM, Potchen EJ. (1990) Direct relationship between proton T2 and exercise intensity in skeletal muscle MR images. *Invest Radiol* 25: 480–485.

Fleckenstein JL, Canby RC, Parkey RW, Peshock RM. (1988) Acute effects of exercise on MR imaging of skeletal muscle in normal volunteers. *AJR* 151: 231–237.

Fleckenstein JL, Bertocci LA, Nunnally RL, Parkey RW, Peshock RM. (1989a) Exercise-enhanced MR imaging of variations in forearm muscle anatomy and use: importance in MR spectroscopy. *AJR* 153: 693–698.

Fleckenstein JL, Peshock RM, Lewis SF, Haller RG. (1989b) Magnetic resonance imaging of muscle injury and atrophy in glycolytic myopathies. *Muscle Nerve* 12: 849.

Fleckenstein JL, Weatherall PT, Parkey RW, Payne JA, Peshock RM. (1989c) Sports related muscle injuries: evaluation with MR imaging. *Radiology* 172: 793–798.

Fleckenstein JL, Shellock FG. (1991) Exertional muscle injuries; Magnetic resonance imaging evaluation. *Top Magn Reson Imaging* 3: 50.

Fleckenstein JL, Weatherall PT, Bertocci LA, et al. (1991a) Locomotor system assessment by muscle magnetic resonance imaging. Magn Reson Q. 7: 79.

Fleckenstein JL, Burns DK, Murphy FK, Jayson HT, Bonte FJ. (1991b) Differential diagnosis of bacterial myositis in AIDS: evaluation with MR imaging. *Radiology* 179: 653–658.

Fleckenstein JL, Haller RG, Bertocci LA, Parkey RW, Peshock RM. (1992) Glycogenolysis, not perfusion, is the critical mediator of exercise-induced muscle modifications on MR images. *Radiology* 183: 25–27.

Fleckenstein JL, Watumull D, Conner KE, et al. (1993) Denervated human skeletal muscle: MR imaging evaluation. *Radiology* 187: 213–218.

Frostick SP, Taylor DJ, Dolecki MJ, Radda GK. (1992) Human muscle cell denervation: the result of a 31-phosphorus magnetic resonance spectroscopy study. *J Hand Surg* 17B: 33–45.

Gordon BA, Martinez S, Collins AJ. (1995) Pyomyositis; characteristics at CT and MR imaging. *Radiology* 197: 279–286.

Greco A, Mc Namara MT, Escher MB, Trifilio G, Parienti J. (1991) Spin-echo and STIR imaging of sports-related muscle injuries at 1.5 T. *J Comput Assist Tomogr* 15: 994–999.

Hernandez RJ, Keim DR, Cenevert TL, Sullivan DB, Aisen AM. (1992) Fat-supressed MR imaging of myositis. *Radiology* 182: 217–219.

Hernandez RJ, Sullivan DB, Chenevert TL, Keim DR. (1993) MR imaging in children with dermatomyositis: musculoskeletal findings and correlation with clinical and laboratory findings. *AJR* 161: 359–366.

Kransdorf MJ, Meis JM, Jelinek JS. (1991) Myositis ossificans: MR appearance with radiologic-pathologic correlation. *AJR* 157: 1243–1248.

Lamminen AE, Hekali PE, Tiula E, Suramo I, Korhola OA. (1989) Acute rhabdomyolysis: evaluation with magnetic resonance imaging compared with computed tomography and ultrasonography. *Br J Radiol* 62: 326–330.

Lauro GR, Kissel JR, Simon SR. (1991) Idiopathic muscular infarction in a diabetic patient. *J Bone Joint Surg (Am)* 73: 301–304.

Levinsohn EM, Bryan PJ. (1979) Computed tomography in unilateral extremity swelling of unusual cause. *J Comput Assist Tomogr* 3: 67–70.

Moore EH, Russell LA, Klein JS, et al. (1995) Bacillary angiomatosis in patients with AIDS: multiorgan imaging findings. *Radiology* 197: 67–72.

Morvan D, Vilgrain V, Arrive L, Nahum H. (1992) Correlation of MR changes with Doppler ultrasound measurements of blood flow in exercising normal muscle. *J Magn Reson Imaging* 2: 645–652.

Noonan TJ, Garrett WE. (1992) Injuries at the myotendinous junction. *Clin Sports Med* 11: 783–806.

Nunez-Hoyo M, Gardner CL, Motta AO, Ashmead JW. (1993) Case report. Skeletal muscle infarction in diabetes: MR findings. *J Comput Assist Tomogr* 17: 986–988.

Nurenberg P, Giddings CJ, Stray-Gundersen J, Fleckenstein JL, Gonyea WJ, Peshock RM. (1992) MR imaging-guided muscle biopsy for correlation of increased signal intensity with ultrastructural changes and delayed-onset muscle soreness after exercise. *Radiology* 184: 865–869.

Palmer EW, Kuong SJ, Elmadbouh HM. (1999) MR imaging of myotendinous strain. *AJR* 173: 703–709.

Paul MA, Imanse J, Golding RP, Kooomen AR, Meijer S. (1991) Accessory soleus muscle mimicking a soft tissue tumor. A report of 2 patients. *Acta Ortho Scand* 62: 609–611.

Polak JF, Jolesz FA, Adams DF. (1988) Magnetic resonance imaging of skeletal muscle prolongation of T1 and T2 subsequent to denervation. *Invest Radiol* 23: 365–369.

Rahmouni A, Chosidow O, Mathieu D, et al. (1994) MR imaging in acute infectious cellulitis. *Radiology* 192: 492–496.

Reimers CD, Schedel H, Fleckenstein JL, et al. (1994) Magnetic resonance imaging of skeletal muscles in ideopathic inflammatory myopathies of adults. *J Neurol* 241: 306–314.

Reimers CD, Vogl TJ. (1996) Myotonic dystrophy. In: Fleckenstein JL, Reimers C, and Crues JV, eds. *Muscle imaging in health and disease*. New York: Springer-Verlag, pp 31–60.

Rodgers WB, Yodlowski ML, Mintzer CM. (1993) Pyomyositis in patients who have the human immunodeficiency virus. *J Bone Joint Surg* 75A: 588–592.

Shabas D, Gerard G, Rossi D. (1987) Magnetic resonance imaging examination of denervated muscle. *Comput Radiol* 11: 9–13.

Shellock FG, Fukunaga T, Mink JH, Edgerton VR. (1991a) Acute effects of exercise on MR imaging of skeletal muscle: concentric vs eccentric actions. *AJR* 156: 765–768.

Shellock FG, Fukunaga T, Mink JH, Edgerton VR. (1991b) Exertional muscle injury: evaluation of concentric versus eccentric actions with serial MR imaging. *Radiology* 179: 659–664.

Suput D, Zupan A, Sepe A, et al. (1993) Discrimation between neurogenic and myopathic muscle disease using MRI. *Acta Neurol Scand* 87: 118.

Zarins B, Ciullo JV. (1983) Acute muscles and tendon injuries in athletes. *Clin Sprts Med* 2: 167–182.

39

Skeletal muscle mass: regional and whole-body measurement methods

Robert Lee, ZiMian Wang and Steven Heymsfield

Introduction

Over one fifth of body mass in the newborn consists of skeletal muscle tissue and the relative amount in the average adult male approaches almost one half of body weight (Table 39.1) (Snyder et al 1975, Gallagher et al 1997). Thereafter, skeletal muscle declines in mass with amounts in men returning to prepubertal levels by the eighth decade. Women experience similar dynamic skeletal muscle mass trends throughout the life span, although most of the currently available information is based on cross-sectional studies (Heymsfield et al 1994).

In addition to a central role in mechanical function, skeletal muscles are intimately involved in metabolic processes in both health and disease. Almost one half of the total body protein pool in men (Table 39.2) and a somewhat similar proportion in women, is found within the skeletal muscle compartment.

The aim of this chapter is to provide the reader with an overview of in vivo skeletal muscle mass measurement methods. The methods reviewed were also described in earlier reports (Gallagher et al 1997, Heymsfield et al 1994, Janssens et al 1994, Heymsfield In Press).

Five-level model

There are over 600 discrete skeletal muscles in humans and each has a definable set of components. Dissection and removal of a discrete skeletal muscle yields "anatomical" skeletal muscle at the Tissue Level (Wang et al 1992). This component includes entrapped adipose tissue, nerves, blood vessels and tendons. The components of anatomic muscle, in turn, can be characterized in terms of Cellular, Molecular and Atomic Level components (Table 39.3 and Fig. 39.1). The fifth body composition level,

Table 39.1 — Proportional contribution of skeletal muscle to the body weight of a man at different stages of development

Stage	% of body weight
Birth	21
Weaning	18
Adolescent	36
Adult	45
Elderly	27

Reprinted with permission from Gallagher et al 1997

Table 39.2 — Distribution of total body protein in the 70 kg Reference Man[a]

Organ/tissue	Protein mass (kg)	% of total body protein
Skeletal muscle	4.8	45.3
Brain	0.11	1.0
Liver	0.32	3.0
Kidney	0.053	0.50
Heart	0.055	0.52
Blood	0.99	9.4
Skin	0.75	7.1
Skeleton	1.9	18.1
Total body	**10.5**	**100**

Reprinted with permission from Gallagher et al 1997
[a]Information based on the Reference Man

Whole Body, is not shown in the figure or table. Each method presented in the following section quantifies skeletal muscle by estimation of one or more of the components that comprise skeletal muscle tissue.

Method organization

Skeletal muscle measurement methods can be organized into four categories based on measurement number and frequency (static and dynamic), location of measurement facility (epidemiological and clinical), anatomical site(s) measured (regional and whole-body), and mathematical prediction function applied (descriptive and mechanistic). The following presentation organizes methods according to mathematical prediction function, although within each section mention will also be made of other relevant measurement characteristics.

Measurement methods

All in vivo methods for measuring skeletal muscle mass can be summarized into the general formula:

$$SM = f(Q)$$

This general formula shows that quantification of skeletal muscle (SM) is dependent on two variables, a measurable quantity (Q) and a mathematical function (f) relating Q to SM. Two main types of mathematical function were identified for in vivo skeletal muscle mass measurement methods: mechanistic and descriptive. Mechanistic methods share in common mathematical functions that are developed based on

Table 39.3—Skeletal muscle composition of Reference Man

Atomic level			Molecular level			Cellular level			Tissue level		
Component	kg	%	Component	kg	%	Component	kg	%	Component	kg	%
Oxygen	21.0	75.0	Water	22.0	78.6	Adipocytes	0.66	2.4	Adipose tissue	0.78	2.8
Carbon	3.0	10.7	Protein	4.80	17.1	Muscle cells	15.0	53.6	Non-AT SM[b]	26.5	94.6
Hydrogen	2.8	10.0	Fat	0.62	2.2	Red cells	0.28	1.0	Blood	0.70	2.5
Nitrogen	0.77	2.75	Ash	0.34	1.2	ECF[b]	12.06	43.1			
Phosphorus	0.050	0.18	Glycogen	0.24	0.86						
Potassium	0.084	0.30									
Sodium	0.021	0.075									
Chlorine	0.0022	0.008									
Calcium	0.0009	0.003									
Sulphur	0.0067	0.024									

[a]Information based on the Reference Man (Snyder et al 1975)
[b]ECF, extracellular fluid; Non-ATSM, non-adipose tissue skeletal muscle

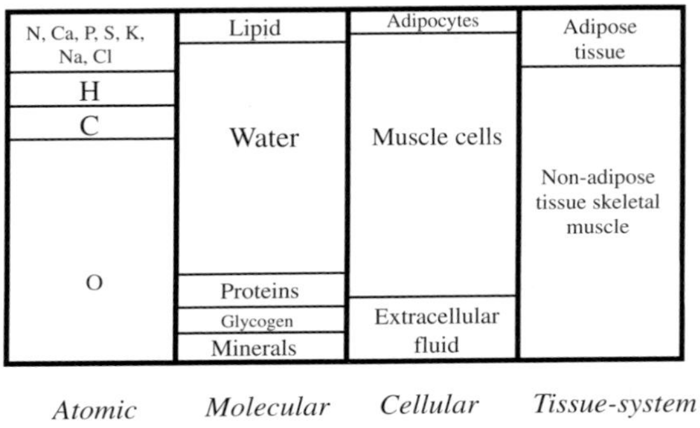

Figure 39.1—Skeletal muscle components at the first four body composition levels. Reprinted from "Skeletal Muscle Markers" by Heymsfield et al. (Gallagher et al 1997). Reprinted with permission.

well-established models that are assumed constant within and between individuals. These models usually represent ratios or proportions of measurable quantities. In contrast, descriptive methods share in common mathematical functions derived by statistical analysis of experimental observations. A reference method is used to estimate SM in a specific population of subjects. Regression analysis is then used to establish the mathematical function (f) between SM and Q to develop the prediction equation.

Mechanistic

Computed tomography

Historically, computerized axial tomography (CT) was the first available imaging method for body composition analysis (Hounsfield 1973). There are now many studies that have examined the validity of CT for estimating the whole body components (Janssens et al 1994, Sjöström 1991, Heymsfield et al 1997). Recently, Mitsiopoulos et al (1998) reported cadaver validation of skeletal muscle measurements by CT. CT estimates of cross-sectional arm and leg skeletal muscle areas were highly correlated with corresponding cadaver values ($R^2 = 0.98$, SEE = 3.8 cm^2, $p<0.001$). The findings support CT as an accurate assessment tool for estimating appendicular skeletal muscle mass in vivo.

At present, imaging methods such as CT are suitable for use as a criterion method when calibrating other body composition methods. CT is capable of detecting small changes in soft tissue composition, and it is an ideal method for quantifying skeletal muscle composition in both cross-sectional and longitudinal studies. Cost, however, is a limiting factor for routine estimation of skeletal muscle mass. Both the high cost of CT scanners and the cost per patient study limit the availability of this method at major medical centres. More importantly, radiation exposure severely limits routine scans or multiple scans over time for subjects, especially children and pregnant women.

Magnetic resonance imaging

Magnetic resonance imaging (MRI) is another important imaging method that offers the advantages of CT but without the risk of radiation exposure. The underlying physical concepts related to MRI were developed as early as 1946, but it was not until 1984 that in vivo images were introduced (Foster et al

1984). Magnetic resonance imaging is based on the interaction between the nuclei of hydrogen atoms in human tissues and the magnetic field generated by the MRI scanner system. An application of a magnetic field to a subject induces the atomic nuclei to align with the field. When a radio frequency (RF) pulse is directed to the body tissues, some nuclei absorb the energy from the magnetic field. Once the RF field is turned off, the energized nuclei release the energy in the form of an RF signal. The computer uses these emitted signals to reconstruct a cross-sectional image. The acquired image is then quantified by various segmentation techniques similar to those described for CT. The whole body MRI imaging protocol is described by Ross (1996).

Studies have demonstrated that MRI estimates of skeletal muscle are in good agreement with those obtained from cadaver sections (Beneke et al 1991, Engstrom et al 1991). Beneke et al (1991) reported a mean error of 1.2% between estimates of skeletal muscle area from MRI with corresponding cadaver cross-sectional area. A high correlation coefficient (R^2 = 0.98) between corresponding MRI and cadaver-skeletal muscle at the proximal thigh was reported by Engstrom et al (1991). More recently, Misiopoulos et al (1998) reported that MRI provides accurate measurements of skeletal muscle cross-sectional area throughout a wide range of values (10–100 cm^2).

The high cost of MRI instrumentation and operation limits the availability of this method for skeletal muscle assessment. In contrast to CT, MRI does not use ionizing radiation, and hence it may be available for scans of children and pregnant women. Imaging methods, such as MRI and CT, are based on measured physical properties and well-established reconstruction formulas. If we assume that the distances between image slices are minimal, there is little question that image-anthropometric muscle mass values can serve as reference values for use in the development of anthropometric models and other methods.

Dual energy X-ray absorptiometry

Although dual-energy X-ray absorptiometry (DEXA) was originally developed for assessing bone mineral content (BMC) and bone density in the study of osteoporosis, this technique has been refined for body composition analysis (Cameron and Sorenson 1963, Lukaski 1996). The DEXA scanner system acquires both body composition and bone data through the attenuation of a X-ray beam at the system's two main energy peaks (Pietrobelli et al 1996). The principle is that as a collimated X-ray beam passes through a

region of the body, the attenuation is determined by the composition of the region, its thickness and the energy of the X-ray. These differing characteristics can be expressed mathematically as a ratio of beam attenuation at the lower energy relative to that at the higher energy (R-value). The software algorithms in the computer first separate the bone mineral from the soft tissue by attenuation characteristics. Soft tissue pixels can be further separated into those for fat and lean soft tissues (Fig. 39.2). In this manner, regional and whole body assessment of fat and bone mineral-free lean soft tissue masses are calculated. The R-values for all lean tissues, including skeletal muscle mass, are similar and they are unrelated to age (Table 39.4) (Pietrobelli et al 1998). The physical concepts of DEXA are described in detail by Pietrobelli et al (Pietrobelli et al 1996). Many studies have supported the use of DEXA in body composition analysis (Kohrt 1995).

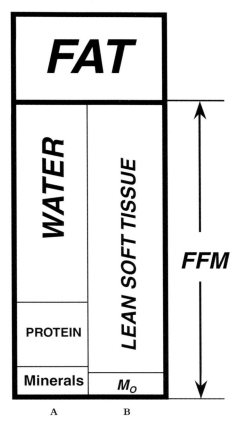

Figure 39.2 — Traditional four component molecular level model (**A**) and three component dual energy X-ray absorptiometry model (**B**). FFM, fat-free body mass; M_o, bone mineral.

Table 39.4— Summary of R-values of various human soft tissues for three age groups

| Soft tissue | Age group | | | p value |
	Newborn	4–7 months	Adults	
Skeletal muscle	1.35237	1.35187	1.35311	n.s
Heart	1.35617	1.35422	1.35400	n.s
Liver	1.35568	1.35333	1.35428	n.s
Kidney	1.35778		1.35971	n.s

Reprinted with permission from Pietrobelli et al 1998

Heymsfield and colleagues first proposed a model to estimate appendicular skeletal muscle mass using dual photon absorptiometry, a method similar to DEXA (Heymsfield et al 1990). The model is as follows:

$$\text{Appendicular skeletal muscle (ASM)} = \text{Appendicular fat-free soft tissue} - \text{Appendicular BMC} \times 1.82$$

Appendicular fat-free (i.e., lean) soft tissue was calculated as the sum of the fat-free soft tissue masses for the arms and legs. According to data for the Reference Man defined as a caucasian being between 20–30 years of age, weighing 70 kg with 170 cm in height, ASM represents 75% of total skeletal muscle mass (Snyder et al 1975). This fraction is assumed to be stable within and between individuals and total body skeletal muscle mass can, therefore, be calculated as:

$$\text{SM (kg)} = \text{ASM} \times 1.33$$

In a recent study, Wang et al compared skeletal muscle estimates in 25 men using CT and DEXA (2). A strong correlation was observed by the investigators between ASM from DEXA and total body skeletal muscle mass from CT ($R^2 = 0.90$, $p<0.001$). Baumgartner et al also reported similar results ($R^2 = 0.95$) comparing DEXA-ASM estimates to total body skeletal muscle mass from MRI.

The DEXA scanner system, however, is limited in its inability to quantify skeletal muscle directly. This method relies on several assumptions in order to calculate total body skeletal muscle mass. For example, one DEXA model assumes (Snyder et al 1975) that skin and bone marrow are negligible in mass. Our group has observed a higher value of skeletal muscle mass derived from the DEXA model compared with corresponding CT measurements (Lukaski 1993). The DEXA model noted earlier (Snyder et al 1975) overestimated skeletal muscle of the calves by 36%, thighs by 27%, forearms by 45% and for all three regions by 31% (all $p<0.01$) (Heymsfield et al 1990). Considerably more progress can be made in developing formulas for the conversion of appendicular lean soft tissue to skeletal muscle and from appendicular muscle to total body muscle. Despite these limitations, DEXA offers a reasonable alternative to CT and MRI for estimating regional and total body skeletal muscle mass. The amount of radiation used with DEXA is far less than with CT, and the cost of purchasing and operating the instrument is considerably less compared to MRI and CT.

In vivo neutron activation/whole body counting

An alternative to CT, MRI and DEXA for estimating skeletal muscle is based on a total body potassium–total body nitrogen (TBK-TBN) model. The model is formulated on TBK measure from ^{40}K whole body counting combined with TBN measured from in vivo neutron activation analysis (IVNA). The isotope ^{40}K, which emits a characteristic gamma ray at 1.46 MeV, is present in the human body at a known natural level (0.012%). Scintillation counters can detect these gamma rays which exit the body. The TBK protocol is described in detail by the International Atomic Energy Agency (1970). Total body nitrogen, an essential component of body protein, can be estimated by IVNA systems. A moderated beam of neutrons is delivered into the subject's tissues that cause the target elements in the body to create unstable isotopes. The unstable isotopes revert to a stable condition by emitting one or more gamma rays of characteristic energy levels. These data can be used to quantify TBN levels. The TBN protocol is described in detail by Vartsky et al (1984).

Conceptually, the body protein mass can be partioned into skeletal muscle and non-skeletal muscle-lean mass. The differences in distribution of potassium and nitrogen in these components allows for this fractionation. Burkinshaw et al proposed the classic model based an assumed constant ratio of K to N in muscle (3.03 mmol/g) and non–muscle–lean (1.33 mmol/g) to develop the following equation (Burkinshaw et al 1978):

$$SM \text{ (kg)} = 0.503 \times TBK - 0.0263 \times TBN$$

Where TBN is measured by prompt gamma neutron activation analysis. This method has been used to document differences in body composition in several studies (Cohn et al 1980a and b).

Whole body ^{40}K, whole body counting and IVNA provide the only non-invasive approach for the estimation of body cell mass and protein. However, the TBK-TBN model for estimating skeletal muscle has several limitations that limit accuracy. The K–N ratio in muscle may not be constant but may vary with age and physical activity levels. In addition there is a long-standing observation that the Burkinshaw model underestimates total body skeletal muscle mass (Burkinshaw 1978). Our previous study with multi-scan CT as the criterion method supports this observation (Wang et al 1996). Compared with CT, the Burkinshaw method underestimated skeletal muscle mass by a mean of 20.1% in healthy subjects. The costs of whole body counters and IVNA systems also limits their use of a few research centres.

Descriptive methods

Anthropometry

The use of anthropometric methods requires the selection of body measurements that relate to either regional or total body skeletal muscle. In general, the same circumferential and skinfold measurement sites used for total body fat prediction are used for skeletal muscle prediction (Heymsfield et al 1982). These sites include mid-upper arm circumference and the corresponding triceps skinfold thickness; mid-thigh circumference and the corresponding thigh skinfold; and mid-calf circumference and corresponding calf skinfold thickness. The limbs are assumed a concentric set of three cylinders (bone, muscle, and subcutaneous adipose tissue). Calculation of limb muscle tissue from anthropometric data requires only two measurements: the limb circumference and the corresponding skinfold thickness. The equation for calculating limb muscle is:

$$C_{muscle} = C_{limb} - \pi \times S$$

Where C_{muscle} is the muscle circumference, C_{limb} is the limb circumference, and S is the skinfold thickness.

There have been relatively few anthropometric models for total body skeletal muscle prediction in the literature (Forbes et al 1988, Matiegka 1921, Martin et al 1990, Doupe et al 1997). Most of the previous approaches either have poor reference methods for estimating skeletal muscle mass (Matiegka 1921) or lack of independent cross validation (Martin et al 1990, Doupe et al 1997).

Martin et al (1990), using the Brussels cadaver study, proposed an anthropometric dimensions and quantified on 12 male cadavers who were then dissected and their muscles weighed. A regional skeletal muscle prediction equation was developed on the 12 men:

$$SM \text{ (g)} = Stat \times (0.0553 \times CTG^2 + 0.0987 \times FG^2 + 0.0331 \times CCG^2) - 2445$$

where Stat is stature in cm, CTG is corrected thigh girth, FG is uncorrected forearm girth and CCG is corrected calf girth. The equation had an R^2 of 0.97 and SEE of 1.53 kg. Both the Martin model and the later Doupe model (1997) were based on data from the Brussels cadaver study that contained a very small sample size (n = 12) of elderly male cadavers (mean age: 68 ± 20 years) (Clarys et al 1984). The descriptive regression equations may, therefore, be highly sample-specific and not applicable for general use. Nevertheless, the Martin model is conceptually interesting, and it may guide investigators in future model development.

Several limitations associated with anthropometry must be emphasised. Calculated arm muscle area overestimates skeletal muscle by 15–25% in non-obese subjects, and the arm muscle area assumptions are inaccurate in obese and elderly subjects (Baumgartner et al 1993, Fried et al 1986). In addition, it is not known whether these or Martin/Doupe anthropometric equations are sensitive enough to monitor small changes in muscle mass caused by weight loss or gain. The potential of developing new anthropometric models now exists because of the development of MRI as a criterion method.

Anthropometry has considerable appeal as a widely used skeletal muscle assessment method despite the lack of cross-validated prediction equations that are widely applicable. Instruments for measuring anthropometric dimensions are portable and inexpensive. Procedures are non-invasive and minimal training is required, thus making anthropometry practical for application in epidemiological and clinical settings.

Ultrasound

Ultrasound methods can be used to estimate regional skeletal muscle thickness (Lukaski 1996). This technique uses high frequency sound waves that are produced by piezoelectric crystals in the transducer probe. Sound waves are directed through the skin surface and reflected off anatomical structures. These reflected sound waves return to the probe as echoes. Two ultrasound system types (A-mode and B-mode) are used. With A-mode systems, tissue interfaces can be identified and the thickness of regional skeletal muscle estimated. The more recent B-mode systems reconstruct cross-sectional images of skeletal muscles from reflected ultrasound sound waves.

Good precision and accuracy (coefficient of reliability >92%) was reported on trunk and appendicular skeletal muscle thickness measured with B-mode systems using a 5 MHz transducer (Ishida et al 1992, Sipila and Suominen 1991). In addition, B-mode systems at 2.4 MHz have been used to measure appendicular cross-sectional areas (Stokes and Young 1986).

Considerable practice is needed to obtain a good image with the ultrasound method. In addition, the transducer needs to be kept directly perpendicular to the skin surface. Additional studies are needed to improve the validity of this method for measuring regional skeletal muscle. The potential exists to measure thickness and cross-sectional areas of muscle in the elderly and during rehabilitation. Lastly, ultrasound systems vary in purchase price with high cost for the best systems.

Bioimpedance analysis

The use of bioimpedance analysis (BIA) is based on the different conductive and dielectric properties of various biological tissues at different frequencies. An alternating current is passed at one or more frequencies via electrodes across a tissue bed and the impedance (Z) or voltage drop is then measured. Tissues that contain electrolytes and high water content such as skeletal muscle are highly conductive whereas fat and bone are highly resistive (Baumgartner 1989). The fluid volume and the length of the electrical pathway in the extremities primarily influence electrical resistance (R) (Chumlea and Guo 1994). To extrapolate impedance to appendicular and total body skeletal muscle, the relationship must be established indirectly by statistical (i.e., descriptive) calibration against criterion methods such as MRI.

Many studies support the use of BIA in assessing appendicular skeletal muscle mass (e.g. Nunez et al 1999, Heymsfield et al 1998, Nunez et al 1996). Recently, our group measured lower limb skeletal muscle mass by DEXA in 94 subjects (Nunez et al 1999). High correlations ($R^2 = 0.79$ for men and

$R^2 = 0.72$ for women) were observed between L^2/R (L, length) and lower limb skeletal muscle mass with age as a covariate. Similar correlation ($R^2 = 0.77$, $p<0.001$) were reported between L^2/Z and arm skeletal muscle estimated by DEXA (Heymsfield et al 1998). Both of these studies suggest the use of a BIA in estimating appendicular skeletal muscle mass.

The BIA method of estimating appendicular skeletal muscle is suitable for epidemiological and field studies. This method offers the advantage of rapid, safe and non-invasive measurements. In addition, BIA instruments are portable and inexpensive. As with most descriptive methods, BIA prediction equations are highly population specific. The potential exists for developing BIA prediction formulas for evaluating muscle compartments of each limb separately.

Urinary creatinine excretion

Endogenous creatinine is produced by the non-enzymatic hydrolysis of creatine, primarily found in skeletal muscle phosphocreatine form (Borsook and Dubnoff 1947). This metabolic end product is excreted in urine and to a lesser extent into the gastrointestinal tract and other secretions (Heymsfield et al 1983). The main concept behind this method is that daily urinary creatinine output is directly proportional to total body skeletal muscle mass. This relation can be expressed mathematically as:

$$SM = k \times Cr$$

where k is a constant ratio referred to as the creatinine equivalence. Many classic studies have attempted to estimate the creatinine equivalence, with k ranging from 16.2 to 17.9 kg/g on ad libitum diets and from 18.6 to 20 kg/g on meat-free diets (Burger 1919, Picou et al 1976, Talbot 1938, Graystone 1968, Kriesberg et al 1970). The variation in k values might be attributed to dietary factors such as exogenous sources of creatine and differing skeletal muscle measurement methods.

The traditional model is not supported by recent experimental observations as the creatinine equivalence is not constant, but varies as a function of skeletal muscle mass (Heymsfield et al 1983). Afting et al (1981) reported that in a paralysed patient with no detectable skeletal muscle, urinary creatinine was still excreted. Non-skeletal muscle sources of creatinine include smooth muscles, brain and other organs. A revised descriptive mathematical function can be expressed as:

$$SM = b \times Cr + a$$

where b is the slope and a is the intercept for the experimentally determined SM-creatinine regression line. Our group studied 12 healthy men on a 7-day meat-free diet (Wang et al 1996). Complete 24-h urine was collected on the last three experimental days and results were averaged. There was a strong correlation between average daily urinary creatinine output and skeletal muscle measured by CT:

$$SM \ (kg) = 18.9 \times Cr + 4.1$$

with $R^2 = 0.85$, SEE = 1.89 kg and $p = 2.55 \times 10^{-5}$. To further explore the validity of this equation in a general population, another 14 subjects were added to develop a new SM prediction equation (Fig. 39.3):

$$SM \ (kg) = 19.4 \times Cr + 2.9$$

with $R^2 = 0.89$. The 26 subjects include 14 men and 12 women, and reference methods for skeletal muscle measurement included CT (n = 12), MRI (n = 11), and DEXA (n = 3). The mean age of the group was 47 ± 22 years with a range of 20–84 years. The lack of a zero intercept for the regression line of both skeletal muscle equations indicates a non-constant ratio of urinary creatinine to skeletal muscle mass.

Despite the strong correlation between urinary creatinine and total body skeletal muscle mass, two factors limit the practical use of the urinary creatinine method. First, subjects should ideally consume a meat-free diet for 7 days in order to eliminate exogenous sources of creatine and creatinine. Second, carefully timed urine collections are needed for accurate estimation of muscle mass.

Urinary 3-methylhistidine excretion

The endogenous excretion of 3-methylhistidine (3-MH) has been proposed as a measure of muscle

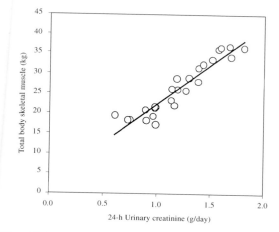

Figure 39.3 — Total body skeletal muscle mass by criterion methods vs 24-h urinary creatinine excretion in subjects ingesting a meat-free diet for one week.

protein breakdown (Young and Munro 1978) and as an index of total body skeletal muscle mass (Lukoski et al 1981). 3-MH is located primarily in skeletal muscle with intermediate concentrations in cardiac and smooth muscle tissues and trace amounts in organs (Elia 1979). The majority of 3-MH is produced by the two muscle-proteins: actin, which is found in all muscle fibres, and myosin, which is found only in white fibres. Studies have shown that the catabolism of actomyosin, the primary skeletal muscle contractile protein, releases 3-MH into the extracellular fluid space and 3-MH is then excreted in urine (Long et al 1975, Long et al 1977, Young et al 1970).

The main concept of this method is that urinary 3-MH is related to the total endogenous skeletal muscle protein pool and hence total skeletal muscle mass. There are relatively few studies in the literature that examine the relationship between endogenous 3-MH and skeletal muscle (Heymsfield In Press). Using the Burkinshaw–Cohn neutron activation model as the reference, Lukaski et al (1981) were the first to propose a skeletal muscle prediction equation from 3-MH,

$$SM \ (kg) = 0.118 \times 3\text{-MH} - 3.45$$

with $R^2 = 0.83$, $p < 0.01$, and SEE = 2.07 kg.

More recently, our group examined 10 healthy adult men on a meat-free diet protocol for 7 days (Wang et al 1998). 3-MH was collected over the last 3 days as consecutive 24-h urine collection. A strong correlation was observed between average daily urinary 3-MH excretion and total body skeletal muscle assessed by CT.

$$SM(kg) = 0.0887 \times 3\text{-MH} + 11.8$$

With $R^2 = 0.77$, $p < 0.001$, and SEE = 2.3 kg. An examination of the two prediction equations based on 3-MH reveals significant intercept differences (−10.2 kg). A possible source of error in the Lukaski model might be the lack of accuracy of the Burkinshaw–Cohn neutron activation model in measuring total body skeletal muscle.

The use of 3-MH as an index of skeletal muscle mass has been hampered by several problems. First, skeletal muscle sources account only for ~75% of the excreted 3-MH (Afting et al 1981). Second, a meat free diet and timed urine collections are essential to estimate 3-MH accurately.

The main features of urinary metabolite methods, including creatinine and 3-MH, are summarized in Table 39.5.

Table 39.5—Main characteristics of urinary metabolite methods

	Method	
	Creatinine	**3-Methylhistidine**
Model	creatinine = $k \times$ [Cr] x SM SM = creatinine ($k \times$ [Cr])	3-MH = $k \times$ [protein] $\times$ SM SM = 3-MH/($k \times$ [protein])
Assumptions Skeletal muscle (SM)	Creatine is almost all within skeletal muscle	Histidine is in two muscle proteins, actin within all muscle fibres and myosin in white fibres.
Creatinine [Cr] and protein [protein]	On a meat-free diet the average concentrations of creatine remains constant; and the total creatine pool remains constant.	On a meat-free diet the average protein concentration in muscle remains constant; and the total muscle protein pool remains constant
Creatinine or muscle protein daily fractional breakdown rate (k)	Creatine is converted to creatinine at a constant daily rate	Muscle protein synthesis and catabolism are in balance and thus 3-MH is produced at a constant daily rate
Urinary creatinine or 3-MH	Creatinine is neither metabolized nor reused in metabolism and completely excreted in urine	3-MH is neither metabolized nor reused in metabolism and completely excreted in urine
Prediction equation	SM = 19.4 $\times$ creatinine + 2.9; $R^2 = 0.89$, $p<0.01$	SM = 0.087 $\times$ 3-MH + 11.8; $R^2 = 0.77$, $p<0.001$

Adapted with permission from Gallagher et al 1997.

Conclusion

Unlike only one decade ago, those interested in quantifying regional and whole body skeletal muscle mass in humans have a wide range of available measurements at their disposal (Table 39.6). Cost, availability, practicality, desired accuracy, and other factors dictate the appropriate choice among these methods (Table 39.7). New insights should be possible when measured skeletal muscle mass, using these methods is combined with other descriptions of muscle biochemical and mechanical function.

Table 39.6—Methods of measuring skeletal muscle mass in vivo

Method	Level	Measures	Whole body	Regional
TBK-TBN	Atomic	ATFSM, SMPro	+	−
ASM by DEXA	Molecular	FFASM	−	+
Creatinine	Cellular	SMCM	+	−
3-MH	Cellular	SMCM	+	−
CT	Tissue-System	Anatomic SM, ATFSM	+	+
MRI	Tissue-System	Anatomic SM, ATFSM	+	+
Anthropometry	Whole body	Anatomic SM	+	+
Ultrasound	Whole body	Anatomic SM	−	+
BIA	Whole body	FFSM	−	+

ASM, appendicular skeletal muscle; ATFSM, adipose tissue-free skeletal muscle; BIA, bioimpedance analyis; Creatinine, 24-hr urinary creatinine excretion; CT, computerized axial tomography; DEXA, dual-energy X-ray absorptiometry; FFSM, fat-free skeletal muscle; 3-MH, 24-hr urinary 3-methylhistidine excretion; MRI, magnetic resonance imaging; SM, total body skeletal muscle; SMCM, skeletal muscle cell mass; SMPro, skeletal muscle protein; TBK, total body potassium; TBN, total body nitrogen. Reprinted with permission from Gallagher et al 1997.

Table 39.7 — Skeletal muscle measurement methods

Technique	Measured quantity	Advantages	Disadvantages
Anthropometry	Skinfolds Circumferences	Non-invasive Applicable to large samples	Poor precision in obese subjects
Ultrasound	Reflected echoes	Cross-sectional images possible	Prone to large measurement error
BIA	Resistance Reactance	Apparatus inexpensive Estimates regional skeletal muscle mass	Population-specific prediction formulas
Creatinine	24-h urinary creatinine	Non-hazardous Inexpensive	Meat-free diet desirable Urine collection accuracy critical Day-to-day variation large
3-Methylhistidine	24-h urinary 3-Methylhistidine	Non-hazardous Inexpensive	Meat-free desirable Urine collection accuracy critical Day-to-day variation large Inaccurate in catabolic states
DEXA	Relative attenuation of two X-ray energies	Estimates appendicular skeletal muscle	Small radiation exposure
MRI	Cross-sectional area measured	Direct visualization of skeletal muscle tissue	Apparatus expensive High cost
CT	Cross-sectional area measured	Direct visualization of skeletal muscle tissue	Apparatus expensive High cost Radiation exposure
Whole body counting/IVNA	Total body nitrogen Total body potassium	Measures cellular muscle component	Apparatus expensive Radiation exposure Model underestimates muscle

BIA, bioimpedance analysis; DEXA, dual X-ray absorptiometry; MRI, magnetic resonance imaging; CT, computerized axial tomography; FFM, fat-free body mass; IVNA, in vivo neutron activation analysis.

References

Afting EG, Bernhard W, Janzen WC, Röthing H-J. (1981) Quantitative importance of non-skeletal muscle N$^\tau$-methylhistidine and creatine in human urine. *Biochem J* 200: 449–452.

Baumgartner RN, Chumlea WC, Roche AG. (1989) Estimation of body composition from bioelectric impedance of body segments. *Am J Clin Nutr* 50: 221–226.

Baumgartner RN, Rhyne RL, Garry PJ, Heymsfield SB. (1993) Imaging techniques and anatomical body composition in aging. *J Nutr* 123: 444–448.

Baumgartner RN, Ross R, Heymsfield SB, et al. Cross-validation of DEXA versus MRI methods of quantifying appendicular skeletal muscle. *Applied Radiat Isot*. In Press.

Beneke R, Neuerberg J, Bohndorf K. (1991) Muscle cross-section measurements by magnetic resonance imaging. *Eur J Appl Physiol* 63: 424–429.

Borsook H, Dubnoff JW. (1947) The hydrolysis of phosphocreatine and the origin of urinary creatine. *J Bio Chem* 168: 493–510.

Burger MZ. (1919) Beiträge zum Kreatininstoffwechsel: I. The meaning of creatinine coefficient for the quantitative measurement of muscle mass and body composition. II. Creatine and creatinine excretion: relationship to muscle mass. *Z Gesamte Exp Med* 9: 361–399.

Burkinshaw L, Hill GL, Morgan DB. (1978) Assessment of the distribution of protein in the human body by in-vivo neutron analysis. In: *International Symposium on Nuclear Activation Techniques in the Life Sciences*. International Atomic Energy Association.

Burkinshaw L. (1987) Models of distribution of protein in the human body. In: Ellis KJ, Yasumura S, Morgan WD, eds. *In vivo body composition studies*. London: Institute of Physical Sciences in Medicine, pp. 15–24.

Cameron JR, Sorenson J. (1963) Measurement of bone mineral in vivo. *Science* 42: 230–232.

Chumlea WC, Guo SS. (1994) Bioelectrical impedance and

body composition: present status and future directions. *Nutr Rev* 52: 123–131.

Clarys JP, Martin AD, Drinkwater DT. (1984) Gross tissue weights in the human body by cadaver dissection. *Hum Bio* 56: 459–473.

Cohn SH, Vartsky D, Yasumura S, et al. (1980) Compartmental body composition based on total-body nitrogen, potassium, and calcium. *Am J Physiol* 39: E524–530.

Cohn SH, Gartenhaus W, Sawitsky A, et al. (1980) Compartmental body composition of cancer patients by measurement of total body nitrogen, potassium and water. *Metabolism* 30: 222–229.

Doupe MB, Martin AD, Searle MS, Kriellaars DJ, Giesbrecht GG. (1997) A new formula for population-based estimation of whole body muscle mass in males. *Can J Appl Physiol* 22: 598–608.

Elia M, Carter A, Smith R. (1979) The 3-methylhistidine content of human tissues. *Br J Nutr* 42: 567–570.

Engstrom CM, Loeb GE, Reid JG, Forrest WJ, Avruch L. (1991) Morphometry of the human thigh muscles: A comparison between anatomical sections and computer tomographic and magnetic resonance images. *J Anat* 176: 139–156.

Forbes GB, Brown MR, Griffiths HJL. (1988) Arm muscle plus bone area: anthropometry and CAT scan compared. *Am J Clin Nutr* 47: 929–931.

Foster MA, Hutchison JMS, Mallard JR, Fuller M. (1984) Nuclear magnetic resonance pulse sequence and discrimination of high- and low-fat tissues. *Mag Res Imaging* 2: 187–192.

Fried AM, Coughlin K, Griffen WO. (1986) The sonographic fat/muscle ratio. *Investigative Radiol* 21: 71–75.

Gallagher D, Visser M, De Meersman RE, et al. (1997) Appendicular skeletal muscle mass: effects of age, gender and ethnicity. *J Appl Physiol* 82 (1): 229–239.

Gallagher D, Heymsfield SB, Wang ZM. (1999) Skeletal muscle. In: The Role of Protein and Amino Acids in Sustaining and Enhancing Performance. Washington, DC: National Academy Press, pp 255–277.

Graystone JE. (1968) Creatinine excretion during growth. In: Cheek DB, ed. *Human growth: body composition cell growth, energy and intelligence*. Philadelphia: Lea & Febinger 12; pp. 182–197.

Heymsfield SB, McManus C, Smith J, Stevens V, Nixon DW. (1982) Anthropometric measurement of muscle mass: revised equations for calculating bone-free arm muscle area. *Am J Clin Nutr* 36: 680–690.

Heymsfield SB, Arteaga C, McManus C, Smith J, Moffitt S. (1983) Measurement of muscle mass in humans: validity of the 24-hour urinary creatinine method. *Am J Clin Nutr* 37: 478–494.

Heymsfield SB, Smith R, Aulet M, et al. (1990) Appendicular skeletal muscle mass: measurement by dual-photon absorptiometry. *Am J Clin Nutr* 52(2): 214–218.

Heymsfield SB, Tighe A, Wang ZM. (1994) Nutritional assessment by anthropometric and biochemical methods. In: Shils ME, Olson JA, Shike M, eds. *Modern nutrition in health and disease. 8th ed*. Philadelphia: Lea & Febiger, pp. 812–841.

Heymsfield SB, Ross R, Wang ZM, Frager D. (1997) Imaging techniques of body composition: Advantages of measurement and new uses. In: *Emerging Technologies for Nutrition Research*. Sydne J, Carlson-Newberry & Rebecca B, Costello, eds. Washington, DC: National Academy Press, pp. 127–150.

Heymsfield SB, Gallagher D, Grammes J, Nunez C, Wang Z, Pietrobelli A. (1998) Upper extremity skeletal muscle mass: potential of measurement with single frequency bioimpedance analysis. *Appl Radiat Isot* 49: 473–474.

Heymsfield SB, Gallagher D, Visser M, Nunez C, Wang ZM. Measurement of skeletal muscle: laboratory and epidemiological methods. *J Gerontol*. In Press.

Hounsfield GN. (1973) Computerized transverse axial scanning (tomography). *Br J Radiol* 46: 1016.

International Atomic Energy Agency. (1970) Directory of whole-body radioactivity monitors, IAEA STI/PUB/213. Vienna: Author.

Ishida V, Carroll ML, Pollock JE, et al. (1992) Reliability of B-mode ultrasound for the measurement of body fat thickness. *Am J Hum Biol* 4: 511–520.

Janssens V, Thys P, Clarys JP, et al. (1994) Post-mortem limitations of body composition analysis by computed tomography. *Ergonomics* 37: 207–216.

Kohrt W. (1995) Body composition by DEXA: tried and true? *Med Sci Sports Exerc* 27: 1349–1353.

Kriesberg RA, Bowdoin B, Meador CK. (1970) Measurement of muscle mass in humans by isotopic dilution of creatine – ^{14}C. *J Appl Physiol* 28: 264–267.

Long CL, Haverbergf LN, Young VR, et al. (1975) Metabolism of 3-methylhistidine in man. *Metabolism* 24: 929–935.

Long CL, Schiller WR, Blakemore WS, et al. (1977) Muscle protein catabolism in the septic patient as measured by 3-methylhistidine excretion. *Am J Clin Nutr* 30: 1349–1352.

Lukaski HC, Mendez J, Buskirk ER, Cohn SH. (1981) Relationship between endogenous 3-methylhistidine excretion and body composition. *Am J Physiol* 240: E302.

Lukaski HC. (1993) Soft tissue composition and bone mineral status: Evaluation by dual energy x-ray absorptiometry. *J Nutr* 123: 438–443.

Lukaski HC. (1996) Estimation of muscle mass. In: Roche

AF, Heymsfield SB, Lohman TG, eds. *Human Body Composition: Methods and Findings*. Champaign: Human Kinetics Publishers, pp. 109–129.

Martin AP, Spenst LF, Drinkwater DT, Clarys JP. (1990) Anthropometric estimation of muscle mass in men. *Med Sci Sports Exerc* 22: 729–733.

Matiegka J. (1921) The testing of physical efficiency. *Am J Phys Anthropol* 4: 223–330.

Mitsiopoulos N, Baumgartner RN, Heymsfield SB, Lyons W, Ross R. (1998) Cadaver validation of skeletal muscle measurement by magnetic resonance imaging and computerized tomography. *J Appl Physiol* 85: 115–122.

Nunez C, Grammes J, Gallagher D, Baumgartner RN, Wang Z, Heymsfield SB. (1996) Appendicular skeletal muscle: estimation by total limb impedance measured with new electrode system. *FASEB J* 10: 3.

Nunez C, Gallagher D, Grammes J. (1999) Bioimpedance analysis: potential for measuring lower limb skeletal muscle mass. *J Parental Enteral Nutr* 32: 96–103.

Picou D, Reeds PJ, Jackson A, Poulter N. (1976) The measurement of muscle mass in children using creatine $-^{15}$N. *Pediatr Res* 10: 184–188.

Pietrobelli A, Formica C, Wang ZM, Heymsfield SB. (1996) Dual energy x-ray absorptiometry body composition model review of physical concepts. *Am J Physiol* 271: E941–E951.

Pietrobelli A, Gallagher D, Baumgartner RN, Ross R, Heymsfield SB, Lean R. (1998) Value for DEXA two-component soft-tissue model: Influence of age and tissue or organ type. *Appl Radiat Isot* 49: 743–744.

Ross R. (1996) Magnetic resonance imaging provides new insight into the characterization of adipose and lean tissue distribution. *Can J Clin Pharmacol* 74: 778–785.

Sipila S, Suominen H. (1991) Ultrasound imaging of the quadriceps muscle in elderly athletes and untrained men. *Muscle Nerve* 14: 527–533.

Sjöström L. (1991) A computer-tomography based multi-component body composition technique and anthropometric predictions of lean body mass, total and subcutaneous adipose tissue. *Int J Obes* 15: 19–30.

Snyder WS, Cook MJ, Nasset ES, Karhausen LR, Howells GP, Tipton IH. (1975) Report of the task group on reference man. Oxford: International Commission on Radiological Protection.

Stokes M, Young A. (1986) Measurement of quadriceps cross-sectional area by ultrasonography: A description of the technique and its application in physiotherapy. *Physiotherapy Practice* 2: 31–36.

Talbot NB. (1938) Measurement of obesity by the creatinine coefficient. *Am J Dis Child* 55: 42–50.

Vartsky D, Ellis KJ, Vaswani AN, et al. (1984) An improved calibration for the in vivo determination of body nitrogen, hydrogen and fat. *Phys Med Biol* 29: 209–218.

Wang ZM, Pierson RN, Jr, Heymsfield SB. (1992) The five level model: a new approach to organizing body composition research. *Am J Clin Nutr* 56: 19–28.

Wang ZM, Visser M, Gallagher D, Kotler D, Heymsfield SB. (1996) *In vivo* measurement of skeletal muscle mass by CT: comparison to skeletal muscle mass estimates by neutron activation and DEXA methods. *J Appl Physiol* 80(3): 824–831.

Wang ZM, Gallagher D, Nelson M, Matthews D, Heymsfield SB. (1996) Urinary 3-methylhistidine excretion: association with total body skeletal muscle mass by computerized axial tomography. *J Parenteral Enteral Nutr* 22: 82–86.

Young VR, Baliga BS, Alexis SD, Munro HN. (1970) Lack of in vivo binding of 3-methylhistidine to transfer RNA by aminoacyl ligases from skeletal muscle. *Biochim Biophys Acta* 199: 297–300.

Young VR, Munro HM. (1978) Nτ-methylhistidine (3-methylhistidine) and muscle protein turnover: An overview. *Fed Proc* 37: 2291–2300.

40

Assessment of muscle function by isometric tests

Greg Wilson

Strength

Isometric tests are commonly used laboratory test to assess strength. Indeed strength is often defined as the force or torque (force multiplied by perpendicular distance to the axis of rotation) generated during a maximal isometric contraction (Atha 1981, Enoka 1994). Perhaps the main reason for the isometric maximum force being a common strength test is due to the fact that the force developed in a concentric contraction is substantially lower than the isometric maximum. More recently, however, it has been observed that greater forces can be recorded during eccentric contractions, however, the traditional standard has tended to be maintained.

Isometric tests are performed against an immovable resistance, which is in series with a strain gauge, cable tensiometer, force platform or similar device whose transducer measures the applied force as a change in voltage. The voltage change is subsequently passed through an analogue to digital converter and recorded as an applied force by a computer or similar device. As with any maximal test, subjects are adequately warmed up prior to performance and are required to give maximal effort over a 3–4 s period.

Research by Viitasalo (1982) has revealed that if, prior to maximum exertion, the muscle is pre-tensed then the maximum force is reduced by approximately 4% compared with a value of zero pre-tension. Hence tests are generally contact from a rested state.

Reliability of the test

Maximal isometric force tests have particularly high test–retest reliability (Viitasalo et al 1980, Bemben et al 1992). Bemben et al (1992) reported that test reliability was greatest when several practice tests were provided prior to data collection and when the data were collected over two days and the values averaged. Christ et al (1994) reported the reliability of maximum isometric force tests for a variety of muscle groups using a testing protocol that involved testing over 3 days and using three trials per day. These researchers reported widely varying values of reliability depending on the muscle group assessed. For example the reliability of the plantar flexors was $r = 0.94$, while for the dorsi flexors the intra-class correlation was 0.55. On the basis of their results the researchers concluded that "Typically more measures (e.g., days, trials) result in greater criterion score reliability, barring the influence of boredom or fatigue" (Christ et al 1994, p. 69). Hortobagyi and Lambert (1992) assessed the reliability of maximum isometric strength of the arm flexors. Two trails of the test were taken over 4 days, interspersed with 3–5 days of no testing. The mean ± SE for each of the four repeat testing occasions were 355 ± 18.9 N, 354 ± 22.9 N, 353 ± 20.4 N and 364 ± 20.8 N.

Limitations of the test

One limitation of the isometric test is that it records the maximal force at only one joint angle and the results gained from this joint angle, are not representative of the strength of the muscle at other positions. Therefore, if information is required regarding force over a range of motion, the test will need to be repeated over a number of positions throughout the range.

Due to the specificity of strength, which implies that individuals can be strong in some muscles but not in others, or even strong in particular ranges of motion but not others, it is important to perform strength tests in positions that are similar to the performance of interest. Indeed, the more specific the test, the more meaningful will be the result.

Relationship to performance

Maximal isometric strength has been observed to be an important predictor of performance in a variety of sports including throwing velocity in water-polo (Bloomfield et al 1990), rowing performance (Secher 1975) and sprinting velocity (Mero et al 1981). In contrast, Considine and Sullivan (1973) reported a low relationship between isometric strength of the knee extensors and vertical jump performance ($r = 0.35$).

Power

An isometric test developed to assess power has been formulated and it is becoming increasingly popular. The test is termed the maximum rate of isometric force development (RFD). In essence, the test aims to quantify the maximum rate at which an individual can develop force in an isometric muscular action. Individuals are required to develop force as quickly, and with as much intensity, as possible against an immovable object, similar to the maximal isometric test. As such the shape of the force–time curve has been thought to describe the intensity of motor unit recruitment and firing during the rapid increasing phase of voluntary contractions (Viitasalo 1982).

Three isometric force–time curves are depicted in Figure 40.1. These theoretical curves represent the force-generating capacity of differing individuals when performing a maximal contraction. Curve 1 represents the force–time characteristics of an individual who is very strong but not particularly powerful, for example a powerlifter. These individuals would be effective in performing strength movements, such as a squat or bench press lift, but less effective in a power event like a high jump or shot put, as they are unable to produce high force levels quickly. Curve 2 represents an individual who has less absolute strength than the individual in Curve 1, however, this individual is able to generate a greater force over a brief period (i.e. 100 ms). Although not capable of lifting as much weight as the strength athlete, this individual may outperform the strength athlete in a dynamic power event such as a high jump. Indeed Hakkinen et al (1984) reported that elite wrestlers develop force more rapidly than elite powerlifters. Curve 3 represents an individual who can produce the available force very rapidly but does not have a high strength level. Consequently this individual is ineffective in both strength and power dominated events.

Rationale of the test

The RFD test is seen to be a particularly important factor in many sports, as the time available for the exertion of force is very limited. For example, in sprinting the ground contact time is typically 80–100 ms. Similarly, during the jumping events, such as high and long jump, the ground contact time is in the order of only 150 ms. Consequently, the ability to rapidly generate force would seem to be of obvious importance.

Quantification of the test

The RFD is quantified in a variety of forms. The most popular is the maximal rate of force development, which is the greatest slope in the RFD curve. This is the maximal change in force over a previously specified period of time. Time periods used have varied from 5 ms (Wilson et al 1993) through to 60 ms (Christ et al 1994). Other methods include determining the time taken to a certain level of absolute force, such as 500 N, or the time taken to a relative force level, such as 30% of maximum force (Viitasalo et al 1980, Hakkinen et al 1985a,b). The latter test is useful if one wishes to study the ability to rapidly develop the available force independent of the level of strength. Alternatively the force or impulse value in a specified time, such as 100 ms, has also been used to quantify speed strength using an isometric test (Baker et al 1994, Wilson et al 1995). These various methods of quantification are outlined in Figure 40.2.

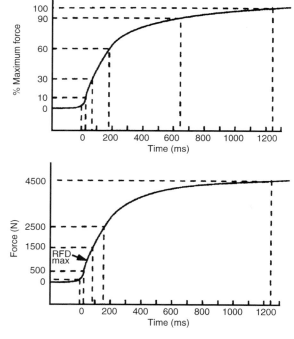

Figure 40.2—Quantification of the isometric force–time curve. Note that several methods are used including calculation of the maximum rate of force development (RFD) and the time taken to achieve an absolute or relative level of force (adapted from Sale 1991).

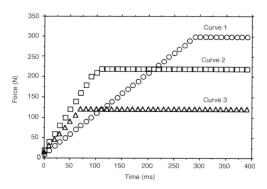

Figure 40.1—Hypothetical force-time curves for individuals of differing strength and power capacities.

Effects of pre-tension

Viitasalo (1982) examined the effect of pre-tension on the maximal isometric force and RFD. This researcher examined pretension levels of 20, 30, 40, 50, 60 and 70% of maximum and reported that maximum RFD decreased dramatically as a function of the pre-tension levels. In fact with a pre-tension level of 20% the maximum RFD decreased from 7338 ± 2938 Ns^{-1} to 4257 ± 944 Ns^{-1}, at 30% of maximum pre-tension the maximum RFD has decreased by half and at 70% maximum pre-tension the maximum RFD was only 21.8% of the value at zero pre-tension. However, the correlations between the various levels of pre-tension were not reported, nor were relationships between performance measures and the RFD values examined. Therefore, the best level of pre-tension to use in RFD tests for muscular assessment is unclear. Given that RFD varies quite dramatically as a function of pre-tension, it may be best to use a level of pre-tension that is similar to the performance of interest. It is quite apparent that RFD will diminish as a function of the initial level of force and, as such, maximum RFD will be achieved when minimum levels of pre-tension are present.

Effect of fatigue

Hakkinen and Myllyla (1990) examined the effect of fatigue on the maximum isometric force and RFD. Comparing endurance, strength and power athletes these researchers reported that the performance of an isometric contraction at a 60% of maximum load for as long as possible significantly reduced the maximum force (from 92.9 to 64.3%) and RFD (from 79.2 to 56.7%). The extent of the decrement in isometric force production varied between the athletes such that the endurance athletes experienced the smallest decrement in both maximum force ($92.9 \pm 7.1\%$) and RFD ($79.2 \pm 20.8\%$), compared with the strength (maximum $65.7 \pm 7.0\%$; RFD, $56.7 \pm 16.0\%$) and power athletes (maximum, $64.3 \pm 8.0\%$; RFD, $74.8 \pm 7.4\%$).

Modification of the rate of force development with training

Hakkinen et al (1985a) reported that while heavy weight training increased maximal isometric force, it did not alter the RFD. However, in a follow-up study Hakkinen et al (1985b) reported that explosive resistance training, in the form of plyometrics, resulted in a smaller increase in maximal isometric force but a greater increase in the maximal rate of force development.

Reliability of the test

The RFD has been shown to be a reliable test (Viitasalo et al 1980, Bemben et al 1992, Christ et al 1994). This reliability is seen in the high correlations achieved when comparing the test results recorded on the same subjects on differing testing occasions. For example, Bemben et al (1992) reported correlations between the maximal RFD, on differing days for a variety of muscles, between 0.92 and 0.98. Christ et al (1994) using a testing protocol involving three testing days with three trials per day reported correlations between the RFD for six muscle groups that varied between 0.83 and 0.94.

Validity of the test

The relationship between the RFD and athletic performance has received various values from differing researchers. Mero et al (1981) did not observe a relationship between maximal isometric RFD and running speed, and they found similar rate of force development values for runners of differing ability. Similarly Wilson et al (1995) reported that the maximal isometric RFD did not appear to be a useful predictor of performance in running or cycling. However, Viitasalo and Aura (1984) reported a strong relationship between the average values of isometric RFD for the quadriceps muscle group and high jumping performance for eight nationally ranked high jumpers. Further, Hakkinen and Myllyla (1990) reported that isometric RFD could distinguish between differing types of athletes. For example, the maximum RFD recorded by power athletes, of $48\,096 \pm 6670$ Ns^{-1}, was significantly higher than the $30\,656 \pm 7998$ Ns^{-1} recorded by endurance athletes. However, these researchers also reported that untrained control subjects recorded maximal RFD values that were greater than strength athletes.

If one examines the force profiles and associated muscular activity of most competitive events, such as running, jumping and so on, it is apparent that force is developed during the eccentric phase of these activities and that during the concentric phase of the movement the force decreases because of the force–velocity relationship of muscle (Fig. 40.3). Consequently, the ability to rapidly develop force during an isometric or concentric contraction does not appear to be a

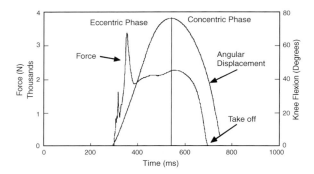

Figure 40.3 — Force- and angle-time curve from the performance of a 40 cm drop jump by an experienced subject (courtesy Wilson et al 1996).

relevant requirement of most sports that involve a dynamic eccentric contraction, as the force is develop during the eccentric phase. Therefore, the validity of the isometric rate of force development test is currently questionable.

Underlying mechanisms for poor validity of isometric tests

Wilson and Murphy (1996) performed a detailed review of the use of isometric tests for the purpose of athletic assessment. On the basis of their review they concluded that: "Because of the large neural and mechanical differences between isometric and dynamic muscular actions, athletic assessment, which is dynamic in nature, is generally most appropriately accomplished using dynamic muscular assessment methods, and in most instances isometric testing should be avoided" (Wilson and Murphy 1996a, p. 20).

There appear to be some fundamental limitations with static testing of the musculature that conceptually would effect the validity and usefulness of such tests, particularly as they relate to dynamic movements. One of the major limitations of isometric testing is that it is not specific to the performance of most human activities because force is only measured statically at one point, and one can not assume that there is a strong relationship between values obtained at differing joint angles in a given movement range. That is, there is no research to suggest that any one point in the range of movement is representative of the entire movement. Indeed research by Murphy et al (1995) examined the effect of joint angle on isometric assess-

ment using bench press tests conducted at elbow angles of 90° and 120°. These authors reported that the correlations between the two angles of both maximum force and RFD were below 0.7, indicating that over 50% of the variance was not common between the various joint angles.

The rationale as to why isometric tests of muscular function appear to be poorly related to dynamic performance appears to be primarily based on the neural and mechanical differences between isometric and dynamic contractions.

Neural

As early as 1960, researchers began to suspect that differences in the force output between static and dynamic contractions may be neuromuscular in origin. For example, Henry and Whitley (1960) reported no correlation's between the force developed in a static movement of the arm compared with a dynamic one. The authors rationalized these results, suggesting that relatively distinct neuromuscular patterns were probably responsible for dynamic and static muscular contractions even though no electromyography (EMG) results were collected. More recently, research has demonstrated distinct differences in activation patterns between isometric and dynamic contractions at the same joint angle (Tax et al 1990, Nakazawa et al 1993). Indeed, Murphy and Wilson (1996), using spectral analysis, have reported significant differences in both the firing characteristics of the motor units and the level of activity of the musculature, between an isometric test and dynamic performance.

In fact, differences in motor unit recruitment have been shown to occur within isometric tasks with changes in the direction of force application or the performance of different tasks of the same muscle (Ter Haar Romeny et al 1982, 1984). A series of studies performed by Ter Haar Romeny et al (1982, 1984), using indwelling needle electrodes, have shown that differing motor units of the same muscle were recruited in isometric contractions depending on the direction of force application. The actual muscle fibres recruited in an activity were, at least in some instances, those which may have more favourable leverage positions for the desired task (Ter Haar Romeny et al 1982). For example, the medially located muscle fibres of the arm flexors were recruited for supination tasks, while the lateral fibres were preferentially recruited for flexion movements.

Further, and being particularly relevant to multi-joint tests, researchers have shown that the relationship between the activation level of synergistic muscle groups varies as a function of joint angle (Hasan and Enoka 1985, Howard et al 1986). In addition, van Zuylen et al (1988) reported results that showed that the activation of muscles varied depending on the mechanical advantage of the muscle during an isometric contraction, such that the muscle with the greater mechanical advantage received the higher neural input. This is particularly relevant because isometric assessment is typically performed at only one arbitrary point in the movement range, and this may not be representative of other points in the movement (Murphy et al 1995).

Consequently, research has demonstrated substantial neural differences between dynamic and isometric contractions, and within isometric contractions under different conditions. Such differences may at least partially account for the poor relationship between isometric assessment and dynamic performance, and they may account for the apparent superiority of the dynamic tests of muscular function compared with isometric tests (Murphy et al 1994, Pryor et al 1994, Wilson et al 1995, Wilson and Murphy 1995). As stated by Wilson and Murphy (1995): "...isokinetic and vertical jump tests may be superior to the isometric tests as they are dynamic in nature and thus would invoke a neural response that was essentially similar to the dynamic performance of interest" (Wilson and Murphy 1995, p. 22).

Mechanical

As well as neural differences, there are also large mechanical differences between isometric and dynamic muscular actions. Dynamic performances that involve stretch shorten cycle actions involve the use of substantial quantities of elastic strain energy (Komi and Bosco 1978, Wilson et al 1991). However, because of the lack of a stretch shorten cycle action, isometric contractions do not benefit to the same degree from the use of elastic strain energy. Further, the maximum force and particularly the RFD produced in isometric tests are heavily dependant on the stiffness of the musculotendinous system. Wilson et al (1994) reported significant correlations between musculotendinous stiffness, quantified using a free oscillation technique, and isometric RFD ($r = 0.72$) and maximum force ($r = 0.63$). However, musculotendinous stiffness was not significantly related to eccentric force production ($r = 0.15$ to 0.27) nor maximum concentric force ($r = 0.38$).

During an isometric contraction the contractile component will contract as the musculotendinous unit

extends. The extent and the rate of contractile component shortening will be proportional to the magnitude of the muscular contraction and the stiffness of the musculotendinous unit. Conceptually a stiffer musculotendinous unit would enhance isometric force production, compared with a more compliant system, because of a reduced contractile component shortening velocity and a relatively longer length of the contractile component throughout the contraction. Further, the musculotendinous unit represents the link between the skeletal system and the contractile component of the muscles (see Fig. 40.4), and as such its stiffness will, to some extent, determine how effectively and rapidly internal forces generated by the contractile component are transmitted through to the skeletal system.

The above mechanisms underlying the relationship between musculotendinous stiffness and performance should operate in both isometric and concentric conditions; however, they will have a greater influence on isometric force production. During the concentric activity the contractile component is shortening dominantly due to the actual movement. In contrast, during an isometric activity, the shortening of the contractile component occurs dominantly due to the extension of the musculotendinous unit. Consequently, while a stiffer musculotendinous unit may serve to reduce the overall length and rate of contractile component shortening, it is not surprising that its effects are more pronounced in isometric compared with concentric activities (Wilson et al 1994).

Consequently, analogous to the neural differences argument outlined above, substantial mechanical differences exist between isometric and dynamic muscular actions. Hence, dynamic tests of muscular function are superior to isometric tests in their relationship to performance, as performance is dynamic in nature and, therefore, involves muscular mechanics, which

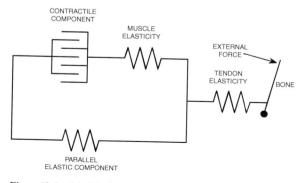

Figure 40.4 — Model of muscle.

are essentially similar to the dynamic muscular function tests that are used in their assessment.

Comparison between testing modalities

Although isometric, isoinertial and isokinetic testing modalities can be used to test the same muscular functions they often result in remarkably differing results. For example, in comparing volleyball players of differing ability Fry et al (1991) reported significant differences between the groups in a range of isoinertial strength measures. However, these differing subjects were not found to differ on a number of sport-specific isometric strength measures, nor on isokinetic strength assessed at 60°, 180° and 300°/s. Hurley et al (1988) compared the peak torque for both the quadriceps and hamstring muscle groups between a group of elite powerlifters and weight-matched untrained control subjects. Despite the powerlifters recording significantly greater isoinertial strength values, the control group recorded isokinetic peak torque values at 30°/s that were significantly greater for both muscle groups. The control group was subsequently trained for 4 months using a variety of isoinertial exercises, which resulted in a significant 40% increase in isoinertial strength; however, after the training period, isokinetic strength was unchanged. Wilson et al (1993) have reported significant changes in athletic performance and isoinertial tests of power as a consequence of resistance training, but no change was apparent in the isometric rate of force development.

Sleivert et al (1995) reported the changes in muscular function associated with performing variable resistance weight training. The training resulted in large increases in weight lifted in the training exercises (43%), significant changes in muscular hypertrophy (13%) and nerve conduction velocity. However, there was little change reported in isometric and isokinetic muscular function. Similar results have also been reported by Sale et al (1992) who reported significant increases in muscle hypertrophy (11%) and weight lifting performance (29%) as a consequence of weight training. However, the training had no effect on muscular function assessed in an isometric testing modality.

Specificity of testing

The above data highlight one of the most important factors in testing: the principle of specificity of testing.

This principle suggests that the testing of muscular function should be very specific to the method of training. When combined with the principle of specificity of training it implies that the training and the testing should be performed in a manner that is specific to each other and the competitive performance. Consequently, athletic performance and training in throwing events are perhaps best assessed by an isoinertial power test that involves throwing or jumping with a load (see Murphy et al 1994). Kicking skills are perhaps best assessed through isokinetic methods set at relatively high speeds.

One of the major problems in the development and use of various test items is that, generally, researchers assess the reliability of the tests, but often the validity of the tests is simply taken for granted and not subjected to the same scrutiny. Further, what the results of the tests actually tell us about functional performance is even less clear. For example, several researchers have assessed the reliability of the isometric rate of force development test and found it reasonably reliable (Viitasalo et al 1980, Bemben et al 1992). However, the validity of the test has been subject to varying reports (Mero et al 1981, Viitasalo and Aura 1984, Wilson et al 1993). Further, the ability to rapidly develop force in an isometric or concentric contraction appears to be of little relevance to the majority of dynamic activities, as the force is developed during the preparatory counter-movement or eccentric phase. Despite this, the isometric rate of force development test is widely used to give specific training recommendations to athletes! Exactly which performance factor this test is actually measuring is not particularly clear at this stage.

Similarly, the popular knee extension/flexion tests are widely used to assess the functional properties of the musculature of the thigh. While this test is well controlled and highly reliable, its lack of specificity to functional movements such as running, jumping and lifting tends to suggest that data from such tests would have very limited application to the real world. For example, we studied an isokinetic squat compared with an isokinetic knee extension; the squat test demonstrated a superior relationship to functional performance compared with the knee extension tests, as well as a greater capacity to discriminate between athletes of differing levels of performance (Wilson et al 1997).

Indeed even in rehabilitation one would have to wonder how functional is the knee extension test? For example if the injured to non-injured knee extension ratio was 70:100% does this necessarily imply that a similar ratio would be applied in an upright closed kinetic chain test such as a squat or upright leg press? I have not seen any research on this topic, but, given the incredible degree of specificity inherent in training adaptations (Wilson et al 1996), I would seriously doubt it. Hence there is little doubt that more functionally specific tests need to be developed. While more research is required, it appears that isometric tests have limited application in functional muscular assessment and hence testing should be dynamic in nature (Wilson and Murphy 1995).

References

Atha J. (1981) Strengthening muscle. In: Miller DI, ed. *Exercise and Sport Science Reviews* Vol. 9, Philadelphia: Franklin Inst Press, pp. 1–73.

Baker D, Wilson G, Carlyon B. (1994) Generality versus specificity: A comparison of dynamic and isometric measures of strength and speed-strength. *Eur J App Physiol* 68(4): 350–355.

Bemben MG, Massey BH, Boileau RA, Misner JE. (1992) Reliability of isometric force-time curve parameters for men aged 20 to 79 years. *J Appl Sport Sci Res* 6(3): 158–164.

Bloomfield J, Blanksby BA, Ackland TR, Allison GT. (1990) The influence of strength training on overhead throwing velocity of elite water polo players. *Austral J Sci Med Sport* 22: 63–67.

Bosco C, Cotelli F, Bonomi R, Mognoni P, Roi GS. (1994) Seasonal fluctuations of selected physiological characteristics of elite alpine skiers. *Eur J Appl Physiol* 69: 71–74.

Brown SL, Wilkinson JG. (1983) Characteristics of national, divisional, and club male alpine ski racers. *Med Sci Sport Exercise* 15(6): 491–495.

Christ CB, Slaughter MH, Stillman RJ, Cameron J, Boileau RA. (1994) Reliability of selected parameters of isometric muscle function associated with testing 3 days X 3 trials in women. *J Strength Conditioning Res* 8(2): 65–71.

Considine W, Sullivan W. (1973) Relationship of selected tests of leg strength and leg power on college men. *Res Quart* 44: 404–415.

Enoka R. (1994) Neurological basis of kinesiology. 2nd ed. Champaign: Human Kinetics.

Fry AC, Kraemer WJ. (1991) Physical performance characteristics of American football players. *J Appl Sport Sci Res* 5: 126–139.

Fry AC, Kraemer WJ, Weseman CA, et al. (1991) Effects of an off-season strength and conditioning program on starters and non-starters in women's collegiate volleyball. *J Appl Sport Sci Res* 5: 174–181.

Hakkinen K, Alen M, Komi PV. (1984) Neuromuscular, anaerobic and aerobic performance characteristics of elite power athletes. *Euro J App Physiol* 53: 97–105.

Hakkinen K, Alen M, Komi PV. (1985a) Electromyographic and muscle fibre characteristics of human skeletal muscle during strength training and detraining. *Acta Physiol Scand* 125: 573–585.

Hakkinen K, Komi PV, Alen M. (1985b) Effect of explosive type strength training on isometric force- and relaxation-time, electromyographic and muscle fibre characteristics of leg extensor muscles. *Acta Physiol Scand* 125: 587–600.

Hakkinen K, Komi PV, Alen M, Kauhanen H. (1987) EMG, muscle fibre and force production characteristics during a one year training period in elite weight-lifters. *Eur J Appl Physiol* 56: 419–427.

Hakkinen K, Myllyla E. (1990) Acute effects of muscle fatigue and recovery on force production and relaxation in endurance, power and strength athletes. *J Sports Med Phys Fitness* 30(1): 5–13.

Hasan Z, Enoka RM. (1985) Isometric torque - angle relationship and movement-related activity of human elbow flexors: implications of the equilibrium-point hypothesis. *Exp Brain Res* 59: 441–450.

Henry FM, Whitley JD. (1960) Relationships between individual differences in strength, speed, and mass of an arm movement. *Res Quart* 31: 24–33.

Hortobagyi T, Lambert NJ. (1992) Influence of electrical stimulation on dynamic forces of the arm flexors in strength-trained and untrained men. *Scand J Med Sci Sport* 2: 70–75.

Howard JD, Hoit JD, Enoka RM, Hasan Z. (1986) Relative activation of two human flexors under isometric conditions: a cautionary note concerning flexor equivalence. *Exp Brain Res* 62: 199–202.

Hurley JM, Hagberg JM, Holloszy BF. (1988) Muscle weakness among elite powerlifters. *Med Sci Sports Exercise* 20: S81.

Kannus P. (1994) Isokinetic evaluation of muscular performance: Implications for muscle testing and rehabilitation. *Int J Sports Med* 15: S11–S18.

Johnson J, Siegal D. (1978) Reliability for an isokinetic movement of the knee extensors. *Res Quart* 49: 88–90.

Komi PV, Bosco C. (1978) Utilization of stored elastic energy in leg extensor muscles by men and women. *Med Sci Sports* 10: 261–265.

Kraemer WJ, Fry AC. (1995) Strength testing: Development and evaluation of methodology. In: *Physiological Assessment of Human Fitness*. Maud PJ, Foster C, eds. Champaign: Human Kinetics, pp. 115–138.

LaFree J, Mozingo A, Worrell T. (1995) Comparison of open chain knee and hip extension to closed kinetic chain leg press performance. *J Sport Rehab* 4: 99–107.

Mero A, Luhtanen P, Viitasalo JT, Komi PV. (1981) Relationship between maximal running velocity, muscle fibre characteristics, force production and force relaxation of sprinters. *Scand J Sports Sci* 3: 16–22.

Murphy AJ, Wilson GJ. (1996) Poor correlations between isometric tests and dynamic performance: relation to muscle activation. *Eur J Appl Physiol* 73: 353–357.

Murphy AJ, Wilson GJ, Pryor JF. (1994) The use of the isoinertial force mass relationship in the prediction of dynamic human performance. *Eur J Appl Physiol* 69(3): 250–257.

Murphy AJ, Wilson GJ, Pryor JF, Newton RU. (1995) Isometric assessment of muscular function: The effect of joint angle. *J Appl Biomechanics* 11: 205–215.

Nakazawa K, Kawakami Y, Fukunaga T, Yano H, Miyashita M. (1993) Differences in activation patterns in elbow flexors during isometric, concentric and eccentric contractions. *Eur J Appl Physiol* 66: 214–220.

Osternig LR. (1986) Isokinetic dynamometry: Implications for muscle testing and rehabilitation. *Exercise Sport Sci Rev* 14: 45–80.

Osternig LR, Sawhill JA, Bates BT, Hamill J. (1982) A method for rapid collection and processing of isokinetic data. *Res Quart Exercise Sport* 53: 252–256.

Pryor JF, Wilson GJ, Murphy AJ. (1994) The effectiveness of eccentric, concentric and isometric rate of force development tests. *J Human Movement Studies* 27: 153–172.

Sale DG. (1991) Testing Strength and Power. In: MacDougall J, Wenger H, Green H, eds. *Physiological Testing of the High Performance Athlete* 2nd ed. Champaign: Human Kinetics, pp. 21–106.

Sale DG, Martin JE, Moroz DE. (1992) Hypertrophy without increased isometric strength after weight training. *Eur J Appl Physiol* 64: 51–55.

Schmidtbleicher D. (1992) Training for power events. In: *Strength and Power Training*. PV Komi ed. Blackwell Science, Oxford pp. 381–395.

Secher NH (1975) Isometric rowing strength of experienced and inexperienced oarsmen. *Med Sci Sports* 7: 280–283.

Sleivert GG, Backus RD, Wenger HA. (1995) The influence of a strength-sprint training sequence on multi-joint power output. *Med Sci Sports Exercise* 27: 1655–1665.

Tax AAM, Denier van der Gon JJ, Erkelens CJ. (1990) Differences in coordination of elbow flexor muscles in force tasks and in movement tasks. *Exp Brain Res* 81: 567–572.

Ter Haar Romeny B, Denier van der Gon J, Gielen C. (1982) Changes in recruitment order of motor units in the human biceps muscle. *Exp Neurol* 78: 360–368.

Ter Haar Romeny BM, Denier van der Gon JJ, Gielen CAM. (1984) Relationship between location of a motor unit in the human biceps brachia and its critical firing levels for different tasks. *Exp Neurol* 85: 631–650.

Van Zuylen EJ, Gielen CM, Denier van der Gon JJ. (1988) Coordination and inhomogeneous activation of human arm muscles during isometric torques. *J Neurophysiol* 60: 1523–1548.

Viitasalo JT. (1982) Effects of pretension on isometric force production. *Int J Sports Med* 3: 149–152.

Viitasalo JT, Aura O. (1984) Seasonal fluctuation of force production in high jumpers. *Can J Appl Sport Sci Res* 9: 209–213.

Viitasalo JT, Saukkonen S, Komi PV. (1980) Reproducibility of measurements of selected neuromuscular performance variables in man. *Electromyography Clin Neurophysiol* 20: 487–501.

Wilson GJ, Lyttle AD, Ostrowski KJ, Murphy, AJ (1995) Assessing dynamic performance: A comparison of rate of force development tests. *J Strength Conditioning Res* 9(3): 176–181.

Wilson GJ, Murphy AJ. (1995) The efficacy of isokinetic, isometric and vertical jump tests in exercise science. *Austral J Sci Med Sport* 27: 62–66.

Wilson GJ, Murphy AJ. (1996a) The Use of Isometric Tests of Muscular Function in Athletic Assessment. *Sport Med* 22(1): 19–37.

Wilson GJ, Murphy AJ. (1996b) Strength diagnosis: the use of test data to determine specific strength training. *J Sport Sci* 14: 167–173.

Wilson GJ, Murphy AJ, Pryor JF. (1994) Musculo-tendinous stiffness: its relationship to eccentric, isometric and concentric performance. *J Appl Physiol* 76(6): 2714–2719.

Wilson GJ, Murphy AJ, Walshe A. (1996) The specificity of strength training: The effect of posture. *Eur J Appl Physiol* 73: 346–352.

Wilson GJ, Newton RU, Murphy AJ, Humphries BJ. (1993) The optimal training load for the development of dynamic athletic performance. *Med Sci Sports Exercise* 25: 1279–1286.

Wilson GJ, Walshe AD, Fisher MR. (1997) The development of an isokinetic squat device: reliability and relationship to functional performance. *Eur J Appl Physiol* 75(5): 455–461.

Wilson GJ, Wood GA, Elliott BC. (1991) Optimal stiffness of the series elastic component in a stretch shorten cycle activity. *J Appl Physiol* 70: 825–833.

41

Dual energy X-ray absorptiometry

José Luis Ferretti, Gustavo R. Cointry, Ricardo F. Capozza, José R. Zanchetta

Introduction

Among the available resources for body composition analysis, the dual-energy X-ray absorptiometry (DEXA) can assess the body mineral, fat and lean compartments with lower radiation exposure, determination time and cost than the multiscan axial CT and MRI (Lukaski 1993) and with a higher precision than the anthropometric and bioimpedance techniques (Clasey et al 1999, Visser et al 1999), even in children (Chan 1992, Lapillone et al 1997). A pitfall is that DEXA provides projectional data that are useful only for mass estimations. This gives no information about the cross-sectional properties of muscles and bones that is relevant for *strength* estimations (Ferretti 1998a, b). In addition, the amount of body fat may induce an underestimation of the lean compartment (Hansen et al 1999).

The absorptiometric principle for DEXA states that the original intensity (I_0) of an X-ray beam passing through a complex substance containing different components "a" and "b" is attenuated proportionally to the material's thickness and composition. The transmitted intensity (I) is given by the attenuation coefficients (u_a, u_b) and the masses (m_a, m_b) of the absorbing components according to $I = I_0 \exp(-u_a.m_a - u_b.m_b)$. The energy attenuation coefficients vary with the X-ray energy and the atomic numbers of the components. The analysis of a given number of substances within the material studied requires an equal number of attenuation measurements. Thus, the availability of two different X-ray energies in DEXA allows separate measurement of only two compartments in each region studied. However, the DEXA measurements can determine no less than *three* different body compartments:

1. bone mineral, rich in calcium and phosphorus

2. fat or lipid, electrolyte-free

3. *lean* (non-fat) *tissues*, containing traces of potassium, chlorine, sulphur and calcium.

First the machine sorts and analyses differently the dense pixels, which correspond to bone, from those which correspond to soft tissue (ST). The ST pixels are analysed for fat (*fat mass*, FM) and fat-free tissue (*lean mass*, LM) as the two materials. The system profits from the fact that variations in the FM/LM composition of the ST produce differences in the respective attenuation coefficients at the two energy levels. Therefore, the automatic calculation of the X-ray attenuation ratio at the two main energy peaks pro-

vides separation of the ST compartment into FM and LM (Peppler and Mazess 1981, Pietrobelli et al 1996).

The composition of the bone-containing pixels is analysed for "*bone mass*" (bone mineral content, BMC) and ST as the two materials. Therefore, the FM/LM mix of the ST component of the bone pixels can not be measured, but only estimated. In relatively homogeneous sites, such as the lumbar region, the ST "hidden" by the bones is assumed to have the same composition as the surrounding pixels containing only ST. The estimation of the ST composition is being continuously improved by the use of calibration standards for fat and lean and the selection of suitable fat-distribution models for the body (Goodsitt 1992).

Assessment of the muscle mass

The LM compartment comprises obviously the *muscle mass* (MM) together with the extraosseous connective tissues, the skin and the visceral mass.

Computational availability in DEXA allows both whole body and regional analyses. For whole body analyses the composition of the LM compartment is rather complex because of the visceral component. Consequently, an indirect estimation of the whole body MM from the LM data would have only a relative value. However, the whole body LM values could be taken as *proportional* indicators of the MM within certain limits (especially in relatively homogeneous samples of non-obese individuals), and as such they have been interpreted in some studies (Ferretti et al 1998a, Mazess et al 1990). For regional, limb analyses the proportions between MM and LM are larger and less variable, and so the accuracy of deriving a MM approach is higher than that offered by the whole body determinations (Mazess et al 1990, Heymsfield et al 1990, Wang et al 1999), especially when the hands and feet are excluded. Good correlations between LM measurements in different limb muscle groups by DEXA and quantitative computed tomography (QCT) (r = 0.86 to 0.96, mean differences lower than 3.9%; Visser et al 1999, Wang et al 1999) or between LM and anthropometric areas (r = 0.82 to 0.92; Heymsfield et al 1990) were reported. New algorithms to improve the DEXA accuracy for the estimation of the actual MM are under development (Wang et al 1999).

We have described the age evolution of the whole body LM values in 1450 normal Caucasian Argentine males and females aged 2 to 87 years with an XR-26 densitometer (Norland Corp., Fort Atkinson, WI; Ferretti et al 1998a; Fig. 41.1A). The values were similar for boys and girls during growth. After puberty a sudden, dramatic increase took place in males until approximately 20 years of age, and the difference over the females was then maintained until the time of menopause. Thereafter, the LM declined smoothly in both genders, slightly faster in males than females.

The simultaneous measurement of the LM and FM by DEXA showed that the allometric proportionality between those variables was quite low, especially after puberty. Little difference was observed between the adult individuals younger (generally leaner) and older than 45 years (Fig. 41.1B and C).

The DEXA estimation of LM has proven useful in analysing changes in body composition after delivery or menopause (Panatopoulos et al 1996, Chou et al

1999), in patients with different nutritional disturbances (Schneider et al 1998) and with many primary or secondary muscle diseases. Although, perhaps the most attractive DEXA application is the simultaneous assessment of the LM and the BMC to analyse the *muscle/bone relationships* for achieving a *biomechanical diagnosis of osteoporosis* (Ferretti et al 1998d).

Analysis of the muscle/ bone interactions

The strains induced on the bone structure by the contractions of the regional muscles are a chief determinant of the bone strength (and indirectly of the bone mass; Ferretti 1998b, Frost et al 1998). Good correlations were reported between BMD and LM ($r^2 = 0.75$ to 0.80; Faulkner et al 1993) or the leg power or strength ($r = 0.41$ to 0.67; Witzke and Snow 1999) with little independent influence of anthropometric parameters. Changes in the endocrine environment of bone tissue can displace the set point of the feedback system that controls that relationship (*bone mechanostat*; Frost 1987), leading to an increased bone mass loss (osteopenia) and eventually inducing a skeletal weakness (osteoporosis).

The diagnosis of osteoporosis is currently based on mere determinations of a reduced bone *mass* (osteopenia) by DEXA (Kanis et al 1994), disregarding the degree of bone *fragility* (which is just empirically deduced from the BMC or its "areal" expression, the bone mineral density, BMD) and the status of the muscle/bone relationships. Tomographic, cross-sectional determinations of bones and muscles obviously give more reliable information for both diagnosis and monitoring (Ferretti 1998a, b). Nevertheless, the universal standardisation of the BMC and MM assessments provided by DEXA supports their provisional use as acceptable indicators of the bone and muscle strength until the new methodologies become widely available.

As evidence of the ability to analyse the muscle/ bone relationships using DEXA, we have described close, linear correlations between the whole body BMC and LM ($r = 0.823$ to 0.908 excluding post-menopausal females) in the Argentine sample (Ferretti et al 1998a; Fig. 41.2A). Practically identical slopes were obtained for boys, girls, young or adult males, and pre- or post-menopausal females. However, significantly higher intercepts of the curves were observed for post- than pre-pubertal individuals, for pre-menopausal females than age-matched men, and for pre-

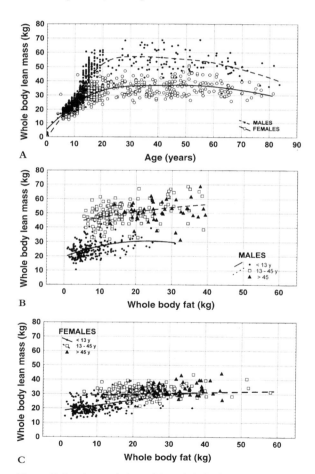

Figure 41.1—Age-evolution of the whole body lean mass (**A**) in 1450 normal Argentine Caucassian males and females (sample description in Ferretti et al 1998a).

than post-menopausal females. Similar results were obtained after adjusting the corresponding BMC values to FM data. Data from newborns (Lapillone et al 1997) fitted the same regression lines. Others have shown:

1. that the LM correlated generally better with the BMC than with the BMD (Hughes et al 1995, Khosla et al 1996)

2. that the FM may play a more important role in post- than in pre-menopausal women (Rico et al 1994, Aloia et al 1995, Khosla et al 1996).

The parallelism of the curves (Fig. 41.2A) evidences the universal nature of the influence of the muscle-induced mechanical stimulation on bone mass as governed by the bone mechanostat in *Homo sapiens*, regardless of age, gender, body habitus or reproductive status. The intercept differences pointed out the *disturbing role* of the endocrine environment on the setpoint of the mechanostat. This factor altered the proportionality of that relationship differently according to the gender and the reproductive status of the individuals.

That striking accumulation of surplus bone mass per unit of "muscle" mass (LM) in the women, proposedly useful for reproductive purposes (fetal skeletal development), was then shown to take place at mechanically little-relevant skeletal sites (metaphyseal trabecular network; Ferretti et al 1998b). This arrangement would avoid its elimination by the bone mechanostat as usually observed with any bone tissue reinforcing the bone structure where there is no specific need for that.

Also strikingly, men were shown to fully compensate for their lower bone/muscle mass proportion by achieving a more efficient distribution of their cortical bone (as assessed by the cross-sectional moment of inertia tomographically determined in the distal radius) than women did (Fig. 41.2B) (Ferretti et al 1998c). As a result of that, the tomographically-assessed bone *strength* (Bone Strength Index; Ferretti et al 1996) of the studied region correlated closely with the dynamometrically-determined regional muscle *strength*, following *a single linear slope* for men and women (Fig. 41.2C) (Schiessl et al 1996). So, it can be said that, over the natural, morphogenetical covariance between bone and muscle masses and the obvious influence of gravity on the weight-bearing skeleton (Arden and Spector 1997, Burr 1997, Nguyen et al 1998, Davis et al 1999, Nordström and Lorentzon 1999), "*bones are what the regional muscles want them to be*".

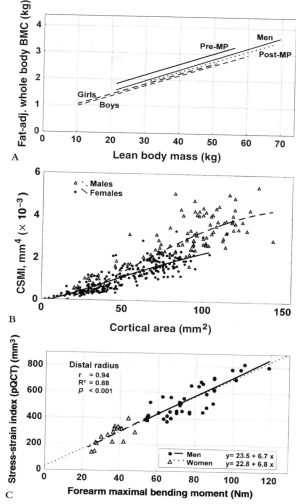

Figure 41.2—Associations between **A** the fat-adjusted, whole body BMC and the whole body LM (DEXA, n = 1450; Ferretti et al 1998a); **B** the tomographically-assessed, ultradistal-radius cross-sectional moment of inertia (CSMI, indicator of the architectural efficiency of the metaphyseal design concerning bending strength) and cortical bone area (indicator of the cortical bone mass) Peripheral Quantitative Computed Tomography (pQCT), n = 370; Ferretti et al 1998b), and **C** the stress-strain index (pQCT) and the forearm maximal bending moment (dynamometry, n = 55; Schiessl et al 1996, Ferretti et al 1998c), in normal Caucassian males and females.

Applications to a biomechanical diagnosis of osteoporosis

The above statement is actually true (central region in Fig. 41.3A) provided that *no endocrine disturbance* alters the bone mechanostat setpoint. If it does, then the muscle/bone relationships may change so as to render the bone mass or strength inadequate with respect to the mass or strength of the regional muscles (right-lower region in Fig. 41.3A). In the first case (muscle/bone adequacy), a relatively low BMC value would correspond to a *physiologic osteopenia*, a condition for which the only treatment should be to increase the mechanical usage of the affected region. Any low BMC value corresponding to the second case would suggest the diagnosis of a *true osteoporosis* with valid, biomechanical criteria (Frost 1997).

After ruling-out ethnicity as a confounding factor (Aloia et al 1999), suitable reference curves (Fig. 41.3B and C) taken from correlation graphs between muscle/bone *mass* (Fig. 41.2A) or strength data (Fig. 41.2C), respectively would do the following:

1. allow adjusting the BMC or BSI data to the muscle mass or strength indicators for inter-group comparisons avoiding confounders such as age, gender or body habitus

2. help to establish whether the bone status is (*osteopenia*) or is not (*osteoporosis?*) adequate to the muscle condition. Two representative cases (A&B) are represented in the figure, showing typical instances in which a BMC value may seem relatively low or high, while the percentiles for the muscle-boner relationships are relatively high and low, respectively. This will provide a diagnosis of a *true osteoporosis* according to valid, biomechanical criteria (Frost 1997).

New developments are coming that will further enhance the wide horizon of application of DEXA analysis of body composition.

References

Aloia JF, Vaswani A, Ma R, Flaster E. (1995) To what extent is bone mass determined by fat-free or fat mass? *Am J Clin Nutr* 61: 1110–1114.

Aloia JF, Vaswani A, Mikhail M, Flaster ER. (1999) Body composition by dual-energy X-ray absorptiometry in black compared with white women. *Osteoporosis Int* 1: 114–119.

Arden NK, Spector TD. (1997) Genetic influences on muscle strength, lean body mass, and bone mineral density: a twin study. *J Bone Miner Res* 12: 2076–2081.

Burr DB. (1997) Muscle strength, bone mass, and age-related bone loss. *J Bone Miner Res* 12: 1547–1551.

Chan GM. (1992) Performance of dual-energy X-ray

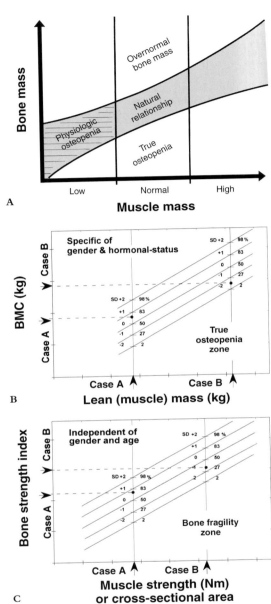

Figure 41.3—**A** Schematic representation of the normal (central region) or systemically-altered regulation (right-lower region) of bone mass by the regional muscle mass (Frost 1997). The same rationale can be applied to muscle/bone *strength* analysis (**C**). **B**, **C** Proposed prototypes for reference charts derived from curves (like those shown in Fig. 41.2A,C, respectively) for evaluating the DEXA-assessed bone mass (BMC) or strength (Bone Strength Indices, BSI) according to the individual's muscle mass (LM) or strength (muscle cross-sections or dynamometric analyses) in order to establish a biomechanical distinction between osteopenias and osteoporoses (Frost 1997). Two hypothetical cases of individuals having relatively low and high values of BMC (cases A&B) are shown, for which the corresponding associations with the muscle indicators give percentile values relatively high and low, respectively.

absorptiometry in evaluating bone, lean body mass, and fat in pediatric subjects. *J Bone Miner Res* 7(4): 369–374.

Chou T-W, Chan GM, Moyer-Mileur L. (1999) Post-partum body composition changes in lactating and non-lactating primiparas. *Nutrition* 15: 481–484.

Clasey JL, Kanaley JA, Wideman L, et al. (1999) Validity of methods of body composition assessment in young and older men and women. *J Appl Physiol* 86: 1728–1738.

Davis JW, Novotny R, Wasnich RD, Ross PD. (1999) Ethnic, anthropometric, and lifestyle associations with regional variations in peak bone mass. *Calcif Tissue Int* 65: 100–105.

Faulkner RA, Bailey DA, Drinkwater DT, Wilkinson AA, Houston CS, McKay HA. (1993) Regional and total-body bone mineral content, bone mineral density, and total-body tissue composition in children 8-16 years of age. *Calcif Tissue Int* 53: 7–12.

Ferretti JL, Capozza RF, Zanchetta JR. (1996) Mechanical validation of a noninvasive (pQCT) index for the non-invasive assessment of rat femur bending strength. *Bone* 16: 97–102.

Ferretti JL. (1998a) Peripheral quantitative computed tomography (pQCT) for evaluating structural and mechanical properties of small bone. In: *Advances in Osteoporosis, Vol. 1.* Lyritis GP, ed. Athens: Hylonome, pp. 53–62.

Ferretti JL. (1998b) Biomechanical properties of bone. In: *Bone Densitometry and Osteoporosis.* Genant HK, Guglielmi G, Jergas M, eds. Berlin: Springer, pp. 143–161.

Ferretti JL, Capozza RF, Cointry GR, et al. (1998a) Gender-related differences in the relationships between densitometric values of whole-body bone mineral content and lean mass in humans between 2 and 87 years of age. *Bone* 22: 683–690.

Ferretti JL, Capozza RF, Cointry GR, et al. (1998b) Menstruating women accumulate bone mineral per unit of muscle mass in skeletal regions of little mechanical relevance. *Bone* 22: 705.

Ferretti JL, Capozza RF, Cointry GR, et al. (1998c) Bone mass is higher in women than men per unit of muscle mass but bone mechanostat would compensate for the difference in the species. *Bone* 23(6S): S471.

Ferretti JL, Schiessl H, Frost HM. (1998d) On new opportunities for absorptiometry. *J Clin Densitom* 1: 41–53.

Frost HM. (1987) The mechanostat: a proposed pathogenetic mechanism of osteoporoses and the bone mass effects of mechanical and nonmechanical agents. *Bone Miner* 2: 73–85.

Frost HM. (1997) Defining osteopenias and osteoporoses: another view (with insights from a new paradigm). *Bone* 20: 385–391.

Frost HM, Ferretti JL, Jee WSS. (1998) Some roles of mechanical usage, muscle strength, and the mechanostat in skeletal physiology, disease, and research. *Calcif Tissue Int* 62: 1–7.

Goodsitt MM. (1992) Evaluation of a new set of calibration standards for the measurement of fat content via DPA and DXA. *Med Phys* 19: 35–44.

Hansen RD, Raja C, Aslani A, Smith RC, Allen BJ. (1999) Determination of skeletal muscle and fat-free mass by nuclear and dual-energy X-ray absorptiometry methods in men and women aged 51–84 y. *Am J Clin Nutr* 70: 228–233.

Heymsfield SB, Smith R, Aulet M, et al. (1990) Appendicular skeletal muscle mass: measurement by dual-photon absorptiometry. *Am J Clin Nutr* 52: 214–218.

Hughes VA, Frontera WR, Dallal GE, Lutz KJ, Fisher C, Evans WJ. (1995) Muscle strength and body composition: associations with bone density in older subjects. *Med Sci Sports Exerc* 27: 967–974.

Kanis JA, Melton J, Christiansen C, Johnston CC, Khaltaev N. (1994) The diagnosis of osteoporosis. *J Bone Miner Res* 9: 1137–1141.

Khosla S, Atkinson E, Riggs BL, Melton LJ. (1996) Relationship between body composition and bone mass in women. *J Bone Miner Res* 11: 857–863.

Lapillone A, Braillon P, Claris O, Chatelain PG, Delmas PD, Salle BL. (1997) Body composition in appropriate and in small for gestational age infants. *Acta Paediatr* 86: 198–200

Lukaski HC. (1993) Soft tissue composition and bone mineral status: evaluation by dual-energy X-ray absorptiometry. *J Nutr* 123: 438–443.

Mazess RB, Barden HS, Bisek JP, Hanson J. (1990) Dual-energy X-ray absorptiometry for total-body and regional bone-mineral and soft-tissue composition. *Am J Clin Nutr* 51: 1106–1112.

Nguyen TV, Howard GM, Kelly PJ, Eisman JA. (1998) Bone mass, lean mass, and fat mass: same genes or same environments? *Am J Epidemiol* 147: 3–16.

Nordström P, Lorentzon R. (1999) Influence of heredity and environment on bone density in adolescent boys: a parent-offspring study. *Osteoporosis Int* 10: 271–277.

Panatopoulos G, Ruiz J-C, Raison J, Guy-Grand B, Basdevant A. (1996) Menopause, fat and lean distribution in obese women. *Maturitas* 25: 11–19.

Peppler WW, Mazess RB. (1981) Total body bone mineral and lean body mass by dual-photon absorptiometry. *Calcif Tissue Int* 33: 353–359.

Pietrobelli A, Formica C, Wang AM, Heymsfield SB. (1996) Dual-energy X-ray absorptiometry body composition model: review of physical concepts. *Am J Physiol* 271 (Endocrinol Metab 34): E941–E951.

Rico H, Revilla M, Villa LF, Ruiz-contreras D, Hernández ER, Alvarez de Buergo M. (1994) The four-compartment models in body composition: data from a study with dual-energy X-ray absorptiometry and near-infrared interactance on 816 normal subjects. *Metabolism* 43: 417–422.

Schiessl H, Ferretti JL, Tysarczyk-Niemeyer G, Willnecker J. (1996) Noninvasive Bone Strength Index as analyzed by peripheral quantitative computed tomography (pQCT). In: Schönau E, ed. *Paediatric Osteology*. Amsterdam: Elsevier, pp. 141–145.

Schneider P, Biko J, Schlamp D, et al. (1998) Comparison of total and regional body composition in adolescent patients with anorexia nervosa and pair-matched controls. *Eating Weight Disord* 3: 179–187.

Visser M, Fuerst T, Lang T, Salamone L, Harris T. (1999) Validity of fan-beam dual-energy X-ray absorptiometry for measuring the fat-free mass and leg muscle mass. *J Appl Physiol* 87: 1513–1520.

Wang W, Wang Z, Faith MS, Kotler D, Shih R, Heymsfield SB. (1999) Regional skeletal muscle measurement: evaluation of a new dual-energy X-ray absorptiometric model. *J Appl Physiol* 87: 1163–1171.

Witzke KA, Snow CM. (1999) Lean body mass and leg power best predict bone mineral density in adolescent girls. *Med Sci Sports Exerc* 31: 1558–1563.

42

Diagnostic electron microscopy

Kyriacos Kyriacou, Theodoros Kyriakides

Introduction

Muscle, being a specialized organ, reacts to noxious stimuli (genetic or acquired) in a limited number of ways. Therefore, ultrastructural abnormalities in isolation are generally not disease specific and they must be interpreted in the correct context. However, certain patterns of ultrastructural changes provide important clues not only in making a diagnosis but also in elucidating pathophysiologic mechanisms.

The aim of this chapter is to give a practical account of the use of electron microscopy in helping today's practising neuropathologist solve diagnostic dilemmas, and not to give an encyclopaedic description of ultrastructural changes in myopathology, which has been so well covered in previous reviews (Schochet and Lampert 1978, Carpenter and Karpati 1984, Sewry 1985, Engel AG and Banker 1994).

Electron microscopy provides the most useful information when the neuropathologist with full knowledge of the clinical problem (and after examining the histology and histochemistry of a case) seeks ultrastructural information to either confirm, refute or supplement his light microscopical assessment.

Muscle biopsy

In many neuromuscular disorders a muscle biopsy is necessary for accurate diagnosis. Details for the selection of the most appropriate muscle to biopsy and the different procedures currently used are described elsewhere in this book.

Preservation of specimens

Electron microscopy

In our laboratory a 2.5% glutaraldehyde solution in 0.1 M phosphate buffer at pH 7.2 is used as a primary fixative. Prior to fixation a strip of muscle, 1.5 cm long and 0.5 cm thick, is pinned at each end at it's natural length on a piece of cork. After a minimum fixation of 30 min this strip is diced into rectangular pieces measuring 1–2 mm in width and 3–4 mm in length. Fixation is continued for a minimum of 4 h to overnight, at 4°C. The tissues are subsequently rinsed in 0.1 M phosphate buffer, postfixed in osmium tetroxide and embedded in epoxy resin according to standard protocols.

Investigation of neuromuscular disorders

Electron microscopy provides essential diagnostic information in only very few neuromuscular disorders. In the majority of cases it supplements or provides confirmatory data for light microscopical observations. Special emphasis will be given to ultrastructural abnormalities that either characterize or are associated consistently with certain neuromuscular diseases.

Congenital myopathies

Congenital myopathies have been defined as a group of slowly evolving or non-progressive myopathies that present in early childhood with generalized muscle weakness and hypotonia. This group of disorders was poorly defined until the advent of frozen section histochemistry, which in combination with electron microscopy, provided important structural criteria for enabling the subclassification of these disorders. Currently, congenital myopathies may be subdivided into five broad categories based on morphological abnormalities (Table 42.1). For some of these morphological entities one or more genetic defects have been identified (Kaplan and Fontaine, 2001).

Normal ultrastructural appearance

This category includes entities such as congenital fibre type disproportion and congenital fibre type predominance (Kyriakides et al 1993). Although these myopathies are diagnosed by enzyme histochemistry, electron microscopy is important in confirming a normal ultrastructure.

Disruption of sarcomeres

Congenital myopathies that belong to this category are those displaying disruption of the normal sarcomere architecture as the predominant ultrastructural abnormality (Bodensteiner 1994). Electron microscopy is highly desirable for confirmation.

Central core myopathy

This myopathy, first described by Shy and Magee in 1956, is characterized by well-circumscribed circular lesions, which tend to extend centrally for most of the length of Type I fibres. These cores are deficient in oxidative enzymes and phosphorylase activity (Dubowicz and Pearse 1960). Central cores are divided into two types:

Table 42.1— Classification of congenital myopathies

Predominant structure involved	Morphological abnormality	Type of myopathy
1. None	Normal	Fibre type disproportion
		Congenital fibre type predominance
2. Sarcomere	Central cores	Central core myopathy
	Multicores / Minicores	Multicore/minicore myopathy
	Trilaminar fibres	Trilaminar myopathy
	Broad A band	Broad A band myopathy
	Interlacing sarcomere	Interlacing sarcomere myopathy
	Central nuclei	Centronuclear myopathy
3. Myonuclei		Myotubular myopathy
	Apoptotic nuclei	Congenital myopathy with apoptotic nuclei
4. Inclusion bodies associated with or derived from pre-existing structures		
Z disk	Nemaline bodies	Nemaline body myopathy
Sarcoplasmic reticulum	Tubular aggregates	Tubular aggregate myopathy
	Microvacuoles	Sarcotubular myopathy
	Spheroid bodies	Spheroid body myopathy
Myofilaments	Aggregates of thin myofilaments	Actin myopathy
5. Inclusion bodies not derived from pre-existing structures	Fingerprint bodies	Fingerprint body myopathy
	Reducing bodies	Reducing body myopathy
	Zebra bodies	Zebra body myopathy
	Cylindrical spirals	Cylindrical spiral myopathy
	Hexagorally cross-linked tubular arrays	Myopathy with hexanolly cross-linked tubular arrays

- structured cores, with relatively well preserved myofibrillar architecture
- unstructured cores, in which the myofibrillar contractile elements are disorganized.

Both types of cores are characterized by lack of mitochondria, decreased glycogen and alterations in the sarcoplasmic reticulum (Neville and Brooke 1971, Hayashi et al 1989).

Multicore/minicore myopathy
The characteristic pathological feature of this myopathy is the finding of multiple areas (Engel AG and Gomez 1966, Engel et al 1971) usually 5–7 μm in width or length, showing loss of cross-striations and reduction in the staining intensity of oxidative enzymes. These minicores consist of disorganized myofibrils accompanied by lack of mitochondria, decreased glycogen and streaming of the Z disks. Minicores are usually detectable by light microscopy, but because of their small size, electron microscopy is desirable for diagnosis (Fig. 42.1).

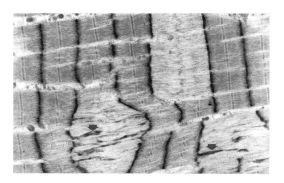

Figure 42.1— Minicore myopathy. Electron micrograph showing the presence of small circumscribed minicores characterized by Z band streaming (arrows), disorganized myofibrils and lack of both myofilaments and mitochondria (×16 200).

Trilaminar myopathy
This is a rare myopathy that is characterized by the presence of fibres with three different tinctorial zones as revealed by the trichrome stain (Ringel et al 1978).

These "trilaminar" fibres have an inner zone, which stains red with Gomori trichrome, an intermediate green-staining zone and an outer purple-staining zone. Ultrastructurally the inner zone consists of mitochondria, vesicles, triads, glycogen and disorganized myofibrils. The intermediate zone appears almost normal, and the outer zone contains randomly arranged filaments, glycogen, ribosomes, mitochondria and lipid. Although light microscopy is characteristic, because of the rarity of this condition, electron microscopy is mandatory.

Broad A band myopathy

This benign congenital myopathy was described in 1996 by Mrak et al. Light microscopy is unremarkable, but ultrastructural examination reveals numerous areas of broadened A bands and loss of distinct I bands, caused by misalignment of thick filaments. The Z band and total sarcomere length appear normal.

Interlacing sarcomere myopathy

This congenital myopathy was described in 1998 by Marbini et al. Ultrastructurally, bands of myofibrils are at right angles or skew to the remaining myofibrils transversing the fibre. In these areas, the sarcomeric structure is preserved apart from lack of Z disks and actin filaments.

Myonuclear abnormalities

Abnormally placed nuclei

Abnormally placed nuclei occur in centronuclear and myotubular myopathies (Spiro et al 1966, Van Wijngaarden et al 1969). Electron microscopy is useful in demonstrating centrally located nuclei surrounded by radial spikes of myofibrils. In myopathies exhibiting internal nuclei as a non-specific feature the latter architectural arrangement is not seen.

Congenital myopathy with apoptotic changes

This myopathy was reported by Ikezoe et al in 2000. By light microscopy, a high proportion of fibres can be seen to have vacuoles, occasionally rimmed, but the most characteristic finding is chromatin condensation and nuclear fragmentation. By electron microscopy, 40% of myonuclei show abnormal morphology. DNA fragmentation in myonuclei can be demonstrated by the TUNEL method (terminal deoxynucleotydil transferase mediated dUTP-digoxigenin nick end labelling).

Inclusion bodies associated with or derived from pre-existing structures

This category encompasses a group of rare myopathies that are characterized by the presence of abnormal inclusions within muscle fibres. Their common feature is that these inclusions are pathologically related to pre-existing structures, such as the Z disk, myofilaments and the sarcoplasmic reticulum. They include nemaline bodies, spheroid bodies and tubular aggregates. Each of these inclusions is not necessarily pathognomonic of a particular disorder, but in the congenital myopathies, they represent the predominant morphological abnormality.

Nemaline body myopathy

Nemaline myopathy, first described by Shy et al (1963), is characterized by the presence of dark red-staining rods, visible with the Gomori trichrome stain. The rods are usually found under the sarcolemma and around nuclei; they measure up to 5 µm in length and up to 1 µm in width (Fig. 42.2). They have a characteristic transverse periodicity with a spacing of 20–25 nm (Gonatas et al 1966, Morris et al 1990), and ultrastructurally they are seen to be associated with actin filaments (Fig. 42.2). Nemaline bodies may be rarely found inside myonuclei (Engel NK and Oberc 1975, Paulus et al 1988, Goebel and Warlo 1997). These structures have also been described in association with polymyositis (Cape et al 1970), in ophthalmoplegia with mitochondrial abnormalities (Fukunaga et al 1980) and in human immunodeficiency virus (HIV) myopathy (Dwyer et al 1992), so clinicopathological correlation is essential.

Tubular aggregate myopathy

This myopathy is characterized by the presence of subsarcolemmal inclusions, consisting of tubules, which probably originate from the sarcoplasmic reticulum (Gruner 1966, Howes et al 1966). Tubular aggregates are stained red with the Gomori trichrome.

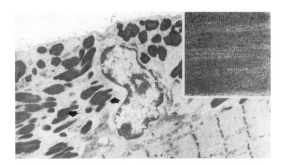

Figure 42.2 — Nemaline myopathy. Electron micrograph showing the presence of numerous cytoplasmic nemaline rods. These are attached to thin filaments of actin, arrows (×11 450). Inset: higher power showing characteristic transverse rod periodicity of 20 nm (×81 000).

Ultrastructurally, the tubules are orientated parallel and perpendicular to the long axis of the myofibrils, and they consist of densely packed double walled tubules 60–80 nm in width (Fig. 42.3). Although this is the main morphological feature in primary tubular aggregate myopathy, similar inclusions have also been found in a variety of disorders including periodic paralysis (Engel WK et al 1970, Kyriacou et al 1997), alcoholic myopathy (Chui et al 1975) and congenital myasthenic syndrome (Engel AG et al 1979).

Sarcotubular myopathy

The characteristic of this myopathy, which was first described by Jerusalem et al (1973), is the presence of small cytoplasmic vacuoles that are thought to be derived from the sarcotubular system. Electron microscopy reveals empty vacuoles that contain traces of amorphous material. Lipid and glycogen are absent, and there is no continuity with the T tubules.

Spheroid body myopathy

This myopathy was first described by Goebel et al in 1978. The muscle of five patients from a large kindred, contained collections of spherical or ovoid masses that stained bluish green on Gomori trichrome. Electron microscopy shows that these inclusions are electron-dense aggregates, measuring 2–15 μm and contain non-membrane bound, granulofilamentous material. High magnification views reveal concentrically and irregularly orientated filaments, which usually vary between 12–15 nm in diameter. Within the core, aggregates of dense Z band material is commonly present. Spheroid bodies are often immunostained by desmin antibodies (Goebel et al 1997a), and they resemble cytoplasmic bodies, which are smaller and which have been described in a variety of other myopathies (MacDonald and Engel 1969, Edstrom

et al 1980, Patel et al 1983). Recent evidence links spheroid body myopathy to a more heterogeneous group of disorders collectively called myofibrillar myopathies (Amato et al 1998).

Congenital myopathy with excess of thin myofilaments (actin myopathy)

Goebel et al (1997b) delineated a new form of congenital myopathy characterized by subsarcolemmal masses of thin myofilaments, which were shown by immunohistochemistry and immunoelectron microscopy to consist of actin. These intracellular masses are bigger and more frequent than the less specific filamentous bodies, also composed of thin myofilaments, which occur as a non-specific feature in many neuromuscular disorders.

Inclusion bodies not derived from pre-existing structures

Some rare congenital myopathies are characterized by the presence of peculiar inclusions whose origin remains unknown. To this category belong fingerprint body myopathy, reducing body myopathy, zebra body myopathy, cylindrical spiral myopathy and myopathy with hexagonally cross-linked tubular arrays.

Fingerprint body myopathy

The fingerprint bodies were first described by Engel AG et al (1972). They appear as dense green inclusions under the sarcolemma with the Gomori trichrome stain. Electron microscopy shows that fingerprint bodies measure 1.0–10.0 μm in length and 0.5–4.00 μm in width; they consist of a complex arrangement of lamellae whose pattern is reminiscent of a fingerprint. They are not membrane bound, and they may also occur in other diverse conditions such as myotonic dystrophy (Tome and Fardeau 1973) and distal myopathy (Borg et al 1991).

Reducing body myopathy

This myopathy is characterized by the presence of reducing bodies, which are subsarcolemmal inclusions staining purple with the Gomori trichrome stain. These bodies have specific reactions, staining for glycogen, RNA, sulfhydryl groups and menadione-linked α-glycerophosphate dehydrogenase (Brooke and Neville 1972). Reducing bodies have unique ultrastructural features: they consist of electron-dense granulofilamentous material, that is not membrane bound (Tome and Fardeau 1975). These abnormal inclusions have not been observed in other myopathies, and their origin remains to be determined. In some instances tubular structures 17 nm in diameter

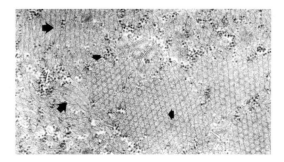

Figure 42.3—Hypokalaemic periodic paralysis. Electron micrograph showing tubular aggregates which have been cut both transversely (small arrows) and longitudinally (large arrows). The tubules are closely packed, double walled with a diameter of 60–80 nm (×58 250).

are seen to be a component of the reducing body (Carpenter et al 1985).

Zebra body myopathy

Zebra body myopathy is a very rare non-progressive muscle disorder (Lake and Wilson 1975, Reyes et al 1987), which is characterized by the presence of zebra-bodies or leptomeres as the predominant pathological feature. These are small inclusions, measuring 2 μm by 0.5 μm, and they can only be recognized by electron microscopy, which shows dense parallel bands resembling Z disks that are interconnected by paler filamentous zones. Zebra bodies are also found in normal muscle near myotendinous junctions (Mair and Tome 1972).

Cylindrical spiral myopathy

This myopathy, first reported by Carpenter et al (1979), is characterized by subsarcolemmal inclusions that appear bright red on Gomori trichrome. On transverse section they consist of 9 to 15 spiralling membranous lamellae, wrapping around a central cytoplasmic core, which contains glycogen and vesicular structures (Carpenter et al 1979, Taratuto et al 1991).

Myopathy with hexagonally cross-linked tubular arrays

This is a new morphological entity characterized by intensely purple cytoplasmic inclusions on the modified Gomori trichrome. Electron microscopy demonstrates pleomorphic, crystalline inclusions, often under the sarcolemma and without a membrane. Perpendicular to their long axis, the inclusions exhibit highly organized round profiles 20 nm in diameter connected by six pairs of spokes, regularly spaced 60° apart (Bourque et al 1999).

Myofibrillar myopathies

A clinically and genetically heterogeneous group of disorders that share common morphological features has recently been delineated and called myofibrillar myopathies (De Bleecker et al 1996, Nakano et al 1996). This group is also known as desminopathies (Goebel and Fardeau 1997) although desmin is only one of several muscle proteins that accumulate in the lesions that characterize these disorders (De Bleecker et al 1996, Amato et al 1998).

There are two major categories of pathological alterations:

- non-hyaline lesions, consisting of myofibrillar destruction associated with Z disk related structures

- hyaline lesions, composed of compacted and degraded myofibrillar elements, including spheroid and cytoplasmic bodies (Nakano et al 1996).

Currently the diagnosis of this group of disorders relies heavily on ultrastructural information as well as on the availability of immunohistochemical data (Goebel and Fardeau 1993, 1997).

Inflammatory myopathies

Inflammatory myopathies form a heterogeneous group of acquired disorders that includes polymyositis, dermatomyositis, inclusion body myositis, parasitic, bacterial and viral myositides. Most of these disorders are idiopathic, and the majority are diagnosed by light microscopy. However, in some, electron microscopy plays an important role in providing ultrastructural confirmatory data.

Inclusion body myositis

The recognition of inclusion body myositis (IBM) as a separate entity is closely related to the application of electron microscopy to myopathology. IBM was first described by Chou (1967), who observed cytoplasmic aggregates of filaments within muscle fibres.

Haematoxylin and eosin staining of frozen sections shows the characteristic features of rimmed vacuoles, containing small basophilic granules, and eosinophilic inclusions, which are usually intracytoplasmic and less commonly intranuclear. Electron microscopy is crucial for characterizing these abnormalities (Carpenter 1996). Most vacuoles appear autophagic, stain positive for acid phosphatase, and contain myeloid bodies, glycogen, filaments and other debris. Ultrastructurally, at high magnification, IBM filaments often have a tubular appearance with an outside diameter of 15–21 nm (Griggs et al 1995; Fig. 42.4). Mitochondrial abnormalities are not uncommon (Santorelli et al 1996).

Dermatomyositis

The endothelial cells of capillaries and arterioles frequently display tubuloreticular inclusions in the cytoplasm (Banker 1975). This is a useful finding since it does not occur in patients with IBM or polymyositis, but it may also be found in systemic lupus erythematosus (SLE) patients and in acquired immunodeficiency syndrome (AIDS) myopathies.

Viral myositis

Electron microscopic examination of patients suffering from viral myositis does not consistently reveal the

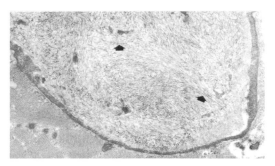

Figure 42.4—Inclusion body myositis. Electron micrograph showing the presence of tubulofilaments having a diameter of 20 nm (arrows) within a myonucleus (×23 300).

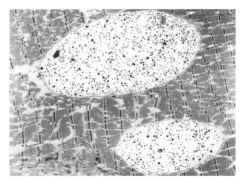

Figure 42.5—Colchicine myopathy. Electron micrograph showing the presence of two large cytoplasmic, membrane-bound vacuoles (autophagosomes) containing a myeloid body (arrow) and other degradation products (×5 300).

presence of virions (Gamboa et al 1979, Farrel et al 1980). HIV infection gives rise to polymyositis (Authier et al 1997), inclusion body myositis (Cupler et al 1996) and acquired nemaline myopathy (Dalakas et al 1987, Feinberg et al 1998). The ultrastructural features of these disorders have been described in other sections of this chapter.

Vacuolar myopathies

Vacuolar myopathies comprise a heterogeneous group of disorders that share as their main pathological feature the presence of vacuoles. A vacuole is defined as an abnormal space within the muscle fibre that appears empty by at least one method of staining (Engel AG 1973). In general vacuoles may be divided into two categories: membrane bound and non-membrane bound, also described as a cytoplasmic space.

A vacuole may contain an excess of normal material, such as glycogen and/or lipid, or an excess of abnormal material such as cytoplasmic degradation products (Fig. 42.5). Although usually no one vacuole is specific for any one disease, certain types of vacuoles tend to be associated with a specific disorder. Electron microscopy provides important information on the characteristics of the vacuoles, which in turn leads to pattern recognition of some of the more common disease entities as shown in Table 42.2.

Metabolic myopathies

Metabolic myopathies encompass disturbances in glycogen and lipid metabolism and mitochondrial myopathies. Often, electron microscopy plays an essential role for the diagnosis of these disorders.

Disturbances in glycogen metabolism

Electron microscopy is useful in demonstrating excess glycogen, which may be either membrane bound (Fig. 42.6) or lie free under the sarcolemma or in between myofibrils (see Table 42.2). In acid maltase deficiency glycogen accumulates in four types of spaces (Engel AG et al 1973). Glycogen may accumulate in non-membrane bound lakes (type 1 space), in membrane bound form (type 2 space), in ordinary autophagosomes with other degradation products (type 3 space) or in transitional forms (type 4 space).

Disturbances in lipid metabolism

Lipid storage myopathy can arise as a result of a variety of metabolic defects. The characteristic electron microscopic finding is the presence of vacuoles, either empty or containing traces of low density material, that lack discernible limiting membranes. Lipid accumulation is usually detected by light microscopy. Electron microscopy is often useful in confirming

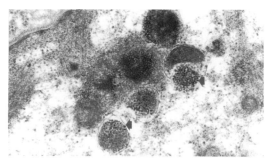

Figure 42.6—Acid maltase deficiency. Electron micrograph showing glycogen sequestration within lysosomes (arrows) (×56 000).

Table 42.2 — Classification of vacuolar myopathies

Type of vacuole	Contents of vacuole	Type of vacuolar myopathy
Membrane bound		
Lysosomal sac	β-particles of glycogen surrounded partly or completely by a single or double membrane	Acid maltase deficiency
Autophagic vacuole	β-particles of glycogen, surrounded by a single or double membrane and including various cytoplasmic degradation products	Acid maltase deficiency
Autophagic vacuole	Myeloid bodies and other cellular degradation products outlined by a single membrane	Chloroquine myopathy, Colchicine myopathy
Autophagic "rimmed" vacuoles	Myeloid bodies, other cytoplasmic degradation products and tubulofilaments 15–21 nm in diameter	Inclusion body myositis, oculopharyngeal dystrophy, distal myopathies, familial inclusion body myopathy
Sarcoplasmic reticulum (SR) and transverse tubular system (T tubules)	Dilated SR and proliferating T tubules containing amorphous material. Appearance of vacuolar contents varies according to stage of maturation	Periodic paralysis
Non-membrane bound		
Cytoplasmic space	β-particles of glycogen and polyglucosan	Non-lysosomal glycogenoses
Cytoplasmic space "rimmed" vacuoles	Tubulofilaments, myeloid bodies	Inclusion body myositis, oculopharyngeal dystrophy, distal myopathies
Lipid	Neutral lipid: electron lucent or slightly electron dense	Lipid storage myopathy

this and in detecting more subtle accumulations of lipid.

Mitochondrial myopathies

The diagnosis of mitochondrial myopathy relies on the presence of ragged red fibres and abnormal histochemistry, with electron microscopy providing evidence of mitochondrial dysmorphology. At the ultrastructural level, the mitochondrial changes that occur in mitochondrial myopathies have been well described (Shy and Gonatas 1964, Shy et al 1966, Stadhouders and Sengers 1987, Sigurd et al 1992, Engel and Banker 1994, Kyriacou et al 1997).

These consist of subsarcolemmal mitochondrial aggregates and/or abnormalities in mitochondrial structure, including the presence of crystalline inclusions (Fig. 42.7) (Morgan-Hughes 1994). However, mitochondrial dysmorphology alone is often not a sufficient criterion for the diagnosis of mitochondrial encephalomyopathies, because several muscle disorders induce secondary mitochondrial morphological abnormalities. We believe that close correlation between light microscopy and electron microscopy is essential in interpreting correctly any mitochondrial abnormalities that are seen. Furthermore, electron microscopy can be especially useful in the diagnosis of paediatric mitochondrial encephalomyopathies, where mitochondrial aggregates large enough to be seen by light microscopy are rarely well developed (Kyriacou et al 1999).

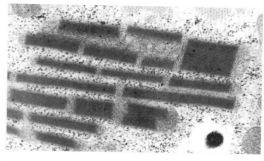

Figure 42.7 — Mitochondrial myopathy. Electron micrograph showing the presence of large rectangular crystalline inclusions within mitochondria (×56 000).

Muscular dystrophies

These disorders are currently diagnosed by immuno-cytochemisry and/or molecular biology techniques. Electron microscopy is not essential for their routine diagnosis, although it provides important information regarding pathophysiological mechanisms. Exemption may be the recent electron microscopic findings of nuclear abnormalities in Emery–Dreifuss muscular dystrophy (Fidzianska et al 1998, Sabatelli et al 2001) and the pathognomonic 8.5 nm intranuclear tubular filaments in oculopharyngeal muscular dystrophy (Tome et al 1997).

Miscellaneous myopathies

Myasthenic syndromes

These diseases are often diagnosed using clinical criteria (Middleton 1997), but electron microscopy has provided important morphological information for diagnosis and understanding of the mechanisms that impair neuromuscular transmission (Engel 1994).

Amyloid myopathy

Muscle involvement in primary systemic amyloidosis is uncommon. Few patients present myopathic symptoms, and ultrastructural examination is useful in improving our understanding of early pathogenic events. In a recent patient, ultrastructural investigations revealed abnormalities in the basal lamina and sarcolemma, which may be an early event leading to myofibre degeneration (Fig. 42.8).

Critical illness myopathy

This recently recognized syndrome, accounting for one of the causes of weakness in the intensive care

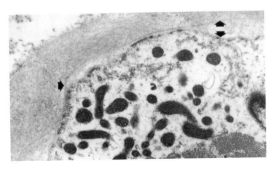

Figure 42.8—Amyloid myopathy. Electron micrograph showing splitting of the basal lamina (arrows) of a myofibre, in juxtaposition to aggregates of amyloid filaments (×33 600).

unit, is characterized by a selective loss of myosin myofilaments in both myofibre types. Electron microscopy is extremely useful in the diagnosis of this condition (Al-Lozi et al 1994).

Trabecular fibre myopathy

Trabecular fibre myopathy is a morphological entity initially described by Bethlem et al (1973) and recently reviewed by Weller et al (1999). It is characterized by maldistribution of mitochondria, presumably a result of an anchoring protein defect, giving rise to trabecular/lobulated fibres. Electron microscopy is useful in confirming the oxidative stains and the normality of mitochondrial structure.

Conclusion

Electron microscopy remains a very useful diagnostic method, especially when applied in conjunction with clinical and light microscopic data. It is of a particular relevance in the diagnosis of congenital, vacuolar and myofibrillar myopathies.

Acknowledgements

We are grateful to Mrs Ch Mikellidou for preparation of the figures and Mrs Ch Hadjiyianni for typing the manuscript.

References

Al-Lozi MT, Pestronk A, Yee WC, et al. (1994) Rapidly evolving myopathy with myosin-deficient muscle fibers. *Ann Neurol* 35: 273–279.

Amato AA, Kagan-Hallet K, Jackson CE, et al. (1998) The wide spectrum of myofibrillar myopathy suggests a multi-factorial etiology and pathogenesis. *Neurology* 51: 1646–1655.

Authier FJ, Chariot P, Gherardi R. (1997) Muscular complications in HIV infection. *Arch Anat Cytol Pathol* 45: 174–178.

Banker BQ. (1975) Dermatomyositis of childhood, ultra-structural alterations of muscle and intramuscular blood vessels. *J Neuropathol Exp Neurol* 34: 46–75.

Bethlem J, Van Wijngaarden GK, De Jong J. (1973) The incidence of lobulated fibers in the facioscapulohumeral type of muscular dystrophy and the limb girdle syndrome. *J Neurol Sci* 18: 351–358.

Bodensteiner JB. (1994) Congenital Myopathies. *Muscle Nerve* 17: 131–144.

Borg K, Tome FM, Edstrom L. (1991) Intranuclear and cytoplasmic filamentous inclusions in distal myopathy (Welander). *Acta Neuropathol* 82: 102–106.

Bourque PR, Lach B, Carpenter S, et al. (1999) Myopathy with hexagonally cross-linked tubular arrays: a new autosomal dominant or sporadic congenital myopathy. *Ann Neurol* 45: 512–515.

Brooke MH, Neville HE. (1972) Reducing body myopathy. *Neurology* 22: 829–840.

Cape CA, Johnson WW, Pitner SE. (1970) Nemaline structures in polymyositis. A nonspecific pathological reaction of skeletal muscles. *Neurology* 20: 494–502.

Carpenter S, Karpati G, Robitaille Y, et al. (1979) Cylindrical spirals in human skeletal muscle. *Muscle Nerve* 2: 282–287.

Carpenter S, Karpati G. (1984) Normal organelles and constituents of skeletal muscle cells and their pathological reactions. In: Carpenter S, Karpati G, eds. *Pathology of skeletal muscle*. New York: Churchill Livingstone, pp. 149–191.

Carpenter S, Karpati G, Holland P. (1985) New observations in reducing body myopathy. *Neurology* 35: 818–827.

Carpenter S. (1996) Inclusion body myositis; a review. *J Neuropathol Exper Neurol* 55: 1105–1114.

Chou SM. (1967) Myxovirus-like structures in a case of human chronic polymyositis. *Science* 158: 1453–55.

Chui LA, Neustein H, Munsat TL. (1975) Tubular aggregates in subclinical alcoholic myopathy. *Neurology* 25: 405–412.

Cupler EJ, Leon-Monzon M, Miller J, et al. (1996) Inclusion body myositis in HIV-1 and HTLV-1 infected patients. *Brain* 119: 1887–1893.

Dalakas MC, Pezeshkpour GH, Flaherty M. (1987) Progressive nemaline (rod) myopathy associated with HIV infection. *N Engl J Med* 317: 1602–1603.

De Bleecker JL, Engel AG, Ertl BB. (1996) Myofibrillar myopathy with abnormal foci of desmin positivity. II. Immunocytochemical analysis reveals accumulation of multiple other proteins. *J Neuropathol Exp Neurol* 55: 563–577.

Dubowitz V, Pearse AGE. (1960) Oxidative enzymes and phosphorylase in central-core disease of muscle. *Lancet* ii: 23–24.

Dwyer BA, Mayer RF, Lee SC. (1992) Progressive nemaline (rod) myopathy as a presentation of human immunodeficiency virus infection. *Arch Neurol* 49: 440.

Edstrom L, Thornell LE, Eriksson A. (1980) A new type of hereditary distal myopathy with characteristic sarcoplasmic bodies and intermediate (skeletin) filaments. *J Neurol Sci* 47: 171–190.

Engel AG, Gomez MR. (1966) Congenital myopathy associated with multifocal degeneration of muscle fibres. *Trans Am Neurol Assoc* 91: 222–223.

Engel AG, Gomez MR, Groover RV. (1971) Multicore disease. A recently recognized congenital myopathy associated with multifocal degeneration of muscle fibers. *Mayo Clin Proc* 46: 666–681.

Engel AG, Angelini C, Gomez MR. (1972) Fingerprint body myopathy. *Mayo Clin Proc* 47: 377–388.

Engel AG. (1973) Vacuolar myopathies: multiple etiologies and sequential structural studies. In: Pearson CM, Mostofi FK, eds. *The striated muscle*. Baltimore: Williams and Wilkins, pp. 301–341.

Engel AG, Gomez MR, Seybold ME, et al. (1973) The spectrum and diagnosis of acid maltase deficiency. *Neurology* 23: 95–106.

Engel AG, Lambert EH, Mulder DM, et al. (1979) Investigations of 3 cases of a newly recognized familial, congenital myasthenic syndrome. *Ann Neurol* 104: 8–12.

Engel AG. (1994) Disturbances of neuromuscular transmission. In: Engel AG, Armstrong CF, eds. *Myology: basic and clinical*. New York: McGraw Hill, pp. 1769–1835.

Engel AG, Banker BQ. (1994) Ultrastructural changes in diseased muscle: In: Engel AG, Armstrong CF, eds. *Myology: basic and clinical*. New York: McGraw Hill, pp. 889–1017.

Engel WK, Bishop DW, Cunningham GG. (1970) Tubular aggregates in type II muscle fibres: ultrastructural and histochemical correlation. *J Ultrastruct Res* 31: 507–525.

Engel WK, Oberc MA. (1975) Abundant nuclear rods in adult onset rod disease. *J Neuropathol Exp Neurol* 34: 119–132.

Farrell MK, Partin JC, Bove KE, et al. (1980) Epidemic influenza myopathy in Cincinnati in 1977. *J Pediatr* 96: 545–551.

Feinberg DM, Spiro AJ, Weidenheim KM. (1998) Distinct light microscopic changes in human immunodeficiency virus-associated nemaline myopathy. *Neurology* 50: 529–531.

Fidzianska A, Toniolo D, Hausmanowa-Petrusewicz I. (1998) Ultrastructural abnormality of sarcolemmal nuclei in Emery-Dreifuss muscular dystrophy (EDMD). *J Neurology Sci* 159: 88–93.

Fukunaga H, Osame M, Igata A. (1980) A case of nemaline myopathy with ophthalmoplegia and mitochondrial abnormalities. *J Neurology Sci* 46: 169–177.

Gamboa ET, Eastwood AB, Hays AP, et al. (1979) Isolation of influenza virus from muscle in myoglobinuric polymyositis. *Neurology* 29: 1323–1335.

Goebel HH, Muller J, Gillen HW, et al. (1978) Autosomal

dominant "spheroid body myopathy". *Muscle Nerve* 1: 14–26.

Goebel HH, Fardeau M. (1993) Desmin in myology. *Neuromusc Disord* 5: 161–166.

Goebel HH, Fardeau M. (1997) Desminopathies. In: Emery AEH, ed. *Diagnostic Criteria for Neuromuscular Disorders.* London: RSM, pp. 75–79.

Goebel HH, Warlo I. (1997) Nemaline myopathy with intranuclear rods – intranuclear rod myopathy. *Neuromusc Disord* 7: 13–19.

Goebel HH, D'Agostino AN, Wilson J, et al. (1997a) Spheroid body myopathy revisited. *Muscle Nerve* 20: 1127–1136.

Goebel HH, Anderson JR, Hubner C, et al. (1997b) Congenital myopathy with excess of thin myofilaments. *Neuromusc Disord* 7: 160–168.

Gonatas NK, Shy GM, Godfrey EH. (1966) Nemaline myopathy: the origin of nemaline structures. *N Engl J Med* 274: 535–539.

Griggs RC, Askanas V, DiMauro S, et al. (1995) Inclusion body myositis and myopathies. *Am Neurol Ass* 705–713.

Gruner JE. (1966) Anomalies of the sarcoplasmic reticulum and proliferation of tubules in the muscle in familial periodic paralysis. *C R Seances Soc Biol Fil* 160: 193–195.

Hayashi K, Miller RG, Brownell AK. (1989) Central core disease: ultrastructure of the sarcoplasmic reticulum and T-tubules. *Muscle Nerve* 12: 95–102.

Howes EL, Jr, Price HM, Blumberg JM, et al. (1966) Hypokalemic periodic paralysis. Electromicroscopic changes in the sarcoplasm. *Neurology* 16: 242–256.

Ikezoe K, Yac C, Momoi T, et al. (2000) A novel congenital myopathy with apoptotic changes. *Ann Neurology* 47: 531–536.

Jerusalem F, Engel AG, Gomez MR. (1973) Sarcotubular myopathy. A newly recognized, benign, congenital, familial muscle disease. *Neurology* 23: 897–906.

Kaplan JC, Fontaine B. (2001) Neuromuscular disorders gene location. *Neuromusc Dis* 11: 680–689.

Kyriacou K, Kassianides B, Hadjisavvas A, et al. (1997) The role of electron microscopy in the diagnosis of nonneoplastic muscle diseases. *Ultrastruct Pathol* 21: 243–252.

Kyriacou K, Mikellidou C, Hadjianastasiou A, et al. (1999) Ultrastructural diagnosis of mitochondrial encephalomyopathis revisited. *Ultrastrct Pathol* 23: 163–170.

Kyriakides T, Silberstein JM, Jongpiputvanich S, et al. (1993) The clinical significance of type 1 fiber predominance. *Muscle Nerve* 16: 418–423.

Lake BD, Wilson J. (1975) Zebra body myopathy; Clinical, histochemical and ultrastructural studies. *J Neurol Sci* 24: 437–446.

MacDonald RD, Engel AG. (1969) The cytoplasmic body: another structural anomaly of the Z-disk. *Acta Neuropathol (Berl)* 14: 99–107.

Mair WG, Tome FM. (1972) The ultrastructure of the adult and developing human myotendinous junction. *Acta Neuropathol* 21: 239–252.

Marbini A, Gemignani F, Badiali L, et al. (1998) Congenital myopathy with mosaic fibers and interlacing sarcomeres: a new structural myopathy. *Acta Neuropathol* 96: 643–650.

Middleton LT. (1997) Congenital myasthenic syndromes. In: Emery AEH, ed. *Diagnostic criteria for neuromuscular disorders.* London: RSM, pp. 91–97.

Morgan-Hughes JA. (1994) Mitochondrial diseases. In: Engel AG, Armstrong CF, eds. *Myology: basic and clinical.* New York: McGraw Hill, pp. 1600–1660.

Morris EP, Nneji G, Squire JM. (1990) The three dimensional structure of the nemaline rod Z-band. *J Cell Biol* 111: 2961–2978.

Mrak RE, Griebel M, Brodsky MC. (1996) Broad A band disease: a new benign congenital myopathy. *Muscle Nerve* 19: 587–594.

Nakano S, Engel AG, Waclawik AJ, et al. (1996) Myofibrillar myopathy with abnormal foci of desmin positivity. I. Light and electron microscopy analysis of 10 cases. *J Neuropathol Exp Neurol* 55: 549–562.

Neville HE, Brooke MH. (1971) Central core fibres: structured and unstructured. In: Kakulas BA, ed. *Basic research in myology.* Amsterdam: Excerpta Medica, pp. 497–511.

Patel H, Berry K, MacLeod P, et al. (1983) Cytoplasmic body myopathy. Report on a family and review of the literature. *J Neurol Sci* 60: 281–292.

Paulus W, Peiffer J, Becker I, et al. (1988) Adult-onset rod disease with abundant intranuclear rods. *J Neurol* 25: 343–347.

Reyes MG, Goldbarg H, Fresco K, et al. (1987) Zebra body myopathy; a second case of ultrastructurally distinct congenital myopathy. *J Child Neurol* 2: 307–310.

Ringel SP, Neville HE, Duster MC, et al. (1978) A new congenital neuromuscular disease with trilaminar muscle fibers. *Neurology* 28: 282–289.

Sabatelli P, Lattanzi G, Ognibene A, et al. (2001) Nuclear alterations in autosomal-dominant Emery–Dreifuss muscular dystrophy. *Muscle Nerve* 24: 826–829.

Santorelli FM, Sciacco M, Tanji K, et al. (1996) Multiple mitochondrial DNA deletions in sporadic inclusion body myositis: a study of 56 patients. *Ann Neurol* 39: 789–795.

Schochet SS, Lampert WD. (1978) Diagnostic electron microscopy of skeletal muscle. In: Trump BF, Jones RT, eds. *Diagnostic electron microscopy.* New York: J. Wiley and Sons, pp. 209–252.

Sewry CA. (1985) Ultrastructural changes in diseased muscle. In: Dubowitz V, ed. *Muscle biopsy: a practical approach.* London: Bailliere-Tindall, pp. 129–183.

Shy GM, Magee KR. (1956) A new congenital non-progressive myopathy. *Brain* 79: 610–621.

Shy GM, Engel WK, Somers JE, et al. (1963) Nemaline myopathy: a new congenital myopathy. *Brain* 86: 793–810.

Shy GM, Gonatas NK. (1964) Human myopathy with giant abnormal mitochondria. *Science* 145: 493–496.

Shy GM, Gonatas NK, Perez M. (1966) Two childhood myopathies with abnormal mitochondria, I: megaconial myopathy; II: pleoconial myopathy. *Brain* 89: 133–158.

Sigurd L, Land I, Torberg T, et al. (1992) Mitochondrial diseases and myopathies: a series of muscle biopsy specimens with ultrastructural changes in the mitochondria. *Ultrastruct Pathol* 16: 263–275.

Spiro AJ, Shy GM, Gonatas NK. (1966) Myotubular myopathy. Persistence of fetal muscle in an adolescent boy. *Arch Neurol* 14: 1–14.

Stadhouders AM, Sengers RC. (1987) Morphological observations in skeletal muscle from patients with a mitochondrial myopathy. *J Inherited Metabol Dis* 10 (Supp. l): 62–80.

Taratuto AL, Matteucci M, Barreiro C, et al. (1991) Autosomal dominant neuromuscular disease with cylindrical spirals. *Neuromusc Disord* 1: 433–441.

Tome FM, Fardeau M. (1973) "Fingerprint inclusions" in muscle fibres in dystrophia myotonic. *Acta Neuropathol* 24: 62–67.

Tome FM, Fardeau M. (1975) Congenital myopathy with "reducing bodies" in muscle fibres. *Acta Neuropathol* 31: 207–217.

Tome FM, Chateau D, Helbling-Leclerc A, et al. (1997) Morphological changes in muscle fibers in oculopharyngeal muscular dystrophy. *Neuromusc Disord* 7(Suppl 11):S63–9.

Van Wijngaarden GK, Fleury P, Bethlem J, et al. (1969) Familial "myotubular" myopathy. *Neurology* 19: 901–908.

Weller B, Carpenter S, Lochmuller H, et al. (1999) Myopathy with trabecular muscle fibers. *Neuromusc Disord* 9: 208–214.

43

Computed tomography as a diagnostic tool for skeletal muscle injury and pathology

Bret H. Goodpaster

Characterization of tissue composition in vivo

Basic principles of computed tomography imaging

Computed tomography (CT) is based on the mathematical principles proving that an accurate image of an object could be produced from a series of projections through that object. From its invention in 1972, CT has been used as a quantitative tool to provide information about the spatial arrangement of tissues and structures within the body. While a detailed explanation of the principles in CT imaging is beyond the scope of this chapter (for a more comprehensive description, see Bushberg et al 1994), a very basic description of CT will aid in the understanding of how it can provide important information about the structure and composition of skeletal muscle. In its fundamental form, a CT scanner involves a large number of X-ray projections around a patient, with multiple detectors and a computer interface to assimilate and compute the image.

The CT image represents a two-dimensional map (slice) of pixels (picture elements) at a location incident to the X-rays. This image corresponds to a three-dimensional section within a patient composed of an equal number of voxels (volume elements). The voxels have the same area as the pixels, but they also include the slice-thickness dimension, so that a given pixel on the image represents the average tissue properties within the voxel. Each pixel in the two-dimensional CT image has a specific number that corresponds to a specific location within the patient. The typical matrix of pixels is 512×512, and the range of numbers is from -1000 to $+3095$ (4096 values). The numerical value of each pixel within the matrix corresponds to a specific level of grey within the image. These values are called *CT numbers* or *Hounsfield Units* (HU), and they correspond to the linear attenuation coefficient which, in turn, depends on physical properties of tissue within the voxel.

CT can differentiate tissues in vivo based on their attenuation characteristics, which further depend on their density (Bushberg et al 1994). Increasing the density of a material within a voxel clearly increases its linear attenuation coefficient. Attenuation values (HU) on CT are based upon a linear attenuation coefficient scale using water as the reference (0 HU). CT can discern fat and muscle primarily because of

their widely different attenuation characteristics. Adipose tissue is less dense than water and displays attenuation values in the negative range (-190 to -30 HU). Muscle is more dense than water and has a positive attenuation (0 to 100 HU), so that areas of adipose tissue are darker, while muscle is lighter on a typical CT image of the lower extremity (Fig. 43.1). Bone has a very high attenuation on CT (>2000 HU) and, therefore, it is very bright on the image. Assuming proper quality control and periodic calibration of individual scanners, tissue attenuation values are highly reproducible within the same subject on the same scanner (Goodpaster et al 2000), given similar image acquisition parameters. Moreover, because of the inherent stability of the attenuation measure and the linear attenuation coefficient scale, the use of external calibration phantoms in CT is usually unnecessary for absolute quantification of attenuation values.

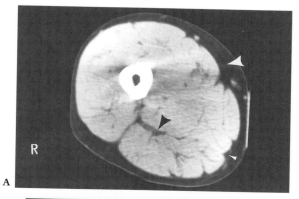

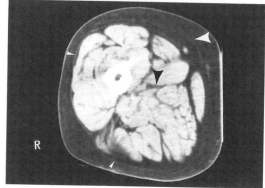

Figure 43.1—Representative mid-thigh computed tomography images in a lean (**A**) and an obese (**B**) volunteer, illustrating compartments of thigh muscle (grey) and adipose tissue (darker). The fascia lata (small white arrowhead) can be seen in these images, dividing subcutaneous (large white arrowhead) from intermuscular adipose tissue (large black arrowhead), which can be seen as pockets of fat infiltrating muscle tissue.

Skeletal muscle composition evaluated by computed tomography

Most CT software has the capability to precisely quantify specific tissue areas because of their inherent attenuation characteristics. For example, by selecting a range of attenuation values between 0 and 100 HU, which is representative of skeletal muscle, the computer simply calculates the number of pixels and the attenuation value for each pixel within this attenuation range. Each pixel has a defined area based on the imaging parameters, i.e. a 512×512 image matrix and 48 cm field of view will display a pixel area of 0.94 mm $\times 0.94$ mm. Therefore, the computer simply calculates the area of tissue represented within this defined range of attenuation values. Most CT scanners in use today have this capability to measure areas of muscle, fat and bone, and CT has been used extensively to measure areas of specific tissues (Borkan et al 1993, Trappe et al 1996, Goodpaster et al 1997, 2000a). In addition, many muscle injuries and diseases can be characterized by structures with particular attenuation characteristics recognizable by CT imaging, ultimately leading to their diagnoses.

The detailed spatial maps of attenuation coefficients within tissue can also be used to calculate the mean tissue attenuation value. The range of attenuation values within muscle may vary within an individual (Jones et al 1983, Nordal et al 1988, Liu et al 1993), and also between individuals (Sipila and Suominen 1995, Goodpaster et al 1997). The variability in muscle attenuation may emanate from alterations in the chemical composition of muscle. Lower muscle attenuation has been interpreted to reflect an increased lipid content within muscle (Jones et al 1983, Nordal et al 1988, Liu et al 1993, Sipila and Suominen 1995, Goodpaster et al 1997, 1999). This concept seems intuitive since adipose tissue is negative on CT, so that an increase in muscle lipid effectively reduces the attenuation of muscle. The findings of a reduced muscle attenuation are consistent with an increased muscle lipid content determined histochemically (Jones et al 1983, Goodpaster et al 2000b). In addition, increasing the lipid content of a chemical phantom by 1% results in a predictable 1 HU decrease in its mean attenuation (Goodpaster et al 2000c). Other muscle properties, such as water content, may influence the muscle attenuation characteristics. In addition, the lipid contained within muscle can not be directly assessed by CT. Nevertheless, as will be discussed more fully later in the chapter, CT represents a non-invasive means to provide valuable information about the composition of skeletal muscle in pathophysio-

logical conditions and in relation to impaired muscle metabolism and function.

Characterization of skeletal muscle injuries and pathologies

Diagnosis of muscle injury by computed tomography

Acute skeletal muscle injury or trauma can usually be identified on a CT image as a physical disruption or tear in the musculature and associated connective tissue. Although these are relatively extreme cases, diagnosis is usually fairly simple with appropriate CT or magnetic resonance imaging (MRI). Less severe muscle injuries, particularly acute muscle strains, can also be diagnosed by CT imaging as areas of hypodensity within muscle, 1–2 days following the injury (Garrett et al 1989). This suggests that acute inflammatory response and oedema are primary components of the injury, rather than bleeding as is often assumed (Garrett et al 1989). Diagnostic CT imaging studies are capable of localizing the muscle injury to specific muscle groups and showing the extent of the injury. Thus, CT may help to define appropriate treatment paradigms for specific injury. Moreover, CT and MRI may also be useful to predict functional outcome and prevention of similar injuries (Sallay et al 1996).

Skeletal muscle injury due to ischaemia has been evaluated with single photon emission CT to quantify the volume of muscle that takes up technetium-99 pyrophosphate above a baseline threshold, i.e. the localization and extent of injury (Forrest et al 1989). This method may help to predict muscle performance and clinical outcome following ischaemic injury (Yip et al 1992). This non-invasive imaging technique may permit accurate documentation of the extent of muscle necrosis or injury, to anticipate the impact of an ischaemia-reperfusion injury and formulate strategies for reducing the extent of post-ischaemic skeletal muscle necrosis.

Plain film and nuclear medicine bone scans are still the traditional imaging modalities used in the evaluation of musculoskeletal infection. However, CT has become critical in the delineation of many types of musculoskeletal infection, in particular, the evaluation of soft tissue infections, including cellulitis, myositis, fasciitis, abscess and septic arthritis (Ma et al 1997). CT has also been used to identify *pyomyositis*, a pyogenic infection in skeletal muscle, in a patient whose clinical symptoms were similar to those of deep venous thrombosis (Wang et al 1997).

Cross-sectional imaging modalities such as MRI or CT are excellent tools to diagnose muscle injury (Garrett et al 1989) and infection (Ma et al 1997) due to their excellent anatomic resolution and soft tissue contrast. However, it should be emphasized that even the most superb CT images, without the experienced radiologist to interpret them, are virtually useless. Indeed, clinical studies demonstrate that experience is not only helpful but indeed necessary in order to correctly identify muscle injury (Brandser et al 1995).

Computed tomography skeletal muscle composition is altered in neuromuscular pathologies

The general appearance of skeletal muscle on CT images is similar for most neuromuscular disorders. Although CT scanning is generally not diagnostic for these pathologies, distinctive skeletal muscle characteristics can be observed in patients presenting with neurologic disease (Nordal et al 1988), postpolio syndrome (Ivanyi et al 1998) or muscular dystrophy (Jones et al 1983, Liu et al 1993). Muscle atrophy is typical in these patients, owing to some primary defect in neuromuscular recruitment, activation or contraction. Another characteristic of muscle in these pathological conditions is a dramatic increase in fatty infiltration around and within muscle (Jones et al 1983, Nordal et al 1988, Liu et al 1993, Ivanyi et al 1998), as well as an alteration in the composition of muscle itself (Liu et al 1993). The alteration in muscle composition has been described in CT studies as muscle possessing lower than normal density or attenuation values. Interestingly, skeletal muscle in elderly individuals shares many similar muscle characteristics with these disease states (Borkan et al 1993, Sipila and Suominen 1995). Regardless of the predisposing factors leading to alterations in muscle structure, these skeletal muscle disorders are associated with diminished muscle function, and most certainly create a vicious cycle of disuse and further derangement unless appropriate interventions are introduced.

Association between altered muscle composition and function

Decreased muscle attenuation has been associated with lower strength (Nordal et al 1988, Liu et al 1993, Sipila and Suominen 1995). CT has been used to determine that symptomatic postpolio patients presented with decreased muscle attenuation compared with asymptomatic patients (Ivanyi et al 1998). In patients with muscular dystrophy, a reduced muscle attenuation is indicative of excess muscle lipid, and it is related to diminished muscular strength (Liu et al 1993). Progression in late polio involves decreased muscle area concomitant with an increase in muscle fatty infiltration and decreased muscle strength (Grimby et al 1996). In addition, recent evidence indicates that decreased muscle attenuation is related to the loss of strength in the elderly (Goodpaster et al 2001). These clinical studies clearly indicate that an altered composition of muscle, namely a decrease in the attenuation and not merely the loss of muscle mass, is a characteristic associated with a loss of strength. The question that, therefore, arises is whether these conditions can be reversed. Indeed, resistance training in elderly women increased both muscle attenuation and strength (Sipila and Suominen 1995), suggesting that the deterioration in muscle composition can be improved by appropriate intervention.

CT may provide information about skeletal muscle that may not be appreciated by simply assessing muscle quantity or function as an integrative measure. The advantage of using CT in assessing muscle composition is that characteristics of multiple muscle groups may be examined non-invasively in the same patient. Moreover, some diseases possess distinct characteristics not shared by other diseases. For example, specific muscle groups may be spared in severe myopathic conditions such as muscular dystrophy. In patients with adult onset acid maltase (Pompes disease) trunk and thigh muscles exhibited decreased attenuation (fatty replacement) whereas muscles of tensor fascia latae, biceps femoris, gracilis and sartorius were relatively spared. Again, the muscles with decreased attenuation were determined to be weaker (de Jager et al 1998). By knowing which muscles are adversely affected in specific myopathic conditions, perhaps more appropriate intervention strategies, such as electrical stimulation or physical therapy, may be applied to those affected areas. CT can identify atrophy or injury of specific muscle groups so that specific muscles may be targeted for restoration of function. The loss of muscle in old age, known as *sarcopenia*, may also benefit from this strategy.

Lower muscle attenuation is associated with impaired metabolic function

Examining the attenuation characteristics of skeletal muscle has also provided novel information about the composition of skeletal muscle in individuals with impaired metabolic function. Kelley et al (1991) found that obese individuals have an increase in muscle area but a reduced mean muscle attenuation. The increased muscle area was a result of an increase in muscle with a reduced density, while the area of muscle with normal density was unaffected by obesity. Skeletal-muscle attenuation, as a marker of increased muscle lipid, is reduced in obesity (Goodpaster et al 1997) and in type 2 diabetes mellitus (Goodpaster et al 2000a), and it is strongly associated with insulin resistance (Goodpaster et al 1997). These findings are consistent with others who found an association between the triglyceride content of skeletal muscle and insulin resistance independent of obesity (Pan et al 1997). Reduced muscle attenuation also is associated with reduced fatty acid oxidation (Kelley et al 1999), oxidative enzyme capacity (Simoneau et al 1995) and low physical fitness (Goodpaster et al 1997).

The alteration in muscle composition observed in these pathophysiological conditions can also be partially reversed. For example, obese individuals participating in a 16 week clinical weight-loss programme had an increase in the mean muscle attenuation (Goodpaster et al 1999), a result congruous with a decrease in lipid contained within their muscle fibres (Goodpaster et al 2000b). In addition, the decrease in muscle area during weight loss in this study was due entirely to a decrease in the area of low-density muscle, while the area of muscle within the normal attenuation range remained unchanged. These studies illustrate how CT can detect individual differences in muscle composition and changes as a result of clinical interventions. Thus, CT has been a valuable tool to advance our understanding of the association between the structure of skeletal muscle and its metabolic and functional capacity.

Advanced computed tomography imaging methods

Recent advances in CT technology have permitted more rapid and detailed examination of the musculoskeletal system. Perhaps the best example of these advances is the advent and application of spiral or helical CT scanning, a method in which ultrafast imaging is conducted, obtaining significantly more information about the structure and composition of tissue in far less time. Spiral CT is a powerful modality for evaluation of the musculoskeletal system (Pretorius and Fishman 1999), particularly when coupled with volume-rendering reconstruction techniques made available to many clinicians through powerful desktop computers. After acquiring a set of axial images, a volume of interest can be reconstructed through interpolation and the appropriate computer algorithm, a process known as volume rendering. In many cases, using volume-rendered spiral CT in routine musculoskeletal imaging protocols can change the approach to management (Pretorius and Fishman 1999). Small fractures and complex injuries may be more obvious on volume-rendered images, and so they can be easily demonstrated to the orthopaedic surgeons. Evaluation of suspected infectious or neoplastic disease is also aided by including volume-rendered imaging in the musculoskeletal spiral CT examination. The extent of disease can be thoroughly evaluated with volume-rendered images, and therapeutic strategies are aided by the anatomic information available from volume-rendered images (Pretorius and Fishman 1999).

Summary

CT is clearly a valuable non-invasive imaging method to examine the quantity, structure and composition of skeletal muscle in vivo. Its widespread availability and relatively low cost make its use practical for the diagnosis of muscle injury and disease. CT has also proven to be a powerful research tool, and it has aided our understanding of the association between the structure of skeletal muscle and its metabolic and functional capacity. This knowledge can ultimately assist in the design of appropriate interventions to improve or prevent deterioration in muscle function.

References

Borkan GA, Hults DE, Gerzof SG, Robbins AH, Silbert CK. (1993) Age changes in body composition revealed by computed tomography. *J Gerontol* 38: 673–677.

Brandser EA, el-Khoury GY, Kathol MH, Callaghan JJ, Tearse DS. (1995) Hamstring injuries: radiographic, conventional tomographic, CT, and MR imaging characteristics. *Radiology* 197: 257–262.

Bushberg JT, Seibert JA, Leidholdt EMJ, Boone JM. (1994) X-ray computed tomography. In: The essentials of medical imaging. Passano WM, ed. Baltimore: Williams & Wilkins, pp. 239–289.

de Jager AE, van der Vliet TM, van der Ree TC, Oosterink BJ, Loonen MC. (1998) Muscle computed tomography in adult-onset acid maltase deficiency. *Muscle Nerve* 21: 398–400.

Forrest I, Hayes G, Smith A, Yip TC, Walker PM. (1989) Identification of clinically significant skeletal muscle necrosis by single photon emission computed tomography. *Can J Surg* 32: 109–112.

Garrett WE, Jr, Rich FR, Nikolaou PK, Vogler JBd. (1989) Computed tomography of hamstring muscle strains. *Med Sci Sports Exercise* 21: 506–514.

Goodpaster BH, Carlson CL, Visser M, et al. (2001) Attenuation of skeletal muscle and strength in the elderly: The Health ABC Study. *J Appl Physiol* 90: 2157–2165.

Goodpaster BH, Kelley DE, Thaete FL, He J, Ross R. (2000) Skeletal muscle attenuation determined by computed tomography is associated with skeletal muscle lipid content. *J Appl Physiol* 89: 104–110.

Goodpaster BH, Thaete FL, Simoneau J-A, Kelley DE. (1997) Subcutaneous abdominal fat and thigh muscle composition predict insulin sensitivity independently of visceral fat. *Diabetes* 46: 1579–1585.

Goodpaster BH, Kelley DE, Wing RR, Meier A, Thaete FL. (1999) Effects of weight loss on regional fat distribution and insulin sensitivity in obesity. *Diabetes* 48: 839–847.

Goodpaster BH, Thaete FL, Kelley DE. (2000a) Thigh adipose tissue distribution is associated with insulin resistance in obesity and in type 2 diabetes mellitus(1). *Am J Clin Nutr* 71: 885–892.

Goodpaster BH, Theriault R, Watkins SC, Kelley DE. (2000b) Intramuscular lipid content is increased in obesity and decreased by weight loss. *Metabolism* 49: 467–472.

Grimby G, Kvist H, Grangard U. (1996) Reduction in thigh muscle cross-sectional area and strength in a 4-year follow-up in late polio. *Arch Phys Med Rehab* 77: 1044–1048.

Ivanyi B, Redekop W, de Jongh R, de Visser M. (1998) Computed tomographic study of the skeletal musculature of the lower body in 45 postpolio patients. *Muscle Nerve* 21: 540–542.

Jones DA, Round JM, Edwards RH, Grindwood SR, Tofts PS. (1983) Size and composition of the calf and quadriceps muscles in Duchenne muscular dystrophy. A tomographic and histochemical study. *J Neurol Sci* 60: 307–322.

Kelley DE, Slasky BS, Janosky J. (1991) Skeletal muscle density: effects of obesity and non-insulin-dependent diabetes mellitus. *Am J Clin Nutrition* 54: 509–515

Kelley DE, Goodpaster B, Wing RR, Simoneau J-A. (1999) Skeletal Muscle Fatty Acid Metabolism in Association with Insulin Resistance, Obesity and Weight Loss. *Am J Physiol (Endocrinol Metab)* 277: E1130–E1141.

Liu M, Chino N, Ishihara T. (1993) Muscle damage progression in Duchenne muscular dystrophy evaluated by a new quantitative computed tomography method. *Arch Phys Med Rehab* 74: 507–514.

Ma LD, Frassica FJ, Bluemke DA, Fishman EK. (1997) CT and MRI evaluation of musculoskeletal infection. [Review: 15 refs]. *Crit Rev Diagnost Imaging* 38: 535–568.

Nordal HJ, Dietrichson P, Eldevik P, Gronseth K. (1988) Fat infiltration, atrophy and hypertrophy of skeletal muscles demonstrated by X-ray computed tomography in neurological patients. *Acta Neurol Scand* 77: 115–122.

Pan DA, Lillioja S, Kriketos AD, et al. (1997) Skeletal muscle triglyceride levels are inversely related to insulin action. *Diabetes* 46: 983–988.

Pretorius ES, Fishman EK. (1999) Volume-rendered three-dimensional spiral CT: musculoskeletal applications. *Radiographics* 19: 1143–1160.

Sallay PI, Friedman RL, Coogan PG, Garrett WE. (1996) Hamstring muscle injuries among water skiers. Functional outcome and prevention. *Am J Sports Med* 24: 130–136.

Simoneau JA, Colberg SR, Thaete FL, Kelley DE. (1995) Skeletal muscle glycolytic and oxidative enzyme capacities are determinants of insulin sensitivity and muscle composition in obese women. *FASEB J* 9: 273–278.

Sipila S, Suominen H. (1995) Effects of strength and endurance training on thigh and leg muscle mass and composition in elderly women. *J Appl Physiol* 78: 334–340.

Trappe SW, Costill DL, Goodpaster BH, Pearson DR. (1996) Calf muscle strength in former elite distance runners. *Scand J Med Sci Sport* 6: 205–210.

Wang KC, Fang CM, Chen WJ, Lee SS, Yang WE, Shih CH. (1997) Pyomyositis of the calf muscles mimicking distal deep venous thrombosis: a case report. *Am J Orthoped* 26: 358–359.

Yip TC, Houle S, Tittley JG, Walker PM. (1992) Quantification of skeletal muscle necrosis in the lower extremities using 99Tcm pyrophosphate with single photon emission computed tomography. *Nuclear Med Comm* 13: 47–52.

44

Biochemical markers of skeletal muscle disease

Stephan Sorichter

Introduction

Skeletal muscle disease can be caused by various factors, for example mutations in the genes that encode components of the striated muscle fibre (i.e., dystrophin–glycoprotein complex). However, skeletal muscle disease or injury more often results from muscular overuse, which produces temporary skeletal muscle damage. This chapter will focus on the diagnostic power of biochemical markers to diagnose skeletal muscle disease induced by muscular overuse. Therefore, a brief review of the pathomechanism of the exercise-induced muscle damage is prefixed.

Exercise-induced muscle injury

After a bout of intensive and unaccustomed exercise, the involved muscles feel weak, and over the next days the muscles also become sore and tender. Additional clinical symptoms are muscle swelling and stiffness (Howell et al 1993), temporary reduction in force production and delayed onset muscle soreness (DOMS; Friden et al 1983, Mair et al 1992, Sorichter et al 1995) which are (patho)-physiological manifestations of skeletal muscle damage.

Exercise-induced muscle fibre damage has been reported after several types of exercise in both animals and humans (Ebbeling and Clarkson 1989, Lieber and Friden 1999), however, there is clear evidence that eccentric biased exercise produces more fibre damage than concentric biased exercise (Stauber 1989). The main reason for this difference is that mechanical, and not metabolic, stress of exercised skeletal muscles is the major contributing factor for inducing muscle damage (Clarkson 1997, Lieber and Friden 1999). Currently, it is well accepted that unaccustomed, high force eccentric action leads to skeletal muscle damage, which can be observed as Z-line streaming and myofibrillar disruption at the cellular level (Friden and Lieber 1992), resulting in structural damage of the contractile apparatus.

Eccentric muscle action is characterized by elongation of the muscle during contraction (Asmussen 1953). This results, at identical forces, in a higher tension per active unit compared with concentric muscle action (Abbott et al 1952, Asmussen 1953). In general, there could be some random variations in sarcomere strength. As the fibre lengthens, some of the weakest sarcomeres will become unable to maintain tension, leaving the passive structures to provide the necessary support. Repeated active lengthening would thus stretch the weak sarcomeres and place stress on the adjacent myofibres leading to sarcomere damage. This is supported by the observations of stretched-out sarcomeres after forced lengthening (Talbot and Morgan 1996) and the increased muscle fibre damage after eccentric muscle actions performed at a long muscle length, compared with exercise at a short length (Newham et al 1988).

This exercise-induced muscle damage activates a cascade of reactions, resulting in an activated skeletal muscle protein metabolism. The initial damage appears to disrupt the cytoskeleton and sarcolemma of the fibre such that there is a loss of the cytoskeletal protein desmin staining from the intracellular area (Lieber et al 1996, Friden and Lieber 1998). Desmin plays a role in the mechanical integration of adjacent myofibrils by connecting them at the Z line. Subsequent damage can then result from increased intracellular calcium (Armstrong 1990) which can activate Ca^{2+} sensitive degradative pathways such as the non-lysosomal cysteine protease calpain. Because calpain cleaves a variety of protein substrates, including cytoskeletal proteins like desmin, α-actinin, vimentin and integrin, and myofibrillar proteins such as troponin and tropomyosin (Saido et al 1994), calpain-mediated degradation is thought to contribute to the changes in muscle structure and function that occur immediately following exercise (Belcastro et al 1998). Therefore, calpain may play a key role in the disassembly and remodelling of the cytoskeletal matrix (Belcastro et al 1998), and reports of the transient and specific removal of Z lines from striated muscle led to the suggestion that calpain initiates the metabolic turnover of myofibril proteins by releasing them from their filamentous structure (Goll et al 1992, Belcastro et al 1994). However, calpain does not degrade proteins to small peptides or amino acids (Belcastro et al 1998). Therefore, it is possible to detect such proteins in peripheral blood after cleavage using specific assays. Examples include troponin I (TnI) and myosin heavy chains (MHC), which are predominantly structurally bound proteins of the contractile apparatus, and which have been described as markers of skeletal muscle injury (Mair et al 1992, Takahashi et al 1996, Sorichter et al 1997a).

A prolonged, complex interaction between protein synthesis and degradation occurs following the initial exercise-induced muscle fibre damage, which was registered by measurement of ^{13}C-leucine after constant infusion and urinary excretion of 3-methylhistidine (3-MEH) (Young and Munro 1978, Fielding et al 1991, Fielding and Evans 1997).

Also infiltration of several types of inflammatory cell into skeletal muscle and secretion of interleukin-1β (IL-1β) occurs after eccentric muscle action (Armstrong et al 1983, Hikida et al 1983). Local IL-6 production, which has been suggested to play a key role in the post-exercise alterations in skeletal muscle, is stimulated within the skeletal muscle following the destruction of muscle fibres (Rohde et al 1997). In addition, it has been shown that muscular heat shock proteins of the highly conserved 70 kD family (i.e., HSP72), stress proteins that guarantee intracellular protein homeostasis, increase during unaccustomed exercise (Puntschart et al 1996) and after intensive training sessions (Liu et al 1999), depending on the exercise intensity (Liu et al 2000). Also HSP72 gene expression increases progressively during prolonged, exhaustive exercise (Febbraio and Koukoulas 2000).

Neutrophil accumulation into striated muscle is the first part of the immunological process, and it appears simultaneously with the morphological changes at the cellular level. This is followed by macrophages that remove debris and, finally, by macrophage subpopulations that are associated with regeneration of fibres (Lowe et al 1995, MacIntyre et al 1995, 1996, 2001, Tidball 1995). It has also been speculated that there is a relationship between Ca^{2+}-stimulated proteolysis and neutrophil accumulation in striated muscle following exercise, and that the calpain system is involved in directing the neutrophilic response with exercise (Raj et al 1998). Prior to the intracellular infiltration, changes in the numbers of inflammatory cells in the peripheral blood can be observed (Malm et al 1999). The repeatedly described exercise-induced leukocytosis with increased numbers of neutrophils, monocytes and lymphocytes is accompanied or induced by changes in cytokines and the neuro-endocrine system. Increases in plasma concentrations of interleukins (IL-1, IL-1β, IL-6) and tumour necrosis factor (TNF-α) have been described after high mechanical load (Cannon et al 1989, 1991, Northoff and Berg 1991, Ullum et al 1994, Smith et al 2000). However, these elevations were modest compared with cytokine levels seen after strenous endurance exercise.

In conclusion, the development of muscle damage after unaccustomed muscle action seems to be a complex network of different mechanisms. To verify muscle damage and to monitor the amount, objective markers of muscle damage are needed. To estimate skeletal muscle damage, measurement of muscle proteins is a common method, and various muscle proteins have been used for this purpose.

Biochemical markers of skeletal muscle damage

Damage to skeletal muscle fibre structures could be documented from a histopathological point of view (Armstrong et al 1983), by biochemical estimators (Sorichter et al 1997a) or, in a non-invasive manner, by using imaging techniques, such as resonance imaging or ultrasonography (Mair et al 1992). Histopathological changes are often absent in the early phase of skeletal muscle fibre damage. Therefore, specific immunohistochemical stainings of certain structural elements of myofibre microarchitecture have proven to be an excellent tool to estimate early muscle fibre damage (Komulainen et al 1998b). Using this technique, specific antibodies against structural proteins such as actin, desmin, dystrophin, fibronectin or nebulin can be utilized, and studies provide evidence that the early phase of myofibre structure disruption plays a central role in the ensuing damage of the skeletal muscle fibre (Huang and Forsberg 1998, Komulainen et al 1998b). Invasive techniques like skeletal muscle biopsies have broadened the insight into the mechanisms of exercise-induced muscle damage. However, these tools are not available for routine diagnosis of skeletal muscle damage; this requires analytic tools that can be used quickly and easily. Measurements of plasma activities or concentrations of certain muscle proteins are common methods for determining muscle fibre damage (Sorichter et al 1999). However, to meet the clinical and/or scientific requirements an ideal marker should:

1. be absolutely muscle fibre specific to allow reliable diagnosis of the skeletal muscle fibre type injury
2. have a broad diagnostic window to allow early as well as late diagnosis
3. be highly sensitive, the marker should detect even small damage
4. be stable and the measurement rapid (a whole-blood assay would be desirable), easy to perform, quantitative and finally inexpensive.

It is also necessary that the marker is not, or barely, detectable in patients without damage of skeletal muscle fibres and that high amounts are present in the skeletal myocytes, which results in a high plasma entry ratio after muscle fibre damage with high diagnostic sensitivity.

A single marker may not fulfil all of these criteria, and, therefore, a combination of markers may be necessary. Some of the currently used markers are given in Table 44.1 and discussed below.

Table 44.1 — Currently used estimators of skeletal muscle damage in blood plasma

Protein[a]	Location	Molecular weight (kD)	Time to peak concentration (h)	Half-life (h)	Specificity for skeletal muscle
CK	Cytoplasm	86	3–12	17	No
Myoglobin	Cytoplasm	17.8	2–6	0.25	No
H–FABP	Cytoplasm	15	2–5	0.3	No
CA III	Cytoplasm	29	2–6	0.3	Yes
MHC	Myofibril	230	24–48	>48	No
TnI	Myofibril	24	3–8	2–4	Yes

[a]CK, creatine kinase; H-FABP, heart type fatty acid binding protein; CA-III, carbonic anhydrase III; MHC, myosin heavy chains; TnI, skeletal troponin I.

Cytoplasmic proteins

Aspartate aminotransferase

Aspartate aminotransferase (ASAT) was the first marker used for the laboratory diagnosis of muscle injury, especially for acute myocardial infarction (AMI; Ladue et al 1954). ASAT lacks muscle fibre type specificity, and it no longer has clinical significance for the diagnosis of muscle fibre injury.

Lactate dehydrogenase

Lactate dehydrogenase (LDH) is an important enzyme of glucose metabolism. Significant LDH activities are found in almost every tissue with its highest activities in skeletal muscle, liver, heart, kidneys, brain, lungs and erythrocytes. LDH exists as a tetramer, which is composed of two different subunits: M (muscle) and H (heart). There are five isoenzymes, and the tissue distribution of LDH isoenzymes and their kinetic properties reflect the metabolic requirements. The expression of the M subunit is an adaptation to enhanced use of anaerobic glycogenolysis for energy supply, because these isoenzymes have their maximal activity at high pyruvate concentrations. Chronically stressed skeletal muscle (chronic muscle disease, recurrent skeletal muscle injury) re-expresses LDH-1 and LDH-2 isoenzymes predominately with H subunits. Slow-twitch skeletal muscle fibres show a relatively constant state of tonic activity, and they have a LDH isoenzyme pattern similar to that of myocardium where LDH-1 is predominant (35–70% of total LDH activity) (Lee and Goldman 1986, Adams et al 1993, Mair et al 1994). Similar to ASAT, LDH has no, or only minor, scientific or clinical significance for the diagnosis of muscle fibre injury.

Creatine kinase

A key enzyme in cellular energetics and in muscular metabolism is Creatine kinase (CK). It catalyses the reversible transfer of a phosphate residue in high energy binding between adenosine triphosphate (ATP) and creatine, and functions mainly as a temporary energy buffer and for the transfer of energy from the mitochondria to the cytosol. There are two forms, cytosolic and mitochondrial CK. Cytosolic CK is a dimeric molecule which is composed of either B subunits (brain form) or M subunits (muscle form); there are three isoenzymes: CKBB (CK-1), CKMB (CK-2), and CKMM (CK-3). Cytosolic CK shows significant binding to myofibrils in skeletal and heart muscle. The mitochondrial form of the enzyme is also a dimer and probably consists of two identical subunits (CK-Mi). Clinically significant amounts of CK activity are found only in skeletal muscle, heart, brain, gut and pregnant uterus, the highest concentration being found in skeletal muscle (Neumaier 1981). CKMM accounts for almost all of the CK activity in skeletal muscle. The CKMB content of skeletal muscle varies depending on the proportion of slow-twitch fibres, which contain up to 5–10% CKMB, whereas fast-twitch fibres contain about 1–3% or less (Neumaier 1981, Ingwall et al 1985). Apple et al have demonstrated a correlation between slow-twitch fibre content and CKMB content in gastrocnemius biopsies of long distance runners, as endurance training accumulates CKMB in skeletal muscle, which may reach myocardial levels (Apple et al 1984). Therefore, elevated CKMB levels after muscular strain in endurance trained athletes should be interpreted as an indicator of skeletal muscle injury. Chronic degeneration and regeneration of skeletal muscle also leads to a marked increase in CKMB content. In chronic muscle injury, such as Duchenne's muscular dystrophy, the CKMB content of skeletal muscle may reach up to 10–50% of total CK activity (Somer et al 1976).

Creatine kinase serum isoforms

One way to increase the diagnostic sensitivity of CK is to determine its isoforms in plasma (Puleo et al 1990). CK serum isoforms are part of the usual clearance process of the CK isoenzymes, and they are present in all human sera. After release from the tissue the carboxy-terminal lysine is cleaved from the subunits by carboxypeptidase (Puleo et al 1990). There are at least two CKMB and three CKMM isoforms. The most frequently applied method for routine measurement is high-voltage electrophoresis, which separates five isoforms. Additional isoforms can be detected by more sophisticated techniques, such as isoelectric focusing. However, these methods are not suitable for the routine laboratory. Immunological methods frequently lack the desirable CK isoform specificity. A MM_3/MM_1 ratio greater than 0.7 in plasma indicates skeletal muscle damage (Mair et al 1995), and the MM_1/MM_3 ratio could be used to indicate periods of release and clearance (Hyatt and Clarkson 1998).

Myoglobin

Myoglobin is an oxygen-binding haem protein of striated muscles, that serves as an oxygen reservoir within the muscle fibre and facilitates oxygen diffusion in striated muscle fibres. It is exclusively found in striated muscles, where it accounts for up to 5–10% of all cytoplasmic proteins. Myoglobin is rapidly released after muscle damage, but it is not muscle fibre type-specific. However, nowadays rapid, quantitative, and automated assays are available (immunonephelometry, immunoturbidimetry, rapid enzymeimmunoassays) to measure myoglobin concentration within a few minutes (Delanghe et al 1990, Mair et al 1992).

Fatty acid binding protein

Fatty acid binding protein (FABP) is involved in the cellular uptake, transport, and metabolism of fatty acids (Glatz and Van 1990, Kleine et al 1992). From the sarcolemmal and the cytoplasmic FABPs, only cytoplasmic FABP was evaluated as a marker for muscle fibre damage. Named after the tissue of their first identification, which in general is the tissue of their greatest abundance, six distinct types (e.g. intestine, liver, heart) of the small (15 kD) cytoplasmic FABP have been identified (Glatz and Van 1990). It was pos-

sible to develop specific monoclonal antibodies against FABP of the heart (H-FABP; Ohkaru et al 1995, Roos et al 1995). However, H-FABPs are also found in considerable amounts in kidneys and skeletal muscle, although with concentrations much lower than in heart (Glatz and Van 1990).

H-FABP shows a similar pattern of release into and clearance from plasma after skeletal muscle injury as myoglobin (Sorichter et al 1998). H-FABP increases rapidly after injury, usually between 2–4 h, in parallel with myoglobin, and peak values occur about 5–10 h later. Lack of muscle type specificity of both markers may be eliminated by the calculation of the myoglobin over H-FABP ratio, as different tissue ratios of myoglobin over H-FABP in heart and skeletal muscle are reflected by differences in ratios of plasma concentrations of both proteins after damage of skeletal (20–70 depending on fibre-type composition) and heart muscle (approximately 4–5) (Van Nieuwenhoven et al 1995).

Carbonic anhydrase

The carbonic anhydrase (CA) is a soluble protein (MW: 29 kD) that efficiently catalyses the hydration of CO_2 to bicarbonate and a proton. Therefore, it is involved in many biochemical processes such as pH regulation, CO_2 and bicarbonate transport, ion transport, and water and electrolyte balance, as well as in ureagenesis, gluconeogenesis and lipogenesis (Jeffery et al 1980, Sly and Hu 1995). Seven CA isoenzymes (I–VII) are encoded by one gene family (Sly and Hu 1995) and these isoenzymes differ in structure, kinetics, subcellular localization and in tissue-specific distribution. The major site of CA-III expression is skeletal muscle (mainly slow-twitch skeletal muscle fibres), but CA-III is not expressed in human myocardium (Jeffery et al 1980, Sly and Hu 1995). Therefore CA-III may gain significance as a marker of skeletal muscle injury, since the diversity among different CA isoenzymes is large enough to produce CA-III specific antibodies (Vaananen et al 1990).

Measurement of CA-III and calculation of the myoglobin over CA-III ratio is another way proposed to increase the muscle type specificity of myoglobin measurements (Beuerle et al 2000).

Structurally bound proteins

The structurally bound contractile and regulatory proteins are among the most abundant proteins in myocytes. These proteins are highly organised in striated muscles, with the sarcomere being the basic structure, which is formed by the geometric arrangement of thick and thin filaments. Thin filaments contain actin and the troponin–tropomyosin regulatory complexes.

Troponin complex

The troponin complex is not present in smooth muscle. It comprises 3 polypeptides (Farah and Reinach 1995).

1. Troponin C (TnC; MW, 18 kD) binds calcium and is responsible for regulating the process of thin filament activation during skeletal and heart muscle contraction (Parmacek and Leiden 1991). TnC can bind up to four calcium ions, and subsequently relieve the inhibition of actin–myosin interaction by inducing a steric shift and reversing the inhibitory activity of troponin I.

2. Troponin I (TnI; MW, 24 kD) is a basic globular protein that prevents contraction in the absence of calcium and TnC, by inhibiting actomyosin ATPase, and thereby blocks myosin movement. This prevents the coupling of actin and myosin.

3. Troponin T (TnT; MW, 37 kD) has a binding site for tropomyosin, and it is thought to be responsible for binding the troponin complex to tropomyosin, thereby positioning the complex onto the thin filaments (Raggi et al 1989).

Myosin

The thick filaments appear to be the major element in energy transduction and strength development. They are composed of myosin molecules. Myosin molecules themselves are highly asymmetric hexametric proteins that consist in their monomeric form of two heavy chains (MHC; MW, approximately 23 kD each) and four light chains (MLC). Both filaments are involved in the sliding filament model of muscle contraction (Cooke 1995), which includes the calcium-mediated regulation of actin–myosin interaction. The functional differences between the muscular types are based on important structural differences. The polymorphic forms of myofibrillar proteins of striated muscle are, among other factors, responsible for the different contractile properties of striated muscle types. For example, the isomyosins are structurally and enzymatically different, and the ATPase activity of myosin is correlated with the speed of muscle shortening. Polymorphic forms of contractile and regulatory proteins are derived from different genes and vary in their tissue distribution, especially between fast-twitch skeletal and cardiac muscle. The tissue-specific isoforms differ in structure and functional properties, and con-

sequently these antigens may be differentiated by immunologic methods. However, gene regulation of contractile proteins is complex. Striking is the degree to which, slow and fast skeletal and cardiac muscle genes are co-expressed or have "overlapping" expression, particularly between myocardium and slow-twitch skeletal muscle fibres. Neither human α- nor β-type MHC are muscle type-specific proteins (Diederich et al 1989, Bredman et al 1991). We found no evidence for a significant soluble MHC pool in the sarcoplasm in skeletal (Sorichter et al 1997a) or heart muscle (Bleier et al 1998), and all MHC of muscle fibres appears to be structurally bound. Therefore, this protein is expected to specifically indicate muscle fibre necrosis. As a consequence of its tissue distribution, all MHC assays described in the literature so far (Larue et al 1991, Simeonova et al 1991), show considerable cross-reaction with MHC from skeletal muscle and cardiac muscle. Increases were found after skeletal and cardiac muscle damage (Mair et al 1994, Sorichter et al 1997a) and a close correlation to changes shown by magnetic resonance imaging (MRI) has been reported (Sorichter et al 2001b). Yet, cardiac MLC, cardiac β-type MHC (the predominant MHC-type in human adult healthy and diseased myocardium), cardiac α-actin, cardiac tropomyosin, as well as cardiac TnC are co-expressed in slow-twitch skeletal muscle fibres (Cummins 1979, Barton et al 1985, Collins et al 1986, Yamauchi-Takihara et al 1989, Parmacek and Leiden 1991, Schwartz et al 1992, Schiaffino and Reggiani 1996, Pette 1998). Therefore, these proteins cannot provide absolute muscle type-specificity despite the application of highly specific monoclonal antibodies in corresponding assays. There remain only two candidates for muscle type-specific markers: TnI and TnT. Both exist in three different isoforms, each with a unique structure—one for slow-twitch skeletal muscle, one for fast-twitch skeletal muscle and one for cardiac muscle (Wilkinson and Grand 1978, Pearlstone et al 1986)—since the isoforms are encoded by three different genes.

Release of biochemical markers after unaccustomed (eccentric) muscle action

Unaccustomed (eccentric) muscle action results in a plasma increase, with a varying delay, of the above mentioned muscle damage markers. This is independent of the exercised muscle group and mass, the intensity of the exercise task, the lengthening of the exercised muscles and the previous individual activity level of the subjects. The small cytoplasmatic proteins myoglobin and H-FABP show a very early increase with a peak after 2 h, followed by a rapid decrease within 24 h after the exercise as they are rapidly cleared from the plasma by the kidneys (Klocke et al 1982). CK, which is bigger than myoglobin and H-FABP, shows a later increase and a delayed decrease over several days. None of these three markers is muscle type specific. Until now, plasma CK activity has been used most frequently. However, there are several observations on the variability of CK activity responses after exercise-induced muscle injury, which preclude a simple interpretation of increased CK activity, especially with regard to the magnitude of injury. This applies also for myoglobin, H-FABP and CA-III. CA-III changes are usually rather similar to those of CK (Komulainen et al 1994a). In addition, LDH activity starts to increase 6–12 h after exercise-induced muscle damage and returns to baseline 8–14 days later due to its slow catabolism. An explanation could be that the exercise-induced release of the predominantly cytoplasmic proteins can be, in principle, caused by either temporary muscle fibre damage accompanied by membrane leakage with subsequent resealing of the membrane, or caused by a final death of the muscle fibre (McNeil and Khakee 1992). In addition, there is a clear influence of gender (Komulainen et al 1999, Sorichter et al 2001a) and race (Schwane et al 2000) on the basal levels and peak values of cytoplasmic muscle proteins. In general, females have lower resting and peak values than male subjects in cytoplasmic proteins. Basal peak values of plasma CK activity in African men is higher compared with the basal values of comparable Caucasian subjects (Schwane et al 2000). However, the plasma CK response is similar to responses of comparable Causacian subjects (Schwane et al 2000). H-FABP and myoglobin allow earlier assessment of exercise-induced muscle damage than does CK, and the simultaneous measurement of both markers could improve the muscle type specificity by calculation of the myoglobin over H-FABP ratio. Therefore, it is suggested that the combination of these two markers could help to avoid over-training and allow early control of specific training sessions, for example, negative workouts (Sorichter et al 1998).

To extend the sensitivity and specificity of tests for detecting skeletal muscle fibre injury, new assays using predominantly structurally bound proteins are being developed. The release of proteins, such as skeletal TnI (sTnI) and MHC, requires both enzymatic degradation and a leaky plasma membrane, which indicate severe damage to muscle fibres. MHC fragments appear in the circulation about 1–3 days after the onset of muscle damage and they are detectable for up to about 10 days (Mair et al 1992) with a monophasic time course. Thus, MHC shows a delayed increase with late peak values in plasma and, therefore, is not suitable for early diagnosis of exercise-induced muscle damage. Additionally, the complexity of MHC isoforms and their expression patterns in striated muscles (Leger et al 1985, Larue et al 1991, Mair et al 1992) makes it difficult to develop an assay that specifically identifies skeletal muscle damage. In contrast to MHC, sTnI is an early marker of exercise-induced muscle injury (Sorichter et al 1997a). The very early release of sTnI after unaccustomed eccentric muscle action may be explained partially by the relatively small cytosolic sTnI pool of 3–4% of the total sTnI content of the skeletal muscle fibres (Sorichter et al 1997a), but other mechanisms must be also involved in its early release in high amounts. In contrast to MHC, sTnI is particularly susceptible to calpain digestion (Belcastro et al 1993, Di Lisa et al 1995), which may contribute to the early increase in sTnI plasma levels after unaccustomed eccentric muscle action. Both markers show a minor influence of gender on basal levels and peak values after unaccustomed exercise (Sorichter et al 2001a). Currently, however, only research assays of sTnI are used to define skeletal muscle damage (Takahashi et al 1996, Sorichter et al 1997a). Simpson et al have shown, using Western blot analysis, that after hypoxaemia-induced muscle damage in canine diaphragm complexes containing sTnI-fragments with higher molecular mass were formed in the stressed muscle (Simpson et al 2000). Therefore, the development of new sTnI or sTnT assays with the possibility of differentiating damage of slow- and fast-twitch fibres, and which exclude cross-reaction with protein-complexes containing sTnI-fragments, will improve the diagnosis of skeletal muscle damage.

Summary

High-force unaccustomed muscle action, especially with eccentric contractions, leads to skeletal muscle damage that can be observed as Z-line streaming and myofibrillar disruption at the cellular level. These changes are accompanied by an increase in muscle-derived proteins in blood plasma, which are useful markers of the skeletal muscle injury. It is certainly of benefit if a plasma marker of exercise-induced skeletal muscle damage can reflect the rapid derangement of the contractile apparatus. Cytosolic proteins such as CK, LDH, myoglobin, H-FABP and CA-III are limited by their weak correlations with histologically quantified muscle fibre damage and, with the exception of CA-III, they are missing muscle fibre-type specificity. The release of predominantly structurally bound proteins, such as sTnI and MHC, requires both enzymatic degradation and a leaky plasma membrane, which indicates severe damage to muscle fibres. Skeletal TnI indicates alterations of the thin–filament troponin complex and has a broad diagnostic window. TnI peaks within 24 h and stays elevated for at least 1–2 days, and it is unique for skeletal muscle. However, currently commercial assays for routine measurement of CA-III, sTnI and MHC are not available. Therefore, measurement of myoglobin (in combination with H-FABP) and CK in plasma are still the currently recommended assays for detecting skeletal muscle damage, monitoring specific training sessions and avoiding over-training.

References

Abbott BC, Bigland B, Ritchie JM. (1952) The physiological cost of negative work. *J Physiol (Lond)* 117: 380–390.

Adams JE, Abendschein DR, Jaffe AS. (1993) Biochemical markers of myocardial injury. Is MB creatine kinase the choice for the 1990s? *Circulation* 88: 750–763.

Apple FS, Rogers MA, Sherman WM, Costill DL, Hagerman FC, Ivy JL. (1984) Profile of creatine kinase isoenzymes in skeletal muscles of marathon runners. *Clin Chem* 30: 413–416.

Armstrong RB. (1990) Initial events in exercise-induced muscular injury. *Med Sci Sports Exerc* 22: 429–435.

Armstrong RB, Ogilvie RW, Schwane JA. (1983) Eccentric exercise-induced injury to rat skeletal muscle. *J Appl Physiol: Respirat Environ Exercise Physiol* 54: 80–93.

Asmussen E. (1953) Positive and negative muscular work. *Acta Physiol Scand* 28: 364–382.

Barton PJ, Cohen A, Robert B, et al. (1985) The myosin alkali light chains of mouse ventricular and slow skeletal muscle are indistinguishable and are encoded by the same gene. *J Biol Chem* 260: 8578–8584.

Belcastro AN, Gilchrist JS, Scrubb J. (1993) Function of skeletal muscle sarcoplasmic reticulum vesicles with exercise. *J Appl Physiol* 75: 2412–2418.

Belcastro AN, Gilchrist JS, Scrubb JA, Arthur G. (1994) Calcium-supported calpain degradation rates for cardiac myofibrils in diabetes. Sulfhydryl and hydrophobic interactions. *Mol Cell Biochem* 135: 51–60.

Belcastro AN, Shewchuk LD, Raj DA. (1998) Exercise-induced muscle injury: a calpain hypothesis. *Mol Cell Biochem* 179: 135–145.

Beuerle JR, Azzazy HM, Styba G, Duh SH, Christenson RH. (2000) Characteristics of myoglobin, carbonic anhydrase III and the myoglobin/carbonic anhydrase III ratio in trauma, exercise, and myocardial infarction patients. *Clin Chim Acta* 294: 115–128.

Bleier J, Vorderwinkler KP, Falkensammer J, et al. (1998) Different intracellular compartmentations of cardiac troponins and myosin heavy chains: a causal connection to their different early release after myocardial damage. *Clin Chem* 44: 1912–1918.

Bredman JJ, Wessels A, Weijs WA, Korfage JA, Soffers CA, Moorman AF. (1991) Demonstration of 'cardiac-specific' myosin heavy chain in masticatory muscles of human and rabbit. *Histochem J* 23: 160–170.

Cannon JG, Fielding RA, Fiatarone MA, Orencole SF, Dinarello CA, Evans WJ. (1989) Increased interleukin 1 beta in human skeletal muscle after exercise. *Am J Physiol* 257: R451–R455.

Cannon JG, Meydani SN, Fielding RA, et al. (1991) Acute phase response in exercise. II. Associations between vitamin E, cytokines, and muscle proteolysis. *Am J Physiol* 260: R1235–R1240.

Clarkson PM. (1997) Eccentric exercise and muscle damage. *Int J Sports Med* 18 Suppl 4: S314–S317.

Collins JH, Theibert JL, Dalla LL. (1986) Amino acid sequence of rabbit ventricular myosin light chain-2: identity with the slow skeletal muscle isoform. *Biosci Rep* 6: 655–661.

Cooke R. (1995) The actomyosin engine. *FASEB J* 9: 636–642.

Cummins P. (1979) The homology of the alpha-chains of cardiac and skeletal rabbit tropomyosin. *J Mol Cell Cardiol* 11: 109–114.

Delanghe JR, Chapelle JP, Vanderschueren SC. (1990) Quantitative nephelometric assay for determining myoglobin evaluated. *Clin Chem* 36: 1675–1678.

Di Lisa F, De Tullio R, Salamino F, et al. (1995) Specific degradation of troponin T and I by mu-calpain and its modulation by substrate phosphorylation. *Biochem J* 308: 57–61.

Diederich KW, Eisele I, Ried T, Jaenicke T, Lichter P, Vosberg HP. (1989) Isolation and characterization of the complete human beta-myosin heavy chain gene. *Human Genetics* 81: 214–220.

Ebbeling CB, Clarkson PM. (1989) Exercise-induced muscle damage and adaptation. *Sports Med* 7: 207–234.

Farah CS, Reinach FC. (1995) The troponin complex and regulation of muscle contraction. *FASEB J* 9: 755–767.

Febbraio MA, Koukoulas I. (2000) HSP72 gene expression progressively increases in human skeletal muscle during prolonged, exhaustive exercise. *J Appl Physiol* 89: 1055–1060.

Fielding RA, Evans WJ. (1997) Aging and the acute phase response to exercise: implications for the role of systemic factors on skeletal muscle protein turnover. *Int J Sports Med* 18 Suppl 1: S22–S27.

Fielding RA, Meredith CN, O'Reilly KP, Frontera WR, Cannon JG, Evans WJ. (1991) Enhanced protein breakdown after eccentric exercise in young and older men. *J Appl Physiol* 71: 674–679.

Friden J, Lieber RL. (1992) Structural and mechanical basis of exercise-induced muscle injury. *Med Sci Sports Exerc* 24: 521–530.

Friden J, Lieber RL. (1998) Segmental muscle fiber lesions after repetitive eccentric contractions. *Cell Tissue Res* 293: 165–171.

Friden J, Sjostrom M, Ekblom B. (1983) Myofibrillar damage following intense eccentric exercise in man. *Int J Sports Med* 4: 170–176.

Glatz JF, Van d V. (1990) Cellular fatty acid-binding proteins: current concepts and future directions. *Mol Cell Biochem* 98: 237–251.

Goll DE, Thompson VF, Taylor RG, Zalewska T. (1992) Is calpain activity regulated by membranes and autolysis or by calcium and calpastatin? *Bioessays* 14: 549–556.

Hikida RS, Staron RS, Hagerman FC, Sherman WM, Costill DL. (1983) Muscle fiber necrosis associated with human marathon runners. *J Neurol Sci* 59: 185–203.

Howell JN, Chleboun G, Conatser R. (1993) Muscle stiffness, strength loss, swelling and soreness following exercise-induced injury in humans. *J Physiol (Lond)* 464: 183–196.

Huang J, Forsberg NE. (1998) Role of calpain in skeletal-muscle protein degradation. *Proc Natl Acad Sci USA* 95: 12100–12105.

Hyatt JP, Clarkson PM. (1998) Creatine kinase release and clearance using MM variants following repeated bouts of eccentric exercise. *Med Sci Sports Exerc* 30: 1059–1065.

Ingwall JS, Kramer MF, Fifer MA, et al (1985) The creatine kinase system in normal and diseased human myocardium. *N Engl J Med* 313: 1050–1054.

Jeffery S, Edwards Y, Carter N. (1980) Distribution of CAIII in fetal and adult human tissue. *Biochem Gen* 18: 843–849.

Kleine AH, Glatz JF, Van Nieuwenhoven FA, Van d V, GJ. (1992) Release of heart fatty acid-binding protein into plasma after acute myocardial infarction in man. *Mol Cell Biochem* 116: 155–162.

Klocke FJ, Copley DP, Krawczyk JA, Reichlin M. (1982) Rapid renal clearance of immunoreactive canine plasma myoglobin. *Circulation* 65: 1522–1528.

Komulainen J, Koskinen SO, Kalliokoski R, Takala TE, Vihko V. (1999) Gender differences in skeletal muscle fibre damage after eccentrically biased downhill running in rats. *Acta Physiol Scand* 165: 57–63.

Komulainen J, Takala TE, Kuipers H, Hesselink MK. (1998b) The disruption of myofibre structures in rat skeletal muscle after forced lengthening contractions. *Pflugers Arch* 436: 735–741.

Komulainen J, Vihko V. (1994a) Exercise-induced necrotic muscle damage and enzyme release in the four days following prolonged submaximal running in rats. *Pflugers Arch* 428: 346–351.

Ladue JS, Wroblewski F, Karmen A. (1954) Serum glutamic oxaloacetic transaminase activity in human acute myocardial infarction. *Science* 120: 497–499.

Larue C, Calzolari C, Leger J, Pau B. (1991) Immuno-radiometric assay of myosin heavy chain fragments in plasma for investigation of myocardial infarction. *Clin Chem* 37: 78–82.

Lee TH, Goldman L. (1986) Serum enzyme assays in the diagnosis of acute myocardial infarction. Recommendations based on a quantitative analysis. *Ann Int Med* 105: 221–233.

Leger JO, Bouvagnet P, Pau B, Roncucci R, Leger JJ. (1985) Levels of ventricular myosin fragments in human sera after myocardial infarction, determined with monoclonal antibodies to myosin heavy chains. *Eur J Clin Invest* 15: 422–429.

Lieber RL, Friden J. (1999) Mechanisms of muscle injury after eccentric contraction. *J Sci Med Sport* 2: 253–265.

Lieber RL, Thornell LE, Friden J. (1996) Muscle cytoskeletal disruption occurs within the first 15 min of cyclic eccentric contraction. *J Appl Physiol* 80: 278–284.

Liu Y, Lormes W, Baur C, et al. (2000) Human skeletal muscle HSP70 response to physical training depends on exercise intensity. *Int J Sports Med* 21: 351–355.

Liu Y, Mayr S, Opitz-Gress A, et al. (1999) Human skeletal muscle HSP70 response to training in highly trained rowers. *J Appl Physiol* 86: 101–104.

Lowe DA, Warren GL, Ingalls CP, Boorstein DB, Armstrong RB. (1995) Muscle function and protein metabolism after initiation of eccentric contraction-induced injury. *J Appl Physiol* 79: 1260–1270.

MacIntyre DL, Reid WD, McKenzie DC. (1995) Delayed muscle soreness. The inflammatory response to muscle injury and its clinical implications. *Sports Med* 20: 24–40.

MacIntyre DL, Reid WD, Lyster DM, Szasz IJ, McKenzie DC. (1996) Presence of WBC, decreased strength, and delayed soreness in muscle after eccentric exercise. *J Appl Physiol* 80: 1006–1013.

MacIntyre DL, Sorichter S, Mair J, Berg A, McKenzie DC. (2001) Markers of Inflammation and myofibrillar proteins following eccentric exercise. *Eur J Appl Physiol* 84: 180–186.

Mair J, Artner-Dworzak E, Lechleitner P, et al. (1992) Early diagnosis of acute myocardial infarction by a newly developed rapid immunoturbidimetric assay for myoglobin. *Br Heart J* 68: 462–468.

Mair J, Koller A, Artner-Dworzak E, et al. (1992) Effects of exercise on plasma myosin heavy chain fragments and MRI of skeletal muscle. *J Appl Physiol* 72: 656–663.

Mair J, Mayr M, Muller E, et al. (1995) Rapid adaptation to eccentric exercise-induced muscle damage. *Int J Sports Med* 16: 352–356.

Mair J, Puschendorf B, Michel G. (1994) Clinical significance of cardiac contractile proteins for the diagnosis of myocardial injury. *Adv Clin Chem* 31: 63–98.

Malm C, Lenkei R, Sjodin B. (1999) Effects of eccentric exercise on the immune system in men. *J Appl Physiol* 86: 461–468.

McNeil PL, Khakee R. (1992) Disruptions of muscle fiber plasma membranes. Role in exercise-induced damage. *Am J Pathol* 140: 1097–1109.

Neumaier D. (1981) Tissue specific distribution of creatine kinase isoenzymes. In: Lang H, ed. *Creatine kinase isoenzymes – pathophysiology and clinical application.* Berlin: Springer-Verlag, pp. 31–83.

Newham DJ, Jones DA, Ghosh G, Aurora P. (1988) Muscle fatigue and pain after eccentric contractions at long and short length. *Clin Sci* 74: 553–557.

Northoff H, Berg A. (1991) Immunologic mediators as parameters of the reaction to strenuous exercise. *Int J Sports Med* 12 Suppl 1: S9–15.

Ohkaru Y, Asayama K, Ishii H, et al. (1995) Development of a sandwich enzyme-linked immunosorbent assay for the determination of human heart type fatty acid-binding protein in plasma and urine by using two different monoclonal antibodies specific for human heart fatty acid-binding protein. *J Immunol Meth* 178: 99–111.

Parmacek MS, Leiden JM. (1991) Structure, function, and regulation of troponin C. *Circulation* 84: 991–1003.

Pearlstone JR, Carpenter MR, Smillie LB. (1986) Amino acid sequence of rabbit cardiac troponin T. *J Biol Chem* 261: 16795–16810.

Pette D. (1998) Training effects on the contractile apparatus. *Acta Physiol Scand* 162: 367–376.

Puleo PR, Guadagno PA, Roberts R, et al. (1990) Early diagnosis of acute myocardial infarction based on assay for subforms of creatine kinase-MB. *Circulation* 82: 759–764.

Puntschart A, Vogt M, Widmer HR, Hoppeler H, Billeter R. (1996) Hsp70 expression in human skeletal muscle after exercise. *Acta Physiol Scand* 157: 411–417.

Raggi A, Grand RJ, Moir AJ, Perry SV. (1989) Structure-function relationships in cardiac troponin T. *Biochim Biophys Acta* 997: 135–143.

Raj DA, Booker TS, Belcastro AN. (1998) Striated muscle calcium-stimulated cysteine protease (calpain-like) activity promotes myeloperoxidase activity with exercise. *Pflugers Arch* 435: 804–809.

Rohde T, MacLean DA, Richter EA, Kiens B, Pedersen BK. (1997) Prolonged submaximal eccentric exercise is associated with increased levels of plasma IL-6. *Am J Physiol* 273: E85–E91.

Roos W, Eymann E, Symannek M, et al. (1995) Monoclonal antibodies to human heart fatty acid-binding protein. *J Immunol Meth* 183: 149–153.

Saido TC, Sorimachi H, Suzuki K. (1994) Calpain: new perspectives in molecular diversity and physiological-pathological involvement. *FASEB J* 8: 814–822.

Schiaffino S, Reggiani C. (1994) Myosin isoforms in mammalian skeletal muscle. *J Appl Physiol* 77: 493–501.

Schiaffino S, Reggiani C. (1996) Molecular diversity of myofibrillar proteins: gene regulation and functional significance. *Physiol Rev* 76: 371–423.

Schwane JA, Buckley RT, Dipaolo DP, Atkinson MA, Shepherd JR. (2000) Plasma creatine kinase responses of 18- to 30-yr-old African-American men to eccentric exercise. *Med Sci Sports Exerc* 32: 370–378.

Schwartz K, Boheler KR, de la Bastie D, Lompre AM, Mercadier JJ. (1992) Switches in cardiac muscle gene expression as a result of pressure and volume overload. *Am J Physiol* 262: R364–R369.

Simeonova PP, Kehayov IR, Kyurkchiev SD. (1991) Identification of human ventricular myosin heavy chain fragments with monoclonal antibody 2F4 in human sera after myocardial necrosis. *Clin Chim Acta* 201: 207–221.

Simpson JA, van Eyk JE, Iscoe S. (2000) Hypoxemia-induced modification of troponin I and T in canine diaphragm. *J Appl Physiol* 88: 753–760.

Sly WS, Hu PY. (1995) Human carbonic anhydrases and carbonic anhydrase deficiencies. *Ann Rev Biochem* 64: 375–401.

Smith LL, Anwar A, Fragen M, Rananto C, Johnson R, Holbert D. (2000) Cytokines and cell adhesion molecules associated with high-intensity eccentric exercise. *Eur J Appl Physiol* 82: 61–67.

Somer H, Dubowitz V, Donner M. (1976) Creatine kinase isoenzymes in neuromuscular diseases. *J Neuro Sci* 29: 129–136.

Sorichter S, Koller A, Haid C, et al. (1995) Light concentric exercise and heavy eccentric muscle loading: effects on CK, MRI and markers of inflammation. *Int J Sports Med* 16: 288–292.

Sorichter S, Mair J, Koller A, et al. (1997a) Skeletal troponin I as a marker of exercise-induced muscle damage. *J Appl Physiol* 83: 1076–1082.

Sorichter S, Mair J, Koller A, et al. (1997b). Skeletal muscle troponin I release and magnetic resonance imaging signal intensity changes after eccentric exercise-induced skeletal muscle injury. *Clin Chim Acta* 262: 139–146.

Sorichter S, Mair J, Koller A, Pelsers MM, Puschendorf B, Glatz JF. (1998) Early assessment of exercise induced skeletal muscle injury using plasma fatty acid binding protein. *Br J Sports Med* 32: 121–124.

Sorichter S, Puschendorf B, Mair J. (1999) Skeletal muscle injury induced by eccentric muscle action: muscle proteins as markers of muscle fiber injury. *Exerc Immunol Rev* 5: 5–21.

Sorichter S, Mair J, Koller A, et al. (2001a) Release of muscle proteins after downhill running in male and female subjects. *Scand J Med Sci Sports* 11: 28–32.

Sorichter S, Mair J, Koller A, et al. (2001b). Relation between Creatine Kinase, Myosin heavy chains and Magnetic Resonance Imaging after eccentric exercise. *J Sports Sci* 19: 687–691.

Stauber WT. (1989) Eccentric action of muscles: physiology, injury, and adaptation. *Exerc Sport Sci Rev* 17: 157–185.

Takahashi M, Lee L, Shi Q, Gawad Y, Jackowski G. (1996) Use of enzyme immunoassay for measurement of skeletal troponin-I utilizing isoform-specific monoclonal antibodies. *Clin Biochem* 29: 301–308.

Talbot JA, Morgan DL. (1996) Quantitative analysis of sarcomere non-uniformities in active muscle following a stretch. *J Muscle Res Cell Motil* 17: 261–268.

Tidball JG. (1995) Inflammatory cell response to acute muscle injury. *Med Sci Sports Exerc* 27: 1022–1032.

Ullum H, Haahr PM, Diamant M, Palmo J, Halkjaer-Kristensen J, Pedersen BK. (1994) Bicycle exercise enhances plasma IL-6 but does not change IL-1 alpha, IL-1 beta, IL-6, or TNF-alpha pre-mRNA in BMNC. *J Appl Physiol* 77: 93–97.

Vaananen HK, Syrjala H, Rahkila P, et al. (1990) Serum carbonic anhydrase III and myoglobin concentrations in acute myocardial infarction. *Clin Chem* 36: 635–638.

Van Nieuwenhoven FA, Kleine AH, Wodzig WH, et al. (1995) Discrimination between myocardial and skeletal muscle injury by assessment of the plasma ratio of myoglobin over fatty acid-binding protein. *Circulation* 92: 2848–2854.

Wilkinson JM, Grand RJ. (1978) Comparison of amino acid sequence of troponin I from different striated muscles. *Nature* 271: 31–35.

Yamauchi-Takihara K, Sole MJ, Liew J, Ing D, Liew CC. (1989) Characterization of human cardiac myosin heavy chain genes. *Proc Natl Acad Sci USA* 86: 3504–3508.

Young VR, Munro HN. (1978) Ntau-methylhistidine (3-methylhistidine) and muscle protein turnover: an overview. *FED Proceed* 37: 2291–2300.

45

Localized muscle impedance measurements

R. Aaron and C. A. Shiffman

Introduction

The use of electrical impedance in physiology and medicine is hardly new, indeed the measurement of body impedance as a useful diagnostic indicator of illness was proposed by King (1901) and the modern impetus to characterize biological structure and function came from Nyober (1950). Hoffer et al (1969) extended this work, showing that impedance was a useful indicator of total body water and thereby establishing the field of Bioelectrical Impedance Analysis (BIA). Figure 45.1A shows the typical electrode setup for conventional BIA measurements. Small, high frequency alternating currents are injected distally at a finger and toe, and the voltage is measured between ankle and wrist. Dividing voltage by current gives the whole body impedance Z, which has two components: the resistance R, associated with tissue hydration, and reactance X, associated with the properties of cell membranes.[1] The magnitude of impedance is

$$Z = (R^2 + X^2)^{1/2}$$

Chertow et al (1997) showed a striking connection between standard whole body impedance data and relative risk of death for a large group of haemodialysis patients. More generally, conventional BIA is widely used to estimate body composition (Lukaski 1987) using statistical relationships between impedance measurements and total body water, body fat, fat free mass, etc, derived using other techniques. However, attempts to understand such relationships in terms of detailed, localized aspects of anatomy and physiology are almost certain to fail, given the complexity of current paths that must traverse essentially the entire body.

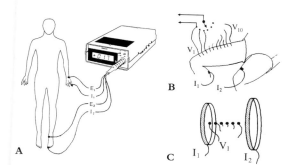

Figure 45.1—Fixed electrode arrangements. Various electrode arrangements used in non-invasive impedance measurements on the body. **A** Conventional whole body BIA. **B** Localized segmental impedance on the thigh. **C** Ring electrode system for measurement of muscle anisotropy and skin-fat layer impedance. (I_1 and I_2 are the current injecting electrodes, while V_1 through V_{10} are voltage sensing electrodes.)

It has been proposed that restricting measurements to individual segments of the body might overcome those interpretive weaknesses (NIH 1996). Figure 45.1B shows a typical setup for the localized segmental studies that are the subject of this chapter.[2] The circuitry is clearly more complicated than for the whole body case, and so are the measurement procedures and analysis, but the concepts are the same. Local measurements are made on limbs such as the thigh or forearm, whose geometric simplicity hopefully allows one to tie the impedance values to the underlying anatomy and physiology.

Resistance and resistivity

For a uniform, isotropic, cylindrical sample of height h and cross sectional area A, the resistance R is given by

$$R = \rho_1 \, h/A$$

and consequently R depends on both the geometry of the sample and microscopic character of the material, whose properties are embodied in the parameter ρ_1, the resistivity. Values of the resistivity encountered in the body range from approximately 1.0 Ωm for plasma to 20 and 200 Ωm for fat and bone respectively. Skeletal muscle is particularly interesting because its bundled fibre structure makes the resistivity for current flowing parallel to the fibres, ρ_{11}, much less than for flow across them. This anisotropy can be put to good use in non-invasive measurements, for example, by making it possible to distinguish the contributions of a particular muscle from that of its neighbours in a segment. Furthermore, ρ_{II} is much less than than the resistivity of fat and bone, so that in limbs almost all the axial current flows through the muscle. Even though blood is a better conductor, the contribution to the overall resistance due to the major blood vessels can usually be ignored, since their cross-sectional areas are such small fractions of the muscle area. Finally, one should note that while Equation 45.2 holds only for the special case of a cylinder, the corresponding formula for R for any shape has the same mathematical structure, i.e ρ_1 times a (sometimes very complicated) function of purely geometrical quantities.

Reactance and phase

If alternating currents are used one must also consider the reactance, X. This is a directly measurable property that (for the uniform cylinder) obeys an equation similar to Equation 45.2, but with ρ_1 replaced by an added material-dependent parameter, ρ_2. Its importance in the present context is that it indicates how the flow of current is affected by cell membranes and by the various facia of the body. In particular, membranes behave like the capacitors of electronic circuits, their layered bilipid structure playing the role of the insulating dielectric. Charges of opposite sign collect on opposing sides, and there are time lags between the voltage and the driving current; for example, the current can reverse direction before the voltage. This effect is characterized by the "Phase angle" θ, defined by $\theta = \arctan X/R$. While R and X depend critically on the size and shape of a segment, this is not necessarily true for θ. General considerations indicate that geometric factors tend to cancel in the ratio X/R, making the phase more universal in character and potentially more useful in clinical applications. Indeed the correlation observed by Chertow et al (1997) is in fact between the *phase* and the relative risk of death.

What follows is an outline of some of our research in applying these ideas to the study of body segments. The reader is referred to our earlier publications for further details and for discussions of the mathematical models used in the analysis of these results. Unless otherwise stated all measurements reported here were performed at a frequency of 50 kHz.

Non–invasive measurements of anisotropy

At virtually every level of organization, skeletal muscle is characterized by quasi-cylindrical symmetry, and electrical transport in muscle is correspondingly anisotropic. Body segments contain muscles with different dominant fibre directions and fibres may change directions within a muscle, complicating the study of anisotropy via non-invasive measurements. Nevertheless *local* anisotropy can be characterized by the resistivites ρ_{II} and $\rho_{\perp}$ for current flow along and transverse to the fibres, respectively. Depending on the distance scale of the measuring technique, then, one can reasonably hope to extract useful average values of those parameters for particular muscles or for the segment as a whole.

Both types of investigations have been done by Aaron et al (1997). An example of a global measurement arrangement is illustrated in Figure 45.1C. Here currents were injected via ring electrodes on the thigh, and potentials were measured using small disk electrodes positioned along a line between the rings at various distances, z, from the lower one. In this way the resistance profile $R(z)$ could be measured and compared with the results of a theoretical model based on the mathematical condition called "homogeneous tensorial anisotropy". The model takes the femur and the skin–fat layer into account, but it assumes perfect cylindrical symmetry and exactly axial alignment of the muscle fibres. Despite these simplifying assumptions, the agreement with experiment was very good.

Furthermore by varying the spacing between the rings one could affect how much of the current flow was perpendicular to he surface of the thigh, making it possible to determine ρ_{sf}, the resistivity of the skin-fat layer, as well as ρ_{II} and $\rho_{\perp}$. A comparison of the results (on a single subject) with those of Rush et al (1963) and Epstein and Foster (1983) is given in Table 45.1. Considering the wide variety of techniques and tissue sources, disagreement between findings is to be expected. It should also be borne in mind that while the muscles of the thigh are oriented more or less parallel to the femur, that is not the case for the *fibres*, which can make substantial angles with that direction. In short, the ring electrode method has the advantage of being non-invasive, but at the price of providing *angle-averaged* values for the resistivities, in particular for ρ_{II}. Nevertheless the value of ρ_{II} obtained here agrees very well with those described below, obtained using an entirely different experimental technique.

An example of more localized measurements is illustrated in Figure 45.2, showing how short, rotatable electrode strips can be used to determine the dominant orientation of the fibres of a particular muscle, in this case the vastus medialis a few centimetres above its attachment at the knee. The theoretical treatment by Shiffman and Aaron (1998) establishes that curves of this type are to be expected on the basis of the same homogeneous tensorial anisotropy condition mentioned above. The details of the mathematics are of no interest here, except to note that the predicted minima depend primarily on the ratio $\rho_{II}/\rho_{\perp}$, vanishing altogether when $\rho_{II} = \rho_{\perp}$ as they must. The model used in this analysis necessarily simplifies the actual anatomy, but there can be little doubt that any substantial change in the properties of cell membranes or intramuscular fascia must alter the anisotropy ratio and hence the size and character of the minima.

Phase and segment shape

The effects of segment shape must be eliminated if one is to extract parameters reflecting the physiological condition of a muscle. This section addresses that issue

Table 45.1— Resistivity measurements

Source	Method	$\rho_{sf}^{\,a}$	$\rho_{\Pi}^{\,b}$	$\rho_{\perp}^{\,c}$	γ^{d}
Rush et al (1963)	Exposed spinal muscles of anaesthetized dogs	25	19	2	9.2
Epstein and Foster (1983)	Exercised skeletal muscles from dogs		13	1.9	6.8
Aaron et al (1997)	Non-invasive average of human mid-thigh	16	7.7	1.5	5.1

[a] Resistivity of the skin–fat layer (Ωm)
[b] Resistivity for current flow along muscle fibres (Ωm)
[c] Resistivity for current flow transverse to muscle fibres (Ωm)
[d] Anisotropy ratio $\rho_{\Pi}/\rho_{\perp}$

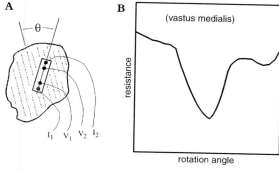

Figure 45.2— Rotating strip electrodes. Rotating-strip electrode system (**A**) and resistance vs angle trace (**B**) for the vastus medialis, with the I_1 electrode fixed several centimetres above the patella.

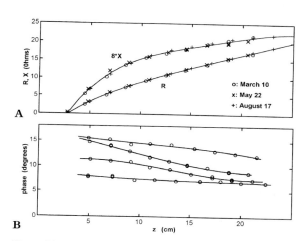

Figure 45.3— Reproducibility and phase. **A** Long term reproducibility of measurements using the electrode arrangement sketched in Figure 45.1B: resistance (R) and reactance (X) as a function of distance along the thigh of an adult male, taken over a period of five months. (The reactance has been multiplied by 8.) **B** Examples of the phase function, $\theta(z) = \arctan X(z)/R(z)$, representing the variety of behaviours found in a sample of 26 adult subjects of various body types. The quantity θ_{avg} defined in the text is obtained by integrating such curves over z, after adjusting for the height of the subject.

as it applies to the thigh, pausing first to demonstrate that the techniques used to obtain R and X give sufficiently reproducible values to justify the analysis that follows. Localized segmental impedance measurements make greater instrumental demands than does standard BIA, and an example of satisfactory overall reproducibility is given in Figure 45.3A. This shows that R and X data taken over a period of 5 months on a healthy adult male are scarcely distinguishable from one another.[3]

Figure 45.3A also makes it very clear that the reactance, $X(z)$, is not simply a scaled version of $R(z)$. This has the consequence that the phase, $\theta = \arctan [X(z)/R(z)]$, is a function of z rather than a single value as in standard BIA. Figure 45.3B shows examples of that function, $\theta(z)$ found in a study of 26 subjects ranging in age from late-teens to mid-sixties and representing a wide variety of body types. The highest and lowest lying curves represent the extremes of the θ behaviour, with the majority displaying curves similar to the middle two.

The distinction between the behaviours of $R(z)$ and $X(z)$ is emphasized by an analysis that attempts to correct for the shape of the thigh by considering only the component of current which is parallel to the z-axis (Shiffman et al 1999). Also, the analysis takes into account the subject's thigh contour and average skin–fat thickness. An example of its use is given in Figure 45.4, with A showing the raw $R(z)$ data and B showing a quantity that in effect is the shape corrected version. The criteria for success are that a least-squares fit of these corrected data to a straight line

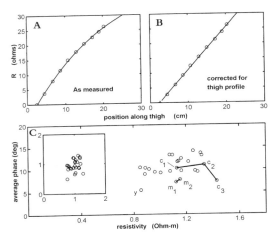

Figure 45.4—Effective resistivity and average phase. **A** Raw $R(z)$ and **B** the same data corrected for thigh profile and skin fat layer. **C** Correlation of the resistivity, ρ_1, obtained from the slope of the corrected data with the z-averaged phase, θ_{avg}. The inset shows the same distribution of ρ_1 and θ_{avg}, now expressed as fractions of their ensemble-averaged values. (See text for discussion of c_1, c_2, c_3, m_1, m_2, y).

should show no evidence of systematic deviations, and that the line should extrapolate to zero at the first voltage electrode (indicated by the extra tick mark in the figure). As one sees, the criteria are very well satisfied, in which case one can find the effective resistivity, ρ_1, directly from the slope.[4]

The analysis predicts similar behaviour for $X(z)$, so one should be able to extract the effective reactivity, ρ_2, in essentially the same way. However the reactance has failed to satisfy the criteria mentioned above in virtually all the cases we have examined. An important clue to the failure for X despite success for R lies in the assumption of negligible transverse current flow, which is strictly true only for cylinders. There must be transverse flow in any tapered shape, and in muscle structures such as the thigh the transverse component must encounter a myriad of facia and cell membranes that lie across its path. These are the anatomical features most directly associated with the reactance and, consequently, with the phase.

Given that θ depends on z in different ways for different individuals, we have adopted its z-averaged value, θ_{avg}, as a simpler pragmatic specification. Figure 45.4C shows the correlations of θ_{avg} with ρ_1 for our subject population, and the inset plots the corresponding values obtained by normalizing these to their ensemble averages. When treated in this way, the standard deviations for phase and resistivity are virtually the same, which lends credence to the overall

procedure—given the very different ways these are derived from the original data. As the inset indicates, the normalized points cluster reasonably tightly, though there are a few that appear to lie significantly low. These are labelled c_3, m_1, m_2 and y in the main figure, and as it happens all have likely clinical associations. The most interesting of these is c_3, part of the sequence (c_1, c_2, c_3) representing an adult female subject who underwent chemotherapy over a 3 month period represented by c_1 and c_2, represented by c_1 and c_2, and who suffered major fluid retention just preceding the c_3 measurement, 2 months later. The steady increase in ρ_1 is undoubtedly significant, but most striking is the 2 standard deviation drop in θ_{avg} between c_2 and c_3. The accompanying girth data showed that almost half of the weight gain was in the thighs, offering *prima facie* evidence that pooling of fluid in the lower extremities was accompanied by changes in the properties of the cell membranes.

The other cases are also interesting. The m_1 and m_2 points represent a clinically anorexic subject (BMI = 15.9) whose flat $\theta(z)$ curve is the lowest one shown in Figure 45.3B. The weak z-dependence and low average phase, coupled with quite normal ρ_1, point to problems with the transverse resistivity and, thereby, to cell membranes once again. (The difference between the m_1 and m_2 points is not experimental scatter; the subject gained 7% in weight in the 52 days between the two measurements). The point y remains a puzzle; θ_{avg} certainly appears to fall outside the "normal" range and yet it pertains to a generally healthy, wiry adult male (BMI = 21), with quite ordinary whole body phase. The subject did suffer a torn Achilles tendon 22 months before these measurements, with surgical correction followed by extensive physical therapy. However the injury was to the *other* leg. The results might point to changes in the healthy leg caused by the effort of protecting the injured one; on the other hand one cannot ignore the possibility that this case simply lies on the tail of the usual Gaussian-type distribution for normal properties in a population.

Impedance changes under static forces

The experiments described previously deal with the impedance of muscle in its nominally relaxed condition, and we now consider the changes that occur when a muscle exerts a force. As before, the connections between impedance and underlying physiology are not well established, but here the important phenomenon of fatigue introduces an additional obstacle to understanding. While there are various definitions of fatigue, irreproducibility at high force levels must certainly be taken as a sufficient condition that a muscle is no longer "fresh". Therefore, an immediate goal must be to establish measurement protocols that yield repeatable data, particularly if the aim is to study the dependence of impedance on force over the full voluntary range.

Localized segmental impedance measurements are well suited to the study of exertion by single muscle or by narrowly defined muscle groups. An example is given in Figure 45.5, showing changes in R and X of the forearm as the subject grips the bar of a Smedley Hand Dynamometer.[5] The inset sketches a resistance-time record as an illustration of the experimental protocol: the subject was directed to exert a constant force, F, for 5–10 s, then increase F to the next level and hold again, and so on. The main figure shows the relative changes in resistance and reactance, $\Delta R/R_o$ and $\Delta X/X_o$, as functions of the force registered by the dynamometer. Here R_o and X_o, are the baseline values of R and X, found with the arm hanging vertically under its own weight and the fingers in a relaxed semi-curled configuration.[6]

These curves represent four sets of measurements separated by 10–20 min rest periods, in the sequence X_1, X_2, R_1, R_2. The coding of points in the figure demonstrates that this scenario guaranteed a reasonable degree of reproducibility. Also it is significant that X (but not R) returned immediately to its baseline when the dynamometer was released at the end of a run, despite "strain" or fatigue. Fatigue was obvious to the subject, and at the largest forces it was clear to others via visible muscle tremors and the struggle to hold F constant. Evidence is also contained in the $R(F)$ and $X(F)$ curves; what appears as grouped pairs or triplets of points usually indicates a failed effort.

As sketched in the introduction, changes in impedance can arise from changes in the nature of conducting medium or from changes in geometrical factors. Ischaemia is a relevant example of the former, while an example of the latter which clearly applies to muscular exertion is contraction. It is important to note that measured ΔR and ΔX are both positive, while independent experiments indicate that changes due to ischaemia should be negative. For example, inducing ischaemia in the forearm using a standard blood pressure cuff shows that the initial effect is to decrease R and X, with increases occurring only for cuff pressures of 200 mmHg and for durations of minutes or more. Furthermore, the shape changes that occur in muscle contraction at zero force must also decrease R and X. As muscles shorten, cross-sectional areas expand, which according to Equation 45.2 should reduce both R and X. The effects of geometry and forces are inextricably tied together, in fact touching the fingers to the palm does cause the impedance to increase. However the range of motion involved in the dynamometer experiments is much smaller than in touching finger to palm, and linearly scaling the results of the touch experiment strongly suggests that the effect of shape change on these results is negligible. It is, therefore, reasonable to conclude that both shape changes and ischaemia are at most secondary factors affecting the signs of the impedance changes, and the general behaviour is shown in Figure 45.5, with the primary effects still to be determined.

The inset emphasizes that R usually overshoots R_o, when the force returns to zero and the cuff experiments offer a simple explanation: muscular contraction produces a mild degree of progressive self-induced ischaemia with consequent reduction in resistance, and overshoot and slow recovery are just the sudden exposure of the hidden ischaemia followed by reperfusion. Accordingly the $R(F)$ curves, while reproducible, probably represent the response of increasingly ischaemic rather than rested muscle. In contrast, the data for the reactance do not appear to suffer appreciably from the overshoot problem, supporting the proposition that X and R are affected (at least in part) by different physiological factors.

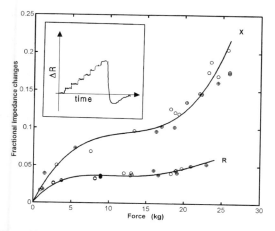

Figure 45.5—Changes under static forces. Changes in resistance and reactance of muscles of the forearm as forces is exerted against a hand dynamometer. The inset sketches a typical resistance vs time curve as the subject increases the force in discrete steps, each of 5–10 s.

Conclusion

The results described here demonstrate that localized segmental measurements have sufficient precision and reproducibility to support the search for more fundamental understanding of the electrical impedance of muscle than has been possible heretofore. They also point to potentially useful new empirical correlations with clinical observables, particularly in longitudinal studies, in which shape idiosyncracies are less troublesome. The chemotherapy case described above is illustrative, but the term "longitudinal" can encompass much shorter time spans; studies of muscle atrophy in microgravity or of strenuous exercise and fatigue are examples. The technique is non-invasive, the apparatus is relatively inexpensive and portable, and the initial results are promising.

Since this chapter was written, sufficient progress has been made in the study of both normal and diseased subjects that some of the conjectures regarding potential usefulness of localized bioimpedance analysis as a clinical tool can now be regarded as largely proven. For example, comparing results using the technique of section 3 on 45 normal subjects and 25 patients with various neuromuscular diseases affecting the quadriceps has demonstrated that low spatially average phase is indeed a distinguishing characteristic for such disease, and that the phase can serve as an excellent indicator of the severity and progress of diseases such as polymyositis and amyaotrophic lateral sclerosis. (Rutkove et al 2001). (The phase was also found to correlate well with standard measures of strength is a subgroup of 11 inclusion body myositis patients.) This study has revealed an even wider variety of shapes for the phase function than shown in figure 3b, some with decidedly positive slope, and theoretical advances have shown that the full range of such features are consequences of the characteristic anisotropy of skeletal muscle tissue (Shiffman et al 2001). We have also shown that connections between the impedance and health status are found in conditions other than neuromuscular disease, for example, changes in impedance that occur subsequent to bone marrow transplants and during hemodialysis (Aaron and Shiffman 2001).

Acknowledgements

The authors are pleased to acknowledge the assistance of T. Pesek and informative discussions with J. R. Libonati.

1 – In mathematical terminology Z is a complex number, with R its real part and X its imaginary part.

2 – The term "segmental bioelectrical impedance analysis (SBIA)" has been applied to studies in which the body is treated as a collection of cylinders representing segments such as trunk, arms and legs (Chumlea et al 1988, Organ et al 1994, Tan et al 1997). These address very different issues from what is discussed here.

3 – Only modest precautions were needed to insure the high degree of reliability shown here, in contrast to the rigorous protocols required to insure reliable results from whole body BIA (Kushner 1992).

4 – This is one of the best examples we have found. In general there are small systematic deviations, reproducible over time for a given subject. This is very much to be expected given the simplifications of the model, in particular the assumption of uniform skin–fat thickness.

5 – Model 56380, Stoelting Co., Wood Dale, IL. Also, the current electrodes were placed on the adductor pollicis brevis and mid lateral biceps and the voltage electrodes were placed on the flexor digitorum sublimis, about 8 cm apart.

6 – R_o was 22 Ω and X_o was 3.5 Ω. These depend on electrode separation, but their ratio provides a good approximation for the phase, 8.9^0. Data for the $R(z)$ and $X(z)$ along a line on the forearm show qualitatively the same curvature as on the thigh, though θ drops much more gradually.

References

Aaron R, Huang M, Shiffman CA. (1997) Anisotropy of human muscle via non-invasive impedance measurements. *Phys Med Biol* 42: 1245–1262.

Aaron R, Shiffman CA. (2000) Using localized impedance measurements to study muscle changes in injury and disease. *Ann NY Acad Sci* 904: 1245–1262.

Chertow GM, Jacobs DO, Lazarus JM, Lew NL, Lowrie EG. (1997) Phase angle predicts survival in hemodialysis patients. *J Renal Nutr* 7: 204–207.

Chumlea WC, Baumgartner RN, Roche AF. (1988) Specific resistivity used to estimate fat-free mass from segmental body measures of bioelectric-impedance. *Am J Clin Nutr* 48: 7–15.

Epstein BR, Foster KR. (1983) Anisotropy in the dielectric properties of skeletal muscle. *Med Biol Eng Comput* 21: 51–55.

Hoffer J, Meadow CK, Simpson DC. (1969) Correlation of whole body impedance with total body water volume. *J Appl Physiol* 27: 531–534.

King WH. (1901) Electricity in medicine and surgery (New York: Bowricke and Runyon Co.)

Kushner RF. (1992) Bioelectrical impedance analysis: A review of principles and applications. *J Amer Col Nutr* 11: 199–209.

Lukaski HC. (1987) Methods for the assessment of human body composition: traditional and new. *Am J Clin Nutr* 46: 537–556.

NIH. (1996) *Bioelectrical Impedance Analysis, Proc. Technology Assessment Conf. (Bethesda, MD, 12-14 December 1994)*. *Am J Clin Nutr* 64(suppl): 424S–432S.

Nyober J. (1950) Impedance Plethysmography. *Medical Physics Vol 2. ed.* Glasser O, (Chicago: Year Book Pub) pp 736–744.

Organ LW, Bradham GB, Gore DT, Lozier SL. (1994) Segmental bioelectrical impedance analysis. *J Appl Physiol* 77: 98–112.

Rush S, Abidskov JA, McFee R. (1963) Resistivity of body tissue at low frequencies. *Circ Res* 12: 40–50.

Rutkove SB, Aaron R, Shiffman CA. (2002) Localized Bioimpedance Analysis in the evaluation of neuromuscular disease. *Muscle and Nerve* (to be published)

Shiffman CA, Aaron R. (1998) Angular dependance of resistance in non-invasive electrical measurements of human muscle. *Phys Med Biol* 43: 1317–1323.

Shiffman CA, Aaron R, Amoss V, Coomler K, Therrien J. (1999) Resistivity and phase in localized BIA. (*submitted to Phys Med Biol*)

Shiffman CA, Aaron R, Altman A. (2001) Spatial dependence of phase in localized bioelectrical impedance analysis. *Phys Med Biol* 46: N97–104.

Tan YX, Nunez C, Sun Y, Zhang K, Wang ZM. (1997) New electrode system for rapid whole-body and segmental bioimpedance analysis. *Med Sci Sports Exerc* 29: 1269–1273.

46

Assessing muscle pain

Dane Cook

Introduction

Muscle pain is a widely recognized phenomenon that is experienced in both clinical and chronic pain populations (e.g., fibromyalgia and chronic fatigue syndrome), as well as in otherwise healthy populations. However, relatively little is known concerning the mechanisms that underlie the experience of *muscle* pain. Indeed, cutaneous nociceptors have been studied most frequently, despite the fact that chronic muscle pain conditions such as low back pain are considered to be the "most expensive benign condition in America" (Mayer et al 1987) afflicting millions of people every year. Therefore, it behoves us as researchers and clinicians to gain a better understanding of muscle pain. Part of the problem stems from the fact that muscle pain is often measured in a narrow and unsophisticated fashion, thus, limiting our ability to gain a deeper understanding of pain. As stated by Turk and Melzack (1992) "The measurement of pain is essential for the study of pain mechanisms and for the evaluation of methods to control pain."

The perception of muscle pain is a complex phenomenon that involves multiple levels of parrallel processing within both the peripheral and central nervous systems. The complexity of the pain processing system contributes to the frequently observed lack of association between the clinical pain, patients subjective rating and objective measures of muscle pain. The sophistication and precision with which pain can be measured is also a barrier to a better understanding of muscle pain. However, much more can be learned with a sophisticated and multidimensional approach to muscle pain measurement. While some researchers prefer objective measures, pain is not an objective phenomenon. For instances, The International Association for the Study of Pain (1979) has defined pain as an unpleasant sensory and emotional experience associated with actual or potential tissue damage, or described in terms of such damage. According to O'Connor and Cook (1999), "Implied in this definition of pain are the ideas that: (a) pain is always a subjective experience, (b) emotions are always an element of pain, and (c) the perception of pain is not always directly related to the amount of tissue damage." Moreover, the definition implies that the measurement of any type of pain, including muscle pain, is inherently difficult, and it should be approached in a well thought out and theoretical manner.

The purpose of this chapter is to provide the reader with an overview of how muscle pain is assessed. First, the chapter will begin with a description of commonly used measures of muscle pain. Second, selected experimental methods used to measure muscle pain will be outlined. Finally, future directions for the measurement of muscle pain, focusing on a multidimensional approach, are recommended.

Commonly used measures of muscle pain

Pain threshold

Pain threshold is defined as the minimum stimulus intensity that is *usually* (e.g., 50% of the time in detection experiments) perceived as painful. Pain threshold has the advantage that it is easily obtained and easily quantified, and it can be obtained for both sensory and emotional dimensions of pain. However, there are several drawbacks to using pain threshold as a primary dependent measure. Pain threshold measures ignore important concerns such as pain intensity, and consequently they only provide limited information to the researcher and clinician. Also, pain threshold measures are unrelated to muscle pain ratings in laboratory experiments (Cook et al 1997), and they fail to predict the type of muscle pain experienced by chronic pain patients (Price and Harkins 1992). Finally, numerous non-sensory factors (e.g., personality, expectations, instructional sets) can bias the reporting of pain (Clark and Goodman 1973, Chapman 1977, Yang et al 1979, Snodgrass et al 1985).

Pain threshold is often measured by simply having the subject (in human studies) indicate (e.g., raising a finger or responding vocally) when he or she feels that the stimulus has changed from one that is not painful to something that is just noticeably painful. Classical psychophysical scaling methods such as the "method of limits" and the "method of constant stimuli" have also been employed to assess pain thresholds (Guilford 1954, Snodgrass et al 1985, Price and Harkins 1992). In the method of limits, the stimulus intensity is either increased or decreased in small steps. In an ascending trial, the intensity is set below pain threshold, and it is increased by small amounts until the stimulus is perceived as painful. In a descending trial, the intensity is set above pain threshold and decreased until the stimulus is no longer perceived as painful. A threshold on any trial is the midpoint between the detected and non-detected stimuli, and the average threshold across trials is taken as the criterion threshold measure. The method of constant stimuli differs from that of the method of limits in that the muscle pain stimulus is presented in a random order of intensity, and several different intensities are presented (Snodgrass et al 1985). More recent techniques using "signal detection methodology" are also available for obtaining threshold measurements. Unlike classical psychophysical approaches, signal detection theory assumes that *no* "true" sensory threshold exists, but that humans operate along a sensory continuum. The complexity and breadth of the signal detection theory approach are beyond the scope of this chapter. However, complete descriptions of both classical psychophysics and signal detection methodology are available to the interested reader (Engen 1971a, 1971b, McNicol 1972, Clark 1974, Snodgrass et al 1985). It is important to note that, even under controlled laboratory conditions, using classical psychophysical measurement approaches, there is substantial intra-individual, and to a greater extent inter-individual, variation on perceptual responses to noxious stimuli (Snodgrass et al 1985). Overall, the high variability, low efficacy for generalization and the susceptibility to response bias observed in pain threshold limits the usefulness of this measure in both laboratory and clinical settings.

Pain tolerance

Pain tolerance can be defined as either the length of time an individual is willing to endure a noxious stimulus or the maximal stimulus intensity that one will endure (O'Connor and Cook 1999). The advantages of using measures of pain tolerance are that they are relatively simple and easily obtained, and, therefore, they can be used for large group data collection. A major disadvantage in measuring pain tolerance in humans is that for most types of noxious stimuli (e.g., noxious pressure, noxious cold or electrical stimulation of the muscle) it is unethical to obtain a true pain tolerance measure because of the potential for extensive tissue damage or permanent injury. For example, in studies involving cold stimulation, compression-ischaemia, noxious pressure or electrical stimulation, a maximal exposure time or a preset intensity cutoff is typically employed. These arbitrary cutoffs serve to truncate the range of possible true tolerance times introducing a "ceiling effect". As with measures of pain threshold, pain tolerance measures are unlikely to generalize to the actual type of muscle pain experienced by the individual (Wolff 1969, Gracely 1994). Additionally, measures of pain tolerance have been shown to be influenced by cultural, social, biological and psychological factors, including both gender (Fillingim and Maixner 1995, Berkley 1997, Cook et al 1998) and the researchers' and the subjects' expectations (Zatrick and Dimsdale 1990, Bayer et al

1998, Ohrbach et al 1998). In sum, true pain tolerance measures cannot be obtained for most experimental pain stimuli. Moreover, measures of pain tolerance are not likely to be externally valid, and several confounding variables can potentially influence these measures. These limitations should be considered when interpreting pain tolerance data.

Ratings of muscle pain

Muscle pain ratings can be defined as verbal reports of stimulus intensities that are above pain threshold, and a variety of scales can be employed to obtain ratings of the perceptions of pain experienced in muscle. A major advantage of obtaining pain ratings during stimuli that evoke muscle pain is that the ratings can be used to examine a persons response to a noxious stimulus in a more complex and multidimensional fashion than either pain threshold or tolerance measures. Moreover, muscle pain ratings may be more likely to represent or generalize to the pain experienced during everyday physical activities such as walking stairs or carrying groceries. This may especially be the case for chronic illnesses such as chronic low back pain, fibromyalgia or chronic fatigue syndrome, where complaints of muscle and joint pain are common in, or central to, the diagnoses of the disease.

After obtaining ratings of muscle pain, psychophysics can be used to make inferences about possible neurophysiological mechanisms underlying muscular pain (Price and Harkins 1992). For example, Bendtsen and colleagues (1997) chose a psychophysical approach to assess pain responses to noxious pressure applied to tender muscle sites in 25 women with fibromyalgia and 25 healthy controls. These investigators examined the stimulus-response functions for muscle pain intensity using a visual analogue scale. The results indicated that pain intensity ratings for tender muscles increased linearly for the fibromyalgia patients while the slope of the function for the controls was a positively accelerating power function. Pain pressure responses for non-tender muscles increased in a positively accelerating manner for both groups. These results suggest that the nociceptive input from tender muscle in fibromyalgia patients is qualitatively different than normal controls and that pain modulatory mechanisms may be dysfunctional in fibromyalgia patients.

While pain ratings represent a more sensitive and complete measure of muscle pain, they are not free from biases such as cultural, social, biological or psychological factors. For example, and with respect to gender differences, Cook et al (1998) reported that females reported higher leg muscle pain intensity ratings than males during cycle ergometry when the data were expressed as a function of the absolute exercise intensity (i.e. 98, 110, 122, 134, 146, 158 W power output). However, when the data were expressed relative to the participants peak power output (i.e. 60%, 70%, 80%, 90%, and 100% of peak power output), females rated the leg muscle pain as significantly less intense than males. The results from this experiment underscore the usefulness of comparing pain ratings relative to a common maximum (i.e. peak power output in Watts), a procedure that is not ethically possible with most types of noxious stimuli.

Measurement tools and techniques

As stated previously, ratings of both muscle pain intensity and emotion can be made using a variety of techniques including category scales, visual analogue scales (VAS), and true psychophysical methods such as magnitude estimation (see Table 46.1). VAS and cate-

Table 46.1 — Commonly used scales and tools for the measurement of muscle pain

Rating and analogue scales:[a]
  Category rating scales
  Numerical rating scales
  Numerical rating scales with verbal descriptors[b]
  Visual analogue scales (VAS)[b]

Ratio scaling techniques:[c]
  Magnitude estimation
  Magnitude production

Multidimensional pain measures:[d]
  McGill pain questionnaire (short and long form)
  Descriptor differential scale

Behavioural measures of pain:[e]
  Facial expressions
  Time to withdrawal from a painful stimulus
  Limping behaviour
  Guarding behaviour
  Pain drawing

[a]For more detailed information refer to Turk and Melzack 1992
[b]See Figures 46.1 and 46.2
[c]For a complete review of ratio scaling techniques see Snodgrass et al 1985
[d]For a more complete description of the McGill Pain Questionnairre refer to Melzack 1975; For a complete description of the Descriptor Differential Scale refer to Gracely and Kwilosz 1988
[e]For a more detailed description of behavioural pain refer to Turk and Melzack 1992

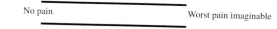

No pain   Worst pain imaginable

No unpleasantness   Most unpleasantness imaginable

Figure 46.1 — Visual analogue scale (VAS) for assessing pain intensity and emotion. Patients or study participants are instructed that the left edge of the line represents "no pain at all" or "no unpleasantness" while the right edge of the line represents the "worst pain imaginable" or "worst unpleasantness imagineable". Individuals are also instructed to make a vertical mark on the 10 cm line that accurately represents current pain intensity at a particular body location. The distance from 0, measured in millimetres, quantifies the pain intensity. (Diagram not to scale)

gory scales, such as those presented in Figures 46.1 and 46.2, are commonly used because they are quick, easy to administer and score and, more importantly, because there is substantial evidence that category and VAS measures of pain are reliable and valid (Revill et al 1976, Jensen et al 1986, Cook et al 1997). Most category scales used to assess muscle pain are limited by "ceiling effects". The 0–10 category pain scale (Fig. 46.2) is designed to overcome these limitations by allowing users to choose a number above 10 when

Pain Intensity Scale

0	No pain at all
$\frac{1}{2}$	Very faint pain (just noticeable)
1	Weak pain
2	Mild pain
3	Moderate pain
4	Somewhat strong pain
5	Strong pain
6	
7	Very strong pain
8	
9	
10	Extremely intense pain (almost unbearable)
●	Unbearable pain

Figure 46.2 — Category-ratio scale for assessing pain. With this scale the subject is free to choose values greater than but relative to 10 (see black dot). For example, if the subject experienced muscle pain that was twice as strong as 10 "extremely intense (almost unbearable), they would respond with the number 20. Reproduced from, and instructions published in, Cook et al 1998.

necessary. It is a category scale not only designed to have ratio properties (i.e., possessing a true zero and unbounded), but it has been shown to perform similarly to ratio scaling methods (Borg 1972, Cook et al 1997).

Alternatively, if a researcher is interested in obtaining a detailed description of an individual's response to pain, classical psychophysical ratio scaling methods such as magnitude estimation and magnitude production can be employed. More comprehensive descriptions of these methods are available elsewhere (Engen 1971a,b). Briefly, with magnitude estimation the participant is instructed to assign a number (any number!) to the first muscle pain stimulus that represent his or her perceived pain intensity. The participants are then instructed that subsequent stimuli are to be judged in relation to the number used in association with the first stimulus. For example, let us assume the first stimulus is given a pain rating of 10. If the test subject judges the second stimulus to be half as painful then the second stimulus is given a pain rating of 5. If a third stimulus is judged to be twice as painful as the first stimulus it would be given a rating of 20. Ratio scaling methods result in muscle pain rating functions with ratio properties because they allow the subject to operate along an unlimited numeric and sensory continuum. However, inter-individual comparisons cannot be made with a magnitude estimation approach. This is because one cannot assume that an individual's assignment of the rating 100 to a pain stimulus is qualitatively the same as another individual's rating 100. Moreover, psychophysical methods are often too cumbersome for use in applied clinical settings. Hence, easily used scales that are qualitatively similar among individuals, and that have established reliability and validity, can be advantageous in both the laboratory and clinical setting. This is especially true, given the evidence that both the VAS (Fig. 46.1) and the category-ratio (Fig. 46.2) scales provide ratio-level measurement (Price 1988, Price and Harkins 1992, Cook et al 1997). Researchers and clinicians should take care to choose a method that best fits his or her practical needs.

While not the focus of this chapter, it is important to note that in clinical settings muscle pain is often assessed in terms of the patient's physical behaviours, such as range of motion, limping, time to withdraw from a noxious stimulus, avoiding the use of (or rubbing) an injured area or quantifying facial expressions indicative of pain (Craig and Patrick 1985, Turk and Melzack 1992). More complete descriptions of behavioural and clinical pain measures are available to the interested reader (Turk and Melzack 1992). These approaches assess pain and provide information that goes beyond its magnitude, and they are very useful in determining appropriate treatment for chronic pain patients. However, behavioural pain tests can vary from clinic to clinic, and they are often conducted in uncontrolled settings. It is, therefore, recommended that clinicians employ standardized muscle pain measures. Moreover, it is important that all investigators interested in examining muscle pain use appropriate instructional sets when assessing muscle pain. Detailed instructions that inform the subject precisely of what is expected of them and that provide anchors in which to operate ensure the collection of interpretable data.

Laboratory methods used in the elicitation and measurement of muscle pain

Laboratory methods for inducing acute pain are advantageous because the environment can be controlled. Moreover, the use of standardized pain stimuli provides the opportunity to attempt to replicate both clinical and experimental findings, which can lead to a better understanding and treatment of muscle pain disorders. A variety of different stimuli, such as noxious chemicals, pressure and electricity, have been used to produce acute muscle pain in the laboratory. Each approach has certain advantages and disadvantages. It is important to recognize that there does not appear to be a strong relationship between people's pain responses to one type of noxious stimulus and their responses to other noxious stimuli (Janal et al 1994). The potential lack of generalizability across noxious stimuli means that investigators interested in measuring muscle pain must carefully decide which noxious stimuli to employ, and they should exercise caution when interpreting results.

Experimental muscle pain

Pressure

Perhaps the most widely used device to assess muscle pain in both clinical research settings is the pressure algometer. Mechanical pressure is commonly used to assess trigger points in myofascial and fibromyalgia pain syndromes (Gerwin 1992, Kosek and Ekholm 1995, Kosek et al 1996, Bendtsen et al 1997), and to assess pain thresholds and tolerances in experimental settings (Forgione and Barber 1971, Brennum et al 1989, Gracely 1994, Cook et al 1997). Mechanical stimuli such as the pressure from a football cleat applied against the anterior tibialis have been used as a pain stimulus in exercise and pain studies (Ryan and Kovacic 1966, Ryan and Foster 1967, Bartholomew et al 1996). The advantages of the newer pressure algometers are that the rate of increase in pressure applied can be precisely controlled. This is important because research has shown that pain responses to mechanical pressure can be influenced by the rate at which the pressure is applied and by the magnitude of the area that is stimulated (Gracely 1994). However, pressure algometry applied to the surface of the skin inevitably stimulates cutaneous, as well as deep, tissue receptors. This may result in either gating of the nociceptive signal or, if the pressure is of sufficient intensity, an exacerbation of the nociceptive input. The potential confound of cutaneous nociceptor stimulation should be considered. Some investigators have employed skin anaesthesia to minimize this problem (Kosek et al 1996).

Electricity

Electricity stimulation has also been used to produce muscle pain. Advantages of this technique are that the stimulus is highly reproducible, and it is relatively easy to control. However, it does not represent a type of stimulus that naturally occurs with normal muscle action. This is because the electrical stimulus excites afferent pathways in an unnatural, synchronized fashion, with the signal bypassing the afferent receptors completely. Moreover, in many cases, the electrical current stimulates both nociceptive and non-nociceptive afferent nerve fibres (Gracely 1994). Thus, it is unclear how well pain rating during electrical stimulation generalize to the pain experienced during a naturally occurring muscle contraction.

Chemical stimuli

Noxious chemicals, such as the intramuscular injection of hypertonic saline, have been used to provoke muscle pain (Graven-Nielsen et al 1997, Matre et al 1998). The stimulus can be controlled by injecting different concentrations (e.g., 10% vs 20%) of saline within the muscle. The type of pain induced by hypertonic saline is described as dull, aching and cramping in nature. Unfortunately, this method is invasive, requiring both the anaesthetic and saline injection. This introduces a potential confound in the pain ratings because the participants perceptions may be influenced by the experimental procedure. Specifi-

cally, pre-exposure to a painful needle stick has the potential to alter subsequent perceptions of pain induced by the hypertonic saline injection (Padawer and Levine 1992). Studies involving microdialysis suggest that pain resulting from intramuscular injection of hypertonic saline is related to increased intramuscular sodium and/or potassium content (Graven-Nielsen et al 1997). However, it is unlikely that this type of hypertonic saline environment is ever encountered in a natural setting such as trigger point flare up in fibromyalgia.

Ischaemia

Compression-ischaemia is a muscle pain stimulus that has been employed in laboratory studies since the 1930s (Lewis et al 1931). The pain is induced by applying supra-systolic pressure with an inflatable cuff around the upper arm and then requiring participants to perform hand-grip exercise. Compression-ischaemia produces pain that increases over time and which is dependent upon the energy expended by the muscle and the contraction frequency (Lewis et al 1931, Mills et al 1982, O'Connor and Cook 1999). One disadvantage of this method is the lack of certainty over whether the mechanical compression or the magnitude of the ischaemia is identical across repeated trials; another is the assumption that the end point of hand exercise during compression-ischaemia is caused by intolerable pain rather than fatigue (Park and Rodbard 1962). Therefore, pain and fatigue ratings should be obtained during this procedure and the contribution of both to subjective tolerance should be assessed.

Muscle actions

Experimental pain stimuli have many advantages for researching muscle pain, and they may have the potential to uncover mechanisms involved in noxious signal transmission. However, in most cases, the pain induced by experimental stimuli is novel, and it is unlikely to generalize to muscle pain that an individual normally experiences. Hence, a potentially useful, and presently under utilized, pain stimulus is that of naturally occurring muscle pain associated with moderate to intense exercise (Dorpat and Holmes 1955, Caldwell and Smith 1966, Hamilton et al 1996, Cook et al 1997, 1998). Exercise models such as moderate-to-high intensity hand-grip exercise and cycle ergometry have been shown to reliably produce forearm and leg muscle pain, respectively (Dorpat and Holmes 1955, Caldwell and Smith 1966, Cook et al 1997). Naturally occurring muscle pain is described as exhausting, intense, sharp, burning, cramping, pulling and rasping (Cook et al 1997). These same descriptors have been used to characterize clinical pain conditions such as menstrual pain, arthritic pain, cancer pain and chronic back pain (Melzack and Katz 1992). Therefore, an advantage of using an exercise model of muscle pain is that it may be more likely to generalize to the pain experienced by chronic pain patients.

Another advantage of naturally occurring muscle pain is that it can be produced transiently, safely and reproducibly. Moreover, the inter-individual pain ratings can be examined relative to each individual's maximum performance. This makes within and between group comparisons potentially more meaningful than if a pre-set maximum is used; as is the case with other noxious laboratory pain stimuli (e.g., pressure, electricity, chemicals).

Moving towards a multidimensional measure of pain

To this point I have described how pain measures are commonly reported and some of the techniques used to elicit and assess muscle pain. For the most part, the assessment and elicitation of pain is measured in terms of the individual's perception of pain intensity. However, intensity is only one aspect of pain. As stated earlier, pain is a complex phenomenon. There are multiple features representative of the pain experience including its location, quality (e.g., stabbing, throbbing, sharp or dull) and how it changes over time.

There are several approaches that can be used to assess pain in a broader dimension (Gracely 1994). For example, the Descriptor Differential Scale was developed to minimize potential response bias. The scale is also designed to provide separate assessments of the sensory and emotional components of pain. It is based on the psychophysical approach of cross-modality matching (Gracely and Kwilosz 1988), and it allows clinical researchers to determine whether pain treatments influence both or only one of these dual pain dimensions. Another simple approach used to assess pain more thoroughly is to examine both the intensity and emotional components of pain with the use of two VAS measures. One VAS is labelled to inquire about the intensity and the other to assess how unpleasant the pain is (Fig. 46.1). Finally, the McGill Pain Questionnaire (MPQ; Melzack 1975, Wilkie et al 1990) has been used extensively to assess three aspects of pain—the sensory quality, the affective quality and an overall evaluation of the pain experi-

ence. Thus, the tools are available for the researcher to assess pain in a multidimensional context that provides information beyond simply quantifying how intense a particular pain stimulus is.

Concluding remarks

A more sophisticated muscle pain assessment approach is necessary for both researchers and clinicians. There are many ways to assess muscle pain and each method has its advantages and disadvantages. Pain threshold and tolerance measures are easy to obtain, but they are often unreliable. Pain intensity ratings provide a more complete assessment of the muscle pain experience, but the ratings can be influenced by external factors such as personality and gender. The tools used to gather pain data also vary in sophistication. Simple category scales are easy to use, but they are less sensitive than true ratio methods. Magnitude estimation and production methods are sensitive, but they do not allow for inter-individual comparisons. Several clinical and experimental tools exist to elicit muscle pain in a controlled fashion. Stimuli such as noxious pressure, electricity, chemicals and ischaemia are controllable, but they may not generalize to the experience of clinical muscle pain. Muscle pain that is produced naturally during muscular contractions may provide a model that is more generalizable to the chronic muscle pain experience, yet is safely and transiently produced. It is recommended, that in addition to the unidimensional measures of pain intensity, researchers and clinicians take a more multidimensional approach addressing the qualities and emotions associated with the pain experience. There are several tools available to assess pain more thoroughly including scales that assess both the intensity and unpleasantness (e.g., the VAS and the Descriptor Differential Scale) and the quality of the muscle pain experience (e.g., the McGill Pain Questionnaire). Thus, the proper use and application of multiple pain measures can lead to a better understanding of both chronic and naturally occurring muscle pain conditions.

References

Bartholomew JB, Lewis BP, Linder DE, Cook DB. (1996) Post-exercise analgesia: replication and extension. *J Sports Sci* 14: 329–334.

Bayer TL, Coverdale JH, Chiang E, Bangs M. (1998) The role of prior pain experience and expectancy in psychologically and physically induced pain. *Pain* 74: 327–331.

Bendtsen L, Norregaard J, Jensen R, Olesen J. (1997) Evidence of qualitatively altered nociception in patients with fibromyalgia. *Arth Rheum* 40: 98–102.

Berkely KJ. (1997) Sex differences in pain. *Beh Brain Res* 20: 371–380.

Borg G. (1972) A ratio scaling method for interindividual comparisons. *Reports from the Institute of Applied Psychology.* The University of Stockholm, 27: 1–8.

Brennum J, Kjeldsen M, Jensen K, Jense TS. (1989) Measurement of human pressure-pain thresholds on fingers and toes. *Pain* 38: 211–217.

Caldwell LS, Smith RP. (1966) Pain and endurance of isometric muscle contractions. *J Engineer Psychol* 5(1): 25–32.

Chapman CR. (1977) Sensory decision theory methods in pain research: A reply to Rollman. *Pain* 3: 295–305.

Clark WC. (1974) Pain sensitivity and the report of pain: An introduction to sensory decision theory. *Anesthesiology* 40: 272–287.

Clark WC, Goodman J. (1973) Effects of suggestion on d' and Cx for pain detection and pain tolerance. *J Appl Psychol* 83: 364–372.

Cleeland CS, Ryan KM. (1994) Pain assessment: Global use of the Brief Pain Inventory. *Ann Acad Med Singapore* 23: 129–138.

Cook DB, O'Connor PJ, Eubanks SA, Smith JC, Lee M. (1997) Naturally occurring muscle pain during exercise: assessment and experimental evidence. *Med Sci Sports Exerc* 29: 999–1012.

Cook DB, O'Connor PJ, Oliver SE, Lee Y. (1998) Sex differences in naturally occurring leg muscle pain and exertion during maximal cycle ergometry. *Intl J Neurosci* 95: 183–202.

Craig KD, Patrick CJ. (1985) Facial expression during induced pain. *J Personal Social Psychol* 48: 1080–1091.

Dorpat TL, Homes TH. (1955) Mechanisms of skeletal muscle pain and fatigue. *A M A Arch Neurol Psychiat* 74: 628–640.

Engen T. (1971a) Psychophysics I: Discrimination and detection. In: Kling JW, Riggs LA, eds. *Experimental Psychology 3rd ed.* New York: Holt pp 11–46.

Engen T. (1971b) Psychophysics II: Scaling methods. In: Kling JW, Riggs LA, eds. *Experimental Psychology 3rd ed.* New York: Holt pp 47–86.

Fillingim RB, Maixner W. (1995) Gender differences in the response to noxious stimuli. *Pain Forum* 4: 209–221.

Forgione AG, Barber TX. (1971) A strain gauge stimulator. *Psychophysiology* 8: 102–106.

Gerwin RD. (1992) The clinical assessment of myofascial pain. In: Turk DC, Melzack R, eds. *Handbook of Pain Assessment.* New York: The Guilford Press, pp. 61–70.

Gracely RH. (1994) Studies of pain in normal man. In: Wall PD, Melzack R, eds. *Textbook of Pain 3rd ed.* New York: Churchill Livingstone, pp. 315–336.

Gracely RH, Kwilosz DM. (1988) The descriptor differential scale: Applying psychophysical principles to clinical pain assessment. *Pain* 35: 279–288.

Graven-Nielsen T, McArdle A, Phoenix J, et al. (1997) In vivo model of muscle pain: Quantification of intramuscular chemical, electrical, and pressure changes associated with saline-induced muscle pain in humans. *Pain* 69: 137–143.

Guilford JP. (1954) *Psychometric Methods.* New York: McGraw-Hill.

Hamilton AL, Killian KJ, Summers E, Jones NL. (1996) Quantification of intensity of sensations during muscular work by normal subjects. *J Appl Physiol* 81: 1156–1161.

Holroyd KA, Holm JE, Keefe FJ, et al. (1992) A multicenter evaluation of the McGill Pain Questionnaire: Results from more than 1700 chronic pain patients. *Pain* 48: 301–311.

International Assocation for the Study of Pain, Subcommittee on Taxonomy. (1979) Pain terms: A list with definitions and notes on usage. *Pain* 6: 249–252.

Janal MN, Glusman M, Kuhl JP, Clark WC. (1994) On the absence of correlation between responses to noxious heat, cold, electrical and ischemic stimulation. *Pain* 58: 403–411.

Jensen MP, Karoly P, Braver S. (1986) The measurement of clinical pain intensity: A comparison of six methods. *Pain* 27: 117–126.

Kemppainen P, Hämäläinen O, Könönen M. (1998) Different effects of physical exercise on cold pain sensitivity in fighter pilots with and without the history of acute in-flight neck pain attacks. *Med Sci Sports Exerc* 30(4): 577–582.

Kosek E, Ekholm J. (1995) Modulation of pressure pain thresholds during and following isometric contraction. *Pain* 61: 481–486.

Kosek E, Ekholm J, Hansson P. (1996) Modulation of pressure pain thresholds during and following isometric contraction in patients with fibromyalgia and in healthy controls. *Pain* 64: 415–423.

Lewis T, Pickering GW, Rothschild P. (1931) Observations upon muscular pain in intermittent claudication. *Heart* 15: 359–389.

MacIntyre DL, Reid WD, McKenzie DC. (1995) Delayed muscle soreness: The inflammatory response to muscle injury and its clinical implications. *Sports Med* 20(1): 24–40.

Matre DA, Sinkjaer T, Svensson P, Arendt-Nielsen L. (1998) Experimental muscle pain increases the human stretch reflex. *Pain* 75: 331–339.

Mayer T, Gatchel R, Mayer H, Kishino N, Keeley J, Mooney V. (1987) A prospective two year study of functional restoration in industrial low back injury, an objective assessment procedure. *JAMA* 258: 1763–1767.

McNicol D. (1972) *A primer of signal detection theory.* London: George Allen & Unwin.

Melzack R. (1975) The McGill Pain Questionnaire: Major properties and scoring methods. *Pain* 1: 277–299.

Melzack R, Katz J. (1992) The McGill Pain Questionnaire: appraisal and current status. In: Turk DC, Melzack R, eds. *Handbook of Pain Assessment.* New York: The Guilford Press, pp. 152–168.

Mills KR, Newham DJ, Edwards RHT. (1982) Force, contraction frequency and energy metabolism as determinants of ischaemic muscle pain. *Pain* 14: 149–154.

O'Connor PJ, Cook DB. (1999) Exercise and pain: the neurobiology, measurement, and laboratory study of pain in relation to exercise in humans. Holloszy JO, Seals DR, eds. *Exercise and Sport Sciences Reviews. Vol. 27.* Baltimore: Williams & Wilkins, pp 119–166.

Ohrbach R, Crow H, Kamer A. (1998) Examiner expectancy effects in the measurement of pressure pain thresholds. *Pain* 74: 163–170.

Padawer WJ, Levine FM. (1992) Exercise-induced analgesia: Fact or artifact? *Pain* 48: 131–135.

Park SR, Rodbard S. (1962) Effects of load and duration of tension on pain induced by muscular contraction. *Am J Physiol* 203(4): 735–738.

Price DD. (1988) *Psychological and Neural Mechanisms of Pain.* New York: Raven Press.

Price DD, Harkins SW. (1992) Psychophysical approaches to pain measurement and assessment. In: Turk DC, Melzack R, eds. *Handbook of Pain Assessment.* New York: The Guilford Press, pp. 111–134.

Revill SI, Robinson JO, Rosen M, Hogg MIJ. (1976) The reliability of a linear analogue for evaluating pain. *Anaesthesia* 31: 1191–1198.

Ryan ED, Foster R. (1967) Athletic participation and perceptual augmentation and reduction. *J Pers Soc Psychol* 6: 472–476.

Ryan ED, Kovacic CR. (1966) Pain tolerance and athletic participation. *Perceptual Motor Skills* 22: 383–390.

Snodgrass JG, Levy-Berger G, Haydon M. (1985) Psychophysical Methods Snodgrass JG, ed. In: *Human Experimental Psychology.* New York: Oxford University Press, pp 58–87.

Turk DC, Melzack R. (1992) The measurement of pain and the assessment of people experiencing pain. In: Turk DC, Melzack R, eds. *Handbook of Pain Assessment.* New York: The Guilford Press, pp. 3–12,

Wilkie DJ, Savedra MC, Holzemer WL, Tesler MD, Paul SM. (1990) Use of the McGill Pain Questionnaire to measure pain: A meta-analysis. *Nursing Res* 39(1): 36–41.

Wolff BB. (1969) Factor analysis of human pain responses: Pain endurance as a specific pain factor. *J Ab Psychol* 78: 292–298.

Yang JC, Clark C, Nagai S, Berkowitz B, Spector S. (1979) Analgesic action and pharmokinetics of morphine and diazepam in man: An evaluation by sensory decision theory. *Anesthesiology* 51: 495–502.

Zatzick DF, Dimsdale JE. (1990) Cultural variations in response to painful stimuli. *Psychosom Med* 52: 544–557.

47

Strategies for increasing optimal function of skeletal muscle in the aged

Ben F. Hurley and Frederick M. Ivey

Introduction

The loss of muscle mass and muscle function with age (sarcopenia) has important health and economic implications because it is related to functional disabilities (Bassey et al 1992, Rantanen and Avela 1997), risk of falling (Lipsitz et al 1994, Lord et al 1994) and a higher rate of outpatient clinic visits in the elderly (Buchner et al 1997). Therefore, this review will start with an overview on the effects of aging on muscle mass, muscular strength and muscle quality. We will then summarize the research literature on the most commonly used interventions for the prevention and possible reversal of sarcopenia. These are strength training and hormone replacement therapy (growth hormone and testosterone administration). A discussion of the effects of these interventions on muscle mass, strength and muscle quality (when information is available) will be followed by a summary of possible risks or side-effects associated with each intervention.

Ageing effects

Muscle mass and muscular strength

There is not much known about the losses in muscle mass with age because most studies on this topic have used cross-sectional designs with indirect measurements of muscle mass that are not accurate or reliable. However, when muscle mass is measured by creatinine excretion in large populations, it follows a similar time course of age-related decline as that of muscular strength (Metter et al 1999). Strength has been reported to reach peak values between the ages of 25–35 years, it is maintained or slightly lower in the forties, and then it decreases by about 12–14% per decade after age 50 (Asmussen and Heeboll-Nielsen 1962, Larsson et al 1979, Lindle et al 1997, Metter et al 1997). Although these age-associated differences in strength are highly correlated with age differences in estimated muscle mass (Maughan et al 1983, Kallman et al 1990, Reed et al 1991), the specific mechanisms for the age-related decline in strength have not yet been identified.

Men are about 30–50% stronger than women in both the arm and leg muscle groups (Asmussen and Heeboll-Nielsen 1962, Frontera et al 1991, Reed et al 1991, Miller et al 1993), and they have a greater proportion of their muscle mass in the arms than women (Miller et al 1993, Kanehisa et al 1994). This has important implications for targeting interventions, because women may be more susceptible to the

adverse consequences and disabilities associated with decrements in strength (Foley et al 1986) and muscle mass, since they typically live a longer time period in infirmity than men (Hing 1987). Results from our group (Lynch et al 1999) confirm previous reports that showed a greater age-related loss of strength in the leg compared with the arm (Viitasalo 1985, Bember et al 1991, Reed et al 1991). A possible explanation for the greater leg strength loss may be greater disuse in the legs, but no physiological or biochemical mechanisms have been identified.

Muscle quality

Although not as well understood as strength, the importance of expressing age-related strength losses in terms of muscle quality was emphasized by a panel of experts at the 1996 National Institutes on Aging (NIA) workshop entitled, "Sarcopenia and Physical Performance in Old Age", in which they concluded that there is a need for more comprehensive evaluations of age-related changes in muscle quality (Dutta et al 1997). The term muscle quality (MQ), also known as specific tension, refers to strength per unit of muscle mass, and it may be a better indicator of muscle function than strength alone (Dutta et al 1997). The impact of age on MQ may depend on the method by which muscle mass is estimated (Frontera et al 1991, Metter et al 1999). For example, Metter et al (1999) observed age-associated losses in both arm and leg muscle groups when muscle mass was estimated using limb cross-sectional areas from anthropometric measurements and when using fat-free mass (FFM) measured by dual energy X-ray absorptiometry (DEXA), but not when muscle mass was estimated by creatinine excretion. Until recently, it was believed that MQ declines with age in men (Viitasalo 1985, Young et al 1985, Kallman et al 1990, Reed et al 1991, Overend et al 1992), but not in women (Young et al 1984). In contrast, we found age-related declines in MQ in the arm and leg musculature in both men and women throughout the adult life span (ages 19–94 years) (Lindle et al 1997, Lynch et al 1999). Leg MQ declined with age at the same rate in men as women, although arm MQ did decline more in men than in women (Lynch et al 1999). The age-related decline in leg MQ was greater than arm MQ in women, whereas arm and leg MQ declined with age at the same rate in men. MQ of the arm was significantly higher than MQ of the leg across the entire adult life span in both genders.

Strength training

Muscle mass

Strength training (ST) has been shown to be a safe (Hurley et al 1995) and effective (Frontera et al 1988, Brown et al 1990, Fiatarone et al 1990, Charette et al 1991, Nichols et al 1993, Nelson et al 1994, Treuth et al 1994, Hurley et al 1995, McCartney et al 1995, O'Hagan et al 1995, Sipilä and Suominen 1995, Phillips and Hazeldene 1996, Welle et al 1997, Tracy et al 1999) intervention for counteracting losses in muscle mass with age. Increases in muscle magnetic resonance imaging (MRI) cross-sectional areas (CSA) of 3 to 15% have been reported in response to ST of varying durations (Frontera et al 1988, Fiatarone et al 1990, 1994, Roman et al 1993, Keen et al 1994, McCartney et al 1995, Welle et al 1997).

Welle et al 1997) concluded that aging reduced the hypertrophic response of muscle when they compared young and older men and women after 3 months of ST using CSA of the elbow flexors, and the knee flexors and extensors. However, Fiatarone et al (1990) demonstrated that even in the very old, significant gains in muscle size, strength and functional mobility could be achieved through ST.

Ivey et al (2000) compared age and gender responsiveness to ST and found that men increase their quadricep muscle volume about twice as much as women (204 ± 20 cm^3 vs 101 ± 13 cm^3) in response to ST, but that older men and women (65–75 years) increase their muscle volume just as much as young men and women (20–30 years; Ivey et al 2000). When men and women stop training, there is a significantly greater loss of muscle volume, after about 6 months of detraining, in men than in women (151 ± 13 cm^3 vs 88 ± 7 cm^3), but again, no significant difference between young and older individuals (Ivey et al 2000). Therefore, in contrast to gender, ageing does not appear to affect the muscle mass response to either ST or detraining.

Muscular strength

Frontera et al (1988) observed large increases (107%) in 1 repetition maximum (RM) values for the knee extensors after 12 weeks of bilateral ST in older subjects. Even greater relative increases in leg strength (174%) were later reported from the same laboratory (Fiatarone et al 1990) after only 8 weeks of training. In another study, women displayed a 93% increase in 1 RM strength after 12 weeks of ST (Charette et al 1991). When these percentage increases are compared

with those reported in young subjects after ST, one might be tempted to conclude that older individuals have substantially greater responses to ST than young subjects, based on the fact that the percentage increases in strength among young subjects are typically less than half of those reported by Frontera et al (1988), Fiatarone et al (1990) and (Charette et al (1991). However, it is more likely that these unusually high increases in strength may be explained by the extremely low baseline strength values (sometimes in the single digits) of the very elderly and the absence of familiarization sessions to control for motor learning effects (Frontera et al 1988, Fiatarone et al 1990, Charette et al 1991). ST-induced increases in strength in both young and older subjects more commonly range from ~30 to 44% (Kauffman 1985, Craig et al 1989, Welle et al 1995, Rall et al 1996).

We recently demonstrated that changes in 1 RM strength in response to both ST and detraining are affected by age, but not by gender (Lemmer et al 2000). In response to 9 weeks of ST, young subjects showed greater increases in 1 RM knee extensor strength compared to the older subjects ($34 \pm 3\%$ vs $28 \pm 3\%$, respectively). In absolute terms the average increases in young subjects amounted to ~24 kg compared with ~16 kg increases in older subjects in 1 RM knee extension strength. The 28% increase in our older subjects represents a reversal of ~30 years of age-associated decline in strength (Lynch et al 1999). ST-induced increases in muscular strength appear to be maintained equally well in young and older men and women during 12 weeks of detraining, and they are maintained above baseline levels even after 31 weeks of detraining in young men, young women and older men (Lemmer et al 2000). However, older subjects show a greater strength loss than young subjects between 12 and 31 weeks of detraining. This, along with another report from our laboratory (Ivey et al 2000), suggests that disuse atrophy does not entirely explain the decreases in muscular strength with advancing age. Nevertheless, the results do reinforce the idea that older individuals can respond well to ST, and maintain ST-induced increases in muscular strength just as well as young individuals for at least 12 weeks after training has ceased.

Muscle quality

Although many investigators have reported greater relative increases in strength than in muscle size after ST in older subjects (Frontera et al 1988, Brown et al 1990, Fiatarone et al 1990, 1994, Roman et al 1993, Treuth et al 1994, Hakkines and Hakkinen 1995,

Welle et al 1997, Hakkinen et al 1998), only a few of them have reported MQ (or specific tension) values before and after training. Welle et al (1997) compared MQ responses to ST in young and older men and women. Both the young and older groups increased their MQ with ST, but there was no difference in response to training between the age groups for most muscle groups tested, with the exception of the knee flexors, which increased to a greater extent in the older group.

Ivey et al (2000) compared MQ response to ST in young men, young women (20–30 years), older men and older women (65–75 years) and found that all four groups increased their MQ significantly with training, but the gain in MQ was significantly greater in the young women compared with the other three groups. After 31 weeks of detraining, MQ values remained significantly elevated above baseline levels in all groups, except the older women. These findings suggest that factors other than muscle mass contribute to strength gains with ST in young and older men and women, but that those other factors may account for a higher portion of the strength gains in young women. These factors continue to maintain strength levels above baseline for up to 31 weeks after cessation of training in young men and women, and in older men. The specific neuromuscular mechanisms responsible for ST-induced increases in MQ are unknown, though increases in motor unit recruitment or discharge rate, increased activation of synergistic muscles and decreased activation of antagonist muscles are possible explanations (Sale 1988, Hakkinen et al 1998). Another factor that could affect changes in MQ with ST is alterations in muscle architecture (Kawakami et al 1993, 1995). Kawakami et al (1993) reported greater pennation angles in subjects with hypertrophied muscles compared with controls.

Risks

We have demonstrated that ST posses very little risk of injury in the elderly (Hurley et al 1995). The risk of injury from strength testing appears to be higher than that of strength training (Pollock et al 1991).

Hormone replacement therapy

In addition to alterations in muscular activity there is a growing body of evidence indicating that age-associated alterations in hormonal status may contribute to sarcopenia (Rudman et al 1981, Carter 1995). Evidence that alterations in these hormonal relationships have a direct impact on the structure and function of skeletal muscle comes from studies investigating the effects of hormone deficiencies in young adults (Cuneo et al 1990, Rutherford et al 1994, Mauras et al 1998).

Given the established link between the hormonal systems and physical frailty, hormone replacement therapy has emerged as a potential intervention strategy for the prevention and possible reversal of sarcopenia. Hence, this portion of the review will focus on growth hormone and testosterone administration, because they are the most commonly studied hormone replacement therapies with regard to their effects on muscle function.

Growth hormone administration

Muscle mass

The impetus behind the current consideration of recombinant human growth hormone (rhGH) as a potential remedy for age-induced physical frailty is the much heralded study by Rudman et al (1990). While short-term experimentation with rhGH in the elderly had previously been undertaken (Marcus et al 1990), the work of Rudman et al (1990) was the first of four placebo-controlled clinical trials that have been completed with older individuals. This group studied 21 healthy men (61–81 years) with low plasma insulin-like growth factor (IGF-1) levels (12 treatment, 9 placebo controls) before and after treatment with rhGH (30 μg rhGH/kg body weight, 3 times per week for 6 months). The administration of rhGH was accompanied by, among other things, an 8.8% increase in estimated lean body mass (potassium-40 counting), and it caused widespread speculation that this form of therapy was a viable means of counteracting sarcopenia, despite the absence of functional outcome measurements. A subsequent clinical trial in 1994 involving 27 healthy elderly women (13 treatment, 14 placebo controls; Holloway et al 1994) conflicted somewhat with the earlier results by Rudman et al (1990) in that measurements of nitrogen balance were unchanged during the treatment period. This implied the absence of any effect on muscle mass. Again, no functional measurements were reported. Two factors that could have accounted for some of the conflicting results were that only women were studied, instead of men, and no baseline IGF-1 level criteria was established for the women (Holloway et al 1994). The results may have been further confounded by oestrogen replacement therapy undertaken by half of the treatment group, since it is unclear whether the two forms of treatment produce synergistic effects.

Muscular strength

Papadakis et al (1996) conducted a similar study to Rudman et al (1990) with respect to population, duration of rhGH treatment (6 months), dosage and IGF-1 deficiency status, but for the first time measured functional outcomes in their elderly subjects. Despite observing a 4.3% increase in lean tissue mass by DEXA, functional ability did not improve in the elderly men (mean age, 75 years; n = 26) receiving rhGH compared with placebo controls (n = 26). Functional ability was ascertained from a battery of tests, which included measurements of muscle strength, aerobic capacity (VO_2 max), and physical performance (e.g., stair climbing ability). At 6 months, the changes in muscle strength were no different between the rhGH and placebo groups with respect to either grip strength or knee extensor strength. Furthermore, neither endurance nor physical performance tests were altered with growth hormone treatment. Further support for the above findings came from Yarasheski and Zachwieja (1996) who observed no improvements in upper or lower body strength, despite significant gains in lean body mass after 4 months of rhGH administration in 60 to 74-year-old men and women.

Despite the virtual absence of evidence for functional benefits to the elderly from rhGH therapy, many still hypothesize that rhGH retains the potential for improving functional outcomes in older individuals based on rhGH trials in younger subjects with organic hypopituitary disorders. Although these growth hormone deficient (GHD) adults have achieved functional gain after rhGH, while elderly individuals have not, the conclusions that can be drawn from these two different population groups are not far apart. For example, in the studies of GHD adults lasting 6 months or less (Jorgensen et al 1989, Salomon et al 1989, Degerblad et al 1990, Cuneo et al 1991, Whitehead et al 1992), rhGH had no effect on muscle strength or endurance capacity despite significant increases in either total lean body mass or regional muscle mass. However, when study durations were expanded to a year or more (Jorgensen et al 1991, 1994, 1996, Johannsson et al 1997, Janssen et al 1999), GHD recipients of rhGH began to show clear signs of functional improvements. In this context, Janssen et al (1999) reported significant increases in quadriceps isometric and isokinetic strength in GHD adults after 1

year of treatment with rhGH. After 3 years in another study (Jorgensen et al 1994), GHD adults nearly normalized their isometric strength and endurance capacity. Therefore, it appears that body composition changes precede functional improvements, which require a much longer period of rhGH administration become apparent. Interestingly, to date, none of the controlled clinical trials using rhGH in the elderly have extended past 6 months. Therefore, there is a real need for placebo controlled rhGH trials of extended duration in the elderly.

Risks

Long-term treatment of elderly individuals with rhGH has so far been limited by a high incidence of side-effects. Among the individuals who continued therapy after the controlled 6 month trial of Rudman et al (1990) had ended, a large percentage were ultimately forced to discontinue treatment because of the severity of the physical problems encountered. Most notable among the adverse reactions were substantial frequencies of carpal tunnel syndrome, gynaecomastia and hyperglycaemia (Rudman et al 1991, Cohn et al 1993). In addition, there are a number of rhGH side-effects arising from sodium and water retention. These include weight gain, dependent oedema and a sensation of tightness in the hands (Mardh et al 1994). It has also been linked to hyperinsulinaemia (Moller et al 1993), hypertension (Salomon et al 1989), cardiovascular complications and headache with tinnitus (Bengtsson et al 1993). Future studies may need to assess the risk to benefit ratio of using lower dosages.

It has been suggested that side-effects arise out of the failure of growth hormone injections to mimic the pulsatile release pattern of natural pituitary secretion. Two proposed methods of augmenting the somatotrophic axis, while at the same time circumventing this problem, have been the administration of GH releasing hormone and GH releasing peptides. While the side-effects associated with these GH secretagogues have so far been few, compared with rhGH, most studies have been too brief (Merriam et al 1997) to determine body composition and functional effects. One alternative has been the administration of recombinant human IGF-1 (rhIGF-1), either alone (Thompson et al 1995) or in combination with rhGH (Sullivan et al 1998). Unfortunately, this form of therapy is similarly accompanied by the physical side-effects of fluid retention, gynaecomastia and orthostatic hypotension when given in high enough doses (Thompson et al 1995, Sullivan et al 1998).

Testosterone

Muscle mass

Less work has been done to investigate the potential of testosterone administration for reversing age-related declines in skeletal muscle mass and function. However, in the few testosterone trials completed in elderly hypogonadal men, the results have been encouraging. The evidence has been virtually unequivocable in support of the ability of testosterone to have a positive impact on muscle mass. Treatment progressively increased lean tissue mass measured by DEXA (Young et al 1993) and potassium-40 counting (Forbes et al 1992), due in large part to observed increases in muscle protein synthesis (Griggs et al 1989).

Strength

The first report in elderly hypogonadal men involved biweekly intramuscular injections of testosterone enanthate (TE) for a period of 3 months (Morley et al 1993). Hand-grip strength was significantly elevated in the group receiving TE, but not in placebo controls. Two years later it was reported that elderly men with low serum levels of testosterone could achieve strength benefits after just 4 weeks of testosterone administration (Urban et al 1995). The isokinetic muscle strength increases, in both right and left hamstring and quadricep muscles, were accompanied by significant changes in the fractional synthetic rate of muscle protein, determined by stable isotope infusion. Interestingly, the testosterone injections were shown to increase IGF-1 mRNA implying a mediating role for the intramuscular IGF-1 system.

Sih et al (1997) examined the effects of year-long testosterone administration (200 mg injected intramuscularly every 2 weeks) on 32 older men (15 placebo, 17 treatment; mean age, 67 years). Testosterone significantly improved bilateral grip strength in contrast with the placebo control group, which showed no change.

Risks

Although Sih et al (1997) concluded that testosterone may have a role in the treatment of frailty in hypogonadal older men, they also advised extreme caution concerning potential risks due to 7 of the 17 having to withdraw prematurely because of an abnormal elevation in haematocrit. However, there were no incidences of a rise in prostate specific antigen (PSA), a side-effect reported by others (Morley et al 1993). Evidence of prostate carcinoma has even been reported during testosterone replacement in some elderly hypogonadal men (Jackson et al 1989). Consequently, if testosterone replacement is ever to be marketed as an appropriate countermeasure for andropause and the accompanying muscular deficits, more research related to the precise dosing and delivery method will need to be undertaken to avoid unnecessary health risks.

Summary

Table 47.1 is a qualitative summary of the benefits and risks associated with strength training, growth hormone administration and testosterone administration, the three most commonly used interventions for sarcopenia. Muscle mass is used as an indicator of muscle structure, whereas strength and muscle quality are indicators of muscle function. Based on the published research to date, it appears that strength training offers a better benefit to risk ratio than the administration of growth hormone or testosterone.

Table 47.1 — Summary of benefits and risks for the most commonly used interventions for sarcopenia

Intervention	Duration of intervention	Muscle mass	Muscle strength	Muscle quality	Risks
Strength training	3–6 months	↑↑	↑↑↑	↑↑	↑
Growth hormone	≤6 months	↑	↔	?	↑↑
	>6 months	↑	↑	?	↑↑↑
Testosterone	≤ 6 months	↑	↑	↑	↑↑

↑, small increase; ↑↑, moderate increase; ↑↑↑, large increase; ↔, no change.

References

Asmussen E, Heeboll-Nielsen K. (1962) Isometric muscle strength in relation to age in men and women. *Ergonomics* 5: 167–169.

Bassey E, Fiatarone M, O'Neil E, Kelly M, Evans W, Lipsitz L. (1992) Leg extensor power and functional performance in very old men and women. *Clin Sci* 82: 321–327.

Bember MG, Massey BH, Bemben DA, Misner JE, Boileau RA. (1991) Isometric muscle force production as a function of age in healthy 20- to 74-yr-old men. *Med Sci Sports Exerc* 11: 1302–1310.

Bengtsson BA, Eden S, Lonn L, et al. (1993) Treatment of adults with growth hormone deficiency with recombinant human GH. *J Clin Endocrinol Metab* 76: 309–317.

Brown A, McCartney N, Sale D. (1990) Positive adaptation to weight-lifting in the elderly. *J Appl Physiol* 69: 1725–1733.

Buchner DM, Cress ME, de Lateur BJ, et al. (1997) The effect of strength and endurance training on gait, balance, fall risk, and health services use in community-living older adults. *J Gerontol Med Sci* 52A: M218–M224.

Carter WJ. (1995) Effect of anabolic hormones ad insulin-like growth factor-I on muscle mass and strength in elderly persons. *Clin Geriat Med* 11: 735–748.

Charette S, McEvoy L, Pyka G, et al. (1991) Muscle hypertrophy response to resistance training in older women. *J Appl Physiol* 70: 1912–1916.

Cohn L, Feller AG, Draper MW, Rudman IW, Rudman D. (1993) Carpal tunnel syndrome and gynaecomastia during growth hormone treatment of elderly men with low gynaecomastia during growth hormone treatment of elderly men with low circulating IGF-1 concentrations. *Clin Endocrinol* 39: 417–425.

Craig B, Everhart J, Brown R. (1989) The influence of high-resistance training on glucose tolerance in young and elderly subjects. *Mechan Aging Development* 49: 147–157.

Cuneo RC, Salmon F, Wiles CM, Sonksen PH. (1990) Skeletal muscle performance in adults with growth hormone deficiency. *Hormone Res* 33: 55–60.

Cuneo RC, Salomon F, Wiles CM, Hesp R, Sonksen PH. (1991) Growth hormone treatment in growth hormone-deficient adults. I. Effects on muscle mass and strength. *J Appli Physiol* 70: 688–694.

Degerblad M, Almkvist O, Grunditz R, et al. (1990) Physical and phsychological capabilities during substitution therapy with recombinant growth hormone in adults with growth hormone deficiency. *Acta Endocrinol* 123: 185–193.

Dutta C, Hadley EC, Lexell J. (1997) Sarcopenia and physical performance in old age: overview. *Muscle Nerve (Suppl)* 5: S5–S9.

Fiatarone M, Marks E, Ryan N, Meredith C, Lipsitz L, Evans W. (1990) High-intensity strength training in nonagenarians. *JAMA* 263: 3029–3034.

Fiatarone M, O'Neill E, Ryan N, et al. (1994) Exercise training and nutritional supplementation for physical frailty in very elderly people. *N Engl J Med* 330: 1769–1775.

Foley DJ, Berkman LF, Branch LG, Farmer ME, Wallace RB. (1986) Physical function. In: *Established Populations for Epidemiologic Studies of the Elderly: Resource Data Book*, Cornoni-Huntley J, Brock DB, Ostfeld AM, Taylor JO, Wallace RB. Bethesda, MD: NIH, (NIH Publication 86–2443) pp. 56–88.

Forbes GB, Porta CR, Herr BE, Griggs RC. (1992) Sequence of changes in body composition induced by testosterone and reversal of changes after drug is stopped. *JAMA* 267: 397–399.

Frontera WR, Hughes VA, Lutz KJ, Evans WJ. (1991) A cross-sectional study of muscle strength and mass in 45- to 78-yr-old men and women. *J Appl Physiol* 71: 644–650.

Frontera WR, Meredith C, O'Reilly K, Knuttgen H, Evans WJ. (1988) Strength condition in older men: skeletal muscle hypertrophy and improved function. *J Appl Physiol* 63: 1038–1044.

Griggs RC, Kingston W, Jozefowicz RF, Herr BE, Forbes GB, Halliday D. (1989) Effect of testosterone on muscle mass and muscle protein synthesis. *J Appl Physiol* 66: 498–503.

Hakkinen K, Kallinen M, Izquierdo M, et al. (1998) Changes in agonist-antagonist EMG, muscle CSA, and force during strength training in middle-aged and older people. *J Appl Physiol* 84: 1341–1349.

Hakkine K, Hakkinen A. (1995) Neuromuscular adaptations during intensive strength training in middle-aged and elderly males and females. *Electromyogram Clin Neurophysiol* 35: 137–147.

Hing E. (1987) *Preliminary data from the 1985 National nursing home survey*. Use of Nursing Homes by the Elderly: (PHS) 87-1250. Hyattsville, MD, US Public Health Service (Generic).

Holloway L, Butterfield GE, Hintz RI. (1994) Effects of recombinant human growth hormone on metabolic indices, body composition, and bone turnover in healthy elderly women. *J Clin Endocrinol Metab* 79: 470–479.

Hurley B, Redmond R, Pratley R, Trueth M, Rogers M, Goldberg A. (1995) Effects of strength training on muscle hypertrophy and muscle cell disruption in older men. *Int J Sports Med* 16: 380–386.

Ivey FM, Tracy BL, Lemmer JT, et al. (2000) Effects of age, gender and myostatin genotype on the hypertrophic response to heavy resistance strength training. *J Gerontol Med Sci* 55A: M641–M648.

Ivey FM, Tracy BL, Lemmer JT, NessAiver M, Metter EJ, Fozard JL, Hurley BF. (2000) Effects of strength training and detraining on muscle quality: age and gender comparisons. *J Gerontol Biol Sci* 55A: B152–B157.

Jackson JA, Waxman J, Spiekerman AM. (1989) Prostate complications of testosterone replacement therapy. *Arch Int Med* 149: 2365–2366.

Janssen YJH, Doornbos J, Roelfsema F. (1999) Changes in muscle volume, strength, and bioenergetics during recombinant human growth hormone (GH) therapy in adults with GH deficiency. *J Clin Endocrinol Metab* 84: 279–284.

Johannsson G, Grimby G, Sunnerhagen KS, Bengtsson BA. (1997) Two years of growth hormone (GH) treatment increase isometric and isokinetic muscle strength in GH-deficient adults. *J Clin Endocrinol Metab* 82: 2877–2884.

Jorgensen JOL, Pedersen SA, Thuesen L, Jorgenson J, Ingemann-Hansen T, Skakkebaek NE, Christiansen JS. (1989) Beneficial effects of growth hormone treatment in GH-deficient adults. *Lancet* 3: 1221–1225.

Jorgensen JOL, Pedersen SA, Thuesen L, et al. (1991) Long-term growth hormone treatment in growth hormone deficient adults. *Acta Endocrinol* 125: 449–453.

Jorgensen JOL, Thuesen L, Muller J, Ovesen P, Skakkebaek NE, Christiansen JS. (1994) Three years of growth hormone treatment in growth hormone-deficient adults: near normalization of body composition and physical performance. *Eur J Endocrinol* 130: 224–228.

Jorgensen JOL, Vahl N, Hansen TB, Thuesen L, Hagen C, Christiansen JS. (1996) Growth hormone versus placebo treatment for one year in growth hormone deficient adults: increase in exercise capacity and normalization of body composition. *Clin J Encocrinol Metab* 70: 519–527.

Kallman DA, Plato SC, Tobin JD. (1990) The role of muscle loss in the age-related decline of grip strength: cross-sectional and longitudinal perspectives. *J Gerontol Biol Sci Med Sci* 45: M82–M88.

Kanehisa H, Ikegawa S, Tsunoda N, Fukunaga T. (1994) Cross-sectional areas of fat and muscle in limbs during growth and middle age. *Int J Sports Med* 15: 420–425.

Kauffman TL. (1985) Strength training effect in young and aged women. *Arch Phys Med Rehab* 66: 223–226.

Kawakami Y, Abe T, Kuno S, Fukunaga T. (1995) Training-induced changes in muscle architecture and specific tension. *Eur J Appl Physiol* 72: 37–43.

Kawakami Y, Abe T, Fukunaga T. (1993) Muscle fiber pennation angles are greater in hypertrophied than in normal muscles. *J Applied Physiol* 74: 2740–2744.

Keen AA, Yue GH, Enoka RM. (1994) Training-related enhancement in the control of motor output in the elderly. *J Appl Physiol* 77: 2648–2658.

Larsson L, Grimby G, Karlsson J. (1979) Muscle strength and speed of movement in relation to age and muscle morphology. *J Appl Physiol* 46: 451–456.

Lemmer JT, Hurlbut DE, Martel GF, Tracy BL, Ivey FM, Metter EJ. (2000) Age and gender responses to strength training and detraining. *Med Sci Sports Exerc* 32: 1505–1512.

Lindle R, Metter E, Lynch N, et al. (1997) Age and gender comparisons of muscle strength in 654 women and men aged 20–93. *J Appl Physiol* 83: 1581–1587.

Lipsitz LA, Nakajima I, Gagnon M, Hirayama T, Connelly CM, Izumo H. (1994) Muscle strength and fall rates among residents of Japanese and American nursing homes: An international cross-cultural study. *J Am Geriat Soc* 42: 953–959.

Lord SR, Ward JA, Williams P, Anstey K. (1994) Physiological factors associated with falls in older community-dwelling women. *J Am Geriat Soc* 42: 1110–1117.

Lynch NA, Metter EJ, Lindle RS, et al. (1999) Muscle Quality I: Age-associated differences in arm vs. leg muscle groups. *J Appl Physiol* 86: 188–194.

Marcus R, Butterfield GE, Holloway L, et al. (1990) Effects of short term administration of recombinant human growth hormone to elderly people. *J Clin Endocrinol Metab* 70: 519–527.

Mardh G, Lundin K, Borg G, Johnsson B, Lindberg A. (1994) Growth hormone. *Endocrinol Metab* 1: 43–49.

Maughan RJ, Watson JS, Weir J. (1983) Strength and cross-sectional area of human skeletal muscle. *J Physiol* 338: 37–49.

Mauras N, Hayes V, Welch S, et al. (1998) Testosterone deficiency in young men: marked alterations in whole body protein kinetics, strength, and adiposity. *J Clin Endocrinol Metab* 83: 1886–1892.

McCartney N, Hicks AL, Martin J, Webber CE. (1995) Long-term resistance training in the elderly: effects on dynamic strength, exercise capacity, muscle, and bone. *J Gerontol Biol Sci Med Sci* 50: B97–B104.

Merriam GR, Buchner DM, Prinz PN, Schwartz RS, Vitiello MV. (1997) Potential applications of GH secretagogs in the evaluation and treatment of the age-related decline in growth hormone secretion. *Endocrinology* 7: 49–52.

Metter EJ, Lynch N, Conwit R, Lindle R, Tobin J, Hurley B. (1999) Muscle quality and age: cross-sectional and longitudinal comparisons. *J Gerontol Biol Sci* 54A: B207–B218.

Metter EJ, Conwit R, Tobin J, Fozard JL. (1997) Age-associated loss of power and strength in the upper extremities in women and men. *J Gerontol Biol Sci Med Sci* 52: B267–B276.

Miller AE, Mac Dougall JD, Tarnopolsky MA, Sale DG. (1993) Gender differences in strength and muscle fiber characteristics. *Eur J Appl Physiol* 66: 245–262.

Moller J, Jorgensen JOL, Lauersen T. (1993) Growth hormone dose regimens in adult GH deficiency: effects on biochemical growth markers and metabolic parameters. *Clin Endocrinol* 39: 417–425.

Morley JE, Perry HM, Kaiser FE, et al. (1993) Effects of testosterone replacement therapy in old hypogonadal males: a preliminary study. *J Am Geriat Soc* 41: 149–152.

Nelson M, Fiatarone M, Morganti C, Trice I, Greenberg R, Evans W. (1994) Effects of high-intensity strength training on multiple risk factors for osteoporotic fractures. A randomized controlled trial. *JAMA* 272: 1909–1914.

Nichols JF, Omizo DK, Peterson KK, Nelson KP. (1993) Efficacy of heavy-resistance training for active women over sixty: muscular strength, body composition, and program adherence. *J Am Geriat Soc* 41: 205–210.

O'Hagan F, Sale D, MacDougall D, Garner S. (1995) Response to Resistance Training in Young Women and Men. *Intl J Sports Med* 16: 314–321.

Overend T, Cunningham D, Paterson D, Lefcoe M. (1992) Thigh composition in young and elderly men determined by computed tomography. *Clin Physiol* 12: 629–640.

Papadakis MA, Grady D, Black D, et al. (1996) Growth hormone replacement in healthy older men improves body composition but not functional ability. *Annu Int Med* 124: 708–716.

Phillips W, Hazeldene R. (1996) Strength and muscle mass changes in elderly men following maximal isokinetic training. *Gerontology* 42: 114–120.

Pollock M, Carroll J, Graves J, et al. (1991) Injuries and adherence to walk/jog and resistance training programs in the elderly. *Med Sci Sports Exerc* 23: 1194–1200.

Rall LC, Meydani SN, Kehayias JJ, Dawson-Hughes B, Roubenoff R. (1996) The effect progressive resistance training in rheumatoid arthritis: increased strength with changes in energy balance or body composition. *Arthritis Rheumatol* 39: 415–426.

Rantanen T, Avela J. (1997) Leg extension power and walking speed in very old people living independently. *J Gerontol Med Sci* 52A: M225–M231.

Reed R, Pearlmutter L, Yochum K, Meredith K, Mooradian A. (1991) The relationship between muscle mass and muscle strength in the elderly. *J Am Geriat Soc* 39: 555–561.

Roman W, Fleckenstein J, Stray-Gundersen J, Alway S, Peshock R, Gonyea W. (1993) Adaptations in the elbow flexors of elderly males after heavy-resistance training. *J Appl Physiol* 74: 750–754.

Rudman D, Feller AG, Cohn L, Shetty KR, Rudman IW, Drape MW. (1991) Effects of human growth hormone on body composition in elderly men. *Hormone Res* 36: 73–81.

Rudman D, Feller AG, Nagraj HS, et al. (1990) Effects of human growth hormone in men over 60 years old. *N Engl J Med* 323: 1–6.

Rudman D, Kutner M, Rogers CM, Lubin MF, Fleming GA, Balbi, V. (1981) Impaired growth hormone secretion in the adult population. *J Clin Invest* 67: 1361–1369.

Rutherford OM, Beshyah SA, Johnston DG. (1994) Quadriceps strength before and after growth hormone replacement in hypopituitary adults: relationship to changes in lean body mass and IGF-1. *Endocrinol Metab* 1: 41–47.

Sale DG. (1988) Neural adaptation to resistance training. *Med Sci Sports Exerc* 20: S135–S145.

Salomon F, Cuneo RC, Hesp R, Sonksen PH. (1989) The effects of treatment with recombinant human growth hormone on body composition and metabolism in adults with growth hormone deficiency. *N Engl J Med* 321: 1797–1803.

Sih R, Morley JE, Kaiser FE, Perry HM, Patrick P, Ross C. (1997) Testosterone replacement in older hypogonadal men: a 12-month randomized controlled trial. *J Clin Endocrinol Metab* 82: 1661–1667.

Sipilä S, Suominen H. (1995) Effects of Strength and Endurance Training on Thigh and Leg Muscle Mass and Composition in Elderly Women. *J Appl Physiol* 78: 334–340.

Sullivan DH, Carter WJ, Warr WR, Williams LH. (1998) Side effects resulting from the use of growth hormone and insulin-like growth factor-I as combined therapy to frail elderly patients. *J Gerontol* 53A: M183–M187.

Tenover JS, Journal of Clinical Endocrinology Metabolism (1992) Effects of testosterone supplementation in the aging male. *J Clin Endocrinol Metab* 75: 1092–1098.

Thompson JL, Butterfield GE, Marcus R, et al. (1995) The effects of recombinant human insulin-like growth factor-I and growth hormone on body composition in elderly women. *J Clin Endocrinol Metab* 80: 1845–1852.

Tracy BL, Ivey FM, Hurlbut D, et al. (1999) Muscle Quality II: Effects of strength training in 65-75 year old men and women. *J Appl Physiol* 86: 195–201.

Treuth M, Ryan A, Pratley R, et al. (1994) Effects of strength training on total and regional body composition in older men. *J Appl Physiol* 77: 614–620.

Urban RJ, Bodenburg YH, Gilkison C, et al. (1995) Testosterone administration to elderly men increases skeletal muscle strength and protein synthesis. *Am J Physiol* 269: E820–E826.

Viitasalo JT. (1985) Muscular strength profiles and anthropometry in random samples of men aged 31-35, 51-55, and 71-75 years. *Ergonomics* 28: 1563–1574.

Welle S, Totterman S, Thornton C. (1997) Effect of age on muscle hypertrophy induced by resistance training. *J Gerontol* 51A: M270–M275.

Welle S, Thornton C, Statt M. (1995) Myofibrillar protein synthesis in young and old human subjects after three months of resistance training. *Am J Physiol* 268: E422–E427.

Whitehead HM, Boreham C, McIlrath EM, et al. (1992) Growth hormone treatment of adults with growth hormone deficiency: results of a 13-month placebo controlled cross-over study. *Clin Endocrinol* 36: 45–52.

Yarasheski KE, Zachwieja JJ. (1996) Effect of growth

hormone administration on muscle strength, protein turnover, and glucose metabolism in the elderly. *FASEB* 10: A754.

Young A, Strokes M, Crowe M. (1984) Size and strength of the quadriceps muscles of old and young women. *Eur J Clin Invest* 14: 282–287.

Young A, Strokes M, Crowe M. (1985) The size and strength of the quadriceps muscles of old and young men. *Clin Physiol* 5: 145–154.

Young NR, Baker HWG, Liu G, Seeman E. (1993) Body composition and muscle strength in health men receiving testosterone enanthate for contraception. *J Clin Endocrinol Metab* 77: 1028–1032.

48

Nutritional therapies for improving skeletal muscle function and recovery in pathologies: an overview

S. C. Dennis and E. W. Derman

Introduction

In this chapter, we review nutritional therapies that may improve the exercise capacity of patients with skeletal muscle disorders. Skeletal muscle disorders can be broadly sub-divided into neuropathies and myopathies (Table 48.1). Neuropathies are caused by damage to the nerves enervating the muscle and myopathies result from defects within the muscle itself. Damage to motor neuronal cell bodies or to their peripheral axons leads to an atrophy of usually both slow (Type I) and fast (Type II) muscle fibres. In contrast, defects within the muscle result in either an atrophy of mainly Type II fibres, a progressive destruction of both Type I and II fibres or an impaired supply of energy from mitochondria.

Classification of neuropathies and myopathies is complicated by large overlaps in muscle disorders. For example, mitochondrial and lipid storage myopathies are only classified separately because mitochondrial myopathies generally reduce the supply of energy for contraction more than disorders of fat metabolism. Defects in mitochondrial myopathies include impairments in the metabolism of pyruvate or in complex I of the electron transport chain. Lipid storage myopathies result from insufficient carnitine or carnitine acyl transferase activity to transport fatty acyl coenzyme A into the mitochondria or a deficiency in the 3-hydroxyacyl CoA dehydrogenases in complex II of the electron transport chain. Complexes I and II are described later under the heading of riboflavin therapy.

Antioxidant therapy

In many of the disorders involving mitochondrial malfunction or muscle degeneration, there is evidence of oxidative "stress". Oxidative stress occurs when the formation of mainly superoxide free-radical ($O_2^{-\bullet}$) by the mitochondrial electron transport chain exceeds their removal by the enzymes, superoxide dismutase and catalase. Unless the excess $O_2^{-\bullet}$ and its related reactive oxygen species (H_2O_2 and OH^-) are "scavenged" by the antioxidant defences, they oxidatively damage proteins and unsaturated lipids in cell membranes. Antioxidant defenses include glutathione (GSH), vitamins E and C, ubiquinol (coenzyme Q_{10}) and the enzymes, glutathione reductase and glutathione peroxidase. Glutathione reductase converts oxidized glutathione (GSSG) back to GSH and glutathione peroxidase breaks down the lipid peroxides formed by free-radical attack.

Whether anti-oxidant therapy is of benefit in the treatment of muscle disorders is debatable (Table 48.2). Whereas Mathews et al (1993) reported that antioxidants were ineffective in the treatment of patients with mitochondrial myopathy, Peluchetti et al (1991) found that high doses of vitamins E and C improved the function of such patients. High doses of vitamins E and C have also been shown to protect against the oxidative damage caused by zidovudine-treatment of human immunodeficiency virus (HIV) infection (de la Asuncion et al 1998). Treatment of HIV patients with zidovudine (formerly called azidothymidine or AZT) causes a mitochondrial and lipid

Table 48.1 — Summary of muscle disorders[a]

Neuropathy		Myopathy			
		Shrinkage of muscle fibres	Destruction of muscle fibres		Impairment of energy supply
Neuronal cell body	Peripheral axon	Atrophic (A)	Inflammatory (A)	Dystrophic (G)	Metabolic (G or A)
Spinal muscular atrophy (G)	Hereditary motor and sensory myopathy (G)	Chronic malignant diseases	Polymyositis	Duchenne,	Mitochondrial myopathy
Amyotrophic lateral sclerosis (A)	Alcohol abuse (A) Diabetes (A) Guillain–Barré (A)	Hypothyroidism Corticosteroids	Dermatomyositis	Becker, Myotonic etc.	Lipid storage myopathy

[a]Data are taken from Jones and Round (1990). (G) and (A) indicate a genetic or an acquired disorder.

Table 48.2— Anti-oxidant treatment of skeletal muscle disorders

Treatment[a]	Muscle disorder	Effect	References
Vitamins E & C + ubiquinol	Mitochondrial myopathy	None	Mathews et al 1993
Vitamins E & C	Mitochondrial myopathy	Improved	Peluchetti et al 1991, de al Asuncion et al 1998
Vitamin E + selenium	Amyotrophic lateral sclerosis	Improved	Apostolski et al 1998
	Myotonic dystrophy	None	Orndahl et al 1986, 1994
	Duchenne muscular dystrophy	None	Backman et al 1988, Jackson et al 1989

[a]Daily doses of vitamin E and selenium were 600–800 mg and 1.6–1.8 mg, respectively.

storage myopathy with carnitine deficiency that is unrelated to the inflammatory polymyositis associated with HIV infection (Dalakas et al 1990, 1994).

Anti-oxidant therapy may also benefit patients with sporadic amyotrophic lateral sclerosis (Table 48.2). Apostolski et al (1998) found that vitamin E and selenium (a micronutrient constituent of glutathione peroxidase) increased the low superoxide dismutase and glutathione peroxidase activities of patients with sporadic amyotrophic lateral sclerosis and slowed the progression of the disease. In contrast, others have reported no affect of vitamin E and selenium supplementation on the oxidative damage and functional deterioration of patients with myotonic dystrophy or Duchenne muscular dystrophy (Table 48.2).

Corticosteroid treatment

High, ≥ 0.75 mg/kg body mass/day, doses of prednisone produce the greatest improvements in patients with Duchenne muscular dystrophy but such doses often have to be reduced to <0.3 mg/kg body mass/day to limit the side-effects of weight gain, cushingoid appearance and excessive hair growth (Mendell et al 1989, Fenichel et al 1991, Griggs et al 1991). Contrary to original opinion, the benefit of prednisone in the treatment of patients with Duchenne muscular dystrophy is probably not due to its suppression of the T-lymphocyte invasion into the diseased muscle (Griggs et al 1993, Kissel et al 1993). Instead, it is more likely that prednisone stabilizes membranes. A membrane stabilizing effect would explain why prednisone treatment also benefits some patients with lipid storage myopathies (Engel and Siekert 1972, Mastaglia et al 1980, Tein et al 1995). In such patients, prednisone is thought to stabilize the attachment of the 3-hydroxyacyl CoA dehydrogenases to the electron transport chain in complex II of the inner mitochondrial membrane.

Riboflavin therapy

Duchenne muscular dystrophy has been more commonly treated with the corticosteroid, prednisone. However, de Visser et al (1986) reported a case of a progressive lipid storage myopathy that did not respond to prednisone treatment. Instead the condition of their patient only improved with riboflavin (vitamin B_2) therapy. Others have also found that a ~100 mg/day intake of riboflavin improved the function of patients with mitochondrial (complex I deficiency) and lipid storage (complex II deficiency) myopathies (Table 48.3). Riboflavin is a constituent of the flavin mononucleotide (FMN) and flavin adenine dinucleotide (FAD) prosthetic groups in complexes I and II of the mitochondrial electron transport chain. FMN transfers hydrogen atoms from NADH dehydrogenase to ubiquinone (coenzyme Q_{10}) in complex I. FAD delivers hydrogen atoms to ubiquinone from the glycerol phosphate dehydrogenase, succinate dehydrogenase and 3-hydroxyacyl CoA dehydrogenase enzymes in complex II.

Carnitine supplementation

Some patients with mitochondrial or lipid storage myopathies also appear to benefit from carnitine supplementation. Several groups have shown that 50–200 mg/kg body mass/day doses of carnitine improve the condition of mitochondrial and lipid storage myopathy patients, irrespective of the presence or absence of a

Table 48.3 — Riboflavin and carnitine treatment of mitochondrial and lipid storage myopathies

Treatment[a]	Muscle disorder	Effect	References
Riboflavin	Mitochondrial myopathy	Improved	Ogle et al 1997
	Lipid storage myopathy	Improved	de Visser et al 1986, Gregersen et al 1986, DiDonato et al 1989, Peluchetti et al 1991, Antozzi et al 1994, Araki et al 1994
Riboflavin + carnitine	Mitochondrial myopathy	Improved	Bernsen et al 1991
Carnitine	Mitochondrial myopathy[b]	Improved	DiDonato et al 1978, Campos et al 1993
	Lipid storage myopathy[b]	Improved	Matsuishi et al 1985
	Lipid storage myopathy[c]	None	de Visser et al 1986, DiDonato et al 1989, Antozzi et al 1994
		Improved	Sengers et al 1980, Snyder et al 1982
	Idiopathic carnitine deficiency	Improved	Shapira et al 1993

[a]Riboflavin (vitamin B$_2$) doses were around 100 mg/day. Carnitine doses ranged from 50 to 200 mg/kg body mass/day.
[b]With and [c]without carnitine deficiency.

carnitine deficiency (Table 48.3). Carnitine supplementation probably increases the transport of long-chain fatty acids (FA) into the mitochondria of patients with lipid storage myopathies. Scholte et al (1987) found that rates of FA oxidation in muscle mitochondria isolated from patients with lipid storage myopathy were more dependent on the concentration of carnitine in the incubation medium than rates of FA oxidation in muscle mitochondria isolated from control subjects. Whereas a 0.5 mM concentration of carnitine was sufficient for maximum rates of FA oxidation in mitochondria from control subjects, rises in carnitine concentration from 0.5 to 5 mM increased the rates of FA oxidation in the mitochondria from the patients with lipid storage myopathy.

Scholte et al (1987) also reported that patients with a primary carnitine deficiency caused by a renal carnitine leak often develop a cardiomyopathy which is reversed by carnitine supplementation. However, others have shown that carnitine ingestion (2 g/day) does not improve the weakened muscle function in carnitine-deficient, chronic renal-failure patients receiving dialysis (Rogerson et al 1989, Derman et al 1995). Carnitine supplementation also has no affect on FA oxidation (Vukovich et al 1994) or exercise performance in healthy subjects (Trappe et al 1994, Massen et al 1995). In normal individuals, the uptake of carnitine from plasma into muscles occurs against a large concentration gradient (40–60 μM vs 3–4 mM) that is not influenced by carnitine availability (Engel and Rebouche 1984, Soop et al 1988).

Caffeine ingestion

Caffeine ingestion may also improve exercise capacity by promoting FA oxidation. In healthy subjects, an intake of 3–10 mg of caffeine per kg body mass elevates plasma catecholamine concentrations (Graham and Spreit 1991, Spriet et al 1992, Graham and Spreit 1995) and accelerates the release of FA from triacylglycerol stores (Costill et al 1978, Essig et al 1980, Powers et al 1983, Sasaki et al 1987, Dodd et al 1991, Spreit et al 1992, Graham and Spreit 1995). However, only one group has reported that caffeine extends endurance by increasing FA oxidation (Costill et al 1978, Essig et al 1980). Others have found little effect of caffeine ingestion on fuel utilization during exercise and have suggested that caffeine probably acts on the central nervous system. Although caffeine ingestion has no effect on near-maximal work rates leading to exhaustion within 10 min, most studies have shown that caffeine extends the time to fatigue in prolonged (30–90 min) sub-maximal exercise by 20–40% in healthy individuals (Table 48.4).

In contrast, it remains to be determined whether caffeine ingestion improves the more limited exercise capacity of patients with muscle myopathies. We could find only one study on the effects of caffeine on exercise tolerance in a diseased population. In that study, Hirsch et al (1989) gave patients with coronary artery disease a random order of beverages containing either 250 mg of caffeine or placebo. Caffeine inges-

Table 48.4— Caffeine ingestion and exercise capacity[a]

Exercise	Effect	References
Peak power in <1 min	None	Collomp et al 1991
	Improved	Anselme et al 1992, Collomp et al 1992
Progressive exercise to exhaustion in 5–10 min	None	Perkins and Williams 1975, Bond et al 1987, Dodd et al 1991
	Improved	Powers et al 1983
Exercise endurance over 30–90 min	None	Butts and Crowell 1985, Sasaki et al 1987
	Improved	Costill et al 1978, Essig et al 1980, Cardarette et al 1982, Graham and Spriet 1991, 1995, Pasman et al 1995

[a]These studies were conducted in healthy individuals. Caffeine doses ranged from 3–10 mg/kg body mass and were usually ingested 60 min before exercise.

tion increased the patients' peak systolic blood pressure from about 150 to 160 mmHg, but it had no effect on their weakened muscle function.

Creatine supplementation

It is more likely that dietary creatine supplementation may be of benefit to patients with muscle wasting diseases. Creatine "shuttles" energy from the mitochondria to the sites of adenosine triphosphate (ATP) utilization in muscle cells. At the mitochondria, creatine is phosphorylated to creatine phosphate by ATP and, at the myofibrils, creatine phosphate is used in the re-synthesis of ATP from adenosine diphosphate (ADP).

Typically, a 70 kg person excretes about 2 g of muscle creatine a day in the form of urinary creatinine. About half of that creatine is replaced by the liver and the remaining 1 g is obtained from the equivalent of about 250 g of meat in the diet. When sporting individuals creatine "load" they generally increase their intake of creatine to 20–25 g/day for 5–7 days and then maintain their elevated muscle creatine and creatine phosphate contents by ingesting ≥2 g of creatine a day. Large doses of creatine monohydrate (5 g, 4–5 times per day) increase the total creatine content of healthy muscle from 120–130 to 140–150 μmol/g dry weight (Harris et al 1992, Greenhaff et al 1994, Hultman et al 1996), particularly when ingested with carbohydrate (Green et al 1996) and without caffeine (Vandenberghe et al 1996).

Increases in the total creatine content of healthy muscle have little affect on sub-maximal exercise lasting >2 min (Table 48.5). Instead, creatine "loading"

mainly improves performances over <30–60 s, where some of the ATP for muscle contraction is re-synthesized by a net breakdown of creatine phosphate to creatine. Most studies have shown that high doses of creatine improve maximum muscle contractions and sprints by 5–15% (Table 48.5).

Such improvements in muscle function could be even greater in patients with muscle wasting diseases. Patients with muscle wasting diseases often retain less creatine and creatine phosphate in their muscles than normal individuals. Lower than normal levels of creatine and creatine phosphate have been found in patients with muscular dystrophies (Fitch 1977) or with atrophic myopathies secondary to chronic pulmonary or cardiovascular disease (Karisson et al 1975, Bergstrom et al 1976, Moller et al 1982, Jakobsson et al 1990, Gertz et al 1997).

One suggestion that oral creatine supplementation may be useful in the treatment of patients with depressed creatine levels comes from studies of patients with gyrate atrophy of the choroid retina. Gyrate atrophy of the choroid retina is attributed to a defect in creatine synthesis, which leads to a progressive constriction of visual fields and an atrophy of fast-twitch (Type II) muscle fibres. Supplementary creatine (1.5 g/day) in the treatment of gyrate atrophy of the choroid retina stabilizes the condition (Sipila et al 1981) and increases the diameter of Type II muscle fibres (Vannas-Sulonen et al 1985). Large (20 g/day) intakes of creatine have also been shown to improve skeletal muscle function in heart failure patients (Gorden et al 1995, Andrews et al 1998). Gordon et al (1995) found that 10 days of creatine supplementation improved knee extensor peak torque by 5%, one-legged repetitive knee extension performance by 21% and two-legged cycling performance by 10%, with no change in the patients' cardiac ejection fractions. Andrews et

Table 48.5 — Creatine ingestion and exercise capacity[a]

Exercise	Effect	References
Exercise lasting >2 min	None	Terrilion et al 1977, Balsom et al 1993b, Stroud et al 1994, Febbraio et al 1995, Burke et al 1996
Sprint(s) lasting <60 s	None	Cooke et al 1995, Dawson et al 1995, Burke et al 1996, Barnett et al 1996, Mujika et al 1996, Odland et al 1997, Cooke and Barnes 1997
	Improved	Greenhaff et al 1993, Balsom et al 1993a, Birch et al 1994, Balsom et al 1995, Dawson et al 1995, Earnest et al 1995, Casey et al 1996, Grindstaff et al 1997, Prevost et al 1997, Kreider et al 1998
Maximum contraction(s)	None	Thompson et al 1996
	Improved	Greenhaff et al 1993, Birch et al 1994, Ernest et al 1995, Vandenberghe et al 1996, 1997, Volek et al 1997, Bosco et al 1997, Kreider et al 1998

[a]These studies were conducted in healthy individuals. Most creatine doses were 20 g/day for 5 days.

al (1998) reported that 5 days of creatine supplementation increased the number of 5 s handgrips their patients were able to complete at 75% of maximum effort from about 8 to 14. Such findings suggest that creatine therapy should be further investigated in diseases where muscle function is impaired.

Cyst(e)ine supplementation

Cyst(e)ine supplementation may also help to reduce the weakness of patients with atrophic myopathies secondary to clinical conditions such as cancer or chronic renal, pulmonary or cardiovascular disease. Patients with conditions leading to skeletal muscle catabolism (or cachexia) have recently been found to possess abnormally low plasma cystine and glutamine levels (Droge and Holme 1997, Hack et al 1997). A "low CG syndrome" in many muscle-wasting diseases has led to a suggestion that an adequate circulating cystine concentration may be required to limit the normal post-absorptive breakdown of skeletal muscle protein (Droge and Holme 1997). If that hypothesis is correct, cyst(e)ine supplementation could help conserve skeletal muscle protein in patients with chronic malignant diseases.

Conclusion

In summary, anti-oxidant therapy appears to benefit patients with mitochondrial myopathy or sporadic amyotrophic lateral sclerosis but not patients with lipid storage myopathy or muscular dystrophy. Patients with lipid storage myopathy or Duchenne muscular dystrophy have been more commonly treated with prednisone. Some patients with lipid storage or mitochondrial myopathies have also benefited from riboflavin and/or carnitine supplementation. In contrast, carnitine ingestion did not improve the weakened muscle function in chronic renal-failure dialysis patients. Instead, it is more likely that dietary creatine and perhaps cyst(e)ine supplementation may be of benefit to patients with atrophic myopathies secondary to cancer or chronic renal, pulmonary or cardiovascular disease.

References

Andrews R, Greenhaff P, Curtis S, Perry A, Cowley AJ. (1998) The effect of dietary creatine supplementation on skeletal muscle metabolism in congestive heart failure. *Eur Heart J* 19: 617–622.

Anselme F, Collomp K, Mercier B, Ahmaidi S, Prefaut C. (1992) Caffeine increases maximal anaerobic power and blood lactate concentration. *Eur J Appl Physiol* 65: 188–191.

Antozzi C, Garavaglia B, Mora M, et al. (1994) Late-onset riboflavin responsive myopathy with combined multiple acyl coenzyme A dehydrogenase and respiratory chain deficiency. *Neurology* 44: 2153–2158.

Apostolski S, Marinkovic Z, Nikolic A, Blagojevic D, Spasic MB, Michelson AM. (1998) Glutathione peroxidase in amyotrophic lateral sclerosis: the effects of selenium supplementation. *J Environ Pathol Toxicol Oncol* 17: 325–329.

Araki E, Kobayashi T, Kohtake N, Goto I, Hashimoto T. (1994) A riboflavin responsive lipid storage myopathy due to multiple acyl-CoA dehydrogenase deficiency: an adult case. *J Neurol Sci* 126: 202–205.

Backman E, Nylander E, Johansson I, Henriksson KG, Tagesson C. (1988) Selenium and vitamin E treatment of Duchenne muscular dystrophy: no effect on muscle function. *Acta Neurol Scand* 78: 429–435.

Balsom P, Ekblom B, Sjodin B, Huitman E. (1993a) Creatine supplementation and dynamic high-intensity exercise. *Scand J Med Sci Sports* 3: 39–93.

Balsom P, Harridge S, Soderlund K, Sjodin B, Ekblom B. (1993b) Creatine supplementation per se does not enhance endurance exercise performance. *Acta Physiol Scand* 149: 521–523.

Balsom P, Soderlund K, Sjodin B, Ekblom B. (1995) Skeletal muscle metabolism during short duration high-intensity exercise: influence of creatine supplementation. *Acta Physiol Scand* 154: 303–310.

Barnett C, Hinds M, Jenkins D. (1996) Effects of oral creatine supplementation on multiple sprint cycle performance. *Aus J Sci Med Sports* 28: 35–39.

Bergstrom J, Bostrom H, Furst P, Hultman E, Vinnars E. (1976) Preliminary studies of energy rich phosphogens in muscle from severely ill patients. *Crit Care Med* 4: 197–204.

Bernsen PL, Gabreels FJ, Ruitenbeek W, Sengers RC, Stadhouders AM, Renier WO. (1991) Successful treatment of pure myopathy, associated with complex I deficiency, with riboflavin and carnitine. *Arch Neurol* 48: 334–338.

Birch R, Noble D, Greenhaff P. (1994) The influence of dietary creatine supplementation on performance during repeated bouts of maximal isokinetic cycling in man. *Eur J Appl Physiol* 69: 268–270.

Bond V, Adams R, Balkissoon B, et al. (1987) Effects of caffeine on cardiorespiratory function and glucose metabolism during rest and graded exercise. *J Sports Med* 27: 47–52.

Bosco C, Tihanyi J, Pucspk J, et al. (1997) Effect of oral creatine supplementation on jumping and running performance. *Intl J Sports Med* 18: 369–372.

Burke L, Pyne D, Telford R. (1996) Effect of oral creatine supplementation on single-effort sprint performance in elite swimmers. *Intl J Sports Nutri* 6: 222–233.

Butts NK, Crowell D. (1985) Effect of caffeine ingestion on cardiorespiratory endurance in men and women. *Res Q Exercise Sport* 56: 301–305.

Cadarette BS, Levine L, Berube CL, Posner BM, Evans WJ. (1982) Effects of varying doses of caffeine on endurance exercise to fatigue. In: Knuttgen HG, Vogel JA, Poortmans J, eds. *Biochemistry of Exercise*. Champaign: Human Kinetics, pp. 871–876.

Campos Y, Huertas R, Lorenzo G, et al. (1993) Plasma carnitine insufficiency and effectiveness of L-carnitine therapy in patients with mitochondrial myopathy. *Muscle Nerve* 16: 150–153.

Casey A, Constantin-Teodosiu D, Howell D, Huitman E, Greenhaff P. (1996) Creatine ingestion favorably affects performance and muscle metabolism during maximal exercise in humans. *Am J Physiol* 271: E31–E37.

Collomp K, Ahmaidi S, Audran M, Chanal JL, Prefaut C. (1991) Effects of caffeine ingestion on performance and anaerobic metabolism during the Wingate test. *Intl J Sports Med* 12: 439–443.

Collomp K, Ahmaidi S, Chatard JC, Audran M, Prefaut C. (1992) Benefits of caffeine ingestion on sprint performance in trained and untrained swimmers. *Eur J Appl Physiol* 64: 377–380.

Cooke W, Barnes W. (1997) The influence of recovery duration on high intensity exercise performance after oral creatine supplementation. *Can J Appl Physiol* 22: 454–467.

Cooke W, Grandjean P, Barnes W. (1995) Effect of oral creatine supplementation on power output and fatigue during bicycle ergometry. *J Appl Physiol* 78: 670–673.

Costill DL, Dalsky GP, Fink WJ. (1978) Effects of caffeine ingestion on metabolism and exercise performance. *Med Sci Sports* 10: 155–158.

Dalakas MC, Ilia I, Pezeshkpour GH, Laukaitis JP, Cohen B, Griffin JL. (1990) Mitochondrial myopathy caused by long-term zidovudine therapy. *N Engl J Med* 322: 1098–1105.

Dalakas MC, Leon-Monzon ME, Bernardini I, Gahi WA, Jay CA. (1994) Zidovudine-induced mitochondrial myopathy is associated with muscle carnitine deficiency and lipid storage. *Ann Neurol* 35: 482–487.

Dawson B, Cutler M, Moody A, Lawrence S, Goodman C, Randall N. (1995) Effects of oral creatine loading on single and repeated maximal short sprints. *Aus J Sci Med Sports* 27: 56–61.

de la Asuncion JG, del Olmo ML, Sastre J, et al. (1998) AZT treatment induces molecular and ultrastructural oxidative damage to muscle mitochondria. Prevention by antioxidant vitamins. *J Clin Invest* 102: 4–9.

de Visser M, Scholte HR, Schutgens RB, et al. (1986) Riboflavinresponsive lipid-storage myopathy and giutaric aciduria type II of early adult onset. *Neurology* 36: 367–372.

Derman KL, Derman EW, Noakes TD. (1995) Ingestion of L-carnitine does not improve exercise tolerance of patients with chronic renal failure undergoing peritoneal dialysis. *Med Sci Sports Exerc* 27: S146 (Abstract).

DiDonato S, Cornelio F, Balestrini MR, Bertagnolio B, Peluchetti D. (1978) Mitochondria-lipid-glycogen myopathy, hyperlactacidemia and carnitine deficiency. *Neurology* 28: 1110–1116.

DiDonato S, Gellera C, Peluchetti D, et al. (1989) Normalization of short-chain acyl coenzyme A dehydrogenase after riboflavin treatment in a girl with multiple acyl coenzyme A dehydrogenase-deficient myopathy. *Ann Neurol Sci* 25: 479–484.

Dodd SL, Brooks E, Powers SK, Tully R. (1991) The effects of caffeine on graded exercise performance in caffeine naive versus habituated subjects. *Eur J Appl Physiol* 62: 424–429.

Droge W, Holme E. (1997) Role of cysteine levels and glutathione in HIV infection and other diseases associated with muscle wasting and immunological dysfunction. *FASEB J* 11: 1077–1089.

Earnest C, Snell P, Rodriguez R, Almada A, Mitchell T. (1995) The effect of creatine monohydrate ingestion on anaerobic power indices, muscular strength and body composition. *Acta Physiol Scand* 153: 207–209.

Engel AG, Rebouche CJ. (1984) Carnitine metabolism and inborn errors. *J Inherited Metab Dis* 7: 38–43.

Engel AG, Siekert RG. (1972) Lipid storage myopathy responsive to prednisone. *Arch Neurol* 27: 174–181.

Essig D, Costill DL, Handel van PJ. (1980) Effects of caffeine ingestion on utilization of muscle glycogen and lipid during leg ergometer cycling. *Ant J Sports Med* 1: 86–90.

Febbraio M, Flanagan T, Snow R, Zhao S, Carey M. (1995) Effect of creatine supplementation on intramuscular Tcr, metabolism and performance during intermittent exercise. *Acta Physiol Scand* 155: 387–395.

Fenichel GM, Florence JM, Pestronk A, et al. (1991) Long-term benefit from prednisone therapy in Duchenne muscular dystrophy. *Neurology* 41: 1874–1877.

Fitch CD. (1977) Significance of abnormalities of creatine metabolism. In: Rowland LP, ed. *Pathogenesis of human muscular dystrophies*. Amsterdam: Excerpta Medica, pp. 328–340.

Gertz I, Hedenstierna G, Hellers G, Wahren J. (1977) Muscle metabolism in patients with chronic obstructive lung disease and acute respiratory failure. *Clin Sci* 52: 395–403.

Gordon A, Hultman E, Kaijser L, et al. (1995) Creatine supplementation in chronic heart failure increase skeletal muscle creatine phosphate and muscle performance. *Cardiovasc Res* 30: 413–418.

Graham TE, Spriet LL. (1991) Performance and metabolic responses to a high caffeine dose during prolonged exercise. *J Appl Physiol* 71: 2292–2298.

Graham TE, Spriet LL. (1995) Metabolic, catecholamine and exercise performance responses to varying doses of caffeine. *J Appl Physiol* 78: 867–874.

Green A, Simpson E, Littlewood J, Macdonald I, Greenhaff P. (1996) Carbohydrate ingestion augments creatine retention during creatine feedings in humans. *Acta Physiol Scand* 158: 195–202.

Greenhaff P, Bodin K, Harris R, Soderland K, Hultman E. (1994) Effect of oral creatine supplementation on skeletal muscle phosphocreatine resynthesis. *Am J Physiol* 266: E725–E730.

Greenhaff P, Casey A, Short A, Harris R, Soderlund K, Hultman E. (1993) Influence of oral creatine supplementation on muscle torque during repeated bouts of maximal voluntary exercise in man. *Clin Sci* 84: 565–571.

Gregersen N, Christensen MF, Christensen E, Kolvraa S. (1986) Riboflavin responsive multiple acyl-CoA dehydrogenation deficiency. Assessment of 3 years riboflavin treatment. *Acta Paediatr Scand* 75: 676–681.

Griggs RC, Moxley RT III, Mendell JR, et al. (1991) Prednisone in Duchenne dystrophy. A randomized, controlled trial defining the time course and dose response, Clinical investigation of Duchenne dystrophy group. *Arch Neurol* 48: 383–388.

Griggs RC, Moxley RT III, Mendell JR, et al. (1993) Duchenne dystrophy. Randomized, controlled trial of prednisone (18 months) and azathioprine (12 months). *Neurology* 43: 520–527.

Grindstaff P, Kreider R, Bishop R, et al. (1997) Effects of creatine supplementation on repetitive sprint performance and body composition in competitive swimmers. *Intl J Sports Nutr* 7: 330–346.

Hack V, Schmid D, Breitkreutz R, et al. (1997) Cystine levels, cystine flux, and protein catabolism in cancer cachexia, HIV/SIV infection, and senescence. *FASEB J* 11: 84–92.

Harris R, Soderlund K, Hultman E. (1992) Elevation of creatine in resting and exercised muscle of normal subjects by creatine supplementation. *Clin Sci* 83: 367–374.

Hirsch AT, Gervino EV, Nakao S, Come PC, Silverman KJ, Grossman W. (1989) The effect of caffeine on exercise tolerance and left ventricular function in patients with coronary artery disease. *Ann Intern Med* 110: 593–598.

Hultman E, Soderlund K, Timmons J, Cederblad G, Greenhaff P. (1996) Muscle creatine loading in man. *J Appl Physiol* 81: 232–237.

Jackson MJ, Coakley J, Stokes M, Edwards RH, Oster O. (1989) Selenium metabolism and supplementation in patients with muscular dystrophy. *Neurology* 39: 655–659.

Jakobsson P, Jorfeldt L, Brundin A. (1990) Skeletal muscle metabolises and fibre types in patients with advanced chronic obstructive pulmonary disease (COPD), with and without chronic respiratory failure. *Eur Respir J* 3: 192–196.

Jones DA, Round JM. (1990) *Skeletal muscle in health and disease*. Manchester: Manchester University Press, pp. 189–215.

Karlsson J, Willerson JT, Leshin SJ, Mullins CB, Mitchell

JH. (1975) Skeletal muscle metabolises in patients with cardiogenic shock or severe congestive heart failure. *Scand J Clin Lab Invest* 35: 73–79.

Kissel JT, Lynn DJ, Rammohan KW, et al. (1993) Mononuclear cell analysis of muscle biopsies in prednisone- and azathioprine-treated Duchenne muscular dystrophy. *Neurology* 43: 532–536.

Kreider R, Ferreira M, Wilson M, et al. (1998) Effects of creatine supplementation on body composition, strength and sprint performance. *Med Sci Sports Exerc* 30: 73–82.

Massen N, Schröder P, Schneider G. (1995) Carnitine does not enhance maximum oxygen uptake and does not increase performance in endurance exercise in the range of one hour. *Intl J Sports Med* 15: 375 (abstract).

Mastaglia FL, Thompson PL, Papadimitriou JM. (1980) Mitochondrial myopathy with cardiomyopathy, lactic acidosis and response to prednisone and thiamine. *Aust NZ J Med* 10: 660–664.

Mathews PM, Ford B, Dandurand RJ, et al. (1993) Coenzyme Q10 with multiple vitamins is generally ineffective in treatment of mitochondrial disease. *Neurology* 43: 884–890.

Matsuishi T, Hirata K, Terasawa K, et al. (1985) Successful carnitine treatment in two siblings having lipid storage myopathy with hypertrophic cardiomyopathy. *Neuropediatrics* 16: 6–12.

Mendell JR, Moxley RT, Griggs RC, et al. (1989) Randomized, double-blind six month trial of prednisone in Duchenne's muscular dystrophy. *N Engl J Med* 320: 1592–1597.

Moller P, Bergstrom J, Furst P, Hellstrom K, Uggla E. (1982) Energy rich phosphagens, electrolytes and free amino acids in leg skeletal muscle of patients with chronic obstructive lung disease. *Acta Med Scand* 21: 187–193.

Mujika I, Chatard J, Lacoste L, Barale F, Geyssant A. (1996) Creatine supplementation does not improve sprint performance in competitive swimmers. *Med Sci Sports Exerc* 28: 1435–1441.

Odland L, MacDougall J, Tarnopolsky M, Elorriage A, Borgmann A. (1997) Effect of oral creatine supplementation on muscle [PCr] and short term maximum power output. *Med Sci Sports Exerc* 29: 216–219.

Ogle RF, Christodoulou J, Fagan E, et al. (1997) Mitochondrial myopathy with tRNA(Leu(UUR)) mutation and complex I deficiency responsive to riboflavin. *J Pediatr* 130: 138–145.

Orndahl G, Grimby G, Grimby A, Johansson G, Wilhelmsen L. (1994) Functional deterioration and selenium-vitamin E treatment in myotonic dystrophy. A placebo-controlled study. *J Intern Med* 235: 205–210.

Orndahl G, Sellden U, Hallin S, Wetterqvist H, Rindby A,

Selin E. (1986) Myotonic dystrophy treated with selenium and vitamin E. *Acta Med Scand* 219: 407–414.

Pasman WJ, Baak van MA, Jeukendrup AE, de Haan A. (1995) The effect of different dosages of caffeine on endurance performance time. *Ant J Sports Med* 16: 225–230.

Peluchetti D, Antozzi C, Roi S, DiDonato S, Cornelio F. (1991) Riboflavin responsive multiple acyl-CoA dehydrogenase deficiency: functional evaluation of recovery after high dose vitamin supplementation. *J Neurol Sci* 105: 93–98.

Perkins R, Williams MH. (1975) Effect of caffeine upon maximal muscular endurance of females. *Med Sci Sports* 7: 221–224.

Powers SK, Byrd RJ, Tulley R, Callender T. (1983) Effects of caffeine ingestion on metabolism and performance during graded exercise. *Eur J Appl Physiol* 50: 301–307.

Prevost M, Nelson A, Morris G. (1997) The effects of creatine supplementation on total work output and metabolism during high-intensity intermittent exercise. *Res Q Exerc Sport* 68: 233–240.

Rogerson ME, Rylance PB, Wilson R, et al. (1989) Carnitine and weakness in haemodialysis patients. *Nephrol Dial Transplant* 4: 366–371.

Sasaki H, Maeda J, Usui S, Ishiko I. (1987) Effect of sucrose and caffeine ingestion on performance of prolonged strenuous running. *Ant J Sports Med* 8: 261–265.

Scholte HR, Luyt-Houwen IE, Vaandrager-Verduin. (1987) The role of the carnitine system in myocardial fatty acid oxidation: carnitine deficiency, failing mitochondria and cardiomyopathy. *Basic Res Cardiol* 82 (Suppl 1): 63–73.

Sengers RC, Bakkeren JA, Trijbels JM, et al. (1980) Successful carnitine treatment in a noncarnitine deficient lipid storage myopathy. *Eur J Pediatr* 135: 205–209.

Shapira Y, Glick B, Harel S, Vattin JJ, Gutman A. (1993) Infantile idiopathic myopathic carnitine deficiency – treatment with L-carnitine. *Pediatr Neurol* 9: 35–38.

Sipila I, Rapola J, Simell O, Vannas A. (1981) Supplementary creatine as a treatment for gyrate atrophy of the choroid retina. *N Engl J Med* 304: 867–870.

Snyder TM, Little BW, Roman-Campos G, McQuillen JB. (1982) Successful treatment of familial idiopathic lipid storage myopathy with L-carnitine and modified lipid diet. *Neurology* 32: 1106–1115.

Soop M, Björkman O, Cederblad G, Hagenfeldt L, Wahren J. (1988) Influence of carnitine supplementation on muscle substrate and carnitine metabolism during exercise. *J Appl Physiol* 64: 2394–2399.

Spriet LL, MacLean DA, Dyck DJ, Huitman E, Cederblad G, Graham TE. (1992) Caffeine ingestion and muscle metabolism during prolonged exercise in humans. *Am J Physiol* 262: E891–E898.

Stroud M, Holliman D, Bell D, Green A, MacDonald I, Greenhaff P. (1994) Effect of oral creatine supplementation on respiratory gas exchange and blood lactate accumulation during steady-state incremental treadmill exercise and recovery in man. *Clin Sci* 87: 707–710.

Tein I, Donner EJ, Hale DE, Murphy EG. (1995) Clinical and neurophysiologic response of myopathy and neuropathy in long-chain L-3-hydroxyacyl CoA dehydrogenase deficiency to oral prednisone. *Pediatr Neurol* 12: 68–76.

Terrilion K, Kolkhorst F, Doigener F, Joslyn F. (1997) The effect of creatine supplementation on two 700-m maximal running bouts. *Intl J Sports Nutr* 7: 138–143.

Thompson C, Kemp G, Sanderson A, et al. (1996) Effect of creatine on aerobic and anaerobic metabolism in skeletal muscle in swimmers. *Br J Sports Med* 30: 222–225.

Trappe SW, Costill DL, Goodpaster B, Vukovich MD, Fink WJ. (1994) The effects of L-carnitine supplementation on performance during interval swimming. *Intl J Sports Med* 15: 181–185.

Vandenberghe K, Gillis N, Van Leemputte M, Van Hecke P, Vanstapel F, Hespel P. (1996) Caffeine counteracts the ergogenic action of muscle creatine loading. *J Appl Physiol* 80: 452–457.

Vandenberghe K, Goris M, Van Hecke P, Van Leemputte M, Vangerven L, Hespel P. (1997) Long-term creatine intake is beneficial to muscle performance during resistance training. *J Appl Physiol* 83: 2055–2063.

Vannas-Sulonen K, Sipila I, Vannas A, Simmell O, Rapola J. (1985) Gyrate atrophy of the choroid retina – a five year follow-up of creatine supplementation. *Ophthalmology* 92: 1719–1727.

Volek J, Kraemer W, Bush J, et al. (1997) Creatine supplementation enhances muscular performance during high-intensity resistance training. *J Am Diet Assoc* 97: 765–770.

Vukovich MD, Costill DL, Fink WJ. (1994) Carnitine supplementation: effect on muscle carnitine and glycogen content during exercise. *Med Sci Sports Exerc* 26: 1122–1129.

49

Endocrine therapies for reducing skeletal muscle wasting: theory and practice

Paul V. Carroll

Introduction

Skeletal muscle is the principal component of lean body mass (LBM) in humans (Forbes et al 1987), and it is intimately involved in amino acid metabolism in health, during starvation and throughout periods of illness (Cahill 1970, Rennie 1985). Muscle mass accounts for ~40% of total body weight in the healthy adult (Cheek 1968) but the total amount and composition of muscle declines with aging, reflected by a selective decrease in Type II muscle fibres (Campbell et al 1973, Aniansson et al 1978, Larsson 1978). The understanding of the mechanisms regulating LBM in health and disease is steadily increasing, resulting in attempts to influence protein catabolism to counteract the skeletal wasting associated with the aging process and specific disease states. Evidence suggests that these strategies are similarly recognized and "abused" by athletes as part of performance enhancing methods. This chapter addresses the theoretical and practical basis of endocrine therapies for reducing skeletal muscle wasting, and it reviews the actions of individual hormones on protein metabolism in health and disease.

Background

Carbohydrate and protein metabolism are integral to muscle health and function, and skeletal tissue is important in both the storage and release of amino acids and the synthesis of protein. Differences in predominant muscle fibre type are important in the regulation of protein metabolism (Saltin et al 1977). Muscles with large amounts of Type I fibres (slow twitch, oxidative) have a higher rate of protein turnover than muscles containing Type II (fast-twitch) fibres (Millward and Waterlow 1978, Furuno and Goldberg 1986).

Total free amino acids are present in higher concentration in skeletal muscle than seen in the circulation (Bergström et al 1974), and muscle stores account for approximately 75% (or 850 g) of whole body free amino acids. The concentrations of free amino acids in muscle are reduced during periods of net anabolism (Waterlow et al 1978), and conversely they are increased during periods of net catabolism. The amino acids alanine, glutamine and glutamate are synthesized in muscle as reflected by their presence at higher levels in the free pool than in skeletal tissue. During periods of severe illness with prolonged catabolism the levels of these amino acids decrease (Fürst et al 1982). Loss of skeletal muscle (wasting) occurs when protein

catabolism exceeds the rate of anabolism, as observed during prolonged starvation, increases in metabolic rate and during periods of illness arising from trauma, burns, sepsis and infection (Rennie 1985).

Physiological regulation of muscle protein metabolism

Effects of nutrition

A variety of techniques have been used to study protein metabolism in both the whole body and specific tissues, including the use of 3-methylhistidine production, arterio-venous differences in amino acid concentrations, muscle ribosome content and radioactive or stable-labelled amino acid tracer techniques (Smith and Rennie 1990).

Several studies employing a variety of techniques have confirmed stimulation of muscle protein synthesis following nutritional intake (Cheng et al 1985, 1987, Rennie 1986, Halliday et al 1988). In addition, decreased protein breakdown in forearm muscle has been demonstrated following feeding (Rennie 1986, Cheng et al 1985, 1987), with the sum of these effects resulting in net protein accumulation.

Prolonged fasting is associated with a depression of protein turnover (Young et al 1973) and decreased protein synthesis (Wernerman et al 1985). Overall restriction of nutritional intake results in decreased protein turnover with reduced protein synthesis. Restoration of adequate caloric and amino acid intake enhances protein synthesis and net gain of LBM.

Effects of hormones

Insulin, growth hormone (GH), and insulin-like growth factor-1 (IGF-1) are the principal hormones regulating protein metabolism in the healthy human. Circulating concentrations of these agents vary with nutritional status, and they are altered in disease states. Several other systemic hormones (cortisol, glucagon, thyroid, androgens and catecholamines) affect protein balance and thus skeletal muscle mass and function. Increasing evidence suggests that locally produced cytokines and inflammatory mediators, including tumour necrosis factor-α and several components of the interleukin superfamily, also influence metabolic processes, including protein metabolism. It has been suggested that these agents are important determinants of the skeletal muscle wasting seen in critical illness (Carroll

1999). The effects of the major endocrine agents are summarized in Table 49.1.

Insulin

In vitro studies indicate that insulin inhibits protein breakdown, stimulates amino acid uptake, and the synthesis of nucleic acids and protein (Saltiel and Cuatrecasas 1988). In humans, the insulin deficiency of type 1 diabetes results in abnormal protein metabolism (Nair et al 1987, Luzi et al 1990), characterized by increased plasma amino acid concentrations and protein flux. Insulin exerts a net anabolic effect on in vivo protein metabolism principally through reducing the rate of protein breakdown (Umpleby et al 1986, Castellino et al 1987, Nair et al 1987), with associated reductions in circulating amino acid levels. There is evidence that this action is enhanced by IGF-1 (Carroll et al 2000).

Growth hormone

As GH administration results in increases in IGF-1 and insulin, it is difficult to be certain in longer-term studies that measured effects are directly attributable to GH activity. GH has anabolic effects on protein metabolism, increasing both growth and muscle mass in GH-deficient children (Cheek and Hill 1970, Tanner et al 1977). GH administration in humans has been shown to reduce nitrogen excretion and increase skeletal muscle ribosome content, indicating an increase in muscle protein synthesis (Kostyo 1964).

More recently GH treatment in GH-deficient adults has been shown to increase LBM and thigh mass (Jorgensen et al 1989, Salomon et al 1989). Studies using stable isotope tracers indicate that these effects occur via GH mediated increases in protein synthesis without effects on protein breakdown (Russell-Jones et al 1993). GH administration results in alterations in body composition characterized by reduced fat stores, particularly truncal fat (Carroll and Christ 1998). These pronounced effects on protein metabolism and body composition have led to the recognition of GH as a potent anabolic agent. Consequently attempts to maintain or increase LBM and skeletal muscle have mostly focused on the potential benefits of GH in a variety of clinical illnesses.

Insulin-like growth factor-1

Initial isotopic studies indicated that an acute infusion of IGF-1 had an insulin-like effect on protein metabolism, with a reduction in proteolysis without effects on protein synthesis (Hussain et al 1993, Laager et al 1993, Boulware et al 1994). These results were surprising, as IGF-1 has been shown to mediate the anabolic actions of growth hormone in vivo (Walker et al 1991). However these studies were performed on fasted subjects, with reduced circulating levels of amino acids. Subsequently Russell-Jones et al (1994) used an amino acid clamp protocol, in which circulating levels of amino acids were maintained with an amino acid infusion, to compare the actions of IGF-1 and insulin on protein metabolism. IGF-1 treatment resulted in an increase in protein synthesis, indicating that IGF-1 has a direct effect on protein synthesis in

Table 49.1 — Effects of the major endogenous hormones on protein metabolism

Agent	Protein flux	Protein breakdown	Protein oxidation	Protein synthesis
GH	↑	↔	↓	↑
IGF-1	↔	↔	↓	↑
Insulin	↓	↓	↓	↔ / ↑
Glucocorticoids	↔ / ?	↔ / ↑	↔	↑
Glucagon	↔	↔	↔	↔
Androgens	↔	↔	↓	↑
Catecholamines	?	↓	↔	↓
Thyroid hormones	↓	↓ / ↔	↓	↓

This table summarizes the available information detailing the physiological actions of endogenous hormones on protein metabolism in humans. The effects may vary with duration of exposure, particularly at pharmacological concentrations. ↑, increased rate; ↓, decreased rate; ↔, unaltered rate; ?, data not available or inconclusive; GH, growth hormone; IGF-1, insulin-like growth factor-1.

the presence of an adequate supply of amino acids. The predominant action of insulin on protein metabolism in this study was suppression of protein breakdown with no effect on the rate of protein synthesis.

Muscle and protein metabolism in disease states

Loss of LBM as a result of trauma was described as far back as 1930 (Cuthbertson 1930). It is now known that increased protein breakdown and increased nitrogen excretion are the hallmarks of the hypermetabolic, catabolic state. Measurement of nitrogen balance has been used as the main measure of outcome in many studies of post-operative patients in which, nutritional regimens (Stehle et al 1989, Larrson et al 1990), hormonal treatments (Jiang et al 1989, Mjaaland et al 1993) and other therapies (Brandt et al 1978, Carli et al 1989) have been evaluated.

Using stable isotope methodology, decreased whole body protein synthesis with unchanged protein breakdown have been shown in subjects following an elective surgical trauma (O'Keefe et al 1974, Crane et al 1977). Following more major surgery and in other groups of intensive care unit (ICU) patients whole body proteolysis is increased (Long et al 1977, Birkhahn et al 1980, Tomkins et al 1983, Jahoor et al 1988, Carli et al 1990, Jackson et al 1999). In these studies protein synthesis was also increased, indicating an increase in the flux rate of total body protein turnover. Figure 49.1 indicates the increase in protein flux seen in critically ill ICU subjects (Jackson et al 1999).

An increased proteolytic rate has also been demonstrated using the 3-methylhistidine flux technique early in the course of sepsis (Sjölin et al 1990). By measuring the density of skeletal muscle ribosome particles Wernerman et al (1985) demonstrated that protein synthesis decreases following surgical trauma and that total parenteral nutrition (TPN) fails to attenuate this decrease (Wernerman et al 1986).

Studies of body composition and the effects of different treatments in critically ill patients have shown that body protein is lost and fat accumulated during the initial 10 days in ICU when subjects received TPN (Streat et al 1987). In addition, it has been shown that, although feeding can restore body weight, changes in composition are not corrected for up to 8 months following recovery from illness (Keys 1950).

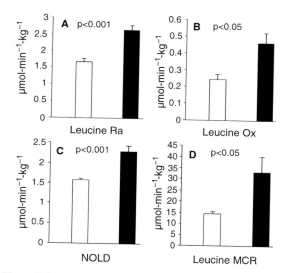

Figure 49.1 — Post-absorptive protein metabolic rates in critically ill (ICU) patients and healthy matched control subjects. **A** Leucine appearance rate (R_a, *protein breakdown*), **B** oxidation rate (Ox, *protein oxidation*), **C** non-oxidative leucine disposal (NOLD, *protein synthesis*), and **D** metabolic clearance rate (MCR) for ICU patients (solid bars) and matched controls (open bars). Values are means ± SE; $n = 7$ in each group. (Taken from Jackson et al 1999)

A variety of techniques, therefore, indicate that illness results in rapid and major changes in protein metabolism. Depending on the nature, severity and duration of the insult these alterations may persist for periods varying from days to months, and evidence suggests that protein catabolism influences outcome in the critically ill patient (Windsor and Hill 1988, Herrmann et al 1992). The major changes are increased rates of whole body proteolysis, with increased amino acid oxidation and in certain circumstances reduced protein synthesis.

Use of anabolic agents to promote maintenance and accumulation of skeletal muscle and LBM

The anabolic effects of GH, IGF-1 and to a lesser extent the androgens, testosterone and DHEA have been studied in a variety of clinical conditions associated with catabolism resulting in loss of skeletal muscle. These include surgery, burns, sepsis and trauma, acquired immunodeficiency syndrome (AIDS) associated wasting and old age. Table 49.2 summarizes

Table 49.2— Summary of the controlled studies investigating the effects of growth hormone administration on protein metabolism in conditions associated with loss of skeletal muscle[a]

Year	n	Method	Patient category	Effect	Significance compared with placebo
1986	14	Nitrogen excretion/ [15]N lysine	Major GI surgery	Increased nitrogen balance, decreased protein oxidation, increased fat oxidation	$p<0.01$
1989	18	Nitrogen balance/ Body composition	Gastrectomy/ colectomy	Increased nitrogen balance/ maintained LBM	$p<0.001$
1991	10	Nitrogen balance/^{15}N lysine isolated limb	Severe burns	Increased nitrogen balance/ increased limb and whole body protein synthesis	$p<0.03$
1992	20	Nitrogen balance	Septic shock (+ TPN)	Increased nitrogen balance	$p<0.05$
1995	18	Nitrogen balance	Non-septic adults	Increased nitrogen balance (transient)	$p<0.05$
1995	20	15N glycine/ Nitrogen balance	Trauma (adults)	Increased nitrogen balance & protein synthesis	$p<0.001$
1996	66	Body composition	HIV[+ve] males	Reduced FM/Increased LBM (unsustained)	NS
1996	20	Nitrogen balance	Post-surgical sepsis	Increased nitrogen retention	$p<0.001$
1996	60	Body composition	LBM in AIDS assoc. wasting	Increased LBM	$p<0.001$
1997	12	[13]C Leucine	Colonic resection (carcinoma)	Increased WB protein synthesis	$p<0.03$
1998	24	DEXA/Body composition	IAA	Increased nitrogen retention, LBM	both <0.001
1999	30	Nitrogen balance	Surgery (GI tract malignancy)	Increased nitrogen balance	$p<0.05$
1999	28	Ribosomal analysis	Elective cholecystectomy	Increased hepatic protein synthesis	$p<0.01$
1999	24	Body composition	Ileo-anal J pouch surgery	Increased LBM	$p<0.05$

[a]The patients in this study received both growth hormone and insulin-like growth factor-1, and many of the changes in body composition were not sustained over 12 weeks; PA, pulmonary artery; AAA, abdominal aortic aneurysm; GI, gastrointestinal; FM, Fat mass; LBM, lean body mass; TPN, total parenteral nutrition; TNF, tumour necrosis factor, IAA, ileo-anal anastamosis, ^{13}C, carbon-13; ^{15}N, nitrogen-15; HIV[+ve], human immunodeficiency virus-positive; AIDS, acquired immunodeficiency syndrome; WB, whole body. Taken from Carroll 1999.

results from studies assessing the effect of GH treatment on protein metabolism in conditions associated with loss of LBM.

Growth hormone in surgery

A large number of investigators, employing a variety of techniques, have assessed the effects of GH administration in subjects undergoing surgical procedures. In elective surgery GH treatment resulted in increased IGF-1 levels, whole body protein flux and resting energy expenditure (REE; Ponting et al 1990). When used in combination with hypocaloric nutritional support GH resulted in positive nitrogen balance (Jiang et al 1989). Peri-operative GH and TPN therapy together have been shown to improve glutamine retention, nitrogen balance and polyribosome concentration (Hammarqvist et al 1992). Similarly unlike TPN alone, TPN with GH has resulted in a net positive nitrogen balance in humans undergoing upper gastrointestinal (GI) resection for malignancy (Berman et al 1999). The addition of combined GH and IGF-1 to glutamine-supplemented TPN has recently been demonstrated, unlike nutritional support alone, to result in net protein gain in critically ill subjects soon after admission to the ICU. The majority of these patients were post emergency surgery (Jackson et al 2000; Fig. 49.2).

A recent study assessed the effects of GH treatment in adults undergoing surgery for ulcerative colitis (Kissemeyer-Nielsen et al 1999). Assessments of total muscle strength, fatigability and body composition were made prior to operation and up to 90 days following

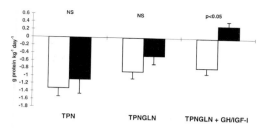

Figure 49.2—Net protein balance in critically ill subjects randomized to receive conventional total parenteral nutrition (TPN; n=7), glutamine supplemented TPN (TPNGLN; n=7) and TPNGLN with combined growth hormone (GH) and insulin-like growth factor-1 (IGF-I; n=5). Data were obtained using ^{13}C leucine and each group was studied initially in the fasting state (open bars) and subsequently following 3 days treatment (solid bars). The data indicate that following both TPN and TPNGLN the subjects remained in net negative protein balance but net protein gain was observed in these critically ill patients during treatment with TPNGLN + GH/IGF-1. (Data unpublished)

surgery. GH treatment (from 2 days before to 7 days after surgery) resulted in preserved LBM, increased muscular strength and decreased post-operative fatigue. These data suggest that the administration of GH can modify protein metabolism following both elective and emergency surgery. When used in conjunction with nutritional support this effect has translated into improved nitrogen balance in most but not all studies.

Growth hormone in burns

In 1961 it was demonstrated that human GH derived from cadavers increased nitrogen balance in severely burned patients (Liljedahl et al 1961). Subsequent studies confirmed this observation and indicated that GH administration increased oxygen consumption and decreased respiratory quotient (Soroff et al 1967), while increasing insulin and glucose levels (Wilmore et al 1974). Using recombinant GH more recent studies have shown that GH treatment increases the rate of healing of graft donor sites (Herndon et al 1990), thereby reducing length of hospital stay in burns patients. Further investigations suggest that GH-mediated increases in protein synthesis may be responsible for this effect (Gore et al 1991a), but provided evidence that GH administration induced insulin resistance in burns patients by decreasing glucose uptake and oxidation (Gore et al 1991b). Recently double-blind placebo-controlled studies have demonstrated effective decreases in donor-site healing following GH treatment in severely burned children (Sherman et al 1989, Gilpin et al 1994).

Growth hormone in sepsis and trauma

Okamura et al (1989) demonstrated that GH treatment increased nitrogen retention without affecting 3-methylhistidine excretion in a rat model of sepsis. This experimental model provided evidence of an effect on protein synthesis with unaltered protein breakdown. A simultaneous study showed increased amino acid uptake into muscle protein following GH treatment in nutritionally deprived patients receiving TPN (Fong et al 1989). Further evidence of GH-mediated increases in protein synthesis without effects on proteolysis were provided by a stable isotope tracer study in trauma patients with sepsis (Douglas et al 1990). In these studies, fat oxidation was increased by GH treatment but leucine oxidation was decreased indicating a preferential use of fat rather than protein as a calorie source. A study of the effects of GH with the addition of TPN in sepsis demonstrated decreased nitrogen production during the treatment period (Voerman et al 1992). Koea et al (1996) studied the effects of 7 days GH in surgical patients with sepsis who were receiving TPN. Both TPN and TPN with GH decreased net protein catabolism, but this effect was greater in subjects randomized to GH.

Overall the evidence indicates that GH treatment alters protein metabolism in sepsis and trauma via an increase in the rate of protein synthesis with largely unchanged rates of protein breakdown.

Growth hormone and insulin-like growth factor-1 in AIDS wasting

AIDS is associated with protein wasting leading to loss of LBM. In an early study reversal of pre-treatment weight loss, increased IGF-I levels, and decreased fat mass and urinary nitrogen excretion were recorded in 10 AIDS patients treated with GH (Krentz et al 1993). Virtually identical effects were seen in a subsequent study of human immunodeficiency virus (HIV) positive men with documented weight loss (19% average) treated with GH over 7 days (Mulligan et al 1993). Combined GH and IGF-1 administration decreased fat mass and increased LBM after 6 weeks treatment in HIV-infected males (Schambelan et al 1996), however these effects were not sustained over 12 weeks treatment. A study of 60 patients with AIDS wasting indicated that both GH and IGF-1 in isolation increased LBM and reduced fat mass, but these changes were greatest in patients who received these agents in combination. No changes were recorded in instruments used to assess quality of life in these patients (Waters et al 1996).

A simultaneous study reported on a larger cohort of 142 subjects, randomized to receive GH and IGF-1 or placebo in a similar protocol lasting 12 weeks (Lee et al 1996). Active treatment was associated with a transient increase in weight and fat free mass but these effects were only observed after 3 weeks and not persistent throughout the 12 week duration, suggesting that combined GH and IGF-1 had no major anabolic effect in HIV-associated wasting (Lee et al 1996). Overall the evidence suggests that GH treatment has effects on reducing weight loss and preserving lean body mass in patients with AIDS-associated weight loss. It remains unclear whether these benefits would be sustained over periods of treatment longer than 3 months, and it is not certain whether the altered protein metabolism would result in clinical benefits.

Insulin-like growth factor-1

As IGF-1 is recognized to mediate many of the actions of GH it has been suggested that IGF-1 administration may provide the anabolic benefits of GH while eliminating the harmful effects associated with GH treatment. A study performed in a rat model of burn injury, where an IGF-1 infusion was provided, indicated maintenance of serum levels of IGF-1, increased body weight and decreased oxygen consumption compared with the sham controls (Strock et al 1990). A more recent study of rodents with liver injury (induced by thioacetamide), comparing the effects of GH and IGF-1 (Inaba et al 1997) demonstrated that both agents resulted in a decrease in nitrogen excretion. Unlike GH, treatment with IGF-1 resulted in reduced gut mucosal atrophy and increased body weight, suggesting that IGF-1 may have greater anabolic potential in this model.

Clemmons compared the effects of IGF-1 and GH on nitrogen balance in healthy adult volunteers in whom moderate hypercatabolism was induced by starvation (Clemmons et al 1991). Both GH and IGF-1 resulted in improved nitrogen balance. GH treatment increased insulin and glucose levels but IGF-1 treatment decreased both of these variables. Using methylprednisolone to induce catabolism in 26 healthy subjects Oehri et al (1996) compared the effects of GH and IGF-1 on protein metabolism. Both GH and IGF-1 decreased leucine oxidation (improving net protein balance). In humans with thermal injury IGF-1 treatment decreased protein oxidation and increased glucose oxidation (Cioffi et al 1994). Lieberman et al (1994) treated AIDS patients with IGF-1 for 10 days. Two doses were used and both resulted in cumulative increases in nitrogen balance over the treatment period.

Goeters et al (1995) reported the effects of IGF-1 administration in post-operative gastric surgery patients receiving TPN. Despite an increase in IGF-1 levels no alterations were observed in nitrogen balance. In this study insulin-like growth factor binding protein (IGFBP-1) levels were elevated by IGF-1 treatment leading to the suggestion that alterations in the levels of the IGFBP[s] following IGF-1 treatment may alter IGF-1 activity.

Combined administration of growth hormone and insulin-like growth factor-1

As IGF-1 is known to have a hypoglycaemic effect, it has been suggested that co-administration of both GH and IGF-1 may maintain blood glucose concentrations and facilitate the anabolic actions of each agent.

In a study of parenterally-fed rats exposed to operative stress although both GH and IGF-1 in isolation resulted in nitrogen retention and weight gain, combined treatment had a synergistic effect and increased fat oxidation (Lo et al 1995). In addition the combined treatment resulted in an additive rather than synergistic effect on weight gain. In these experiments TPN was provided and hypoglycaemia was not observed. A recent study has investigated the effects of combined treatment with GH and IGF-I in addition to glutamine supplemented TPN in critically ill humans (Jackson et al 2000). Using stable isotopes, the findings indicate that this combined approach results in net protein gain in critically ill subjects without a major effect on whole body glutamine plasma flux.

Growth hormone treatment in aging

A number of studies have addressed the effects of GH administration in aging humans. GH given to healthy older men for a period of 6 months resulted in a gain in LBM (3.7 kg) with an associated reduction in fat mass (2.4 kg) compared with controls (Rudman et al 1990). These effects were sustained over 12 months (Rudman et al 1991). In a similar placebo-controlled trial active treatment resulted in an increase in LBM (3.3 kg), together with significant gains in muscle strength for knee flexion and extension (Welle et al

1996). These studies have used doses of GH comparable to, or even higher than, those used in the treatment of adult GH-deficiency, resulting in a high incidence of GH related side-effects leading to the withdrawal of large numbers of subjects.

In elderly subjects undergoing total hip replacement, peri-operative GH administration resulted in preservation of thigh muscle area on computed tomography (CT) scans, and gain in hip abductor strength. This appeared to be largely a result of preoperative gain in muscle mass, negating the catabolic effects of surgery (Weissberger et al 1997). Similarly, in older patients undergoing renal dialysis treated with GH, active treatment resulted in significantly greater increase in serum albumin, fat-free mass and calf muscle area (Ahlmen et al 1997). Much remains unclear with regard to the possible interaction between GH and gonadal steroids in both men and women. Administration of testosterone has been shown to increase IGF-1 levels in normal men (Hobbs et al 1993), and in older women taking oestrogen as hormone replacement therapy (HRT); oral oestrogens have been shown to enhance GH secretion (Friend et al 1996). Overall, the preliminary data in older subjects suggest that GH treatment may help maintain or increase skeletal muscle bulk and strength. Although considerable interest exists it remains uncertain whether such a treatment will have clinical application.

Conclusions

Advances in recombinant techniques leading to the widespread availability of peptide hormones, including GH and IGF-1, have resulted in studies assessing the potential of these agents in promoting anabolism in a variety of clinical conditions. Patients with catabolic skeletal muscle disorders have received particular attention and include those with AIDS, sepsis, burns, trauma and patients undergoing surgery.

Several well-conducted studies have been performed and these indicate that both GH and IGF-1, alone or in combination, result in positive nitrogen balance and net protein gain in different conditions using a variety of techniques. The majority of these trials have included selected patients, and investigations have been performed over short periods. Not surprisingly, significant benefits in body composition, muscle function and long-term clinical outcome have yet to be identified. Smaller studies have addressed the effects of other growth promoting agents in disease states. It is unlikely that testosterone, DHEA or anabolic steroids (including stanozolol, nandrolone and oxandrolone) will have therapeutic applications in disorders associated with loss of skeletal muscle. Newer agents include oral GH-secretagogues, which are being assessed in elderly subjects, and modulators of cytokine activity, which are currently undergoing development.

The studies of critically ill ICU patients reported in 1999 (Takala et al 1999) provide clear evidence that GH used in unselected ICU subjects with acute illness results in major increases in morbidity and mortality. Although the mechanisms responsible remain poorly understood, these findings have had a significant impact on both clinical practice and research activities investigating the potential of anabolic agents.

Anabolic treatments have been shown to alter protein metabolism and result in net protein gain in health and in a variety of disease states. It is likely that the effects are most pronounced when combined with appropriate provision of nutrition. Early evidence indicates that the use of several anabolic treatments simultaneously may have synergistic effects on protein gain. Little information is available regarding the long-term use of these treatments, and whether the use of growth promoting agents will result in improved clinical outcome is not clear. Importantly, the widespread use of GH in acute illness results in increased mortality, and current recommendations are that anabolic treatments should not be used in this setting. Ongoing research will address many of the outstanding issues relating to hormonal treatments for the promotion of protein gain. It remains to be seen whether anabolic agents will have a useful and safe therapeutic role in specific illnesses.

References

Ahlmen J, Johansson G, Johansson A, Bengtsson B-A. (1997) Beneficial effects of growth hormone treatment in elderly patients on dialysis. *Endocrinol Metab* 4 (Suppl A): 18.

Aniansson A, Grimby G, Hedberg M, et al. (1978) Muscle function in old age. *Scand J Rehab Med* 6: 43–49.

Bergström J, Fürst P, Nòree L-O, Vinnars E. (1974) Intracellular free amino acid concentration in human muscle tissue. *J Appl Physiol* 36: 693–697.

Berman RS, Harrison LE, Pearlstone DB, Burt M, Brennan MF. (1999) Growth hormone alone and in combination with insulin, increases whole body and skeletal muscle protein kinetics in cancer patients after surgery. *Ann Surg* 229: 1–10.

Birkhahn RH, Long CL, Fitkin D, et al. (1980) Whole-body protein metabolism due to trauma in man as estimated by 1-(1, 14C)- leucine. *Surgery* 88: 294–300.

Boulware SD, Tamborlane WV, Rennert NJ, Gesundheit N, Sherwin RS. (1994) Comparison of the metabolic effects of recombinant human insulin-like growth factor-I and insulin: dose-response relationships in healthy young and middle-aged adults. *J Clin Invest* 93: 1131–1139.

Brandt MR, Fernandes A, Mordhorst R, Kehlet H. (1978) Epidural analgesia improves postoperative nitrogen balance. *Br Med J* 1: 1106–1108.

Cahill GF. (1970) Starvation in man. *N Engl J Med* 282: 668–675.

Campbell MJ, McComas AJ, Pepito F. (1973) Physiological changes in ageing muscles. *J Neurol Neurosurg Psychiat* 36: 171–182.

Carli F, Emery PW, Freemantle CAJ. (1989) Effect of peroperative normothermia on postoperative protein metabolism in elderly patients undergoing hip arthroplasty. *Br J Anaesth* 63: 276–282.

Carli F, Webster J, Ramachandra V, et al. (1990) Aspects of protein metabolism after elective surgery in patients receiving constant nutritional support. *Clin Sci* 78: 621–628.

Carroll PV, Christ ER. (1998) GH-deficieny in adulthood and the effects of GH replacement. A review. *J Clin Endocrin Metab* 83: 382–395.

Carroll PV. (1999) Protein metabolism and the use of growth hormone and insulin-like growth factor-I in the critically ill patient. *Growth Hormone IGF Res* 9: 400–413.

Carroll PV, Christ ER, Umpleby AM, et al. (2000) IGF-I replacement in adults with type 1 diabetes mellitus-effects on glucose and protein metabolism in both the fasting state and during a hyperinsulinaemic euglycaemic amino acid clamp. *Diabetes* 49: 789–796.

Castellino P, Luzi L, Simonson DC, Haymond M, DeFronzo RA. (1987) Effect of insulin and plasma amino acid concentrations on leucine metabolism in man. *J Clin Invest* 80: 1784–1793.

Cheek DB. (1968) Muscle cell growth in normal children. In: Cheek DB, ed. *Human Growth.* Philadelphia: Lea & Febiger, pp. 337–351.

Cheek DB, Hill DE. (1970) Muscle and liver cell growth. Role of hormone and nutritional factors. *Federation Proc* 29: 1503–1509.

Cheng KN, Dworzak F, Ford GC, et al. (1985) Direct determination of leucine metabolism and protein breakdown in humans using L-[1-13C, 15N]- leucine and the forearm model. *Eur J Clin Invest* 15: 349–354.

Cheng KN, Pacy PJ, Dworzak F, et al. (1987) Influence of fasting on leucine and muscle protein metabolism across the human forearm determined using L-[13C, 15N]-leucine as the tracer. *Clin Sci* 73: 241–246.

Cioffi WG, Gore DC, Rue LC, et al. (1994) Insulin-like growth factor-I lowers protein oxidation in patients with thermal injury. *Ann Surg* 220: 310–319.

Clemmons DR, Smith-Banks A, Underwood LE. (1991) Reversal of diet-induced catabolism by infusion of recombinant insulin-like growth factor-I in humans. *J Clin Endocrin Metab* 75: 234–238.

Crane CW, Picou D, Smith R, Waterlow JC. (1977) Protein turnover in patients before and after elective orthopaedic operations. *Br J Surg* 64: 129–133.

Cutherbertson DP. (1930) Disturbance of metabolism produced by bony and non-bony injury, with notes on certain abnormal conditions of bone. *Biochem J* 24: 1244–1263.

Douglas RG, Humberstone DA, Haystead A, Shaw JH. (1990) Metabolic effects of recombinant human growth hormone: isotopic studies in the postabsorptive state and during total parenteral nutrition. *Br J Surg* 77: 785–790.

Fong Y, Rosenbaum M, Tracey KJ, et al. (1989) Recombinant growth hormone enhances muscle myosin heavy chain mRNA accumulation and amino acid accrual in humans. *Proc Nat Acad Sci USA* 86: 3371–3374.

Forbes GB. (1987) *Human Body Composition: Growth, Aging, Nutrition and Activity.* New York: Springer-Verlag, p. 171.

Friend KE, Hartman ML, Pezzoli SS, Clasey JL, Thorner MO. (1996) Both oral and transdermal oestrogen increase growth hormone release in post-menopausal women – a clinical research center study. *J Clin Endocrin Metab* 81: 2250–2256.

Fürst P, Elwyn DH, Askanazi J, Kinney JM. (1982) Effects of nutrition and catabolic stress on intracellular branched-chain amino acids. In: Wesdorp RIC, Soeters PB, eds. *Clinical Nutrition '81,* Edinburgh: Churchill Livingstone, p. 10.

Furuno K, Goldberg AL. (1986) The activation of protein degradation in muscle by Ca2+ or muscle injury does not involve a lysosomal mechanism. *Biochem J* 237: 859–864.

Gilpin DA, Barrow RE, Rutan RL, Broemeling L, Herndon DN. (1994) Recombinant human growth hormone accelerates wound healing in children with large cutaneous burns. *Ann Surg* 220: 19–24.

Goeters C, Mertes N, Tacke J, et al. (1995) Repeated administration of recombinant human insulin-like growth factor-I in patients after gastric surgery. *Ann Surg* 222: 646–653.

Gore DC, Honeycutt D, Jahoor F, et al. (1991a) Effect of exogenous growth hormone on whole body and isolated limb protein kinetics in burned patients. *Arch Surg* 126: 38–43.

Gore DC, Honeycutt D, Jahoor F, et al. (1991b) Effect of exogenous growth hormone on glucose utilisation in burn patients. *J Surg Res* 51: 518–523.

Halliday D, Pacy PJ, Cheng KN, et al. (1988) Rate of protein synthesis in skeletal muscle of normal man and patients with muscular dystrophy: a reassessment. *Clin Sci* 74: 237–240.

Hammarqvist F, Strömberg C, von der Decken A, et al. (1992) Biosynthetic growth hormone preserves both muscle protein synthesis and the decrease in muscle-free glutamine, and improves whole-body nitrogen economy after operation. *Ann Surg* 216: 184–191.

Herndon DN, Barrow RE, Kunkle KR, Broemeling L, Rutan L. (1990) Effects of recombinant human growth hormone on donor site healing in severely burned children. *Ann Surg* 212: 424–429.

Herrmann FR, Safran C, Levkoff SE, Minaker KL. (1992) Serum albumin level on admission as a predictor of death, length of stay, and readmission. *Arch Intl Med* 152: 125–130.

Hobbs CJ, Plymate SR, Rosen CJ, Adler RA. (1993) Testosterone administration increases IGF-I in normal men. *J Clin Endocrin Metab* 77: 776–779.

Hussain MA, Schmitz O, Mengel A, et al. (1993) Insulin-like growth factor-I stimulates lipid oxidation, reduces protein oxidation and enhances insulin sensitivity in humans. *J Clin Invest* 95: 2249–2256.

Inaba T, Saito H, Fukushima R, et al. (1997) Insulin-like growth factor I has beneficial effects, whereas growth hormone has limited effects on postoperative protein metabolism, gut integrity, and splenic weight in rats with chronic mild liver injury. *J Parenteral Enteral Nutr* 21: 55–62.

Jackson NC, Carroll PV, Russell-Jones DL, Sönksen PH, Treacher DF, Umpleby AM. (1999) The metabolic consequences of critical illness: acute effects on glutamine and protein metabolism. *Am J Physiol* 276: E163–E170.

Jackson NC, Carroll PV, Russell-Jones DL, Sönksen PH, Treacher DF, Umpleby AM. (2000) Effects of glutamine supplementation, GH and IGF-I on glutamine metabolism in critically ill patients. *Am J Physiol* 278: E226–E233.

Jahoor F, Desai M, Herndon DN, Wolfe RR. (1988) Dynamics of the protein metabolic response to burn injury. *Metabolism* 37: 330–337.

Jiang ZM, He GZ, Zhang SY, et al. (1989) Low-dose growth hormone and hypocaloric nutrition attenuate the protein-catabolic response after major operation. *Ann Surg* 210: 513–524.

Jorgensen JOL, Pedersen SA, Thuesen L, et al. (1989) Beneficial effects of growth hormone treatment in GH-deficient adults. *Lancet* i: 1221–1225.

Keys A, Brozek J, Henschel A, et al. (1950) *The biology of human starvation*. Minneapolis: University of Minnesota Press.

Kissmeyer-Nielsen P, Jensen MB, Laurberg S. (1999) Perioperative growth hormone treatment and functional outcome after major abdominal surgery: a randomized, double-blind, controlled study. *Ann Surg* 229: 298–302.

Koea JB, Breier BH, Douglas RG, Gluckman PD, Shaw JH. (1996) Anabolic and cardiovascular effects of recombinant human growth hormone in surgical patients with sepsis. *Br J Surg* 83: 196–202.

Kostyo JL. (1964) Separation of the effects of GH on muscle amino acid transport and protein synthesis. *Endocrinology* 75: 113–119.

Krentz AJ, Koster FT, Crist DM, et al. (1993) Anthropometric, metabolic, and immunological effects of recombinant human growth hormone in AIDS and AIDS-related complex. *J Acquired Immunodeficiency Syndromes* 6: 245–251.

Laager R, Ninnis R, Keller U. (1993) Comparison of the effects of recombinant human insulin-like growth factor-I and insulin on glucose and leucine kinetics in humans. *J Clin Invest* 92: 1903–1909.

Larsson L. (1978) Morphological and functional characteristics of ageing skeletal muscle in man. *Acta Physiol Scand* 457: 1–36.

Larrson J, Lennmarken C, Mårtennson J, et al. (1990) Nitrogen requirements in severely injured patients. *Br J Surg* 77: 413–416.

Lee PD, Pivarnik JM, Bukar JG, et al. (1996) A randomized, placebo-controlled trial of combined insulin-like growth factor I and low dose growth hormone therapy for wasting associated with human immunodeficiency virus infection. *J Clin Endocrin Metab* 81: 2968–2975.

Lieberman SA, Butterfield GE, Harrison D, Hoffman AR. (1994) Anabolic effects of recombinant insulin-like growth factor-I in cachectic patients with the acquired immunodeficiency syndrome. *J Clin Endocrinol Metab* 78: 404–410.

Liljedahl S, Gemzell C, Plantin L, Birke G. (1961) Effect of human growth hormone in patients with severe burns. *Acta Chir Scand* 122: 1–14.

Lo HC, Hinton PS, Peterson CA, et al. (1995) Simultaneous treatment with IGF-I and growth hormone additively increases anabolism in parenterally fed rats. *Am J Physiol* 269: E368–E376.

Long CL, Jeevanandam M, Kim BM, Kinney JM. (1977) Whole body protein synthesis and catabolism in septic man. *Am J Clin Nutr* 30: 1340–1344.

Luzi L, Castellino P, Simonson DC, Petrides AS, DeFronzo RA. (1990) Leucine metabolism in IDDM. *Diabetes* 39: 38–48.

Millward DJ, Waterlow JC. (1978) Effect of nutrition on protein turnover in skeletal muscle. Federation Proceedings. *Fed Am Soc Exp Biol* 37: 2283–2290.

Mjaaland M, Unneberg K, Larsson J, et al. (1993) Growth hormone after gastrointestinal surgery: attenuated forearm glutamine, alanine, 3-methylhistidine and total amino acid efflux in patients treated with total parenteral nutrition. *Ann Surg* 217: 413–422.

Mulligan K, Grunfeld C, Hellerstein MK, Neise RA, Schambelan M. (1993) Anabolic effects of recombinant human growth hormone in patients associated with human immunodeficiency virus infection. *J Clin Endocrinol Metab* 77: 956–962.

Nair KS, Ford GC, Halliday D. (1987) Effect of intravenous insulin treatment on in-vivo whole-body leucine kinetics and oxygen consumption in insulin-deprived type 1 diabetic patients. *Metabolism* 36: 491–495.

Nair KS, Garrow JS, Ford C, Mehler RF, Halliday D. (1993) Effect of poor diabetic control and obesity on whole body protein metabolism in man. *Diabetologia* 25: 400–403.

Oehri M, Ninnis R, Girard J, Frey FJ, Keller U. (1996) Effects of growth hormone and IGF-I on glucocorticoid-induced protein catabolism in humans. *Am J Physiol* 270: E552–E558.

Okamura K, Okuma T, Tabira Y, Miyauchi Y. (1989) Effect of administered growth hormone on protein metabolism in septic rats. *J Parenteral Enteral Nutr* 13: 450–454.

O'Keefe SJ, Sender PM, James WP. (1974) "Catabolic" loss of body nitrogen in response to surgery. *Lancet* 2: 1035–1038.

Ponting GA, Ward HC, Halliday D, Teale JD, Sim AJW. (1990) Protein and energy metabolism with biosynthetic growth hormone in patients on full intravenous nutritional support. *J Parenteral Enteral Nutr* 14: 437–441.

Rennie MJ, Edwards RHT, Halliday D, et al. (1982) Muscle protein synthesis measured by stable isotope techniques in man: the effects of feeding and fasting. *Clin Sci* 63: 519–523.

Rennie MJ. (1985) Muscle protein turnover and the muscle wasting due to injury and disease. *Br Med Bull* 41: 257–264.

Rennie MJ. (1986) Metabolic insights from the use of stable isotopes in nutritional studies. *Clin Nutr* 5: 1–7.

Rudman D, Feller AG, Nagraj HS, et al. (1990) Effects of human growth hormone on men over 60 years old. *N Engl J Med* 323: 1–6.

Rudman D, Feller AG, Cohn L, Shetty KR, Rudman IW, Draper MW. (1991) Effects of human growth hormone on body composition in elderly men. *Hormone Res* 36: 73–81.

Russell-Jones DL, Weissberger AJ, Bowes SB, et al. (1993) The effects of growth hormone on protein metabolism in adult growth hormone deficient patients. *Clin Endocrinol* 38: 427–431.

Russell-Jones DL, Umpleby AM, Hennessy TR, et al. (1994) Use of a leucine clamp to demonstrate that IGF-I actively stimulates protein synthesis in normal humans. *Am J Physiol* 267: E591–E598.

Salomon F, Cuneo RD, Hesp R, Sönksen PH. (1989) The effects of treatment with recombinant human growth hormone on body composition and metabolism in adults with growth hormone deficiency. *N Engl J Med* 321: 1797–1803.

Saltiel AR, Cuatrecasas P. (1988) In search of a second messenger for insulin. *Am J Physiol* 255: C1–11.

Saltin B, Henriksson J, Nygaard E, Andersen P. (1977) Fiber types and metabolic potentials of skeletal muscles in sedentary man and endurance runners. *Ann NY Acad Sci* 301: 3–29.

Schambelan M, Mulligan K, Grunfeld C, et al. (1996) Recombinant human growth hormone in patients with HIV-associated wasting. A randomized, placebo-controlled trial. *Ann Intern Med* 125: 873–882.

Sherman SK, Demling RH, LaLonde C, et al. (1989) Growth hormone enhances re-epithelialization of human split skin graft donor sites. *Surg Forum* 40: 37–39.

Sjölin J, Stjernström H, Friman G, et al. (1990) Total and net muscle protein breakdown in infection determined by amino acid effluxes. *Am J Physiol* 258: E856–E863.

Smith K, Rennie MJ. (1990) Protein turnover and amino acid metabolism in human skeletal muscle. In: Harris JB, Turnbull DM, eds. *Muscle Metabolism, Clinical Endocrinology and Metabolism*. London: Baillière Tindall, WB Saunders, pp. 461–498.

Soroff HS, Rozin RR, Mooty JM, Lister J. (1967) Role of human growth hormone in the response to trauma: 1. Metabolic effects following burns. *Ann Surg* 166: 739–752.

Stehle P, Mertes N, Puchstein C, et al. (1989) Effect of parenteral glutamine peptide supplements on muscle glutamine loss and nitrogen balance after major surgery. *Lancet* 1: 231–233.

Streat SJ, Beddoe AH, Hill GL. (1987) Aggressive nutritional support does not prevent protein loss despite fat gain in septic intensive care patients. *J Trauma* 27: 262–266.

Strock LL, Singh H, Abdullah A, et al. (1990) The effect of insulin-like growth factor-I in post-burn hypermetabolism. *Surgery* 108: 161–164.

Takala J, Ruokonen E, Webster NR, et al. (1999) Increased mortality associated with growth hormone treatment in critically ill adults. *N Engl J Med* 341: 785–792.

Tanner JM, Hughes PCR, Whitehouse RH. (1977) Comparative rapidity of response of height, limb muscle and limb fat to treatment with human GH in patients with and without GH deficiency. *Acta Endocrinol* 184: 681–696.

Tomkins AM, Garlick PJ, Scholfield WN, Waterlow JC.

(1983) The combined effects of infection and malnutrition on protein metabolism in children. *Clin Sci* 65: 313–324.

Umpleby AM, Boroujerdi MA, Brown PM, Carson ER, Sönksen PH. (1986) The effect of metabolic control on leucine metabolism in type-1 (insulin-dependent) diabetic patients. *Diabetologia* 29: 131–141.

Voerman HJ, Strack van Schijndel RJ, Groeneveld AB, et al. (1992) Effects of recombinant human growth hormone in patients with severe sepsis. *Ann Surg* 216: 648–655.

Walker JL, Ginalska-Malinowska M, Romer TE, Pucilowska J, Underwood LE. (1991) Effects of infusion of IGF-I in a child with growth hormone insensitivity syndrome (Laron Dwarfism). *N Engl J Med* 24: 1483–1488.

Waterlow JC, Garlick PJ, Millward DJ. (1978) *Protein turnover in Mammalian Tissues and in the Whole Body.* Amsterdam: Elsevier–North Holland.

Waters D, Danska J, Hardy K, et al. (1996) Recombinant human growth hormone, insulin-like growth factor-I, and combination therapy in AIDS associated wasting. A randomized, double-blind, placebo-controlled trial. *Ann Intern Med* 125: 865–872.

Weissberger AJ, Anastasiadis AD, Sturgess I, Martin FC, Smith MA, Sönksen PH. (1997) Recombinant human growth hormone (GH) treatment in elderly patients undergoing total hip replacement: effects on muscle mass and strength. *Endocrinol Metab* 4 (Suppl A): 18.

Welle S, Thornton C, Stott M, McHenry B. (1996) Growth hormone increases muscle mass and strength but does not rejuvenate myofibrillar protein synthesis in healthy subjects over 60 years old. *J Clin Endocrinol Metab* 83: 3239–3244.

Wernerman J, von der Decken A, Vinnars E. (1985) Size distribution of ribosomes in biopsy specimens of human skeletal muscle during starvation. *Metabolism* 34: 665–669.

Wernerman J, von der Decken A, Vinnars E. (1986) Protein synthesis in skeletal muscle after abdominal surgery: the effect of total parenteral nutrition. *J Parenteral Enteral Nutr* 10: 578–582.

Wilmore DW, Moylan JA, Bristow BF, Mason Jr AD, Pruitt Jr BA. (1974) Anabolic effects of human growth hormone and high-caloric feedings following thermal injury. *Surg Gynecol Obstet* 138: 875–884.

Windsor JA, Hill GA. (1988) Risk factors of postoperative pneumonia: the importance of protein depletion. *Ann Surg* 208: 209–214.

Young VR, Haverberg LN, Bilmazes C, Munro HN. (1973) Potential use of 3-methylhistidine excretion as an index of pregressive reduction in muscle protein catabolism during starvation. *Metabolism* 22: 1429–1436.

50

Dynamic myoplasty

Pierre A. Grandjean

Introduction

"Passive" myoplasty encompasses a variety of clinical procedures involving the transfer of skeletal muscle for replacement or enhancement of body parts. Typical uses have been for filling of facial defects and for breast reconstruction after mastectomy. In "dynamic" myoplasty procedures, the addition of electrical stimulation allows the transferred skeletal muscle also to provide a contractile function. The two major applications presently in clinical use or investigation are *dynamic cardiomyoplasty* for the treatment of heart failure and *dynamic graciloplasty* for the treatment of faecal and urinary incontinence.

Dynamic cardiomyoplasty was the first clinical application in which a skeletal muscle was transferred, stimulated and trained to provide a function different from its original one (Carpentier and Chachques 1985). In this procedure, the latissimus dorsi (LD) skeletal muscle is transferred and wrapped around the ventricles to support the myocardium contractions. Other cardiac assist approaches form pumping chambers called "skeletal muscle ventricles" connected at points along the aorta (Acker et al 1986) or involve a direct wrap of the ascending or descending aorta. These different approaches and clinical status have been recently reviewed in a book "Cardiac Bioassist", edited by Carpentier et al (1997).

For these cardiac assist applications, the transferred muscle is stimulated cyclically in such a way as to synchronize its contraction with a selected portion of the cardiac cycle, and it is subjected to a conditioning protocol to sustain this demanding new function without fatigue.

For the treatment of faecal or urinary incontinence, the gracilis muscle(s) is wrapped around the anus, urethra or bladder neck to form a neosphincter. After conditioning, the muscle is stimulated continuously except when the patient interrupts it to defecate or urinate. This chapter briefly reviews the technical and clinical experience with these various clinical applications of dynamic myoplasty procedures.

Dynamic cardiomyoplasty

Dynamic cardiomyoplasty is a procedure aimed at treating patients with chronic heart failure, refractory to medical therapy, that severely limits their daily life: a Class III or intermittent Class IV condition, according to the New York Heart Association (NYHA) classification. Cardiomyoplasty is the only method of skeletal muscle cardiac assistance currently in clinical use or clinical evaluation (in the USA). Because this method uses autologous tissue, there are no rejection problems, and so no need for immunosuppressive drugs (as for heart transplants) and no need for an external power source (as for mechanical pumps).

The major limitation in the initial application of dynamic cardiomyoplasty (and other skeletal muscle powered concepts) was the early onset of muscle fatigue as soon as a skeletal muscle was activated at cardiac rates. Pioneering work by Salmons and Vrdová (1969) and Pette et al (1973) showed that the composition of muscle fibres and resulting physiologic and metabolic properties (e.g., force, fatigue resistance, contraction and relaxation duration) depend on neural activity. By electrically controlling nerve and muscle activation with functional neuromuscular stimulation (FNS), Peckham et al (1976) produced increased force and improved fatigue resistance of atrophied paralysed muscle in quadriplegic patients (with intact lower motoneurons), confirming clinically the plasticity of skeletal muscles.

The possibility of combining knowledge gained in the FNS field with anatomical and surgical considerations suggested two solutions to the problem of early muscle fatigue in cardiomyoplasty: an innovative progressive muscle stimulation protocol (Carpentier et al 1991); and the choice of the latissimus dorsi muscle (Chachques et al 1982). This muscle is used in cardiomyoplasty, as done today, because of its wide muscle size, it is not necessary for normal activity, and it can be easily transferred into the thorax. The LD muscle has its neuromuscular pedicle in its proximal part, making its transfer to the heart possible without major disturbance of the nerve and main blood supply.

Skeletal muscle conditioning for cardiomyoplasty

Cardiac and skeletal muscle differ in their response to electrical stimulation. A single electrical pulse above a given threshold will cause an action potential to propagate through the entire cardiac muscle mass, producing a smooth muscle contraction. On the other hand, the magnitude and duration of the skeletal muscle contraction varies with the characteristics of the electrical pulses: amplitude, width and interpulse interval (or pulse frequency). Pulse train stimulation grades the magnitude and duration of evoked muscle force by varying the rate of motor unit excitation (temporal summation). Only a train of pulses spaced to produce summation will result in a prolonged (>50 ms) and forceful contraction. The fatigue resistance of stimulated muscles depend on fibre composition, metabolism, stimulus parameters and duty cycle (Grandjean et al 1991).

By the 1970s, three groups (Salmons et al 1969, Pette et al 1973, Peckham et al 1976) had shown that the fatigue resistance of skeletal muscle could be increased by several weeks of low-frequency electrical stimulation. To understand the source of this aerobic capacity, Clark et al (1988) studied the bioenergetic correlates of fatigue resistance in conditioned canine latissimus dorsi muscle using phosphorus-31 nuclear magnetic resonance spectroscopy. This study indicated that the markedly enhanced resistance to fatigue of the conditioned muscle is in part due to the result of its increased capacity for oxidative phosphorylation.

Oxygen consumption was also measured directly in conditioned muscles. It was found that electrically transformed muscle is capable of generating more isometric work while consuming less oxygen per amount of tension developed than its contralateral control muscle (Clark et al 1988). More recently, muscle conditioning pre- and post-transfer has been shown to be very important to optimize muscle use for cardiac assist. Salmons (1998) has shown that a 2 week pre-transfer in situ stimulation (2 Hz) of the LD muscle enables its convertion to intermediate fibre types (IIB) while making it less susceptible to ischaemic injury. Chekanov et al (1998a and b) and Carraro et al (1998)

have shown that a less strenuous duty cycle (e.g., stopping stimulation at night or during periods of low activity) enable the maintenance of more forceful muscle fibres with faster contraction/relaxation times. Carraro et al (1998) also developed a non-invasive method to monitor the LD muscle condition after transfer and documented clinically the benefits of "intermittent" stimulation. Other means of improving muscle status includes surgically ligating main perforators for 2 weeks prior to transfer (Tobin et al 1995).

Surgical procedure

Cardiomyoplasty surgery (Fig. 50.1) begins with the patient in the lateral position. Through an oblique incision the latissimus dorsi muscle is freed from its distal insertions; it is lifted and the stimulation electrodes inserted near the nerve branches of the muscle (proximal LD; Carpentier et al 1991). The muscle is then inserted into the thorax through a 6 cm window made by resection of part of the second rib. The second phase of the surgery is carried out in the supine position via a vertical sternotomy. The LD muscle is brought under the heart and wrapped around both ventricles and sutured to the myocardium or the pericardium sack. Patients with chronic heart failure usually have very dilated ventricles and the heart coverage the muscle can provide is sometimes insufficient.

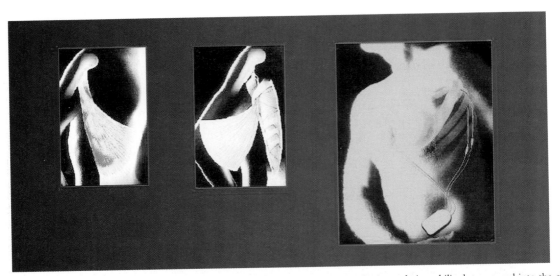

Figure 50.1—Dynamic Cardiomyoplasty procedure. In cardiomyoplasty, the latissimus dorsi muscle is mobilised, transposed into the chest through a window in the second rib, and wrapped around the ventricles of the heart. The muscle is then stimulated in synchrony with the heart contractions to augment its pumping function (with permission of Medtronic Inc.).

In such cases, a piece of pericardium is used to complete the wrapping. The procedure is done in different ways depending on the nature of the heart failure. If the heart is only dilated, the muscle is used as a reinforcement; this type of surgery is done without the use of circulatory support, and it is carried out in 4–5 h. If the patient exhibits a large aneurysm, the aneurysm can be resected and the muscle used as patch, taking care that a non-thrombogenic surface (usually pericardium) is placed between the muscle and the blood to prevent clotting problems.

Stimulation device

The stimulation device is an implantable two-channel pulse train generator ("cardiomyostimulator"), which provides muscle stimulation synchronized on cardiac activity (Fig. 50.2). It is powered by a lithium battery and sealed in a titanium case. The heart channel senses ventricular rhythm and paces it if necessary (bradycardia episodes). Ventricular sensing/pacing is achieved via an epicardial or endocardial lead placed on or in the left or right ventricle The signal from the cardiac channel is processed via a synchronization circuit which, after a synchronization delay, initiates the muscle stimulation pulse train. Muscle stimulation is usually achieved via a pair of intramuscular electrodes placed near nerve branches. Perineural electrodes have also been used by some researchers. As these are in direct contact with the nerve fibres, this approach carries a greater risk of irreversible nerve injury.

Therefore, the intramuscular type has been favoured for clinical application.

Triggering of the muscle by the heart alone may create problems, because most of these heart failure patients have a high resting heart rate (90–100 beats per min). Stimulating the muscle at this rate could lead to muscle fatigue and, consequently, muscle damage. This problem has been addressed in the Medtronic Model 4710 cardiomyostimulator by providing means to programme the device within the following parameters (Grandjean and Leinders 1997):

- synchronization ratio: enables augmentation or reduction of muscle activity by synchronizing the muscle on different heart beats (e.g., every 3 heart beats)
- muscle upper rate: enables programming the maximum muscle contraction rate allowed
- synchronization upper rate: enables programming a cardiac upper rate above which the muscle stimulation is disabled
- adaptive burst duration: enables the pulse train duration to automatically adapt to heart rate (burst length decreases as heart rate increases).

In addition, cardiac channel sensitivity, refractory period and synchronization delay (time from cardiac event to muscle burst initiation) are programmable to adjust muscle activation to ventricular contraction.

Many characteristics of the stimulator are adjustable (muscle on/off, pulse amplitude, pulse width, interpulse interval, number of pulses/burst)

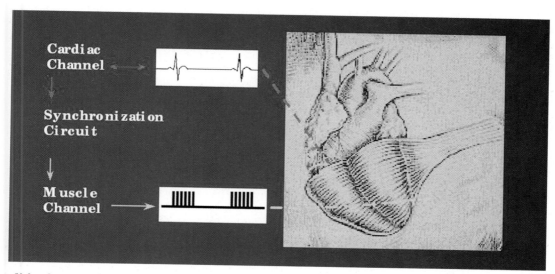

Figure 50.2—Operation of the cardiomyostimulator. In response to signals from the heart, the cardiomyostimulator stimulates the muscle grafted to the heart with trains of impulses (with permission of Medtronic Inc.).

At standard muscle settings (5 V, 6 pulses/burst, 1:2 synchronization rate), the Medtronic Model 4710 will last 6 years.

Clinical outcome

More than 1000 cardiomyoplasty clinical procedures have been performed world-wide, 75% of them with the Medtronic systems. About 80% of patients have shown clinical improvement after the procedure, averaging 1.6 NYHA class improvement (Carpentier et al 1997). The hospital mortality was less than 10% in most centres despite the severity of these patients condition prior to surgery. More invasive haemodynamic studies using sophisticated conductance techniques have been carried out in some centres (Kass et al 1995, Schreuder et al 1997). They have documented a progressive and significant decrease of heart size at 6, 12 and 24 month follow-up, a process called "reverse remodelling" of the heart, suggesting a significant recovery of myocardium function. Other studies have documented a decrease in myocardial oxygen consumption during LD synchronous muscle stimulation, a prevention of further ventricular dilatation and a cross vascularization from the LD muscle to the myocardium.

To elucidate the benefits of cardiomyoplasty compared with more conventional medical treatments, the cardiomyoplasty procedure is under clinical evaluation under a multicentre FDA-approved randomized protocol (C-SMART: Cardiomyoplasty- Skeletal Muscle Assist Randomised Trial). This prospective randomization protocol compares medical treatment alone with medical treatment with cardiomyoplasty. To date, more than 100 patients (NYHA Class III) have been randomized. Despite the severity of cardiac condition, hospital mortality of the cardiomyoplasty group has been below 2%. Single-centre data show better clinical condition after cardiomyoplasty, and they also suggest a survival benefit for the cardiomyoplasty group at 6, 12 and 18 months (Keogh 1998, Silver 1998). However, data from the interim analysis of the multicentre study (~200 patients) are needed before making firm conclusions.

Improvements

With any of the cardiac assist approaches that rely on skeletal muscle power, close attention needs to be given to improvement of pre-operative skeletal muscle condition. This is further amplified by the fact that, with the ongoing improvement of medical treatments for heart failure, patients referred to surgery are older than before, with a larger number of heart failure symptoms, and, usually, in a more severe heart failure condition.

Short and long-term muscle graft function may be improved by better muscle preparation (pre-operative, e.g., voluntary or evoked exercising, passive and active stretch, perforator ligation, pharmacological support) and peri-operative handling (e.g., to prevent episodes of ischaemia). Muscle status and activation needs to be monitored closely to evaluate the benefits of such preparations. To this end, research is being performed to monitor graft function by fluoroscopy, computer tomography and magnetic resonance scans, echo-Doppler imaging and more recently by mechanogram. The activation pattern should maximize power output while minimizing energy expenditure (i.e. minimizing fatigue), aiming first at customizing muscle training to adjust to patient muscle condition and then to prevent overuse of muscle at long term. For cardiomyoplasty, improving muscle energy transfer to the heart may require better heart coverage by the transplanted muscle, improved muscle heart coupling and improved tissue interface characteristics.

Applications of new "minimally invasive" video-assisted surgical techniques (Mesana 1997, Mesana et al 1998, Carpentier et al 1998) is opening new opportunities to reduce surgical trauma as well as facilitating muscle preparation under local anaesthesia.

Finally, the major role played by arrhythmic events (ventricular tachycardia and fibrillation, atrial fibrillation) as well as conduction disturbance (right and left bundle branch blocks) in this patient population strongly supports the combination of defibrillators with cardiomyostimulators as well as more recent multi-site cardiac stimulation modalities.

Dynamic gracioplasty for faecal and urinary incontinence

Faecal incontinence

Faecal incontinence is an underreported condition that affects 2.5% of the population (Madoff et al 1992). The anal sphincter mechanism consists of the internal sphincter (smooth muscle that provides 80% of resting sphincter pressure), the external sphincter (voluntary muscle) and the puborectalis muscle (voluntary muscle). In addition to adequate sphincter function, normal continence depends on mental function, stool volume and consistency, colonic transit, rectal distensibility, anorectal sensation and reflexes. Thus, even if the sphincter itself is normal, other abnormalities can cause faecal incontinence. Among people with normal pelvic floor, causes of incontinence are diarrhoea states, overflow due to impaction or neoplasm, and a wide range of neurologic conditions. Among people with abnormal pelvic floor, causes of incontinence include anorectal malformation and trauma iatrogenic injury to pudendal nerves (due to childbirth or habitual straining). A third group of patients become incontinent following anorectal resection for removal of malignancy. In this group, dynamic graciloplasty may be done in conjunction with perineal colostomy to approximate the function of the anus.

If there is sphincter injury, surgical repair is effective in restoring continence for solids in about 80% of patients. If the sphincter is intact, biofeedback training has reduced episodes of incontinence by 90% (Madoff et al 1992). If these therapies are unsuccessful, colostomy is an effective option, but many patients will not accept it.

In the 1950s, surgeons developed a passive wrap of gracilis muscle around the anal canal (Pickrell 1952). Patients were, however, unable to maintain the necessary contraction of the muscle voluntarily. For this reason, the electrically stimulated muscle neosphincter (ESMNS) was developed as a new option for patients whose conditions were not amenable to standard available therapy (Fig. 50.3). The ESMNS procedure adds to the passive muscle wrap a neural or intramuscular electrode to stimulate the muscle (Baeten et al 1991, Williams et al 1991). Conditioning with electrical stimulation increases its content of Type I fibres, thus improving its fatigue resistance. When conditioned, the muscle is continuously stimulated to achieve continence. When a person wishes to defecate, he or she uses a magnet to turn the stimulator off and then back on afterwards.

Surgical procedure

Dynamic myoplasty for faecal incontinence uses the gracilis muscle because it is easily transposable and not essential to lower limb function. It is a long, thin, ribbon-like muscle whose nerve and blood supply enter proximally. The muscle is mobilized up to that point. Through multiple incisions, the muscle is wrapped around the anal canal, and its tendon is secured to the ischial tuberosity. Muscle stimulation is facilitated by either nerve electrode (Williams et al 1991) or intramuscular electrodes (Baeten et al 1991) connected to implantable neuromuscular stimulators

(e.g., Medtronic Itrel Model 7224). Both methods provide muscle stimulation at low voltage that remain stable over the long term. The neuromuscular stimulator is programmable to adjust muscle contraction magnitude as well as to facilitate muscle conditioning.

Clinical outcome

To date, more than 800 dynamic graciloplasty clinical procedures have been performed in many parts of the world. Overall faecal incontinence has been achieved in 75% of patients submitted to surgery, resulting in a significant improvement in quality of life of patients.

Urinary incontinence

The success of dynamic graciloplasty for faecal incontinence led some investigators to explore similar approach to restore urinary continence (Janknegt et al 1992, Williams 1993). Because this technique involves more complex phenomena that influence the efficacy of muscle contraction (e.g., muscle wrap technique, location, low urinary viscosity), several surgical techniques have been explored: bladder neck graciloplasty and bulbous urethral graciloplasty. Some clinical cases have been peformed and have proven the clinical feasibility of these approaches. In two patients, urethral graciloplasty was even combined with dynamic graciloplasty to treat both urinary and faecal incontinence problems (Geerdes et al 1997).

The place of dynamic utinary graciloplasty in the range of treatment options still remains to be defined, and it is the goal of an ongoing multicentre study.

Improvements

Improvement in the efficacy and outcome of dynamic graciloplasty procedures could result from research and developments in the following areas:

- muscle: • improvement of muscle condition e.g. vascular delay
  - choice of muscle (gracilis, sartorius, gluteus), multiple muscles ?
- surgical procedure: • whether or not to create a stoma
  - wrap configuration
- stimulation regime: • customized conditioning protocol (i.e to minimize muscle damage)
  - contraction sensor feedback (i.e. to optimize functional outcome)
  - closed loop control.

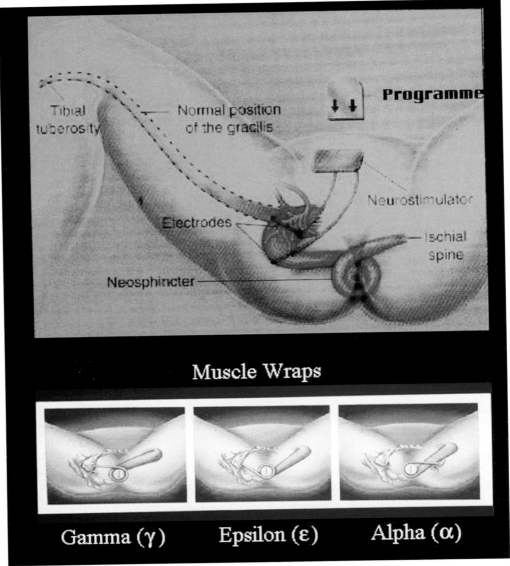

Figure 50.3—Dynamic graciloplasty for faecal incontinence. In dynamic graciloplasty to treat faecal incontinence, the gracilis muscle is transferred and wrapped around the anal canal. Three different wrap configurations are shown. After a conditioning period, the gracilis muscle(s) is then stimulated continuously to achieve continence. When wishing to defecate, the patient turns the stimulator off with the help of a small patient programmer (with permission of Medtronic Inc.).

Conclusion

Dynamic myoplasty procedures share in common the transfer and stimulation of skeletal muscles. Both dynamic cardiomyoplasty for cardiac assistance and dynamic graciloplasty for faecal incontinence have been shown to be efficacious procedures at short and long term (>10 years). However, basic studies of transferred muscle and fibre conversion/adaptation will continue to be important to the refinement of these procedures. The inherent force capacity of a transferred muscle is reduced by 30% when the tendon is cut (Kadhiresan et al, 1993). In addition, depending on conditioning protocol and stimulation regimen, force capacity may also be lost if the muscle fibres convert to Type I (Brooks and Faulkner 1991). This stresses the importance of improving surgical techniques for muscle preparation, muscle monitoring and stimulation optimization. A better understanding of the phenomena involved as well as means to restore or maintain muscle fitness in an ageing population are needed in order to realize the full potential of these dynamic myoplasty procedures.

References

Acker MA, Hammond RL, Mannion JD, Salmons S, Stephenson LW. (1986) An autologous biological pump. *J Thorac Cardiovasc Surg* 92: 733–746.

Baeten CMGI, Konsten J, Spaans F, et al. (1991) Dynamic gracioplasty for treatment of faecal incontinence. *Lancet* 338: 1163–1165.

Brooks SV, Faulkner JA. (1991) Force and power of slow and fast skeletal muscles in mice during repeated contractions. *J Physiol* 436: 701–710.

Carpentier A, Chachques JC. (1985) Myocardial substitution with a stimulated skeletal muscle: first successful clinical case. *Lancet* June 1 8440: 1267.

Chachques JC, Grandjean PA, Carpentier A, et al, eds. (1991) *Cardiomyoplasty.* New York: Futura Publishings.

Carpentier A, Chachques JC, Grandjean PA, et al eds. (1997) *Cardiac Bioassist.* New York: Futura Publishings.

Carpentier A, et al. (1998) Minimally invasive videoassisted cardiomyoplasty. Basic and Applied Myology: Cardiomyoplasty Symposium, Padova Jan. 98. *Basic Appl Myol* 8(1) suppl. IWDC98 Abstracts: 6.

Carraro U, Docali G, Bariero M, Brunazzi C, Gealow K, Casarotto D, Muneretto C, et al. (1998) Demand dynamic cardiomyoplasty. Improved clinical benefits by non-invasive monitoring of LD flap and long-term tuning of its dynamic contractile characteristics by activity-rest regime. *Basic Appl Myol* 8(1): 11–16.

Chachques JC, et al. (1982) Evolution expérimentale du muscle grand dorsal pédiculé, transposé dans le thorax du chien. In: Magalon G, Mitz V, eds. *Soc Franc Chirurgie Plastique.* Paris.

Chachques JC, Carpentier A, Zakine G, D'Atellis N. (1998) Minimally invasive video-assisted cardiomyoplasty. *Basic Appl Myol* 8(1)suppl IWDC 98: 6.

Chekanov VS, Nikolaychik VN, Rieder MA, Tchekanov GV, Smith LM, Schmidt H, et al. (1998) Improving cardiomyoplasty results. Introduction of an integrated five-step approach for overcoming its weak points. Basic and Applied Myology: Cardiomyoplasty Symposium,

Padova Jan. 98. *Basic Appl Myol* 8(1) suppl. IWDC98 Abstracts: 4.

Chekanov VS, Nikoloaychik VN, Rieder MA, Schmidt DH, et al. (1998) Partial cardiac assistance begun immediately after Latissimus Dorsi muscle mobilization and cardiomyoplasty. *Basic Appl Myol* 8(1): 27–34.

Clark BJ, Acker MA, McCully K, et al. (1988) In vivo P-NMR spectroscopy of chronically stimulated canine skeletal muscles. *Am J Physiol* 254: C258–C266.

Geerdes BP, Heesakkers JP, Heineman E, Spaans F, Janknegt RA, Baeten CG. (1997) Simultaneous treatment of faecal and urinary incontinence in children with spina bifida using double dynamic bracioplasty. *Br J Surg* vol 84: pp 1002–1003.

Grandjean PA. (1991) Electrical stimulation of skeletal muscles. In: Cardiomyoplasty. Carpentier A, Chachques JC, Grandjean P, eds. New York: Futura Publishings pp. 39–62.

Grandjean PA, Leinders R. (1997) A new stimulation system for cardiomyoplasty. In: Cardiac Bioasist. Carpentier A, Chachques JC, Grandjean PA, eds. New York: Futura Publishings pp. 277–286.

Janknegt RA, Baeten CGMI, Weil F, Spaans F. (1992) Neuromuscular Gracilis sphincter: a new concept in the treatment of sphincter in incontinence. 10th Congress of European Association of Urology vol 10: 287.

Kadhiresan VA, Guelinckx PJ, Faulkner JA. (1993) Tenotomy and repair of latissimus dorsi muscles in cats: implications to transposed muscle grafts. *J Appl Physiol* 75(3): 1294–1295.

Kass D, Baugham KC, Pak PH, et al. (1995) Reverse remodelling after dynamic cardiomyoplasty. *Circulation* 91(9): 2314–2318.

Keogh. (1998) Preliminary results of randomised cardiomyoplasty study. Cardiac Society of Australia and New Zealand Meeting. Perth, Aug. 98.

Madoff RD, Williams JG, Caushaj PF, et al. (1992) Faecal incontinence. *N Engl J Med* 326(15): 1002–1007.

Mesana T. (1997) Minimally invasive cardiomyoplasty and aortomyoplasty: experimental study. Minimally invasive surgery Congress. Marseille Sept. 97.

Mesana TG, Mouly-Bandinin A, Ferzoco SJ, et al. (1998) Dynamic aortomyoplasty: clinical experience and thoracoscopic surgery feasibility study. *J Card Surg* 13: 60–69.

Peckham PH, Marsolais EB, Mortimer JT, et al. (1976) Alteration in the force and fatigability of skeletal muscles in quadriplegic humans following exercise induced by electrical stimulation. *Clin Orthop* 114: 326–334.

Pette D, Schmidt ME, Staudte HW, Vrbová G, et al. (1973) Effects of long-term electrical stimulation on contractile and metabolic characteristics of fast rabbit muscles. *Pflugers Arch* 338: 257–272.

Pickrell KL. (1952) Construction of a rectal sphincter and restoration of anal continence by transplanting the gracilis muscle: a report of 4 cases in children. *Ann Surg* 135: 853–863.

Salmons S, Vrobvá G. (1969) The influence of activity on some contractile characteristics of mammalian fast and slow muscles. *J Physiol* 201: 535–549.

Salmons S. (1998) Preserving the viability of the graft. Basic and Applied Myology: Cardiomyoplasty Symposium, Padova Jan. 98. *Basic Appl Myol* 8(1) suppl. IWDC98 Abstracts: 8.

Schreuder JJ, van der Veen FH, van der Velde ET, et al. (1997) Left ventricular Pressure-Volume relationships before and after cardiomyoplasty in patients with heart failure. *Circulation* 96: 2978–2986.

Silver M. (1998) Surgical outcome of randomised cardiomyoplasty trial. 71st American Heart Association Conference. Nov. 1998.

Tobin GR, Keelen PC, Barker JH, Frank JM, Anderson GL, et al. (1995) Latissimus Dorsi flap loss in cardiomyoplasty: anatomic basis and prevention by delay. In: Carpentier A. *Proceedings of the World Symposium on Cardiomyoplasty*. Paris June 1995.

Williams NS, Patel J, George BD, Hallan RI, Watkins ES, et al. (1991) Development of an electrically stimulated neoanal sphincter. *Lancet* 338: 1166–1169.

Williams NS, Fowler CG, George BD, Blandy JP, Badenoch DF, Patel J. (1993) Electrically stimulated gracolis sphincter for bladder incontinence. *Lancet* 8837: 115-116.

51

Therapeutic effects of exercise in heart disorders

Roy J. Shephard

Introduction

For many years, cardiac physicians advocated prolonged rest for the majority of their patients. Inevitably, this led to a wasting of both skeletal and cardiac muscle, with a progressive loss of functional capacity. However, this thinking has undergone a complete revolution since the 1970s. Exercise programmes are now prescribed not only for the prevention of cardiac disease (Shephard 1981), but also as a major component of treatment following myocardial infarction (Pollock and Schmidt 1995), angioplasty and coronary bypass surgery (Foster et al 1998), cardiac transplantation (Shephard 1998), and in congenital heart disease (Galioto 1990) and stable congestive heart failure (Kavanagh et al 1996, Shephard 1997a). Moreover, the traditional aerobic programme has been expanded to include resistance exercise that will reverse muscle wasting, weakness and an omnipresent fatigue that impairs the overall quality of life of the patient.

The therapeutic value of exercise in the management of cardiac disorders is now well accepted. Nevertheless, many of the benefits that are associated with a progressive exercise regimen reflect interactions between muscle strength and myocardial function rather than a direct modification of skeletal muscle function. It seems appropriate, therefore, to note changes in myocardial function briefly before discussing more specific disorders of skeletal muscle function and their resolution through progressive resistance training.

Exercise programmes and myocardial function

Participation in a regular exercise programme has both indirect and direct effects on the cardiovascular system, both of which can enhance functional capacity and reduce the likelihood of future cardiac problems.

Indirect effects

Important indirect benefits of exercise include a strengthening of the skeletal muscles, a reduction of obesity, an optimization of the lipid profile (Williams et al 1982), a reduction in the risk of maturity-onset diabetes (Helmrich et al 1991) and a change in certain aspects of life style, particularly a reduction of stress (Shephard 1997b).

Muscle strength has an important influence on myocardial function. When a muscle contracts vigorously, a high intramuscular pressure tends to occlude the local blood supply, and peripheral chemoreceptors induce a compensating increase of systemic blood pressure. The increased after-loading of the heart limits cardiac ejection fraction and stroke volume. Occlusion of the local blood supply begins when the muscles are contracting at about 15% of their maximal voluntary force, and it becomes complete when contractions reach some 70% of maximal force (Kay and Shephard 1969). In many patients with heart disease, the peak muscle force has been weakened by bed rest and/or the administration of corticosteroids. A given physical task is, therefore, performed at a high fraction of peak muscle force, increasing the extent of vascular occlusion and after-loading of the heart. However, if muscle strength can be restored by an appropriate regimen of resistance exercises, there will be a corresponding improvement in peak cardiac performance. Initially, training-related gains of strength reflect mainly an improved coordination of skeletal muscle contraction, but as an exercise programme continues, some hypertrophy of the active muscle usually occurs, with a restoration of lean tissue mass.

The body weight must be supported and/or displaced in most forms of physical activity. Consequently, the energy cost of most activities (and the resultant strain on both cardiac and skeletal muscle) is closely related to the individual's body mass (Godin and Shephard 1973). If the patient's body mass can be reduced by a training programme, the functional capacity of the heart and skeletal muscles will be enhanced, even if there are no anatomical or biochemical changes in cardiac or skeletal muscle. An increase of daily energy expenditure through a programme of regular moderate-intensity physical activity is one of the most effective methods of correcting obesity (Hill and Peters 1995). An important advantage of exercise over a simple dietary regimen is that body fat content can generally be reduced without a parallel loss of skeletal muscle mass (Ballor and Keesey 1991).

Direct benefits

The direct cardiovascular effects of regular physical activity include a slowing of resting heart rate, an increase of peripheral venous tone and an expansion of plasma volume with a resultant increase in cardiac pre-loading, a reduction of blood pressure and thus cardiac after-loading, and an increase of myocardial contractility. There may also be increases in coronary blood flow and the threshold for the development of ventricular fibrillation.

Resting bradycardia

A decrease in resting heart rate is an obvious response to regular physical activity. Underlying mechanisms include an increase of stroke volume (below) and an altered autonomic balance. There is an increase of parasympathetic nerve activity, possibly reflecting a resetting of the arterial baroreceptors (Gwirtz et al 1990). The intrinsic rate of contraction of the atria is also reduced (Smith et al 1989) and there may be a downregulation of beta-adrenergic receptors (Jost et al 1989). Perhaps most importantly in our present context, if the exercise programme has restored muscle strength, perfusion of the active tissues is enhanced. We might, therefore, anticipate a reduced drive from peripheral chemoreceptors during vigorous exercise (Mitchell and Schmidt 1983); moreover, there is some evidence that in patients with congestive heart failure the discharge of the muscle metaboreceptors is decreased during static exercise (Sterns et al 1991).

Training also reduces the heart rate at any given intensity of submaximal exercise. This increases cardiac reserve and thus boosts the individual's functional capacity. The relative lengthening of the diastolic phase of the cardiac cycle also facilitates myocardial perfusion. For the coronary-prone patient, an even more important advantage is a decrease in the double-product at any given rate of working. This decreases the myocardial oxygen consumption and thus reduces the risk of myocardial ischaemia during effort.

Reduction of resting blood pressure

There is now a consensus that regular physical activity will induce a small but therapeutically useful fall in resting blood pressures, both in normotensive (−3/−3 mmHg) and in hypertensive (−10/−8 mmHg) individuals (Fagard and Tipton 1994). Pressures at any given absolute intensity of exercise are also lower after training, this trend being augmented by strengthening of the skeletal musculature and a reduced drive from the peripheral chemoreceptors.

After-loading of the left ventricle is thereby reduced, with an increase of ejection fraction and stroke volume. Peak cardiac output is augmented, and there is an associated gain in functional capacity. Perhaps more importantly from the viewpoint of the coronary-prone patient, the lower systolic pressure yields a corresponding reduction in double-product and thus a reduction in the risk of exercise-induced myocardial ischaemia at any given rate of submaximal exercise.

Increased peripheral venous tone

Venous return depends on a combination of peripheral venous tone and the pumping action of the skeletal muscles. An aerobic training programme increases peripheral venous tone (Holmgren 1967), in part because of a shift in autonomic balance and in part because a fitter individual can perform a given task with a smaller increase in core temperature. If the programme also includes resistance training, a strengthening of the skeletal muscles contributes to the enhancement of venous return.

The increase of peripheral venous tone has the effect of increasing central blood volume, and thus ventricular preloading; cardiac stroke volume is augmented and the likelihood of hypotension following a bout of exercise is reduced. These changes again have importance for the coronary-prone patient, since heart attacks are commonly precipitated by the sudden fall in blood pressure at the end of exercise. One preventive measure is to enhance action of the muscle pump, but the main remedies are a substantial cooldown and the avoidance of hot showers immediately following exercise.

Plasma volume expansion

A training-induced expansion of plasma volume contributes to an increase of cardiac stroke volume. However, it may also cause a decrease in the haemoglobin content of unit volume of blood, so that oxygen transport per litre of cardiac output actually diminishes after training (Green et al 1987). Moreover, at least in theory, the expansion of plasma volume could have a negative impact on the patient with congestive heart failure.

Increased myocardial contractility

Training induces some increase in myocardial contractility (Morris et al 1990). This contributes to the increase in stroke volume. The greater contractility increases myocardial oxygen consumption, but it also reduces the average dimensions of the heart; this reduces the tension in the ventricular wall and facilitates perfusion of the critical endocardial zone by perforating branches of the coronary artery.

Increased stroke volume

Training may increase cardiac stroke volume by 20% or more, both at rest and during vigorous exercise. Mechanisms include an increase of preloading (increased peripheral venous tone and plasma volume expansion), and a reduction of after-loading (strengthening of the skeletal muscles and a reduction of systolic pressures). In addition, there is an increase of myocardial contractility and (if training is strenuous and prolonged) ventricular hypertrophy (Rost and Hollmann 1992).

Coronary blood supply

Recent evidence supports the view that vigorous training can increase the coronary flow reserve, as demonstrated by dipyramidole (Czernin et al 1993) and the vasodilatory response to nitroglycerine (Haskell et al 1993). The maximum tolerated rate–pressure product is also increased (Hagberg 1991), and quantitative cineangiography confirms an improved coronary perfusion (Gould et al 1992). However, benefit could reflect a development of collateral vessels, a reduction of lesions in the main coronary vessels, or simply an effect arising from a relative prolongation of the diastolic phase of the cardiac cycle.

Fibrillation threshold

Treadmill training can also increase the ventricular fibrillation threshold, although the mechanism of this change remains unclear (Noakes et al 1983).

Skeletal muscles and cardiac disease

Prevention

The direct role of the skeletal muscles in the prevention of cardiac disease is relatively limited. Nevertheless, there is now good evidence that an enhancement of lean tissue mass, by a programme that combines aerobic and resistance exercise, is helpful in enhancing glucose and insulin homeostasis, thus reducing an important risk factor for myocardial infarction and peripheral vascular disease (Schwartz 1997). Likewise, a strengthening of the skeletal muscles reduces the fraction of maximal muscle force that must be exerted when performing a heavy physical task. As explained above, this reduces the exercise-induced rise in blood pressure, and thus it reduces the cardiac work-rate and the risk of relative myocardial ischaemia while the task is being completed.

Treatment

The contribution of skeletal muscle abnormalities to the weakness, fatigue and impairment of aerobic power in cardiac disease is gaining increased recognition (see also Ch. 10). Problems may arise in both the chest and the limb muscles.

Skeletal muscle abnormalities can develop after myocardial infarction, but they have received particular attention in the context of congestive heart failure (Shephard 1997a), where physical activity has often been limited for many years, and in cardiac transplantation, where the tendency to a negative energy balance and loss of lean tissue is exacerbated by the administration of corticosteroids. Many cardiac patients show a substantial loss of lean tissue mass in response to a lack of normal physical activity (Mancini et al 1992a) and high plasma concentrations of tumour necrosis factor (Levine et al 1990). Studies of skeletal muscle reveal wasting and loss of strength and endurance, with an increase of peripheral vascular resistance (Davies and Lipkin 1992, Reading et al 1993), although this last change may be a response to the limited cardiac output rather than a consequence of the muscle weakness (Yamabe et al 1992). The proportion of fast-twitch, Type II muscle fibres is increased in the cardiac patient (Lipkin et al 1988, Mancini et al 1989, Sullivan et al 1990), but paradoxically this is accompanied by a decrease in both muscle strength (Buller et al 1991) and endurance (Minotti et al 1992, Wilson et al 1992). Mitochondrial volume is decreased, and a low activity of aerobic enzymes leads to an increased drop of pH during exercise (Lipkin et al 1988, Katsuki et al 1995, Wilson 1995). The respiratory muscles also show weakness and susceptibility to fatigue (Hammond et al 1990, Mancini et al 1992b) in the face of an increased oxygen cost of breathing (Kraemer et al 1993).

All of these adverse changes have the potential to impair physical performance. Many can be reversed by an appropriate training programme, although it is less clear how far the reversal of muscle abnormalities contributes to a restoration of functional capacity. One frequently observed response to training is a lesser accumulation of lactate at any given intensity of effort. This has been linked to an improved perfusion of the working muscles and an enhanced activity of aerobic enzymes (Coats 1993, Stratton et al 1994, Bellardinelli et al 1995, Hambrecht et al 1995). Specific training of the respiratory muscles may also increase peak respiratory pressures and ventilatory capacity and thus reduce the perception of dyspnoea (Mancini et al 1995). Lean tissue mass was not increased by 4 weeks of single-arm training (Minotti et al 1992), but local gains were seen with 30 days of handgrip exercises (Sinoway et al 1987). Others have increased both the strength and endurance of key muscles by appropriate muscle building regimens (Kelemen et al 1986, Stewart et al 1988, Ghilarducci et al 1989, Sparling et al 1990, Koch et al 1992, Mancini et al 1992a). Metabolic studies have noted a restoration of oxidative enzyme activity in the muscles, with better maintenance of creatine phosphate reserves (Sullivan et al 1990, Minotti et al 1992, Adamopoulos et al 1993, Stratton et al 1994), and increases in both the total volume density of the mitochondria and the volume density of cytochrome-*c*-oxidase positive mitochondria (Hambrecht et al 1995).

A full reversal of the skeletal muscle abnormalities does not seem essential to a restoration of aerobic power or capacity. For example, Kavanagh et al (1996) found that a 12-month programme of progressive aerobic training yielded a substantial increase of aerobic power in patients with stable congestive heart failure, despite the absence of any increase in muscle strength or lean tissue mass. Nevertheless, there was a decrease in the ventilatory equivalent for oxygen and carbon dioxide, perhaps linked to the training-related increases in aerobic enzyme activity that others have described (Minotti et al 1990, Adamopoulos et al 1991, Coats 1993). Moreover, there is no guarantee that a simple restoration of aerobic power will assure the muscle strength needed for a good quality of life.

Longitudinal studies following cardiac transplantation have noted that in the first post-operative year, there is no change in muscle fibre type distribution, but there is an increase in lean tissue mass (Kavanagh et al 1988). A 35–39% increase in the cross-sectional area of the muscle fibres has been described in parallel with an increase in aerobic power (Bussières et al 1997). The number of capillaries per muscle fibre remains unchanged, but, as in congestive heart failure, training leads to increases in both glycolytic and oxidative enzymes. The activities of phosphofructokinase, citrate synthase and beta-hydroxyacyl coenzyme A dehydrogenase increase by 26, 47 and 63%, respectively (Bussières et al 1997). Magnetic resonance studies also demonstrate an enhanced phosphocreatine resynthesis and a trend to higher phosphocreatine reserves 15 months after cardiac transplantation (Stratton et al 1994).

Prescribing exercise for patients with cardiac disorders

For most of the sedentary population, any form of physical activity is better than none, and the prognosis is substantially better for those who begin to exercise than for those who do not. This aphorism applies at least equally to the typical patient with cardiac disease.

It might, therefore, be thought unnecessary and even counter-productive to suggest the need for a detailed clinical and laboratory examination, together with fitness testing and a detailed exercise prescription, before undertaking a moderate increase in habitual physical activity. The health of the average patient is quite well-served if a little more aerobic and muscular exercise is performed than during the previous week, and much of this physical activity can be incorporated into normal daily life—for instance, a walk to the store and gardening with hand rather than power tools. Assuming that a person feels no more than pleasantly tired a few hours following such exercise, then the aim should be to do a little more in each successive week until the desired level of cardiovascular and muscular fitness has been attained.

Nevertheless, many patients with established cardiac disease feel insecure if they are provided with such generalized advice. For such individuals, it is desirable to make more specific recommendations concerning the type, intensity, frequency and duration of exercise.

Type

Traditional exercise prescriptions for the cardiac patient have tended to avoid resistance (muscle-building) exercise. This was because of a generally unsubstantiated belief that static contractions would provoke a decrease in venous return and a large, sudden rise in blood pressure, thus placing an undesirable load on the heart and increasing the risk of a cardiac event (Lind and McNicol 1967, Painter and Hanson 1984). Some early reports suggested that isometric exercise caused a reduction in left ventricular ejection fraction, regional wall motion abnormalities and a variety of dysrhythmias, particularly in patients who had a poor ventricular function (Atkins et al 1976, Painter and Hanson 1984). However, other investigations have shown that, provided contractions are not held against a closed glottis for a prolonged period, well-selected patients can undertake resistance exercise safely, without an excessive rise of blood pressure (DeBusk et al 1978), myocardial ischaemia or dysrhythmia (Ferguson et al 1981, Stewart et al 1988, Ghilarducci et al 1989, Squires et al 1991).

Increments of systolic pressure with a well-designed programme of resistance exercise are no greater than with aerobic exercise (Lewis et al 1985). There may be some increase in diastolic pressure, but this helps to increase myocardial perfusion (Kerber et al 1975, Sheldahl et al 1985, Bertagnoli et al 1990, Graves and

Pollock 1993). Indeed, the current consensus is that in view of the skeletal muscle abnormalities discussed above, and the tendency for pure aerobic activity to lead to a further loss of lean tissue (Pollock et al 1987), resistance exercise is a highly desirable component of the exercise prescription for a cardiac patient.

For most patients, the preferred mode of aerobic exercise is fast walking progressing to jogging. The resistance component should include a variety of 8 to 10 muscle strengthening activities, covering most of the major muscle groups of the body. Because of the risk of left ventricular decompensation, dynamic forms of exercise such as heavy lifting are preferred to static muscle contractions (Painter and Hanson 1984). In the early (Phase II) portion of a rehabilitation programme, exercise may be provided simply by use of 2–3 kg dumb-bells, but in later phases it is convenient to use multistation weight machines if these are available to the patient. Other potential options include the use of free weights and dumb-bells, wall pulleys, inner tubes and stretch elastic bands (American Association of Cardiovascular and Pulmonary Rehabilitation 1995).

The possible impact of the Valsalva manoeuvre (expiration against a closed glottis) on blood pressure changes during various forms of resistance exercise is controversial (Ewing et al 1976, Lentini et al 1993). However, to avoid any harmful effects of breath-holding, the weight should be lifted slowly and smoothly over a 2-s interval, while exhaling, and lowered over the following 4 s, while inhaling.

Intensity

For many years, it was held that, in order to induce an aerobic training response, the intensity of effort must lie in the target zone—60–70% of the individual's maximal oxygen intake. More recently, it has been suggested that, in sedentary older adults, aerobic fitness can be enhanced by exercise at intensities as low as 50% of maximal oxygen intake; this is particularly true if functional capacity has been restricted by disease and bed rest (Blair et al 1989). It is further argued that some health benefits (for instance, reduction in body fat and enhancement of the lipid profile) may be realized even if the intensity of effort is insufficient to augment aerobic power (Blair et al 1989). Attempts to reach the previously proposed "target zone" are likely to discourage the cardiac patient because of discomfort or lack of success. The initial recommendation should, therefore, be for a moderate intensity of effort such as brisk walking.

The intensity of resistance training is prescribed relative to the patient's one-repetition (1-RM) maximal voluntary force for a given muscle group, or the maximum force that can be sustained two or three times (90% of the 1-RM). Depending on the patient's condition, individual contractions should begin at 30–50%, but later progress to 60% of the 1-RM value, as muscle strength improves. In terms of Borg's categoric rating of perceived exertion (RPE), the score should initially be no greater than 13 ("somewhat hard"), but it can progress to an RPE of 15–16 ("hard") as condition improves. One or two "sets" of 8–12 repetitions should be undertaken for each muscle group on any given day, taking care that the time allocated to resistance training does not lead to either poor compliance or inadequate performance of the aerobic component of the exercise prescription. Individual efforts should not be held for more than 5–6 s, to avoid an increase of cardiac overloading.

Frequency

Aerobic exercise should be performed on most days of the week, although once physical condition has been restored, fitness can probably be sustained by undertaking at least three sessions of aerobic activity per week. It may be possible to build much of the necessary activity into the daily routine—for example, a walk to and from the commuter station—and such an approach is helpful in countering the usual excuse for poor compliance ("a lack of time").

The processes leading to muscle hypertrophy have a slower time course. Protein synthesis is enhanced for 2–3 days following an exercise session, and the skeletal muscles are, therefore, best strengthened by carrying out two sessions of resistance exercise each week.

Duration

A minimum of 30 min of aerobic exercise per day is required. Cardiac patients may initially find difficulty in sustaining moderate activity for 30 min, but almost equal benefit can be obtained if the activity session is split into two or even three parts (US Surgeon General 1996).

Dangers of excessive exercise

Excessive exercise, whether aerobic or muscle-building, can precipitate muscle injury and even sudden death. The Type A person, who has sustained a myocardial infarction, may be tempted to indulge in excessively intense or competitive exercise, in the belief that this will speed the recovery process. However, a more common risk for most patients with cardiac disease is that the volume of activity undertaken will be too small to enhance physical condition or correct the abnormalities of muscle function.

There are now clear guidelines concerning preliminary clinical examination, contra-indications to exercising and indications to halt an exercise or test session for patients with a diagnosis of myocardial infarction, congestive heart failure or cardiac transplantation (American College of Sports Medicine 2001).

Exercise and specific heart disorders

Myocardial infarction

The principles of aerobic exercise for the patient who has sustained a myocardial infarction are well recognized and described (American Association of Cardiovascular and Pulmonary Rehabilitation 1995, American College of Sports Medicine 1995, Pollock and Schmidt 1995).

Resistance training is an important component of Phase II programmes; it should be introduced 3 to 6 weeks after infarction or surgery (Stewart et al 1988, Gordon et al 1989). Particular attention should be directed to muscle groups that will contribute to the patient's job performance. Gains in strength depend to some extent on initial condition, but, in general, the response to resistance training seems much as in healthy individuals who undertake a programme of similar intensity (Verrill et al 1989). One early study of circuit weight training carefully monitored heart rate and blood pressure, keeping values at less than 60% of those observed during maximal effort; nevertheless, muscle strength increased by an average of 24% (Kelemen et al 1986). Other reports found that strength gains of 12 to 53% were realized without clinical problems (Stewart et al 1988, Ghilarducci et al 1989, Sparling et al 1990).

Contra-indications to resistance training include an abnormal haemodynamic response to exercise, a poor left ventricular function, ischaemic changes at a rate–pressure product less than that developed during the muscle-building programme, uncontrolled hypertension or dysrhythmias, and a low peak exercise capacity (American Association of Cardiovascular and Pulmonary Rehabilitation 1995). A useful measure is the metabolic equivalent (MET; expressed as a ratio to basal metabolism); 1 MET corresponds to an oxygen consumption of approximately 3.5 ml/(kg.min). Some have recommended restricting resistance exercise to those with a peak power greater than 6 METS, but this would eliminate a large fraction of those who

would profit from muscle building; certainly, the approach must be progressively more cautious in those with a peak power below this threshold. If the patient is recovering from thoracic surgery, care must also be taken to avoid exercises that place undue stress on the thoracic cage.

In the early phases of rehabilitation, the patient should be monitored for an excessive rise of heart rate or blood pressure, dysryhthmias and excessive ST segmental depression of the electrocardiogram; blood pressures should be measured at a non-moving site (for example, the lower limbs during arm exercises). It is important to establish that the double-product during the resistance exercises does not exceed the safe ceiling as determined by a progressive treadmill test. The individual's ability to monitor the intensity of effort in terms of RPE should also be assured. Warning signs to terminate an exercise session include dizziness, dysrhythmias, anginal pain and excessive dyspnoea.

Progress should be monitored in terms of the 1-RM, or the force developed on an isokinetic dynamometer at varying rates of muscle contraction.

Congestive heart failure

Exercise programmes should be limited to those whose condition has remained stable for at least a 1-month period, and regular clinical monitoring is important to ensure that condition is improving rather than worsening. Severe dyspnoea or an increased use of medications are indications for careful re-evaluation. The initial peak aerobic power, as measured by a treadmill test with direct determination of oxygen intake, should be at least 3 METS (10.5 ml/(kg.min)). The cardiac ejection fraction should also reach a minimum of 20%, and a favourable response to training is unlikely if there is also exercise-induced ischaemia or dysrhythmia.

Probably because many patients are treated by a combination of digoxin and diuretics, serum potassium and serum magnesium levels tend to be low, and a careful watch must be kept for hypotension and malignant dysryhthmias.

Cardiac transplantation

Light aerobic exercise should begin as soon as possible following surgery, often within the first week, with progressive increases in intensity and volume as condition improves. Resistance exercises may be added after 3–6 weeks.

The prescription of an appropriate intensity of either aerobic or resistance exercise for the patient who has undergone a cardiac transplantation is complicated by the limited heart rate response to physical activity. The intensity of aerobic effort is best regulated by a combination of oxygen consumption measurements (a load is set at 60–70% of peak oxygen intake, just below the individual's anaerobic threshold) and the corresponding ratings of perceived exertion and dyspnoea. The RPE is also more useful than heart rate in regulating the intensity of resistance exercise. Because normal cardiac innervation is lacking, the heart rate on- and off-transients are substantially prolonged during aerobic exercise, and a longer than normal time must be allowed for both "warm-up" and "cool-down" from exercise. It is particularly important to monitor blood pressures after cardiac transplantation, from several perspectives. Hypertension is a common side-effect of the immunosuppressant drug cyclosporin, administered to this class of patients. Because of cardiac denervation, there are no warning signs of myocardial ischaemia, and this is a relatively common complication since atherosclerosis develops more rapidly than normal in a transplanted heart. Abnormal blood pressure responses may also provide an early warning of transplant rejection episodes; if rejection is confirmed by cardiac biopsy, this is an indication to moderate and often to halt the training programme, depending on the severity of the rejection episode. Further complications are introduced by the liberal prescription of prednisone or other corticosteroids; from the viewpoint of the exercise programme, hazards include sodium and fluid retention, increased excretion of potassium ions, muscle wasting and osteoporosis. Fractures may result if the exercise programme places excessive loads on the skeleton.

Conclusions

Patients with cardiac disease show a variety of manifestations of impaired skeletal muscle function. These arise mainly from disuse. Cardiac rehabilitation programmes initially had a purely aerobic focus. However, experience accumulated since the 1970s has shown that the majority can participate safely in a programme of graded resistance exercises, and that such training is important to a full restoration of function. Progressive resistance exercise restores muscle strength, enhancing the individual's quality of life, and, in the case of myocardial infarction, it often allows a return to demanding occupations. Moreover, once strength has been normalized, physically demanding activities can be performed at a smaller fraction of maximal voluntary force, with a corresponding decrease in the strain imposed upon the damaged heart. Rehabilitation programmes for the cardiac patient should always include a resistance component, except in the presence of specific contra-indications.

References

Adamopoulos S, Brunotte F, Coats A, et al. (1991) Skeletal muscle metabolism in experimental heart failure: effects of infarct size and physical training. *J Am Coll Cardiol* 17 (Suppl. A): 158A.

Adamopoulos S, Coats AJS, Brunotte F, et al. (1993) Physical training improves skeletal metabolism in patients with chronic heart failure. *J Am Coll Cardiol* 21: 1101–1106.

American Association of Cardiovascular and Pulmonary Rehabilitation. (1995) *Guidelines for Cardiac Rehabilitation Programs*. Champaign, IL.: Human Kinetics Publishers.

American College of Sports Medicine. (2001) *Guidelines for Graded Exercise Testing and Exercise Prescription*. Baltimore, MD.: Williams & Wilkins.

Atkins JM, Mathews OA, Blomqvist CG, et al. (1976) Incidence of arrhythmias induced by isometric and dynamic exercise. *Br Heart J* 38: 465–471.

Ballor DL, Keesey RE. (1991) A meta-analysis of the factors affecting exercise-induced changes in body mass, fat mass, and fat-free mass in males and females. *Intl J Obesity* 15: 717–726.

Bellardinelli R, Georgiou D, Scocco V, et al. (1995) Low intensity exercise training in patients with chronic heart failure. *J Am Coll Cardiol* 26: 975–982.

Bertagnoli K, Hanson P, Ward A. (1990) Attenuation of exercise-induced ST depression during combined isometric and dynamic exercise in coronary artery disease. *Am J Cardiol* 65: 314–317.

Blair SN, Kohl HW, Paffenbarger RS, et al. (1989) Physical fitness and all-cause mortality: A prospective study of healthy men and women. *JAMA* 262: 2395–2401.

Buller NP, Jones D, Poole-Wilson PA. (1991) Direct measurement of skeletal muscle fatigue in patients with chronic heart failure. *Br Heart J* 65: 20–24.

Bussières LM, Pflughelder PW, Taylor AW, et al. (1997) Changes in skeletal muscle morphology and biochemistry after cardiac transplantation. *Am J Cardiol* 79: 630–634.

Coats AJS. (1993) Exercise rehabilitation in chronic heart failure. *J Am Coll Cardiol* 22 (Suppl. A): 172A–177A.

Czernin J, Barnard RJ, Sun K, et al. (1993) Beneficial effect of cardiovascular conditioning on myocardial blood flow and coronary vasodilator capacity. *Circulation* 88: 1–51 (abstract).

Davies SW, Lipkin DP. (1992) Exercise physiology and the role of the periphery in cardiac failure. *Curr Opin Cardiol* 7: 389–396.

DeBusk RF, Valdez R, Houston N, et al. (1978) Cardiovascular responses to dynamic and static effort soon after myocardial infarction. Application to occupational work assessment. *Circulation* 58: 368–375.

Ewing DJ, Kerr F, Leggett R. (1976) Interaction between cardiovascular responses to sustained handgrip and Valsalva manoeuvre. *Br Heart J* 38: 483–490.

Fagard RH, Tipton CM. (1994) Physical activity, fitness and hypertension. In: Bouchard C, Shephard RJ, Stephens T, eds. *Physical Activity, Fitness and Health*. Champaign, IL.: Human Kinetics Publishers, pp. 633–655.

Ferguson RJ, Cote P, Bourassa MG, et al. (1981) Coronary blood flow during isometric and dynamic exercise in angina pectoris patients. *J Card Rehabil* 1: 21–26.

Foster C, Meyer K, Hector LL. (1998) Exercise prescription in the rehabilitation of patients following coronary artery bypass graft surgery and percutaneous transluminal coronary angioplasty. In: Shephard RJ, Miller H, eds. *Exercise and the Heart in Health and Disease*. New York, NY.: Marcel Dekker, pp. 341–353.

Galioto FM. (1990) Exercise rehabilitation programs for children with congenital heart disease: a note of enthusiasm. *Pediatr Exerc Sci* 2: 197–200.

Ghilarducci LE, Holly RG, Amsterdam EA. (1989) Effects of high resistance training in coronary artery disease. *Am J Cardiol* 64: 866–870.

Godin G, Shephard RJ. (1973) Body weight and the energy cost of activity. *Arch Environ Health* 27: 289–293.

Gordon NF, Kohl HW, Villegas JA, et al. (1989) Effect of real interval duration on cardiorespiratory responses to hydraulic resistance circuit training. *J Cardiopulm Rehab* 9: 325–330.

Gould KL, Ornish D, Kirkeeide R, et al. (1992) Improved stenosis geometry by quantitative coronary arteriography after vigorous risk factor modification. *Am J Cardiol* 69: 845–853.

Graves JE, Pollock ML. (1993) Exercise testing in cardiac rehabilitation: Role in prescribing exercise. *Cardiol Clin* 11: 253–266.

Green HJ, Jones LL, Hughson RL, et al. (1987) Training-induced hypervolemia: Lack of an effect on oxygen utilization during exercise. *Med Sci Sports Exerc* 19: 202–206.

Gwirtz PA, Brandt MA, Mass HJ, et al. (1990) Endurance training alters arterial baroreflex function in dogs. *Med Sci Sports Exerc* 22: 200–206.

Hagberg JM. (1991) Physiological adaptations to prolonged high intensity training in patients with coronary artery disease. *Med Sci Sports Exerc* 23: 661–667.

Hambrecht R, Niebauer J, Fiehn E, et al. (1995) Physical training in patients with stable chronic heart failure: effects on cardiorespiratory fitness and ultrastructural abnormalities of leg muscles. *J Am Coll Cardiol* 25: 1239–1249.

Hammond MD, Bauer KA, Sharp JT, et al. (1990) Respiratory muscle strength in congestive heart failure. *Chest* 98: 1091–1094.

Haskell WL, Sims C, Myll J, et al. (1993) Coronary artery size and dilating capacity in ultradistance runners. *Circulation* 87: 1076–1082.

Helmrich SP, Ragland DR, Leung RW, et al. (1991) Physical activity and reduced occurrence of non-insulin dependent diabetes mellitus. *N Engl J Med* 325: 147–152.

Hill JO, Peters JC. (1995) Exercise and macronutrient balance. *Intl J Obesity* 19 (Suppl. 4): S88–S92.

Holmgren A. (1967) Cardiorespiratory determinants of cardiovascular fitness. *Can Med Assoc J* 96: 697–702.

Jost J, Weiss M, Weicker H. (1989) Comparison of sympatho-adrenergic regulation at rest and of the adrenoceptor system in swimmers, long-distance runners, weight-lifters, and untrained men. *Eur J Appl Physiol* 58: 596–604.

Katsuki T, Yasu T, Ohmura N, et al. (1995) Role of skeletal muscle metabolism in exercise capacity of patients with myocardial infarction studied by phosphorus 31 nuclear magnetic resonance. *Jap Circ J* 59: 315–322.

Kavanagh T, Myers MG, Baigrie RS, et al. (1996) Quality of life and cardiorespiratory function in chronic heart failure: effects of 12 months' aerobic training. *Heart* 76: 42–49.

Kavanagh T, Yacoub MH, Mertens DJ, et al. (1988) Cardiorespiratory responses to exercise training after orthotopic cardiac transplantation. *Circulation* 77: 162–171.

Kay C, Shephard RJ. (1969) On muscle strength and the threshold of anaerobic work. *Int Z Angew Physiol* 27: 311–328.

Kelemen MH, Stewart KJ, Gillilan RE, et al. (1986) Circuit weight training in cardiac patients. *J Am Coll Cardiol* 7: 38–42.

Kerber RE, Miller RA, Naijar SM. (1975) Myocardial ischemic effects of isometric, dynamic and combined exercise in coronary artery disease. *Chest* 67: 388–394.

Koch M, Douard H, Broustet J-P. (1992) The benefit of graded exercise in chronic heart failure. *Chest* 101: 231S–235S.

Kraemer MD, Kubo SH, Rector TS, et al. (1993) Pulmonary and peripheral vascular factors are important determinants of peak exercise oxygen uptake in patients with heart failure. *J Am Coll Cardiol* 21: 641–648.

Lentini AC, McElvie RS, McCartney N, et al. (1993) Left ventricular response in healthy young men during heavy intensity weight-lifting. *J Appl Physiol* 75: 2703–2710.

Levine B, Kalman J, Mayer L, et al. (1990) Elevated circulating levels of tumor necrosis factor in severe chronic heart failure. *N Engl J Med* 323: 236–244.

Lewis SF, Snell PG, Taylor WF, et al. (1985) Role of muscle mass and mode of contraction in circulatory responses to exercise. *J Appl Physiol* 58: 146–151.

Lind AR, McNicol GW. (1967) Muscular factors which determine the cardiovascular responses to sustained and rhythmic exercise. *Can Med Assoc J* 96: 706–713.

Lipkin DP, Jones DA, Round JM, et al. (1988) Abnormalities of skeletal muscle in patients with chronic heart failure. *Intl J Cardiol* 18: 187–195.

Mancini D, Coyle E, Coggan A, et al. (1989) Contribution of intrinsic skeletal muscle changes to 31P NMR skeletal muscle metabolic abnormalities in patients with chronic heart failure. *Circulation* 80: 1338–1346.

Mancini DM, Walter G, Reichek N, et al. (1992a) Contribution of skeletal muscle atrophy to exercise intolerance and altered muscle metabolism in heart failure. *Circulation* 85: 1364–1373.

Mancini DM, Henson D, LaManca J. (1992b) Respiratory muscle function and dyspnea in patients with chronic congestive heart failure. *Circulation* 86: 909–919.

Mancini DM, Henson D, LaManca J, et al. (1995) Benefit of selective respiratory muscle training on exercise capacity in patients with congestive heart failure. *Circulation* 91: 320–329.

Minotti JR, Johnson EC, Hudson TL, et al. (1990) Skeletal muscle response to exercise training in congestive heart failure. *J Clin Invest* 86: 751–758.

Minotti JR, Pillay P, Chang L, et al. (1992) Neurophysiological assessment of skeletal muscle fatigue in patients with congestive heart failure. *Circulation* 86: 903–908.

Mitchell JH, Schmidt RF. (1983) Cardiovascular reflex control by afferent fibers from skeletal muscle receptors. In: Shepherd JT, Abboud FM, eds. *Handbook of Physiology: Vol. 3. Circulation, part 2.* Bethesda, MD.: American Physiological Society, pp. 623–658.

Morris GS, Baldwin KM, Lash JM, et al. (1990) Exercise alters cardiac myosin isozyme distribution in obese Zucker and Wistar rats. *J Appl Physiol* 69: 380–383.

Noakes TD, Higginson L, Opie LH. (1983) Physical training increases ventricular fibrillation thresholds of isolated rat hearts during normoxia, hypoxia, and regular ischemia. *Circulation* 67: 24–30.

Painter P, Hanson P. (1984) Isometric exercise: Implications for the cardiac patient. *Cardiovasc Res Rep* 5: 261–279.

Pollock ML, Foster C, Knapp D, et al. (1987) Effect of age and training on aerobic capacity and body composition of master athletes. *J Appl Physiol* 62: 725–731.

Pollock ML, Schmidt DH. (1995) *Heart Disease and Rehabilitation.* Champaign, IL.: Human Kinetics Publishers.

Reading JL, Goodman JM, Plyley MJ, et al. (1993) Vascular conductance and aerobic power in sedentary and active subjects and heart failure patients. *J Appl Physiol* 74: 567–573.

Rost R, Hollmann W. (1992) Cardiac problems in endurance in sports. In: Shephard RJ, Åstrand PO, eds. *Endurance in Sport.* Oxford, UK.: Blackwell Scientific Publishers, pp. 438–452.

Schwartz RS. (1997) Physical activity, insulin resistance and diabetes. In: Leon AS, ed. *Physical Activity and Cardiovascular Health.* Champaign, IL.: Human Kinetics Publishers, pp. 104–111.

Sheldahl LM, Wilke NA, Tristani FE. (1985) Response of patients after myocardial infarction to carrying a graded series of weight loads. *Am J Cardiol* 52: 698–703.

Shephard RJ. (1981) *Ischemic Heart Disease and Exercise.* London: Croom Helm Publishing.

Shephard RJ. (1997a) Exercise for patients with congestive heart failure. *Sports Med* 23: 75–92.

Shephard RJ. (1997b) Exercise and relaxation in health promotion. *Sports Med* 23: 211–217.

Shephard RJ. (1998) How important is exercise-centered rehabilitation following cardiac transplantation? *Crit Rev Rehab Med* 10: 101–121.

Sinoway LI, Shenberger J, Wilson J, et al. (1987) A 30-day forearm work protocol increases maximal forearm blood flow. *J Appl Physiol* 62: 1063–1067.

Smith MJ, Hudson DL, Gratitzer HM, et al. (1989) Exercise training bradycardia: the role of autonomic balance. *Med Sci Sports Exerc* 21: 40–44.

Sparling PB, Cantwell JD, Dolan CM, et al. (1990) Strength training in a cardiac rehabilitation program: a six-month follow-up. *Arch Phys Med Rehab* 71: 148–152.

Squires RW, Muri AJ, Anderson LJ, et al. (1991) Weight training during Phase II (early outpatient) cardiac rehabilitation: Heart rate and blood pressure responses. *J Card Rehab* 11: 360–364.

Sterns DA, Ettinger SM, Gray KS, et al. (1991) Skeletal muscle metaboreceptor exercise responses are attenuated in heart failure. *Circulation* 84: 2034–2039.

Stewart KJ, Mason M, Kelemen MH. (1988) Three year participation in circuit weight training improves muscular strength and self-efficacy in cardiac patients. *J Card Rehab* 8: 292–296.

Stratton JR, Dunn JF, Adamopoulos S, et al. (1994) Training partially reverses skeletal muscle abnormalities during exercise in heart failure. *J Appl Physiol* 76: 1575–1582.

Stratton JR, Graham JK, Daly RC, et al. (1994) Effects of cardiac transplantation on bioenergetic abnormalities of skeletal muscle in congestive heart failure. *Circulation* 89: 1624–1631.

Sullivan MJ, Green HJ, Cobb FR. (1990) Skeletal muscle biochemistry and histology in ambulatory patients with long-term heart failure. *Circulation* 81: 518–527.

US Surgeon General. (1996) *Physical Activity and Health: A Report of the Surgeon General*. Atlanta, GA.: US Dept. of Health & Human Services, Centers for Disease Control and Prevention.

Verrill D, Shoup E, McElveen G, et al. (1989) Resistive exercise training in cardiac patients. *Sports Med* 13: 171–193.

Williams PT, Wood PD, Haskell WL, et al. (1982) The effect of running mileage and duration on plasma lipoprotein levels. *JAMA* 247: 2672–2679.

Wilson JR. (1995) Exercise intolerance in heart failure: Importance of skeletal muscle. *Circulation* 91: 559–561.

Wilson JR, Mancini DM, Simpson M. (1992) Detection of skeletal muscle fatigue in patients with heart failure using electromyography. *Am J Cardiol* 70: 488–493.

Yamabe H, Itoh K, Yasaka Y, et al. (1992) The distribution of the blood flow during exercise in chronic heart failure–compensatory mechanism to the decrease in cardiac output. *Jap Circ J* 56: 494–499.

52

Management of muscle pathology in the critically ill (sepsis and multiple organ failure)

R. D. Griffiths

Introduction

A patient enters intensive care because of the failure of one or more of their organ systems, and this usually means that without support death would be likely. Understandably cardio-respiratory dysfunction predominates in the first instance. Therefore, the problems of skeletal muscle pathology do not rank commonly among the first issues that an intensive care specialist has to deal with, except rarely when muscle weakness is the primary cause of the respiratory failure. However, the most frequent causes of a prolonged critical illness are as the result of major trauma, burns, and severe sepsis, the latter commonly either respiratory or intra-abdominal. This chapter takes a clinical view of muscle pathology in the critically ill and where therapeutic options, if any, are taking us.

Lean tissue and skeletal muscle wasting

Increased nitrogen excretion as a consequence of protein breakdown has been recognized as the metabolic response to injury since the 1930s (Cuthbertson 1930). Following elective abdominal surgery, nitrogen loss only accounts for a proportion of the energy deficit but, as the severity of injury and sepsis increases, loss of lean tissue predominates. Confirmation of this loss, especially from skeletal muscle in the critically ill patient, has come from detailed whole body composition studies made possible by siting the measuring equipment adjacent to an intensive care unit. Over a

Table 52.1—Summary of changes seen over 21 days in severe sepsis (from Plank et al 1998)

1. No change in total body fat mass
   Tissue fat oxidation occurs when inadequate energy intake

2. Initial 12.5 l positive fluid balance
   Body weight loss at 0.5 kg/day (79 kg down to 66 kg)
   7.8 l extracellular fluid lost over 21 days

3. 1.2 kg (13.1%) protein lost over 21 days
   Skeletal muscle mass loss of ≈ 3 kg tissue (19.9 kg down to 16.6 kg)
   67% protein loss is from skeletal muscle in first 10 days
   Later protein loss is from visceral mass ≈ 3 kg tissue

21 day period following either severe trauma or sepsis, progressive losses of 17% total body water, 16% total body protein and 19% total body potassium have been documented (Finn et al 1996). Sequential studies in severely septic patients with peritonitis over 21 days (see Table 52.1; Plank et al 1998) show that they initially gained about 12 l body water in the first couple of days of resuscitation, but this was then steadily lost. Patients lost about 1.21 kg of protein (13%), of which two thirds came from skeletal muscle in the first 10 days alone, but later more was lost from the viscera. The total loss of skeletal muscle mass was estimated to be 3 kg. These losses of lean body mass (whole body water and protein), ranging from 0.5 to 1.0% per day, is far greater than that caused by bed rest alone.

Provision of nutrition and muscle wasting in the critically ill

It should be remembered that the losses of protein occur in the context of apparent full provision of nutritional support, and they are not related to starvation. In sepsis, providing protein in excess of 1.5 g per kilogram of body weight per day does not improve the nitrogen balance. In eight septic ventilated patients, despite receiving parenteral nutrition of 2700 kcal and 22.6 g nitrogen, sophisticated neutron activated analysis of whole body composition showed a loss of 1.5 kg protein and gain of 2.2 kg fat and glycogen over 10 days (Streat et al 1987). A consistent feature seen in all these studies is that body fat could be preserved by adequate calorie provision. In those patients with multiple organ failure, the extent of muscle wasting appears to have little relationship to whether the patient is nutritionally in positive energy or nitrogen balance (Green et al 1995). Retrospective examination of nutrient provision tentatively suggest that giving more than even the modest amount of 1.0 g protein/day/kg body weight does nothing to reduce this loss of protein (Ishibashi et al 1998). The almost obligatory nature of this protein loss from skeletal muscle has been recognized for many years, but it is the rapidity and extent of the catabolic muscle wasting in the critically ill that has not been fully appreciated. Muscle biopsy studies show losses of muscle protein approaching 2% per day (Gamrin et al 1997) and equivalent degrees of progressive fibre atrophy, even resulting in cell necrosis (Helliwell et al 1991). The functional consequences of this loss only become apparent as the patient starts to recover and has to breathe for him or herself and is ambulant again. The diaphragm and the other skeletal muscles of the respiratory system are not protected from this process in keeping with that seen in malnutrition (Arora and Rochester 1982). More recent work, however, shows that despite a 35–50% decline in respiratory and skeletal muscle function there is no loss of cardiac mass or function in critically ill patients over the first 3 weeks once cardiovascular stability has been established (Hill et al 1997). This is consistent with the sustained increased cardiac output usually observed.

Protein synthesis and degradation in the critically ill

The resulting net muscle wasting is a balance between protein synthesis and protein degradation. After modest surgery, there is a decrease in whole body protein synthesis rather than breakdown (Crane et al 1977), similar to the decrease in skeletal muscle protein synthesis seen with short-term starvation (Essen et al 1992). Trauma and major surgery increase synthesis and degradation, the later being more enhanced (Birkhahn et al 1980). In multiple organ failure increased whole body protein breakdown predominates over increased protein synthesis (Arnold et al 1993). The various tissues and organs respond differently, and they also change during the course of an illness, with the liver and immune system showing marked protein synthesis early following trauma. Tissue protein synthesis in the critically ill has now been characterized (Wernerman et al 1996, Essen et al 1998). Muscle protein synthesis is varied corresponding to metabolic status, and it can be increased as well as decreased. The rate of protein synthesis in peripheral blood lymphocytes is increased, and, along with the recognized acute phase protein production in the liver, contrary to popular belief albumin synthesis is also increased. There is clearly a metabolic demand by many tissues for substrates involved in protein synthesis, with the supply coming predominantly from skeletal muscle such that the factors leading to muscle catabolism are overwhelming.

Neuromuscular pathology

Apart from the wasting and protein loss described in the muscle, it is now recognized that the nerves are also involved in multiple organ failure and sepsis (Table 52.2). Workers in Canada (Bolton et al 1984) and France (Coronel et al 1990) described a critical illness polyneuropathy that involves a primary axonal degeneration of motor and sensory pathways, although a combination of pathologies have been described. This is recognized later in the intensive care unit (ICU) stay, is associated with sepsis and multiple organ failure, and is more usually described in those patients who have been ventilated for more than 2 weeks. While the first descriptions suggested that the abnormalities were related to the use of steroids or neuromuscular blocking agents, it has become clear that it is more generally related to sepsis, a prolonged illness and ventilatory support. Furthermore, during the ICU stay a combination of pathologies ranging from purely motor to mixed motor and sensory pathologies can be detected, but there is no clear pattern and relationship to the wide range of histological abnormalities seen in the muscle (Latronico et al 1996, Coakley et al 1998). Although patients may be admitted with respiratory failure caused by a demyelinating condition, its development during the ICU stay is unusual. The relative incidence of a critical illness myopathy and the critical illness polyneuropathy varies among studies; this reflects differences in populations, inclusiveness and timing of the studies (Lacomis et al 1998). With a generalized systemic inflammatory response syndrome (SIRS), it may well be that there is a common endothelial and vascular pathology that leads to both the nerve and muscle damage. It is likely that distal nerve injury coexists with muscle fibre damage. In a retrospective review of treatment with immunoglobulin early in sepsis, Mohr et al (1997) suggested a reduced incidence of the critical illness neuropathy, but this has not been prospectively examined in a randomized study.

The electrophysiological abnormalities usually take a few weeks to appear, but changes due to fibre atrophy in muscle are evident within the first few days, with necrosis being an unusual late event (Helliwell et al 1998a). Although Type II fibre atrophy is well known to occur with inactivity, in the very severely ill serial biopsies in the first 10 days show that the mean daily decrease in the fibre area is 4% in Type II fibres but also 3% for Type I fibres. It should be realized that the biopsies having the largest fibres show the greatest atrophy. The muscles show the early differential changes that occur in contractile and structural proteins (loss of myosin but relative preservation of actin and the structural proteins such as desmin) as well as increased lysosomal and ubiquitin proteolysis. Electron microscopy shows loss of myosin filaments with the accumulation of cellular debris in lysosome-like particles. Myosin

Table 52.2—Muscle histology and electrophysiological features seen in the septic critically ill patient

Abnormal muscle histology and reduced amplitude of the compound muscle action potential on electrophysiology are seen early, within first 10 days. Early on there is discrepancy between histology and other electrophysiological findings.

Muscle histology
    Lipid accumulations in Type I fibres
    Enlargement of subsarcolemmal nuclei
    Degeneration seen in fibres frequently
      (Focal cytoplasmic features with retention of dystrophin immunolabelling)
    Fibre necrosis in only a few fibres, but seen more often later
      (Complete loss of cytoplasmic structure and break in labelling of dystrophin)
    Generalized fibre atrophy of Type I and II fibres early
      Daily fibre decrease 4% Type II, 3% Type I in first 10 days
      More common in fibres showing degeneration, independent of necrosis
    Rare to see typical denervation atrophy of scattered fibres

Muscle and capillary ultrastructure
    Contraction system disorganization
    Loss of myosin filaments
    Abnormalities of mitochondria
    Membranous debris and lysosome like bodies
    Broken neuromuscular contacts
    Isolated segmental necrosis
    Endothelial cell swelling
    Thickened capillary basement membrane

Electrophysiological abnormalities
    Concordance with histological features seen only after several weeks of illness
    After 1–3 weeks fibrillation potentials and positive sharp waves suggest denervation
    Motor unit potentials reduced in amplitude and polyphasic consistent with myopathic features
    Nerve recordings usually show low amplitude signals with normal latency consistent with axonal degeneration.
    Axonal neuropathy seen on histology increases with duration of sepsis and is a feature of a prolonged ICU stay of several weeks
      Motor axonal neuropathy most common
      Mixed motor-sensory neuropathy
      Sensory axonal neuropathy less frequently
    Demyelinating neuropathy on admission, but seen less often later.
    Defects in neuromuscular transmission rarely detected in sepsis.

retians its immunoreactivity, but loses its filamentous structure, suggesting that the myosin filaments disaggregate before undergoing extensive proteolysis. The early loss of mysosin with the retention of the structural proteins may imply that these fibres have the potential to recover.

Microvascular pathology in muscle

There is good evidence of widespread and profound capillary endothelial activation (Helliwell et al 1998b) with an increase in thickness of the endothelial cell and basement membrane without, however, any reduction in the capillary lumen or evidence for vascular occlusion. There was a significant 65% increase in the endothelial and basement membrane thickness, which might compromise the blood–tissue interface. Deposition of the complement membrane attack complex (C5-9MAC) was present in many capillaries, perhaps reflecting immune complex or endotoxin activation. The endothelial swelling was characterized by increased von Willebrand factor (vWF) staining consistent with the increased vWF levels observed in the plasma in the critically ill (McGill et al 1998). These all point to the generalized involvement of muscle during sepsis and multiorgan failure.

Muscle proteolysis in sepsis

The pathway responsible for the increased proteolysis in catabolic conditions is now recognized to be the ubiquitin-proteasome pathway that requires ATP and which is stimulated by fasting, acidosis, trauma, sepsis, cancer or denervation (Mitch and Goldberg 1996). The increase in activity occurs within hours of the injection of endotoxin. It would appear that gluco-corticoids are important in this process not only in regulating and increasing the proteolysis in muscle but also enhancing the utilization of the resulting amino acids in the liver. The chief factor opposing the cata-bolic effect of glucocorticoids is insulin (Wing and Goldberg 1993). The response to sepsis or injury and the signal cascade of tumour necrosis factor (TNF) and interleukins from activated macrophages and endothe-lial cells also stimulate the ubiquitin-proteasome path-way in muscle, probably involving multiple cytokine signals and, in cancer, also some novel glycoproteins (Todorov et al 1996). Normally during prolonged starvation, after the initial mobilization of amino acids for gluconeogenesis, protein breakdown decreases as increased energy is derived instead from fat metabolism. This important control, preserving muscle protein, is lost in the face of sustained stimulation of protein breakdown in sepsis and inflammation (Hasselgren and Fischer 1998).

Inactivity and muscle pathology

A feature common to severely ill patients is the marked inactivity of their muscle. In healthy subjects immobilization of a limb results in muscle atrophy. In part this can be ameliorated by activity or letting the muscle undergo electrically stimulated contractions (Gibson et al 1988). Bouletreau et al (1986) suggested that muscle wasting in the severely ill could be reduced by similar means. What is not clear is whether it is the muscle contraction per se or the forces and stresses induced in the muscle that prevent atrophy. Studies where normal volunteers lay for 30 days in head down tilt, as a pseudo-weightlessness model to imitate a reduction in gravitational stress, has shown a number of structural changes in human skeletal muscle that imitate some of the features seen in the critically-ill (Hikida et al 1989).

Passive stretching of muscle

The question whether passive stretching of muscle alone could alter the structural and biochemical processes in the critically ill patient has been examined (Griffiths et al 1995). One leg was passively stretched and the other leg acted as the control for all the gen-eral metabolic and nutritional influences. To exclude the effect of voluntary contractile activity the patients received neuromuscular blocking agents so that any forces on the muscle were strictly passive and not influenced either by central drive or stretch reflex activation. There was preservation of muscle architec-ture with reduced protein loss and less fibre atrophy. However this was not by a mechanism involving stim-ulation of protein synthesis (as measured by ribosomal analysis), implying instead that the proteolytic activity was reduced. The striking preservation of the archi-tectural structure of the muscle suggests a reduced activity of the proteolytic processes discussed earlier. From a clinical perspective the passive stretch study underlines the importance of preventing immobility, and that as far as the recovery of skeletal muscle is concerned every effort must be taken to re-establish mobility and the positive effects of load and stress that this has on muscle. The suggested mechanisms that translate mechanical force into cellular activity are listed in Table 52.3 (Bishop et al 1995). With these mechan-ical responses are associated increased growth factors, and it has been suggested that the changes in muscle may partly be mediated by the autocrine/paracrine action of insulin-like growth factor-1 (IGF-1; Millward 1995).

Table 52.3 — Mechanisms that may translate mechanical force into cellular activity (from Bishop et al 1995)

1. Integrin receptors on the cell surface and the associated intracellular cytoskeletal microtubular system may permit direct transmission of the mechanical force from the extracellular matrix to intracellular protein synthesis (ribosomal or nuclear).

2. Influx of Na^+ and Ca^{2+} through stretch activated ion channels with intracellular signals may initiate mechanotransduction.

3. Second messengers, especially adenylate cyclase and phospholipase C from membrane bound enzyme complexes, may stimulate early gene and cell replication.

Muscle growth promotors in the critically ill

Although the potential therapies of testosterone, anabolic steroids or β_2-agonists to promote muscle growth exist there is no clinical evidence in the critically ill period. The anabolic steroid nandrolone decanoate has been given in a placebo-controlled trial, with and without nutrition supplements, to malnourished patients with chronic obstructive pulmonary disease (Schols et al 1995). By 8 weeks those patients given nutrition supplements and the anabolic steroid had improvements in fat free mass and respiratory muscle function. During the recovery phase, after the hypermetabolism due to severe burns has settled, giving oxandrolone has been shown to increase protein intake and improve the rate of restoration of the lost weight (Demling and DeSanti 1997).

The potential role of recombinant growth hormone (rhGH) as an anti-catabolic agent has received the greatest attention (Ross et al 1993). The role of these growth factors in catabolism has been reviewed in detail by Botfield et al (1997). During critical illness the basal levels of growth hormone (GH) are generally increased, but the pulsatility is lost (Ross et al 1991). Circulating IGF-1 and the IGF binding proteins (IGFBP)-3 decline with an increase in the protease directed at this protein (Timmins et al 1996). IGFBP-1 levels rise in the critically ill. The metabolic consequences are that the indirect anabolic actions of GH mediated by IGF-1 are reduced and the fall in circulating IGF-1 may promote catabolism, with the resultant release of metabolic fuels from peripheral muscle. This is consistent with the increased liver synthesis and hyperglycaemia. The raised basal GH promotes lipolysis and insulin antagonism.

Many studies have shown improved nitrogen retention in catabolic patients treated with supraphysiological doses of growth hormone. Among the problems limiting the use of GH as an anti-catabolic or anabolic treatment are the side-effects of carbohydrate intolerance and fluid retention. A resistance to its effect develops such that the more severely ill the patients are, the poorer the IGF-1 response is to the administration of GH. Giving GH in combination with IGF-1 avoids the hyperglycaemia and may have synergistic effects (Kupfer et al 1993). Studies of GH in the less severely ill have shown preservation of muscle strength (Jiang et al 1989) with GH and better healing of donor skin sites during recovery in children

with burn injury (Herndon et al 1990). An open non-randomized study of surgical ICU patients "failing" to wean from the ventilator at 18 days suggested a better survival than predicted (Knox et al 1996), although an improvement in respiratory function is suggested, this study lacks a proper control group for comparison. In contrast, in a randomised, controlled and blinded study giving GH to ICU patients requiring prolonged ventilation despite a significant increase in IGF-1 and a positive cumulative nitrogen balance, Pichard et al (1996) were unable to show any benefit in muscle function or ventilatory function. Multicentre European study of GH in ICU patients has had to be discontinued following interim analysis showing excess mortality in the treatment group (Takala et al 1999). It may well be that, early on in critical illness, the mobilization of important fuels for the immune system (such as glutamine from skeletal muscle) is important for survival, and GH administration has been shown to reduce the release of glutamine (Biolo et al 2000).

Muscle changes and glutamine

Following trauma or surgery there is a consistent and similar pattern of amino acid changes that occur in skeletal muscle that occurs promptly and takes many days to recover (Askanazi et al 1980). There is marked depletion of non-essential amino acids, notably glutamine (Gln), with an increase in the essential amino acids. The most marked rise is in the branch chain amino acids (precursors of glutamine): phenylalanine, tyrosine and methionine. The same pattern over time has been described in ICU patients (Gamrin et al 1997) with intramuscular glutamine reduced some 75% (Palmer et al 1996).

Glutamine accounts for nearly two thirds of the free intracellular amino acid pool; glutamine concentration is typically 0.6 mmol/l in plasma, but about 20 mmol/l in intracellular water in skeletal muscle. In stress it is released from skeletal muscle through activation of a special transport system-N (Rennie et al 1994) and acts as an inter-organ nitrogen and carbon transporter. It is an important energy source directly to many cells and indirectly as a player in glycogen metabolism (Nurjhan et al 1995). Recent work in exercise physiology suggests that protein and amino acid derived carbon is exported primarily in the form of glutamine and not as alanine. Alanine is the source of carbon that comes from blood glucose and muscle glycogen (Fig. 52.1; Wagenmakers 1998). This implies that

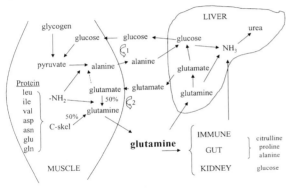

Figure 52.1—Interrelationship of skeletal muscle with glutamine, glucose and amino acid metabolism. In the glucose-alanine cycle (1) the carbon of alanine derives from glucose metabolism with the α-amino group coming from the major amino acids metabolized in muscle; this provides one non-toxic transport pathway for ammonia out of muscle during exercise. In contrast the amino-acid derived carbon is primarily exported from muscle in the form of glutamine. This implies that glutamine is quantitatively more important than alanine as a precursor for gluconeogenesis to provide additional glucose. Glutamine is the primary precursor for gluconeogenesis in the kidney. The immune and gastrointestinal systems utilize glutamine and produce a number of intermediate precursors that return to the liver along with ammonia. The glutamate–glutamine cycle (2) may account for as much as 50% of glutamine production and release, and it contributes to another pathway for ammonia transport from muscle (adapted from Wagenmakers 1998).

glutamine is quantitatively more important than alanine in gluconeogenesis from protein breakdown. Glutamine donates nitrogen for the synthesis of purines, pyrimidines, nucleotides and amino sugars. Glutamine is also an important substrate for the synthesis of glutathione, which is abundant in muscle and acts as an endogenous scavenger with the ability to counteract oxidative injury from oxygen free radicals. Depletion of tissue glutathione has also been shown in the critically ill muscle (Hammarqvist et al 1997), and it appears closely related to low glutamine levels. Important consumers of glutamine are the kidney, liver and small intestine, but it is the liver and immune system where glutamine plays a major role in protein synthesis and immune modulation (Wilmore and Shabert 1998). Since skeletal muscle provides the bulk of glutamine production, this suggests a link between muscle and the immune system (Newsholme and Calder 1997). Further evidence points to a regulatory role for glutamine in arginine–nitric oxide metabolism (Roth 1998) such that glutamine plays a more global regulatory role by modifying the endogenous inflammatory response and/or by upregulating anti-inflammatory factors (Wilmore 1997).

Provision of glutamine in nutrition

Conventional parenteral nutrition (PN) does not contain glutamine. Supplemental parenteral glutamine administration in the less severely ill, through a wealth of clinical studies, has shown benefits to intestinal integrity, immune function and can counteract the fall in muscle glutamine and protein synthesis following surgery. There are few studies in the critically ill. Fully replenishing the low plasma and intramuscular glutamine in the critically ill patient in the first 5 days of glutamine PN has proved difficult (Palmer et al 1996). If the endogenous glutamine supply from muscle is a limiting factor in the critically ill, the benefit of its exogenous replacement would be seen by the prevention of deaths late in the ICU stay. These deaths are often caused by second episodes of sepsis after the mortality risk of the initial illness has been overtaken by the risks of a sustained ICU stay. This hypothesis was examined using a prospective randomized, double-blind controlled study in 84 critically ill adult patients intolerant of enteral nutrition (Griffiths et al 1997), and reviewed by Wernerman (1998). Over three quarters of the patients had major sepsis, with intra-abdominal causes the most common. Survival at 6 months was significantly better with glutamine (57%) compared with controls (33%, $p = 0.049$). In those patients who were receiving parenteral nutrition for more than 10 days there was a significantly greater mortality in patients dependent on the control (glutamine deficient) formulation compared with those receiving a glutamine containing feed ($p = 0.03$). Differences in mortality increased with time on parenteral nutrition, and they were related only to the presence or absence of glutamine and not related to age, illness severity or total amount of nutrition received. A low body mass index is an independent predictor of excess mortality in multiple organ failure and this becomes evident at about 25 days into the illness (Galanos et al 1997). Similarly, the excess death in the control group occurred after 21 days, consistent with the time scales of the loss of lean body mass resulting from muscle wasting discussed earlier and this suggests that endogenous glutamine supply had become critical to survival.

Conclusion

The longer the ICU stay the more profound will be the muscle wasting, myopathy and polyneuropathy, and this will prolong convalescence (Leijten et al 1995). Only in the severest axonopathy, however, is prognosis guarded. Otherwise the outlook is more promising, based upon personal experience over the last 10 years of following the recovery of patients who have stayed a long time on ICU. It is reassuring that if the patient survives to leave hospital there is considerable return of nerve and muscle function, although it may take more than a year if the weakness was profound. The muscle wasting in the critically ill has many causes that are multi-factorial, which include inadequate nutrition, neuropathic and myopathic processes, problems secondary to sepsis and intense cytokine stimulation, neurohumoral disturbances and drug therapy, all combined with inactivity. That muscle serves an important physiological nutrient store should not be underestimated. From a clinical standpoint the critically ill patient must get better and move in order to restore lost muscle. Particularly with an increasing ageing population, the critically ill patient has an outcome clock ticking away that is related to their starting mass of muscle. The more you have, the greater the insult and the longer you can suffer before a critical protein reserve is reached. Measures such as nutrition support have so far done little to slow this process, but the addition of glutamine may ameliorate the consequences of a deficient supply from a declining muscle pool. As we start to understand the complex interactions in the severely ill patient, it is likely that combinations of treatments more carefully related to the phases of the illness will hold a better prospect of benefit.

References

Arnold J, Campbell IT, Samuels TA, et al. (1993) Increased whole body protein breakdown predominates over increased whole body protein synthesis in multiple organ failure. *Clin Sci* 84: 655–661.

Arora NS, Rochester DF. (1982) Respiratory muscle strength and maximum voluntary ventilation in undernourished patients. *Am Rev Resp Dis* 126: 5–8.

Askanazi J, Carpentier YA, Michelsen CB, et al. (1980) Muscle and plasma amino acids following injury; influence of intercurrent infection. *Ann Surg* 192: 78–85.

Biolo G, Iscra F, Bosutti A, et al. (2000) Growth hormone decreases muscle glutamine production and stimulates protein synthesis in hypercatabolic patients. *Am J Physiol Endocrinol Metab* 279: E323–E332.

Birkhahn RH, Long CL, Fitkin D, Geriger JW, Blakemore WS. (1980) Effects of major skeletal trauma on whole body tunrover in man measured by L-1, 14C-leucine. *Surgery* 88: 294–300.

Bishop JE, Butt RP, Low RB. (1995) The effect of mechanical forces on cell function:implications for pulmonary vascular remodelling due to hypertension. In: *Pulmonary Vascular remodelling*, Bishop J, Reeves J, Laurent G, eds. London: Portland Press, pp. 213–239.

Bolton CF, Gilbert JJ, Hahn AF, Sibbald WJ. (1984) Polyneuropathy in critically ill patients. *J Neurol Neurosurg Psychiatry* 47: 1223–1231.

Botfield C, Ross RJM, Hinds CJ. (1997) The role of IGFs in catabolism. *Bailliere's Clin Endocrinol Metab* 11: 679–697.

Bouletreau P, Patricot MC, Saudin F, Guiraud M, Mathian B. (1986) Effets des stimulations musculaires intermittentes sur le catabolisme musculaire des malades immobilises en reanimation. *Ann Fr Anesth Reanim* 54: 376–380.

Coakley JH, Nagendran K, Yarwood GD, Honavar M, Hinds CJ. (1998) Patterns of neurophysiological abnormality in prolonged critical illness. *Intensive Care Med* 24: 801–807.

Coronel B, Mercatella A, Couturier J-C, et al. (1990) Polyneuropathy: potential cause of difficult weaning. *Crit Care Med* 18: 486–489.

Crane CW, Picou D, Smith R, Waterlow JC. (1997) Protein turnover in patients before and after elective orthopaedic operations. *Br J Surgery* 64:129–133.

Cuthbertson DP. (1930) The disturbance of metabolism produced by bony and non-bony injury with notes on certain abnormal conditions of bone. *Biochem J* 24: 1244–1263.

Demling RH, DeSanti L. (1997) Oxandrolone, an anabolic steroid, significantly increases the rate of weight gain in the recovery phase after major burns. *J trauma-injury infection crit care* 43: 47–51.

Essen P, McNurlan MA, Gamrin L, et al. (1998) Tissue protein synthesis rates in critically ill patients. *Crit Care Med* 26: 92–100.

Essen P, McNurlan MA, Wernerman J, Milne E, Vinnars E, Garlick PJ. (1992) Short term starvation decreases skeletal muscle protein synthesis rate in man. *Clin Physiol* 12: 287–299.

Finn PJ, Plank LD, Clark MA, Connolly AB, Hill GL. (1996) Progressive cellular dehydration and proteolysis in critically ill patients. *Lancet* 347: 654–656.

Galanos AN, Pieper CF, Kussin PS, et al. For the SUPPORT investigators. (1997) Relationship of Body Mass Index to subsequent mortality among seriously ill hospitalised patients. *Crit Care Med* 25: 1962–1968.

Gamrin L, Andersson K, Hultman E, Nilsson E, Essen P, Wernerman J. (1997) Longitudinal changes of biochemical parameters in muscle during critical illness. *Metabolism* 46: 756–762.

Gibson JNA, Smith K, Rennie MJ. (1988) Prevention of

disuse atrophy by means of electrical stimulation: maintenance of protein synthesis. *Lancet* ii: 767–770.

Green CJ, Campbell IT, McClelland P, et al. (1995) Energy
and nitrogen balance and changes in midupper-arm circumference with multiple organ failure. *Nutrition* 11:
739–746.

Griffiths RD, Jones C, Palmer TEA. (1997) Six-month outcome of critically ill patients given glutamine supplemented parenteral nutrition. *Nutrition* 13: 295–302.

Griffiths RD, Palmer TEA, Helliwell T, Maclennan P,
Macmillan RR. (1995) Effect of passive stretching on the
wasting of muscle in the critically ill. *Nutrition* 11:
428–432.

Hammarqvist F, Luo JL, Cotgreave IA, Andersson K,
Wernerman J. (1997) Skeletal muscle glutathione is
depleted in critically ill patients. *Crit Care Med* 25: 78–84.

Hasselgren PO, Fisher JE. (1998) Sepsis: Stimulation of
energy-dependent protein breakdown resulting in protein
loss in skeletal muscle. *World J Surg* 22: 203–208.

Helliwell TR, Coakley JH, Wagenmakers AJM, et al.
(1991) Necrotizing myopathy in critically ill patients. *J
Pathol* 164: 307–314.

Helliwell TR, Wilkinson A, Griffiths RD, McClelland P,
Palmer TEA, Bone MJ. (1998a) Muscle fibre atrophy in
patients with multiple organ failure is associated with the
loss of myosin filaments and the presence of lysosomal
enzymes and ubiquitin. *Neuropathol Appl Neurobiol* 24:
507–517.

Helliwell TR, Wilkinson A, Griffiths RD, Palmer TEA,
McClelland P, Bone JM. (1998b) Microvascular endothelial activation in the skeletal muscles of patients with
multiple organ failure. *J Neurol Sci* 154: 26–34.

Herndon DN, Barrow RE, Kunkel KR, Broemeling L,
Rutan RL. (1990) Effect of recombinant human growth
hormone on donor-site healing in severely burned children. *Ann Surg* 212: 424–429.

Hikida RS, Gollnick PD, Dudley GA, Covertino VA,
Buchanan P. (1989) Structural and metabolic characteristics of human skeletal muscle following 30 days of
simulated microgravity. *Aviation Space Environ Med* 60:
664–670.

Hill AA, Plank LD, Finn PJ, et al. (1997) Massive Nitrogen
loss in critical surgical illness. Effect on cardiac mass and
function. *Ann Surg* 226: 191–197.

Ishibashi N, Plank LD, Sando K, Hill GL. (1998) Optimal
protein requirements during the first 2 weeks after the
onset of critical illness. *Crit Care Med* 26: 1529–1535.

Jiang ZM, He GZ, Zhang SY, et al. (1989) Low-dose growth
hormone and hypocaloric nutrition attenuate the protein-
catabolic response after major operation. *Ann Surg* 210:
513–525.

Knox JB, Wilmore DW, Demling RH, Sarraf P, Santos AA.
(1996) Use of growth hormone for postoperative respiratory failure. *Am J Surg* 171: 576–580.

Kupfer SR, Underwood LE, Baxter RC, Clemmons DR.
(1993) Enhancement of the anabolic effects of GH and
IGF-1 by use of both agents simultaneously. *J Clin Invest*
91: 391–396.

Lacomis D, Petrella JT, Guiliani MJ. (1998) Causes of neuromuscular weakness in the intensive care unit: a study of
ninety-two patients. *Muscle Nerve* 21: 610–617.

Latronico N, Fenzi F, Recupero D, et al. (1996) Critical
Illness myopathy and neuropathy. *Lancet* 347: 1579–1582.

Leijten FS, Harinck-de Weerd JE, Poortvliet DC, de Weerd
AW. (1995) The role of polyneuropathy in motor convalescence after prolonged mechanical ventilation. *JAMA*
274: 1221–1225.

McGill SN, Ahmed NA, Christou NV. (1998) Increased
plasma von Willebrand factor in the systemic inflammatory
response syndrome is derived from generalised endothelial cell activation. *Crit Care Med* 26: 296–300.

Millward DJ. (1995) A protein-stat mechanism for regulation of growth and maintenance of the lean body mass.
Nutr Res Rev 8: 93–120.

Mitch WE, Goldberg AL. (1996) Mechanisms of muscle
wasting: The role of the ubiquitin-proteasome pathway.
New Engl J Med 335: 1897–1905.

Mohr M, Englisch L, Roth A, Burchardi H, Zielmann S.
(1997) Effects of early treatment with immunoglobulin
on critical illness polyneuropathy following multiple
organ failure and gram-negative sepsis. *Intens Care Med*
23: 1144–1149.

Newsholme EA, Calder PC. (1997) The proposed role of
glutamine in some cells of the immune system and speculative consequences for the whole animal. *Nutrition* 13:
728–730.

Nurjhan N, Bucci A, Perriello G, et al. (1995) Glutamine: A
major gluconeogenic precursor and vehicle for interorgan
carbon transport in man. *J Clin Invest* 95: 272–277.

Palmer TEA, Griffiths RD, Jones C. (1996) Effect of
parenteral l-glutamine on muscle in the very severely ill.
Nutrition 125: 316–320.

Pichard C, Kyle U, Chevrolet JC, et al. (1996) Lack of
effects of recombinant growth hormone on muscle function in patients requiring prolonged mechanical ventilation: a prospective, randomized, controlled study. *Crit
Care Med* 24: 403–413.

Plank LD, Connolly AB, Hill GL. (1998) Sequential
changes in the metabolic response in severely septic
patients during the first 23 days after the onset of peritonitis. *Ann Surg* 228: 146–158.

Rennie MJ, Tadros L, Khogal S, Ahmed A, Taylor PM.

(1994) Glutamine transport and its metabolic effects. *J Nutr* 124: 1503S–1508S.

Ross RJ, Miell JP, Freeman E, et al. (1991) Critically ill patients have high basal GH levels with attenuated oscillatory activity associated with low levels of IGF-1. *Clin Endocrinol* 35: 47–54.

Ross RJM, Rodriguez-Arnao J, Bentham J, Coakley JH. (1993) The role of insulin, growth hormone and IGF-1 as anabolic agents in the critically ill. *Intens Care Med* 19: S54–S57.

Roth E. (1998) L-argine-nitric oxide metabolism. Glutamine: a new player in this metabolic game? *Clin Nutr* 17: 1–2.

Schols AM, Soeters PB, Mostert R, Pluymers RJ, Wouters EF. (1995) Physiologic effects of nutritional support and anabolic steroids in patients with chronic obstructive pulmonary disease. A placebo-controlled randomized trial. *Am J Respir Crit Care Med* 152: 1268–1274.

Streat SJ, Beddoe AH, Hill GL. (1987) Aggressive nutritional support does not prevent protein loss despite fat gain in septic intensive care patients. *J Trauma* 27: 262–266.

Takala J, Ruokonen E, Webster NR, Nielsen MS, Zandstra DF, Vundelinck G, Hinds CJ. (1999) Increased mortality associated with growth hormone treatment in critically ill patients. *N Engl J Med* 341: 785–792.

Timmins AC, Cotterill AM, Hughes SC, et al. (1996) Critical illness is associated with low levels of IGF-1 and -II, alterations in IGFBPs and induction of an IGFBP-3 protease. *Crit Care Med* 24: 1460–1466.

Todorov P, Cariuk P, McDevitt T, Coles B, Fearon K, Tisdale M. (1996) Characterisation of a cancer cachectic facture. *Nature* 379: 739–742.

Wagenmakers AJ. (1998) Muscle amino acid metabolism at rest and during exercise: role in human physiology and metabolism. *Exerc Sport Sci Rev* 26: 287–314.

Wernerman J, Hammarqvist F, Gamrin L, Essen P. (1996) Protein metabolism in critical illness. *Baillieres Clin Endocrinol Metab* 10: 603–615.

Wernerman J. (1998) Glutamine-containing TPN: a question of life and death for intensive care unit-patients? *Clin Nutr* 17: 3–6.

Wilmore DW (1997) Glutamine saves lives! What does it mean? *Nutrition* 13: 375–376.

Wilmore DW, Shabert JK. (1998) Role of glutamine in immunologic responses. *Nutrition* 14: 618–626.

Wing SS, Goldberg AL. (1993) Glucocorticoids activate the ATP-ubiquitin-dependent proteolytic system in skeletal muscle during fasting. *Am J Physiol* 264: E668–E676.

53

Immunomodulation in skeletal muscle disease

Kanneboyina Nagaraju

Introduction

A number of muscle diseases—such as polymyositis, dermatomyositis, inclusion body myositis, myasthenia gravis, Lambert–Eaton myasthenic syndrome, Guillain–Barre syndrome, acquired myotonia and amyotropic lateral sclerosis—have been recognized to have an autoimmune component in their aetiopathogenesis (Sinha et al 1991, Kawamata et al 1992, Link et al 1992, Hohlfeld and Engel 1994, Yi et al 1994, Drachman et al 1995, Hafer-Macko et al 1996, Dalmau et al 1999). In order to better understand the role of immune system and immunomodulation in muscle disease, it is helpful to review the principles of immune response. This chapter will provide an overview of the general cellular and cytokine networks during an immune inflammatory response and the possible communication networks between the immune system and muscle cells. On the basis of these premises, I will discuss the possible levels of immunomodulatory interventions directed against autoimmune cells and their activation receptors, along with common agents used to diminish inflammation in the target tissue.

Generally, when microorganisms invade the host, the pathogen is cleared through an orchestrated immune response. This involves coordination of multiple effector cells of the immune system and the resident target cells in the microenvironment. Many of the components involved in the cellular cooperation and communication are molecules that are expressed or produced by the cells, which bind to the receptors on other cells; some of these are membrane bound antigens and others are soluble secretory factors. These receptors facilitate signalling not only among cells of the immune system but also of the neuroendocrine system, and this, in turn, produces factors that can modulate immune, neural and endocrine responses. Understanding this cellular cross-talk is important in designing strategies for effective modulation of the immune response.

To elicit a productive immune response, a determined minimum set of stimuli is required. Interaction of lymphocytes with cells not expressing minimum set of co-stimulatory molecules (non-professional antigen-presenting cells (APC)) will result in an abortive immune response. Apart from cell–cell interactions, lymphocytes also communicate with a variety of receptors for soluble factors such as cytokines, chemokines, growth factors, prostaglandins, leukotrines, hormones and neurotransmitters. Thus, the outcome of an immune response is an extremely complex process involving both contact dependent and soluble factor-mediated signals.

Communication among immune cells through direct cell-cell contact

Generation of an effective immune response requires professional antigen presentation to T cells and cross-talk between T helper cells and B cells through various receptors. For example, T and B cells constantly receive signals via functionally distinct receptors including through the T cell receptors (TCR) and B cell receptors (BCR). Ligation of the antigen receptor can trigger the TCR or BCR complex to transduce an intracellular signalling cascade. The strength and the time course of these interactions determine the final lymphocyte response. At least in the case of TCR, it appears possible that the overall shape of the trimolecular complex (major histocompatibility complex (MHC)/peptide:TCR) not only determines the quantitative outcome of TCR triggering, but it can influence the qualitative outcome of a T cell response (anergy verses response). In addition to these, lymphocytes have several other invariant coreceptors that detect the presence of costimuli provided by antigen presenting cells. Some of the important receptors and ligands and their functions are listed in Table 53.1. Among the costimulatory receptors, CD28/CTLA-4 on T cells and CD40 on B cells have recently been recognized as key costimulatory receptors that act as checkpoints for the response to antigen receptor activation, often controlling the choices between cellular proliferation, tolerance induction or apoptosis (Fig. 53.1). Strategies have been developed to successfully target these and other molecules to abort an undesirable immune response in autoimmune diseases.

MHC/peptide: TCR and costimulatory interactions

Generally mononuclear phagocytes, Langerhans-dendritic cells and B cells act as APCs (Janeway et al 1987, Steinman RM 1991). Other cell types, such as skeletal muscle cells, can be made to function as facultative APCs under special conditions. Antigen presentation is an obligatory step in the recognition of protein antigens by the T cell lineage. The APCs bearing MHC class I and class II molecules bind peptides

Table 53.1 — Molecules involved in antigen presenting cell–T cell interaction

APC	T cell	Functions
MHC class I	TCR and CD8	T cell activation
MHC class II	TCR and CD4	T cell activation
CD80/CD86	CD28	Costimulation
CD80/CD86	CTLA-4	Inhibition
CD40	CD40L	B cell activation
LFA-3	CD2	Costimulation
LFA-1	CD54	Adhesion/costimulation
CD72	CD5	Adhesion
CD22	CD45	Adhesion
VCAM-I	VLA-4	Adhesion

APC, antigen presenting cell; LFA, leukocyte function associate antigen; MHC, major histocompatibility complex; TCR, T cell receptor; VCAM, vascular cell adhesion molecule 1; VLA, very late antigen.

APCs (Macrophage/Skeletal muscle/endothelial cells)

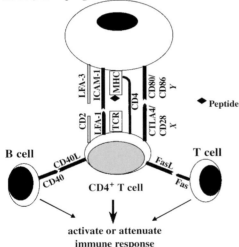

Figure 53.1 — Schematic diagram of cellular interactions of immune response. Antigen presenting cell (APC)–T cell interactions are initiated by the presentation of MHC/peptide complexes to the T cell receptor. Macrophage, B cells and under certain conditions non-lymphoid cells such as skeletal muscle cells and endothelial cells may act as APC. A variety of additional receptors expressed on APC (ICAM-1, LFA-3, CD80/CD86 and unknown receptor, Y), bind to the counter-receptor (LFA-1, CD2, CTLA-4/CD28 and unknown counter-receptor, X) on T cells. These interactions facilitate adhesion and costimulation. A lack of these additional receptors or inhibition of signalling through these receptors would appear to play a crucial role in tolerance induction. T cell-B cell interactions are facilitated by the engagement of CD40 on B cells with its ligand, CD40L on activated T cells results in B cell proliferation, immunoglobulin secretion and isotype switching in the presence of IL-4 and IL-5. The engagement of Fas by its receptor FasL results in the induction of apoptosis and downsizing the magnitude of immune response.

resulting from intracellular processing of proteins. The MHC peptide complexes constitute the antigenic determinants (i.e., the epitopes that engage the TCR). Class I molecules serve to select primarily, but not exclusively, peptides (8 or 9 amino acid residues in length) derived from cytoplasmic proteins, and the class II molecules select peptides (8–30 amino acid residues in length) from proteins found in the vesicular system (Rotzschke et al 1990, Chicz et al 1992). In this form, the lymphocytes recognize products from viruses and self-antigens by way of the MHC class I system and products of endocytosed and phagocytosed antigens by the class II MHC system.

The strength of interactions between MHC/peptide and TCR determine the responsiveness of T cells. But the mere engagement of T cell receptor with MHC/peptide in the absence of other costimulatory receptors can result in the development of clonal antigen-specific unresponsiveness or anergy (Schwartz 1996). The CD28 and CTLA-4 molecules on T cells and their counter-receptors, CD80 (B7.1) and CD86 (B7.2), on APCs constitute an important costimulatory pathway for immune response to antigens (Linsley and Ledbetter 1993). CD28 and CTLA-4 are positive and negative regulators of T cell activation, respectively, and CTLA-4 is critical for the induction of peripheral tolerance and deletion of autoreactive T cells (van Parijs et al 1998). Accordingly, CTLA-4 deficient mice develop severe lymphoproliferative disease that is characterized by multi-focal lymphocyte infiltrate and spontaneous proliferation of lymph node cells (Tivol et al 1995). Unlike CD28, CTLA-4 is expressed only transiently on the cell surface, immediately after T cell activation, implying that T cell activation is regulated by the net balance between on and off switches. The counter-receptors, CD80 and CD86, are members of immunoglobulin gene superfamily having V- and C-like extra cellular domains. These molecules share only 27% amino acid identity in their extracellular domains, which is surprising since both molecules bind the same CD28 and CTLA-4 receptors (Azuma et al 1993, Freeman et al 1993). Although both CD80 and CD86 have similar potencies in inducing T cell proliferative response, they show differences in expression patterns: CD86 is constitutively expressed on unstimulated dendritic cells and blood monocytes, whereas CD80 is generally absent in unstimulated cells. CTLA-4 has a greater than 400-fold higher avidity for the B7 receptors than CD28, but it is expressed at low levels on the cell surface. It is proposed that, following activation, the T cell expresses CTLA-4 and CD28 and, with moderate to high levels of B7, both are engaged, with the stimulatory CD28 response dominating. As B7 expression declines to low levels, all available B7 is engaged by higher avidity CTLA-4, and CTLA-4 signalling leads to downregulation of the T cell response (Linsley et al 1994).

Apart from these, several additional receptors and ligands are required to physically stabilize interactions between collaborating pairs of T cells–APCs, T cells–B cells, and to bring effector cells such as cytotoxic T cells and NK cells into close apposition with their target cells. Intercellular adhesion molecules ICAM-1 (CD54), ICAM-2 (CD102) and ICAM-3 (CD50) interact with their counter-receptors, the β_2-integrins, LFA-1 (CD11a and CD18), Mac-1 (CD11b/CD18), and p105/95 (CD11c/CD18). ICAMs are expressed on all leukocytes and a wide variety of non-haematopoietic cells, including endothelial and epithelial cells. The basal levels of ICAM expression are typically low, and they are highly inducible by proinflammatory cytokines such as interleukin-1 (IL-1), tumour necrosis factor-α (TNF-α) and interferon-γ (IFN-γ). ICAMs are shown to have costimulatory signalling properties, and this is consistent with their role as adhesion and accessory molecules. The counter-receptors, integrins, are metalloproteins requiring divalent cations Mg^{2+} and Ca^{2+} for activity. β_2-integrins are present in cytoplasmic granules and they are rapidly translocated to the membrane following exposure of myeloid cells to inflammatory stimuli such as cytokines and chemokines. The ICAM-1, -2 and -3 recognized by the β_2-integrin LFA-1 may serve as ligands in different situations. ICAM-3 is highly expressed by naïve T cells and on APCs; ICAM-2 is expressed on endothelial cells; and ICAM-1 is induced at high levels by inflammatory stimuli, and it provides the strongest interaction with LFA-1. In addition to promoting the intercellular collaborations, the binding of the ICAMs with the β_2-integrins also plays a key role in leukocyte transendothelial migration during normal circulation and trafficking and in the specialized localization of leukocytes in the vasculature and subsequent transendothelial migration into inflamed tissue.

Likewise, the involvement of CD2 in T lymphocyte adhesion and activation is well-documented (Holter et al 1996). CD2 is a glycoprotein expressed primarily on non-B cells in humans and on B cells and macrophages in rodents. CD2 binds to ubiquitously expressed cell surface glycoprotein CD58 (LFA-3), which is present on many human cell types including APCs and endothelial cells. Among the accessory T cell molecules examined so far, CD2 appears to be unique in its ability to participate in the reversal of anergy (Boussiotis et al 1994). In addition to providing accessory signals for T cell receptor-mediated activation of lymphocytes, CD2 has been shown to play a role in potentiating T cell responses to the cytokines IL-1, IL-6 and IL-12 and it is also involved in the regulation of T cell anergy.

Another major communication among immune cells is the interaction between T cells and B cells, and these interactions are dependent on CD40/CD40L receptors. CD40 antigen is a tumour necrosis factor receptor (TNF-R) family member expressed by multiple haematopoietic (B cells, plasma cells, monocytes and some T cells) and non-haematopoietic cells (endothelial cells, fibroblasts, and epithelial cells). The low constitutive expression of CD40 on monocytes can be unregulated by cytokines such as GM-CSF, IL-3 and IFN-γ. The CD40L is a member of the TNF family, and it is readily expressed on CD4$^+$ and CD8$^+$ T cells after activation through pathways that are inhibited by cyclosporin. Basophils, eosinophils and activated B cells have also been reported as expressing CD40L. CD40 ligation of monocytes and dendritic cells results in the secretion of multiple cytokines, including IL-1, IL-6, IL-8, IL-10, IL-12, TNF-α, and MIP-1α, which may act as autocrine and paracrine growth and differentiation factors (Banchereau et al 1994). The critical role of CD40 and CD40L interactions *in vivo* came from discovery that hyper IgM syndrome, an X-linked immunodeficiency, is due to genetic alteration of the CD40L. This disease is characterized by a severe impairment of T cell dependent antibody responses with no B cell memory, no circulating IgG, IgA and IgE, and no somatic hypermutation because of the lack of germinal centres within the secondary lymphoid organs (Kroczek et al 1994). The signalling pathways between CD40 and CD28 are interconnected, for example CD40 signalling induces B7 expression and CD28 signalling induces CD40L expression. The signal transduction through costimulatory receptors during the antigen-dependent activation promotes not only cell proliferation, but also cell survival (Boise et al 1995, Vella et al 1997). Thus, B7/CD28 and CD40/CD40L pathways cross-talk to reinforce an effective immune activation.

Generally, uncontrolled immune activation leads to autoimmunity. Therefore, it is essential for the immune system to downsize its population of activated cells through Fas and FasL interactions; the clonal amplification of activated cells is partly regulated by Fas and FasL interactions. Fas is a TNF-R family member expressed by a wide variety of cells including T cells, B cells, NK cells, neutrophils and thyrocytes. Fas expression can be upregulated by IFN-γ or in combination with TNF-α. The Fas ligand is a member of TNF ligand family. Like the other members of the family, membrane FasL is cleaved by metalloprotease into a soluble form that is biologically active, and this can mediate its effects both locally and systemically. Although Fas is expressed by many tissues and cell types, the expression of FasL is relatively restricted. CD8[+], CD4[+] T cells, NK cells and LAK cells express functional FasL and are capable of inducing apoptosis in Fas-expressing target cells. There is a clear evidence that Fas plays a role in the inactivation and removal of self-reactive T cells in the periphery that have escaped thymic deletion. These peripheral self-reactive cells are thought to die through the process of activation-induced cell death, whereby previously activated T cells that are stimulated through the TCR undergo apoptosis (Ju et al 1995). It was also shown that Fas/FasL interactions are responsible for the maintenance of immune-privileged sites such as sertoli cells in testis and cornea, and retinal pigment epithelium in the eye (Green and Ware 1997). Natural mutations in Fas and FasL genes result in the development of progressive lymphoadenopathy and splenomegaly. Thus, the cognate interactions between Fas/FasL are involved in peripheral deletion of autoreactive lymphocytes and limiting the magnitude of an immune response by clonal downsizing (Lynch et al 1995). Several agents that interfere with the interactions between immune receptors were successfully used to modulate the long-term outcome of autoimmunity and transplantation tolerance in experimental models of human disease.

The cellular communications during the immune response are much more complicated than the above simple descriptions. The intent here is to highlight important molecules that are critical for eliciting an effective immune response. However, there are many other known and unknown molecules that have a role in modifying signals in immune cells, such as the CD19/CD20 complex, CD22 and CD45, which have been shown to regulate signals through BCR.

Communications between immune cells and muscle cells through direct cell–cell contact

To effectively intervene at any of the stages in skeletal muscle inflammation, one needs to examine the existence of such cell–cell interactions in inflammatory myopathies. Indeed, infiltration of skeletal muscle by inflammatory cells has been reported in a number of chronic pathologic conditions including autoimmune inflammatory myopathies, muscular dystrophies, post-poliomyelitis progressive muscular atrophy and Graves' disease. The cells are usually activated T cells, B cells, macrophages and occasionally NK cells (Behan et al 1987, Arahata and Engel 1988, Karpati et al 1988, Zuk and Fletcher 1988, Emslie-Smith et al 1989). To elicit an immune inflammation, these cells communicate either through direct cell–cell contact or through cytokine networks at the inflammatory site. The principal players in this process are lymphocytes, macrophages, endothelial cells and skeletal muscle cells. Skeletal muscle cells are both targets and effectors of immune inflammation. Normal human skeletal myoblasts constitutively express low levels of class I MHC antigens. Proinflammatory cytokines (IL-1α, IL-1β, TNF-α and IFN-γ and C-C chemokine MIP-1α upregulate class I MHC expression on myoblasts and myotubes. In the absence of added proinflammatory cytokines, class II MHC and ICAM-1 expression was not detected, IFN-γ induced high levels of class II expression and other cytokines induced low levels of class II MHC expression (De Bleecker and Engel 1994, Hohlfeld and Engel 1994, Nagaraju et al 1998). Costimulatory molecules of the B7 family, BB-1, were shown to be expressed on IFN-γ stimulated myoblasts and in polymyositis (PM) and sporadic IBM patients biopsies, whereas CD86 (B7-2) was seen occasionally on regenerating/degenerating muscle fibres in some dermatomyositis (DM) biopsy specimens (Behrens et al 1998, Murata Ky and Dalakas 1999, Nagaraju et al 1999). These observations and the evidence that IFN-γ stimulated myoblasts are fully capable of presenting T cell dependent antigens to CD4[+] T cell lines suggest that muscle cells under proinflammatory conditions may act as facultative APCs (Goebels et al 1992). Recent studies demonstrate that the infiltrating immune cells in the biopsies of inflammatory myopathies also show the presence of costimulatory molecules, such as CTLA-4, CD28 and CD40, suggesting that the muscle cells are actively engaged in the initiation and perpetuation of immune inflammation in myositis (Behrens et al 1998, Murata Ky and Dalakas 1999, Nagaraju et al 1999). Under certain conditions, exogenous antigens can be presented in the context of MHC class I (Bohm et al 1995, Schirmbeck et al 1995). Consequently, presentation may occur by protein transfer from transfected muscle cells to a professional APC. Although professional APCs are required for the generation of an antigen-specific immune response, cells not normally capable of antigen presentation may acquire MHC class I and class II and ICAM-1 along with costimulatory molecules after induction by inflammatory cytokines such as IFN-γ (Tews and Goebel 1995). Thus, facultative APC-like activated muscle cells may be responsible for increasing immune-mediated inflammation.

Within muscle tissue, professional APCs are sparse; they are recruited to the muscle usually in response to injury (Austyn et al 1994, Pardoll and Beckerleg 1995). It is possible that during an inflammatory response, activated endothelial cells also may act as facultative APCs (Cunningham et al 1997). The potential of activated endothelial cells to act as APCs is not surprising, since the pattern of various antigens expressed on activated endothelial cells is reminiscent of mononuclear phagocytes. There is also evidence that MHC and costimulatory molecules are also present on the endothelial cells of the blood vessels and capillaries in myositis biopsies, indicating their role either directly or indirectly in the process of antigen processing and presentation during muscle inflammation (Higuchi et al 1991, Pedrol et al 1995). Numerous experimental systems have shown that presentation of antigens by non-professional APCs, which lack appropriate costimulatory molecules, is more likely to tolerize than stimulate T cells, but in certain situations the non-professional APCs, such as transfected fibroblasts, are able to induce a MHC class I and MHC class II restricted lymphoproliferative response (Smythe et al 1999). This implies that the antigen presentation and costimulation do not need to be provided by the same cell as long as it is done in an appropriate local environment. Thus it is possible that cytotoxic T cells could receive the first signal from the peptide/MHC class I complex expressed by endothelial cells or muscle cells and the second signal from haematopoietic antigen presenting cells recruited during the inflammatory process in myositis. Several studies conducted on the biopsies of patients with inflammatory myopathies showed that the cells and surface molecules needed for transducing signal one (MHC/Peptide:TCR) and signal two (CD80/CD86:CD28/CTAL4) are abundant and they may be responsible for auto-amplification of the inflammatory response in skeletal muscle. The infiltrating mononuclear cells express MHC class I (HLA A, B, and C), MHC class II (HLA DP, DQ, and DR), ICAM-1, B7.1 and B7.2 antigens, suggesting the presence of professional APCs in myositis (Higuchi et al 1991, Bernasconi et al 1998, Nagaraju et al 1999).

Probably the magnitude of the immune response in muscle inflammation is controlled by the expression of molecules like Fas. Several studies showed that the muscle fibres of myositis patients, but not the controls, express increased levels of Fas receptor (Behrens et al 1997, Inukai et al 1997, Olive et al 1997). Varying proportions of infiltrating lymphocytes showed both Fas and FasL expression. These observations suggest that there are potential interactions through Fas and FasL between and among muscle cells and lymphocytes, which could lead to Fas and FasL induced cell death in muscle cells and lymphocytes, reversing signalling through FasL, leading to maximal activation and proliferation of CD8[+] lymphocytes (Suzuki and Fink 1998) in the inflammatory milieu, and the induction of fibrosis in the inflamed muscle as has been shown in pulmonary fibrosis model (Kuwano et al 1999). In theory, FasL expressed on lymphocytes could engage abundantly expressed Fas receptor on the muscle fibres and induce apoptosis of muscle fibres. In myositis, where apoptosis is absent, signalling through Fas receptor may contribute to the control of the amplification of autoreactive T cells, and thus regulate the magnitude of the immune response.

Communication through cytokines secreted by the cells in the inflammatory milieu

Cytokines are low molecular weight protein mediators involved in cell growth, inflammation, immunity, differentiation and tissue repair. A majority of cytokines mediate their effects locally. Some cytokines such as IL-6 and IL-1 do have systemic effects, but the major physiological role of cytokines is over a short range—within a few cell diameters. In an immune inflammation, many lymphocytes (Th1 and Th2), monocyte/macrophage lineage, and other non-immune cells (fibroblasts, skeletal muscle cells and nerve cells) outside the immune system also produce wide variety of cytokines. Cytokines are typically pleiotropic, meaning that they have multiple effects on different cells. Cytokines mediate their effects after binding to high affinity receptors on the surface of the target cells, and they are subject to a variable degree of upregulation upon cell activation. Since cytokines have potent effects, it is clearly important that their action be limited to avoid pathogenic effects. For this purpose, many cytokines have receptors that have natural antagonists (e.g., interleukin-1 receptor agonist; IL-1Ra) and circulating inhibitors (Hannum et al 1990, Symons et al 1995). Cytokines form extremely complex communication networks; they have multiple physiological roles during normal as well as inflammatory situations, but overlapping sets of functions on cells present in the inflammatory milieu. For example, vascular cells and skeletal muscle are both a source and a target for cytokines. These soluble polypeptide mediators serve to communicate with leukocytes, as well as other target tissues or organs in the inflammatory milieu (Arai et al 1990; Fig. 53.2). Many cytokines are produced locally in the inflamed organ and affect a wide variety of cells and their functions. These may be broadly classified into the following groups:

- proinflammatory cytokines
- immunoregulatory cytokines
- anti–inflammatory cytokines and inhibitors
- chemokines.

Proinflammatory cytokines

Interleukin-1 family

The IL-1 family consists of IL-1α, IL-1β and IL-1Ra. These polypeptides are structurally related, with IL-1α and IL-1β having agonist, and IL-1Ra antagonist, properties. IL-1 is produced by numerous cells, including macrophages, monocytes, neutrophils, lymphocytes, endothelial cells, synovial lining cells, fibroblasts, astrocytes, microglia and dendritic cells (Dinarello 1991). IL-1 mediates its biological activity mainly through Type I receptors, which are expressed on the majority of the cells, including T cells, fibroblasts and endothelial cells. The Type II receptor found on neutrophils, monocytes, B cells and bone marrow

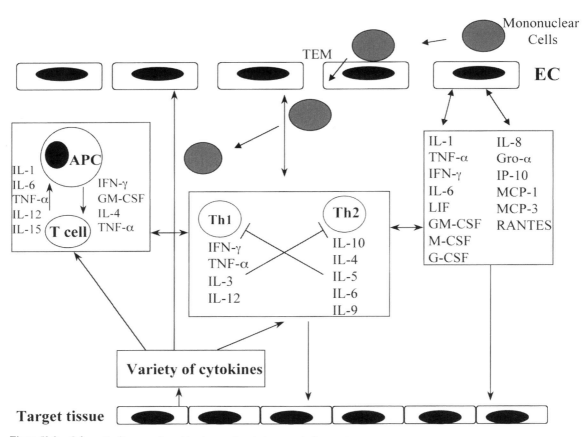

Figure 53.2 — Schematic diagram of cytokine interactions in immune inflammation. During the inflammatory process the immune cells migrate to the site of inflammation and secrete various cytokines and chemokines. These, in turn stimulate various immune cells, target tissue cells, e.g., skeletal muscle cells and endothelial cells to synthesize a variety of cytokines and chemokines. The balance between the pro and anti–inflammatory cytokines partly determine the course of immune activation particularly, APC–T cell interactions, Th1/Th2 cytokine predominance and finally the progression of inflammatory process. APC: antigen presenting cells; TEM: transendothelial migration; EC: endothelial cells.

progenitor cells acts as a decoy receptor since it has no signal transduction function (Colotta et al 1994). IL-1β stimulates non-specific host defences to infection by stimulating the recruitment and the release of neutrophils and macrophages from the bone marrow and also stimulating the natural killer cells. It also causes B cell proliferation, increases antibody production, promotes leukocyte migration to sites of inflammation and increases adhesion by up-regulating the synthesis of leukocyte adhesion molecules. The activated T cells, B cells, macrophages, and NK cells (Engel and Arahata 1986, Karpati et al 1988, Emslie-Smith et al 1989) are capable of secreting a variety of cytokines, and, in fact, various cytokines and chemokines have been found in muscle biopsies of inflammatory myopathies by a variety of techniques (Lundberg et al 1995, Tews and Goebel 1996, Adams et al 1997). The source and the effects of these local cytokines, however, are not known. Muscle biopsies from patients with inflammatory myopathies show expression of IL-1α and IL-1β on the mononuclear inflammatory cells and on endothelial cells (Lundberg et al 1995, 1997) as well as on muscle fibres (Tews and Goebel 1996). IL-1α in particular was detected both on the endothelial cells of the endomysial capillaries and in perifasicular arterioles and venules, as well as in mononuclear infiltrates (Lundberg et al 1997). The IL-1β mRNA expression in cultured skeletal muscle cells could be induced by combination of proinflammatory cytokines (Nagaraju et al 1998).

Tumour necrosis factor

TNF is produced by numerous cells, including monocytes, tissues macrophages, lymphocytes, neutrophils and endothelial cells as a 26 kDa procytokine of 233 amino acid residues. The biological effects result from free TNF binding to specific receptors that occur on almost all cells. Two distinct membrane associated receptors, termed TNF-R1 (55 kDa) and TNF-R2 (75 kDa) have been recognized (Tartaglia and Goeddel 1992). Stimulation of TNF-R1 results in cytotoxicity, expression of adhesion molecules on endothelial cells and keratinocytes and activation of sphingomyelinase with formation of ceramide and activation of NF-kB. Stimulation of TNF-R2 results in a proliferative response in mouse thymocytes, cytotoxic T cells fibroblasts and natural killer (NK) cells. These receptors also interact with other TNF-related cytokines to produce distinctive cellular responses that usually overlap one another, resulting in an extremely complex system. Like IL-1, TNF also influences a number of leukocyte functions and promotes leukocyte con-

gregation, adherence, migration through endothelial surfaces and chemotaxis to the site of inflammation (Gamble et al 1985, Moser et al 1989, van der Poll et al 1992). IL-1 reproduces many effects of TNF alone and strongly potentiates the effects of TNF when given in combination (Espevik and Waage 1988). TNF-α was detected in the muscle biopsies of myositis and Duchenne muscular dystrophy patients. Expression has been shown both on the infiltrating mononuclear cells and on the muscle fibres (Tews and Goebel 1996, Adams et al 1997, Lundberg et al 1997). The TNF-R2 receptor was found to be expressed strongly on endothelial cells in the midst of inflammatory infiltrates in PM, DM, and IBM patients whereas TNF-R1 was strongly expressed on the myonuclei of regenerating muscle fibres (De Bleecker et al 1999). Cultured skeletal muscle cells do not constitutively express TNF-α; its mRNA expression was readily induced by many proinflammatory cytokines (Nagaraju et al 1998).

Other interleukins

IL-6 is a pleiotropic cytokine involved in a wide variety of functions including a major role in inflammation. IL-6 is produced by several immune cells, fibroblasts, epithelial cells, endometrial cells and various tumour cells. IL-6 binds to IL-6 receptor and triggers signal transduction by activating the gp130 protein. The gp130 protein also serves as a signal transducer for leukaemia inhibitory factor, oncostatin M and ciliary neurotrophic factor showing many overlapping shared functions for these cytokines (Kishimoto et al 1992). Dysregulated production of IL-6 has been associated with chronic inflammatory conditions like rheumatoid arthritis and cancer. IL-6 expression was detected in the muscle biopsies of myositis and Duchenne muscular dystrophy patients (Tews and Goebel 1996, Adams et al 1997, Lundberg et al 1997). Cultured skeletal muscle cells express low levels of IL-6 constitutively and proinflammatory cytokines (IL-1α, IL-1β, TNF-α, and IFN-γ) induce IL-6 expression in a dose and time dependent manner (Bartoccioni et al 1994, Nagaraju et al 1998).

IL-12 was originally found through its costimulatory activity on NK and T cells. IL-12 protein is composed of two polypeptide chains (IL-12p40 and IL-12p35) linked by one disulphide bridge. Macrophage and dendritic cell lineage cells are the major producers of this protein. The regulation of IL-12 synthesis is complex because it is controlled by two independent genes, which have to be coexpressed in the same cell. The major cell types that respond to

IL-12 are NK cells and T cells (CD4[+], CD8[+] and γ/δT cells). The responsiveness of IL-12 is in part controlled by IL-12R expressed on activated lymphocytes. IL-12 is important for stimulation of innate immunity and the development of the protective Th1 type of immune response (Trinchieri and Scott 1999). Cultured skeletal muscle cells do not express IL-12 constitutively or in response to proinflammatory cytokines (Nagaraju et al 1998).

IL-16 is a proinflammatory cytokine implicated in the pathogenesis of asthma and other conditions characterized by recruitment of CD4[+] T cells to sites of the disease. IL-16 is a natural ligand for CD4 receptor, and it is known to modulate the APC and T lymphocyte functions (Hermann et al 1999). It was also shown that it is a chemoattractant for CD4[+] T cells and inhibits mixed lymphocyte reaction (Cruikshank et al 1998).

Likewise, IL-17 is a newly recognized member of the proinflammatory cytokines produced by CD4[+] activated memory cells (CD45[+]RO) T cells. It was also suggested that IL-17 might be a soluble factor by which T cells induce or contribute to the inflammation. In fact this cytokine has been shown to be spontaneously secreted by rheumatoid synovial cultures. IL-17 has been shown to interact with other cytokines within the inflammatory site, for example, it potentiates the effect of IL-1 on IL-6 and LIF production by synoviocytes. Moreover, IL-1 and IL-17 have been demonstrated to upregulate IL-6 production in a synergistic manner. The effects of IL-17 are inhibited by the Th2 cytokine, IL-4 (Chabaud et al 1999, Kotake et al 1999). The presence of these new members of proinflammatory cytokines (IL-16 and IL-17) in muscle disease remains to be seen.

Immunoregulatory cytokines

Interleukin-2

IL-2 is a growth factor for T cells and NK cells, where it induces G1–S phase progression, and a differentiation factor for B cells, where it induces immunoglobulin secretion. The high affinity IL-2 receptor is found on activated lymphocytes and consists of a α:β:γc trimeric complex. As this receptor complex generates a proliferative response at low concentrations of IL-2, it is thought to represent the physiologically relevant IL-2R for in vivo responses. IL-2 is required to maintain the growth and viability of T cells in vitro, and it may be required to limit the magnitude of immune response and prevent the development of certain forms of autoimmunity in vivo (Theze et al 1996). The expression of IL-2 along with IL-1α, IL-1β was

reported in several muscle diseases (Isenberg et al 1986, Tews and Goebel 1996, Adams et al 1997).

Interferon-gamma (IFN-γ) is an important immunoregulatory cytokine produced mainly by lymphoid cells (NK, T and B cells) upon activation. All the biological actions of IFN-γ require binding of IFN-γ specific cell surface receptors, expressed on virtually all types of cells. It plays a major role in the activation of monocytes or macrophages, and it enhances antigen presentation by upregulating MHC and costimulatory molecules. IFN-γ is a hallmark of the Th1 response. IFN-γ alone or in combination with TNF-α induces chemokine secretion by endothelial cells and monocytes. It is also involved in the regulation of apoptosis in lymphoid cells (Boehm et al 1997). IFN-γ is not a prominent cytokine present in the biopsies of inflammatory myositis (Lundberg et al 1995).

Interleukin-15

IL-15 is a recently discovered T cell growth factor, which interacts with the subunits of IL-2 (Grabstein et al 1994). By virtue of its tertiary structure, IL-15 belongs to the helix bundle peptide family of cytokines and growth factors. Members of these bioactive peptides are not homologous by sequence, but they bind to the receptors with similar structures and include growth hormone and proliferin (Horseman and Yu-Lee 1994). Recently a possible role for IL-15 in the pathogenesis of rheumatoid arthritis (RA) has been suggested; IL-15 is present in the synovial fluids of RA patients, where it might contribute to the recruitment of T cells (McInnes and Liew 1998). Northern blot analysis of an array of human tissues and cells indicated that the IL-15 is highly expressed in skeletal muscle tissue compared with most other tissues (Grabstein et al 1994). The mRNA for IL-15 is found both in normal as well as myositis biopsy specimens. It was further suggested that IL-15 might have similar functions to IL-2 as it shares the IL-2 receptor (Adams et al 1997).

Anti-inflammatory cytokines and inhibitors

Interleukin-4

IL-4 is a pleiotropic cytokine produced by several subsets of activated lymphoid cells; Th2 cells are an important source of this cytokine as they are critical for initiating humoral immunity against extracellular pathogens. IL-4 receptor complexes exist in two forms: type 1 receptors consist of IL-4α and the γc, and type II receptors consists of IL-4α and the low affinity IL-13Rα. In addition to regulating B cell growth and immunoglobulin secretion, IL-4 also affects T cells. In vitro, IL-4 promotes T cell growth, and it can potentially induce cytolytic T cell activities. IL-4 and IL-12 exert antagonizing effects on T cell differentiation (Keegan et al 1994). IL-4 expression was detected in the muscle biopsies of myositis and Duchenne muscular dystrophy patients (Lundberg et al 1995, Tews and Goebel 1996).

Interleukin-10

IL-10, also known as cytokine synthesis inhibitory factor, is produced by a wide variety of immune cells including activated T cells, monocytes, B cells as well as non-haematopoietic sources, such as keratinocytes and melanoma cells (Moore et al 1993). In humans, Th2 cells are the major source of this cytokine. The IL-10 receptor is mainly found on haematopoietic cells. Like most other cytokines, IL-10 exerts multiple effects upon the function of various cell lineages, including lymphocytes, monocytes, NK cells and dendritic cells. IL-10 specifically inhibits Th1 cell cytokine synthesis, particularly when macrophages are used as APCs. IL-10 has been demonstrated to have inhibitory effects on the proliferation, survival and cytokine production of human T cells. It has been shown to effectively inhibit the synthesis and gene expression of IL-1, TNF-α, IL-6, IL-8 and colony stimulating factors (Vieira et al 1991). The peripheral blood mononuclear cells of myositis patients showed an increase in IL-10 expression, whereas its presence in the biopsies of myositis patients was sparse (Adams et al 1997).

Transforming growth factor-beta

Transforming growth factor-β (TGF-β) is produced by a multitude of cells including T and B cells and macrophages. The pleiotropic effect of TGF-β induced strong growth enhancing as well as growth inhibiting properties depending on the type of the cell and the presence of other growth factors. Mice deficient for TGF-β develop multifocal inflammation and autoimmunity. It completely suppresses the proliferative response of the CD4+ or CD8+ T cells to IL-2 and blocks the generation of cytotoxic T cells, thus down-regulating cell-mediated and humoral immunity through the inhibition of IFN-γ expression. TGF-β1 is elevated in the skeletal muscle of Duchenne muscular dystrophy patients and to a lesser extent in Becker muscular dystrophy, leading to the suggestion that the fibrosis in the Duchenne muscular dystrophy may be regulated by the TGF-β1 (Yamazaki et al 1994,

Bernasconi et al 1995). TGF-β is prominently expressed in the blood vessels, mononuclear infiltrates and interstitial tissues of myositis biopsies; there is no difference in the expression pattern of TGF-β1, TGF-β2, and TGF-β3 among DM, PM and IBM patients (Lundberg et al 1995, Confalonieri et al 1997).

Chemokines

Chemokines are small, soluble, structurally-related cytokines that mediate rapid triggering of integrin-mediated adhesion and selectively induce the directional migration of various leukocyte subsets both in vivo and in vitro. These molecules play a critical role in haematopoiesis, angiogenesis and cellular activation, as well as in a variety of acute and chronic inflammatory disease states (Schwarz and Wells, 1999). Chemokines are divided into α and β subfamilies; typically α-chemokines (IL-8, IP-10, Gro-α) induce neutrophil, but not monocyte migration, while β-chemokines (MIP-1α, MIP-1β, MCP-1, MCP-2, MCP-3, and RANTES) predominantly act on monocytes and macrophages with no activity on neutrophils. Chemokine receptors are members of the rhodopsin receptor superfamily, and they are expressed on a wide variety of cells. Both the groups also activate a wide range of other cells such as keratinocytes, endothelium, smooth muscle cells and fibroblasts. Many of their biological properties contribute not only to their immunological role in inflammation but also to their physiological roles in tissue repair and cell growth/differentiation (Taub and Oppenheim 1994). A predominance of β-chemokines in inflammatory myopathies was reported (Adams et al 1997, Liprandi et al 1999). MIP-1α and MIP-1β were detected in a majority of the myositis biopsies, whereas RANTES was detected less frequently. MCP-1 was also shown to be expressed by macrophages, lymphocytes, and endothelial cells of myositis biopsies (Liprandi et al 1999).

We investigated the capabilities of human skeletal muscle cells to express cytokines under stimulated and unstimulated conditions in culture. We found that normal unstimulated human muscle cells in vitro constitutively express IL-6 and TGF-β, suggesting that these cytokines have a role in muscle homeostasis. Indeed, IL-6 and TGF-β have been shown to induce neuronal differentiation and to inhibit myogenesis (Florini et al 1986). The proinflammatory cytokines increased secretion of both IL-6, which may help differentiation of B cells and activation of T cells in the inflammatory milieu (Randall et al 1993) and TGF-β, which has the opposite effect. The increased TGF-β levels may promote fibrosis by stimulating the synthesis of extracellular matrix (Engel et al 1994). In addition to IL-6 and TGF-β, cultured human myoblasts and myotubes secreted GM-CSF under inflammatory conditions (Nagaraju et al 1998).

The synthesis of mRNAs for IFN-α, TNF-α, MIP-1α, and IL-1β was also detected, but the meaning of this finding is unclear since secreted proteins were not detected. They may be translated while remaining cell-bound, or they may be secreted below the level of detection. Under no test conditions did we detect any IL-1α, IL-4, IL-10, IL-12 and IFN-γ synthesis by human skeletal myoblasts (Nagaraju et al 1998).

There is limited data regarding the actual detection of cytokine proteins secreted by muscle cells. One report showed constitutive and TNF-α and/or IFN-γ induced expression of IL-6 by human myoblasts (Bartoccioni et al 1994). In our study, we also detected the presence of TGF-β and GM-CSF proteins in culture supernatants (Nagaraju et al 1998). The cytokine proteins for IFN-α, TNF-α and MIP-1α were not detected by enzyme-linked immunosorbant assay (ELISA) even after ten-fold concentration of culture supernatants (Nagaraju et al 1998).

As explained earlier in this chapter, the T cells that receive co-stimulatory signals produce cytokines, thus permitting the proliferation of an expanded population of cells capable of mediating a sustained immune response. Muscle cells actively participate in this process, and they have the inherent ability to express and respond to a variety of cytokines and chemokines depending on the inflammatory stimuli. Moreover, the apparently important upregulation of MHC class I, class II, costimulatory molecule BB-1 and ICAM-1 in inflamed muscle may be influenced by the secreted products of the stimulation. Such interactions may be responsible for the perpetuation of autoimmune inflammatory myopathies and contribute to the rejection of transplanted myoblasts. Designing interventions directed against these processes may help to effectively treat inflammatory muscle diseases. Some of the immunomodulatory interventions commonly used to block the above-described interactions are discussed in the next section.

Immunomodulatory interventions

The complex pathways, with numerous receptors, ligands and their signals, would appear to be an ideal target to be modified by pharmacological manipulation, provided that the correct balance can be achieved. These pathways have become a major area of research in many immunologically mediated diseases, and, currently, many therapeutic agents acting at all levels of the inflammatory response are being developed. A number of muscle diseases have been recognized to have an autoimmune component in their aetiopathogenesis, a clear knowledge regarding the immunopathogenetic mechanisms of these muscle diseases is still lacking. Therefore, currently, most therapies used in autoimmune disorders are nonspecific immune interventions aimed at suppressing the activated immune system. In this section, I will overview some of the current and potential immunotherapies useful for treating muscle diseases as follows:

1. conventional immunosuppressive chemicals

2. immunotherapies directed against APC–T cell interactions

3. conventional and non-conventional immunological agents, such as antibodies, cytokines, cytokine inhibitors and soluble receptors used in various animal models of human autoimmune diseases.

Few immunotherapeutic interventions have been tried in inflammatory myopathies because of the lack of experimental models for these diseases and also the lack of clear understanding of the immunopathogenetic events, the nature and type of relevant immune cells and their receptors. Therefore, the descriptions in the second part of this section are some of the novel therapeutic experimental approaches that might be useful once the cell types, receptors and peptides involved in the myositis are better known.

Non-selective immunosuppressive agents

The use of non-selective immunosuppressive agents forms the mainstay of conventional treatment of chronic immune-inflammatory diseases. The basis for this mode of therapy is to repress the formation of precursor cells, destroy or blockade immunocompetent cells, and suppress proliferation and differentiation of lymphocytes and monocytes by inhibiting the of biosynthesis of nucleic acids and proteins during immune response. However, the use of non-specific drugs, that is, drugs whose action is not limited to immunocompetent cells, remains hazardous. This is because they act by indiscriminately blocking or damaging all cells that happened to be in mitosis, in particular normally functioning cells that are important to the survival of the host. Therefore, the next stage of the development of lymphocytotoxic drugs or methods focused on the elimination of the immuno-competent cells, mainly lymphocytes. Corticosteroids fall into this group, and they have potent lympho-cytolytic activity, particularly with respect to T lympho-cytes. Corticosteroids not only intervene at many points of the immune response, such as preventing lymphocyte recirculation and generation of antibody producing and cytotoxic effector cells, but they also posses a remarkable anti-inflammatory potency by in-hibiting neutrophil adherence to vascular endothelium. High-dose steroids are immunosuppressive, and they are used to induce remission in myositis. Low doses are used for maintenance therapy, often in combina-tion with other immunosuppressive drugs. Combina-tions of different agents is intended to produce maximal suppression while keeping the side-effects as few as possible (Villalba et al 1995). Corticosteroids have several side-effects affecting the gastrointestinal, musculoskeletal, cutaneous and central nervous sys-tem; these are dose and duration dependent.

More recent therapies are directed to defined sub-populations of immunocompetent cells. Cyclosporin, FK506, and rapamycin are the major drugs in this group. These agents have more selective action than other immunosuppressive drugs. They act by inhibit-ing the activation of T cells and the secretion of cytokines. The overall effect is to prevent the prolifer-ation and differentiation of activated T cells and B cells. Drugs such as cyclosporin have major adverse effects such as nephrotoxicity and hypertension. Cyclosporin and FK506 has been used in myositis (Griggs 1994, Oddis et al 1999), and myasthenia gravis (Tindall et al 1993). Other immunosuppressive agents such as azathioprine, cyclophosphamide, chlorambucil and methotrexate are used with varying degrees of success in myasthenia gravis and inflammatory myo-pathies (Drachman 1996, Mastaglia et al 1997, Villalba et al 1998). Apart from these several newer anti-inflammatory agents (e.g. selective inhibitors of cyclo-oxygenase-2, inhibitors of matrix metalloproteinases and antagonists of leukotrienes) with diverse actions are being tested for their efficacy in various animal models of human autoimmune diseases. Several com-monly used immunosuppressents and their mecha-nisms of action are listed in Table 53.2.

Immunotherapies directed against APC–T cell interactions

Since the majority of the drugs described in the previ-ous section are not selective, intense efforts are being made to achieve the selective interference of immune activation through various immunological methods. The major goal of these immunological interventions is to reduce selectively the unwanted immune response while retaining protective immune responses without serious adverse effects. To do this effectively we need to know the antigens responsible for the initiation and perpetuation of the immune response. With the possible exceptions of myasthenia gravis and type 1 diabetes mellitus, the antigens which initiate and perpetuate the inflammatory process in most human diseases have not been identified. Therefore, the current methods are directed against processes involved in the initiation (APC–T cell interaction) and progression (cytokines) of an immune response to

Table 53.2 — Non-selective immunosuppressive agents used in autoimmune diseases

Drug	Mechanism of action	Diseases
Methotrexate	Inhibits purine synthesis	Myositis
Azathioprine	Inhibits purine synthesis	Myositis, MG
Corticosteroids	Inhibits cytokine gene expression	Myositis, MG
Cyclosporin	Inhibits T cell activation	Myositis, MG
Cyclophosphamide	Inhibits DNA replication	MG
Chlorambucil	Inhibits DNA replication	Myositis
FK506	Inhibits T cell activation	Myositis
Leflunomide	Inhibits pyrimidine synthesis	RA, EAE
Rapamycin	Inhibits T cell activation	RA, SLE models
Mycophenolate	Inhibits IMP dehydrogenase synthesis	Psoriasis, RA
Thalidomide	Immunosuppressive agent	MG

MG, Myasthenia gravis; RA, Rheumatoid arthritis; EAE, Experimental allergic encephalomyelitis, SLE, systemic lupus erythematosus.

an antigen. The available evidence at least in inflammatory myopathies suggests that there is ongoing immune activation in the inflamed muscle, and it might be possible to intervene these processes in a variety of ways. Table 53.3 briefly summarizes various immunological interventions and their mechanisms of action tested in experimental animal models and human patients with autoimmune diseases. Depletion of T helper cells using anti-CD4 antibodies has led to some clinical improvement in myasthenia patients (Ahlberg et al 1994). Similarly, a moiety of IL-2 was coupled to diphtheria toxin to eliminate the IL-2R-expressing activated T cells in the experimental autoimmune myasthenia gravis (EAMG) model with some success. Intervention using CTLA-4Ig in the EAMG model showed significant inhibition of both cellular and antibody responses to acetylcholine receptor, with decreased IL-2 production and T cell proliferation (McIntosh et al 1998). Even though the positive results are encouraging, the inhibitory effects of CTLA-4Ig are not complete. Therefore, a combination of IL-2 toxin and CTLA-4Ig was tested in this model with some beneficial effects (McIntosh et al 1998). A combination of immunosuppressive agents may be a suitable method to achieve antigen-specific immunosuppression. Several other methods developed to intervene in cell–cell interactions of the immune system such as anti-CD3, anti-CD4, anti-MHC and anti-TCR interventions are being tested in various autoimmune disease models with varying degrees of success.

The potential advantages of immunologically active agents in the treatment of immune mediated diseases include rapid onset and increased specificity of the effect without concomitant immunosuppression. However, the apparent specificity evident in animal models of disease and in vivo assays has rarely been translated into meaningful clinical effects in established disease. This failure reflects the redundancy of the immunological and cytokine networks. There are some disadvantages to the use of these newer biologically active agents. Products targeted to specific aspects of the immune response may be less toxic but the initial clinical benefits may be for a short duration and not maintained with readministration or chronic therapy. Some of these treatments also result in manifestation of autoimmune disease symptoms, similar to the experience reported following IL-2, IFN and G-CSF treatments of cancer or after transplantation (Perez et al 1991). From the experience with monoclonal antibodies against T cell surface antigens (CD5 immunoconjugates, anti-CD4 mAb), it is clear that prospective randomized, placebo-controlled clinical trials are of critical importance in identifying the potential clinical benefit of these agents (van der Lubbe et al 1995).

Table 53.3 — Immunotherapeutic interventions used in autoimmune diseases

Immunotherapy	Disease/model	Mechanism of action	Reference
Anti-CD3	NOD mice	Depletion	(Chatenoud et al 1994)
Anti-CD4	Arthritis	Interfere with Th function	(Levitt et al 1992)
	MG		(Ahlberg et al 1994)
Anti-CD5	RA	Depletion of T cells	(Olsen et al 1996)
Anti-ICAM-1	RA	Inhibit cell adhesion	(Kavanaugh et al 1994)
CD52	RA	Lymphocyte lysis	(Matteson et al 1995)
IL-2R fusion toxin	RA	Eliminate activated T cells	(Sewell et al 1993)
	MG		(McIntosh et al 1998)
CTLA-4Ig	Lupus mice	Block costimulation	(Finck et al 1994)
	EAMG		(McIntosh et al 1995)
Immunotoxins	EAMG	Specific lymphocyte lysis	(Killen and Lindstrom 1984)
	EAMG		(McIntosh et al 1998)
Anti-MHC class II	EAE	Block Ag presentation	(Steinman L 1991)
Copolymers-1	MS	Lymphocyte suppression	(Arnon et al 1996)
Anti-TCR	EAE	Interfere with specific T cells	(Zaller et al 1990)

MG, Myasthenia gravis; RA, Rheumatoid arthritis; EAMG, Experimental autoimmune myasthenia gravis; EAE, Experimental autoimmune encephalitis; MS, Multiple sclerosis; Ag, antigen; Ig, immunoglobulin; MHC, major histocompatibility complex; TCR, T cell receptor; NOD, Non-obese diabetic mice

Conventional and unconventional immunobiological agents

Cytokines and cytokine inhibitors

Inhibition of a proinflammatory cytokine by prevention of either receptor binding or effector cell function may offer transient clinical benefit. Several methods have been developed to inhibit the effector functions of cytokines. These include receptor antagonist proteins (IL-1Ra), soluble receptors (sIL-1R) and several monoclonal antibodies to the cytokines or their receptors. In general IL-1, TNF-α, and IL-6 are considered proinflammatory, and they are implicated in many of the pathogenic processes underlying autoimmunity. For example, cytokines such as TNF-α play an important role in the pathogenesis of rheumatoid arthritis and many other inflammatory conditions. Treatment with chimeric or humanized anti-TNF-α antibodies demonstrated significant clinical response with concordant reductions in malaise, fatigue, serum IL-6 and CRP levels. The clinical benefit is rapid in onset and continues with readministration. The development of autoantibodies to double stranded DNA and cardiolipin after the anti-cytokine treatment were unexplained side-effects seen after treatment with anti-TNF antibodies (Feldmann et al 1996). Several soluble receptor proteins (sTNF-RI and sTNF-RII) are also under various stages of testing. Based on the experience in the animal models of other autoimmune diseases and in some human trials, targeting proinflammatory cytokines may have some beneficial effects. For example, it is likely that the treatments that effectively inhibit proinflammatory cytokine such as IL-1 may have significant benefit in the treatment of chronic inflammatory myopathies (Lundberg and Nyberg 1998). Several cytokines such as TGF-β, IL-10, and IL-4 have anti-inflammatory properties. These cytokines have been effectively used to treat chronic inflammatory conditions. Table 53.4 shows some of the cytokine inhibitors currently used in human patients and in experimental models of chronic inflammatory conditions.

Intravenous immunoglobulins

Intravenous immunoglobulins are normal polyspecific immunoglobulin preparations from plasma pools of large number of healthy individuals. They probably mediate their immunomodulatory anti-inflammatory activities at least in part through Fc and F (ab)2 components of the immunoglobulin (Dalakas 1998a, Jordan et al 1998; Fig. 53.3). These were initially developed as replacement therapy for patients with antibody deficiencies, but the discovery of their beneficial effects on idiopathic thrombocytopenic purpura demonstrated their efficacy in treating autoimmune diseases. Intravenous immunoglobulins(IVIgs) are being explored in haematological (idiopathic thrombocytopenic purpura), autoimmune (myositis), neurological (myasthenia gravis, Guillain–Barre syndrome) and endocrine (insulin-dependent diabetes mellitus, thyroid opthalmopathy) disorders. The proposed mechanisms of action are depicted in Fig. 53.3. One or several of these mechanisms may be operating to yield the therapeutic benefits of IVIg. As depicted, some of these mechanisms are dependent on interactions between the Fc portions of IgG and the Fc receptors on phagocytes and lymphocytes. Others may be primarily dependent on the F(ab)2 region of infused antibodies. Although IVIg is an expensive drug, this therapy provides an alternative temporizing measure in muscle diseases like myasthenia gravis. Several studies with IVIg were done in myositis patients and the beneficial effects were mainly described for the treatment resistant PM or DM cases

Table 53.4— Interventions using cytokines or their inhibitors

Cytokines/inhibitors	Disease	Mechanism of action	Reference
IL-1Ra	CA	Block IL-1 actions	(Joosten et al 1996)
IFN-γ	RA	Inhibit IL-1/Th2 cytokines	(Obert and Hofschneider 1985)
sIL-1R	RA	Inhibit IL-1 actions	(Drevlow et al 1996)
anti-TNF	RA	Inhibit inflammation	(Elliott et al 1997)
sTNF-R	RA	Inhibit TNF induced damage	(Moreland et al 1999)
TGF-β	EAE	Immunosuppressive effects	(Racke et al 1991)
IL-4	EAE	Antagonize Th1 inflammation	(Racke et al 1994)

CA, collagen induced arthritis; RA, rheumatoid arthritis; EAE, experimental allergic encephalomyelitis; IL, interleukin; IFN, interferon; TNF, tumour necrosis factor.

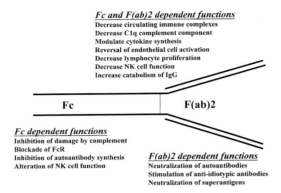

Fc and F(ab)2 dependent functions
Decrease circulating immune complexes
Decrease C1q complement component
Modulate cytokine synthesis
Reversal of endothelial cell activation
Decrease lymphocyte proliferation
Decrease NK cell function
Increase catabolism of IgG

Fc | **F(ab)2**

Fc dependent functions
Inhibition of damage by complement
Blockade of FcR
Inhibition of autoantibody synthesis
Alteration of NK cell function

F(ab)2 dependent functions
Neutralization of autoantibodies
Stimulation of anti-idiotypic antibodies
Neutralization of superantigens

Figure 53.3— Mechanisms of action of intravenous immunoglobulins (Igs). (Fc: fragment that crystallizes; F(ab)2: antigen binding fragment; FcR: Fc receptor; NK: natural killer cells).

where IVIg was given together with corticosteroids or other immunosuppressive drugs, whereas IVIg as a primary monotherapy was less successful (Cherin et al 1991, Cherin et al 1994, Dalakas 1997, Dalakas 1998b).

Oral tolerance

Several studies suggest that orally administered auto-antigens may be able to suppress experimental models of autoimmune diseases such as experimental allergic encephalomyelitis (EAE), collagen-induced arthritis (CIA), adjuvant arthritis (AA), uveitis, myasthenia gravis, diabetes, thyroiditis and colitis (Singh and Nagaraju 1996). The mechanism of suppression in these models depends on the dose administered. For example, in Lewis rats, high doses of Myelin basic protein (MBP) result in clonal anergy (Whitacre et al 1991) whereas lower doses induce transferable cellular suppression (Lider et al 1989). In the nervous system of animals fed with low doses, the inflammatory cytokines such as TNF-α and IFN-γ are downregulated (Khoury et al 1992, Miller A et al 1992). Oral MBP partially suppressed the serum antibody responses especially at higher doses. Even though the muscle disease in myasthenia gravis is antibody mediated, oral and nasal administration of the Torpedo acetylcholine receptor to Lewis rats prevented or delayed the onset of the disease (Wang et al 1995). This procedure is likely to be of limited use for treatment of other inflammatory muscle diseases. Identification of target autoantigens is a prerequisite for the use of not only oral tolerance but also of the other interventions such as altered peptide ligands, T cell vaccination or T cell peptide vaccination described in the subsequent sections.

Altered peptide ligands

It is known that TCR can interact with a spectrum of ligands, and that these ligands deliver different signals to the T cells, which result in a wide range of outcomes. For example agonist peptides will induce full T cell activation (proliferation and cytokine secretion), whereas the change of a few amino acid residues in an agonist peptide generates antagonists and partial antagonists peptides that either stop T cell activation altogether or produce partial activation (e.g., secretion of certain cytokines). Exploitation of interactions between TCR and variant ligands has been suggested as a mode of therapy for autoimmune diseases (Wraith et al 1989). In an MBP–TCR transgenic model, Ac1–11 (Myelin basic protein peptide Ac1–11) and its analogues can produce T cells with different phenotypes. Administration of a soluble analogue peptide for a T cell clone can prevent disease induced with a second encephalitogenic clone or line, by a mechanism that is blocked by the administration of IL–4. All these effects appear to depend on direct interaction with a specific TCR. However, it is possible that APLs can recruit a different population of T cells from the naïve repertoire in vivo (Wucherpfennig et al 1995). This mode of therapy has good potential even though the human T cell responses are more complex than the T cell responses observed in EAE model because of bystander effects (Nicholson et al 1997). Except in a rare variant of PM where monoclonal γ/δ T cells recognize a 65 kDa heat shock protein as a candidate autoantigen, for the majority of these conditions the autoantigens and peptides responsible for the initiation of autoimmune process in myositis are not known, and hence testing this mode of treatment in inflammatory myopathies is not possible at this time.

T cell vaccination

Suppression of potentially autoreactive clones could be achieved by immunization with attenuated auto-reactive T cells. This concept of T cell vaccination relies on the injection of autoantigen-specific T cell clones, which must be isolated from the prospective recipient, cultured and expanded, attenuated or inactivated in vitro and readministered as a vaccine (Ben-Nun and Cohen 1981). This method has been used with some success in patients and in an experimental model of multiple sclerosis, but the studies in RA with T cell vaccination were not successful (van Laar et al 1993a, b) partly because of the heterogeneous nature of the clones used in these studies. Nevertheless, these studies demonstrate that toxicity related to the subcutaneous vaccination of attenuated autologous T cells does not seem to be a major problem. Administration of inactivated T cells is well tolerated in humans, and it has no adverse effects. Analysis of T cell receptor family revealed a limited TCR repertoire in muscle inflammation (Mantegazza et al 1993, Lindberg et al 1994) of PM patients compared with that in DM patients (O'Hanlon et al 1995). Using inverse-polymerase chain reaction (PCR) and immunocytochemistry, it was shown that there is dissociation between TCR usage of autoinvasive and interstitial T cells (Bender et al 1995). Therefore, the available evidence in inflammatory myopathies (PM and IBM) suggests that T cells are oligoclonal and may recognize a limited number of MHC class I associated antigenic peptides. Therefore, the preferential usage of some of these combinations in myositis may be related to the recognition of a specific autoantigen in the muscle tissue, and this mode of therapy has not been explored in inflammatory myopathies so far. More recently, peptides of the antigen-specific TCR from autoreactive T cells, rather than whole T cells, have been used for TCR peptide vaccination in other autoimmune diseases (Vandenbark et al 1998).

Gene therapies

Both humoral and cell-mediated immune responses are implicated in autoimmune muscle diseases such as polymyositis and dermatomyositis. Skeletal muscle cells might be genetically altered to protect themselves during an autoimmune attack by ectopic expression of immunoregulatory molecules such as FasL, IL-4 or IL-10 to reduce the immune inflammation and the symptoms of autoimmune attack. Syngenic myoblasts that expressed FasL protected allogeneic islets of Langerhans from immune rejection when co-transplanted under the kidney capsule (Lau et al 1996). The presumed immune privilege conferred by exogenous expression of FasL in this system appeared to be similar to the naturally occurring immune protection described in the anterior chamber of the eye (Griffith et al 1995), in rodent testis (Bellgrau et al 1995) and in malignant melanoma (Hahne et al 1996), all of which express endogenous FasL. It was also shown that genetically engineered FasL-expressing myoblasts could function as killers of solid tumours in vivo. Transfer of myoblasts expressing various anti-inflammatory molecules offers a convenient way of modulating inflammation in muscle disease. The potential of this method is yet to be explored in autoimmune muscle diseases.

Very heterogeneous procedures such as plasmapheresis, total lymphoid irradiation, thoracic duct drainage, splenectomy, thymectomy, anti-lymphocyte serum or globulins are used to achieve the goal of immunosuppression in myasthenia gravis and inflammatory myopathies with variable effect. Plasmapheresis has been used successfully for the short-term treatment of severe myasthenia gravis, and early in Guillain–Barre syndrome (McKhann et al 1988), but does not work in myositis (Miller et al 1992). Since the depletion of pathogenic antibodies is only temporary, treatment with other immunosuppressive agents is essential in chronic autoimmune disease conditions.

Despite significant advances in understanding the immunopathogenesis of other autoimmune diseases, the basic research on the immunopathogenetic mechanisms for inflammatory muscle diseases has progressed slowly because of the lack of an experimental animal model. Therefore, currently the most effective way to treat these disorders is to use non-specific immunosuppressive agents, despite their serious side-effects. Studying basic immunological mechanisms in muscle diseases should provide new clues in designing effective therapeutic interventions in future.

Acknowledgements

I would like to thank Dr. Paul Plotz and Dr. Michael Centola for their valuable comments and suggestions. I am also thankful to Paul J. Rochon for his tremendous editorial help, comments and suggestions at various stages during the preparation of this manuscript. I am also thankful to Tomasina Parker for her typographical help. Furthermore, I would like to thank my wife and newly born daughter for their patience during the preparation of this manuscript.

References

Adams EM, Kirkley J, Eidelman G, Dohlman J, Plotz PH. (1997) The predominance of beta (CC) chemokine transcripts in idiopathic inflammatory muscle diseases. *Proc Assoc Am Physicians* 109: 275–285.

Ahlberg R, Yi Q, Pirskanen R, et al. (1994) Treatment of myasthenia gravis with anti-CD4 antibody: improvement correlates to decreased T-cell autoreactivity. *Neurology* 44: 1732–1737.

Arahata K, Engel AG. (1988) Monoclonal antibody analysis of mononuclear cells in myopathies IV: Cell-mediated cytotoxicity and muscle fibre necrosis. *Ann Neurol* 23: 168–173.

Arai KI, Lee F, Miyajima A, Miyatake S, Arai N, Yokota T. (1990) Cytokines: coordinators of immune and inflammatory responses. *Annu Rev Biochem* 59: 783–836.

Arnon R, Sela M, Teitelbaum D. (1996) New insights into the mechanism of action of copolymer 1 in experimental allergic encephalomyelitis and multiple sclerosis. *J Neurol* 243: S8–13.

Austyn JM, Hankins DF, Larsen CP, Morris PJ, Rao AS, Roake JA. (1994) Isolation and characterization of dendritic cells from mouse heart and kidney. *J Immunol* 152: 2401–2410.

Azuma M, Phillips JH, Lanier LL. (1993) CD28- T lymphocytes. Antigenic and functional properties. *J Immunol* 150: 1147–1159.

Banchereau J, Briere F, Liu YJ, Rousset F. (1994) Molecular control of B lymphocyte growth and differentiation. *Stem Cells (Dayt)* 12: 278–288.

Bartoccioni E, Gallucci S, Scuderi F, et al. (1994) MHC class I, MHC class II and intercellular adhesion molecule-1 (ICAM-1) expression in inflammatory myopathies. *Clin Exp Immunol* 95: 166–172.

Behan WM, Behan PO, Durward WF, McQueen A. (1987) The inflammatory process in polymyositis: monoclonal antibody analysis of muscle and peripheral blood immuno-regulatory lymphocytes. *J Neurol Neurosurg Psychiatry* 50: 1468–1474.

Behrens L, Bender A, Johnson MA, Hohlfeld R. (1997) Cytotoxic mechanisms in inflammatory myopathies. Co-expression of Fas and protective Bcl-2 in muscle fibres and inflammatory cells. *Brain* 120: 929–938.

Behrens L, Kerschensteiner M, Misgeld T, Goebels N, Wekerle H, Hohlfeld R. (1998) Human muscle cells express a functional costimulatory molecule distinct from B7.1 (CD80) and B7.2 (CD86) in vitro and in inflammatory lesions. *J Immunol* 161: 5943–5951.

Bellgrau D, Gold D, Selawry H, Moore J, Franzusoff A, Duke RC. (1995) A role for CD95 ligand in preventing graft rejection [see comments] [published erratum appears in *Nature* (1998) 394(6689):133]. *Nature* 377: 630–632.

Ben-Nun A, Cohen IR. (1981) Vaccination against autoimmune encephalomyelitis (EAE): attenuated autoimmune T lymphocytes confer resistance to induction of active EAE but not to EAE mediated by the intact T lymphocyte line. *Eur J Immunol* 11: 949–952.

Bender A, Ernst N, Iglesias A, Dornmair K, Wekerle H, Hohlfeld R. (1995) T cell receptor repertoire in polymyositis: clonal expansion of autoaggressive CD8+ T cells. *J Exp Med* 181: 1863–1868.

Bernasconi P, Confalonieri P, Andreetta F, Baggi F, Cornelio F, Mantegazza R. (1998) The expression of co-stimulatory and accessory molecules on cultured human muscle cells is not dependent on stimulus by pro-inflammatory cytokines: relevance for the pathogenesis of inflammatory myopathy. *J Neuroimmunol* 85: 52–58.

Bernasconi P, Torchiana E, Confalonieri P, et al. (1995)

Expression of transforming growth factor-beta 1 in dystrophic patient muscles correlates with fibrosis, Pathogenetic role of a fibrogenic cytokine. *J Clin Invest* 96(2): 655–656.

Boehm U, Klamp T, Groot M, Howard JC. (1997) Cellular responses to interferon-gamma. *Annu Rev Immunol* 15: 749–795.

Bohm W, Schirmbeck R, Elbe A, et al. (1995) Exogenous hepatitis B surface antigen particles processed by dendritic cells or macrophages prime murine MHC class I-restricted cytotoxic T lymphocytes in vivo. *J Immunol* 155: 3313–3321.

Boise LH, Minn AJ, Thompson CB. (1995) Receptors that regulate T-cell susceptibility to apoptotic cell death. *Ann NY Acad Sci* 766: 70–80.

Boussiotis VA, Freeman GJ, Griffin JD, Gray GS, Gribben JG, Nadler LM. (1994) CD2 is involved in maintenance and reversal of human alloantigen-specific clonal anergy. *J Exp Med* 180: 1665–1673.

Chabaud M, Durand JM, Buchs N, et al. (1999) Human interleukin-17: A T cell-derived proinflammatory cytokine produced by the rheumatoid synovium. *Arthritis Rheum* 42: 963–970.

Chatenoud L, Thervet E, Primo J, Bach JF. (1994) Anti-CD3 antibody induces long-term remission of overt autoimmunity in nonobese diabetic mice. *Proc Natl Acad Sci USA* 91: 123–127.

Cherin P, Herson S, Wechsler B, et al. (1991) Efficacy of intravenous gammaglobulin therapy in chronic refractory polymyositis and dermatomyositis: an open study with 20 adult patients. *Am J Med* 91: 162–168.

Cherin P, Piette JC, Wechsler B, et al. (1994) Intravenous gamma globulin as first line therapy in polymyositis and dermatomyositis: an open study in 11 adult patients [see comments]. *J Rheumatol* 21: 1092–1097.

Chicz RM, Urban RG, Lane WS, et al. (1992) Predominant naturally processed peptides bound to HLA-DR1 are derived from MHC-related molecules and are heterogeneous in size. *Nature* 358: 764–768.

Colotta F, Dower SK, Sims JE, Mantovani A. (1994) The type II 'decoy' receptor: a novel regulatory pathway for interleukin 1. *Immunol Today* 15: 562–566.

Confalonieri P, Bernasconi P, Cornelio F, Mantegazza R. (1997) Transforming growth factor-beta 1 in polymyositis and dermatomyositis correlates with fibrosis but not with mononuclear cell infiltrate. *J Neuropathol Exp Neurol* 56: 479–484.

Cruikshank WW, Kornfeld H, Center DM. (1998) Signaling and functional properties of interleukin-16. *Int Rev Immunol* 16: 523–540.

Cunningham AC, Zhang JG, Moy JV, Ali S, Kirby JA. (1997) A comparison of the antigen-presenting capabilities of class II MHC-expressing human lung epithelial and endothelial cells. *Immunology* 91: 458–463.

Dalakas MC. (1997) Intravenous immune globulin therapy for neurologic diseases. *Ann Intern Med* 126: 721–730.

Dalakas MC. (1998a) Mechanism of action of intravenous immunoglobulin and therapeutic considerations in the treatment of autoimmune neurologic diseases. *Neurology* 51: S2–8.

Dalakas MC. (1998b) Controlled studies with high-dose intravenous immunoglobulin in the treatment of dermatomyositis, inclusion body myositis, and polymyositis. *Neurology* 51: S37–45.

Dalmau J, Gultekin HS, Posner JB. (1999) Paraneoplastic neurologic syndromes: pathogenesis and physiopathology. *Brain Pathol* 9: 275–284.

De Bleecker JL, Engel AG. (1994) Expression of cell adhesion molecules in inflammatory myopathies and Duchenne dystrophy. *J Neuropathol Exp Neurol* 53: 369–376.

De Bleecker JL, Meire VI, Declercq W, Van Aken EH. (1999) Immunolocalization of tumor necrosis factor-alpha and its receptors in inflammatory myopathies. *Neuromuscul Disord* 9: 239–246.

Dinarello CA. (1991) Interleukin-1 and interleukin-1 antagonism. *Blood* 77: 1627–1652.

Drachman DB. (1996) Immunotherapy in neuromuscular disorders: current and future strategies. *Muscle Nerve* 19: 1239–1251.

Drachman DB, Fishman PS, Rothstein JD, et al. (1995) Amyotrophic lateral sclerosis. An autoimmune disease? *Adv Neurol* 68: 59–65.

Drevlow BE, Lovis R, Haag MA, et al. (1996) Recombinant human interleukin-1 receptor type I in the treatment of patients with active rheumatoid arthritis. *Arthritis Rheum* 39: 257–265.

Elliott MJ, Woo P, Charles P, Long-Fox A, Woody JN, Maini RN. (1997) Suppression of fever and the acute-phase response in a patient with juvenile chronic arthritis treated with monoclonal antibody to tumour necrosis factor-alpha (cA2). *Br J Rheumatol* 36: 589–593.

Emslie-Smith AM, Arahata K, Engel AG. (1989) Major histocompatibility complex class I antigen expression, immunolocalization of interferon subtypes, and T cell-mediated cytotoxicity in myopathies. *Hum Pathol* 20: 224–231.

Engel AG, Arahata K. (1986) Mononuclear cells in myopathies: quantitation of functionally distinct subsets, recognition of antigen-specific cell-mediated cytotoxicity in some diseases, and implications for the pathogenesis of the different inflammatory myopathies. *Hum Pathol* 17: 704–721.

Engel AG, Hohlfeld R, Banker BQ. (1994) The Polymyositis and Dermatomyositis Syndromes. In: Engel AG,

Franzini-Armstrong C, eds. *Myology*. New York: McGraw-Hill, pp. 1335–1383.

Espevik T, Waage A. (1988) The involvement of tumor necrosis factor-alpha (TNF-alpha) in immunomodulation and in septic shock. *Dev Biol Stand* 69: 139–142.

Feldmann M, Brennan FM, Maini RN. (1996) Role of cytokines in rheumatoid arthritis. *Annu Rev Immunol* 14: 397–440.

Finck BK, Linsley PS, Wofsy D. (1994) Treatment of murine lupus with CTLA4Ig. *Science* 265 1225–1227.

Florini JR, Roberts AB, Ewton DZ, Falen SL, Flanders KC, Sporn MB. (1986) Transforming growth factor-beta. A very potent inhibitor of myoblast differentiation, identical to the differentiation inhibitor secreted by Buffalo rat liver cells. *J Biol Chem* 261: 16509–16513.

Freeman GJ, Gribben JG, Boussiotis VA, et al. (1993) Cloning of B7-2: a CTLA-4 counter-receptor that costimulates human T cell proliferation [see comments]. *Science* 262: 909–911.

Gamble JR, Harlan JM, Klebanoff SJ, Vadas MA. (1985) Stimulation of the adherence of neutrophils to umbilical vein endothelium by human recombinant tumor necrosis factor. *Proc Natl Acad Sci USA* 82: 8667–8671.

Goebels N, Michaelis D, Wekerle H, Hohlfeld R. (1992) Human myoblasts as antigen-presenting cells. *J Immunol* 149: 661–667.

Grabstein KH, Eisenman J, Shanebeck K, et al. (1994) Cloning of a T cell growth factor that interacts with the beta chain of the interleukin-2 receptor. *Science* 264: 965–968.

Green DR, Ware CF. (1997) Fas-ligand: privilege and peril [see comments]. *Proc Natl Acad Sci USA* 94: 5986–5990.

Griffith TS, Brunner T, Fletcher SM, Green DR, Ferguson TA. (1995) Fas ligand-induced apoptosis as a mechanism of immune privilege [see comments]. *Science* 270: 1189–1192.

Griggs RC. (1994) Developing new treatments for muscle disease: prospects and promise. *Curr Opin Neurol* 7: 422–426.

Hafer-Macko CE, Sheikh KA, Li CY, et al. (1996) Immune attack on the Schwann cell surface in acute inflammatory demyelinating polyneuropathy. *Ann Neurol* 39: 625–635.

Hahne M, Rimoldi D, Schroter M, et al. (1996) Melanoma cell expression of Fas(Apo-1/CD95) ligand: implications for tumor immune escape [see comments]. *Science* 274: 1363–1366.

Hannum CH, Wilcox CJ, Arend WP, et al. (1990) Interleukin-1 receptor antagonist activity of a human interleukin-1 inhibitor. *Nature* 343: 336–340.

Hermann E, Darcissac E, Idziorek T, Capron A, Bahr GM. (1999) Recombinant interleukin-16 selectively modulates surface receptor expression and cytokine release in macrophages and dendritic cells. *Immunology* 97: 241–248.

Higuchi I, Nerenberg M, Ijichi T, et al. (1991) Vacuolar myositis with expression of both MHC class I and class II antigens on skeletal muscle fibres. *J Neurol Sci* 106: 60–66.

Hohlfeld R, Engel AG. (1994) The immunobiology of muscle. *Immunol. Today* 15: 269–274.

Holter W, Schwarz M, Cerwenka A, Knapp W. (1996) The role of CD2 as a regulator of human T-cell cytokine production. *Immunol Rev* 153: 107–122.

Horseman ND, Yu-Lee LY. (1994) Transcriptional regulation by the helix bundle peptide hormones: growth hormone, prolactin, and hematopoietic cytokines. *Endocr Rev* 15: 627–649.

Inukai A, Kobayashi Y, Ito K, et al. (1997) Expression of Fas antigen is not associated with apoptosis in human myopathies. *Muscle Nerve* 20: 702–709.

Isenberg DA, Rowe D, Shearer M, Novick D, Beverley PC. (1986) Localization of interferons and interleukin 2 in polymyositis and muscular dystrophy. *Clin Exp Immunol* 63: 450–458.

Janeway CA, Jr, Ron J, Katz ME. (1987) The B cell is the initiating antigen-presenting cell in peripheral lymph nodes. *J Immunol* 138: 1051–1055.

Joosten LA, Helsen MM, van de Loo FA, van den Berg WB. (1996) Anticytokine treatment of established type II collagen-induced arthritis in DBA/1 mice. A comparative study using anti-TNF alpha, anti-IL-1 alpha/beta, and IL-1Ra. *Arthritis Rheum* 39: 797–809.

Jordan SC, Tyan D, Czer L, Toyoda M. (1998) Immunomodulatory actions of intravenous immunoglobulin (IVIG): potential applications in solid organ transplant recipients. *Pediatr Transplant* 2: 92–105.

Ju ST, Panka DJ, Cui H, et al. (1995) Fas(CD95)/FasL interactions required for programmed cell death after T-cell activation [see comments]. *Nature* 373: 444–448.

Karpati G, Pouliot Y, Carpenter S. (1988) Expression of immunoreactive major histocompatibility complex products in human skeletal muscles. *Ann Neurol* 23: 64–72.

Kavanaugh AF, Davis LS, Nichols LA, et al. (1994) Treatment of refractory rheumatoid arthritis with a monoclonal antibody to intercellular adhesion molecule 1. *Arthritis Rheum* 37: 992–999.

Kawamata T, Akiyama H, Yamada T, McGeer PL. (1992) Immunologic reactions in amyotrophic lateral sclerosis brain and spinal cord tissue. *Am J Pathol* 140: 691–707.

Keegan AD, Nelms K, Wang LM, Pierce JH, Paul WE. (1994) Interleukin 4 receptor: signaling mechanisms. *Immunol Today* 15: 423–432.

Khoury SJ, Hancock WW, Weiner HL. (1992) Oral tolerance to myelin basic protein and natural recovery from experimental autoimmune encephalomyelitis are associated with downregulation of inflammatory cytokines and differential upregulation of transforming growth factor beta, interleukin 4, and prostaglandin E expression in the brain. *J Exp Med* 176: 1355–1364.

Killen JA, Lindstrom JM. (1984) Specific killing of lymphocytes that cause experimental autoimmune myasthenia gravis by ricin toxin-acetylcholine receptor conjugates. *J Immunol* 133: 2549–2553.

Kishimoto T, Akira S, Taga T. (1992) IL-6 receptor and mechanism of signal transduction. *Intl J Immunopharmacol* 14: 431–438.

Kotake S, Udagawa N, Takahashi N, et al. (1999) IL-17 in synovial fluids from patients with rheumatoid arthritis is a potent stimulator of osteoclastogenesis. *J Clin Invest* 103: 1345–1352.

Kroczek RA, Graf D, Brugnoni D, et al. (1994) Defective expression of CD40 ligand on T cells causes "X-linked immunodeficiency with hyper-IgM (HIGM1)". *Immunol Rev* 138: 39–59.

Kuwano K, Hagimoto N, Kawasaki M, et al. (1999) Essential roles of the Fas-Fas ligand pathway in the development of pulmonary fibrosis. *J Clin Invest* 104: 13–19.

Lau HT, Yu M, Fontana A, Stoeckert CJ, Jr. (1996) Prevention of islet allograft rejection with engineered myoblasts expressing FasL in mice [see comments]. *Science* 273: 109–112.

Levitt NG, Fernandez-Madrid F, Wooley PH. (1992) Pristane induced arthritis in mice. IV. Immunotherapy with monoclonal antibodies directed against lymphocyte subsets. *J Rheumatol* 19: 1342–1347.

Lider O, Santos LM, Lee CS, Higgins PJ, Weiner HL. (1989) Suppression of experimental autoimmune encephalomyelitis by oral administration of myelin basic protein. II. Suppression of disease and in vitro immune responses is mediated by antigen-specific CD8+ T lymphocytes. *J Immunol* 142: 748–752.

Lindberg C, Oldfors A, Tarkowski A. (1994) Restricted use of T cell receptor V genes in endomysial infiltrates of patients with inflammatory myopathies. *Eur J Immunol* 24: 2659–2663.

Link H, Xu ZY, Melms A, et al. (1992) The T-cell repertoire in myasthenia gravis involves multiple cholinergic receptor epitopes. *Scand J Immunol* 36: 405–414.

Linsley PS, Ledbetter JA. (1993) The role of the CD28 receptor during T cell responses to antigen. *Annu Rev Immunol* 11: 191–212.

Linsley PS, Peach R, Gladstone P, Bajorath J. (1994) Extending the B7 (CD80) gene family. *Protein Sci* 3: 1341–1343.

Liprandi A, Bartoli C, Figarella-Branger D, Pellissier JF, Lepidi H. (1999) Local expression of monocyte chemo-attractant protein-1 (MCP-1) in idiopathic inflammatory myopathies. *Acta Neuropathol (Berl)* 97: 642–648.

Lundberg I, Brengman JM, Engel AG. (1995) Analysis of cytokine expression in muscle in inflammatory myopathies, Duchenne dystrophy, and non-weak controls. *J Neuroimmunol* 63: 9–16.

Lundberg I, Ulfgren AK, Nyberg P, Andersson U, Klareskog L. (1997) Cytokine production in muscle tissue of patients with idiopathic inflammatory myopathies. *Arthritis Rheum* 40: 865–874.

Lundberg IE, Nyberg P. (1998) New developments in the role of cytokines and chemokines in inflammatory myopathies. *Curr Opin Rheumatol* 10: 521–529.

Lynch DH, Ramsdell F, Alderson MR. (1995) Fas and FasL in the homeostatic regulation of immune responses [see comments]. *Immunol Today* 16: 569–574.

Mantegazza R, Andreetta F, Bernasconi P, et al. (1993) Analysis of T cell receptor repertoire of muscle-infiltrating T lymphocytes in polymyositis. Restricted V alpha/beta rearrangements may indicate antigen-driven selection. *J Clin Invest* 91: 2880–2886.

Mastaglia FL, Phillips BA, Zilko P. (1997) Treatment of inflammatory myopathies. *Muscle Nerve* 20: 651–664.

Matteson EL, Yocum DE, St Clair EW, et al. (1995) Treatment of active refractory rheumatoid arthritis with humanized monoclonal antibody CAMPATH-1H administered by daily subcutaneous injection. *Arthritis Rheum* 38: 1187–1193.

McInnes IB, Liew FY. (1998) Interleukin 15: a proinflammatory role in rheumatoid arthritis synovitis. *Immunol Today* 19: 75–79.

McIntosh KR, Linsley PS, Bacha PA, Drachman, DB. (1998) Immunotherapy of experimental autoimmune myasthenia gravis: selective effects of CTLA4Ig and synergistic combination with an IL2-diphtheria toxin fusion protein. *J Neuroimmunol* 87: 136–146.

McIntosh KR, Linsley PS, Drachman DB. (1995) Immunosuppression and induction of anergy by CTLA4Ig in vitro: effects on cellular and antibody responses of lymphocytes from rats with experimental autoimmune myasthenia gravis. *Cell Immunol* 166: 103–112.

McKhann GM, Griffin JW, Cornblath DR, Quaskey SA, Mellits ED. (1988) Role of therapeutic plasmapheresis in the acute Guillain-Barre syndrome. *J Neuroimmunol* 20: 297–300.

Miller A, Lider O, Roberts AB, Sporn MB, Weiner HL. (1992) Suppressor T cells generated by oral tolerization to myelin basic protein suppress both in vitro and in vivo immune responses by the release of transforming growth factor beta after antigen-specific triggering. *Proc Natl Acad Sci USA* 89: 421–425.

Miller FW, Leitman SF, Cronin ME, et al. (1992) Controlled trial of plasma exchange and leukapheresis in polymyositis and dermatomyositis [see comments]. *N Engl J Med* 326: 1380–1384.

Moore KW, O'Garra A, de Waal Malefyt R, Vieira P, Mosmann TR. (1993) Interleukin-10. *Annu Rev Immunol* 11: 165–190.

Moreland LW, Schiff MH, Baumgartner SW, et al. (1999) Etanercept therapy in rheumatoid arthritis. A randomized, controlled trial. *Ann Intern Med* 130: 478–486.

Moser R, Schleiffenbaum B, Groscurth P, Fehr J. (1989) Interleukin 1 and tumor necrosis factor stimulate human vascular endothelial cells to promote transendothelial neutrophil passage. *J Clin Invest* 83: 444–455.

Murata KY, Dalakas MC. (1999) Expression of the costimulatory molecule BB-1, the ligands CTLA-4 and CD28, and their mRNA in inflammatory myopathies. *Am J Pathol* 155: 453–460.

Nagaraju K, Raben N, Merritt G, Loeffler L, Kirk K, Plotz P. (1998) A variety of cytokines and immunologically relevant surface molecules are expressed by normal human skeletal muscle cells under proinflammatory stimuli. *Clin Exp Immunol* 113: 407–414.

Nagaraju K, Raben N, Villalba ML, et al. (1999) Costimulatory markers in muscle of patients with idiopathic inflammatory myopathies and in cultured muscle cells. *Clin Immunol* 92: 161–169.

Nicholson LB, Murtaza A, Hafler BP, Sette A, Kuchroo VK. (1997) A T cell receptor antagonist peptide induces T cells that mediate bystander suppression and prevent autoimmune encephalomyelitis induced with multiple myelin antigens. *Proc Natl Acad Sci USA* 94: 9279–9284.

O'Hanlon TP, Dalakas MC, Plotz PH, Miller FW. (1995) The alpha beta T-cell receptor repertoire in idiopathic inflammatory myopathies: distinct patterns of gene expression by muscle-infiltrating lymphocytes in different clinical and serologic groups. *Ann NY Acad Sci* 756: 410–413.

Obert HJ, Hofschneider PH. (1985) [Interferon in chronic polyarthritis. Positive effect in clinical evaluation]. *Dtsch Med Wochenschr* 110: 1766–1769.

Oddis CV, Sciurba FC, Elmagd KA, Starzl TE. (1999) Tacrolimus in refractory polymyositis with interstitial lung disease [letter]. *Lancet* 353: 1762–1763.

Olive M, Martinez-Matos JA, Montero J, Ferrer I. (1997) Apoptosis is not the mechanism of cell death of muscle fibres in human muscular dystrophies and inflammatory myopathies. *Muscle Nerve* 20: 1328–1330.

Olsen NJ, Brooks RH, Cush JJ, et al. (1996) A double-blind, placebo-controlled study of anti-CD5 immunoconjugate in patients with rheumatoid arthritis. The Xoma RA Investigator Group [published erratum appears in *Arthritis Rheum* (1996) 39(9): 1575]. *Arthritis Rheum* 39: 1102–1108.

Pardoll DM, Beckerleg AM. (1995) Exposing the immunology of naked DNA vaccines. *Immunity* 3: 165–169.

Pedrol E, Grau JM, Casademont J, et al. (1995) Idiopathic inflammatory myopathies. Immunohistochemical analysis of the major histocompatibility complex antigen expression, inflammatory infiltrate phenotype and activation cell markers. *Clin Neuropathol* 14: 179–184.

Perez R, Padavic K, Krigel R, Weiner L. (1991) Anti-erythrocyte autoantibody formation after therapy with interleukin-2 and gamma-interferon. *Cancer* 67: 2512–2517.

Racke MK, Bonomo A, Scott DE, et al. (1994) Cytokine-induced immune deviation as a therapy for inflammatory autoimmune disease. *J Exp Med* 180: 1961–1966.

Racke MK, Dhib-Jalbut S, Cannella B, Albert PS, Raine CS, McFarlin DE. (1991) Prevention and treatment of chronic relapsing experimental allergic encephalomyelitis by transforming growth factor-beta 1. *J Immunol* 146: 3012–3017.

Randall TD, Lund FE, Brewer JW, Aldridge C, Wall R, Corley RB. (1993) Interleukin-5 (IL-5) and IL-6 define two molecularly distinct pathways of B-cell differentiation. *Mol Cell Biol* 13: 3929–3936.

Rotzschke O, Falk K, Deres K, et al. (1990) Isolation and analysis of naturally processed viral peptides as recognized by cytotoxic T cells [see comments]. *Nature* 348: 252–254.

Schirmbeck R, Melber K, Reimann J. (1995) Hepatitis B virus small surface antigen particles are processed in a novel endosomal pathway for major histocompatibility complex class I-restricted epitope presentation. *Eur J Immunol* 25: 1063–1070.

Schwartz RH. (1996) Models of T cell anergy: is there a common molecular mechanism? [comment]. *J Exp Med* 184: 1–8.

Schwarz MK, Wells TN. (1999) Interfering with chemokine networks – the hope for new therapeutics. *Curr Opin Chem Biol* 3: 407–417.

Sewell KL, Parker KC, Woodworth TG, Reuben J, Swartz W, Trentham DE. (1993) DAB486IL-2 fusion toxin in refractory rheumatoid arthritis. *Arthritis Rheum* 36: 1223–1233.

Singh VK, Nagaraju K. (1996) Experimental autoimmune uveitis: molecular mimicry and oral tolerance. *Immunol Res* 15: 323–346.

Sinha S, Newsom-Davis J, Mills K, Byrne N, Lang B, Vincent A. (1991) Autoimmune aetiology for acquired neuromyotonia (Isaacs' syndrome) [see comments]. *Lancet* 338: 75–77.

Smythe JA, Fink PD, Logan GJ, Lees J, Rowe PB, Alexander IE. (1999) Human Fibroblasts Transduced with CD80 or CD86 Efficiently trans-Costimulate CD4+ and CD8+ T Lymphocytes in HLA-Restricted Reactions: Implications for Immune Augmentation Cancer Therapy and Autoimmunity. *J Immunol* 163: 3239–3249.

Steinman L. (1991) The development of rational strategies for selective immunotherapy against autoimmune demyelinating disease. *Adv Immunol* 49: 357–379.

Steinman RM. (1991) The dendritic cell system and its role in immunogenicity. *Annu Rev Immunol* 9: 271–296.

Suzuki I, Fink PJ. (1998) Maximal proliferation of cytotoxic T lymphocytes requires reverse signaling through Fas ligand. *J Exp Med* 187: 123–128.

Symons JA, Young PR, Duff GW. (1995) Soluble type II interleukin 1 (IL-1) receptor binds and blocks processing of IL-1 beta precursor and loses affinity for IL-1 receptor antagonist. *Proc Natl Acad Sci USA* 92: 1714–1718.

Tartaglia LA, Goeddel DV. (1992) Two TNF receptors. *Immunol Today* 13: 151–153.

Taub DD, Oppenheim JJ. (1994) Chemokines, inflammation and the immune system. *Ther Immunol* 1: 229–246.

Tews DS, Goebel HH. (1995) Expression of cell adhesion molecules in inflammatory myopathies. *J Neuroimmunol* 59: 185–194.

Tews DS, Goebel HH. (1996) Cytokine expression profile in idiopathic inflammatory myopathies. *J Neuropathol Exp Neurol* 55: 342–347.

Theze J, Alzari PM, Bertoglio J. (1996) Interleukin 2 and its receptors: recent advances and new immunological functions [see comments]. *Immunol Today* 17: 481–486.

Tindall RS, Phillips JT, Rollins JA, Wells L, Hall K. (1993) A clinical therapeutic trial of cyclosporine in myasthenia gravis. *Ann NY Acad Sci* 681: 539–551.

Tivol EA, Borriello F, Schweitzer AN, Lynch WP, Bluestone JA, Sharpe AH. (1995) Loss of CTLA-4 leads to massive lymphoproliferation and fatal multiorgan tissue destruction, revealing a critical negative regulatory role of CTLA-4. *Immunity* 3: 541–547.

Trinchieri G, Scott P. (1999) Interleukin-12: basic principles and clinical applications. *Curr Top Microbiol Immunol* 238: 57–78.

van der Lubbe PA, Dijkmans BA, Markusse HM, Nassander U, Breedveld FC. (1995) A randomized, double-blind, placebo-controlled study of CD4 monoclonal antibody therapy in early rheumatoid arthritis. *Arthritis Rheum* 38: 1097–1106.

van der Poll T, van Deventer SJ, Hack CE, et al. (1992) Effects on leukocytes after injection of tumor necrosis factor into healthy humans. *Blood* 79: 693–698.

van Laar JM, de Vries RR, Breedveld FC. (1993a) T cell vaccination in humans: the experience in rheumatoid arthritis. *Clin Exp Rheumatol.* 11 Suppl 8: S59–62.

van Laar JM, Miltenburg AM, Verdonk MJ, Leow A, Elferink BG, Daha MR, Cohen IR, de Vries RR, Breedveld FC. (1993b) Effects of inoculation with attenuated autologous T cells in patients with rheumatoid arthritis. *J Autoimmun* 6: 159–167.

van Parijs L, Perez VL, Abbas AK. (1998) Mechanisms of peripheral T cell tolerance. *Novartis Found Symp* 215: 5–14; discussion 14–20.

Vandenbark AA, Chou YK, Whitham R, Bourdette DN, Offner H. (1998) Effects of vaccination with T cell receptor peptides: epitope switching to a possible disease-protective determinant of myelin basic protein that is cross-reactive with a TCR BV peptide. *Immunol Cell Biol* 76: 83–90.

Vella AT, Mitchell T, Groth B, et al. (1997) CD28 engagement and proinflammatory cytokines contribute to T cell expansion and long-term survival in vivo. *J Immunol* 158: 4714–4720.

Vieira P, de Waal-Malefyt R, Dang MN, et al. (1991) Isolation and expression of human cytokine synthesis inhibitory factor cDNA clones: homology to Epstein-Barr virus open reading frame BCRFI. *Proc Natl Acad Sci USA* 88: 1172–1176.

Villalba L, Hicks JE, Adams EM, et al. (1998) Treatment of refractory myositis: a randomized crossover study of two new cytotoxic regimens. *Arthritis Rheum* 41: 392–399.

Villalba ML, Hicks JE, Thornton B, et al. (1995) A combination of oral methotrexate and azathioprine is more effective than high dose intravenous methotrexate with leucovorin rescue in treatment-resistant myositis. *Arthritis Rheum* 38, s307(Abstract).

Wang ZY, He B, Qiao J, Link H. (1995) Suppression of experimental autoimmune myasthenia gravis and experimental allergic encephalomyelitis by oral administration of acetylcholine receptor and myelin basic protein: double tolerance. *J Neuroimmunol* 63: 79–86.

Whitacre CC, Gienapp IE, Orosz CG, Bitar DM. (1991) Oral tolerance in experimental autoimmune encephalomyelitis. III. Evidence for clonal anergy. *J Immunol* 147: 2155–2163.

Wraith DC, Smilek DE, Mitchell DJ, Steinman L, McDevitt HO. (1989) Antigen recognition in autoimmune encephalomyelitis and the potential for peptide-mediated immunotherapy. *Cell* 59: 247–255.

Wucherpfennig KW, Hafler DA, Strominger JL. (1995) Structure of human T-cell receptors specific for an immunodominant myelin basic protein peptide: positioning of T-cell receptors on HLA- DR2/peptide complexes. *Proc Natl Acad Sci USA* 92: 8896–8900.

Yamazaki M, Minota S, Sakurai H, et al. (1994) Expression of transforming growth factor-beta 1 and its relation to endomysial fibrosis in progressive muscular dystrophy. *Am J Pathol* 144: 221–226.

Yi Q, Ahlberg R, Pirskanen R, Lefvert AK. (1994) Acetylcholine receptor-reactive T cells in myasthenia gravis: evidence for the involvement of different subpopulations of T helper cells. *J Neuroimmunol* 50: 177–186.

Zaller DM, Osman G, Kanagawa O, Hood L. (1990) Prevention and treatment of murine experimental allergic encephalomyelitis with T cell receptor V beta-specific antibodies. *J Exp Med* 171: 1943–1955.

Zuk JA, Fletcher A. (1988) Skeletal muscle expression of class II histocompatibility antigens (HLA-DR) in polymyositis and other muscle disorders with an inflammatory infiltrate. *J Clin Pathol* 41: 410–414.

54

Treatment of myasthenia gravis

Mark B. Bromberg

Introduction

Myasthenia gravis (MG) is an autoimmune disorder with autoantibodies to epitopes on and around the neuromuscular junction. Treatment of MG largely follows the principles of immunosuppression for other autoimmune disorders, but there are several unique treatment options available for MG. These include acetylcholine esterase inhibitors that improve neuromuscular junction transmission without altering the immune system, the ability to remove antibodies by therapeutic plasma apheresis and the surgical removal of the thymus gland. Many of the therapeutic options are derived from other autoimmune disorders, and it is important to consider efficacy data derived specifically from trials in MG. Accordingly, this chapter will focus on data from randomized and controlled trials in MG when available, and it will include less robust data when necessary. This chapter will begin with a brief review of the underlying pathophysiology and immunologic mechanisms in MG as an aid to understanding and selecting therapies, but the reader is referred to other chapters in this volume for detailed descriptions of these issues.

Pathophysiology of myasthenia gravis

Normal neuromuscular junction transmission is the faithful conversion of nerve fibre action potentials to muscle fibre action potentials. Transmission is mediated by the release of acetylcholine from presynaptic terminals. Acetylcholine diffuses across the synaptic cleft and interacts with acetylcholine receptors on the postsynaptic membrane. The acetylcholine receptor is a ligand-gated sodium channel that opens and closes in a binary fashion to allow inward sodium currents leading to an excitatory end plate potential. The resultant depolarization opens nearby voltage-gated sodium channels that further increase the inward flow of sodium ions. When the excitatory end-plate potential reaches a threshold level of depolarization, a muscle fibre action potential is initiated. The neuromuscular junction is located at the middle portion of muscle fibres, and the action potential travels along the muscle fibres in both directions. The action potential initiates excitation–contraction coupling along the muscle fibre, resulting in generation of force.

Under normal circumstances, there is more than enough acetylcholine released to interact with the large number of acetylcholine receptors, in order to generate an excitatory end–plate potential that exceeds the threshold for initiation of a muscle fibre action potential. The excess acetylcholine released is called the neuromuscular junction "safety factor", and it accounts for the essentially 100% reliability of transmission under normal circumstances. In MG, there are several antibody-mediated processes that can reduce the safety factor by reducing the number of acetylcholine receptors. When a nerve action potential is not converted into a muscle fibre action potential that muscle fibre does not generate force. A muscle will be clinically weak when a sizable fraction of muscle fibres are not activated. Malfunction of neuromuscular junctions in MG can be very patchy in distribution with a normal junction within 300 μm of a failed neuromuscular junction.

Clinically, MG can be divided into two classes, antibody positive and antibody negative. These designations are operational in that both forms are believed to be mediated primarily by IgG antibodies, but, at this time, antibodies can be detected in 75% to 85% of MG patients (Sanders et al 1997). The preferred terms are seropositive and seronegative MG.

The immunologic aetiology of MG is unknown, but the loss of T cell tolerance is believed to occur in the thymus gland (Sprent and Kishimoto 1998). There are myoid cells in the thymus, and this may account for the organ specificity of antibodies in MG compared with other autoimmune diseases. The process of making autoantibodies involves both the cellular and humoral arms of the immune system.

Principles of therapy

In managing MG patients, it is helpful to keep in mind that the disease has both natural and iatrogenic-induced variability. Some exacerbations are precipitated by infection, others by reduction in medication, but a number occur for unclear reasons. Remissions may occur naturally, following treatment of infections or after treatment specific for MG. The natural history of untreated MG is not well described. However, early reviews indicate that exacerbations can be severe and approximately one quarter to one third of patients died from respiratory failure. Another quarter experienced transitory remissions. One fifth had complete remissions, while a smaller number had mild residual weakness (Grob et al 1981, Oosterhuis 1989). A feature of MG is that patients will experience their most severe exacerbation within 3 to 5 years after onset of their disease (Grob et al 1981, Oosterhuis 1989).

The goal in treating MG is a complete remission, which is defined as no symptoms, no signs and taking no medication. In working toward this goal, several principles can be kept in mind. First, the clinical manifestations of MG vary markedly among patients. Accordingly, treatment regimens also vary. Some patients will require no medication or minimal medication, and the management of others can tax the most experienced clinician. A more realistic treatment goal is to keep the patient at the highest level of function with the least amount of medication. The second principle is that MG is a chronic disease and, for an individual patient, several agents and procedures may be needed at different times. The third principle is to understand the mode of action and duration of the individual therapies to aid in selecting the appropriate agents to optimize strength.

The fourth principle relates to care of patients in crisis, and that is to monitor respiration and support it artificially if necessary. There is no accurate measure of pulmonary function (forced vital capacity, maximum pressures) that will predict failure, and it remains a clinical decision (Rieder et al 1995). Respiratory support will allow time for a careful assessment of factors causing the exacerbation and choice of optimum therapeutic programme. Indeed, the greatest advancement in the treatment of MG is a two-thirds reduction in mortality related to the development of positive pressure ventilation and respiratory intensive care units (Grob et al 1981).

Types of therapy

Acetylcholine esterase inhibitors

Acetylcholine esterase is an enzyme located near acetylcholine receptors, which very rapidly hydrolyses acetylcholine into acetyl Co-A and choline. Acetylcholine esterase inhibitors slow the enzymatic degradation of acetylcholine and increase the chance that acetylcholine molecules will interact with acetylcholine receptors. Acetylcholine esterase inhibitors do not alter the antibody-mediated disease process, but they have the advantage of rapid onset of action. Acetylcholine esterase is also present at autonomic ganglia, and transmission along these fibres can become enhanced with administration of acetylcholine esterase inhibitors.

Removal of antibodies

It has been shown that serum antibodies from both seropositive and seronegative MG patients can directly impair neuromuscular junction transmission (Toyka et al 1977, Burges et al 1994). Conversely, removal of antibodies by therapeutic plasma apheresis can be effective in reversing these antibody-mediated actions. The process of plasma apheresis consists of removing whole blood from the patient, separating the cellular component from the plasma portion and returning the cellular component, along with fluids and albumin, to the patient (Chopek and McCullough 1980). The plasma fraction contains gammaglobulin (IgG), and, during the apheresis procedure, a percentage of the patient's IgG fraction is removed. Approximately 45% of IgG is intravascular, and after apheresis there will be an equilibration with extravascular IgG. Accordingly, more IgG will be removed by a series of aphereses. Plasma apheresis probably does not alter the underlying process of antibody production, but lowering the concentration of acetylcholine antibodies may alter their catabolism. After removal, the time for antibody concentration to return to baseline levels is 4 to 5 weeks (Wood and Jacobs 1986).

Infusion of antibodies

The regulation of antibody production and the pathologic action of autoantibodies in MG is poorly understood. However, there is empiric evidence that infusing exogenous antibodies from pooled donors in the form of intravenous immunoglobulin (IVIg) can be effective in reversing symptoms in MG. The mechanisms of action are speculative, and they include binding of infused anti-idiotypic antibodies to pathogenic antibodies to neutralize them or block their pathogenic activities, or downregulation of B cell production (Dalakas 1998). A recently proposed mechanism is based on IgG catabolism (Yu and Lennon 1999). IgG may normally escape degradation by binding to intracellular receptors that the Fc end of the antibody recognizes (Fc receptors). These receptors become saturated by IVIg leading to an increased rate of endogenous IgG catabolism. In this model, the 28 day half-life of infused immunoglobulins leaves progressively more Fc receptors available, resulting in a return to the slower intrinsic rate of catabolism.

Immunosuppression

The most important treatment modality for MG is immunosuppression. This can be achieved by immunomodulating agents and immunosuppressive agents. Immunomodulating agents are corticosteroids. A number of immunosuppressive agents have been used in MG, primarily as steroid-sparing agents. The mechanisms of action are not clear for MG, but presumably they reduce the production of autoantibodies.

Removal of the thymus gland

Thymic hyperplasia and thymomas are associated with MG. Although the pathophysiologic relationship between the thymus and MG has not been fully clarified, thymectomy has been performed for the treatment of MG since 1934. It has been argued that the effects of removing the thymus gland may take years to become clinically evident. Accordingly, thymectomy is not a surgical cure for MG, and other therapeutic agents may be necessary in the interim.

Specific therapies

When considering therapy for MG, it is important to keep in mind that only a few agents have been subjected to randomized controlled trials for MG. For the majority of agents used in MG, efficacy data are from uncontrolled trials and clinical experience. The interpretation of uncontrolled data may be confounded by the concurrent use of multiple therapeutic agents and natural remissions.

Acetylcholine esterase inhibitors

Historically, acetylcholine esterase inhibitory drugs were the first treatment used for MG (1935). The most commonly used esterase inhibitor is pyridostigmine. It is available in several oral and parenteral forms, as a 60 mg scored tablet, a 180 mg time release capsule, and a syrup (60 mg/5 ml). The half-life of oral pyridostigmine is just under 2 h, with onset of action within 45 min (Riggs 1982). Effective doses begin at 30 mg Q4h. The optimal dosage of pyridostigmine varies among patients, and few derive added benefit above 150 mg at each dose. Most patients do well upon awakening without medication during the night. If clearly necessary, the time capsule can be given at night. Absorbtion of the time release capsules is erratic, and this form is usually not given during the day.

Pyridostigmine is also available in parenteral form when severe bulbar impairment prevents swallowing oral forms. Absorbtion of the oral form is poor (bioavailability 5–10%), and the dose of the parenteral form is approximately 1/30th of the oral form. The half-life of the parenteral form is 90 min. An alternative to frequent intravenous dosing is continuous infusion (Saltis et al 1998). A solution of pyridostigmine (25 mg in 100 ml of 5% dextrose in water) can be infused at 2 mg/h and gradually increased by 0.5 to 1.0 mg/h to a maximum of 4 mg/h.

There is concern for possible over-medication with acetylcholine esterase inhibitors, which could lead to a cholinergic crisis and greater clinical weakness than that due to MG. This is based on the fact that when too many molecules of acetylcholine are present in the synaptic cleft, the quantal release of acetylcholine from the next nerve impulse will be ineffective at generating a muscle fibre action potential. Although a cholinergic crisis is possible, it is extremely rare and most patients with impending respiratory failure have a myasthenic crisis (Rowland 1980, Thomas et al 1997). When the question of a cholinergic crisis arises, it is clinically prudent to stop pyridostigmine, support respiration if necessary and thoroughly evaluate the patient.

There are other acetylcholine esterase inhibitors for special circumstances. Neostigmine is available in oral and parenteral forms. It is more potent but has a shorter half-life than pyridostigmine (50 min versus 2 h). There are no clear advantages of neostigmine over pyridostigmine. Edrophonium is only available in parenteral form and has a half-life of 3 min. Accordingly, it is used as an aid in the diagnosis of MG, or as a test to determine if a very weak MG patient is under-medicated (myasthenic crisis) or over-medicated (cholinergic crisis) with esterase inhibitors. The usual dose of edrophonium is 10 mg in 1 ml. The testing procedure is to give a 2 mg (0.2 ml) test dose to determine if the patient will have muscarinic side-effects of bradycardia and excess bronchial secretions. Atropine (0.4 mg) should be available to counteract these. If the test dose is tolerated, the remaining 8 mg can be injected and its clinical effects observed. For an edrophonium test to be considered positive, during either a diagnostic evaluation or investigation of a crisis, an unequivocal clinical change should be apparent.

The side-effects of pyridostigmine are more troublesome than severe. Direct effects at the neuromuscular junction are increased frequency of fasciculations. Indirect effects are a result of increased autonomic nervous system activity, most commonly as gastro-intestinal cramping and diarrhoea, and less commonly as increased oral secretions and increased sweating. Diarrhoea is transient, occurring during peak blood levels, and can be treated with atropine sulphate (0.4 mg PO QD or BID), glycopyrronium bromide (1 to 2 mg PO BID to TID) or propantheline (2 mg PO QD or BID).

There have been no formal controlled trials of acetylcholine esterase inhibitors in MG, but the edrophonium test is frequently performed using a test syringe and a placebo syringe and the effect monitored by a blinded observer (Riggs 1982). Although efficacy of pyridostigmine in MG is not in doubt, the response varies among patients (Rowland 1980). Some gain good strength from a dose and can detect a wearing off when a dose is missed. Patients may find that an extra tablet before physical activity is beneficial. Other patients derive little benefit from pyridostigmine. For unclear reasons, acetylcholine esterase inhibitors appear to be less effective for ocular and bulbar weakness than for limb weakness.

In review, pyridostigmine is a reasonable initial drug for MG because it has rapid onset of therapeutic action. A clear response helps confirm the diagnosis of a disorder of neuromuscular transmission. The dosage can easily and quickly be increased to maximum effect. If a patient remains functionally disabled with optimum use of pyridostigmine, other therapeutic modalities need to be considered. At some point, the efficacy of pyridostigmine should be reassessed and discontinued if no longer effective.

Therapeutic plasma apheresis

Therapeutic plasma apheresis usually consists of a series of aphereses, but the optimum number has not been established. It is common to give four to six, but there are data to suggest that two aphereses may be as effective (Mantegazza et al 1987). A QOD schedule is used to allow time for fibrinogen and other clotting factors to return to a reasonable level. The first two aphereses can be performed on consecutive days without clotting problems, or fresh frozen plasma can be given to rapidly restore clotting factors, but QD aphereses are not clinically necessary.

There are no randomized and controlled trials for plasma apheresis in MG. Clinical experience with objective measures of strength and respiratory function shows a rapid improvement in strength when apheresis is the sole treatment (Milner-Brown and Miller 1982, Antozzi et al 1991, Goti et al 1995, Gajdos et al 1997). The clinical response to plasma apheresis can be within the same day, but usually occurs within 1 to 2 weeks after the start of a series of aphereses (Milner-Brown and Miller 1982). The response to apheresis is usually limited, from weeks to months. Accordingly, plasma apheresis is most commonly used in MG to rapidly improve strength in the treatment of crisis, to maximize strength prior to surgery, or as part of a maintenance regimen in a patient who is resistant to more conventional maintenance therapies (Dau 1980). In these rare circumstances, apheresis schedules are based on patient response, and they may be as frequent as every 10 days.

Plasma apheresis is well tolerated. The most common side-effects are hypotension, dizziness and perioral tingling (Therapeutics and Technology Assessment Subcommittee 1996). Risks of disease transmission are not an issue if only albumin is used as the replacement fluid. The greatest potential for complications comes from vascular access. When the use of peripheral veins is limited, the need for a central venous line can be associated with improper placement, infection and damage to nerves in the neck.

In review, plasma apheresis is an effective treatment for severe weakness in MG, but its effect is temporary. There are two other practical issues with plasma apheresis. One is accessibility to the appropriate machine. Apheresis should be performed on a machine specifically designed for the procedure, although haemodialysis machines can be modified to perform apheresis. This makes plasma apheresis most commonly available in large medical centres. A second issue is cost. Each apheresis, in the US, costs between $1000 and $2000, and a series will range from $5000 to $10 000. This expense should be balanced against the costs of respiratory failure and intensive care costs.

Intravenous immune globulin

IVIg is the gammaglobulin fraction pooled from several thousand donors, and contains immunoglobulins of all classes. Approximately one in a thousand individuals has a selected IgA immune deficiency, but only one third will have anti-IgA antibodies. A small percentage of these, most commonly in patients with common variable immunodeficiency, will have an anaphylactic reaction (Burks et al 1986). It is prudent to perform quantitative immunoglobulin testing before administering IVIg. The plasma extraction process is regulated, and the risk of infection is very low. There have been no cases of transmission of the human immunodeficiency virus. There have been cases of possible hepatitis C transmission, but the treatment process has been modified since that time and is now believed safe (Dalakas 1998).

A sound protocol for IVIg therapy has not been determined. It is common to initiate therapy with a high dose and use a lower dose for maintenance. The customary initial dose is 2 g/kg administered in divided doses over 2 to 5 consecutive days. Dividing the dose reduces the hyperviscosity effect of the infused immunoglobulins, which is preferable in the elderly who are more likely to have cerebrovascular disease and in patients with renal disease. A lower maintenance dose of 1 g/kg over 1 day can be given based on a schedule or to treat a relapse.

There are no randomized and controlled trials of IVIg in MG. IVIg has been used to treat myasthenic crisis and as maintenance therapy. In one trial, 87 patients were randomized to receive plasma apheresis (three) or IVIg (0.4 g/kg per day for 3 to 5 days (Gajdos et al 1997). Patients were assessed at 15 days, with a functional scale. Apheresis and IVIg were equally effective. Sixty-one per cent of patients receiving 3 days of IVIg responded, but curiously, only 39% who received 5 days of IVIg responded (not statistically significant). Although the long-term efficacy of IVIg was not assessed in this study, it appears that there is no added benefit to higher dose and longer duration therapy.

Most reports of IVIg in MG are case series. A review of published reports enrolling 10 or more patients has been made (van der Meché and van Doorn 1997). Many patients were taking other drugs concurrently for MG. The overall response rate for IVIg was 76% (range 48–92%, median 87%), with improvement beginning in the first week and lasting from 2 to 9 weeks. There are little clinical data to guide the interval of IVIg as maintenance therapy. One approach is to taper the initial dose by keeping the interval at 1 month (the half-life of IVIg) and lowering the dosage. The specific taper rate can be determined by patient response.

IVIg is well tolerated. The most common side-effects are myalgias, arthalgias and headache. These can largely be prevented by premedication with diphenhydramine 25 to 50 mg PO and ibuprofen 400 mg PO before and Q4 h for the next 24 h. Aseptic meningitis may be prevented by pretreatment with ibuprofen. Rare side-effects include stroke in patients with cerebral vascular disease and acute renal failure in patients with preexisting renal disease (Dalakas 1998).

In review, the response to IVIg is variable among MG patients and less predictable than plasma apheresis. It is best considered as part of the armamentarium. It is expensive for routine treatment without good reasons, such as the medical need for a steroid-sparing agent or for a patient in a crisis who has insufficient venous access for plasma apheresis. An infusion of 2 g/kg in the US costs between $2000 and $4000. Over the past few years IVIg has been used for a larger number of conditions and there has been an increase in the demand leading to shortages. One advantage of IVIg therapy is that it can be performed anywhere, including in the patient's home. Infusion requires the presence of an experienced nurse, and it is customary to give the first infusion in a clinical setting (hospital or office) to determine if it is well tolerated.

Corticosteroids

Corticosteroids have been used to treat MG since 1935. They are frequently considered to be the initial immunomodulating agent if symptoms can not be managed by acetylcholine esterase inhibitors alone. Oral prednisone, or prednisolone, is usually started at a high dose and then tapered. A common starting dose of prednisone is 40–60 mg PO QAM for 4 to 6 weeks. There are many taper schedules, and the goal is to reduce prednisone before side-effects become problematic, but not so rapidly as to induce a relapse. Many taper schedules include an early shift from QD to QOD dosage because it is believed that side-effects are reduced on a QOD schedule (Frey and Frey 1990). The dosage is decreased by 5–10 mg every 2 weeks. The rate of taper frequently slows when doses of 20 mg QOD are reached. Some patients will relapse when the taper reaches zero, but will be maintained at doses of 5–10 mg QOD (Pascuzzi et al 1984).

There is a concern that an MG patient who is naïve to corticosteroids may experience transient weakness, which may include respiratory failure, developing within 2 weeks of starting high-dose prednisone (60 mg QD) (Pascuzzi et al 1984). To prevent this, the dose can be raised to 60 mg in steps over 4 to 6 days (20 mg for 2 days, 40 mg for 2 days, and then 60 mg), or the patient should be watched in the hospital.

The side-effects of long-term corticosteroids have been described (Pascuzzi et al 1984). The most common one is weight gain, more from increased appetite than from fluid. Others include the onset or worsening of diabetes melitis, demineralization of bone, and gastric or duodenal haemorrhage. It is prudent to emphasize the use of calcium (1500 mg PO QD), and an initial evaluation for bone density if the patients is at risk of osteoporosis. There is also a concern of steroid myopathy with long-term administration. It can be difficult to differentiate between myasthenic weakness and myopathy. When this is an issue, quantitative electrophysiological testing can be helpful. For example, the initial severity of MG can be assessed by the amount of decrement to repetitive nerve stimulation or by the amount of jitter from single fibre electromyography (EMG). Initial values can be compared with values obtained during treatment; improved electrophysiological testing suggests a myopathy while worsening electrophysiological testing suggests an exacerbation of MG.

There have been no randomized and controlled trials of corticosteroids in MG. However, empiric data from case series have confirmed its efficacy. In a review of 116 MG patients followed for up to 17 years who received prednisone (60 to 80 mg QD with a subsequent taper to QOD schedule), 80% had a satisfactory outcome defined as marked improvement or remission (Pascuzzi et al 1984). Clinical improvement began in the majority by 3 weeks after starting therapy, and maximal improvement was achieved by 6 months. The minimum maintenance dose was established by trial, with 60% requiring a maintenance dose of 5 to 50 mg QOD, and 40% in remission on no prednisone. In another retrospective study, 60 patients received prednisone at varying starting doses followed by a taper (Sghirlanzoni et al 1984). Five per cent were in complete remission, 37% were without symptoms but required steroids and 30% were improved.

High-dose intravenous methylprednisolone has been used in place of long-term oral prednisone to reduce side-effects. In a randomized and placebo controlled trial, 20 MG patients were randomized to receive methylprednisolone (2 g QD for 2 days) or placebo (Lindberg et al 1998). The endpoint measure was improvement in a muscle fatigue test. Improvement was observed in 80% of patients receiving methylprednisolone and in 10% of patients receiving placebo. Improvement lasted from 4 to 14 weeks. High-dose intravenous methylprednisolone has also been used in an uncontrolled trial to bring about a rapid reversal of a severe exacerbation (Arsura et al 1985). Fifteen patients with impending respiratory failure received methylprednisolone (2 gm IV) every 5 days until a response was observed or to a maximum of three treatments. A satisfactory response was observed in 10 patients after two doses, and in two additional patients after a third dose. Most patients in this series were naïve to corticosteroids, and oral prednisone was started at the same time.

In review, corticosteroids are the mainstay of therapy in MG patients who can not be maintained on pyridostigmine alone. It is reliable when an initial high dose is given, followed by a slow taper, but patients frequently require a low maintenance dose. Corticosteroids are relatively safe, but long-term side-effects are of concern.

Azathioprine

Azathioprine may be given as a fixed dose of 2 to 3 mg/kg QD or titrated upward until blood cell indices change (an elevation in the mean corpuscular volume or a fall in the total while cell count). The drug is usually started at 50 mg PO QD and raised to the final BID dose over several weeks. During dose escalation, biweekly haematologic monitoring for early blood cell suppression is recommended. Liver transaminase levels may also rise, and these should also be monitored. An occasional patient will experience a white cell count drop after a period of stability, and twice yearly haematologic monitoring is recommended after a stable dose has been achieved (Kissel et al 1986).

Azathioprine is well tolerated by most patients, but 15–20% experience an idiosyncratic reaction within the first 3 weeks after starting the drug (Kissel et al 1986, Hohlfeld et al 1988). The reaction is characterized by influenza-like symptoms with arthralgias and myalgias, fever and a high erythrocyte sedimentation rate. Symptoms resolve promptly with stoppage of the drug. Occasionally re-challenging with the drug at a lower starting dose is successful. There is a long-term concern for an increased incidence of lymphomas. Data from patients taking azathioprine for other diseases shows a greater than chance increased incidence of this type of tumour 15 to 20 years later (Krueger et al 1985). The teratogenic effects of azathioprine are unknown and the drug should be used with caution in patients of either gender when pregnancy is a possibility (Seybold 1998).

Azathioprine has been used as the sole immunosuppressive agent or as a steroid-sparing agent. There has been one randomized and controlled trial comparing azathioprine (2.5 mg/kg) to prednisone (60 mg QD for 6 weeks followed by a taper) as the first and sole immunosuppressive drug in 10 MG patients (Bromberg et al 1997). Patients were followed for 1 year and a disability scale was the endpoint measure. Of the five patients who were randomized to azathioprine, two had idiosyncratic reactions, two completed 1 year on azathioprine with little improvement and were crossed over to prednisone with a good response, and one patient had a satisfactory response.

In another trial, 41 patients were randomized to azathioprine (3 mg/kg QD) or prednisone (1 mg/kg QD for 1 month followed by a taper) (Myasthenia Gravis Clinical Study Group 1993). It must be noted that patients randomized to azathioprine also received prednisone (1 mg/kg) for the first month. Patients were followed an average of 30 months and clinical deterioration was the endpoint. Nine out of 21 patients on azathioprine deteriorated, compared with 12 out of 20 patients on prednisone (not significant). There were significantly more treatment failures in the group taking prednisone.

There has been a non-randomized trial of azathioprine as the sole drug in 32 patients who had slow progression of disease (Mantegazza et al 1988). Patients were followed for 1 year. Seventy-five per cent of patients responded to some degree and 25% had a complete remission. Patients who did not respond to azathioprine did respond to other medications (prednisone). In another non-randomized study, eight of 24 patients showed a response to azathioprine alone (Witte et al 1984).

The long-term need for azathioprine has been assessed in a prospective study (Hohlfeld et al 1985). Fifteen patients who were receiving azathioprine alone or in combination with methylprednisolone had their azathioprine stopped abruptly and methylprednisolone tapered over 1 month. Eight of 15 patients experienced a relapse within 11 months of stopping their medication, and seven remained stable for 20 to 40 months.

There has been a randomized and controlled trial of the steroid-sparing action of azathioprine (Palace et al 1998). Patients were randomized to receive either azathioprine (2.5 mg/kg QD) with prednisolone (1.5 mg/kg QOD followed by a taper to the minimal dose required to sustain remission) or prednisolone alone. The study showed no difference in prednisolone dose between the two groups after 1 year, but after 2 years there was a significant reduction in the dose of prednisolone required to sustain remission in the group taking azathioprine.

In review, azathioprine is less effective as a first line immunosuppressive drug for MG and more effective as a corticosteroid-sparing agent. However, it takes up to 2 years for maximum efficacy to become apparent, and consideration for starting the drug should be given early in the treatment with corticosteroids. A percentage of patients will not tolerate azathioprine, and another group should not receive it because of potential teratogenic effects.

Ciclosporin

There have been two randomized and controlled trials of ciclosporin in MG. In the first, 20 patients who were taking only acetylcholine esterase inhibitory therapy were randomized to ciclosporin (6 mg/kg QD in a single dose) or placebo (Tindall et al 1987). At 6 months and 12 months, patients taking ciclosporin had significantly less disability and no treatment failures compared to the placebo group. Nephrotoxicity occurred in three patients but was reversible with dose reduction. In the second trial, 39 patients who had prominent symptoms despite moderate to high doses of corticosteroid therapy were randomized to BID ciclosporin in an effort to increase trough serum levels but reduce peak levels and nephrotoxicity (Tindall et al 1993). Ciclosporin was initiated at 5 mg/kg in divided dosage and adjusted to trough levels of 300 to 500 ng/ml. A rapid steroid taper was begun after 2 months. The endpoint at 6 months was failure to complete the steroid taper, measured by respiratory failure or bulbar weakness that did not respond to increasing steroids. At 6 months the ciclosporin group had significantly fewer symptoms and greater strength, but patients were not able to significantly reduce their steroid needs compared with the placebo group. There has also been an open label trial of ciclosporin in severe MG (Bonifati and Angelini 1997). Patients were treated with cyclosporine 5 to 6 mg/kg BID or TID initially and tapered to approximately 4 mg/kg. Concurrent treatment with azathioprine was stopped and corticosteroids were tapered. Patients were followed for 16 to 36 months and there was an average reduction of steroid dosage from 53 mg QD to 17 mg QD.

In review, ciclosporin may be effective in MG. Its side-effects and cost make it a drug primarily for difficult to treat MG patients.

Thymectomy

Thymectomy is the most controversial issue in the treatment of MG. There are many variables that are difficult to factor into the interpretation of the literature, including the surgical approach, the follow-up time interval and whether immunosuppressive or modulating drugs were used to help control the disease during the follow-up period. It is worthwhile reviewing the major factors. The surgical removal of the thymus gland is a straight forward procedure with minimal mortality and little morbidity. There is, however, a debate on which surgical procedure gives optimal access to the gland. Thymic tissue is intermixed with mediastinal fat, and rests of thymic tissue may be found from the diaphragm into the neck (Jaretzki 1997). The least invasive procedure is video-assisted thoracoscopic thymectomy where the thymus is observed with an endoscope and tissue is removed by instrumentation. Another less invasive approach is to enter the mediastinum through a cervical incision. A more direct approach is to open the sternum, either by a partial sternotomy or a full sternotomy. The most complete procedure is to explore all areas where thymic tissue has been found, from the diaphragm to the neck, by opening both the sternum and at the neck (Jaretzki 1997). It is the surgeon who usually makes the choice.

There are no randomized and controlled trials of thymectomy in MG, and most studies compare surgical results with historic controls. A computer-assisted case control study of the effects of thymectomy has been carried out (Buckingham et al 1976). Eighty MG patients who had a thymectomy were matched with 80 patients treated medically based on age, gender and severity and duration of disease. A complete remission was experienced in 35% of the thymectomy patients compared with 8% of the medically treated group. One third of the surgical group experienced an improvement compared with 17% in the medical group.

Most case series favour a better long-term outcome after thymectomy (Rowland 1980), but there are exceptions. An extensive review of MG treatment from one clinic under the direction of the same clinician affords the chance to compare patient response over a long period (Grob et al 1987). From 1940–1985, 1487 MG patients were followed for an average of 18 years each. Patients who had a thymectomy between 1940 and 1957 had a higher rate of remission than patients who were treated medically. Patients who had a thymectomy between 1958 and 1985 did not fair better than medically treated patients. It was felt that during the period 1958 to 1985 both the thymectomy and medically treated patients owed their general improvement to the use of corticosteroids.

The greatest success with thymectomy has been reported with an en bloc transcervical–transsternal procedure (Jaretzki et al 1988). The results in 75 patients followed for 6 to 89 months revealed that 96% derived benefit, 79% were symptom free, 46% were in complete remission and 33% were symptom free while receiving only pyridostignime. However, a recent comparison has been made for the long-term outcome of complete remission between the transcervical approach and other operative procedures. There were no significant differences for the various procedures.

Thymectomy and the surgical procedure will remain controversial because of the inability to perform sham operations, the use of immunosuppressive and modulating therapy during the follow-up period, and the natural history of MG. Exacerbations and remissions in MG may be spontaneous, caused by other medical conditions, such as infections, or related to adjustments in treatment. Further, the effects of thymectomy are thought to take years to become fully manifest. Accordingly, one must be conservative in interpreting patient series reports.

In review, there remains a consensus, at least in North America, that thymectomy increases the chances that a patient will achieve a complete remission or a favourable long-term outcome. There is a question of whether it is appropriate for patients who are seronegative. The decision to perform a thymectomy must be tempered with the general physical state of the patient and the degree of weakness. Thymectomy is appropriate when a thymoma is suspected. There have been concerns that thymectomy may be less effective if the duration between MG symptom onset is long or the patient is older. The analysis of several case series indicates no significant differences (Buckingham et al 1976).

Treatment of myasthenia gravis in children

This review has largely focused on data from treatment trials in adults. Juvenile acquired MG should be distinguished from congenital MG, a family of genetic disorders of the neuromuscular junction. The clinical spectrum of juvenile MG is similar to adult MG, but there may be differences in the long-term outcome based on race and whether the symptoms began before or after puberty (Andrews et al 1994).

There have been no randomized and controlled treatment trials in juvenile MG. In a case series of 32 children, pyridostigmine controlled symptoms in 41%, and prednisone was required in the remaining patients (Snead et al 1980). Plasma apheresis was effective but temporary in one patient. In another patient series, 149 juvenile MG patients were followed for a mean of 17 years (Rodriguez et al 1983). Twenty-two patients had a spontaneous remission rate. In this series, 57% received a thymectomy based on severity of disease and 40% of these had a remission within 3 years. Twenty-four per cent of patients who had a thymectomy required corticosteroids; they were effective in 30%, and lack of efficacy in some of the remaining may have been due to inadequate corticosteroid dosage. Data from the side-effects of long-term corticosteroid therapy in children are derived from treatment of other medical disorders, but they indicate that low doses for shorter intervals and QOD dose schedules are associated with fewer adverse effects on growth and other side-effects (Seybold 1998).

The question of the efficacy of thymectomy in children has been approached by reviewing five published juvenile case series (Seybold 1998). The review suggests that the remission rate may be as high as 57% among patients operated within the first 2 years after MG onset, 25% among patients operated after the first 2 years, and 20% among patients treated medically (spontaneous remission). The concern for adverse effects on the immune system related to thymectomy in children has not been born out.

In review, the overall treatment of MG is similar for children as for adults (Andrews 1998). Children have a better chance for a spontaneous remission and a better outcome after early thymectomy. Concern for side-effects includes growth retardation.

Summary

The treatment of MG must be tailored to the individual because the disease varies marked among patients. However, general guidelines can be proposed from clinical experience and with data from clinical trials (Keesey 1998a and b). First, the diagnosis must be secure. This may be problematic if the symptoms are very mild and acetylcholine receptor antibodies are normal, for false positive diagnoses have been described. Second, initial treatment with pyridostigmine is reasonable because the clinical response occurs rapidly. In a small number of patients, pyridostigmine may control symptoms and can be used as the sole agent. Conversely, it may be withdrawn without worsening symptoms in a surprisingly large number of patients after starting treatment with other modalities. Plasma apheresis or IVIg may be used when a patient is very weak or experiencing an acute exacerbation. An alternative treatment is high-dose intravenous methylprednisolone. The majority of MG patients will require immunomodulation or suppression. Prednisone is the most reliable, with initial doses of 60 mg QD for approximately 1 month followed by a slow taper reaching levels of 20 to 30 mg QOD over 6 months. Patients may require a low maintenance prednisone dose to prevent an exacerbation. Azathioprine may be started concomitant with prednisone to improve the chances of achieving better control with less or no steroids after 2 years. Ciclosporin may be used in challenging patients. A chest computed tomography (CT) scan should be obtained in all MG patients at time of diagnosis. If the thymus is enlarged, a thymectomy should be performed because it may harbour a thymoma. If the thymus is not enlarged, consideration should be given to a thymectomy because it will optimize the likelihood for a remission. Some patients with severe disease are clinically challenging. Although they can usually be helped, they may require multiple treatment modalities and close evaluation.

References

Andrews P. (1998) A treatment algorithm for autoimmune myasthenia gravis in childhood. *Ann NY Acad Sci* 841: 789–802.

Andrews P, Massey J, Howard J, Sanders D. (1994) Race, sex, and puberty influence onset, severity, and outcome in juvenile myasthenia gravis. *Neurology* 44: 1208–1214.

Antozzi C, Gemma M, Regi B, et al. (1991) A short plasma exchange protocol is effective in severe myasthenia gravis. *J Neurol* 238: 103–107.

Arsura E, Brunner N, Namba T, Grob D. (1985) High-dose intravenous methylprednisolone in myasthenia gravis. *Arch Neurol* 42: 1149–1153.

Bonifati D, Angelini C. (1997) Long-term cyclosporine treatment in a group of severe myasthenia gravis patients. *J Neurol* 244: 542–547.

Bromberg M, Wald J, Forshew D, Feldman E, Albers J. (1997) Randomized trial of azathioprine or prednisone for initial immunosuppressive treatment of myasthenia gravis. *J Neurol Sci* 150: 59–62.

Buckingham J, Howard F, Bernatz P, et al. (1976) The value of thymectomy in myasthenia gravis: A computer-assisted matched study. *Ann Surg* 184: 453–457.

Burges J, Vincent A, Molenaar P, Newsom-Davis J, Peers C, Wray D. (1994) Passive transfer of seronegative myasthenia gravis to mice. *Muscle Nerve* 17: 1393–1400.

Burks A, Sampson H, Buckley R. (1986) Anaphylactic reactions after gamma globulin administration in patients with hypogammaglobulinemia. *N Engl J Med* 314: 560–564.

Chopek M, McCullough J. (1980) Protein and biochemical changes during plasma exchange: American Association of Blood Banks.

Dalakas M. (1998) Mechanisms of action if intravenous immunoglobulin and therapeutic considerations in the treatment of autoimmune neurologic diseases. *Neurology* 51 (Suppl 5): S2–S8.

Dau P. (1980) Plasmapheresis therapy in myasthenia gravis. *Muscle Nerve* 3: 468–482.

Frey B, Frey F. (1990) Clinical pharmacokinetics of prednisone and prednisolone. *Clin Pharmacokinetics* 19: 126–146.

Gajdos P, Chevret S, Clair B, Tranchant C, Chastang C, Group MGS. (1997) Clinical trial of plasma exchange and high-dose intravenous immunoglobulin in myasthenia gravis. *Neurology* 41: 789–796.

Goti P, Spinelli A, Marconi G, et al. (1995) Comparative effects of plasma exchange and pyridostigmine on respiratory muscle strength and breathing pattern in patients with myasthenia gravis. *Thorax* 50: 1080–1086.

Grob D, Asura E, Brunner N, Namba T. (1987) The course of myasthenia gravis and therapies affecting outcome. *Ann NY Acad Sci* 505: 472–499.

Grob D, Brunner N, Namba T. (1981) The natural course of myasthenia gravis and effect of therapeutic measures. *Ann NY Acad Sci* 377: 652–669.

Hohlfeld R, Michels M, Heininger K, Besinger U, Toyka K. (1988) Azathioprine toxicity during long-term immunosuppression of generalized myasthenia gravis. *Neurology* 38: 258–261.

Hohlfeld R, Toyka K, Besinger U, Gerhold B, Keininger K. (1985) Myasthenia gravis: Reactivation of clinical disease and of autoimmune factors after discontinuation of long-term azathioprine. *Ann Neurol* 17: 238–242.

Jaretzki A. (1997) Thymectomy for myasthenia gravis: Analysis of the controversies regarding technique and results. *Neurology* 48 (Suppl): S52–S63.

Jaretzki A, Penn A, Younger D, et al. (1988) "Maximal" thymectomy for myasthenia gravis. *J Thoracic Cardiovasc Surg* 95: 747–757.

Keesey J. (1998) A treatment algorithm for autoimmune myasthenia in adults. *Ann NY Acad Sci* 841: 753–768.

Keesey J. (1998) Myasthenia gravis. *Arch Neurol* 55(5): 746–746.

Kissel J, Levy R, Mendell J, Griggs R. (1986) Azathioprine toxicity in neuromuscular disease. *Neurology* 36: 35–39.

Krueger J, Tallent M, Richie R, Johnson H, MacDonnel R, Turner B. (1985) Neoplasia in immunosuppressed renal transplant patients: A 20-year experience. *Southern Med J* 78: 501–505.

Lindberg C, Andersen O, Lefvert A. (1998) Treatment of myasthenia gravis with methylprednisolone pulse: a double blind study. *Acta Neurol Scand* 97: 370–373.

Mantegazza R, Antozzi C, Peluchetti D, Sghirlanzoni A, Cornelio F. (1988) Azathioprine as a single drug or in combination with steroids in the treatment of myasthenia gravis. *J Neurol* 235: 449–453.

Mantegazza R, Bruzzone E, Regi B, et al. (1987) Single donor plasma in therapeutic plasma exchange in myasthenia gravis. *Intl J Artificial Organs* 5: 315–318.

Milner-Brown H, Miller R. (1982) Time course of improved neuromuscular function following plasma exchange alone and plasma exchange with prednisone/azathioprine in myasthenia gravis. *J Neurol Sci* 57: 357–368.

Myasthenia Gravis Clinical Study Group. (1993) A randomized clinical trial comparing prednisone and azathioprine in myasthenia gravis. Results of the second interim analysis. *J Neurol Neurosurg Psychiat* 56: 1157–1163.

Oosterhuis H. (1989) The natural course of myasthenia gravis: a long term follow up study. *J Neurol Neurosurg Psychiat* 52: 1121–1127.

Palace J, Newsom-Davis J, Lecky B, Group MGS. (1998) A randomized double-blind trial of prednisolone alone or with azathioprine in myasthenia gravis. *Neurology* 50: 1778–1783.

Pascuzzi R, Coslett B, Johns T. (1984) Long-term corticosteroid treatment of myasthenia gravis: Report of 116 patients. *Ann Neurol* 15: 291–298.

Rieder P, Louis M, Jolliet P, Chevrolet J-C. (1995) The repeated measurement of vital capacity is a poor predictor of the need for mechanical ventilation in myasthenia gravis. *Intens Care Med* 21: 663.

Riggs J. (1982) Pharmacologic enhancement of neuromuscular transmission in myasthenia gravis. *Clin Neuropharmacol* 5: 277–292.

Rodriguez M, Gomez M, Howard F, Taylor W. (1983) Myasthenia gravis in children: Long-term follow-up. *Ann Neurol* 13: 504–510.

Rowland L. (1980) Controversies about the treatment of mysthenia gravis. *J Neurol Neurosurg Psychiat* 43: 644–659.

Saltis L, Martin B, Traeger S, Bonfiglio M. (1998) Continuous infusion of pyridostigmine in the management of myasthenic crisis. *Crit Care Med* 21: 938.

Sanders D, Andrews P, Howard J, JM M. (1997) Seronegative myasthenia gravis. *Neurology* 48(Suppl): S40–S45.

Seybold M. (1998) Thymectomy in childhood myasthenia gravis. *Ann NY Acad Sci* 841: 731–741.

Sghirlanzoni A, Peluchetti D, Mantegazza R, Fiacchino F, Cornelio F. (1984) Myasthenia gravis: Prolonged treatment with steroids. *Neurology* 34: 170–174.

Snead O, Benton J, Dwyer D, et al. (1980) Juvenile myasthenia gravis. *Neurology* 30: 732–739.

Sprent J, Kishimoto H. (1998) T cell tolerance in the thymus. *Ann NY Acad Sci* 841: 236–245.

Therapeutics and Technology Assessment Subcommittee. (1996) Assessment of plasmapheresis. *Neurology* 47: 840–843.

Thomas C, Mayer S, Gungor Y, et al. (1997) Myasthenic crisis: Clinical features, mortality, complications, and risk factors for prolonged intubation. *Neurology* 48: 1253–1260.

Tindall R, Phillips J, Rollins J, Wells L, Hall K. (1993) A clinical therapeutic trial of cyclosporine in myasthenia gravis. *Ann NY Acad Sci* 681: 539–551.

Tindall R, Rollins J, Phillips J, Greenlee R, Wells L, Belendiuk G. (1987) Preliminary results of a double-blinded, randomized, placebo-controlled trial of cyclosporine in myasthenia gravis. *N Engl J Med* 316: 719–724.

Toyka K, Drachman D, Griffin D, et al. (1977) Myasthenia gravis: study of humoral immune mechanisms in passive transfer to mice. *N Engl J Med* 296: 125–131.

van der Meché F, van Doorn P. (1997) The current place of high-dose immunoglobulins in the treatment of neuro-muscular disorders. *Muscle Nerve* 20: 136–147.

Witte A, Cornblath D, Parry G, Lisak R, Schatz N. (1984) Azathioprine in the treatment of myasthenia gravis. *Ann Neurol* 15: 602–605.

Wood L, Jacobs P. (1986) The effect of serial therapeutic plasmapheresis on platelet count, coagulation factors, plasma immunoglobulin, and complement levels. *J Clin Apheresis* 3: 124–128.

Yu Z, Lennon V. (1999) Mechanism of intravenous immune globulin therapy in antibody-mediated auto-immune diseases. *N Engl J Med* 340: 227–228.

55

Pharmacological preconditioning of skeletal muscle against infarction

Cho Y. Pang and Christopher R. Forrest

Introduction

Skeletal muscle is routinely subjected to warm global ischaemia in many clinical situations such as autogenous muscle transplantation and application of vascular clamps or tourniquets in vascular and musculoskeletal reconstructive surgery. Human skeletal muscle is known to tolerate warm (room temperature) global ischaemia for up to 2.5 h with minimal risk of irreversible ischaemic injury (Blaisdell et al 1978, Sjostrom et al 1982, Rutherford 1987, Eckert and Schnackerz 1991). However, prolonged or repeated ischaemic insults to skeletal muscles sometimes occur in these clinical situations as a result of unexpected intra- and/or postoperative complications. Although reperfusion is established, various amounts of irreversible muscle damage (infarction) may occur (Blaipdell et al 1978, Matsen and Krugmire 1978, Haimovici 1979a, Hollier 1983, Tawes et al 1985), and this phenomenon is known as ischaemia/reperfusion injury (Walker 1986). Muscle infarction causes considerable morbidity, and it may require additional surgery and hospitalization. Occasionally, life threatening hyperkalaemia, acidosis, myoglobinurea and renal failure can occur if muscle infarction is extensive (Blaisdell et al 1978, Haimovici 1979b, McCarron et al 1979, Rakowski and Cerasaro 1979). In recent years, much effort has been directed to studying the mechanism of postischaemic microvascular dysfunction and skeletal muscle reperfusion injury, with the ultimate goal of identifying effective pharmacological agents for the prevention of muscle necrosis. This area of research has been reviewed in detail (Rubin et al 1996). However, ischaemia/reperfusion injury occurs during sustained ischaemia as well as postischaemic reperfusion. Therefore, in our opinion, pharmacological intervention of skeletal muscle ischaemia/reperfusion injury should be directed at mitigation of injury occurring during ischaemia. The pathogenic mechanisms of ischaemia and reperfusion injury are interrelated and mitigation of ischaemic injury by increasing ischaemic tolerance will most likely reduce reperfusion injury. The purpose of this review is to discuss the efficacy, mechanism and potential clinical application of acute ischaemic preconditioning of skeletal muscle, for induction of ischaemic tolerance as a new alternative approach for preventation of skeletal muscle from ischaemia/reperfusion injury.

Evidence of cytoprotective effect of acute ischaemic preconditioning in skeletal muscle

Our idea of augmentation of ischaemic tolerance for prevention of ischaemic injury in skeletal muscle is derived from the phenomenon of ischaemic preconditioning of myocardium against infarction in the dog (Murry et al 1986). Specifically, it was observed that ischaemic preconditioning (IPC) of dog myocardium with four cycles of 5-min ischaemia and 5-min reperfusion reduced myocardial infarction when the myocardium was subsequently subjected to 40 min of sustained ischaemia and 4 days of reperfusion. Further studies from the same laboratory showed that myocardial IPC in the dog was associated with preservation of high energy phosphate production capacity, and reduction of the cellular load of metabolites (Murry et al 1990). Subsequently, other investigators reported that one brief cycle of IPC was effective to induce myocardial ischaemic tolerance in the rat (Yellon et al 1992), rabbit (Van Winkle et al 1991), dog (Li et al 1990) and pig (Schulz et al 1994). In 1992, we demonstrated for the first time the phenomenon of IPC against infarction in skeletal muscle in the pig (Mounsey and Pang 1992). Subsequently, we also demonstrated in pig lattisimus dorsi (LD) and gracilis muscles that the threshold of IPC against infarction was higher in the skeletal muscle than in the cardiac muscle. Specifically, a minimum of three cycles of 10-min ischaemia/reperfusion were required to induce significant anti-infarction effect in pig LD and gracilis muscles subjected to 4 hours of global ischaemia and 48 hours of reperfusion. The infarct size was reduced by 40% and 60% in LD and gracilis muscles, respectively, compared with the ischaemic control (Pang et al 1995). This infarct protective effect was diminished when the sustained ischaemic time was increased to 5 hours (unpublished data). We also observed that the anti-infarction effect of IPC was independent of systemic mean arterial blood pressure and local muscle blood flow (Pang et al 1995). Subsequently, other investigators also demonstrated the cytoprotective effect of IPC in skeletal muscle in other species of laboratory animals. Specifically, it was reported that:

- IPC attenuated microvascular ischaemic/reperfusion injury in dog gracilis muscle (Jerome et al 1995)
- IPC augmented viability of muscle and musculocutaneous flaps in the rat (Caroll et al 1997, Zahir et al 1998)
- IPC improved postischaemic skeletal muscle functional recovery in the rat (Gürke et al 1995a b, Lee et al 1996)
- IPC of skeletal muscle induced myocardial protection (i.e. remote protection) in the rabbit (Birmbaum et al 1997), and protection against reperfusion tachyarrhythmia in the rat (Oxman et al 1997).

Mechanism of ischaemic preconditioning against infarction in skeletal muscle

It is important to investigate the cellular/molecular mechanism of IPC against infarction because understanding the mechanism will permit the development of potential therapeutic agents (IPC mimetics) for augmentation of skeletal muscle ischaemic tolerance. Observations made from cardiac muscle thus far indicate that the mechanism of IPC against myocardial infarction may involve three major components:

1. initiator (adenosine, noradrenaline (norephine-phrine), bradykinase, opioids)

2. intermediate (postreceptor) signal transduction pathway (receptor coupled inhibitory G protein, protein kinase C/D, tyrosine kinase)

3. effector (ATP-sensitive potassium channels).

The importance of each component and the endogenous substances thereof seems to vary with species of animal. The mechanism of myocardial IPC have been reviewed by various groups of investigators (Cohen and Downey 1996, Kloner et al 1998, Przyklenk and Kloner 1998, Yellon et al 1998). Hereafter, discussion will be focused mainly on the mechanism of IPC in skeletal muscle.

Initiator

We have demonstrated that 10-min preischaemic local intra-arterial infusion of adenosine or the adenosine-1

(A_1) receptor agonist N^6-1-(phenyl-2R-isopropyl) adenosine (PIA) reduced the muscle infarct size to the similar extent as IPC (3 cycles of 10-min ischaemia/reperfusion) in pig LD muscles subjected to 4 h of warm (room temperature) global ischaemia and 48 h of reperfusion (Fig. 55.1). In addition, the infarct-limiting effect of IPC and preischaemic adenosine treatment was completely blocked by pretreatment with local intra-arterial infusion of the A_1 receptor antagonist 8-cyclopentyl-1,3-dipropylxanthine (DPCPX). Preischaemic treatment with DPCPX or postischaemic treatment with adenosine alone did not have any effect on muscle infarct size (Fig. 55.1). Local intra-arterial infusion of adenosine, PIA, or DPCPX also did not affect the systemic mean arterial blood pressure or local muscle blood flow (Forrest et al 1997, Pang et al 1997b). The infarct-limiting effect of adenosine was confirmed in pig gracilis muscles (Forrest et al 1997). These observations were taken to indicate that adenosine, mediated by A_1 receptors, most likely plays an important role in triggering the acute infarct protective effect of IPC in pig skeletal muscle.

At the present time, the phenomenon of infarct-limiting effect of IPC has not been studied in human skeletal muscle. However, in a preliminary study, we observed that about 50% of cultured human skeletal muscle myocytes were irreversibly damaged after 4 h of warm (room temperature) ischaemia and 3 h of reperfusion, and preischaemia exposure of muscle cells

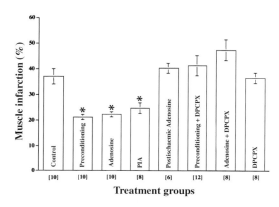

Figure 55.1 — Role of adenosine in triggering the anti-infarction effect of ischaemic preconditioning in pig latissimus dorsi muscles. Values are mean ± SEM. Numbers in brackets indicate the number of muscles contributing to the corresponding mean value. Means with an asterisk are similar and are significantly ($p<0.05$) different from ischaemic control. Mean values without an asterisk are similar to the control. Drugs were delivered to each muscle by 10-min local intra-arterial infusion: adenosine, 0.5 mg; N^6-1-(phenyl-2R-isopropyl) adenosine (PIA), 0.75 mg; 8-cyclopentyl-1,3-dipropylxanthine (DPCPX), 3 mg. (Data from Pang et al 1997b.)

to 100 μM adenosine for 30 min reduced irreversible cell damage to less than 10% (unpublished data). This same dose of adenosine also mimicked the cytoprotective effect of IPC in cultured human myocardiocytes subjected to 90 min of ischaemia and 30 min of reperfusion (Ikonomidis et al 1997).

There is evidence to indicate that both A_1 and A_3 receptors are involved in the infarct protective effect of IPC in rabbit myocardium and cardiomyocytes (Armstrong and Ganoate 1994, Liu et al 1991, 1994) and in human isolated atrial muscle (Carr et al 1997). However, it is most likely that the adenosine-mediated component of myocardial IPC is preferentially mediated by A_1 rather than A_3 receptors due to the selectivity of adenosine for A_1 receptor subtype (Hill et al 1998). The role of A_3 receptors in IPC of skeletal muscle has not been studied.

Postreceptor signal transduction pathway

We used protein kinase C (PKC) inhibitors, chelerythrine (Chel.) and polymyxin B (Poly B) and PKC activators, phorbal-12-myristate-13-acetate (PMA) and 1-oleoy-2-acetyl glycerol (OAG) as probes to investigate the role of PKC in mediation of IPC against infarction in pig LD muscles. These drugs were also delivered to the muscle by 10-min local intra-arterial infusion. It was observed that IPC or preischaemic treatment with adenosine, PMA or OAG significantly ($p < 0.01$) reduced the infarct size of pig LD muscles subjected to 4 h of ischaemia and 24 h of reperfusion by 40, 50, 48 and 52% respectively, compared with the ischaemic control. The anti-infarction effect of IPC and adenosine was completely blocked by Chel. or Poly B. However, Chel. or Poly B alone did not have any effect on muscle infarct size, mean arterial blood pressure or muscle blood flow (Hopper et al 1996, Hopper 1997). Taken together, these observations indicate that activation of PKC is important in the post-adenosine receptor signal transduction pathway in IPC of pig skeletal muscle against infarction. The exact action of PKC is not known. It is possible that the activated PKC in the cytosol is translocated to cell membrane to phosphorylate the effector proteins responsible for the infarct protective effect of IPC (Cohen and Downey 1996). To test this hypothesis, we investigated cytosol to sarcolemma PKC translocation in pig LD muscles preconditioned with three cycles of 10-min ischaemia/reperfusion (Hopper et al 1997). Muscle biopsies were harvested before IPC and at various time-points after IPC. Muscle biopsies were fractionated into cytosol and sarcolem-

mal membrane components and were screened for PKC isoforms of conventional (cPKCs, α, β_I, β_{II}, and γ), novel (nPKCs δ, ϵ, η, and θ), and atypical (aPKCs ζ, ι and λ) types by Western blot analysis using commercially available antibodies. The apparent molecular weights of all bands ranged from 64 to 90 kD. We observed that nPKCε was the only PKC isoform that demonstrated a progressive increase in immunoblot band density in purified sarcolemmal membrane fraction within 15 min of sustained global ischaemia following IPC. On the other hand, the band densities in the cytosol fraction decreased significantly ($p < 0.05$) during this period of time (Hopper et al 1997). These observations seem to reveal cytosol to sarcolemmal membrane PKCε translocation during sustained ischaemia following IPC in pig LD muscle. It must be mentioned that PKCε isoform may also have been translocated to other locations (e.g., cytoskeleton, mitochondria) that we did not study. We are investigating if PKC cytosol to sarcolemmal membrane translocation can occur following IPC but prior to sustained ischaemia.

The role of PKC in IPC of skeletal muscle against infarction has not been investigated in other species of laboratory animals. It is important to point out that evidence for involvement of PKC in IPC of myocardium has not extended to all species and controversy has developed even within a species. For example, PKC inhibitors, Chel., Poly B and staurosporine blocked the infarct-protective effect of preconditioning in rabbit and rat myocardium (Liu et al 1994, Speechly-Dick et al 1994, Ytrehus et al 1994, Kitakage et al 1996). Conversely, PKC activators, phorbol esters and diacylglycerol analogues, provided an infarct-protective effect similar to that afforded by IPC (Speechly-Dick 1994, Ytrechus 1994). Using protein tyrosine kinase inhibitors (genistein or lavendustin A) and activator (anisomycin) and the PKC activator PMA as probes, it was also demonstrated that PKC is linked downstream to protein tyrosine kinase in IPC of rabbit myocardium (Baines et al 1998). In addition, IPC-induced cytosol to membrane translocation of PKCδ isoform was seen in rat myocardium using immunohistochemical technique (Michell et al 1995), and, translocation of PKCε and PKCη isoforms in rabbit myocardium using immunoblotting technique (Ping et al 1997). Furthermore, it was also observed that PKC inhibitors Chel. and calphostin C blocked and the PKC activator PMA mimicked the cytoprotective effect of IPC in cultured human cardiomyocytes (Ikonomidis 1997). On the other hand, there is negative evidence for an important role of PKC in myocardial IPC. It has been reported that PKC inhibitors failed to attenuate myocardial anti-infarction effect of IPC in the dog (Przyklank et al 1995) and pig (Vahlhaus et al 1996), whereas brief preischaemic infusion of PMA did not limit infarct size in pig myocardium (Vahlhaus et al 1996). Biochemical quantitation of tissue PKC activity failed to detect PKC translocation induced by IPC in rabbit and dog myocardium (Przyklank et al 1995, Simkhovich 1996), and fluorescence focal microscopy failed to detect IPC-induced PKC translocation in dog myocardium as well (Przyklank et al 1995). At the present time, it is not known if these negative findings result from differences in species, drug dose, non-specific effects of drugs of limitation of chemical analysis (Brooks and Hearse 1996).

Effector

Gross et al (1994) speculated that the activated PKC in the sarcolemma may prolong or enhance opening of ATP-sensitive potassium (K_{ATP}) channels by phosphorylation of the sarcolemmal protein involved in maintaining K_{ATP} channel opening. Sustained opening of K_{ATP} channels may cause an increase in efflux of K^+, membrane hyperpolarization, shortening of action potentials and decrease of Ca^{2+} influx through voltage regulated Ca^{2+} channels. All these activities may contribute to reduction in contractility and energy metabolism and increase in ischaemic tolerance. This speculation led us to investigate the role of K_{ATP} channels in IPC of skeletal muscle against infarction. In a preliminary study, we observed that the anti-infarction effect of PKC activators PMA and OAG in pig LD muscles subjected to 4 h of ischaemia and 24 h of reperfusion was completely blocked by pretreatment with the K_{ATP} channel blocker sodium 5-hydroxydecanoate (5-HD), independent of systemic mean arterial blood pressure and local muscle blood flow (Hopper 1996). This observation was taken to indicate that K_{ATP} channels are linked downstream to PKC and they may be involved in the mechanism of IPC against infarction in skeletal muscle. Therefore, we proceeded to investigate the role of K_{ATP} channels in IPC of pig LD muscles against infarction (Pang et al 1997a). Specifically, we compared the anti-infarction effect of the K_{ATP} channel opener lemakalim with IPC (3 cycles of 10-min ischaemia/reperfusion) and preischaemic adenosine treatment. We also investigated the antagonistic effect of the K_{ATP} channel blockers 5-HD and glybenclamide (glyben.) on the infarct protective effect of IPC and adenosine in pig LD muscles subjected to 4 h of global ischaemia and 24 h of reperfu-

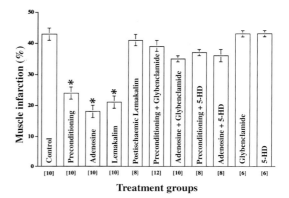

Figure 55.2—Role of ATP-sensitive potassium channels in ischaemic preconditioning of pig latissimus dorsi muscles against infarction. Values are mean ± SEM. Numbers in brackets indicate the number of muscles contributing to the corresponding mean value. Means with an asterisk are similar and are significantly ($p < 0.05$) different from the ischaemic control. Mean values without an asterisk are similar to the control. The following drugs were delivered to each muscle by 10-min local intra-arterial infusion: adenosine, 0.5 mg; lemakalim, 0.18 mg; 5-hydroxydecanoate (5-HD), 27 mg. Glybenclamide (0.3 mg/kg) was given intravenously over 10 min. (Data from Pang et al 1997a.)

sion. We observed that the muscle infarct size was similar among the IPC (24 ± 2%), adenosine (18 ± 2%) and lemakalim (21 ± 2%) groups and the infarct size of these three groups was smaller than the ischaemic control (43 ± 2%) (Fig. 55.2). Glyben. or 5-HD completely blocked the anti-infarction effect of IPC and adenosine. Lemakalim given at the onset of reperfusion and glyben. or 5-HD given prior to sustained ischaemia did not affect the muscle infarct size (Fig. 55.2). These observations are interpreted to indicate that K_{ATP} channels are central to IPC against infarction in pig skeletal muscle.

There is also a large body of evidence supporting an important role of K_{ATP} channels in IPC of myocardium against infarction. For example, it has been reported that K_{ATP} channel blockers such as glyben. or Chel. abolished the cardioprotective effect of IPC in rats (Qian et al 1996, Schultz et al 1997), rabbits (Toombs et al 1993, Hide and Thiemermann 1996, Kouchi et al 1998), dogs (Auchampach and Groer 1992, Grover et al 1992) and pigs (Schulz et al 1994). Conversely, treatment with a K_{ATP} channel opener mimicked the myocardial infarct protective effect in rabbits (Kouchi et al 1998) and dogs (Mizumura et al 1995).

Effect of ischaemic preconditioning on high energy phosphate metabolism in skeletal muscle

It is important to understand how IPC increases the ischaemic tolerance in skeletal muscle. Therefore, we investigated the effect of IPC, adenosine and lemakalim on energy metabolism in pig LD muscles (Pang et al 1995, 1997a, 1997b). Drugs were delivered to LD muscles, prior to 4 h of sustained global ischaemia, by 10 min of local intra-arterial infusion. Muscle biopsies were obtained before and at the end of 2 and 4 h of warm global ischaemia and 1.5 h of reperfusion. Muscle contents of high energy phosphates were measured using high performance liquid chromatography and muscle contents of lactate were assayed by a fluorimetric technique. We observed that the muscle content of ATP at the end of 4 h of ischaemia and 1.5 h of reperfusion was higher for the IPC, adenosine and lemakalim groups than the time-matched ischaemic control (Fig. 55.3). The muscle contents of ATP among the IPC, adenosine and lemakalim groups were similar at the end of 4 h of ischaemia and 1.5 h of reperfusion (Fig. 55.3).

The muscle adenylate charge potential (ECP=ATP + 0.5 × ADP/(ATP + ADP + AMP)) was calculated to gain insight into the energy store of the adenylate

system in LD muscles. The ECP in preconditioned muscles and in muscles treated with preischaemic adenosine or lemakalim was higher than the time-matched control at the end of 2 and 4 h of ischaemia and 1.5 h of reperfusion (Fig. 55.4). Within each time-point studied, the muscle ECP was similar among these three treatment groups. It is of interest to note that although IPC resulted in a decrease in muscle content of ATP and muscle ECP compared with the control prior to sustained ischaemia, the muscle content of ATP and muscle ECP were higher in the IPC group than in the control at the end of 4 h of sustained ischaemia (Fig. 55.4).

We also observed that the preischaemic muscle contents of lactate were similar among the control, IPC, adenosine and lemakalim groups (Fig. 55.5). However, the muscle contents of lactate in precondi-

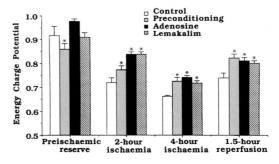

Figure 55.4— Muscle energy charge potential in pig latissimus dorsi muscles. Values are mean ± SEM; n=6 muscles. Means with an asterisk are significantly ($p < 0.05$) different from the time-matched ischaemic control. Adenosine (0.5 mg/muscle) and lemakalim (0.18 mg/muscle) were delivered to the muscle by 10 min of local intra-arterial infusion. (Data from Pang et al 1997a, 1997b.)

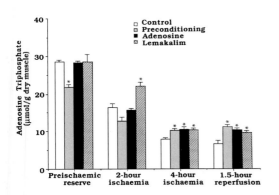

Figure 55.3— Muscle content of adenosine triphosphate (ATP) in pig latissimus dorsi muscles. Values are mean ± SEM; n=6 muscles. Means with an asterisk are significantly ($p < 0.05$) different from the time-matched ischaemic control. Adenosine (0.5 mg/muscle) and lemakalim (0.18 mg/muscle) were delivered to the muscle by 10 min of local intra-arterial infusion. (Data from Pang et al 1997a, 1997b.)

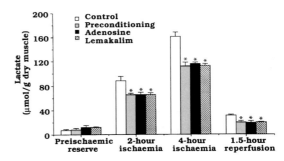

Figure 55.5— Muscle content of pig latissimus dorsi muscles. Values are mean ± SEM; n=6 muscles. Mean values with an asterisk were significantly ($p < 0.05$) different from the time-matched control. Adenosine (0.5 mg/muscle) and lemakalim (0.18 mg/muscle) were delivered to the muscle by 10 min of local intra-arterial infusion. (Data from Pang et al 1997a, 1997b.)

tioned muscles and in muscles pretreated with adeno-sine or lemakalim were significantly lower than the time-matched ischaemic control at the end of 2 and 4 h of sustained ischaemia and 1.5 h of reperfusion (Fig. 55.5). These observations on skeletal muscle high energy phosphate metabolism (Figs 55.3 and 55.4) and lactate accumulation (Fig. 55.5) seem to indicate that IPC of skeletal muscle prior to sustained ischaemia is associated with slowing of high-energy phosphate depletion and metabolite accumulation and this energy sparing effect of IPC can be mimicked by 10 min of preischaemic treatment of adenosine or the K_{ATP} channel opener lemakalim.

Effect of ischaemic preconditioning on postischaemic neutrophil accumulation in skeletal muscle

There is the perception from published data that adenosine not only plays an important role in initiat-ing the protective effect of IPC, but it may also serve as an effector of IPC in skeletal muscle (Akinitsu et al 1996). Using intravital microscopy, it was observed in murine cremaster muscles that topical application of adenosine before 60 min of sustained ischaemia (i.e., adenosine preconditioning) and throughout 60 min of ischaemia and reperfusion was as effective as IPC in attenuation of neutrophil adhesion in postischaemic cremaster muscles. However, only partial reduction of neutrophil adhesion was achieved when topical adenosine was applied before or during reperfusion only. Conversely, the inhibitory effect of IPC on neutrophil adhesion was completely blocked when adenosine deaminase (ADA), an adenosine degrada-tion enzyme, was applied topically before and during 60 min of ischaemia and reperfusion. Topical applica-tion of ADA during IPC or reperfusion alone only partially blocked the anti-neutrophil adhesion effect of IPC. Taken together, these investigators speculated that IPC in murine cremaster muscles caused increased release of adenosine during IPC and reperfusion and adenosine may act as initiator and effector, respectively, in IPC of murine skeletal muscle (Akinitsu et al 1996).

We performed an in vivo study to investigate the effect of IPC and 10-min preischaemic adenosine treatment on neutrophilic myeloperoxidase (MPO) activities in pig LD muscles subjected to 4 h of global

ischaemia and 16 h of reperfusion (Pang et al 1997b). We observed that IPC or preischaemic adenosine treatment reduced neutrophil accumulation as indi-cated by a lower muscle neutrophilic activity during 16 h of reperfusion in IPC and preischaemic adenosine treated LD muscles, compared with the time-matched ischaemic control (Fig. 55.6). However the observa-tions from our model did not indicate that adenosine may have played an effector role in attenuation of neutrophil accumulation during reperfusion because preischaemic adenosine treatment alone was sufficient to cause a reduction in muscle neutrophilic MPO activity to the similar extent as IPC (Fig. 55.6). In addition, we observed previously that IPC did not increase muscle content of adenosine during sustained ischaemia or reperfusion (Pang et al 1995, 1997b) and the same dose of adenosine given at the onset of reper-fusion did not attenuate reperfusion injury (Fig. 55.1). Our explanation for the effect of IPC on attenuation of muscle neutrophil accumulation is that IPC or preischaemic adenosine treatment increased ischaemic tolerance, thus reducing muscle injury and inflamma-tory reaction during 4 h of global ischaemia, com-pared with the ischaemic control. Reduction in local muscle inflammatory reaction decreased neutrophil activation, recruitment and accumulation during reper-fusion, thus resulting in attenuation of reperfusion injury. We have also demonstrated previously that the neutrophil but not the xanthine oxidase/dehydro-genase system is the main source of oxyradicals in reperfusion injury in pig and human skeletal muscle (Dorion et al 1993).

Other investigators also observed in dog gracilis muscles that IPC or preischaemic treatment with the

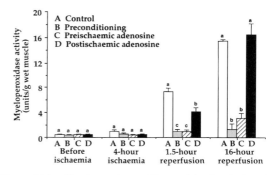

Figure 55.6—Muscle myeloperoxidase activity in pig latissimus dorsi muscle. Values are mean ± SEM; n=6 muscles. Within each time-point, means without a common lower case letter are signifi-cantly ($p < 0.05$) different. Adenosine (0.5 mg/muscle) was deliv-ered to the muscle by 10 min of local intra-arterial infusion. (Data from Pang et al 1997b.)

K_{ATP} channel opener pinacadil prior to 4 hours of sustained ischaemia reduced the extent of postischaemic capillary no reflow compared with the ischaemic control and this protective effect was reversed by the K_{ATP} channel blocker glyben (Jerome et al 1995). These observations were interpreted to indicate that IPC limited the extent of capillary no-reflow in post-ischaemic skeletal muscle by a mechanism that involves activation of K_{ATP} channels. Since the development of postischaemic capillary no-reflow is critically dependent on the neutrophil accumulation, we decided to investigate the role of IPC and K_{ATP} channels on neutrophil accumulation during reperfusion of ischaemic pig LD muscles (Pang et al 1997a). We observed that IPC or 10-min preischaemic treatment with the K_{ATP} channel opener lemakalim reduced muscle neutrophilic MPO activity during 16 h of reperfusion, compared with the ischaemic control (Fig. 55.7). However, observations from our pig LD muscles did not indicate that opening of K_{ATP} channels in IPC plays a direct role in prevention of postischaemic muscle neutrophil accumulation because postischaemic treatment with lemakalim did not reduce muscle neutrophilic MPO activity assessed at 16 h of reperfusion (Fig. 55.7) or muscle infarction assessed at 24 h of reperfusion (Fig. 55.2). We believe that the key role of the K_{ATP} channel was not directly on the recruitment/accumulation of neutrophils. Instead, opening of the K_{ATP} channel in IPC most likely contributed to the augmentation of ischaemic tolerance as in the case of IPC and adenosine treatment, resulting in decrease in muscle ischaemic injury and inflammatory reaction. Reduction in inflammatory reaction would attenuate recruitment/and accumulation, and postischaemic capillary no-reflow.

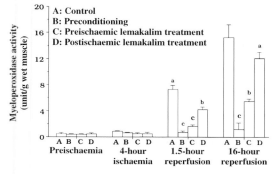

Figure 55.7—Muscle myeloperoxidase activity in pig latissimus dorsi muscle. Values are mean ± SEM; n=6–8 muscles. At each time-point, means without a common lower case letter are significantly ($p < 0.05$) different. Lemakalim (0.18 mg/muscle) was delivered to the muscle by 10 min of local intra-arterial infusion. (Data from Pang et al 1997a.)

Delayed (second window) protection of ischaemic preconditioning against infarction

The phenomenon of IPC against infarction discussed thus far is known as acute IPC because it was observed in cardiac muscle that the infarct protective effect of IPC was lost when the sustained ischaemic insult was started beyond 2 h after IPC (Van Winkle et al 1991). However, two laboratories later independently observed in the myocardium of the rabbit (Marber et al 1993) and dog (Kuzuya et al 1993) that protection against infarction appeared again 24 h after IPC, and this is known as the second window of protection. Subsequently, the phenomenon of the second window of protection in IPC was also reported in cardiomyocytes of the rat (Zhou et al 1996) and human (Arstall et al 1998). Recent work suggests that the second window of protection in myocardium extends over a period of 24–72 h after IPC (Baxter et al 1997). There is evidence to indicate that the mechanism of the second window of protection in IPC may involve A_1 receptors (Baxter et al 1994, 1997), induction of nitric oxide synthase (Takano et al 1998), activation of PKC (Baxter 1997), increase in expression of heat shock protein (Marber et al 1993) and increase in superoxide dismutase activity (Yamashita et al 1994). It should be mentioned that other investigators failed to demonstrate a myocardial infarct-reduction effect in the second window of protection in the rat (Jagasia et al 1996), rabbit (Tanaka et al 1994) and pig (Qiu et al 1997).

If the phenomenon of the second window of protection could be induced by IPC of skeletal muscle, it should have important clinical application in vascular and musculoskeletal reconstructive surgery. Specifically, muscles are subjected to sustained global ischaemia during vascular anastomosis in autogenous muscle transplant or during application of vascular clamp or tourniquets in vascular or musculoskeletal reconstructive surgery. This is known as the primary ischaemic insult. However, suture-line thrombosis or other vascular complications can occur within the first 48 h of reperfusion resulting in interruption of blood supply to the muscles. This is known as the secondary ischaemic insult (Zelt et al 1986). Obviously, a second window of protection in IPC would offer ischaemic tolerance to skeletal muscle undergoing secondary ischaemic insult until the vascular problem is resolved surgically. So far, we have not been able to demonstrate the phenomenon of second window of protection against infarction of pig LD muscles preconditioned with 4–6 cycles of 10-min ischaemia/reperfusion or treated with local intra-arterial infusion of adenosine (0.5–1 mg/muscle) in LD muscle before subjecting to 4 h of ischaemia and 6 h of reperfusion (unpublished data). Other investigators have reported that the second window of protection preserved capillary reperfusion in rat extensor digitorum longus muscles subjected to 2 h of ischaemic insult, but IPC did not afford second window of protection against vascular parenchyma injury (Pudupakkam et al 1998). Therefore, a model of second window of protection in IPC of skeletal muscle against infarction remains elusive at the present time.

Future research in ischaemic preconditioning of skeletal muscle against infarction

Experimental evidence discussed thus far supports our speculation that it is possible to develop pharmacological preconditioning strategies for acute and perhaps also second window of protection against skeletal muscle infarction in vascular and musculoskeletal surgery, in which skeletal muscle may be subjected to unexpected prolonged and/or repeated ischaemic results. This acute prophylactic pharmacological treatment may also be useful in cardiomyoplasty, where skeletal muscle ischaemia/reperfusion injury is a common clinical complication. However, we believe that the following areas of research should be pursued before clinical trials can be realized.

Efficacy and mechanism in human skeletal muscle cells

It is important to demonstrate that the cytoprotective phenomenon of acute and second window protection in IPC are relevant to human skeletal muscle, and to understand the mechanism underlying these two phenomenon in human skeletal muscle. To this end, isolated primary skeletal muscle myocytes should be used to study the efficacy of acute and second window

of protection in IPC against ischaemia/reperfusion injury, and to identify the initiator, mediator (post-receptor signal transduction pathway) and effector mechanism. Human primary cardiomyocytes have already been used to study acute and second window of protection in IPC (Arstall et al 1998), and this technique can be modified for human skeletal muscle myocytes.

In vivo studies on the role of protein kinase C

There is the need to use large animal models to elucidate the A_1-receptors–PKC–K_{ATP} channel-linked mechanism in acute protection of skeletal muscle against infarction. Special emphasis should be placed on the location of PKC translocation and phosphorylation and tyrosine kinase activation.

In vivo studies on the role of K_{ATP} channels

The earlier hypothesis that opening of sarcolemmal K_{ATP} (sar.K_{ATP}) channels in IPC results in reducing muscle contractility, energy metabolism and infarction (Gross et al 1994) cannot explain the more recent observation that the infarct protective effect of IPC can also be induced in a non-contracting muscle. For example, IPC with three cycles of 10-min ischaemia/reperfusion or 10-min preischaemic treatment with the K_{ATP} channel opener lemakalim afforded an infarct protective effect in surgically denervated and non-contracting pig LD muscles subjected to 4 h of global ischaemic and 24 h of reperfusion (Pang et al 1997a). In addition, the K_{ATP} channel opener diazoxide, which is known to have no effect on the sar.K_{ATP} channel in skeletal muscle cells of the mouse (Weik and Neumcke 1990) and rat (Barrett-Jolley and McPherson 1998), is effective in mimicking the anti-infarction effect of IPC in surgically denervated and non-contracting pig LD muscles subjected to 4 h of ischaemia and 24 h of reperfusion (Pang et al 1998). Furthermore, a low dose of the K_{ATP} channel opener bimakalim induced cardioprotection in the dog without any effect on the sarcolemmal action potential (Yao and Gross 1994). Last but not least, the cytoprotective effect of IPC could be induced in non-contracting cultured human myocardiocytes (Iknonomidias et al 1997). These observations seem to indicate that the sar.K_{ATP} channel may not be the effector of acute IPC in both skeletal and cardiac muscles. Recently, emerging experimental evidence indicates that K_{ATP} channels also exist in mitochondrial (mito.) membrane of cardiomyocytes (Garlid et al 1996, 1997). Using the selective mito.K_{ATP} channel opener diazoxide and blocker 5-HD as probes, it was demonstrated that mito.K_{ATP} channels were involved in myocardial IPC in the rat (Garlid et al 1997) and rabbit (Liu et al 1998) and the mito.K_{ATP} channel was linked to PKC in the rabbit cardiomyocyte (Sato et al 1998). Therefore, future in vivo studies are required to investigate the acute infarct protective effect of the mito.K_{ATP} channel in skeletal muscle and to study how enhancing or sustaining opening of mito.K_{ATP} channels can induce energy sparing and anti-infarction effects in skeletal muscle.

Summary

Experimental evidence cumulated from our laboratory thus far has led us to hypothesize that the protective mechanism of acute IPC against skeletal muscle infarction involves the A_1 receptor–PKC–K_{ATP} channel-linked events as summarized in Fig. 55.8. Briefly described, brief cycles of ischaemia/reperfusion results in stepwise metabolism of ATP to ADP, AMP and adenosine, which in turn activates A_1/A_3 membrane receptors. The activated A_1/A_3 receptors couple to Gi-protein, resulting in activation of phospholipase C/D (PLC/PLD). Activated PLC degrades membrane phosphatidylinositol-4,5-biphosphate (PIP_2) to inositol-1,4,5-triphosphate (IP_3) and diacyl glycerol (DAG) while activated PLD degrades membrane phosphatidylcholine to phosphadic acid (PA) which is then hydrolysed by PA phosphohydrolase to DAG as well. DAG is a co-factor for translocation and activation of PKC. The activated PKC may:

1. phosphorylate cytoskeleton structures to tolerate ischaemic injury

2. phosphorylate metabolic enzyme to preserve energy

3. phosphorylate proteins responsible for enhancement of sustained opening of sar.K_{ATP} and/or mito.K_{ATP} channels which are reponsible for energy sparing and anti-infarction effect of acute IPC.

At the present time, it is not know how opening of mito.K_{ATP} channels can contribute to energy preservation and reduced infarction. There is the possibility that opening of mito.K_{ATP} channels can:

1. preserve mitochondrial function by prevention of Ca^{2+} overload

2. reduce rate of anaerobic glycolysis, energy depletion, metabolite accumulation and eventually muscle infarction

3. preserve mitochondrial ATPase and adenine nucleotide translocase activities for rapid restoration of high energy phosphate in the early stage of reperfusion.

At the present time, little is known about the efficacy and mechanism of the second window of protection in IPC of skeletal muscle. In conclusion, the experimental evidence presented by us thus far should provide a mandate for further investigation aimed at elucidating the cellular/molecular mechanism of acute and second window of protection against infarction in IPC and translating this knowledge into effective therapeutic strategies for augmentation of skeletal muscle ischaemic tolerance in vascular and musculo-skeletal reconstructive surgery and cardiomyoplasty.

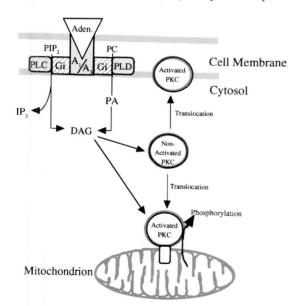

Figure 55.8—Proposed mechanism for acute protection of ischaemic preconditioning against skeletal muscle infarction. A_1/A_3, adenosine$_{1/3}$ receptors; Gi, inhibitory G protein; PLC/PLD, phospholipase C/D; PIP_2, phosphatidylinositol-4,5-biphosphate; IP_3, insositol-1,4,5-triphosphate; DAG, diacylglycerol; PKC, protein kinase C; PA, phosphadic acid.

Acknowledgements

This research project is supported by an operating grant from the Medical Research Council (MRC) of Canada (MT 12148). Christopher R. Forrest is an MRC scholar.

References

Akinitsu T, Gute DC, Korthuis RJ. (1996) Ischaemic pre-conditioning attenuates postischemic leukocytes adhesion and emigration. *Am J Physiol* 271: H2052–H2059.

Armstrong S, Ganote CE. (1994) Adenosine receptor speci-ficity in preconditioning of isolated rabbit cardiomyo-cytes: evidence of A3 receptor involvement. *Cardiovasc Res* 28: 1049–1056.

Arstall MA, Zhao Y-Z, Hornberger L, et al. (1998) Human ventricular myocytes in vitro exhibit both early and delayed preconditioning responses to simulated ischemia. *J Mol Cell Cardiol* 30: 1019–1025.

Auchampach JA, Groer GJ. (1992) Blockage of ischemic preconditioning in dogs by the novel ATP-dependent potassium channel antagonist sodium 5-hydroxyde-canoate. *Cardiovasc Res* 26: 1054–1062.

Baines CP, Wang L, Cohen MV, Downey JM. (1998) Protein tyrosine kinase is downstream of protein kinase C for ischemic preconditioning's anti-infarct effect in the rabbit heart. *J Mol Cell Cardiol* 30: 383–392.

Barrett-Jolley R, McPherson GA. (1998) Characterization of K_{ATP} channels in intact mammalian skeletal muscle fibres. *Br J Pharmacol* 123: 1103–1110.

Baxter GF. (1997) Ischemic preconditioning of myo-cardium. *Ann Med* 29: 345–352.

Baxter GF, Marber MS, Patel VC, Yellon DM. (1994) Adenosine receptor involvement in a delayed phase of myocardial protection 24 hours after ischemic precondi-tioning. *Circulation* 90: 2993–3000.

Baxter GF, Zaman MJS, Kerac M, Yellon DM. (1997) Protection against global ischaemia in the rabbit isolated heart 24 hours after transient adenosine A_1 receptor acti-vation. *Cardiovasc Drug Ther* 11: 83–85.

Birmbaum Y, Hal SL, Kloner RA. (1997) Ischemic precon-ditioning at a distance. Reduction of myocardial infarct size by partial reduction of blood supply combined with rapid stimulation of the gastrocnemius muscle in the rabbit. *Circulation* 96: 1641–1646.

Blaisdell FW, Steel M, Allen RE. (1978) Management of acute lower extremity arterial ischaemia due to embolism and thrombosis. *Surgery* 84: 822–834.

Brooks A, Hearse DJ. (1996) Role of protein kinase C is ischemic preconditioning: player or spectator? *Circ Res* 79: 627–630.

Caroll CMA, Carrol SM, Overgoor MLE, Tokin G, Barker JH. (1997) Acute ischemic preconditioning of skeletal muscle prior to flap elevation augments muscle flap sur-vival. *Plast Reconstr Surg* 100: 58–64.

Carr CA, Hill RJ, Kennedy SP, et al. (1997) Evidence for a role of both adenosine A_1 and A_3 receptors in protection of isolated human atrial muscle against ischemia. *Cardiovasc Res* 36: 52–59.

Cohen M, Downey JM. (1996) Myocardial preconditioning promises to be a novel approach to the treatment of ischemic heart disease. *Annu Rev Med* 47: 21–29.

Dorion D, Zhong A, Chiu C, Forrest CR, Boyd B, Pang CY. (1993) Role of xanthine oxidase in reperfusion injury of ischemic skeletal muscles in the pig and human. *J Appl Physiol* 75: 246–255.

Downey JM, Liu Y, Ytrehus K. (1994) Adenosine and the artifact effects of preconditioning. In: *Ischaemic precondi-tioning: the concent of endogenous cardioprotection*. Prazyklenk K, Klona RA, Yellon DM, eds. Boston: Kluwer Academic Publishers, pp. 137–152.

Eckert P, Schnackery K. (1991) Ischaemic tolerance of human skeletal muscle. *Ann Plast Surg* 26: 77–84.

Forrest CR, Neligan P, Zhong A, He W, Yang RZ, Pang CY. (1997) Acute adenosine treatment is effective in augmentation of ischemic tolerance in muscle flaps in the pig. *Plast Reconstr Surg* 95: 177–182.

Garlid KD, Paucek P, Yarov-Yarovoy V, et al. (1997) Cardioprotective effect of diazoxide and its interaction with mitochondrial ATP-sensitive K^+ channels. Possible mechanism of cardioprotection. *Circ Res* 81: 1072–1082.

Garlid KD, Paucek P, Yarov-Yarovoy V, Sun X, Schindler PA. (1996) Mitochondrial K_{ATP} channel receptor for potassium channel opener. *J Biol Chem* 271: 8796–8799.

Gross GJ, Yao Z, Auchampach JA. (1994) Role of ATP-sensitive potassium channels in ischemic preconditioning. In: *Ischemic preconditioning: the concept of endogenous cardio-protection*. Przyklenk K, Kloner RA, Yellon DM, eds. Boston: Kluwer Academic Publishers, pp. 123–135.

Grover GJ, Sleph PG, Dzwonczyk S. (1992) Role of myo-cardial ATP-sensitive potassium channels in mediating preconditioning in the dog heart and their possible inter-action with adenosine A_1 receptors. *Circulation* 86: 1310–1316.

Gürke EL, Marx A, Sutter PM, Salm T, Harder F, Herberer M. (1995a) The efficacy of ischemic preconditioning of skeletal muscle depends on the number of precondition-ing cycles. *Surgical Forum* XLVI: 601–602.

Gürke EL, Marx A, Sutter PM, Frentzel A, Harder F, Herber M. (1995b) Ischemic preconditioning improves function but not ATP-levels in postischemic skeletal muscle ischemic tissue reperfusion injury. (Abstract) *FASEB J* 9: 3792.

Haimovici HJ. (1979a) Muscular, renal and metabolic com-plication of acute arterial occlusions: Myonephropathic metabolic syndrome. *Surgery* 85: 461–468.

Haimovici HJ. (1979b) Metabolic complication of acute arterial occlusions. *J Cardiovasc Surg (Torino)* 20: 349–357.

Hide EJ, Thiemermann C. (1996) Limitation of myocardial infarct size in the rabbit by ischemic preconditioning is abolished by sodium 5-hydroxydecanoate. *Cardiovasc Res* 31: 941–946.

Hill RJ, Oleynek JJ, Magee W, Knight DK, Tracey WR. (1998) Relative importance of adenosine A_1 and A_3 receptors in mediating physiological or pharmacological protection from ischaemic myocardial injury in the rabbit heart. *J Moll Cell Cardiol* 30: 579–585.

Hollier LH. (1983) Principles and techniques of surgical treatment of occlusive arterial diseases of the lower extremities. In: *Clinical Vascular Disease*. Vol. 13. Spittell JA Jr, ed. Philadelphia: F.A. Davis Co., pp. 37–48.

Hopper RA. (1997) The role and cellular mechanism of protein kinase C in ischemic preconditioning of porcine skeletal muscle against infarction. M.Sc. Thesis. Department of Medical Science, University of Toronto, Toronto, Ontario, Canada.

Hopper R, Forrest CR, Zhong A, He W, Pang CY. (1996) In vivo evidence for a link between protein kinase C and ATP-sensitive K+ channels in ischemic preconditioning against infarction. (Abstract) *Circulation* 94(8): I–549.

Hopper RA, Forrest CR, Xu H, et al. (2000) Role and mechanism of PKC in ischemic preconditioning of pig skeletal muscle against infarction. *Am J Physiol* 279: R666–R676.

Hu K, Duan D, Li GR, Nattel S. (1996) Protein kinase C activates ATP-sensitive K^+ current in human and rabbit ventricular myocytes. *Circ Res* 78: 492–498.

Ikonomidis JS, Shirai T, Weisel RD, et al. (1997) Preconditioning cultured human pediatric myocytes require adenosine and protein kinase C. *Am J Physiol* 272: H1220–H1230.

Jagasia D, Whiting JM, McNulty PH. (1996) Ischemic preconditioning fails to produce a second window of protection of 24hrs later in the rat. (Abstract) *Circulation* 94(Suppl.1): 1–184.

Jerome SN, Akinitsu T, Gute DC, Korthuis RJ. (1995) Ischemic preconditioning attenuates capillary no-reflow induced by prolonged ischemia and reperfusion. *Am J Physiol* 268: H2063–2067.

Kitakaze M, Node K, Minamuio T, et al. (1996) Role of activation of protein kinase C in the infarct size-limiting effect of ischemic preconditioning through activation of ecto-5'-nucleotidase. *Circulation* 93: 781–791.

Kloner RA, Bolli R, Marban E, Reinlib L, Braunwald E. (1998) Medical and cellular implications of stunning, hibernation, and preconditioning. An NHLB1 workshop. *Circulation* 97: 1848–1867.

Kouchi I, Murakami T, Nawada R, Akao M, Sasyama S. (1998) K_{ATP} channels are common mediators of ischemic and calcium preconditioning in rabbits. *Am J Physiol* 274: H1106–1112.

Kuzuya T, Hoshida S, Yamashida N, et al. (1993) Delayed effects of sabbatical ischemia on the acquisition of tolerance to ischemia. *Circ Res* 72: 1293–1299.

Larrson J, Hultman E. (1979) The effect of long-term arterial occlusion on energy metabolism of the human quadriceps muscle. *Scand J Clin Invest* 12: 69–79.

Lee HT, Schroeder CA, Shah PM, Babu SC, Thompson CI, Belloni FL. (1996) Preconditioning with ischaemia or adenosine protects muscle from ischemic tissue reperfusion injury. *J Surg Res* 63: 29–34.

Li GC, Vasquez JA, Gallagher KP, Lucchesi BR. (1990) Myocardial protection with preconditioning. *Circulation* 82: 609–619.

Liu Y, Gao WD, O'Rourke B, Marban E. (1996) Synergetic modulation of ATP-sensitive K^+ currents by protein kinase C and adenosine. Implications for ischemic preconditioning. *Circ Res* 78: 443–454.

Liu Y, Cohan MU, Downey JM. (1994) Chelerythrine, a highly selective protein kinase C inhibitor, blocks the anti-infarct effect of ischemic preconditioning in rabbit hearts. *Cardiovasc Drug Ther* 8: 881–882.

Liu GS, Richard RA, Olsson K, Mullane K, Walsh RS, Downey JM. (1994) Evidence that the adenosine A_3 receptor may mediate the protection afforded by preconditioning in the isolated rabbit heart. *Cardiovasc Res* 28: 1057–1061.

Liu Y, Sato T, O'Rourke B, Marban E. (1998) Mitochondrial ATP-dependent potassium channels. Novel effectors of cardioprotection? *Circulation* 97: 2463–2469.

Liu GS, Thornton J, Van Winkle DM, Stanley AWH, Olsson RA, Downey JM. (1991) Protection against infarction afforded by preconditioning is mediated by A_1 adenosine receptors in the rabbit heart. *Circulation* 84: 350–356.

Marber MS, Latchman DS, Walker JM, Yellon DM. (1993) Cardiac stress protein elevation 24 hours after brief ischaemia or heat stress is associated with resistance to myocardial infarction. *Circulation* 88: 1264–1272.

Matsen FA, Krugmire RB. (1978) Compartment syndrome. *Surg Gynecol Obstet* 147: 943–949.

McCarron DA, Elliot WC, Rose JS. (1979) Severe mixed metabolic acidosis secondary to rhabdomyolysis. *Am J Med* 67: 905–908.

Michell MB, Meng X, Ao L, Brown JM, Harker AH, Banerjee A. (1995) Preconditioning of isolated rat heart mediated by protein kinase C. *Circ Res* 76: 73–81.

Mizumura T, Nithipatikom K, Gross GJ. (1995) Bimakalim, an ATP-sensitive potassium channel opener, mimics the effects of ischemic preconditioning to reduce infarct size, adenosine release and neutrophil function in dogs. *Circulation* 92: 1236–1245.

Mounsey R, Pang CY. (1992) Augmentation of skeletal muscle survival in the latissimus dorsi porcine model using acute ischaemic preconditioning. *J Otalaryngology* 21: 315–320.

Murry CE, Jennings RB, Reimer KA. (1986) Preconditioning with ischemia: A delay of lethal cell injury in ischemic myocardium. *Circulation* 74: 1124–1136.

Murry CE, Richard VJ, Reimer KA, Jennings RB. (1990) Ischemic preconditioning slows energy metabolism and delays ultrastructural damage during a sustained ischemic episode. *Cir Res* 66: 913–931.

Oxman T, Arad M, Klein R, Auzor N, Rabinowitz B. (1997) Limb ischemia preconditions the heart against reperfusion tachyarrhythmia. *Am J Physiol* 273: H1707–H1712.

Pang CY, Neligan P, Xu H, et al. (1997a) Role of ATP-sensitive K+ channels in ischaemic preconditioning of skeletal muscle against infarction. *Am J Physiol* 273: H44–H51.

Pang CY, Neligan P, Zhong A, He W, Xu H, Forrest CR. (1997b) Effector mechanism of adenosine in acute ischemic preconditioning of skeletal muscle against infarction. *Am J Physiol* 273: R887–R895.

Pang CY, Yang RZ, Zhong A, Xu N, Boyd B, Forrest CR. (1995) Acute ischemic preconditioning protects against skeletal muscle infarction in the pig. *Cardiovasc Res* 29: 782–788.

Pang CY, Neligan P, Zhong A, Xu H, Forrest CR. (1998) In vivo infarct protective effect of diazoxide (Abstract). *Circulation* 98(17): I–343.

Ping P, Zhang J, Qui Y, et al. (1997) Ischemic preconditioning induces selective translocation of PKC isoform ε and η in the heart of conscious rabbits without subcellular redistribution of total protein kinase C activity. *Circ Res* 81: 404–414.

Przyklenk K, Klona A. (1998) Ischemic preconditioning: exploring the paradox. *Proc Cardiovasc Dis* 40: 517–547.

Przyklenk K, Sussman MA, Simkhovich BZ, Kloner RA. (1995) Does ischemic preconditioning trigger translocation of protein kinase C in the canine model? *Circulation* 92: 1546–1557.

Pudupakkam S, Harris KA, Jamieson WG, et al. (1998) Ischemic tolerance in skeletal muscle: role of nitric oxide. *Am J Physiol* 275: H94–H99.

Qian YZ, Levasseur JE, Yoshida K-I, Kukreja RC. (1996) K_{ATP} channel in rat heart: blockage of ischemic and acetylcholine-mediated preconditioning by glibenclamide. *Am J Physiol* 271: H23–H28.

Qiu Y, Tang XL, Park SW, Sun JZ, Kalya A, Bolli R. (1997) The early and late phases of ischemic preconditioning: a comparative analysis of their effects on infarct size, myocardial stunning and arrhythmias in conscious pigs undergoing a 40-minute coronary occlusion. *Circ Res* 80: 730–742.

Rakowski TA, Cerasaro TS. (1979) Myoglobinuria. *Am Fam Physician* 20: 129–134.

Rubin B, Romaschin A, Walker PM, Gute DC, Korhius RJ. (1996) Mechanisms of postischemic injury in skeletal muscle: intervention strategies. *J Appl Physiol* 80: 369–387.

Rutherford RJ. (1987) Nutrient bed protection during lower extremity arterial reconstruction. *J Vasc Surg* 5: 529–554.

Sato T, O'Rourke B, Margan E. (1998) Modulation of mitochondrial ATP-dependent K^+ channels by protein kinase C. *Circ Res* 83: 110–114.

Schultz JET, Qian YZ, Gross GJ, Kukreja RC. (1997) The ischaemia-sensitive K_{ATP} channel antagonist, 5-hydroxy-decanoate, blocks ischaemic preconditioning in the rat heart. *J Mol Cell Cardiol* 29: 1055–1060.

Schulz R, Rose J, Heusch G. (1994) Involvement of activation of ATP-dependent potassium channels in ischemic preconditioning in swine. *Am J Physiol* 267: H1341–H1352.

Simkhovich BZ, Przyklenk K, Hale SL, Patterson M, Kloner RA. (1996) Direct evidence that ischaemic preconditioning does not cause protein kinase C translocation in rabbit heart. *Cardiovasc Res* 32: 1064–1070.

Sjostrom M, Friden J, Eklof B. (1982) Human skeletal muscle metabolism and morphology after temporary incomplete ischemia. *Eur J Clin Invest* 12: 69–79.

Speechly-Dick ME, Mocanu MM, Yellon DM. (1994) Protein kinase C. Its role in ischemic preconditioning in the rat. *Circ Res* 75: 586–590.

Takano H, Manchikalapudi S, Tang X-L, et al. (1998) Nitric oxide synthase is the mediator of late preconditioning against myocardial infarction in conscious rabbits. *Circulation* 98: 441–449.

Tanaka M, Fujiwara H, Yamusaki K, et al. (1994) Ischaemic preconditioning elevates but does not limit infarct size 24 or 48 hours later in rabbits. *Am J Physiol* 267: H1476–H1482.

Tawes RL Jr, Harris EJ, Brown WH, et al. (1985) Arterial thromboembolism. A 20-year perspective. *Arch Surg* 120: 595–599.

Toombs CF, Moore TL, Shebuski RJ. (1993) Limitation of infarct size in the rabbit by ischemic preconditioning is reversible with glybenclamide. *Cardiovasc Res* 27: 617–622.

Tountas CP, Bergman RA. (1997) Touriquet ischemia: Ultrastructural and histochemical observations of ischemic human muscle and of monkey muscle and nerve. *J Hand Surg* 2: 31–37.

Vahlhaus C, Schulz R, Post H, Onallah R, Heusch G. (1996) No prevention of ischemic preconditioning by the protein kinase C inhibitor staurosporine in swine. *Circ Res* 79: 407–414.

Van Winkle DM, Thornton D, Downey JM. (1991) The natural history of preconditioning: cardioprotection depends on duration of transient ischemia and time to subsequent ischemia. *Coronary Artery Disease* 2: 613–619.

Walker PM. (1986) Pathophysiology of acute arterial occlusion. *Can J Surg* 29: 340–342.

Weik R, Neumcke B. (1990) Effects of potassium channel openers on single potassium channels in mouse skeletal muscle. *Naumyn-Schmeideberg's Arch Pharmacol* 342: 258–263.

Yamashita N, Nishida M, Hoshida S, et al. (1994) Induction of manganese superoxide dismutase in rat cardiac myocytes increases tolerance to hypoxia 24 hours after preconditioning. *J Clin Invest* 94: 2193–2199.

Yao Z, Gross GJ. (1994) Effect of K_{ATP} channel opener bimakalim on coronary blood flow, monophasic action potential, and infarct size in dogs. *Circulation* 89: 1769–1775.

Yellon DM, Alkhulaifi AM, Browne EE, Pugsley WB. (1992) Ischemic preconditioning limits infarct size in the rat heart. *Cardiovasc Res* 26: 983–987.

Yellon DM, Baxter GF, Garcia-Dorado D, Heusch G, Sumeray. (1998) Ischemic preconditioning: present position and future directions. *Cardiovasc Res* 37: 21–33.

Ytrehus K, Liu Y, Downey JM. (1994) Preconditioning protects ischemic rabbit heart by protein kinase C activation. *Am J Physiol* 266: H1145–1152.

Zahir KS, Syed SA, Zink JR, Restifo RJ, Thomson JG. (1998) Ischemic preconditioning improves the survival of skin and myocutaneous flaps in a rat model. *Plast Reconstr Surg* 102: 140–151.

Zhou X, Zhai X, Ashraf M. (1996) Direct evidence that initial oxidative stress triggered by preconditioning contributes to second window of protection by endogenous antioxidant enzyme in myocytes. *Circulation* 93: 1177–1184.

Zelt RG, Olding M, Kerrigan CL, Daniel RK. (1986) Primary and secondary critical ischemic times of myocutaneous flaps. *Plast Reconstr Surg* 78: 498–503.

56

Management of skeletal muscle after stroke

Louise Ada and Colleen Canning

Introduction

This chapter discusses adaptations to skeletal muscle that occur as a result of immobility imposed by stroke. The main adaptations that interfere with function are length-associated changes where muscles lose their extensibility, and disuse-associated changes where muscles atrophy. Although these problems are secondary to the primary neurological impairments of loss of strength and dexterity, they influence outcome because they impose an additional obstacle to recovery. If these adaptations are allowed to develop, intervention to correct them will need to be implemented in order for the relearning of everyday tasks to occur. Therefore, the focus of this chapter is on preventing these maladaptations in the first instance. This involves anticipating which muscles are most at risk of length- and disuse-associated changes. Implementing effective preventative strategies also requires an understanding of the contribution of neurological and environmental factors to the development of secondary musculoskeletal problems after stroke.

Adaptions of skeletal muscle after stroke and their effect on function

Length-associated changes

Animal studies provide insight into the mechanism behind length-associated changes in muscle. When muscles are kept in a shortened position, they lose their extensibility as a result of a decrease in both length and compliance, i.e., they become shorter and stiffer. Essentially, they respond by losing sarcomeres (Tabary et al 1972, Hayat et al 1978, Williams and Goldspink 1978, Huet de la Tour et al 1979, Witzmann et al 1982). The change in sarcomere number appears to happen so that there is a myosin–actin overlap suitable for the new length (Williams and Goldspink 1978). Recently, decreases in the length and compliance of the tendon, which will contribute to the overall decrease in length of the muscle–tendon unit, have also been reported (Heslinga and Huijing 1993, Herbert and Crosbie 1997). Connective tissue is also remodelled. There is a relative increase in the amount of connective tissue, which will contribute to the increase in stiffness in immobilized muscles (Williams et al 1988). This increase is especially pronounced when muscles have been left in a shortened position

(Williams and Goldspink 1984). For more detailed information, see Gossman et al (1982), Herbert (1988, 1993a) and Goldspink and Williams (1990).

After stroke, if the person is effectively immobilized as a result of loss of strength, then muscles adapt to their new resting position. A decrease in muscle length, clinically referred to as contracture, results in a loss of joint range, which has a detrimental effect on function. For example, short calf muscles, in particular the gastrocnemius muscle, reduce ankle dorsiflexion, which interferes with the ability to walk. During stance phase, the forward movement of the shank over the fixed foot is necessary to allow forward translation of the body. With the foot flat on the floor and the knee straight, a short gastrocnemius muscle prevents forward movement of the shank. The only way the body mass can be moved forward in this situation is by flexing at the hip, a commonly observed walking strategy after stroke. The increased stiffness throughout the range of a muscle that accompanies a decrease in length poses an additional problem for function. Stiffness is the ratio of tension developed to the amount of lengthening that occurs, in this case, during passive stretching. An increase in stiffness throughout range, in human muscles with contracture following stroke, has been measured (O'Dwyer et al 1996). Stiffer muscles mean that more force has to be developed by opposing muscles to passively lengthen the stiff muscles.

Changes in muscle length also result in a shift in the active length–tension curve. When muscles become short, their length–tension curve shifts so that peak tension occurs at a shorter length (Williams and Goldspink 1978). This means that the greatest amount of force is generated nearer to inner range than normal. However, this change may not interfere with function as much as the adaptation that occurs in the antagonist muscles. When muscles are held in a lengthened position, they add sarcomeres, which has the effect of moving the length–tension curve so that peak tension occurs nearer to outer range than normal. This means that muscles that are antagonist to muscles with contracture not only generate the greatest amount of force nearer to outer range than normal but they may not be able to generate adequate force in the inner range. For example, short shoulder adductors opposed by long shoulder abductors may interfere with elevation of the arm. If the deltoid muscle has added sarcomeres as a result of the weak arm resting by the side of the body, lifting the arm to shoulder height will be difficult, not only as a result of weakness but also as a result of the adapted muscle's inability to generate force in that shortened position.

Disuse-associated changes

When muscles are not used, they generate less force as a result of atrophy, i.e., they become weaker. In the case of disuse-associated changes, studies on human as well as animal muscle have provided insight into the mechanism behind the behavioural change. Essentially, muscles that are not used reduce protein synthesis (Goldspink 1977, Booth and Seider 1979) and increase protein degradation (Goldspink 1977). This leads to a decrease in cross-sectional area, which in turn leads to a decrease in the ability of the muscle to generate tension. However, when a muscle is not used and it rests in its shortened position, the effects are magnified (Simard et al 1982). For more detailed information see Rose and Rothstein (1982), Halkjaer-Kristensen and Ingemann-Hansen (1985), St Pierre and Gardiner (1987), Goldspink and Williams (1990) and Herbert (1993b).

After stroke, if the person is effectively immobilized as a result of loss of strength, then muscles adapt by atrophying. A decrease in muscle mass caused by lack of use will result in a reduction in the muscle's ability to generate force, clinically referred to as disuse weakness. Loss of strength in elbow, knee and ankle muscles can be estimated at about 35% after 3 weeks of immobilization due to bed rest or casting in non-neurologically-impaired patients (see Herbert 1993b). However, it is hard to gauge the effect of this secondary adaptation on function after stroke because one of the main primary impairments interfering with function is loss of strength. While disuse weakness may ultimately contribute to long-term disability (Hachisuka et al 1997), weakness as a result of the lesion is the primary problem immediately after stroke. Bohannon and Smith (1987) reported loss of strength at 60–73% in upper limb muscles after stroke.

Factors affecting adaption of skeletal muscle after stroke

Obviously, it is beneficial if maladaptive changes can be prevented so that their detrimental effects on function do not occur. In order to prevent them, an understanding of the neural and environmental factors that contribute to their development is required. The stimulus for muscles to shorten appears to result from the imposed length change rather than from the movement deprivation imposed by immobilization. In animals, muscles immobilized in neutral do not markedly change in length or stiffness (Tabary et al 1972). In contrast, the stimulus for muscles to atrophy appears to result from lack of activity. Disuse results from a decrease in movement (hypokinesia) as well as a decrease in force production (hypodynamia). After stroke, muscles are effectively immobilized as a result of loss of strength. The affected limbs will, therefore, spend long periods of time in one position without moving, thereby fulfilling both criteria for disuse weakness—hypokinesia and hypodynamia. Furthermore, those muscles resting in their shortened range will develop contracture. For example, in sitting, if the foot cannot be moved back because of lack of strength and dexterity in the knee flexors and the dorsiflexors, the ankle assumes a position of plantarflexion. In addition to secondary disuse weakness of all the lower limb muscles, this combination of events produces short calf muscles, which will then interfere with everyday activities involving the lower limbs such as standing up and walking.

The effect of the environment (i.e., interaction with people and objects) can reinforce the effect of immobility on the development of contracture and disuse weakness. For example, early after stroke, if the arm is immobilized because of loss of strength and dexterity, it spends most of the time resting in the lap. In this position, muscles such as the shoulder adductors and internal rotators, the forearm pronators and wrist flexors are predisposed to developing contracture as they are resting in their shortened position. Unlike the lower limb, it is more possible to function one-handed than it is one-legged. Stroke patients who are not encouraged to keep trying to elicit muscle activity in the arm exhibit "learned non-use". Originally described by Taub (1980), deafferented monkeys "learned" not to use their limb after unsuccessful attempts. Similar behaviour observed after stroke leads to the arm being left resting in the lap, which in turn leads to length- and disuse-associated changes in upper limb muscles. Learned non-use will be further reinforced by a rehabilitation environment that is organized to cope with one-handedness, by staff either performing activities for patients or providing one-handed implements.

As well as immobility caused by loss of strength and dexterity after stroke, spasticity has been viewed as having a role in the development of contracture. The experimental model that best approximates muscle overactivity produced as a result of hyperactive stretch reflexes in spasticity is that of electrical stimulation. In animals, when immobilization in a shortened position is combined with electrical stimulation so that the muscles are made to chronically contract, the muscles become more short more quickly than with immobilization alone (Huet de la Tour et al 1979, Tabary et al 1981). It would, therefore, be expected that people exhibiting spasticity after stroke would develop marked contractures quickly. Although contracture and spasticity are often present simultaneously after stroke, there is no direct evidence that spasticity causes contracture (for review see O'Dwyer and Ada 1996). However, the reduction in muscle stiffness following the administration of spasticity-reducing drugs is accompanied by an increase in joint range (Albright et al 1993, Hesse et al 1994) suggesting that spasticity and contracture are linked.

Management of skeletal muscle after stroke— prevention of contracture and disuse weakness

The main aims of stroke rehabilitation can be summarized as:

1. maximizing potential function

2. minimizing secondary disability.

One of the difficulties in meeting these aims is that people after stroke have so many actions affected making intervention very costly in terms of time. Therefore, it is important to carry out the second aim as efficiently as possible. This can be done by designing intervention strategies that address both aims simultaneously. For example, improvement in function and prevention of contracture can both be addressed during task-specific training that emphasizes the use of muscles at risk of developing contracture in their lengthened range. Additionally, task-specific training that emphasizes using body weight to load muscles addresses improvement in function at the same time as prevention of disuse weakness.

Maintaining muscle length

After stroke, whenever patients are not being assisted to move, they tend to spend their time sitting in a chair (Fig. 56.1). In this position, the hips and knees are flexed and the ankles are usually slightly plantarflexed, the arm rests in the lap with the shoulder in internal rotation, the elbow, wrist and fingers in

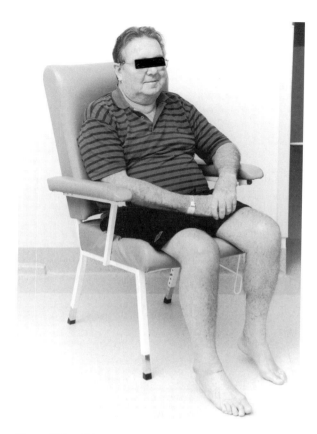

Figure 56.1 — This man is effectively immobilized as a result of a recent stroke. With his affected arm resting in his lap, the shoulder internal rotators, the elbow, wrist and fingers flexors, the forearm pronators and the thumb adductors are in their shortened range, and they are, therefore, susceptible to developing contractures. The chair is too high for him so that his feet are not flat on the floor and, therefore, the calf muscles of his affected ankle are also likely to shorten.

flexion, the forearm in pronation and the thumb in adduction. The muscles resting in a shortened part of their range are at risk of developing contracture. Given that it may be too time consuming and, therefore, not possible to prevent contracture in all muscles, attention should be focused on those muscles that, if short and stiff, will most interfere with function. This depends mostly on how important a small decrease in range is to the performance of everyday tasks. For example, reaching even slightly to the side relies on almost full external rotation at the shoulder and so a decrease in range of 10–20° will interfere with this movement, whereas a 10–20° decrease in shoulder flexion range will have very little effect on function. Muscles in which a small decrease in range will have a large effect on function include the shoulder internal rotators, the wrist flexors, the web space of the hand and the calf muscles. Therefore, prevention of contractures in these muscles is a priority.

Animal studies show that muscles immobilized in a shortened position lose up to 40% of their sarcomeres, and muscles immobilized in a lengthened position add up to 25% of their sarcomeres, within 3 weeks (Tabary et al 1972, Williams and Goldspink 1978). Animal studies suggest that 15 min of stretch every 2 days only partially prevents muscle shortening whereas 30 min every day prevents it entirely (Williams 1990). Little is known about the length of time needed to be spent in the lengthened position to prevent contractures in human muscle. Clinical studies have found that 2 h of low-load, prolonged stretch is more effective at increasing joint range than high-load, brief stretch (Light et al 1984) in frail elderly and that 2 × 20 min of positioning the shoulder in external rotation reduces

contracture in the internal rotators after stroke, although not significantly (Dean et al 2000). Currently, a reasonable clinical guideline seems to be that muscles at risk of developing contracture should spend at least 20–30 min in their longest position, either as the result of active contractions by the patient or passive positioning by staff.

Muscle length may be effectively maintained if training in everyday tasks includes exercises that place at-risk muscles in lengthened positions. For example, eccentric control by the calf muscles at the end of stance phase to decelerate the shank over the fixed foot is an important component of relearning to walk. In standing, moving the body mass forward over a fixed foot places the affected ankle in dorsiflexion. The gastrocnemius muscle is working eccentrically, and it is being lengthened at the same time (Fig. 56.2).

Active motor training may have to be supplemented by passive positioning where active training does not

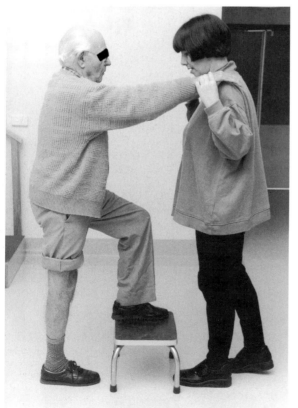
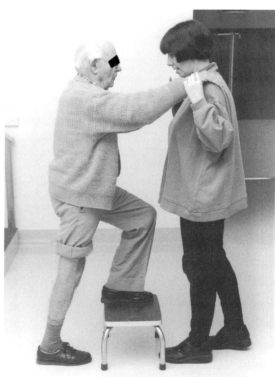

A

B

Figure 56.2—**A** This man after stroke is practicing weight-bearing through his affected right leg in preparation for the single support part of the stance phase of walking. **B** With his knee extended, he extends his hip and dorsiflexes at his ankle to shift his weight forward. This exercise requires that he lengthen his plantarflexors eccentrically to control the forward rotation of the shank on the fixed foot. His intact left leg rests on a stool and his hands rest on the therapists shoulders for balance.

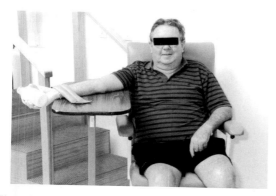

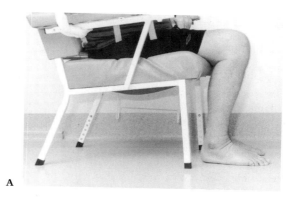

A

Figure 56.3— This man is undergoing his daily 30 min routine of passive lengthening of the upper limb muscles at risk of shortening after stroke. The arm rests on a table adjusted to shoulder height so that the shoulder is in horizontal abduction and external rotation. A sandbag holds the forearm in supination. The hand rests over the edge of the table so that the wrist is extended. A large cylindrical object is taped into the hand to stretch the web space and the finger flexors.

keep the at-risk muscles in a lengthened position for sufficient time. This is especially the case in people who are very weak after stroke so that there is little or no antagonist muscle activity opposing the at-risk muscles. The use of a position that lengthens several at-risk muscles at once is time efficient. For example, supporting the affected arm at shoulder height in abduction and external rotation, with the wrist extended and the hand positioned around a large jar lengthens the shoulder internal rotators, adductors and extensors, the forearm pronators and the wrist flexors as well as stretches the web space between the thumb and first finger (Fig. 56.3).

The process of positioning will be more efficient if it is incorporated into routine ward protocols. For example, if part of providing an environment tailored to individual patients is to adapt a height-adjustable chair to just below knee height in order to make standing up an achievable task, then this should also include the responsibility by staff to ensure that the affected foot is back behind the knee, not only during standing up but also when sitting (Fig. 56.4a). Adoption of this protocol should help maintain the length of the soleus and, to a lesser extent, the gastrocnemius muscle and, therefore, have a beneficial effect on lower limb functions involving dorsiflexion. Similarly, positioning the arm in some external rotation on a gutter splint or lap board when sitting (Fig. 56.4b) should assist in maintaining the length of the internal rotators of the shoulder.

Muscle length needs to be measured every couple of weeks to monitor whether a contracture is devel-

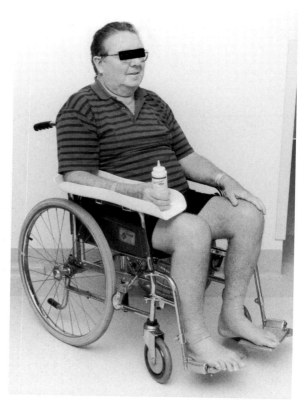

B

Figure 56.4— When not in therapy, part of ward procedure should be that patients sit so as to minimize the risk of contracture. **A** When sitting on the ward, a height adjustable chair is adjusted so that the feet rest flat on the floor with the ankle in maximum dorsiflexion. **B** When being transported in a wheelchair, the arm rests on an arm support so that the arm is not in internal rotation and the forearm not in pronation.

oping. It is important to note that if a contracture is minor in extent it may still be possible to achieve a normal range of motion by the application of sufficient force. For example, Halar et al (1978) applied a force of 178 N and achieved similar magnitudes of ankle dorsiflexion on the affected and unaffected sides of hemiplegic patients, even in the presence of "clinical" contracture. Consequently, in order to assess the magnitude of joint motion, it is important not only to standardize the force applied but also not to exceed the magnitude of force that is normally sufficient to stretch the muscles through the joint range. In addition, if a multi-joint muscle is being assessed, it is important to standardize the position of the joint not being measured. Measurement procedures that are simple, use gravity to apply a standardized force and measure the limit of several joints simultaneously are the best option. Furthermore, the limb should be moved slowly to avoid exciting hyperactive reflexes, which, in spasticity, are velocity-sensitive (Lance 1980).

Training muscle strength

Atrophy begins quickly after immobilization and human studies show a 14–17% decrease in muscle fibre size after only 3 days of immobilization in a shortened position (Lindboe and Platoe 1984). Loss of strength in elbow, knee and ankle muscles can be estimated at about 35% after 3 weeks of immobilization due to bed rest or casting in non-neurologically-

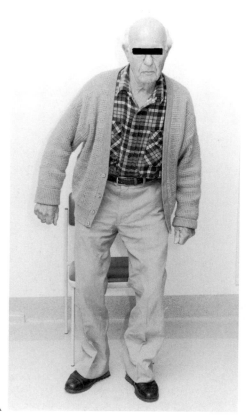
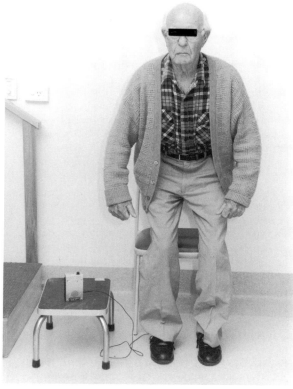

A

B

Figure 56.5—**A** When this man stands up from sitting, he favours his intact left leg. **B** A limb load monitor[#] has been calibrated to 50% of his body weight and the pressure-sensitive footpad placed in his right shoe. As he stands up and sits down, he receives auditory feedback if he keeps 50% of his body weight through his affected right leg. Loading of the affected lower limb extensors in this way will prevent disuse weakness as well as assist his ability to stand up. Further improvement in strength can be promoted by increasing the amount of body weight taken through the affected leg ([#] Electronic Quantification Inc, Philadelphia).

impaired patients (see Herbert 1993b). If addressing the primary problem of weakness includes exercises that require muscles to work under reasonable loads during the training of everyday tasks, then disuse weakness may be largely avoided.

When some ability to activate the muscles is present, this ability needs to be challenged. For example, patients after stroke commonly compensate for loss of strength in the lower limb extensors by standing up with most of their body weight through their intact lower limb (Fig. 56.5a). If they are forced to stand up with more weight through their affected limb, achieved either through manual guidance from the therapist or by feedback from an electronic device such as a limb load monitor, then strength training of the lower limb extensors is being carried out at the same time as training functional recovery (Fig. 56.5b). Similarly, Taub et al (1993) found an increase in function of the affected upper limb following a period of forced use of the affected upper limb in patients after stroke.

It is difficult to prevent disuse weakness in situations where patients are paralysed and so cannot exercise their muscles actively. Electrical stimulation has been shown to reduce muscle atrophy by the mechanism of prevention of a fall in protein synthesis (Goldspink and Goldspink 1986, Gibson et al 1988). Even though electrical stimulation has been shown to increase strength after stroke (Glanz et al 1996), it is not clinically feasible to apply it to all muscles. However, it may be beneficial to apply electrical stimulation in situations where loss of muscle strength will have serious consequences. For example, electrical stimulation to the supraspinatus and posterior deltoid muscles for up to 6 h per day has been shown not only to increase muscle strength but also to reduce subluxation of the humerus in the gleno-humeral joint (Faghri et al 1994).

Summary

The main adaptations to skeletal muscle that interfere with function after stroke are length-associated changes where muscles lose their extensibility, and disuse-associated changes where muscles atrophy. Preventing the development of contracture and disuse weakness involves not only anticipating which muscles are most at risk of length- and disuse-associated changes but also understanding the contribution of both neurological and environmental factors to the development of secondary musculoskeletal problems after stroke. Strategies that involve passive positioning

and electrical stimulation of muscle may be needed to supplement voluntary contraction of muscle.

References

Albright AL, Barron WB, Fasick MP, Polinko P, Janosky J. (1993) Continuous intrathecal baclofen infusion for spasticity of cerebral origin. *JAMA* 270 (20): 2475–2477.

Bohannon RW, Smith MB. (1987) Assessment of strength deficits in eight upper extremity muscle groups of stroke patients with hemiplegia. *Phys Ther* 67: 522–525.

Booth FW, Seider MJ. (1979) Early change in skeletal muscle protein synthesis after limb immobilisation in rats. *J Appl Physiol* 47: 974–977.

Dean CM, Mackey FH, Katrak P. (2000) Examination of shoulder positioning after stroke. A randomised controlled pilot trial. *Aust J Physiother* 46(1): 35–40.

Faghri PD, Rodgers MM, Glaser RM, Bors JG, Ho C, Akuthota P. (1994) The effects of functional electrical stimulation on shoulder subluxation, arm function recovery, and shoulder pain in hemiplegic stroke patients. *Arch Phys Med Rehab* 75(1): 73–79.

Gibson JNA, Smith K, Rennie MJ. (1988) Prevention of disuse muscle atrophy by means of electrical stimulation: maintenance of protein synthesis. *Lancet* 2(8614): 767–770.

Glanz M, Klawansky S, Statson W, Berkey C. (1996) Functional electrostimulation in poststroke rehabilitation: a meta-analysis of the randomised controlled trials. *Arch Phys Med Rehab* 77: 549–533.

Goldspink DF, Goldspink G. (1986) The role of passive stretch in retarding muscle atrophy. In: Nix WA, Vrbova G, eds. *Electrical Stimulation and Neuromuscular Disorders.* Berlin: Springer–Verlag pp 91–100.

Goldspink DF. (1977) The influence of immobilization and stretch on protein turnover of rat skeletal muscle. *J Physiol* 264: 267–282.

Goldspink G, Williams PE. (1990) Muscle fibre and connective tissue changes associated with use and disuse. In: Ada L, Canning C, eds. *Foundations for practice. Key issues in neurological physiotherapy.* London: Heinemann, pp. 197–218.

Gossman MR, Sahrmann SA, Rose SJ. (1982) Review of length-associated changes in muscle. Experimental evidence and clinical implications. *Phys Ther* 62: 1799–1808.

Hachisuka K, Umezu Y, Ogata H. (1997) Disuse muscle atrophy of lower limbs in hemiplegic patients. *Arch Phys Med Rehab* 78: 13–18.

Halar EM, Stolov WC, Venkatesh B, Brozovich FV, Harley JD. (1978) Gastrocnemius muscle belly and tendon length in stroke patients and able-bodied persons. *Arch Phys Med Rehab* 59: 476–484.

Halkjaer-Kristensen J, Ingemann-Hansen T. (1985) Wasting of the human quadriceps muscle after knee ligament injuries. *Scand J Rehab Med Suppl* 13: 5–55.

Hayat A, Tardieu C, Tabary JC, Tabary C. (1978) Effects of denervation on the reduction of sarcomere number in cat soleus muscle immobilised in shortened position during seven days. *J Physiol (Paris)* 74: 563–567.

Herbert R. (1993a) Preventing and treating stiff joints. In: Crosbie J, McConnell J, eds. *Key Issues in Musculoskeletal Physiotherapy*. Oxford: Butterworth-Heinemann, pp. 114–141.

Herbert R. (1993b) Human strength adaptations - implications for therapy. In: Crosbie J, McConnell J, eds. *Key Issues in Musculoskeletal Physiotherapy*. Oxford: Butterworth-Heinemann, pp. 142–171.

Herbert R. (1988) The passive mechanical properties of muscle and their adaptations to altered patterns of use. *Aust J Physiother* 34: 141–149.

Herbert RD, Crosbie J. (1997) Rest length and compliance of non-immobilised and immobilised rabbit soleus muscle and tendon. *Eur J Appl Physiol* 76(5): 472–480.

Heslinga JW, Huijing PA. (1993) Muscle length-force characterisics in relation to muscle architecture: A bilateral study of gastrocnemius medialis muscles of unilaterally immobilized rats. *Eur J Appl Physiol* 66(4): 289–298.

Hesse S, Lücke D, Malezic M, et al. (1994) Botulinum toxin treatment for lower limb extensor spasticity in chronic hemiparetic patients. *J Neurol Neurosurg Psychiatry* 57: 1321–1324.

Huet de la Tour E, Tabary JC, Tabary C, Tardieu C. (1979) The respective roles of muscle length and muscle tension in sarcomere number adaptation of guinea-pig soleus muscle. *J Physiol (Paris)* 75: 589–592.

Lance JW (1980): Symposium synopsis. In: Feldman RG, Young RR, Koella WP, eds. *Spasticity: Disordered motor control*. Chicago/Miami: Symposia Specialists, pp. 485–494.

Light KE, Nuzick S, Personius W, Barstrom A. (1984) Low-load prolonged stretch vs. high-load brief stretch in treating knee contractures. *Phys Ther* 64: 330–333.

Lindboe CF, Platoe CS. (1984) Effect of immobilisation of short duration on the muscle fibre size. *Clin Physiol* 4: 183–188.

O'Dwyer NJ, Ada L, Neilson PD. (1996) Spasticity and muscle contracture following stroke. *Brain* 119: 1737–1749.

O'Dwyer NJ, Ada L. (1996) Reflex hyperexcitability and muscle contracture in relation to spastic hypertonia. *Curr Opin Neurol* 9: 451–455.

Rose SJ, Rothstein JM. (1982) Muscle mutability. Part 1. General concepts and adaptations to altered patterns of use. *Phys Ther* 62(12): 1773–1787.

Simard CP, Spector SA, Edgerton VR. (1982) Contractile properties of rat hindlimb muscles immobilised at different lengths. *Exp Neurol* 77: 467–482.

St Pierre D, Gardiner PF. (1987) The effect of immobilisation and exercise on muscle function: a review. *Physiother Can* 39(1): 24–36.

Tabary JC, Tardieu C, Tardieu G, Tabary C. (1981) Experimental rapid sarcomere loss with concomitant hypoextensibility. *Muscle Nerve* 4: 198–203.

Tabary JC, Tabary C, Tardieu C, Tardieu G, Goldspink G. (1972) Physiological and structural changes in the cat's soleus muscle due to immobilisation at different lengths by plaster casts. *J Physiol (Lond)* 224: 231–244.

Taub E. (1980) Somatosensory deafferentation research with monkeys: implications for rehabilitation medicine. In: Ince LP, ed. *Behavioral Psychology in Rehabilitation Medicine: Clinical Implications*. Baltimore: Williams and Wilkins, pp. 371–401.

Taub E, Miller NE, Novack TA, et al. (1993) Technique to improve chronic motor deficit after stroke. *Arch Phys Med Rehab* 74: 347–354.

Williams PE. (1990) Use of intermittent stretch in the prevention of serial sarcomere loss in immobilised muscle. *Ann Rheum Dis* 49: 316–317.

Williams PE, Goldspink G. (1978) Changes in sarcomere length and physiological properties in immobilized muscle. *J Anat* 127: 459–468.

Williams PE, Goldspink G. (1984) Connective tissue changes in immobilised muscle. *J Anat* 138: 343–350.

Williams PE, Catanese T, Lucey E, Goldspink G. (1988) The importance of stretch and contractile activity in the prevention of connective tissue accumulation in muscle. *J Anat* 158: 109–114.

Witzmann FA, Kim DH, Fitts RH. (1982) Hindlimb immobilisation: length-tension and contractile properties of skeletal muscle. *J Appl Physiol* 53(2): 335–345.

57

Skeletal muscle relaxants

Leo Booij

Introduction

Muscle relaxants are used clinically to induce reliable and reproducible relaxation to facilitate endotracheal intubation and surgical procedures, and to relieve hypertonicity and spasms. Their mechanism of action is by interruption of neuromuscular transmission. Nerve depolarization causes pre-junction release of acetylcholine; this diffuses across the junctional cleft and binds to postsynaptic ligand-gated nicotinergic acetylcholine receptors, which act as sodium channels. Activation causes muscle membrane depolarization and contraction of the muscle. Prevention of acetylcholine binding prevents receptor activation and leads to paralysis.

Pharmacodynamic characteristics of neuromuscular blockade

The pharmacodynamic behaviour of muscle relaxants is described by a number of parameters based on nerve stimulation and measuring the contraction force of the muscle:

- Potency: percentage decrease in force of muscle contraction in relation to the dose
- Onset: time from injection until maximal effect
- Clinical duration (duration$_{25}$): time from injection until 25% recovery of contraction force
- Total duration (duration$_{90}$): time from injection until 90% recovery
- Recovery rate: time from 25 to 75% recovery.

Because these pharmacodynamic parameters depend on the dose administered, they are in general related to a dose causing 95% block (ED$_{95}$). For endotracheal intubation, a dose equal to two times this ED$_{95}$ is generally used. When the muscle contraction force is less than 25% of normal, excellent surgical operation conditions exist. When muscle contraction force has recovered above 75% of normal, the ability for spontaneous breathing is adequate. The effect of relaxants differs between muscles. Therefore, for comparison, the same muscle must be examined (Donati et al 1991, Engbaek and Roed 1992). Because the effect also depends on the rate of nerve stimulation, traditionally a constant current single twitch supra-maximal stimulation at a rate of 0.1–0.15 Hz is employed.

Neuromuscular blockers are characterized by a wide interindividual variability (Katz 1967).

Onset of neuromuscular blockade

One of the major concerns during anaesthesia, and other situations where relaxants are used, is the loss of airway patency. This increases the risk of regurgitation and aspiration of gastric contents, and development of the highly mortal Mendelson's syndrome. Therefore, the trachea is intubated as soon as possible, which demands sufficient relaxation.

Suxamethonium has long been the first choice because of its very rapid onset. However, because of its many side-effects, its use has been questioned, and its replacement by non-depolarizers has been advocated. Most non-depolarizers, however, have a slow onset, and a variety of methods to diminish this delay have been promoted. One of the most frequently employed methods is an increase in the dose. This results in a higher incidence of side-effects. Pancuronium for example will lead to tachycardia and hypertension. Benzylisoquinolines, but not steroids, cause histamine release. A major problem in the administration of large dosages is a prolonged effect, and the risk of undetected residual curarization at the end of the procedure. This is more pronounced with longer acting relaxants, which demand almost routine administration of reversal agents. Administration of anticholinesterases, however, increases the risk for muscarinic complications such as bradycardia, increased bowel motility, nausea and vomiting.

Depolarizing muscle relaxants

Depolarizing muscle relaxants bind to acetylcholine receptors, exert intrinsic activity, and keep them occupied so that further binding of acetylcholine cannot occur. If 25% of the receptors is occupied, the ion-channel opens up, resulting in an uncoordinated depolarization and muscle contraction (fasciculations). Depolarizers do not compete with acetylcholine for the receptor, and the blockade can not, therefore, be reversed pharmacological. The block is terminated by dissociation of the depolarizer from the receptor and its subsequent degradation by plasma cholinesterase in the blood. Prolonged exposure of acetylcholine receptors to depolarizers can cause refractoriness of the receptors to additional application of agonist; this effect is called desensitization. When desensitization occurs, the neuromuscular block changes its characteristics from a phase I (no fade in response to tetanic stimulation) into a long phase II blockade (fading). Although a phase II block can be antagonized with neostigmine, such reversibility is not predictable.

Suxamethonium

Suxamethonium is the only depolarizing relaxant in clinical use. It is not selective for the nicotinic acetylcholine receptors at the neuromuscular junction, but also binds to nicotinergic receptors in the autonomic ganglia (sympathetic and parasympathetic) and muscarinic receptors (parasympathetic) in a number of organs, including the heart. This results in many adverse effects, such as bradycardia, hypertension and cardiac arrest (Robinson et al 1996). It has the potential to increase intra ocular, intracranial and intragastric pressure (Minton et al 1986, Frankville and Drummond 1987, Warner et al 1989). The increase in intra ocular pressure is manifest 1 min after administration, and it peaks at 2–4 min. It is partly due to increased choroidal blood flow and decreases in absorption of aqueous humour from its cycloplegic action (Kelly et al 1993). Also extra ocular muscle contractions contribute to the intra ocular pressure. The use of suxamethonium in patients with an open eye globe remains questionable. The increase in intragastric pressure is partly due to muscle contractions and partly to a muscarinic effect on the intestines. This increases the risk of silent regurgitation and aspiration. However, the rapid onset of action makes rapid intubation possible, and thus counteracts this risk. Suxamethonium changes the electroencephalogram (EEG) in the same way as muscle afferent activity does. The cerebral effects of suxamethonium are mediated by muscle afferent activity, which is abolished during deep anaesthesia or cerebral ischaemia. In a number of situations (extensive burns, cold injury, spinal cord injury, sepsis, neuromuscular diseases, peripheral nerve injury and neuropathy) suxamethonium leads to cardiac arrest and other arrhythmias, presumably through massive potassium release and subsequent hyperkalemia (Martyn et al 1986). The development of extrajunctional acetylcholine receptor sites plays a role in this phenomenon. In patients with muscle diseases, especially Duchenne's muscular dystrophy, suxamethonium can provoke rhabdomyolyis.

Eighty per cent of suxamethonium is normally hydrolysed by plasma cholinesterase before it reaches the neuromuscular junction. With quantitative or qualitative decreases in cholinesterase activity, the effect of suxamethonium is enhanced and its duration prolonged (Vanlinthout et al 1992, Jensen and Viby-Mogensen 1995). The production of cholinesterase in the liver is controlled by genetic expression. Variants in genetic expression may result in decreased activity (Ritter et al 1988, Whittaker and Britten 1987). In patients with plasma cholinesterase deficiency an extremely prolonged neuromuscular blockade occurs. During pregnancy the cholinesterase activity decreases by 25–30% (Robson et al 1986). After cardiopulmonary bypass the activity is decreased for more than 7 days (Shearer and Russell 1993, Collard et al 1996). Also with malignancies, burn trauma and sepsis the activity of cholinesterase decreases (Blanloeil et al 1996). In chronic exposure to insecticides a decrease is also present. Repeated plasma exchange decreases plasma cholinesterase activity, as do some drugs, such as ecothiopate, bambuterol, corticosteroids, cytotoxics, anticonceptives and oestrogens.

In susceptible patients suxamethonium can evoke malignant hyperthermia (hyperthermia, rigidity, acidosis, hyperkalemia, dysrhythmia, hypercapnia, myoglobinuria). The masseter muscle, especially in children, can show spasm in 0.01–1% of cases after administration of suxamethonium (Smith et al 1989). The contracture may be enhanced by halothane anaesthesia. This causes an inability to open the mouth for as long as 10 minutes, and prevents endotracheal intubation. It is surprising that a large difference in incidence exists between the US and Europe. Although many have indicated that there is a relationship between masseter muscle rigidity and malignant hyperthermia, this has never been proven (VanderSpek et al 1990, O'Flynn et al 1994).

It frequently is stated that suxamethonium provides better safety in cases where the trachea cannot be intubated. This is based on the believe that patients start breathing within 5 min after suxamethonium administration. However, the duration of action of suxamethonium after a clinical dose of 0.75–1 mg/kg is approximately 8–15 min, with more cases in the region of 15 min than of 8 min. Such a period of time is sufficient to cause hypoxic brain damage, which is no different from that caused by non-depolarizing relaxants.

Non-depolarizing relaxants

Non-depolarizing relaxants bind to acetylcholine receptors, but they do not have an intrinsic effect. When approximately 75% of the receptors are occupied muscle contraction force starts to decrease and at 90%, full paralysis is present. Such receptor binding is characterized by a constant association and dissociation of drug. The rate of receptor association (association constant) and dissociation (dissociation constant) determine the receptor affinity, and, therefore, they are important factors in the "onset" and "offset" of blockade. As long as there is relaxant in the vicinity of the receptor, occupation can occur. Thus, the concentration of relaxant in the biophase determines the degree of neuromuscular blockade (Shanks et al 1979). This concentration is determined by the plasma concentration and the physical-chemical characteristics of the relaxant. There is competition with acetylcholine and, therefore, anticholinesterases can reverse the blockade.

The clinical muscle relaxants presently available all have side-effects (Clarke and Mirakhur 1994). Cardiovascular effects are the result of several mechanisms. Histamine release is another important effect (Lien et al 1995).

The clinically used non-depolarizers can be roughly divided into a benzylisoquinoline group and a group with a steroidal structure. All have a wide variability in effect for reasons such as interindividual variation in body size and composition, muscular maturity (age), gender and variability in plasma cholinesterase activity. Other factors include interaction with concurrent medication, disorders such as hepatic and renal failure, acid–base imbalance, electrolyte shift and neuromuscular diseases. Non-depolarizers have no effect on intraocular pressure (Robertson et al 1994).

Benzylisoquinoline type relaxants

The development of clinical muscle relaxants began with the examination of the arrow poison produced from *Chondodendron* and *Strychnos* plant species by Indian tribes in the northern part of South America. Alkaloids (respectively chondocurine and toxiferine I) were extracted from them, and these served as the basis for the development of the benzylisoquinoline-type

relaxants (tubocurarine, metocurine, nortoxiferine, atracurium, cisatracurium, doxacurium, mivacurium) (Wintersteiner and Dutcher 1943). The compounds contain two benzylisoquinoline groups, as in most drugs connected to each other with a flexible ester bridge. The bridge contains one or more chiral points, which leads to the existence of several stereoisomers. The benzylisoquinolines, with exceptions of d-tubocurarine and metocurine, are metabolized by ester hydrolysis. Common characteristics of this group of compounds are lack of vagolytic effect, dose related histamine release and reversibility by anticholinesterases (Booij et al 1980, North et al 1987, Stellato et al 1991). The individual compounds have a different time course of action (see Table 57.1). Tubocurarine, a monoquarternary compound, is the oldest benzylisoquinoline relaxant and causes marked histamine release. Atracurium exists in a racemic mixture of 10 stereoisomers, most of which are pharmacologically active (Amaki et al 1985). The main disadvantage of atracurium is its histamine release. Slow administration and avoiding high doses largely overcomes this problem. It was initially thought that the metabolism was by temperature- and pH-dependent Hofmann degradation into laudanosine, an acrylate, and a monoquarternary ester. This ester is further degraded into a second laudanosine molecule and an acrylate ester (Hughes and Chapple 1981). However, because the plasma concentration of laudanosine is highest immediately after injection of atracurium, which is incompatible with spontaneous (Hofmann) degradation, rapid but limited hydrolysis must also be present. Through this mechanism, a large fraction of atracurium is rapidly degraded in the plasma, and so it does

Table 57.1 — Pharmacodynamic characteristics of clinically used muscle relaxants

Drug	ED_{95} (mg/kg)	Intub dose (mg/kg)	Onset (min)	Duration$_{25}$ (min)	Duration$_{95}$ (min)	Rec. rate (min)
Suxamethonium	0.35	1.00	1	5–7	10–12	3
Atracurium	0.25	0.50	6	25–30	35–45	12
Cisatracurium	0.30	0.6	7	25–30	35–45	12
Doxacurium	0.03	0.07	7.5	70–90	120–150	50
Mivacurium	0.08	0.2	4	20–30	30–40	7
Pancuronium	0.06	0.1	5	30–45	60–90	35
Vecuronium	0.05	0.15	4.5	30–45	30–50	20
Rocuronium	0.4	0.8	2.5	30–40	30–50	20
d-Tubocurarine	0.5	0.6	10	90–100	120–180	45

ED_{95}, dose causing 95% block; Intub. dose, dose used for intubation; Onset, time from injection to maximal effect; Duration$_{25}$, Duration$_{95}$, time from injection to 25% and 90%, recovery, respectively; Rec. rate, time from 25–75% recovery.

not reach the acetylcholine receptors in the biophase. Cisatracurium is one of the 10 atracurium stereoisomers (Belmont et al 1995). It causes increase in plasma histamine concentration, but, in clinical dosages does not lead to clinical signs of histamine release or related cardiovascular effects. Metabolism is similar to that of atracurium. Mivacurium has three stereoisomers, and its short duration of action is explained by metabolism through plasma cholinesterase into a pharmacological inactive quaternary mono-ester, a quaternary amino alcohol and dicarboxylic acid (Savarese et al 1988). Duration of action varies with plasma cholinesterase activity, and a number of cases showing prolonged mivacurium effects have been published (Petersen et al 1993, Diefenbach et al 1995). Although cardio-pulmonary bypass decreases cholinesterase activity by 60%, mivacurium during and after this procedure in normothermic conditions is not prolonged. However, a case has been reported where, in a patient with dermatomyositis and low plasma cholinesterase activity, prolonged paralysis and inability to reverse with edrophonium was demonstrated (Mangar et al 1993). More cases with prolonged effect and difficult reversibility have been published (Ostergaard et al 1992, Goudsouzian et al 1993, Maddineni and Mirakhur 1993). Doxacurium is hydrolysed by plasma cholinesterase at a rate 60% that of suxamethonium, and 40% is excreted unchanged in the urine with small amounts in the bile (Basta et al 1988). Doxacurium does not cause haemodynamic effects (Maddineni et al 1992).

Aminosteroidal type of relaxants

In Africa, paralysing poisons were produced from *Malouetia bequaertiana*. From these poisons Malouétine was extracted, and this served as the basis for the steroidal relaxants (pancuronium, pipecuronium, vecuronium, rocuronium; Huu-Lainé and Pinto-Scognamiglio 1964). The basic structure contains an androstan skeleton to which two acetylcholine-like moieties at the A and the D ring are introduced (Buckett et al 1973). The acetylcholine-like moiety at the D ring is apparently responsible for binding to the nicotinic acetylcholine receptor at the neuromuscular junction sites, and the acetylcholine-like moiety at the A ring for binding to muscarinic receptors at other sites (Marshall et al 1980, Appadu and Lambert 1994). The compounds differ in their pharmacodynamic profile (see Table 57.1). The steroids neither have an effect on intra ocular pressure, nor do they cause histamine release (Robertson et al 1983). Most depend on organ function for their excretion. Pancuronium is one of the most frequently used bis-quaternary non-depolarizing muscle relaxants (Krieg et al 1980). It is metabolized mainly by deacetylation in the liver, and is, thereafter, excreted in the urine. The metabolites (3-OH, 17-OH, and 3,7-di-OH) are considerably less potent relaxants (Miller et al 1978). Pancuronium increases heart rate, arterial pressure, and cardiac output. Vecuronium is a mono-quaternary non-depolarizing relaxant without cardiovascular effects. Hepatic uptake lowers its blood concentration, with subsequent deacetylation and renal excretion (Fahey et al 1981). Rocuronium is a rapid onset intermediate-acting mono-quaternary relaxant (Wierda et al 1990, Booij and Knape 1991, Huizenga et al 1992). Its plasma clearance is mainly through liver uptake and bile excretion (Szenohradszky et al 1992). It causes pain on injection and a slight increase in heart rate (McCoy et al 1993).

The pharmacokinetics of muscle relaxants

The pharmacokinetic behaviour of most muscle relaxants can be described in a two or three compartment model. The drug is administered in, and excreted from, the central compartment. Onset and offset of effect is determined by the concentration in the biophase, which is in equilibrium with the plasma concentration (Shanks 1993). There is a rapid distribution phase, followed by a slower elimination phase, with bio-transformation and excretion. The initial volume of distribution is limited to between 80 and 150 ml/kg, due to the water solubility. The volume of distribution in the steady state is between 200 and 450 ml/kg, somewhere between the extracellular water volume and the total body water. Some pharmacokinetic parameters of the individual relaxants are given in Table 57.2. The volumes of distribution and the body clearance of the relaxants can be severely affected by disease states. Protein binding of these relaxants varies between 30 and 85%.

Interaction between relaxants and concurrent diseases

Many diseases interfere with either the pharmacodynamics or the pharmacokinetics of muscle relaxants, resulting in an altered sensitivity and a change in the time course of action (Booij 1989). Some diseases

Table 57.2 — Pharmacokinetic parameters of clinically used muscle relaxants

Drug	VDc (l/kg)	VDss (l/kg)	Clp (ml/kg/min)	$T_{1/2}\beta$ (min)	Protein binding (%)
Atracurium	0.05	0.20	6.6	21	80
Doxacurium		0.22	2.76	99	30–35
Mivacurium		0.11	70	16	
Pancuronium	0.10	0.26	1.8	132	85
Vecuronium	0.07	0.27	5.2	71	70
Rocuronium	0.04	0.21	3.7	97	
d–Tubocurarine	0.03	0.25	2.4	84	35–55

VDc = volume distribution central compartment, VDss = volume distribution steady rate, Clp = plasma clearance, $T_{1/2}\beta$ = half life time elimination phase

Table 57.3 — Percentage and route of elimination of relaxants over 24 h

Drug	Elimination		
	% renal	% hepatic	Metabolism
Suxamethonium	0	0	100% plasma-cholinesterase hydrolysis
Atracurium	6–10	0	90% Hofmann degradation + hydrolysis
Cisatracurium	6–10	0	90% Hofmann degradation + hydrolysis
Doxacurium	25–50		25–20% hydrolysis
Mivacurium	0	0	100% hydrolysis
Pancuronium	60–90	20–30	35% liver
Vecuronium	20–30	50–60	35% liver
Rocuronium	20–30		35% liver
d–Tubocurarine	45–60	10–60	–

interfere with the generation and conductance of motor nerve stimuli, other diseases with acetylcholine synthesis, mobilization, release or metabolism, or with the number of postjunctional acetylcholine receptors available.

Effect of renal and hepatic diseases on muscle relaxants

Most relaxants are water soluble, ionized, quaternary ammonium compounds, and, therefore, depend on glomerular filtration, tubular excretion and tubular reabsorption for their rate of body clearance (see Table 57.3). Others are metabolized and/or glucuronidated in the liver, and then excreted via the kidneys. The liver plays a minor role in the excretion of the maternal compounds. In renal diseases most relaxants show a prolonged time course of action. Also, altered fluid status, metabolic imbalance, electrolyte shift, acid–base imbalance and concurrent administration of drugs are then involved. With most relaxants the initial volume of distribution (central compartment) is not different in patients with renal failure, but the elimination half-life is longer (see Table 57.4). This is because of a larger volume of distribution and a reduced plasma clearance. Protein binding only contributes minimally because relaxants are not highly protein bound (40–50%). Alpha-1-globulin binding is the major component in protein binding.

Because drug metabolism is only affected in the later stages of cirrhosis, this disease, in general, does not influence the duration of neuromuscular blockade. In cholestasis, however, the uptake of relaxants in the liver is decreased, which decreases plasma clearance and leads to prolonged effect (Westra et al 1981). In patients with liver disease the concentration of plasma cholinesterase, on which the metabolism of suxamethonium and mivacurium is dependent, is frequently decreased.

Table 57.4— Pharmacokinetic data of muscle relaxants in patients with and without renal failure, and in cirrhosis

Drug	VDss (l/kg)			Clp (ml/kg/min)			$t_{1/2}\beta$ (min)		
	Normal	Renal	Cirrhosis	Normal	Renal	Cirrhosis	Normal	Renal	Cirrhosis
Atracurium	0.18	0.22	0.28	6.1	6.7	8.0	21	24	25
Doxacurium	0.22	0.27	0.29	2.66	1.6	2.33	96	221	115
Mivacurium	0.11	0.15	0.12	70.3	76.5	33.2	18	34	34
Pancuronium	0.15	0.24	0.42	1.0	0.3	1.5	100	489	208
Vecuronium	0.20	0.24	0.35	5.3	3.1	2.7	53	83	84
Rocuronium	0.21	0.21	0.24	3.7	2.1	2.4	97	104	96
d-Tubocurarine	0.25	0.25	–	2.4	1.5	–	84	132	–

VDss = volume distribution steady state, Clp = plasma clearance, $t_{1/2}\beta$ = half life time elimination phase

Effect of acid–base balance disturbances on muscle relaxants

Acid–base disturbances interfere with muscle relaxation through various mechanisms, such as alteration in protein binding, changes in electrolyte distribution and in acetylcholine release. Suxamethonium is antagonized by acidosis, while alkalosis potentiates its effect. In vitro studies have demonstrated that acidosis potentiates mono-quaternary relaxants (tubocurarine, rocuronium and vecuronium) but antagonizes bis-quaternary relaxants (metocurine and pancuronium) (Ono et al 1990). Respiratory acidosis and metabolic alkalosis decrease the reversing effect of the anticholinesterases.

Effects of neurological and neuromuscular diseases on muscle relaxants

In patients with neurological and neuromuscular diseases there is, in general, a higher sensitivity to muscle relaxants with a longer effect than in normal patients. Administration of suxamethonium in such patients is accompanied by massive potassium release, resulting in hyperkalemia (Fiacchino et al 1991). Non-depolarizers can after long administration, especially in patients with a disturbed blood–brain barrier, reach considerable concentrations in the brain and cause excitatory central nervous system effects (Peduto et al 1989).

Motor neurone lesions

Central motor neurone lesions are associated with resistance to non-depolarizers at the afflicted side, and with hyperkalemia following suxamethonium administration (Moorthy and Hilgenberg 1980). This occurs 2 days after the beginning of the hemiplegia, as a result of sprouting of remaining axons with concomitant spread of extrajunctional acetylcholine receptors (Greenawalt 1992). This has also been described in patients with diffuse intracranial lesions, ruptured cerebral aneurysm and closed head injury. In lower and peripheral motor neurone lesions, however, increased response to non-depolarizers is observed at the afflicted site (Rosenbaum et al 1971). There is supersensitivity to suxamethonium, which leads to hyperkalemia, again as a result of increases in extrajunctional receptors; this has even been reported after transient paraplegia. Muscular contractures may occur spontaneously or following suxamethonium administration in peripherally denervated muscles. In peripheral denervation a normal response to non-depolarizers occurs.

Myotonia

In myotonia (dystrophic, congenita and paramyotonia), suxamethonium can induce myotonic crisis with hyperkalemia and inability to intubate the trachea (Mitchell et al 1978). Also rhabdomyolysis may occur. The effect of non-depolarizers is normal in some patients and enhanced in others (Nightingale et al 1985). Reversal with neostigmine, or use of a nerve stimulator, may also result in sustained muscle contraction.

Muscular dystrophy

In Duchenne's muscular dystrophy the administration of suxamethonium may lead to rhabdomyolysis (Boltshauser et al 1980). Also acidosis and hyperkalemia occur and may even lead to the death of the patient. Patients are easily paralysed from non-depolarizers, and so titration with monitoring of neuromuscular transmission is advocated. Suxamethonium can induce hyperkalemia in apparently healthy children and adolescents, who were subsequently found to have myopathies (Genever 1971). In 50% of cases it caused mortality. Administration of suxamethonium in patients with mitochondrial myopathy may induce malignant hyperthermia (Ohtani et al 1985). Antagonists can induce myotonic crisis (Buzello et al 1982).

Peripheral polyneuropathy

Patients with peripheral polyneuropathy of all origins (diabetes, alcoholism, vascular insufficiency, vitamin deficiencies, tumours, heavy metal poisoning, etc.) are extremely sensitive to non-depolarizing muscle relaxants and resistant to succinylcholine. In Guillain–Barré syndrome suxamethonium can induce hyperkalemia (Feldman 1990, Reilly and Hutchinson 1991).

Myasthenic syndromes

In myasthenia gravis an increased sensitivity for nondepolarizing relaxants exists, strongly related to the titres of individual anti-acetylcholine-receptor antibodies. When, however, equipotent dosages are given the duration of blockade is not different (Nilsson and Meretoja 1990). Patients with "cured myasthenia gravis" remain more sensitive. There is resistance to suxamethonium, and on repeated doses progressive prolongation of blockade occurs and phase II block easily develops (Eisenkraft et al 1988, Vanlinthout et al 1994). When, however, patients receive anticholinesterase treatment, a decrease in plasma–cholinesterase may occur with increased sensitivity to suxamethonium and mivacurium (Baraka 1992).

In myasthenic syndrome (Lambert–Eaton syndrome) the amount of acetylcholine released is diminished. It is the result of production of auto-antibodies against neuronal voltage-operated prejunctional calcium channels and against synaptotagmin (Takamori et al 1995). The patients have an exaggerated response both to suxamethonium and non-depolarizing relaxants (Wise 1962).

The effect of temperature on muscle relaxants

Hypothermia decreases the muscle contraction force, even without the presence of relaxants, when measured with mechanomyography, but it increases muscle contraction force when measured with electromyography (Buzello et al 1986). Hypothermia causes an increase in potency and a prolongation in the duration of relaxants (Buzello et al 1985). The effect of hypothermia is reversed upon rewarming.

Muscle relaxants and drug interactions

More than 250 drugs have an effect on the neuromuscular transmission and, hence, interfere pharmacodynamically with muscle relaxants (Argov and Mastaglia 1979). Some drugs interfere with the metabolism or excretion of the relaxants and, thus, interact pharmacokinetically, others have a pharmacodynamic effect (Lambert et al 1983).

The effect of suxamethonium is enhanced by drugs interfering with plasma cholinesterase activity (i.e., ecothiopate, mono-aminoxidase inhibitors, lidocaine, procaine). The effect of non-depolarizers is potentiated by antibiotics of the aminoglycoside, lincosamide, polypeptide, and tetracycline series (Booij et al 1978, Sokoll and Gergis 1981). These compounds can cause curarization when administered up to 4–6 h after complete recovery of the neuromuscular blockade, even when antagonized with neostigmine or pyridostigmine. The blockade itself is difficult to reverse.

Patients with epilepsy are chronically treated with anti-epileptics. Resistance toward non-depolarizing relaxants (i.e., pancuronium, vecuronium and metocurine) has been described in patients receiving carbamazepine or phenytoine. There seems to be no affect on atracurium. In a prospective study, however, resistance to atracurium in 23 patients chronically treated with phenytoin was also found (Tempelhoff et al 1990).

The use of relaxants at the extremes of age

Shortly after birth neuromuscular transmission is not yet matured. As demonstrated from a spontaneous fade after tetanic stimulation, there is less acetylcholine than in adults. The postjunctional acetylcholine receptors have a different structure, with more receptors located at the extrajunctional membrane in newborn babies. These differences have an effect on the action of the neuromuscular blocking agents.

Besides the pharmacokinetic behaviour of muscle relaxants being different in the various age groups, neonates and infants frequently have a decreased plasma clearance and a prolonged elimination half-life, resulting in prolonged paralysis. The initial volume of distribution in children is larger than in neonates and infants, leading to resistance as indicated from the rate of infusion to maintain a constant block (Brandom et al 1986).

There are several reasons why the pharmacokinetic behaviour of relaxants is altered in elderly compared with younger adults. In general a decrease in total body water, lean body mass and protein binding, resulting in alteration of the volume of distribution and/or the plasma clearance, causes a prolonged and more pronounced effect of relaxants. Also, the number of motor units per muscle is decreased in the elderly, and muscular atrophy occurs. A decrease in cardiac output and increased circulation time lead to a delay in the onset of drugs, including muscle relaxants (Matteo et al 1991). Dehydration and change in body composition result in an apparently increased sensitivity to relaxants (Lien et al 1991), although there is no difference in receptor affinity for the relaxants or the concentration at which a particular degree of blockade occurs (Duvaldestin et al 1982, Bell et al 1989). For example, the dose-response relationship of the new relaxant rocuronium is not different in elderly and younger patients (Bevan et al 1993).

Chronic administration of relaxants

Although relaxants were originally developed for administration during surgery, they are nowadays being used for up to several weeks in the intensive care unit (Willatts 1985). Development of muscle areflexia, atrophy and sensory impairment in patients with multiorgan failure have been attributed to such prolonged administration of relaxants (Gooch et al 1991, Heckmatt et al 1993). In up to 50% of the patients, there is delayed weaning from artificial ventilation as a result of polyneuropathy-induced muscle weakness. However, signs of polyneuropathy are also observed in other critically ill patients that have not received relaxants (critical illness neuropathy). In one study up to 70% of the intensive care patients with sepsis and multiple organ failure had symptoms of this syndrome. In 50% of the patients with critical illness, neuropathy with fibre necrosis has been demonstrated and thus myopathy ensues (Helliwell et al 1991, Kupfer et al 1992). As well as motor function deficits sensory deficits are also present, whereas electromyography (EMG) readings do not demonstrate neuromuscular transmission disorders (Zochodne et al 1994). It is concluded that this disease entity is more characteristic of a myopathy than of a neuropathy.

Relaxants, and other drugs like corticosteroids, aminophylline, and antibiotics that are usually administered to this type of patient, can lead to neuromuscular and muscular abnormalities (Barohn et al 1994).

Relaxant-induced neuropathy is usually symmetrical, and it does not involve the sensory system; EMG readings resemble those in Guillain–Barré syndrome or myonecrosis, but they also resemble readings resulting from residual neuromuscular blockade. Most patients are female and have metabolic acidosis, renal failure and some hepatic dysfunction. The steroidal relaxants mainly seem to cause prolonged muscle weakness (Op de Coul et al 1985, Griffin et al 1992). However, it must be realized that steroids are far more frequently used in intensive care than benzylisoquinolines. The syndrome is also observed with atracurium (Manthous and Chatila 1994, Meyer et al 1994).

Contrary to cases of prolonged weakness, during long administration, cases are reported with development of resistance for pancuronium, vecuronium, and atracurium (Hunter 1991). This is related to increased extrajunctional sensitivity to acetylcholine and/or receptor up-regulation as a result of long neuromuscular blockade (Hogue et al 1992, Dodson et al 1995).

Antagonism of neuromuscular blockade

The effect of non-depolarizers can be reversed with anticholinesterase drugs. However, reversing agents increase the acetylcholine concentration at all cholinergic receptors, and thus exert many side-effects.

It has been demonstrated that too small a dose of neostigmine leads to residual relaxation and that too large a dose leads to neostigmine-induced neuromuscular blockade. With repeated dosages of anticholinesterases, neuromuscular block may occur from transient depolarization of the receptors and blockade of open confirmation channels (Maselli and Leung 1993). Antagonists should, therefore, be titrated with close monitoring of the neuromuscular function. The amount of reversing agent that has to be administered depends on the type of anaesthetic administered, the type of relaxant used and the degree of spontaneous recovery of the neuromuscular blockade (Beemer et al 1991). In renal failure the effect of the reversal agents is prolonged. Reversing agents have a longer effect in elderly patients (Young et al 1988).

Administration of anticholinesterases carries the risk of induction of a central cholinergic syndrome.

References

Amaki Y, Waud BE, Waud DR. (1985) Atracurium-receptor kinetics: simple behavior from a mixture. *Anesth Analg* 64: 777–780.

Appadu BL, Lambert DG. (1994) Studies on the interaction of steroidal neuromuscular blocking drugs with cardiac muscarinic receptors. *Br J Anaesth* 72: 86–88.

Argov Z, Mastaglia FL. (1979) Disorders of neuromuscular transmission caused by drugs. *N Engl J Med* 301: 409–413.

Baraka A. (1992) Suxamethonium block in the myasthenic patient. Correlation with plasma cholinesterase. *Anaesthesia* 47: 217–219.

Barohn RJ, Jackson CE, Rogers SJ, Ridings LW, McVey AL. (1994) Prolonged paralysis due to nondepolarising neuromuscular blocking agents and corticosteroids. *Muscle Nerve* 17: 647–654.

Basta SJ, Savarese JJ, Ali HH, et al. (1988) Clinical pharmacology of Doxacurium chloride. *Anesthesiology* 69: 478–486.

Beemer GH, Bjorksten AR, Dawson PJ, Dawson RJ, Heenan BJ, Robertson BA. (1991) Determinants of the reversal time of competitive neuromuscular block by anticholinesterases. *Br J Anaesth* 66: 469–475.

Bell PF, Mirakhur RK, Clarke RSJ. (1989) Dose-response studies of atracurium, vecuronium and pancuronium in the elderly. *Anaesthesia* 44: 925–927.

Belmont MR, Lien CA, Quessy S, et al. (1995) The clinical neuromuscular pharmacology of 51W89 in patients receiving nitrous oxide/opioid/barbiturate anesthesia. *Anesthesiology* 82: 1139–1145.

Bevan DR, Fiset P, Balendram P, Law-Min JC, Ratcliffe A, Donati F. (1993) Pharmacodynamic behaviour of rocuronium in the elderly. *Can J Anaesth* 40: 127–132.

Binkley K, Cheema A, Sussman G, et al. (1992) Generalized allergic reactions during anesthesia. *J Allergy Clin Immunol* 89: 768–774.

Blanloeil Y, Delaroche O, Tequi B, Gunst JP, Dixneuf B. (1996) Apnee prolongee apres administration au cours de choc toxique staphylococcique. *Ann Fr Anesth Reanim* 15: 189–191.

Boltshauser E, Steinmann B, Meyer A, Jerusalem F. (1980) Anaesthesia induced rhabdomyolysis in Duchenne muscular dystrophy. *Br J Anaesth* 52: 559.

Booij LHDJ, Miller RD, Crul JF. (1978) Neostigmine and 4-aminopyridine antagonism of lincomycin-pancuronium neuromuscular blockade in man. *Anesth Analg* 57: 316–321.

Booij LHDJ, Krieg NN, Crul JF. (1980) Intradermal histamine releasing effect caused by Org-NC 4.) A comparison with pancuronium, metocurine and d-tubocurarine. *Acta Anaesthesiol Scand* 24: 393–394.

Booij LHDJ. (1989) Muscle relaxants and medical status of the patient. *Curr Opin Anaesthesiol* 2: 488–492.

Booij LHDJ, Knape JTA. (1991) The neuromuscular blocking effect of Org 9426. *Anaesthesia* 46: 341–343.

Brandom BW, Stiller RL, Cook DR, Woelfel SK, Chakravorti S, Lai A. (1986) Pharmacokinetics of atracurium in anaesthetized infants and children. *Br J Anaesth* 58: 1210–1213.

Buckett WR, Hewet CL, Savage DS. (1973) Pancuronium bromide and other steroidal neuromuscular blocking agents containing acetylcholine fragments. *J Med Chem* 16: 1116–1124.

Buzello W, Krieg N, Schlickewei A. (1982) Hazards of neostigmine in patients with neuromuscular disorders. *Br J Anaesth* 54: 529–534.

Buzello W, Schluermann D, Schindler M, Spillner G. (1985) Hypothermic cardiopulmonary bypass and neuromuscular blockade by pancuronium and vecuronium. *Anesthesiology* 62: 201–204.

Buzello W, Pollmaecher T, Schluermann D, Urbanyi B. (1986) The Influence of hypothermic cardiopulmonary bypass on neuromuscular transmission in the absence of muscle relaxants. *Anesthesiology* 64: 279–281.

Clarke RSJ, Mirakhur RK. (1994) Adverse effects of muscle relaxants. *Adv Drug React Toxicol Rev* 13: 23–41.

Collard CD, Baker BW 3rd, Johnson D, Bressler R, Harati Y. (1996) Cumulative reduction in serum cholinesterase following repeated therapeutic plasma exchange. *J Clin Anesth* 8: 44–48.

Diefenbach C, Abel M, Rump AFE, Grond S, Korb H, Buzello W. (1995) Changes in plasma cholinesterase activity and mivacurium neuromuscular block in response to normothermic cardioplumonary bypass. *Anesth Analg* 80: 1088–1091.

Dodson BA, Kelly BJ, Braswell LM, Cohen NH. (1995) Changes in acetylcholine receptor number in muscle from critically ill patients receiving muscle relaxants: an investigation of the molecular mechanism of prolonged paralysis. *Crit Care Med* 23: 815–821.

Donati F, Meiselman C, Plaud B. (1991) Vecuronium neuromuscular blockade at the adductor muscles of the larynx and the adductor pollicis. *Anesthesiology* 74: 833–837.

Duvaldestin P, Saada J, Berger JL, D'Hollander A, Desmonts JM. (1982) Pharmacokinetics, pharmacodynamics and dose-response relationships of pancuronium in control and elderly subjects. *Anesthesiology* 56: 36–40.

Eisenkraft JB, Book WJ, Mann SM, Papatestas AE, Hubbard M. (1988) Resistance to succinylcholine in myasthenia gravis : a dose response study. *Anesthesiology* 69: 760–763.

Engbaek J, Roed J. (1992) Differential effect of pancuronium at the adductor pollicis, the first dorsal interosseous and the hypothenar muscles. An electromyographic and mechano-myographic dose-response study. *Acta Anaesthesiol Scand* 36: 664–669.

Fahey MR, Morris RB, Miller RD, Nguyen TL, Upton RA. (1981) Pharmacokinetics of Org NC45 (Norcuron) in patients with and without renal failure. *Br J Anaesth* 53: 1049–1053.

Feldman JM. (1990) Cardiac arrest after succinylcholine administration in a pregnant patient recovering from Guillain-Barré syndrome. *Anesthesiology* 72: 942–944.

Fiacchino F, Gemma M, Bricchi M, Giombini S, Regi B. (1991) Sensitivity to curare in patients with upper and lower motor neurone dysfunction. *Anaesthesia* 46: 980–982.

Frankville DD, Drummond JC. (1987) Hyperkalemia after succinylcholine administration in a patient with closed head injury without paresis. *Anesthesiology* 67: 264–266.

Genever EE. (1971) Suxamethonium-induced cardiac arrest in unsuspected pseudohypertrophic muscular dystrophy. *Br J Anaesth* 984–986.

Gooch JL, Suchyta MR, Balbierz JM, Petajan JH, Clemmer TP. (1991) Prolonged paralysis after treatment with neuromuscular junction blocking agents. *Crit Care Med* 19: 1125–1131.

Goudsouzian NG, d'Hollander AA, Viby-Mogensen J. (1993) Prolonged neuromuscular block from mivacurium in two patients with cholinesterase deficiency. *Anesth Analg* 77: 183–185.

Greenawalt III, JW. (1992) Succinylcholine-induced hyperkalemia 8 weeks after a brief paraplegic episode. *Anesth Analg* 75: 294–295.

Griffin D, Fairman N, Coursin DB, Rawsthorne L, Grossman JE. (1992) Acute myopathy during treatment of status asthmaticus with corticosteroids and steroidal relaxants. *Chest* 102: 510–514.

Heckmatt JZ, Pitt MC, Kirkham F. (1993) Peripheral neuropathy and neuromuscular blockade presenting as prolonged respiratory paralysis following critical illness. *Neuropediatrics* 24: 123–125.

Helliwell TR, Coakley JH, Wagenmakers AJM, et al. (1991) Necrotizing myopathy in critically-ill patients. *J Pathol* 164: 307–314.

Hogue CW, Jr, Ward JM, Itani MS, Martyn JAJ. (1992) Tolerance and upregulation of acetylcholine receptors follow chronic infusion of d-tubocurarine. *J Appl Physiol* 72: 1326–1331.

Hughes R, Chapple DJ. (1981) The pharmacology of atracurium: a new competitive neuromuscular blocking agent. *Br J Anaesth* 53: 31–44.

Huizenga ACT, Vandenbrom RHG, Wierda JMKH, Hommes FDM, Hennis PJ. (1992) Intubating conditions and onset of neuromuscular block of rocuronium (ORG 9426); a comparison with suxamethonium. *Acta Anaesthesiol Scand* 36: 463–468.

Hunter JM. (1991) Resistance to non-depolarising neuromuscular blocking agents. *Br J Anaesth* 67: 511–514.

Huu-Lainé FK, Pinto-Scognamiglio W. (1964) Activité curarisante du dichlorure de 3β-20α bistrimethylammonium 5α-prègnane (malouétine) et de ses stéréoisomères. *Arch Int Pharmacodyn Thér* 147: 209–219.

Jensen ES, Viby-Mogensen J. (1995) Plasma cholinesterase and abnormal reaction to succinylcholine: twenty years experience with the Danish Cholinesterase research Unit. *Acta Anaesthesiol Scand* 39: 151–156.

Katz RL. (1967) Neuromuscular effects of d-tubocurarine, edrophonium and neostigmine in man. *Anesthesiology* 28: 327–336.

Kelly RE, Dinner M, Turner LS, Haik B, Abramson DH, Daines P. (1993) Succinylcholine increased intraocular pressure in the human eye with the extraocular muscles detached. *Anesthesiology* 79: 948–952.

Krieg N, Crul JF, Booij LHDJ. (1980) Relative potency of Org NC45, pancuronium, alcuronium and tubocurarine in anaesthetized man. *Br J Anaesth* 52: 783–788.

Kupfer Y, Namba T, Kaldawi E, Tessler S. (1992) Prolonged weakness after long-term infusion of vecuronium bromide. *Ann Int Med* 117: 484–486.

Lambert JJ, Durant NN, Henderson EG. (1983) Drug-induced modifications of ionic conductance at the neuromuscular junction. *Ann Rev Pharmacol Toxicol* 23: 505–539.

Lien CA, Matteo RS, Ornstein E, Schwartz AE, Diaz J. (1991) Distribution, elimination, and action of vecuronium in the elderly. *Anesth Analg* 73: 39–42.

Lien CA, Belmont MR, Abalos A, et al. (1995) The cardiovascular effects and histamine-releasing properties of 51W89 in patients receiving nitrous oxide/opioid/barbiturate anesthesia. *Anesthesiology* 82: 1131–1138.

Maddineni VR, Cooper R, Stanley JC, Mirakhur RK, Clarke RSJ. (1992) Clinical evaluation of doxacurium chloride. *Anaesthesia* 47: 554–557.

Maddineni VR, Mirakhur RK. (1993) Prolonged neuromuscular block following mivacurium. *Anesthesiology* 71: 227–231.

Mangar D, Kirchhoff GT, Rose PL, Castellano FC. (1993) Prolonged neuromuscular block after mivacurium in a patient with end-stage renal disease. *Anesth Analg* 76: 866–867.

Manthous CA, Chatila W. (1994) Prolonged weakness after the withdrawal of atracurium. *Am J Crit Care Med* 150: 1441–1443.

Marshall IG, Agoston S, Booij LHDJ, Durant NN, Foldes FF. (1980) Comparison of the cardiovascular actions of Org.NC45 with those produced by other non-depolarizing neuromuscular blocking agents in experimental animals. *Br J Anaesth* 52: 21S–32S.

Martyn J, Goldhill DR, Goudsouzian NG. (1986) Clinical pharmacology of muscle relaxants in patients with burns. *J Clin Pharmacol* 26: 680–685.

Maselli RA, Leung C. (1993) Analysis of anticholinesterase-induced neuromuscular transmission failure. *Muscle Nerve* 16: 548–553.

Matteo RS, Ornstein E, Schwartz AE, et al. (1991) Pharmacokinetics and pharmacodynamics of Org 9426 in elderly surgical patients. *Anesthesiology* 75: A1065.

McCoy EP, Maddineni VR, Elliot P, Mirakhur RK, Caroon IW, Cooper RA. (1993) Haemodynamic effects of rocuronium during fentanyl anaesthesia: comparison with vecuronium. *Can J Anaesth* 408: 703–708.

Meyer KC, Prielipp RC, Grossman JE, Coursin DB. (1994) Prolonged weakness after infusion of atracurium in two intensive care unit patients. *Anesth Analg* 78: 772–774.

Miller RD, Agoston S, Booij LHDJ, Kersten UW, Crul JF, Ham J. (1978) The comparative potency and pharmacokinetics of pancuronium and its metabolites in anesthetized man. *J Pharmacol Exp Ther* 207: 539–543.

Minton MD, Grosslight K, Stirt JA, Bedford RF. (1986) Increases in intracranial pressure from succinylcholine: prevention by prior nondepolarising blockade. *Anesthesiology* 65: 165–169.

Mitchell MM, Ali HH, Savarese JJ. (1978) Myotonia and neuromuscular blocking agents. *Anesthesiology* 49: 44–48.

Moorthy SS, Hilgenberg JC. (1980) Resistance to non-depolarizing muscle relaxants in paretic upper extremities of patients with residual hemiplegia. *Anesth Analg* 59: 624–627.

Nightingale P, Healy TEJ, McGuinness K. (1985) Dystrophia myotonica and atracurium. A case report. *Br J Anaesth* 57: 1131.

Nilsson E, Meretoja OA. (1990) Vecuronium dose-response and maintenance requirements in patients with myasthenia gravis. *Anesthesiology* 73: 28–32.

North FC, Kettelkamp N, Hirshman CA. (1987) Comparison of cutaneous and in vitro histamine release by muscle relaxants. *Anesthesiology* 66: 543–546.

O'Flynn RP, Shutack JG, Rosenberg H, Fletcher JE. (1994) Masseter muscle rigidity and malignant hyperthermia susceptibility in pediatric patients. *Anesthesiology* 80: 1228–1233.

Ohtani Y, Miike T, Ishitsu T, Matsuda I, Tamari H. (1985) A case of malignant hyperthermia with mitochondrial dysfunction. *Brain Development* 7: 249–253.

Ono K, Nagano O, Ohta Y, Kosaka F. (1990) Neuromuscular effects of respiratory and metabolic acid-base changes in vitro with and without non-depolarizing muscle relaxants. *Anesthesiology* 73: 710–716.

Op de Coul AAW, Lambregts PCLA, Koeman J, van

Puyenbroek MJE, Ter Laak HJ, Gabreëls-Festen AAWM. (1985) Neuromuscular complications in patients given Pavulon (pancuronium bromide) during artificial ventilation. *Clin Neurol Neurosurg* 887: 17–22.

Ostergaard D, Jensen FS, Jensen E, Skovgaard LT, Viby-Mogensen J. (1992) Influence of plasma cholinesterase activity on recovery from mivacurium-induced neuromuscular blockade in phenotypically normal patiens. *Acta Anaesthesiol Scand* 36: 702–706.

Peduto VA, Gungii P, Di Martino MR, Napoleone M. (1989) Accidental subarachnoid injection of pancuronium. *Anesth Analg* 69: 516–517.

Petersen RS, Bailey PL, Kalameghan R, Ashwood ER. (1993) Prolonged neuromuscular block after mivacurium. *Anesth Analg* 76: 194–196.

Reilly M, Hutchinson M. (1991) Suxamethonium is contraindicated in the Guillain–Barré syndrome. *J Neurol Neurosurg Psych* 54: 1018–1019.

Ritter DM, Rettke SR, Ilstrup DM, Burritt MF. (1988) Effect of plasma cholinesterase activity on the duration of action of succinylcholine in patients with genotypically normal enzyme. *Anesth Analg* 67: 1123–1126.

Robertson EN, Fragen RJ, Booij LHDJ, Crul JF. (1983) Intradermal histamine release by 3 muscle relaxants. *Acta Anaesthesiol Scand* 27: 203–205.

Robertson EN, Hull JM, Verbeek AM, Booij LHDJ. (1994) A comparison of rocuronium and vecuronium: the pharmacodynamic, cardiovascular and intra-ocular effects. *Eur J Anaesthesiol* 11, suppl. 9: 116–121.

Robinson AL, Jerwood DC, Stokes MA. (1996) Routine suxamethonium in children: a regional survey of current usage. *Anaesthesia* 51: 874–878.

Robson N, Robertson I, Whittaker M. (1986) Plasma cholinesterase changes in the puerperium. *Anaesthesia* 41: 243–249.

Rosenbaum KJ, Neigh JL, Strobel GE. (1971) Sensitivity to non-depolarizing muscle relaxants in amyotrophic lateral sclerosis: report of two cases. *Anesthesiology* 35: 638–641.

Savarese JJ, Ali HH, Basta SJ, et al. (1988) The clinical neuromuscular pharmacology of Mivacurium chloride (BW B1090U). *Anesthesiology* 68: 723–732

Shanks CA. (1993) The pharmacokinetics of onset and offset of neuromuscular block. *Anaesth Pharmacol Rev* 1: 20–33.

Shanks CA, Somogyi AA, Triggs EJ. (1979) Dose-response and plasma concentration-response relationship of pancuronium in man. *Anesthesiology* 51: 111–118.

Shearer ES, Russell GN. (1993) The effect of cardio-pulmonary bypass on cholinesterase activity. *Anaesthesia* 48: 293–296.

Smith CE, Donati F, Bevan DR. (1989) Effects of succinylcholine at the masseter and adductor pollicis muscle in adults. *Anesth Analg* 69: 159–162.

Sokoll MD, Gergis SD. (1981) Antibiotics and neuromuscular function. *Anesthesiology* 55: 148–159.

Stellato C, dePaulis A, Cirillo R, Mastronardi P, Mazzarella B, Marone G. (1991) Heterogeneity of human mast cells and basophils in response to muscle relaxants. *Anesthesiology* 74: 1078–1086.

Szenohradszky J, Fisher DM, Segredo V, Caldwell JE, Bragg P, Sharma ML. (1992) Pharmacokinetics of rocuronium bromide (Org 9426) in patients with normal renal function or patients undergoing cadaver renal transplantation. *Anesthesiology* 77: 899–904.

Takamori M, Takahashi M, Yasukawa Y, et al. (1995) Antibodies to recombinant synaptotagmin and calcium channel subtypes in Lambert–Eaton myasthenic syndrome. *J Neurol Sci* 133: 95–101.

Tempelhoff R, Modica PA, Jellish WS, Spitznagel EL. (1990) Resistance to atracurium-induced neuromuscular blockade in patients with intractable seizure disorders treated with anticonvulsants. *Anesth Analg* 71: 665–667.

VanderSpek AFL, Reynolda PI, Fang WB, Ashton-Miller JA, Stohler CS, Schork MA. (1990) Changes in resistance to mouth opening induced by depolarizing and non-depolarizing neuromuscular relaxants. *Br J Anaesth* 64: 21–27.

Vanlinthout LEH, van Egmond J, De Boo T, Lerou JGC, Wevers RA, Booij LHDJ. (1992) Factors affecting magnitude and time course of neuromuscular block produced by suxamethonium. *Br J Anaesth* 69: 29–35.

Vanlinthout LEH, Robertson EN, Booij LHDJ. (1994)

Response to suxamethonium during propofol-fentanyl-N2O/O2 anaesthesia in a patient with active myasthenia gravis receiving chronic anticholinesterase therapy. *Anaesthesia* 49: 509–511.

Warner LO, Brener DL, Davidson PJ, Rogers GL, Beach TP. (1989) Effects of lidocaine, succinylcholine, and tracheal intubation on intraoccular pressure in children anaesthetized with halothane-nitrous oxide. *Anesth Analg* 69: 687–690.

Westra P, Keulemans GTP, Houwertjes MC, Hardonk MJ, Meijer DKF. (1981) Mechanisms underlying the prolonged duration of action of muscle relaxants caused by extrahepatic cholestasis. *Br J Anaesth* 53: 217–227.

Whittaker M, Britten JJ. (1987) Phenotyping of individuals sensitive to suxamethonium. *Br J Anaesth* 59: 1052–1055.

Wierda JMKH, de Wit APM, Kuizinga K, Agoston S. (1990) Clinical observations on the neuromuscular blocking action of Org 9426, a new steroidal non-depolarizing agent. *Br J Anaesth* 64: 521–523.

Willatts SM. (1985) Paralysis for ventilated patients? Yes or No? *Intens Crit Care Digest* 4: 9–10.

Wintersteiner O, Dutcher JD. (1943) Curare alkaloids from Chondodendron tomentosum. *Science* 97: 467–470.

Wise RP. (1962) A myasthenic syndrome complication in bronchial carcinoma. *Br J Anaesth* 17: 488.

Young WL, Matteo RS, Ornstein E. (1988) Duration of action of neostigmine and pyridostigmine in the elderly. *Anesth Analg* 67: 775–778.

Zochodne DW, Ramsay DA, Saly V, Shelley S, Moffatt S. (1994) Acute necrotizing myopathy of intensive care: electrophysiological studies. *Muscle Nerve* 17: 285–292.

58

Gene transfer in skeletal muscle

Johnny Huard

Abstract

As the molecular basis of an expanding number of inherited disorders has been discovered, increasing focus has been placed on gene therapy as a potential approach for the treatment of patients. Skeletal muscle has been extensively studied as a target tissue for gene transfer, both for the production of proteins that may be therapeutic for muscle disorders and the systemic delivery of non-muscle proteins. Although the engineering of new mutant vectors has reduced the problems associated with viral cytotoxicity and immune rejection, the inability of viral vectors to efficiently transduce mature muscle fibres has remained a major barrier to the application of gene transfer to skeletal muscle. In this review, we will summarize recent research which has been aimed at:

- defining the molecular basis of this maturation-dependent viral transduction
- the development of methods that circumvent this major hurdle facing the application of viral gene transfer to skeletal muscle.

The long-term goal of these studies is to develop strategies to achieve an efficient dystrophin delivery to alleviate the muscle weakness in Duchenne Muscular Dystrophy (DMD) patients as well as to enable efficient application of muscle-based gene therapy for other inherited and acquired diseases and conditions of the musculoskeletal system.

Background

Somatic gene therapy, through the transferring of a functional gene into a particular tissue to alleviate a biochemical deficiency, has emerged as a novel and exciting form of molecular medicine. Due to a number of properties, skeletal muscle has been suggested as a promising target for gene therapy. First, since skeletal muscle is composed of multi-nucleated, post-mitotic myofibres, it may allow high and long-term persistence of transgene expression. Second, the mono-nucleated myogenic precursor cells (satellite cells), which are located between the extracellular matrix and the plasma membrane of myofibres, can be relatively easily isolated, cultivated in vitro and efficiently transduced using either viral or non-viral vectors. In addition, the ability of the myogenic cells to stably fuse together or with, myofibres in vivo has established them as promising gene delivery vehicles. Finally, the high level of vascularization of muscle tissue may facilitate the systemic delivery of potentially therapeutic, non-muscle products, such as growth factors, factor IX or erythropoietin (see Blau and Springer 1995, Svensson et al 1996).

To date, most of the studies for gene transfer into muscle cells have been aimed at therapy for DMD. This common X-linked recessive muscular dystrophy is caused by a deficiency of dystrophin—an important component of the plasma membrane cytoskeleton of muscle fibres (Hoffman et al 1987, Arahata et al 1988, Bonilla et al 1988, Watkins et al 1988, Zubryzcka-Gaarn et al 1988). Dystrophin deficiency leads to a continuous loss of muscle fibres with progressive muscle weakness and the early death of patients in their second decade of life. Effective gene therapy for DMD will require the transfer of adequate copies of either the full-length dystrophin gene or dystrophin mini-genes (Ascadi et al 1991, Dunckley et al 1992, 1993, Ragot et al 1993, Vincent et al 1993) into affected muscle to restore adequate production of dystrophin for compensation of the weakness.

Strategies for gene transfer into muscle

Both myoblast transplantation and gene transfer have been investigated to deliver genes to skeletal muscle. The transplantation of normal myoblasts into dystrophin-deficient muscle, to create a reservoir of dystrophin-producing myoblasts capable of fusing with dystrophic myofibres, has been studied extensively in both mdx mice (an animal model for DMD) and DMD patients (for review see Partridge 1991). Although studies showed transient restoration of dystrophin in dystrophic muscle, the limited success of myoblast transplantation has been related to immune-rejection, and the poor survival and spread of injected myoblasts post-transplantation (Morgan et al 1988, 1990, 1993, Partridge et al 1989, Karpati et al 1989, 1992, Tremblay et al 1993, Beauchamps et al 1994, Huard et al 1991a, b, 1992a, b, 1994a, b, c, Mendell et al 1995, Gussoni et al 1992, 1997, Kinoshita et al 1994; Vilquin et al 1995). Although approaches are being developed to improve the efficiency of myoblast transplantation (Guerette et al 1997, Qu et al 1998), recent research has increasingly focused on the application of gene delivery using viral or non-viral vectors.

The intramuscular injection of non-viral vectors (plasmid DNA) to deliver genes to muscle has shown the advantages of low toxicity and immunogenicity

(Wolff et al 1992). An initial disadvantage has been the relatively low transfection efficiency, despite the use of large amounts of plasmid DNA (Ascadi et al 1991, Danko et al 1993). However, multiple studies have shown improved transfection efficiencies in muscle, with an increased accessibility of DNA to the myo-fibres, following: pre-treatment with a myonecrotic agent, such as cardiotoxin; pre-injection of large volumes of hypertonic sucrose; or injection at the myo-tendinous junction (Davis et al 1993a, b, Doh et al 1997). Alternatively, the use of non-targeted lipo-somes and/or polylysine-condensed plasmid DNA has also improved plasmid transfection efficiencies in skeletal muscle (Vitiello et al 1996). In particular, the recent development of ligand (e.g. transferrin)-directed DNA–liposome complexes capable of transducing myogenic cells in a receptor-dependent manner (Feero et al 1997a) is promising.

Strategies of delivering genes to skeletal muscle using viral vectors based on retrovirus, adenovirus, herpes simplex virus or adeno-associated virus have evolved rapidly. Retroviral vectors are relatively safe, and they can infect dividing myoblasts (progenitors of mature muscle) with a high efficiency (Barr and Leiden 1991, Dhawan et al 1991, Dunckley et al 1992, 1993, Salvatori et al 1993). In addition, the ability of retroviruses to become stably integrated into the host cell genome can provide long-term, stable expression of the delivered gene. However, retro-viruses remain incapable of infecting post-mitotic cells (Miller et al 1990). Muscle cells become post-mitotic very early in their development, and the mature muscle tissue has no actively dividing cells unless injured or affected by a genetic dystrophy. Therefore, skeletal muscle shows a dramatic loss of retroviral transduction during maturation. Other limitations to the use of retroviruses are the limited gene-insert capacity (less than 7 kb), the relatively low titres (10^5–10^6 pfu/ml), and the risk of insertional mutagenesis.

Adenoviral vectors (AdV) can infect both mitotic myoblasts and post-mitotic immature myofibres (Quantin et al 1992, Ragot et al 1993, Vincent et al 1993, Acsadi et al 1994a,b 1996, Huard et al 1995a, b), and they can be prepared at high titres (10^9–10^{11} pfu/ml). However, the stability and long-term expression of transgenes delivered to skeletal muscle using first generation adenoviral vectors have been mainly limited by the immune-rejection. The low gene insert capacity (<8 kb) of first generation adenoviral vectors has been overcome by the development of new mutant adenoviral vectors lacking all viral genes and having an expanded insert capacity (Kochanek et al 1996, Kumar-Singh and Chamberlain 1996,

Haecker et al 1996). These adenoviral vectors have been capable of inserting up to 28 kb of exogenous DNA, including the full-length dystrophin and β-galactosidase, and they promise to dramatically reduce immunogenicity.

Viral vectors derived from the herpes simplex virus type 1 (HSV-1) are naturally capable of carrying large DNA fragments, such as the 14 kb dystrophin cDNA, and they have been studied for their ability to trans-duce muscle cells (Huard et al 1995c, 1996, 1997a, b). Herpes simplex viral vectors, which can persist in the host cell in a non-integrated state and be prepared at adequately high titres (10^7–10^9 pfu/ml), have shown efficient transduction of myoblasts, myotubes and immature myofibres, but they remain incapable of efficiently transducing mature myofibres. The rela-tively high cytotoxicity, which hampers the long-term transgene expression, has been identified as a major disadvantage of first generation herpes simplex viral vectors. In attempts to overcome this hurdle, deletion of multiple viral immediate–early (IE) genes from the mutant vectors has been shown to reduce cytotoxicity in muscle cells (Huard et al 1997b).

Recombinant adeno-associated viral vectors (rAAV) have also been used as gene delivery vehicles for muscle cells. Although long-term transgene expression (up to 18 months) and a high efficiency of mature myofibre transduction have been observed in mouse skeletal muscle (Xiao et al 1996, Fisher et al 1997, Clark et al 1997), the application of adeno-asso-ciated viral vectors for gene therapy purposes may be limited by their restrictive gene insert capacity (<5 kb) especially for DMD.

Limitations associated with gene delivery systems to muscle

Different systems have been investigated to achieve an efficient gene delivery to skeletal muscle, but many of them have been found incapable of achieving stable transgene expression in the injected skeletal muscle. Myoblast transplantation has been hindered primarily by immune rejection problems, inefficient spread of the injected cells and poor survival of the injected myoblasts post-implantation. The main limitation associated with gene transfer based on non-viral vectors remains the inefficiency of gene delivery to muscle cells. Gene transfer mediated by viral vectors (AdV, HSV-1) has also been hindered by immune rejection problems, cellular cytotoxicity due to viral transduction and a poor level of viral transduction in adult muscle in contrast to that observed in newborn muscles. As the immunological barriers and the viral cytotoxicity are characterized and almost overcome, it becomes paramount to address the inability of viral vectors to efficiently transduce mature muscle fibres.

Barriers to viral gene transfer of mature myofibres

Although the further engineering of viral vectors and the use of appropriate immunosuppressive agents can overcome the barriers associated with host cell immune responses and viral cytotoxicity, the inability of viral vectors to efficiently transduce mature myofibres still remains a major hurdle facing the widespread application of viral gene transfer to muscle. Retroviral, AdV and HSV-1 vectors fail to efficiently transduce mature, fully differentiated myofibres in contrast to newborn muscle. In this section, we review recent research aimed at defining the molecular basis of the maturation-dependent retroviral, AdV and HSV-1 transduction of skeletal muscle and propose strategies that have been implemented in an attempt to circumvent this barrier.

Post-mitotic muscle cells

Muscle is a highly developed and organized tissue in which the constituent myofibres become post-mitotic early in fetal life. However, mitotically active myoblasts are known to be capable of fusing with pre-existing post-mitotic myofibres. Therefore, viral transduction during skeletal muscle maturation may require mitotically active myoblasts. This hypothesis is valid for the retrovirus, which is known to require dividing cells (i.e., myoblasts) for genomic integration and gene expression (Miller et al 1990). Retroviruses likely transduce myofibres indirectly via the fusion of transduced myoblasts with existing host myofibres. Since AdV and HSV-1 vectors have been shown to transduce post-mitotic, immature myofibres in vitro and in vivo (Quantin et al 1992, Ragot et al 1993, Acsadi et al 1994a, Huard et al 1996, 1997a,b, Feero et al 1997b), other factors are more likely to be involved in the poor level of viral transduction of mature myofibres.

Development of immune system during muscle maturation

The reduced viral transduction during maturation of muscle may be related to the maturation of the immune system in adult mice, which consequently generates a stronger and/or quicker immune-rejection of transduced myofibres, when compared with that in neonatal mice. The inability of AdV and HSV-1 vectors to efficiently transduce mature myofibres in adult immunodeficient SCID mice (Acsadi et al 1996, Huard et al 1997a, b) has demonstrated that the low level of transduction in mature muscle using these viral vectors is not directly associated with the host immune system.

Receptor-dependent transducibility of muscle

The interaction between viral targeting peptides and host cell attachment/internalization receptors has been shown to determine the viral transducibility of muscle cells. AdV transduction has been markedly better in myoblasts than in myotubes. This differential transducibility can be explained in part by the level of the $\alpha_v\beta_3/\beta_5$-integrin internalization receptor, which is more abundant in myoblasts than myotubes (Acsadi et al 1994b). Similarly, the attachment receptors of the adenovirus have been identified, and a low level of expression has been reported in skeletal muscle (Tomko et al 1997). In contrast, HSV-1 vectors can infect myoblasts, myotubes and immature myofibres with comparable transduction efficiencies (Huard et al 1996, 1997a, b). These vectors use the heparan sulfate proteoglycan receptors, which are expressed abundantly in most cell types at all developmental stages, for attachment. High concentrations of these receptors have been found in both immature and mature myofibres (Huard et al 1996). To improve adenoviral gene delivery to different cell types, genetically modified adenoviral vectors have been engineered to carry particular motifs in their viral fibre coat proteins that target the binding to alternative attachment receptors at the surface of the host cells (e.g., AdVpK vectors targeted to heparan-containing receptors; Wickham et al 1996). These adenoviral vectors with enhanced attachment properties might significantly improve gene transfer efficiencies in mature skeletal muscle. Although we have observed that they display a better transduction than first generation adenovirus, these viruses remain incapable of efficiently transducing mature myofibres (van Deutekom et al 1999).

The extracellular matrix of mature myofibres acts as a physical barrier

It has been proposed that the extracellular matrix acts as a physical barrier to HSV-1 mediated gene delivery to mature myofibres (Huard et al 1996, 1997a, b). Co-localization of collagen IV, a component of the extracellular matrix, and HSV-1 particles by immunohistochemistry has revealed that the viral particles are blocked by the extracellular matrix, and thus remain in the interstitial space between the mature myofibres in both normal and immunodeficient mice. In contrast, HSV-1 particles are capable of penetrating myofibres isolated from neonatal mice, suggesting that the immature and probably rudimentary extracellular matrix is more permeable to viral penetration in newborn muscle tissue.

Since the extracellular matrix of mature myofibres contains pores estimated to be 40 nm in size (Yurchenco 1990), it may protect the myofibres against penetration by the 120–300 nm in diameter HSV-1 particles. In the dystrophic dy/dy mouse, an abnormal myofibre extracellular matrix is present as a result of a merosin deficiency (Arahata et al 1993, Sunada et al 1994, Xu et al 1994a, b). HSV-1 particles have been found to be capable of efficiently penetrating and transducing mature myofibres of dy/dy mice in vitro (Feero et al 1997b) and in vivo (Huard et al 1996). These data support the hypothesis that the extracellular matrix acts as a physical barrier to HSV-1 penetration of mature muscle fibres.

Since the diameter of AdV particles ranges between 70 nm and 100 nm, the extracellular matrix might also be a barrier to AdV penetration of mature myofibres. Consistent with this hypothesis, adenoviral transduction has been detected in mature muscle of dy/dy mice, while AdV failed to transduce skeletal muscle from normal adult, age-matched mice (van Deutekom et al 1998a, b). These results indicate that the extracellular matrix of mature myofibres is acting as a physical barrier against both HSV-1 and AdV penetration, and it may play a dominant role in the maturation-dependent viral transduction of muscle. Finally, the small size of the adeno-associated viral particles (20 nm) and the ability of these viral particles to penetrate and consequently transduce mature myofibres further support the hypothesis that the sizes of AdV and HSV-1 particles are too large to penetrate the pore size of the extracellular matrix.

Myoblast-mediated viral transduction

While the extracellular matrix appears to hamper viral transduction during muscle maturation, other factors may still be involved. Myoblasts are abundantly present in immature muscle tissue, where they actively fuse with developing myofibres, but they are generally quiescent in mature muscle. Hence, myoblasts may serve as intermediaries in the viral transduction of neonatal myofibres. The loss of actively fusing myoblasts as the muscle matures could explain the reduced viral transducibility of mature myofibres. Dystrophic muscle (mdx mice) shows a high activity of muscle degeneration and regeneration throughout the development of skeletal muscle; thus, it should contain a constant reservoir of mitotically active myoblasts. Indeed, injection of AdV vectors, retrovirus and HSV-1 vectors in mature mdx muscle has demonstrated a substantially better transduction efficiency when compared with normal muscle (van Deutekom et al 1998a, b). Gamma-irradiation of mouse neonatal muscle in vivo has demonstrated the inactivation of myoblasts and the substantial reduction of AdV transduction of neonatal myofibres (van Deutekom et al 1998a, b, Cao et al 2001). These findings are consistent with the hypothesis that myoblasts mediate some of the viral transduction of neonatal myofibres, as well as that the reduced transducibility of skeletal muscle throughout maturation is at least partially caused by the progressive loss of mitotically active myoblasts.

Approaches to overcome the poor level of viral transduction of mature myofibres

Permeating the extracellular matrix

The extracellular matrix has been shown to play an important role in protecting mature myofibres against viral penetration. Enzymatic permeation of this extracellular matrix prior to viral injection might enlarge the pore sizes and allow a better viral penetration in mature myofibres. To date, different enzymes, such as streptokinase, gelatinase, urokinase or dispase, have been tested to permeate the extracellular matrix of isolated mature myofibres in vitro. Preliminary results have shown a high level of HSV-1 transduction of isolated mature myofibres treated with 5 units of streptokinase for 1 h prior to infection (van Deutekom et al 1998a, b). In addition, since the extracellular matrix also appears to partially prevent AdV transduction in mature muscle in vivo, an artificial enzymatic permeation of the extracellular matrix of myofibres prior to AdV infection also remains under investigation. Indeed, pre-treatment of adult muscle with 5 units of streptokinase significantly improves adenoviral gene transfer to mature myofibres when compared with non-treated muscle. The application of this strategy to increase viral transduction efficiencies in mature muscle in vivo is currently being evaluated. Eventually, viral vectors may be engineered to carry the genes encoding those enzymes shown to be successful in permeating the extracellular matrix and facilitating viral penetration in mature myofibres.

The use of new viral vectors

Although adeno-associated virus has been found capable of efficiently penetrating and transducing mature myofibres, the small insert capacity of the viral vector may limit its use for delivering genes to skeletal muscle. In fact, large genes, including full-length dystrophin and merosin, are not compatible with the size insert capacity of AAV; consequently, AAV can not be used to deliver these genes to dystrophic muscle. The use of a truncated (mutated) version of these genes that is capable of protecting the muscle against degeneration may eventually allow AAV to insert and deliver the modified genes into skeletal muscle.

Similarly, the use of modified shortened fibre shaft adenovirus displaying a reduction in the size of the viral particles may help to circumvent the maturation-dependent adenoviral transduction of mature skeletal muscle. These new adenoviral vectors display a reduction of up to 25% in the size of the viral particles, and they may become small enough to penetrate the extracellular matrix pores (40 nm) and allow an efficient adenoviral transduction in mature myofibres.

Artificial induction of muscle regeneration

The intermediate levels of viral transduction in regenerating muscle tissue of adult mdx mice suggest that viral transduction in muscle is partially mediated by myoblasts. Therefore, artificial induction of muscle regeneration using myonecrotic agents, such as notexin, bupivacaine, or cardiotoxin, to enhance gene transfer in mature muscle has been studied (Davis et al 1993a, Danko et al 1994, Vitadello et al 1994). Muscle tissue of adult mice treated by an intramuscular injection of cardiotoxin at 1 to 4 days prior to an injection of a retroviral vector carrying the LacZ reporter gene has shown a high level of retroviral transduction in comparison with non-treated mature muscle (van

Deutekom et al 1998a, b). Since retrovirus can only infect dividing myoblasts, this high level of transduction in cardiotoxin-treated muscle clearly demonstrates the ability of myoblasts to mediate retroviral gene transfer in mature myofibres. Similarly, AdV and HSV-1 transduction of mature muscle have shown dramatic improvement after induction of regeneration by cardiotoxin treatment in comparison with the non-treated muscle (van Deutekom et al 1998a, b).

The myotendinous junction provides a privileged site for viral entry in mature myofibres

To date, the majority of gene therapy approaches mediated via viral and non-viral vectors have been performed in the muscle belly. In vertebrate muscle fibres, the myotendinous junction (MTJ) is the site where new sarcomeres are inserted during longitudinal fibre growth (Williams and Goldspink 1971). Moreover, Dix and Eisenberg (1990) have observed that in stretching muscles the majority of cells present at the myotendinous junction were myotubes or immature muscle fibres. These myotubes are expected to fuse with, and become extensions of, existing fibres, similar to that observed during muscle development (Moss and Leblond 1971, Williams and Goldspink 1971). The extracellular matrix (basal lamina) is structurally and functionally unique at the myotendinous junction: the surface of the muscle fibre is thrown into elaborate invaginations into which the basal lamina and collagen fibrils extend, altering the composition of the basal lamina (Nakao 1976, Trotter et al 1981, 1983, Bozyczko et al 1989, Tidball and Lin 1989).

It has recently been observed that injection of non-viral vectors at the MTJ leads to a higher level of gene transfer than observed with the same injection at the muscle belly (Doh et al 1997). Based on this observation, we hypothesize that this altered structure may allow virus to penetrate and transduce mature myofibres. In addition, this site may remain highly myogenic, even in mature myofibres, and it may represent an attractive entry site for viral based vectors in adult muscle fibres.

We have recently shown that adenovirus appears to show increased transduction of mature muscle when the direct injection of the virus is performed at the MTJ in comparison with similar injections at the muscle belly. In fact, the injection of 40 μl of 1×10^9 pfu/ml adenovirus leads to a higher number of transduced myofibres when injected at the MTJ (distal tendon) rather than the muscle belly. Visualization of the transduced myofibres, at high magnification and counterstained with hematoxylin-eosin, shows that transduced myofibres are non-regenerating myofibres. The termini of muscle fibres at the tendon may remain immature even at the adult stage, and a high myogenic capacity may be preserved at this site throughout the muscle development, leading to efficient adenoviral transduction in mature muscle.

Myoblast-mediated ex vivo gene transfer approach

The ex vivo gene transfer approach is a promising combination of cell therapy and gene therapy utilizing autologous transplantation of isogenic myoblasts, which are virally transduced in vitro. Application of the ex vivo approach in mature muscle using retroviral, AdV and HSV-1 vectors has demonstrated improved levels of transduction (Booth et al 1997, Floyd et al 1997, 1998) in comparison with direct viral injections of the same number of viral particles (Booth et al 1997, Floyd et al 1997, 1998, van Deutekom et al 1998a, b). Therefore, the ex vivo strategy is a promising approach to overcome the maturation-dependent viral transduction of skeletal muscle with the different viral vectors. Although we have observed an improvement of adenovirus, retrovirus and HSV-1 transduction in mature myofibres when the ex vivo approach is used, 95% of the injected myoblasts still died rapidly following injection (Huard et al 1994c). The development of approaches capable of improving cell survival post-transplantation will eventually further enhance the ex vivo gene transfer of viral vectors in mature muscle.

The poor survival of the injected myoblasts clearly limits the efficiency of the myoblast-mediated ex vivo gene transfer of viral vectors in mature muscle. It has recently been found that the poor survival of the injected myoblasts is partially related to inflammatory reactions (Guerette et al 1997, Merly et al 1998, Tremblay and Guerette 1997). We have investigated whether inflammation is the only factor involved in the poor survival of the injected myoblasts. Advances in cellular and molecular biology have identified interleukin-1 receptor antagonist protein (IL-1Ra) and soluble receptors for tumour necrosis factor-α (TNF-α) as promising proteins to inhibit the inflammation and the progression of arthritis (Bandara et al 1993, Doherty 1995). The extremely wide range of biological activities of IL-1Ra may improve the cell survival by blocking the action of the inflammatory cytokine interleukin-1 (IL-1).

A myoblast cell line was engineered to express IL-1Ra. We observed that engineered myoblasts expressing IL-1Ra allow a better survival rate of the injected myoblasts at 48 h post-injection. The non-engineered myoblast cell line displayed poor survival of the injected cells, but in the same cell line expressing IL-1Ra there was a significant improvement in the survival rate of the injected cells at 48 h post-injection, as observed by a local expression of an anti-inflammatory substance (Qu et al 1998).

Inflammation is probably not the only factor involved in the rapid loss of the injected myoblasts post-implantation. An improvement in the survival rate of the injected myoblasts has been obtained through the use of anti-inflammatory drugs (anti-LFA-1), but there is still some loss of the injected myoblasts (Guerette et al 1997, Tremblay and Guerette 1997). Similarly, we have noted that a substantial reduction in the loss of the injected myoblasts has been achieved with the IL-1Ra-expressing cells, but loss of approximately 20% is observed at 48 hours post-injection. We have, therefore, evaluated whether the use of different populations of muscle-derived cells can help to circumvent the poor survival of the injected myoblasts post-transplantation.

In order to evaluate this hypothesis, an mdx myoblast cell line, pure myoblasts isolated from myofibres and primary myoblasts at different purities have been injected into adult mdx muscle. We have characterized different populations of primary muscle cell cultures isolated from gastrocnemius muscle containing different amounts of cells expressing desmin (Qu et al 1998). In fact, the first preplate (PP) obtained contains 5–10% desmin-positive cells and the last preplate contains over 80% desmin-positive cells (Qu et al 1998).

These various myoblast populations have been adenovirally transduced, and the early fate of the injected cells has been evaluated at different time points post-injection (0.5, 12, 24, 48 h and 5 days). When the same number of cells derived from different populations of muscle-derived cells (PP#1 versus PP#6) were injected into mature muscle, we observed an 83% loss for PP#1 and 124% gain for PP#6 in the transgene expression compared with the non-injected transduced cells (Qu et al 1998). This observation suggests that the isolation of specific populations of muscle-derived cells can totally overcome the rapid loss of the injected cells without blocking the inflammation, and this may further improve the efficiency of the myoblast mediated ex vivo gene transfer approach. Although the percentage of desmin-positive cells can explain the differential survival observed between the earlier and later preplates (PP#1 and PP#6), the inability of desmin-positive cells obtained from both the isolated myofibres and the myoblast cell line to survive suggests that other factors influence cell survival post-injection (Qu et al 1998).

We have characterized whether the source of muscle-derived cells may have a primordial role in the early survival of the injected myoblasts. In fact, a great difference in the content of satellite cells has already been observed between slow- and fast-twitch muscles (Schmalbruch and Hellhammer 1977, Kelly 1978, Gibson and Schultz 1982). The type of satellite cells isolated from these muscles may also possibly display a differential fate post-transplantation. It has been reported that transplantation of L6 rat myoblasts expressing the type II myosin heavy chain isoform (fast MyHCs) in vitro predominantly fuse together into myotubes or with host myofibres expressing the same myosin isoform (Pin and Merrifield 1997). In contrast, a very low percentage of these L6 myoblasts have been found capable of fusing with myofibres expressing slow MyHC when injected into soleus, plantaris and medial gastrocnemius (Pin and Merrifield 1997). Although C_2C_{12} and cloned satellite cells have been found capable of fusing with all fibre types encountered (Hughes and Blau 1992), both populations of cells have been capable of expressing both fast and slow MyHCs in vitro, and they may represent a population of multipotential myoblast stem cells (Edom et al 1994).

We have observed that PP#6 muscle-derived cells have the ability to fuse with myofibres expressing both the slow and fast myosin isoforms (Qu et al 1998) in contrast to myoblasts obtained from isolated single myofibres, which either fused together or with host myofibres showing the absence of slow MyHC (Qu et al 1998). The inability of myoblasts obtained from isolated single myofibres to fuse with myofibres expressing slow MyHC may be involved with the differential survival of the injected myoblasts, since the injected muscle (gastrocnemius and soleus) contains a mixture of myofibres expressing fast and slow myosin isoforms. The injected myoblasts that are less able to fuse with some specific types of host myofibres are likely to display poor survival at the injection site.

We consequently investigated whether cells displaying the best survival also led to a better gene transfer when compared with cells that rapidly die post-transplantation. The primary myoblasts (PMb; PP#6) and the myoblasts from single fibres (FMb; PP#1) were infected with adenoviral vectors carrying the LacZ reporter gene, injected into mdx hindlimb muscle and monitored for the level of gene transfer in soleus (slow) and gastrocnemius (fast). We then observed that

PMb, which displayed the best survival among all the cells tested, led to a greater gene transfer than FMb, and myoblast cell line in the hindlimb muscle (Qu et al 2000). The PMb cells, which partly expressed both slow- and fast-MyHCs in vivo, were detected in the soleus and gastrocnemius white muscles (70% and 0% of fibres containing slow-MyHC respectively) and showed a larger scale fusion with host muscle fibres (fast/slow). In contrast, the FMb cells only expressed fast-MyHCs; when injected in the gastrocnemius, they fused with host muscle fibres expressing the same myosin isoform (Qu et al 2000). This data suggested that the types of myogenic cells and of host muscle fibres both play an important role in the cell survival and, consequently, the myoblast-mediated gene transfer to skeletal muscle.

Acknowledgements

I wish to thank Drs van Deutekom, Zhuqing Qu and Bao Hong Cao (post-doctoral fellows) for their work on the maturation dependent viral transduction of myofibres, Marcelle Pellerin and Ryan Pruchnic for their technical assistance and Megan Mowry and Dana Och for assistance with the manuscript. This work was supported by grants to Dr Johnny Huard from the National Institute of Health (POI AR 45925) the Parent Project (USA/Netherlands), Muscular Dystrophy Association (MDA, USA) and Children's Hospital of Pittsburgh.

References

Arahata K, Ishiura S, Ishiguro T, et al. (1988) Immunostaining of skeletal and cardiac muscle surface membrane with antibody against Duchenne Muscular Dystrophy peptide. *Nature* 333: 861–863.

Arahata K, Hayashi YK, Koga R, et al. (1993) Laminin in animal models for Duchenne Muscular Dystrophy: defect of laminin M in skeletal and cardiac muscles and peripheral nerve of the Homozygous dystrophic dy/dy mice. *Proc Japan Acad* 69 ser B: 259–264.

Acsadi G, Dickson G, Love DR, et al. (1991) Human dystrophin expression in mdx mice after intramuscular injection of DNA constructs. *Nature* 352: 815–818.

Acsadi G, Jani A, Massie B, et al. (1994a) A differential efficiency of adenovirus-mediated in vivo gene transfer into skeletal muscle cells at different maturity. *Hum Mol Gen* 3: 579–584.

Acsadi G, Lochmuller H, Jani A, et al. (1996) Dystrophin expression in muscles of mdx mice after adenovirus-mediated in vivo gene transfer. *Hum Gene Ther* 7: 129–140.

Acsadi G, Jani A, Huard J, et al. (1994b) Cultured human myoblasts and myotubed show markedly different transducibility by replication-defective adenovirus recombinants. *Gene Ther* 1: 338–340.

Bandara G, Mueller GM, Galea-Lauri J, et al. (1993) Intraarticular expression of biologically active interleukin-1 receptor antagonist protein by ex vivo gene transfer. *Proc Natl Acad Sci USA* 90: 10764–10768.

Barr E, Leiden JM. (1991) Systemic delivery of recombinant proteins by genetically modified myoblasts. *Science* 254: 1507–1509.

Beauchamps JR, Morgan JE, Pagel CN, Partridge TA. (1994) Quantitative studies of the efficacy of myoblast transplantation. *Muscle Nerve* 18: S261.

Blau HM, Springer ML. (1995) Molecular medicine: muscle-based gene therapy. *N Engl J Med* 333: 1554–1556.

Bonilla ECE, Samitt AF, Miranda AP, et al. (1988) Duchenne Muscular Dystrophy: deficiency of dystrophin at the muscle cell surface. *Cell* 54: 447–452.

Booth DK, Floyd SS, Day CS, Glorioso JC, Kovesdi I, Huard J. (1997) Myoblast-mediated ex vivo gene transfer to mature muscle. *Tiss Eng* 3(2): 125–133.

Bozyczko D, Decker C, Muschler J, Horwitz AF. (1989) Integrin on developing and adult skeletal muscle. *Exp Cell Res* 183: 72–91.

Clark RK, Sferra TJ, Johnson PR. (1997) Recombinant adeno-associated viral vectors mediated long-term transgene expression in muscle. *Hum Gene Ther* 8: 659–669.

Cao B, Pruchnic R, Ikezawa M, et al. (2001) The role of receptors in the maturation-dependent adenoviral transduction of myofibers. *Gene Ther* 8: 627–637.

Danko I, Fritz JD, Jiao S, Hogan K, Latendresse JS, Wolff JA. (1994) Pharmacological enhancement of in vivo foreign gene expression in muscle. *Gene Ther* 1: 114–121.

Danko I, Fritz JD, Latendresse JS, Herweijer H, Schultz E, Wolff JA. (1993) Dystrophin expression improves myofibre survival in mdx muscle following intramuscular plasmid DNA injection. *Hum Mol Genet* 2(12): 2055–2061.

Davis H, Demeneix BA, Quantin B, Coulombe J, Whalen RG. (1993a) Plasmid DNA is superior to viral vectors for direct gene transfer into adult mouse skeletal muscle. *Hum Gene Ther* 4: 733–740.

Davis HL, Whalen RG, Demeneix BA. (1993b) Direct Gene Transfer into skeletal muscle in vivo: Factors affecting efficiency of transfer and stability of expression. *Hum Gene Ther* 4: 151–159.

Dhawan J, Pan LC, Pavlath GK, Travis MA, Lanctot AM, Blau HM. (1991) Systemic delivery of human growth hormone by injection of genetically engineered myoblasts. *Science* 254: 1509–1512.

Dix DJ, Eisenberg BR. (1990) Myosin mRNA accumulation and myofibrillogenesis at the myotendinous junction of stretched muscle fibres. *J Cell Biol* 111: 1885–1894.

Doh SG, Vahlsing J, Hartikka J, Liang X, Manthorpe M. (1997) Spatial-temporal patterns of gene expression in mouse skeletal muscle after injection of LacZ plasmid DNA. *Gene Ther* 4: 648–663.

Doherty PJ. (1995) Gene therapy and Arthritis. *J Rheum* 22(7): 1220–1223.

Dunckley MG, Davies KE, Walsh FS, Morris GE, Dickson G. (1992) Retroviral-mediated transfer of a dystrophin minigene into mdx mouse myoblasts in vitro. *FEBS Lett* 296(2): 128–134.

Dunckley MG, Wells DJ, Walsh FS, Dickson G. (1993) Direct retroviral-mediated transfer of dystrophin minigene into mdx mouse muscle in vivo. *Hum Mol Genet* 2: 717–723.

Edom F, Mouly JP, Barbet MY, Fiszman MY, Butler-Browne GS. (1994) Clones of human satellite cells can express in vitro both fast and slow myosin heavy chains. *Dev Biol* 164: 219–229.

Feero WG, Li S, Rosenblatt JD, et al. (1997a) Selection and use of ligands for receptor-mediated gene delivery to myogenic cells. *Gene Ther* 4: 664–674.

Feero WG, Rosenblatt JD, Huard J, et al. (1997b) Single fibres as a model system for viral gene delivery to skeletal muscle: Insights on maturation-dependant loss of fibre infectivity. *Gene Ther* 4: 371–380.

Fisher KJ, Jooss K, Alston J. (1997) Recombinant adeno-associated virus for muscle directed gene therapy. *Natl Med* 3: 306–312.

Floyd SS, Booth DK, van Deutekom JCT, Day CS, Huard J. (1997) Autologous myoblast transfer: A combination of myoblast transplantation and gene therapy. *Basic Appl Myol* 7: 241–250.

Floyd SS, Clemens PR, Ontell MR, et al. (1998) Ex vivo gene transfer using adenovirus-mediated full length dystrophin delivery to dystrophic muscles. *Gene Ther* 5: 19–30.

Gibson MC, Schultz E. (1982) The distribution of satellite cells and their relationship to specific fibre types in soleus and extensor digitorum longus muscles. *Anat Rec* 202: 329.

Guerette B, Asselin I, Skuk D, Entman M, Tremblay JP. (1997) Control of inflammatory damage by anti-LFA-1: Increase success of myoblast transplantation. *Cell Trans* 6(2): 101–107.

Gussoni E, Pavlath PK, Lanctot AM, et al. (1992) Normal dystrophin transcripts detected in DMD patients after myoblast transplantation. *Nature* 356: 435–438.

Gussoni E, Blau HM, Kunkel LM. (1997) The fate of individual myoblasts after transplantation into muscles of DMD patients. *Natl Med* 3: 970–977.

Haecker SE, Stedman HH, Balice-Gordon RJ, et al. (1996) In vivo expression of full-length human dystrophin from adenoviral vectors deleted of all viral genes. *Hum Gene Ther* 7: 1907–1914.

Hoffman EP, Brown J, Kunkel LM. (1987) Dystrophin: the protein product of the Duchenne Muscular Dystrophy locus. *Cell* 51: 919–928.

Huard J, Labrecque C, Dansereau G, Robitaille L, Tremblay JP. (1991a) Dystrophin expression in myotubes formed by the fusion of normal and dystrophic myoblasts. *Muscle Nerve* 14: 178–182.

Huard J, Bouchard JP, Roy R, et al. (1991b) Myoblast transplantation produced dystrophin-positive muscle fibres in a 16-year-old patient with Duchenne muscular dystrophy. *Clin Science* 81: 287–288.

Huard J, Bouchard JP, Roy R, et al. (1992a) Human myoblast transplantation: preliminary results of 4 cases. *Muscle Nerve* 15: 550–560.

Huard J, Roy R, Bouchard JP, Malouin F, Richards CL, Tremblay JP. (1992b) Human Myoblast transplantation between immunohistocompatible donors and recipients produces immune reactions. *Transpl Proc* 24(6): 3049–3051.

Huard J, Guerette B, Verreault S, et al. (1994a) Human myoblast transplantation in immunodeficient and immunosuppressed mice: Evidence of rejection. *Muscle Nerve* 17: 224–234.

Huard J, Verreault S, Roy R, Tremblay M, Tremblay JP. (1994b) High efficiency of muscle regeneration following human myoblast clone transplantation in SCID mice. *J Clin Invest* 93: 586–599.

Huard J, Acsadi G, Jani A, Massie B, Karpati G. (1994c) Gene transfer into skeletal muscles by isogenic myoblasts. *Hum Gene Ther* 5: 949–958.

Huard J, Lochmuller H, Acsadi G, Jani A, Massie B, Karpati G. (1995a) The route of administration is a major determinant of the transduction efficiency of rat tissues by adenoviral recombinants. *Gene Ther* 2: 107–115.

Huard J, Lochmueller H, Jani A, et al. (1995b) Differential short-term transduction efficiency of adult versus newborn mouse tissues by adenoviral recombinants. *Exp Mol Pathol* 62: 131–143.

Huard J, Goins B, Glorioso JC. (1995c) Herpes Simplex virus type 1 vector mediated gene transfer to muscle. *Gene Ther* 2: 1–9.

Huard J, Feero WG, Watkins SC, Hoffman EP, Rosenblatt DJ, Glorioso JC. (1996) The basal lamina is a physical barrier to HSV mediated gene delivery to mature muscle fibres. *J Virol* 70(11): 8117–8123.

Huard J, Akkaraju G, Watkins SC, Cavalcoli MP, Glorioso JC. (1997a) LacZ gene transfer to skeletal muscle using a replication defective Herpes Simplex virus type 1 mutant vector. *Hum Gene Ther* 8: 439–452.

Huard J, Krisky D, Oligino T, et al. (1997b) Gene transfer to muscle using herpes simplex virus-based vectors. *Neuromus Disorders* 7: 1–15.

Hughes SM, Blau HM. (1992) Muscle fibre pattern is independent of cell lineage in post-natal rodent development. *Cell* 68: 659–671.

Karpati G, Pouliot Y, Zubrzycka-Gaarn EE, et al. (1989) Dystrophin is expressed in mdx skeletal muscle fibres after normal myoblast implantation. *Am J Pathol* 135: 27–32.

Karpati G, Worton RG. (1992) Myoblast transfer in DMD: problems and interpretation of efficiency. *Muscle Nerve* 15:1209.

Kelly AM. (1978) Satellite cells and myofibre growth in rat soleus and extensor digitorum longus muscle. *Dev Biol* 65: 1.

Kinoshita I, Vilquin JT, Guerette B, Asselin I, Roy R, Tremblay JP. (1994) Very efficient myoblast allotransplantation in mice under FK506 immunosuppression. *Muscle Nerve* 17: 1407–1415.

Kochanek S, Clemens PR, Mitani K, Chen HH, Chan S, Caskey CT. (1996) A new adenoviral vector: Replacement of all viral coding sequences with 28 kb of DNA independently expressing both full-length dystrophin and beta–galactosidase. *Proc Natl Acad Sci USA* 93: 5731–5736.

Kumar-Singh R, Chamberlain JS. (1996) Encapsidated adenovirus minichromosomes allow delivery and expression of a 14 kb dystrophin cDNA to muscle cells. *Hum Mol Genet* 5: 913–921.

Mendell JR, Kissel JT, Amato AA, et al. (1995) Myoblast transfer in the treatment of Duchenne's muscular dystrophy. *N Engl J Med* 333: 832–838.

Merly F, Huard C, Asselin I, Robbins PD, Tremblay J. (1998) Anti-inflammatory effect of transforming growth factor-b1 in myoblast transplantation. *Transplantation* 65: 793–799.

Miller DG, Adam MA, Miller AD. (1990) Gene transfer by retrovirus vectors occurs only in cells that are actively replicating at the time of infection. *Mol Cell Biol* 10: 4239–4242.

Morgan JE, Watt DJ, Slopper JC, Partridge TA. (1988) Partial correction of an inherited defect of skeletal muscle by graft of normal muscle precursor cells. *J Neurol Sci* 86: 137–147.

Morgan JE, Hoffman EP, Partridge TA. (1990) Normal myogenic cells from newborn mice restore normal histology to degenerating muscle of the mdx mouse. *J Cell Biol* 111: 2437–2449.

Morgan JE, Pagel CN, Sherrat T, Partridge TA. (1993) Long-term persistence and migration of myogenic cells injected into pre-irradiated muscles of mdx mice. *J Neurol Sci* 115: 191–200.

Moss FP, Leblond CP. (1971) Satellite cells as the source of nuclei in muscle of growing rats. *Anat Rec* 70: 421–436.

Nakao T. (1976) Some observations on the fine structure of the myotendinous junction in myotomal muscles of the tadpole tail. *Cell Tissue Res* 166: 241.

Partridge TA, Morgan JE, Coulton GR, Hoffman EP, Kunkel LM. (1989) Conversion of mdx myofibres from dystrophin negative to positive by injection of normal myoblasts. *Nature* 337: 176–179.

Partridge TA. (1991) Myoblast transfer: A possible therapy for inherited myopathies. *Muscle Nerve* 14: 197–212.

Pin CL, Merrifield PA. (1997) Developmental potential of rat L6 myoblasts in vivo following injection into regenerating muscles. *Dev Biol* 188: 147–166.

Qu Z, Balkir L, van Deutekom JCT, Robbins PD, Pruchnic R, Huard J. (1998) Development of approaches to improve cell survival in myoblast transfer therapy. *J Cell Biol* 142 (5): 1257–1267.

Qu-Peterson Z, Huard J. (2000) The Influence of Muscle Fiber Type in Myoblast-Mediated Gene Transfer to Skeletal Muscles. *Cell Trans* 9: 503–517.

Quantin B, Perricaudet LD, Tajbakhsh S, Mandell JL. (1992) Adenovirus as an expression vector in muscle cells in vivo. *Proc Natl Acad Sci USA* 89: 2581–2584.

Ragot T, Vincent M, Chafey P, et al. (1993) Efficient adenovirus mediated gene transfer of a human mini-dystrophin gene to skeletal muscle of mdx mice. *Nature* 361: 647–650.

Salvatori G, Ferrari G, Messogiorno A, et al. (1993) Retroviral vector-mediated gene transfer into human primary myogenic cells lead to expression in muscle fibres in vivo. *Hum Gene Ther* 4: 713–723.

Schmalbruch H, Hellhammer, U. (1977) The number of nuclei in adult rat muscle with special reference to satellite cells. *Anat Rec* 189: 169.

Sunada Y, Bernier SM, Kozak CA, Yamada Y, Campbell KP. (1994) Deficiency of merosin in dystrophic dy mice and genetic linkage of laminin M chain gene to dy locus. *J Biol Chem* 269(19): 13729–13732.

Svensson EC, Tripathy SK, Leiden JM. (1996) Muscle based gene therapy: realistic possibilities for the future. *Mol Med Today* 2: 166–172.

Tidball JG, Lin C. (1989) Structural changes at the myogenic cell surface during the formation of myotendinous junction. *Cell Tiss Res* 257: 89.

Tomko RP, Xu R, Philipson L. (1997) HCAR and MCAR: The human and mouse cellular receptors for subgroup C adenovirus and group B coxsackieviruses. *Proc Natl Acad Sci USA* 94: 3352–3356.

Tremblay JP, Malouin F, Roy R, et al. (1993) Results of a blind clinical study of myoblast transplantations without immunosuppressive treatment in young boys with Duchenne Muscular Dystrophy. *Cell Trans* 2: 99–112.

Tremblay JP, Guerette B. (1997) Myoblast Transplantation: a brief review of the problems and of some solutions. *Basic Appl Myol* 7: 221–230.

Trotter JA, Corbet K, Avner BP. (1981) Structure and function of the murine muscle-tendon junction. *Anat Rec* 293–302.

Trotter JA, Eberhard S, Samora A. (1983) Structure domains of the muscle-tendon junction. 1. The internal lamina and the connecting domain. *Anat Rec* 207: 573.

van Deutekom JCT, Hoffman EP, Huard J. (1998a) Muscle Maturation: implications for gene therapy. *Mol Med Today* 4(5): 214–220.

van Deutekom JCT, Floyd SS, Booth DK, et al. (1998b) The development of approaches to improve viral gene delivery to mature skeletal muscle. *Neuromus Disorders* 8: 135–148.

Van Deutekon JCT, Cao B, Pruchnic R, Wickham TJ, Kovesdi I, Huard J. (1999) Extended Tropism of an Adenoviral Vector does not circumvent the Maturation-dependent Transducibility of Mouse Skeletal Muscle. *J Gene Med* 1: 393–399.

Vilquin JT, Wagner E, Kinoshita I, Roy R, Tremblay JT. (1995) Successful histocompatible myoblast transplantation in dystrophin-deficient mdx dystrophin. *J Cell Biol* 131(4): 975–988.

Vincent M, Ragot T, Gilgenkrantz H, et al. (1993) Long-term correction of mouse dystrophic degeneration by adenovirus-mediated transfer of a mini-dystrophin gene. *Nature Genet* 5: 130–134.

Vitadello M, Schiaffino MV, Picard A, Scarpa M, Schiaffino S. (1994) Gene transfer in regenerating muscle. *Hum Gene Ther* 5: 11–18.

Vitiello L, Chonn A, Wasserman JD, Duff C, Worton RG. (1996) Condensation of plasmid DNA with polylysine improves liposome-mediated gene transfer into established and primary muscle cells. *Gene Ther* 3: 396–404.

Watkins SC, Hoffman EP, Slayter HS, Kunkel LM. (1988) Immunoelectron microscopic localization of dystrophin in myofibres. *Nature* 333: 863–866.

Wickham TJ, Roelvink PW, Brough DE, Kovesdi I. (1996) Adenovirus targeted to heparin-containing receptors increases its gene delivery efficiency to multiple cell types. *Nature Biotech* 14: 1570–1573.

Williams PA, Goldspink G. (1971) Longitudinal growth of striated muscle fibres. *J Cell Sci* 751–767.

Wolff JA, Ludtke JJ, Acsadi G, Williams P, Jani A. (1992)

Long-term persistence of plasmid DNA and foreign gene expression in mouse muscle. *Hum Mol Genet* 1: 363–369.

Xiao X, Li J, Samulski RJ. (1996) Efficient long-term gene transfer into muscle tissue of immunocompetent mice by adeno-associated virus vector. *J Virol* 70: 8098–8108.

Xu H, Christmas P, Wu XR, Wewer UM, Engvall E. (1994a) Defective muscle basement membrane and lack of M-laminin in the dystrophic dy/dy mouse. *Proc Natl Acad Sci USA* 91: 5572–5576.

Xu H, Wu XR, Wewer UM, Engvall E. (1994b) Murine muscular dystrophy caused by a mutation in the laminin a2 (Lama2) gene. *Nature Genet* 8: 297–302.

Yurchenco PD. (1990) Assembly of basement membranes. *Ann NY Acad Sci* 580: 195–213.

Zubryzcka-Gaarn EE, Bulman DE, Karpati G, et al. (1988) The Duchenne Muscular Dystrophy gene is localized in the sarcolemma of human skeletal muscle. *Nature* 333: 466–469.

Index